AF868806

Stefano Bottacchiari

COMPOSITE INLAYS AND ONLAYS

Structural, periodontal, and endodontic aspects

Quintessenza Edizioni

Milan, Berlin, Chicago, Tokyo, Barcelona,
Istanbul, London, Moscow, New Delhi, Paris,
Beijing, Prague, Sao Paulo, Seoul, Warsaw

Copyright © 2016 by
Quintessenza Edizioni S.r.l.
via Ciro Menotti, 65 - 20017 Rho (MI) Italy
Tel.: +39.02.93.18.08.21 - Fax: +39.02.93.18.61.59
E-mail: info@quintessenzaedizioni.it
www.quintessenzaedizioni.com

ISBN 88-7492-019-9
978-88-7492-019-8

All rights reserved
The book and all its parts are copyrighted. Any use or sale outside the copyright limits without the publisher's consent is illegal and subject to prosecution. This applies in particular to photostatic reproductions, copies, circulars, duplications, translations, microfilms, electronic processing and data collection.

Printed in Italy

To my son Filippo
and those who love me

TABLE OF CONTENTS

Acknowledgments

My sincere thanks go to the following dentists for their invaluable contributions, each within their own specialties: Sergio De Paoli and Luca Bergamo for periodontology, Marco Forestali for endodontics, Paolo Ferrari for conservative diagnosis, Marco Nicastro for occlusion, and Lorenzo Breschi for adhesion.

I would like to express enormous gratitude to dental technicians Andrea Angelelli, Cristian Orlando, and Lanfranco Manzotti, who made every single inlay and onlay. I learned a lot from them—thank you.

A big thank you naturally also goes to Mrs Cristina Reina of Quintessenza Edizioni, who not only went the extra mile to help me but, above all, so patiently endured my bad temper and the many concerns that I offloaded on her.

Heartfelt thanks also go to my friend Lauro Dusetti, Head of Quintessenza Edizioni, who was always there to offer support on the many occasions that I was at the point of giving up.

Lastly, I would like to thank a special person, Dr Lavinia Landi, because I would have struggled to finish this book without her help. She helped me out with her humility, perseverance, intelligence, discipline, and friendship and made a crucial and significant contribution at the end of the work, sacrificing time she could have spent with her family and her partner, Massimo. To understand Lavinia's qualities, all one must do is look at the quality of her clinical cases, achieved after the shortest imaginable learning curve.
Thanks, Lavi!

Stefano Bottacchiari

Foreword

When we were students in Geneva, resin fillings were still experimental and unstable because they were subject to unsightly shrinkage and did not adhere to the cavity walls. The best-quality fillings were inevitably gold fillings and inlays or onlays. The former were difficult to implement and used in small occlusal or buccal cavities with solid walls. The latter were widely used since they represented the ultimate in filling quality and were durable and safe. The only drawbacks were the need to sacrifice healthy tooth tissue in order to ensure retention and avoid fracturing unsupported cusps and, of course, their unsightly appearance.

The advent of composite material that was structurally solid and above all adhered to the dental structures meant that fewer and fewer of the decidedly unsightly gold fillings were seen. The new materials were also easy to work with. The one risk that did remain, that of post-polymerization shrinkage, could be eliminated only by ensuring that the shrinkage took place outside the mouth, in other words, by producing a composite inlay or onlay that was subsequently cemented using adhesive. This is easy to say but much less easy to achieve: it requires proper preparation of the cavity, precise and accurate impression technique, and perfect finishing.

This is the province of Stefano Bottacchiari, who gained his sound training background in Geneva. In this very fine book he explains how it is possible to perform 3,200 inlays and onlays using a precise yet simple method and obtain secure, durable fillings through the application of proper periodontal practice, allowing the reconstruction of teeth that are fractured or affected by extensive loss of dental tissue.

The author covers all aspects of the subject in six chapters: a clear discussion of implementation technique, the proper choice of adhesives, the use of appropriate periodontal surgery to allow good hygiene of the filling edges, and thorough medium- and long-term follow-ups. All this is complemented by truly exceptional illustrations.

During his lectures, I have had the opportunity to admire his technique and fine photographs. I congratulate Stefano for his great efforts and for having produced a useful and practical book that is bound to meet with the success it deserves.

Guido Goracci

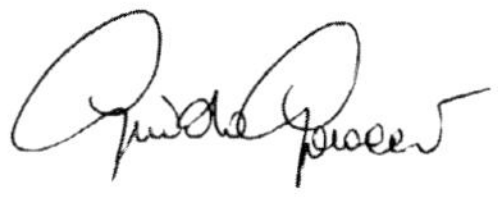

Foreword

I have known Dr Bottacchiari (Botti to his friends) since I was young—for very many years, in other words. Our relationship began as that of colleagues and slowly grew into friendship with time. Our first bond was mutual respect.
He is quite a character and certainly not an easy person to get to know.
In the words of the great Italian journalist Montanelli, it is not common for people who are characters to get along with everyone.
He is very generous, perhaps too generous, and few people have his sense of friendship: If he offers his friendship it is forever. Like all such people, he has few friends. But his friends are true friends.
He loves women, good food, and good wine.
Apart from women, good food, and good wine, he also loves composite inlays and onlays.
He has a fanatical, physical relationship with inlays and onlays. They are perfect, but that is not enough for him. Like everyone else, he naturally shows off photographs of his inlays and onlays. For him, however, the esthetic result goes without saying; for him it goes without saying that a tooth with an inlay or onlay will be totally indistinguishable from the adjacent teeth. The thing he looks at with an absolutely critical eye is the radiograph. The emergence profile is perfect, identical to that of a natural tooth, and his respect for biologic width is absolute. The different radiolucency of the inlay or onlay is the only thing that makes them radiographically distinguishable from the adjacent teeth.
I have no fear of being accused of exaggeration—the huge array of photographs in the book with follow-ups taken years later will bear out the truth of my claims.

Gianfranco Vignoletti

Preface

I wrote this book in the hope of being able to set out a simple, rigorous, and multidisciplinary protocol that could be used to achieve relatively satisfactory results in routine practice.
Why inlays and onlays, and why in composite?
Inlays and onlays, because they allow a significant conservation of sound tooth structure without undermining the tooth's mechanical and physical properties. Composite, because I believe that this extraordinary material offers many specific features, including two that are crucial: the opportunity for correction before and during cementation and, most important of all, long-term reparability.
Another key area that I want to emphasize is the multidisciplinary aspect.
Cooperation with periodontists and endodontists, particularly if you have the good fortune to work with excellent specialists in these areas, makes it possible to achieve predictable and maintainable results. Another thing that prompted me to write this book was the opportunity to provide clinical documentation based on everyday work, with the inevitable imperfections and shortcomings that are typical of routine work.
For example, after cementing inlays or onlays, rubber dam may not be clean and may show some tearing, speckles of blood, or fragments of composite used as cement. This happens because during the initial finishing under rubber dam, the special tools, abrasive strips, and ultrasonic and subsonic burs inevitably touch the flaps of the periodontal surgery performed 3 or 4 days earlier if not on the same day.
For my own self-respect and for that of those who are good enough to read this book, I believed it unrealistic to replace used dam with clean dam simply to present a sanitized image and instead decided to represent the true picture.
I hope my approach will be appreciated.

The text is divided into six chapters that span the entire process from diagnosis to treatment, examining individual steps specifically.
Chapter 1 is devoted to the philosophy of adhesive techniques, showing clinical cases with long-term follow-up. Typically, when considering clinical cases in this book I deliberately chose not to dwell on specific topics such as the physical and mechanical properties of materials, adhesion, and curing but instead to spend more time on the protocol that is integral to my daily work.
The basic principles have been covered superlatively by Dr Mauro Cattaruza in his excellent book and also by Prof Lorenzo Breschi in his innumerable scientific publications.
Thus Chapter 1 covers, amongst other things, the approach to the patient; diagnosis; the importance of radiographic examinations; indications for the current use of amalgam; and respect for dental structure, pulp, and periodontium, always as part of a multidisciplinary approach.
Chapter 2 covers current adhesive systems, considering their advantages and disadvantages and, of course, their clinical application.
Chapter 3 addresses the issue of cavity preparation, removal of decay, analysis of the healthy remaining tooth, buildup, and the different types of preparation, including reconstruction of teeth endodontically treated using Dr Marco Forestali's impeccable technique.
The cementation stage is very important, and I believe that this represents the biggest challenge in terms of adhesive technique.
Chapter 4 concentrates on relationships between the periodontium and the restoration and demonstrates

surgical procedures step-by-step, emphasizing the enormous immediate and long-term advantages of margins that are readily accessible. These greatly facilitate strictly operational stages while also making it easier for hygienists and practitioners to manage these supragingival margins. It is essential for patients to be able to carry out routine oral hygiene. All this was made possible, above all, by the knowledge and technical skill of Dr Sergio De Paoli and Dr Luca Bergamo.

In Chapter 5 I felt it was appropriate to explain all the steps that our dental technicians perform when creating inlays and onlays.

I also give due consideration to the clinical steps necessary to achieve arches with proper occlusal contacts.

Chapter 6, the section dearest to my heart, tackles the much-debated topic of enamel-dentin fracture lines. I found it very difficult to talk about these fracture lines: the predictability of prognosis is shrouded in uncertainty. The clinical case samples are small: patients often present with parafunctions and painful symptoms, demanding guarantees of healing.

Also in this case, I deal with the problem by applying a strict protocol. Above all I seek the cooperation of the patient, explaining that alternative therapies are still possible, but none are so conservative. And often, more often than not, patients place their trust in us!

Medium- and long-term follow-ups show that very many cases are solved simply by using inlays and onlays, which may or may not cover the cusps, often maintaining the vitality of the pulp with very few complete fractures and even fewer tooth extractions.

Stefano Bottacchiari

Partial-coverage composite restorations 1

First visit

The tone of the first visit often provides patients an image of their practitioner that will influence all subsequent interactions (Fig 1); if an unsatisfactory impression is created at this initial stage, it will be very difficult to change it later. Many factors have an impact on a favorable relationship between practitioners and patients, such as practitioners' ability to listen to patients' concerns, their genuine interest in patients' problems, and even their appearance, because patients might believe that practitioners who look sloppy and untidy will be equally disinterested in the details of diagnosis and treatment.

Collecting a full and accurate medical history from patients themselves provides important information on the mindset, background, and emotional state of the person sitting in the dental chair. By the end, the clinician must have identified the problem, the main condition, and the history of the disease in progress. It is unnecessary to stress the importance of radiographic examinations (eg, bitewing, full-mouth, and panoramic radiographs and additional imaging specific to orthodontics and implants) (Fig 2), which, when considered together with the clinical examination, allow the clinician to make the all-important diagnosis before continuing to the treatment planning stage. This next stage may be extremely varied and affected by many factors, including the patient's needs, motivation, time availability, and, last but not least, financial position (Figs 3 to 8). A whole book could be written on these topics, given their importance, but a personal observation immediately springs to mind: the best treatment plan is the one clinicians would offer to their own children.

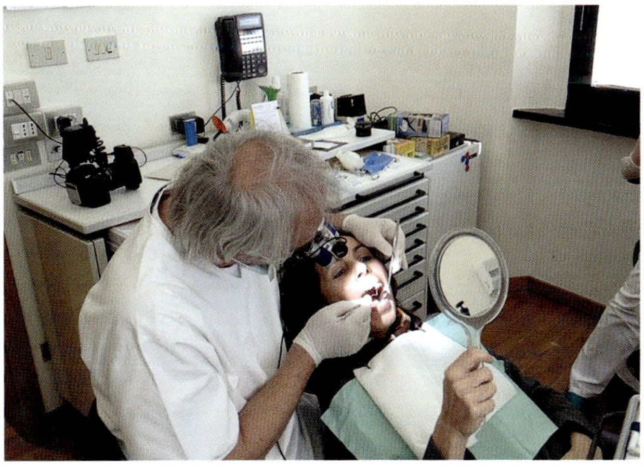

Fig 1 First clinical examination of the patient.

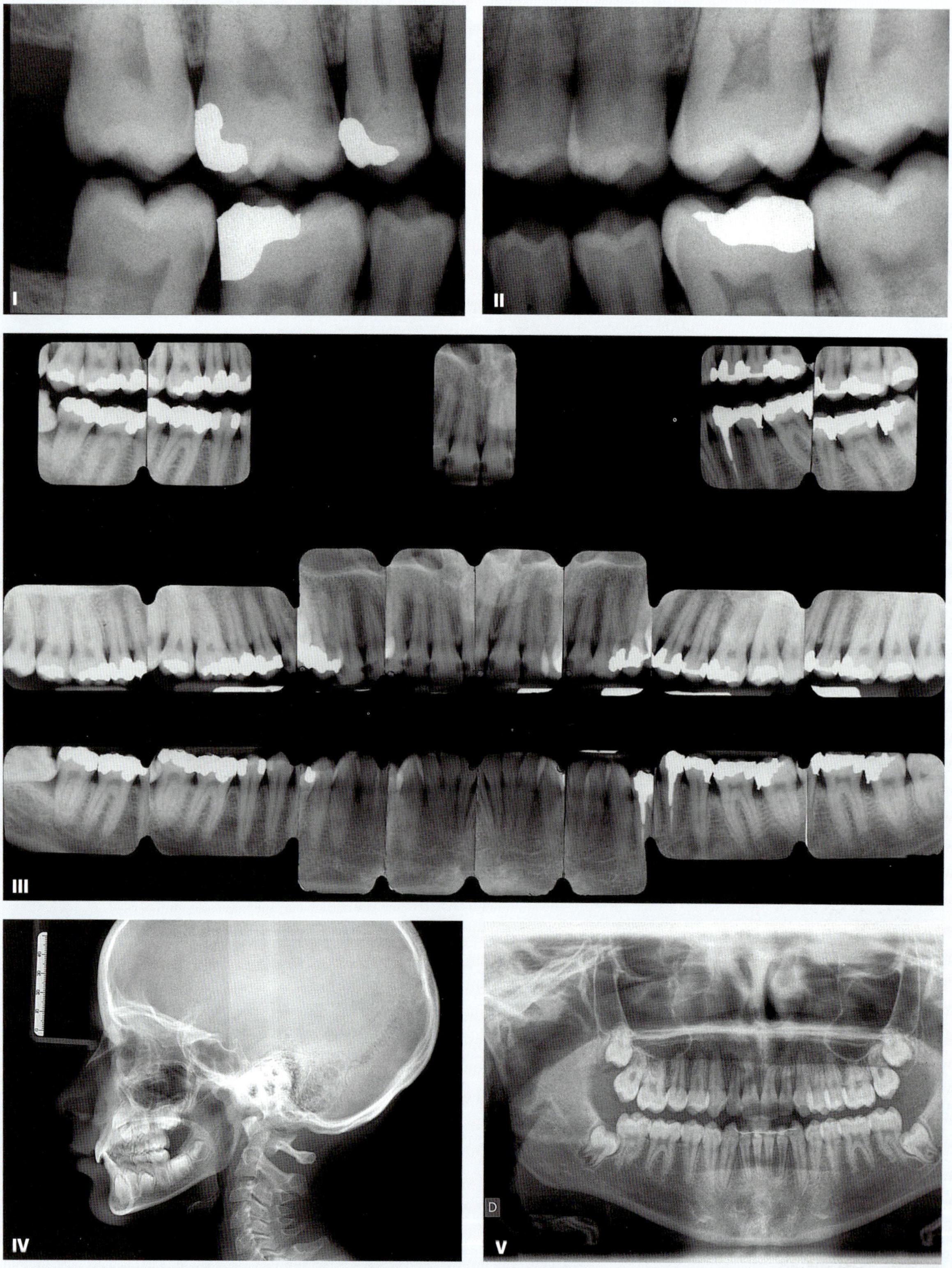

Fig 2 Specific radiographic examinations in dentistry. Bitewing radiograph specific for diagnosing decay *(I, II)*. Full-mouth radiographs providing a full overview of all important elements: the clinical crown, root, bony ridge, and tooth support structures *(III)*. Lateral cephalometric radiograph *(IV)* and panoramic radiograph *(V)* specific to orthodontics. Computed tomography scans necessary for three-dimensional evaluation of alveolar bone and the adjacent structures of the maxillary sinus and mandibular canal for implant dentistry *(VI, VII)*.

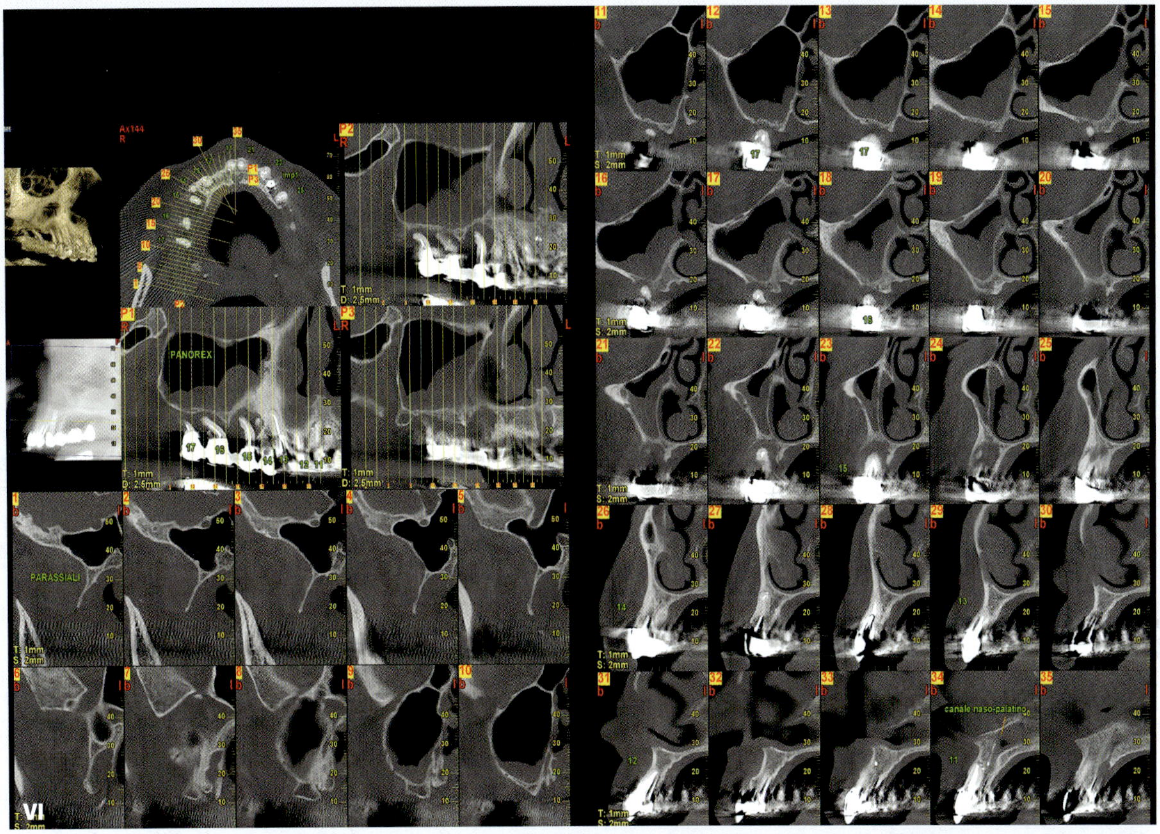
PANOREX
PARASSIALI
canale naso-palatino
VI

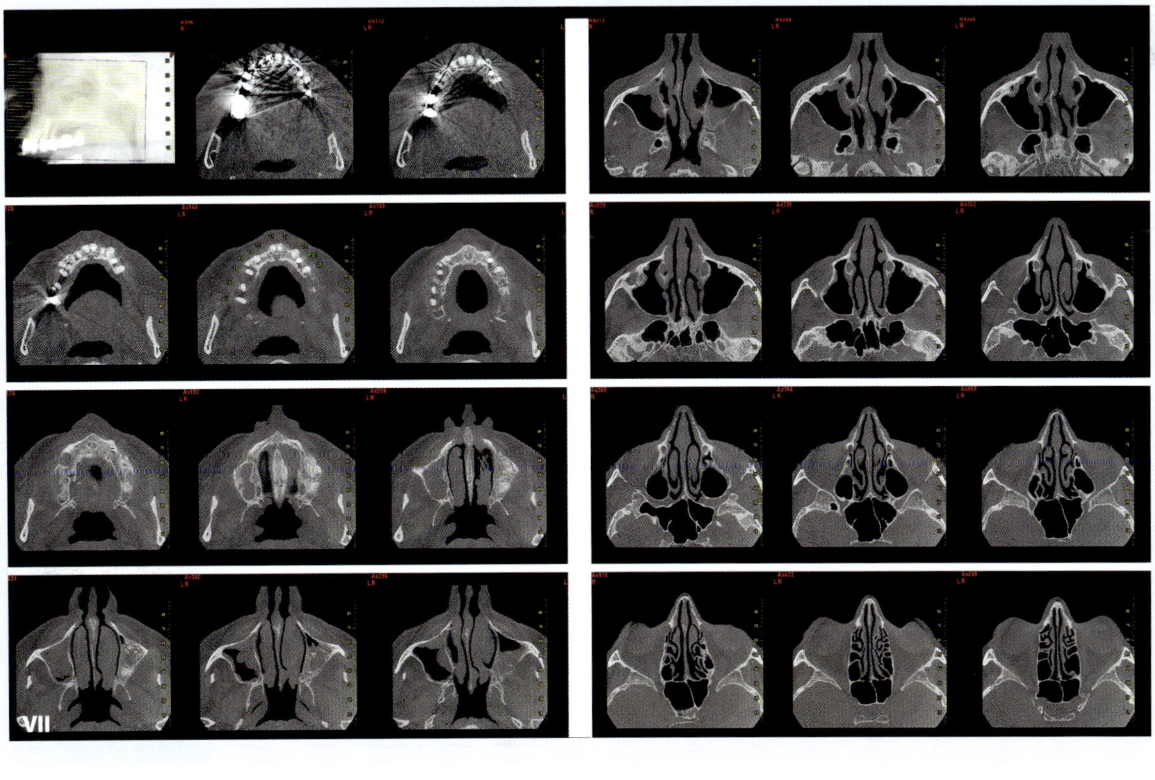
VII

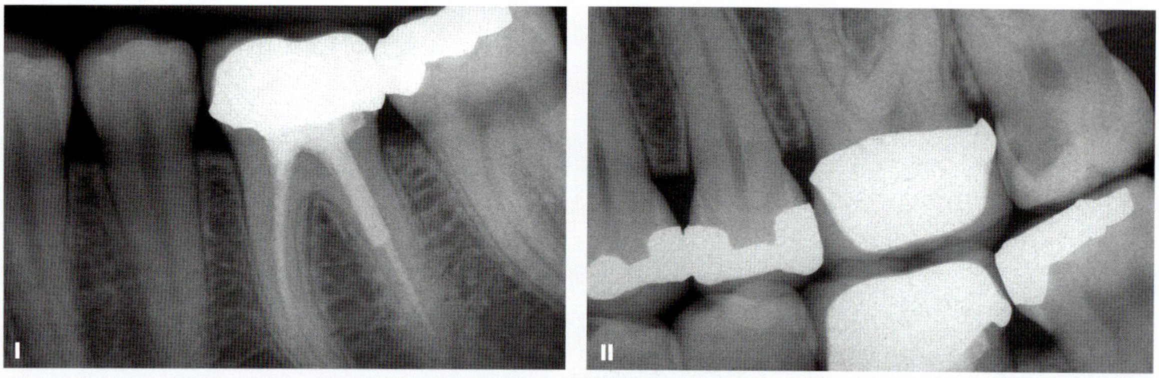

Fig 3 The patient presents with painful symptoms in the third quadrant. A radiograph of the third quadrant *(I)* is insufficient, and a bitewing radiograph *(II)* is required in order to make an accurate diagnosis, ie, pulpitis of the maxillary left second molar.

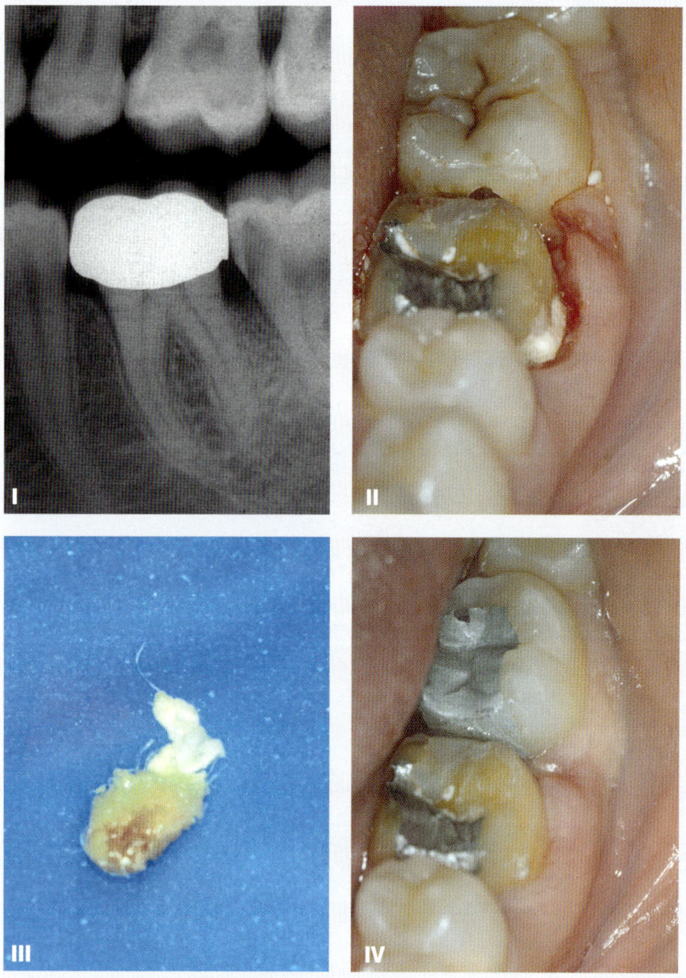

Fig 4 The patient complained of continuous discomfort in the third quadrant. Imperfect sealing of the prosthetic crown margins, without the typical signs of pulpitis that could potentially indicate decay of the mandibular left second molar, led the treatment team to remove the crown and make the correct diagnosis: inflammation of the soft tissues of the adjacent first molar caused by cotton wool and cement present in the gingival sulcus. The immediate treatment of the decay of second molar is an obvious requirement.

Ethics and of course training, professionalism, and intellectual honesty should be the natural ingredients in a proper treatment plan.

Acting in accordance with the instructions of Professor Holz, the author likes to take as long as necessary to educate patients because time spent during this sensitive stage will be of great help at later stages of treatment. Teaching patients to read their own radiographs allows them to be able to interpret the black

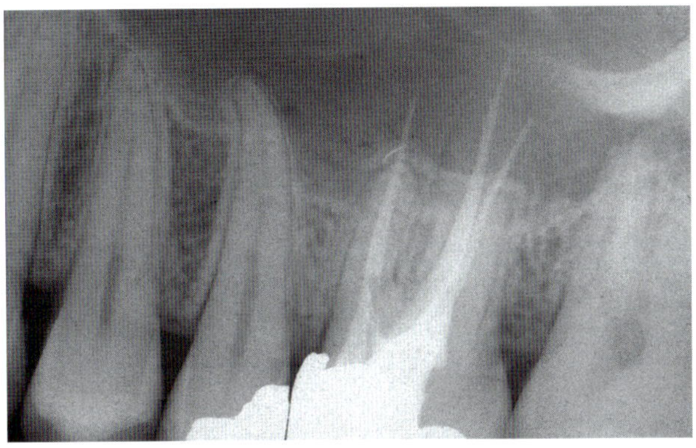

Fig 5 The pain is caused by an invasion of the biologic space by the amalgam restoration with consequent inflammation of the periodontal tissues, and not by the gutta-percha beyond the apex in all the canals.

Fig 6 Differential endodontic-periodontal diagnosis. Absence of periodontal probing leads to the diagnosis of a lesion of endodontic origin and consequently to re-treatment of the root canal.

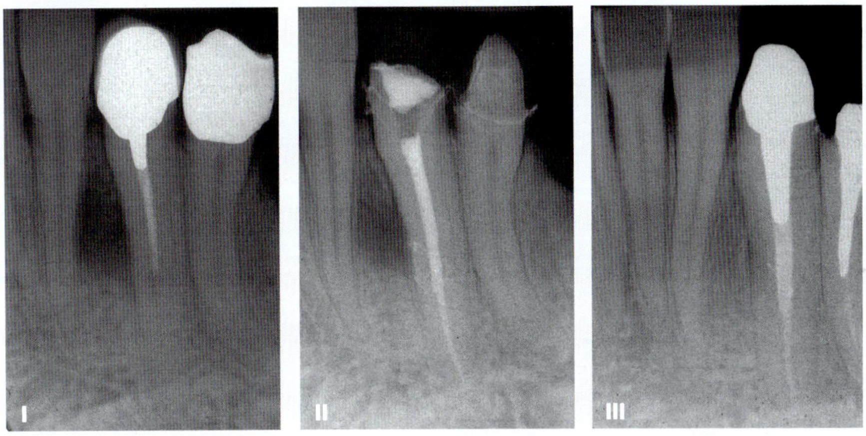

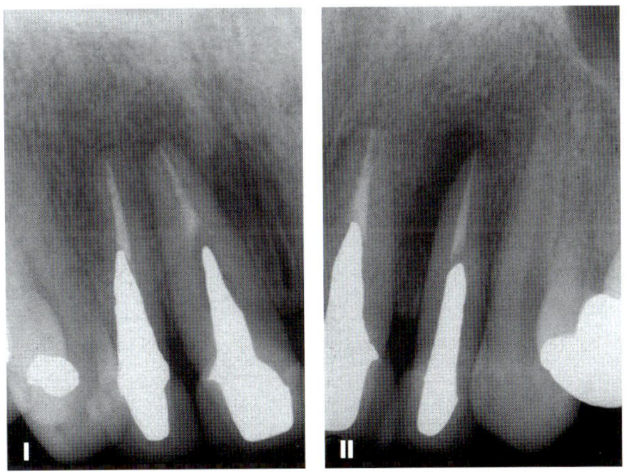

Fig 7 Vertical fracture of the root of the maxillary left lateral incisor caused by the presence of an oversized post.

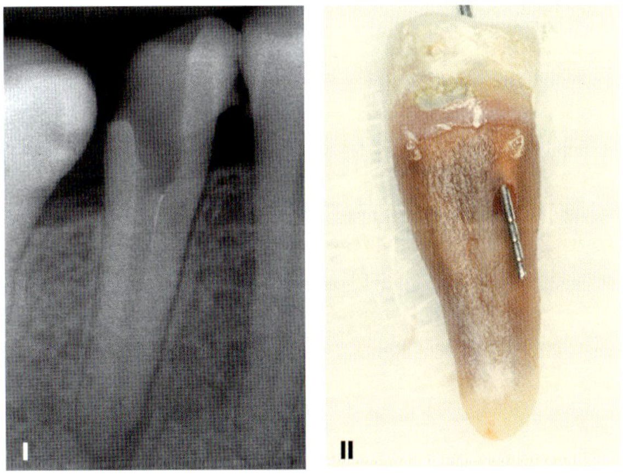

Fig 8 Root perforation caused by incorrect endodontic procedures.

spot breaking the continuity of the white line that they know is the enamel and to "self-diagnose" decay when they attend hygienist appointments. In the same way, they will also be able to recognize an apical lesion, a fracture line in dentin, a situation of periodontal involvement, and occlusal and articular dysfunctions. They will be able to recognize all of these things because they will have been shown everything on the computer before any type of treatment is carried out (Figs 9 and 10).

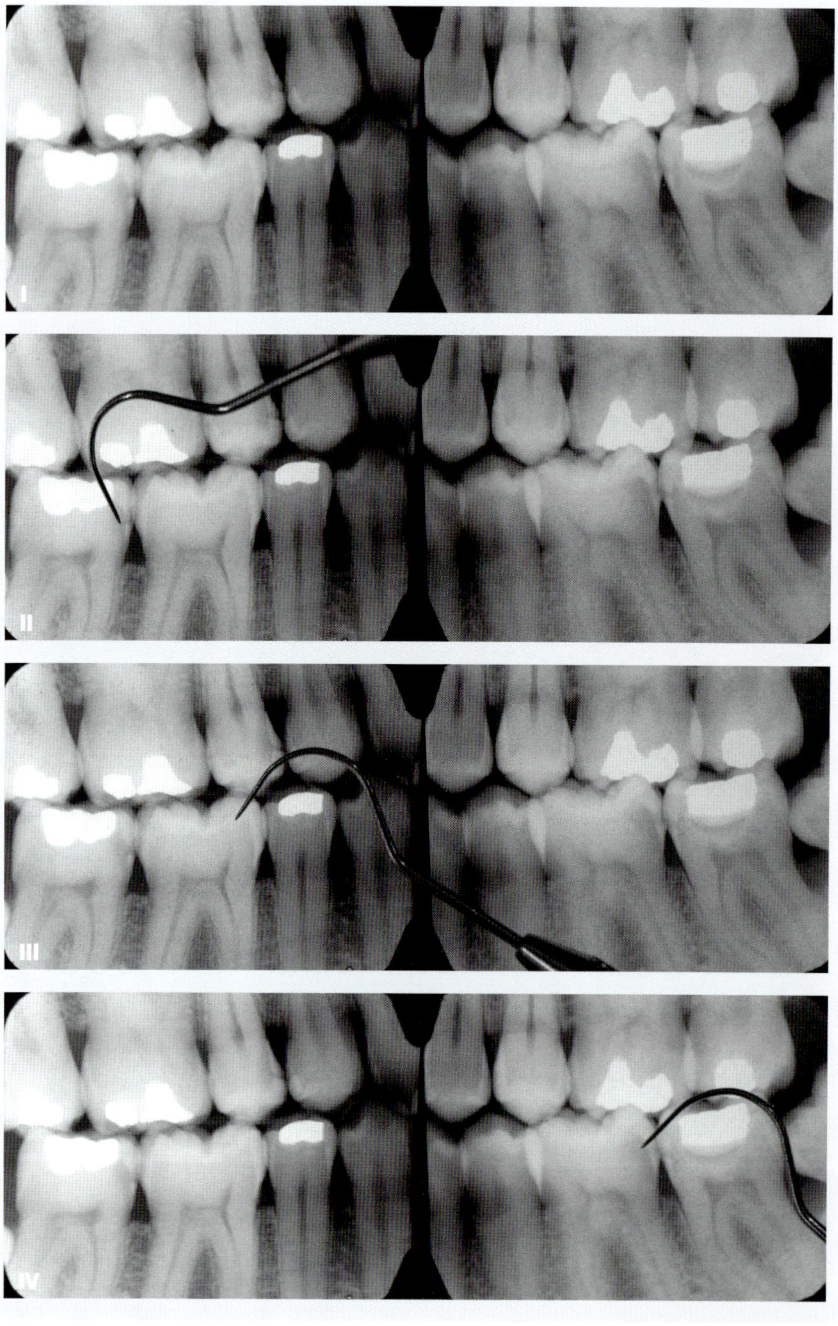

Fig 9 The practitioner teaches the patient to interpret the radiographic differences between healthy and decayed enamel and dentin.

The patient will be aware, for example, that two bitewing radiographs are essential for diagnosing caries lesions, because the practitioner has spent a few minutes explaining this. Above all, the clinician will have explained that caries lesions between teeth are often inaccessible for clinical examination and that these two radiographs therefore must be carried out at least once a year (Figs 11 to 14).

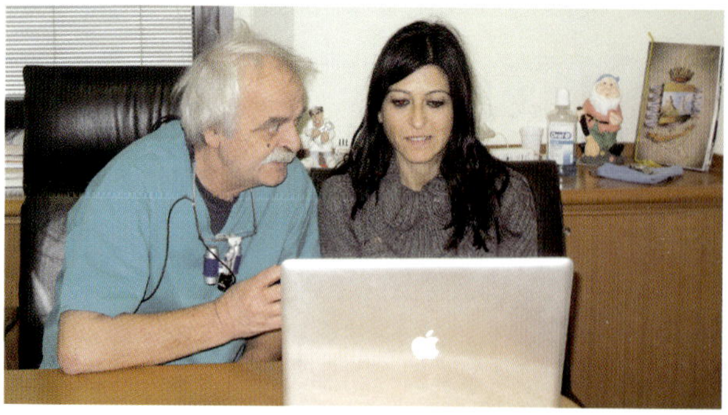

Fig 10 The practitioner shows the patient all the treatment steps to be performed.

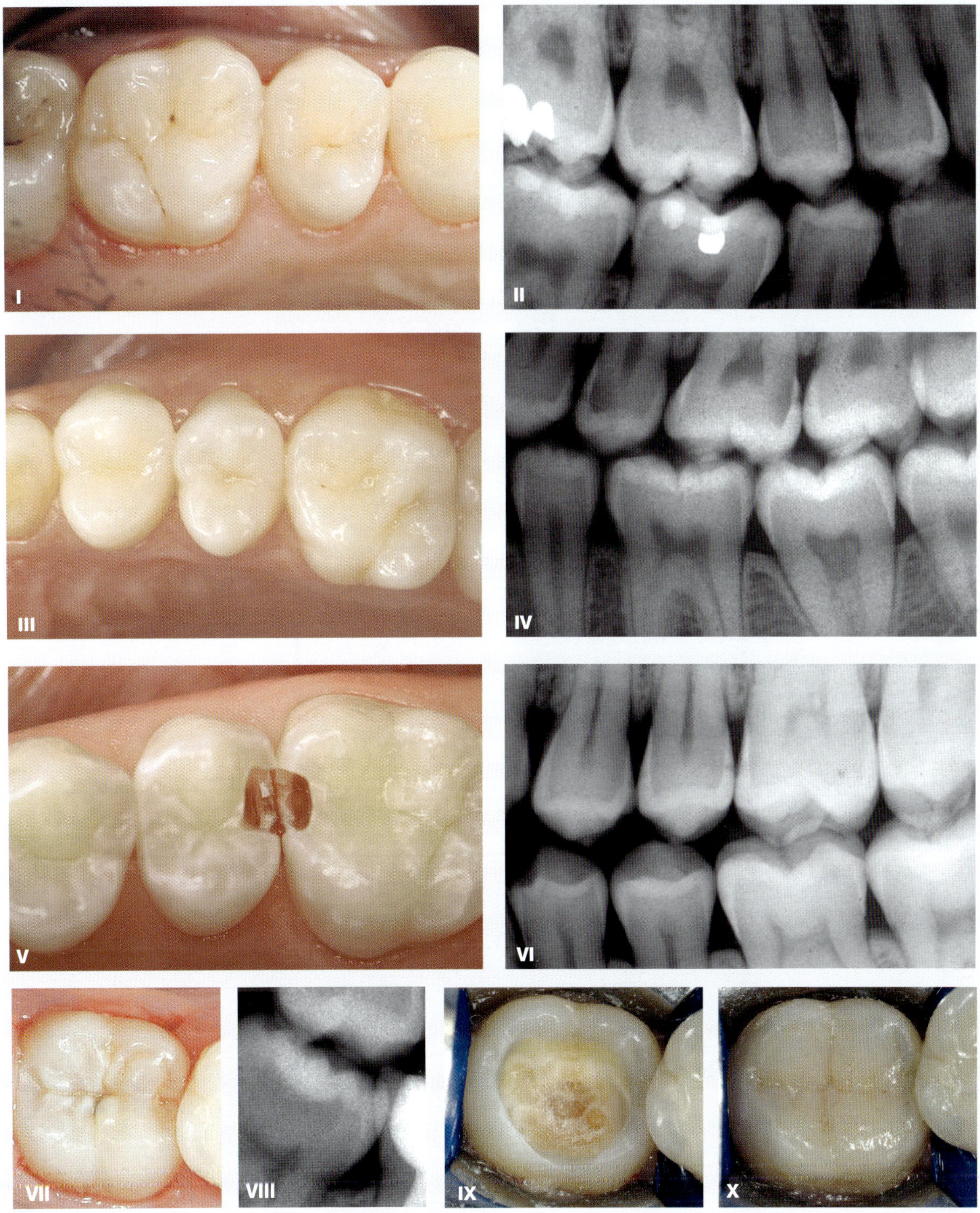

Fig 11 A clinical examination is insufficient to make a diagnosis without the support of radiographs.

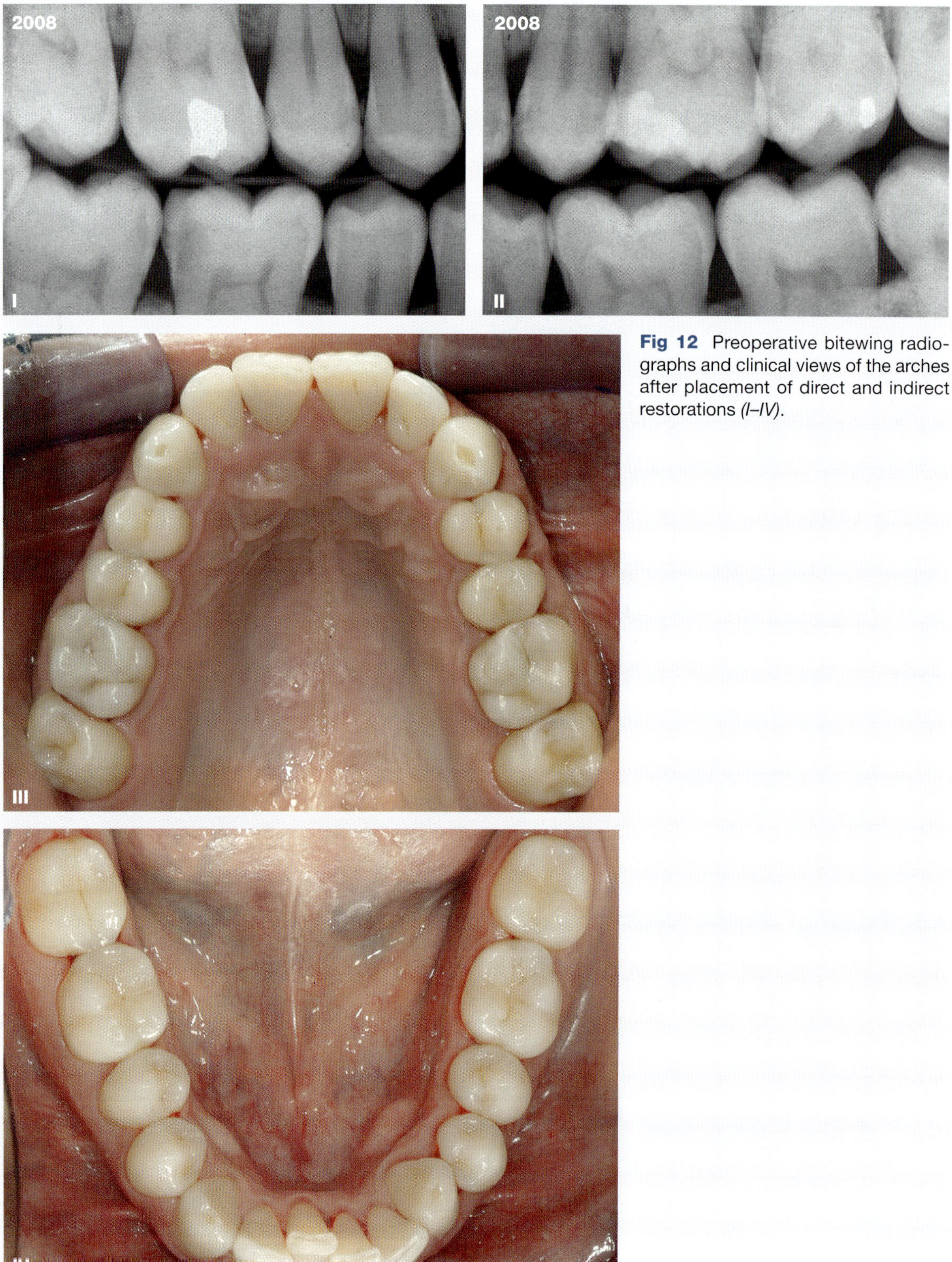

Fig 12 Preoperative bitewing radiographs and clinical views of the arches after placement of direct and indirect restorations *(I–IV)*.

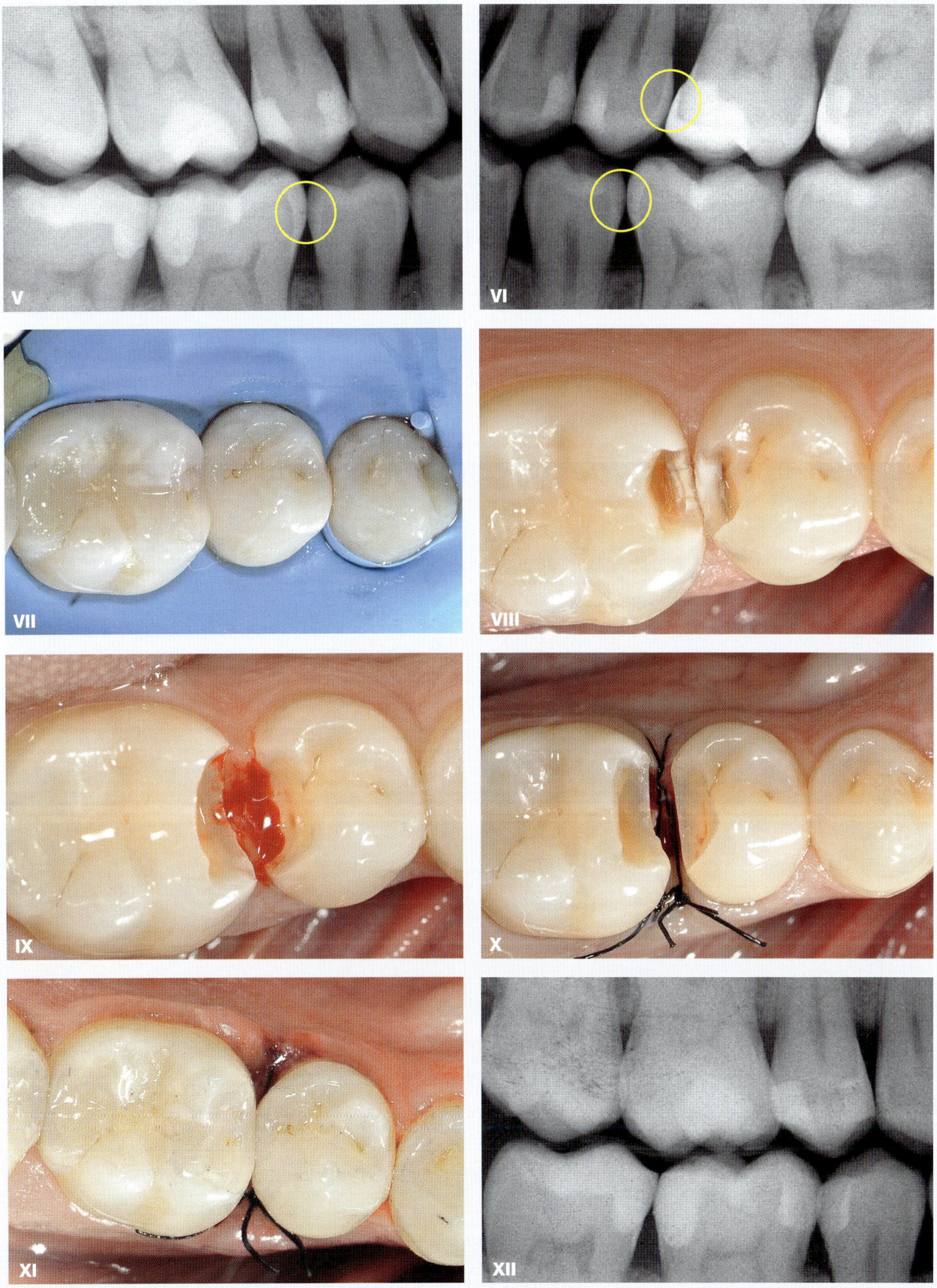

Fig 12 (*continued*) Follow-up radiographs 2 years later. The patient, who is obviously not very motivated, shows caries lesions *(V, VI)*. Restoration of the mandibular right second premolar and first molar with follow-up radiograph *(VII–XII)*.

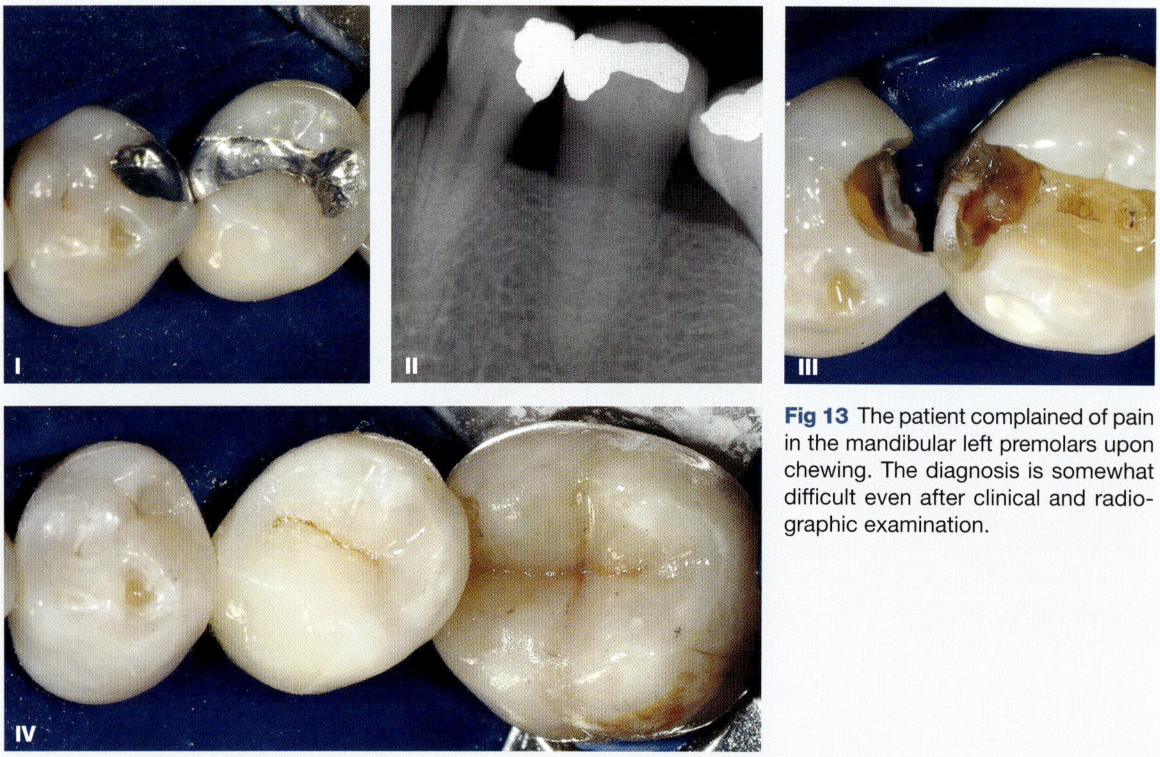

Fig 13 The patient complained of pain in the mandibular left premolars upon chewing. The diagnosis is somewhat difficult even after clinical and radiographic examination.

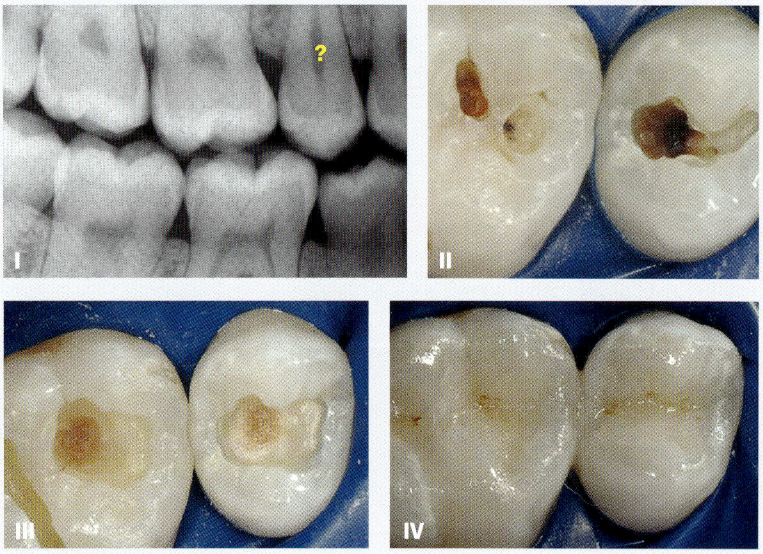

Fig 14 Direct restorative treatment of deep caries of the maxillary right second molar that cannot be diagnosed from a bitewing view.

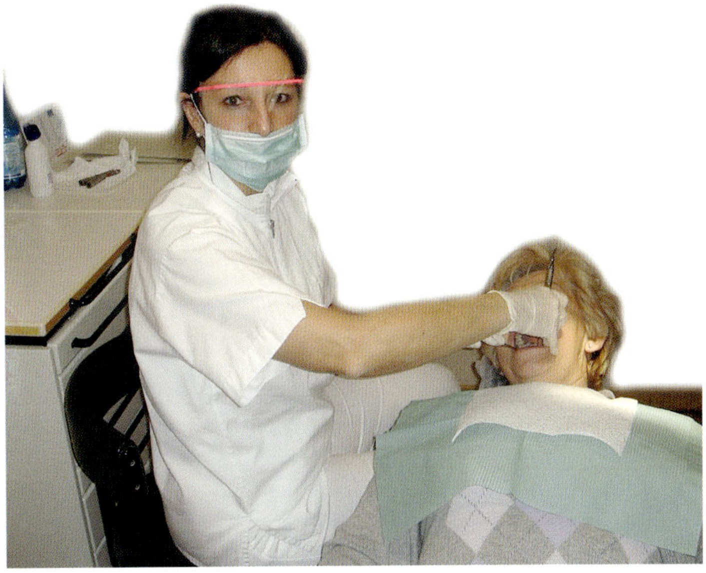

Fig 15 The dental hygienist at work to remove tissue inflammation.

Patients will also be aware that if they are protected in accordance with protocol, these essential radiographic examinations are practically harmless.

This leads to the all-important role of dental hygienists (Figs 15 to 18). An objective definition of their role would be that they are specialists in preventing diseases of the teeth and oral cavity, preventing decay, and providing nonsurgical periodontal treatment. If they perform their job responsibly, they treat patients individually in accordance with their needs and make a significant contribution to promoting oral health through the motivation and associated information that they convey—sometimes with great effort, it must be said—to their patients. A much more subjective definition of their role would

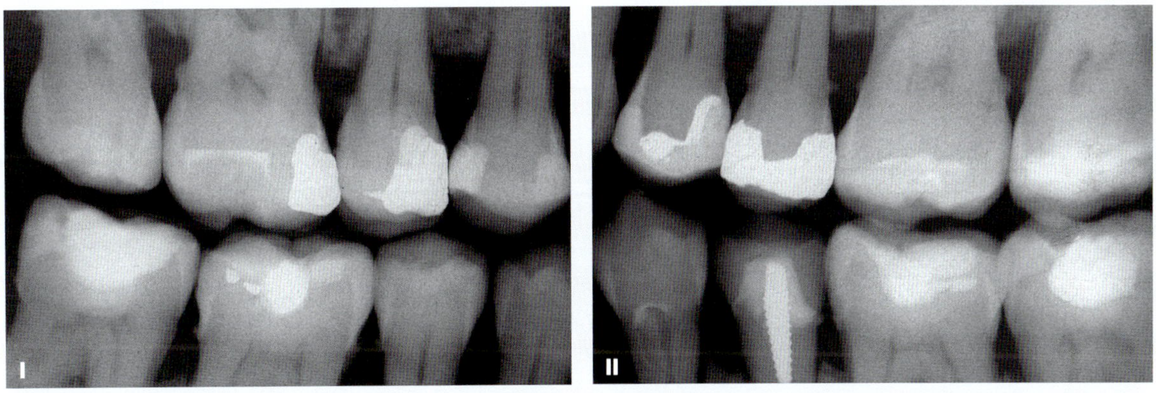

Fig 16 The hygienist can easily identify and remove visible buildup of tartar with the help of bitewing radiographs.

Fig 17 When hygienists notice an entirely abnormal situation, as shown in this image, they become alarmed and immediately alert the dentist so that an examination can be performed.

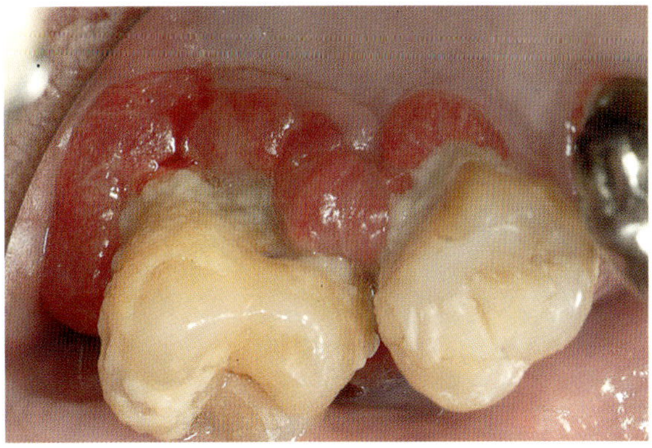

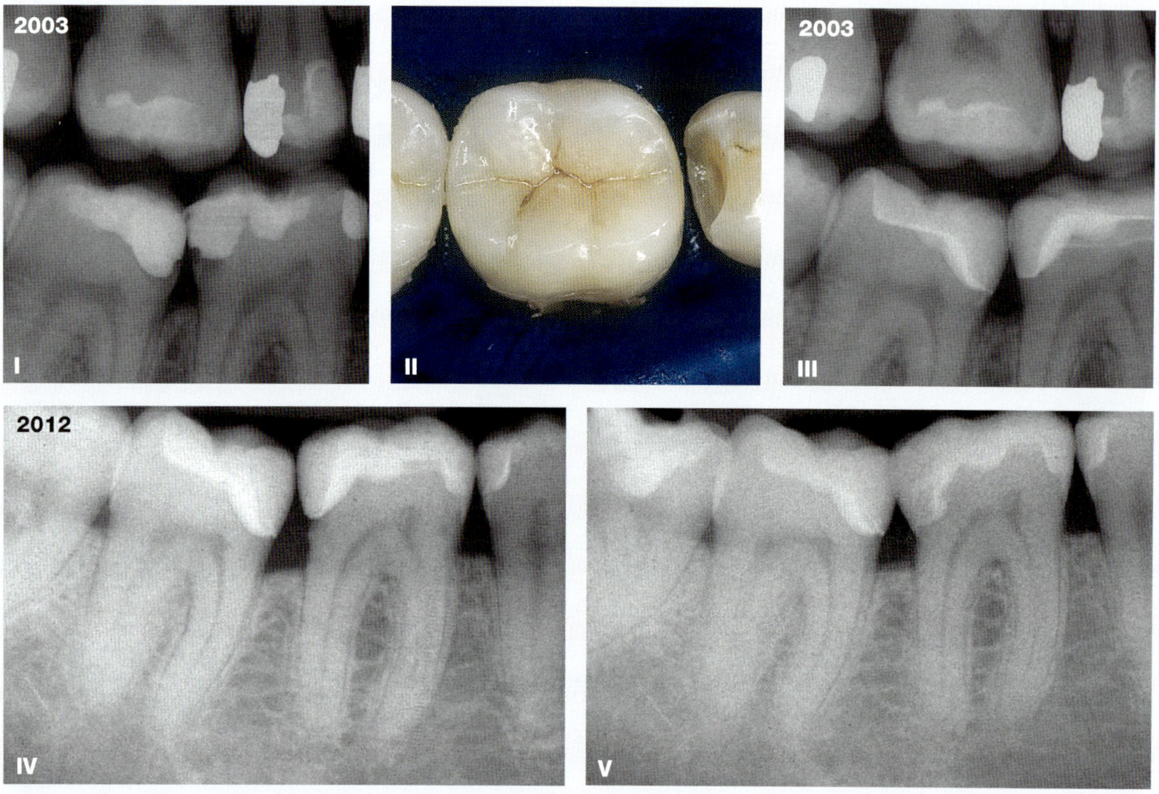

Fig 18 The fundamental task of the hygienist is motivation, and the goal is to check the patient at least once yearly. Failure to carry out consistent exams and removal of inflammation in healthy or restored teeth may naturally lead to a caries lesion or, as in this clinical case, a recurrence after not attending maintenance visits for 9 years.

be that they are an essential part of the team: during the 60 minutes that they treat the patient two, three, or four times a year, according to need, they succeed in establishing a personal relationship that becomes even more valuable when the patient makes the transition to the dentist's chair. Patients who have been motivated and informed that a problem is endodontic rather than periodontal or that they have multiple caries lesions or have been shown in the mirror a crack in a marginal ridge or a particularly abnormal probing will have been properly primed for the practitioner and will find it much less difficult to understand a diagnosis and treatment plan.

In the hour or two that they devote to the patient, according to circumstances, they are able to remove plaque (Fig 19) and tartar, polish the teeth, and take the radiographs that are essential to ensuring that the clinician's work is effective. Above all, however, they understand patients' needs and state of mind at their particular stage of life and gain the trust that will subsequently be a great help to the clinician.

In order to achieve these outcomes, the author believes that it is essential to organize meetings attended by dentists, hygienists, and assistants, where paramedical staff are thoroughly informed of the latest techniques so that they are able to convey the information discussed to the patient. Full knowledge of all these aspects is also a great help to administrative staff when they are communicating with patients on the phone and responding to requests for explanations and confirmations and, last but not least, complaints.

The role of the dental nurse is so important that it transcends mere words: all the author can do is give enormous thanks to his nurses, Alessia and Martina, and all the other nurses who help his colleagues in the practice (Fig 20).

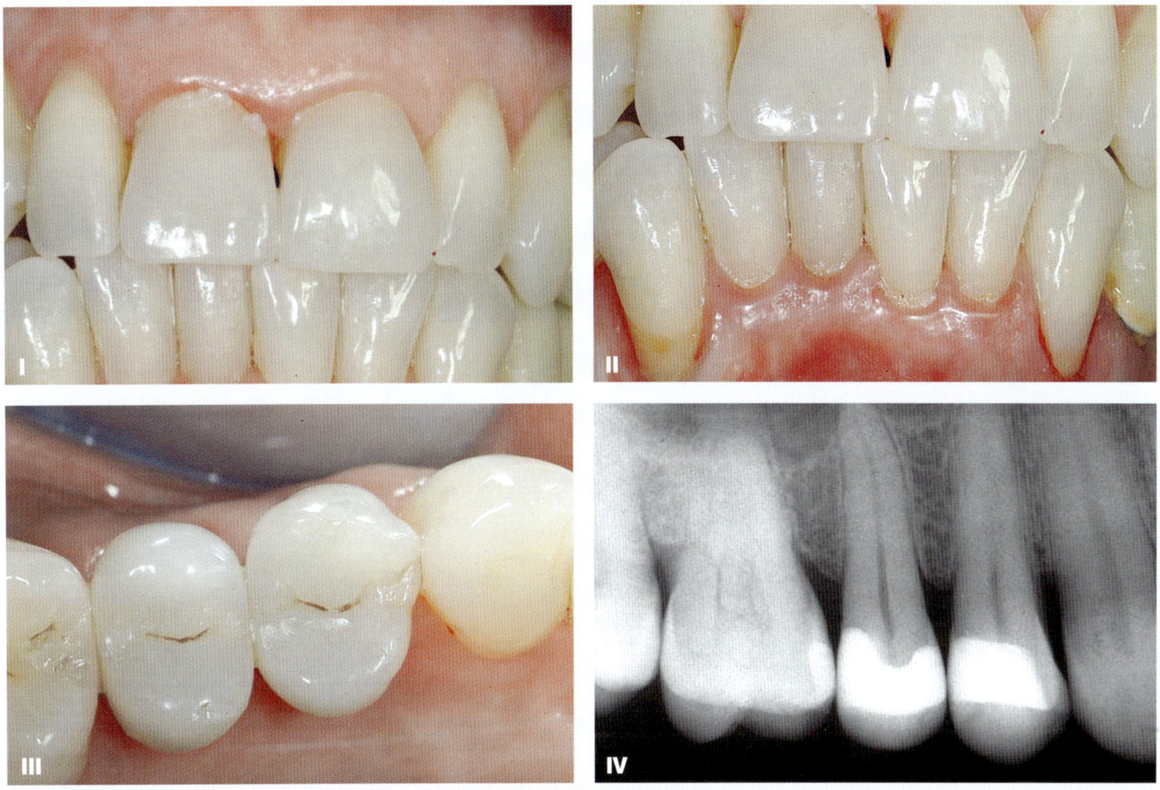

Fig 19 Despite far from assiduous control of bacterial plaque, the clinical and radiographic images 7 years after indirect restoration of the maxillary right premolars is absolutely satisfactory.

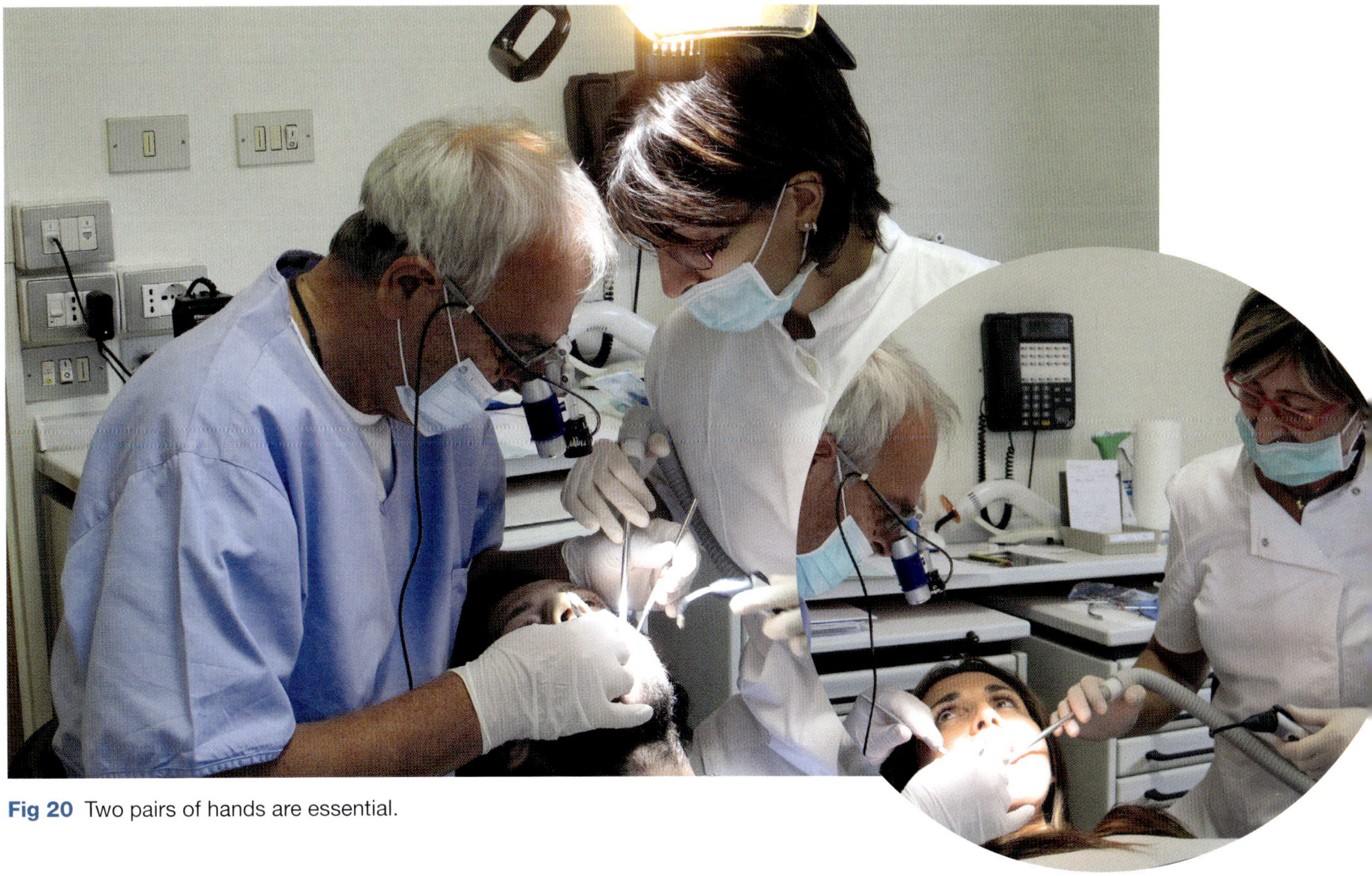

Fig 20 Two pairs of hands are essential.

Diagnosis in conservative dentistry

It is useful to provide a proper definition of dental caries. According to the World Health Organization, dental caries is a localized, posteruptive pathologic process of external origin, involving softening of hard tooth tissue and proceeding to the formation of a cavity.

CLINICAL CLASSIFICATION OF CARIES (University of Geneva)

Initial caries	No cavitation, appears as a whitish, rough, and chalky spot lesion involving only the enamel; the only type of caries that can be reversed by fluoride
Superficial caries	Extends beyond the dentinoenamel junction and therefore initiates dentin invasion
Deep caries	Extends apically and affects the dentinal body of the tooth
Penetrating caries	Causes a reaction of the dentin-pulp complex with formation of tertiary dentin
Perforating caries	Entails exposure of the pulp.

As in all other branches of medicine, a diagnosis (identification of a disease on the basis of signs, symptoms, medical history, and laboratory tests) is a fundamental stage of dentistry and must precede any therapeutic action since it makes it possible to define a proper treatment plan, which is, in turn, followed by a maintenance and follow-up stage (Fig 21).

A satisfactory treatment plan therefore must involve a thorough diagnostic examination that provides a full assessment of the multidisciplinary problems present, without limiting itself to an analysis of the individual tooth. Pure dental evaluation, an integral part of a wider diagnosis, considers the structural, endodontic, and periodontal problems of individual teeth, using traditional methods combined with increasingly sophisticated instruments for examination. Within the more restrictive field of reconstructive dentistry, it is essential to examine the diagnosis of caries in greater depth.

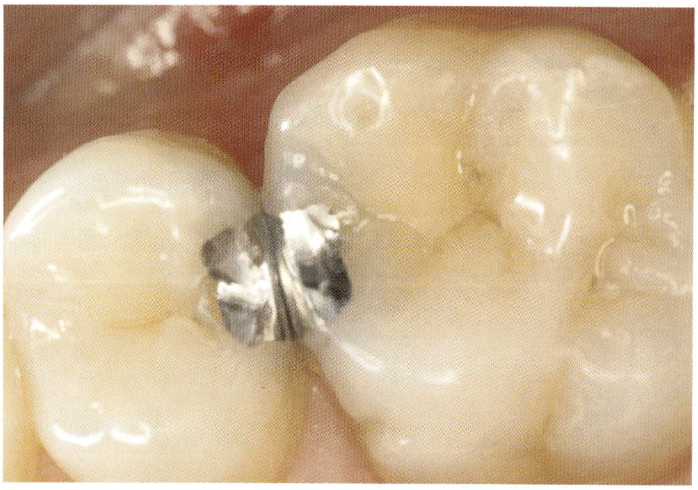

Fig 21 Early diagnosis allows preservation of as much healthy tooth structure as possible. This image shows 16-year follow-up of re-polished amalgam restorations.

A diagnostic evaluation of caries may be divided into three essential stages[1,2]

- Diagnosis of presence
- Diagnosis of activity
- Diagnosis of risk

Diagnosis of presence

The first stage, which must demonstrate the actual presence of caries lesions within individual teeth, is still based on traditional procedures, namely visual and tactile physical assessment and instrumental examination in the form of radiographic, digital, or classic examinations, which are now supported by new, increasingly advanced technologies.

A classic physical examination involves direct inspection of the accessible tooth surfaces once they have been thoroughly cleaned, dried, and illuminated with the aim of evaluating the enamel color and the presence of any cavitation involving the dentin. The use of a magnifying system makes this procedure much easier. Tactile examination using a sharp probe should make it possible to identify cavitated lesions by evaluating the extent to which the instrument sinks into the tooth. Some authors believe that this action is not ideal because excessive pressure on grooves and fissures could lead to a high risk of iatrogenic lesions with cavitation of decalcified enamel.[3] Considering the difficulty in standardizing the pressure exercised by the instrument, it is advisable to restrict the use of probes to those that are fine but not excessively sharp in the evaluation of dentinal hardness at root level, excluding occlusal and interproximal surfaces.[4]

The classic instrumental examinations used to diagnose the presence of decay are radiographs and transillumination.

A thorough radiographic examination, whether traditional or digital, should be considered essential for the proper diagnosis of caries, particularly at the interproximal level. Some authors believe that without properly executed radiographs there is a potential risk of failing to diagnose 80% of lesions.[5,6] Bitewing radiography is the most recommended technique for diagnosis and also for making decisions regarding the need for intervention. A radiographically evident caries lesion justifies the need for swift intervention, while treatment based on long-term prevention and reassessment would certainly be more recommendable in the absence of such signs.[2,4]

Radiographs also represent an essential instrument when checking existing restorations (Fig 22).

Transillumination is a noninvasive procedure that is recommended for the assessment of interproximal regions, particularly in the anterior teeth. The principle is based on the physical effect of attenuating a light beam generated by a special lamp that passes through the calcified dental tissue; the caries lesion is clearly evident as a dark area[2] (Fig 23).

The most advanced instrumental diagnostic techniques that have appeared recently are based on the principle of evaluating changes in the physical characteristics of demineralized tissues. Some authors believe

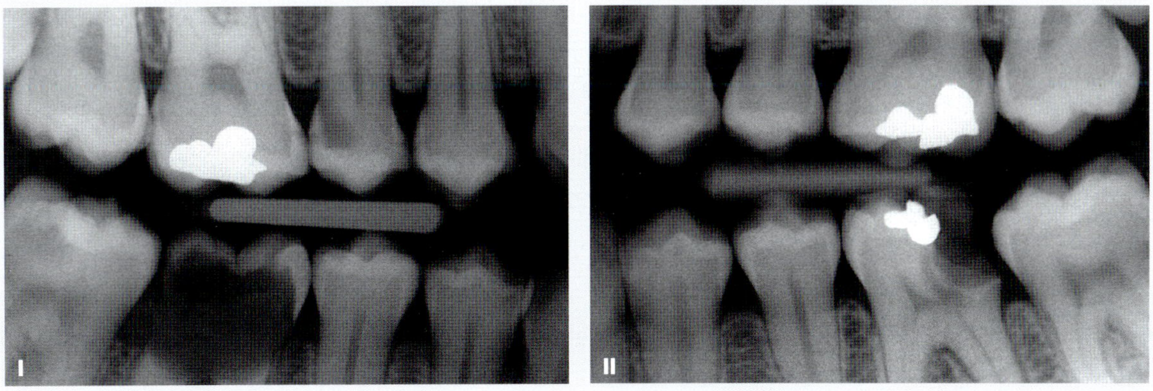

Fig 22 Bitewing radiographs allowing diagnosis of interdental caries lesions with different levels of dentinal involvement.

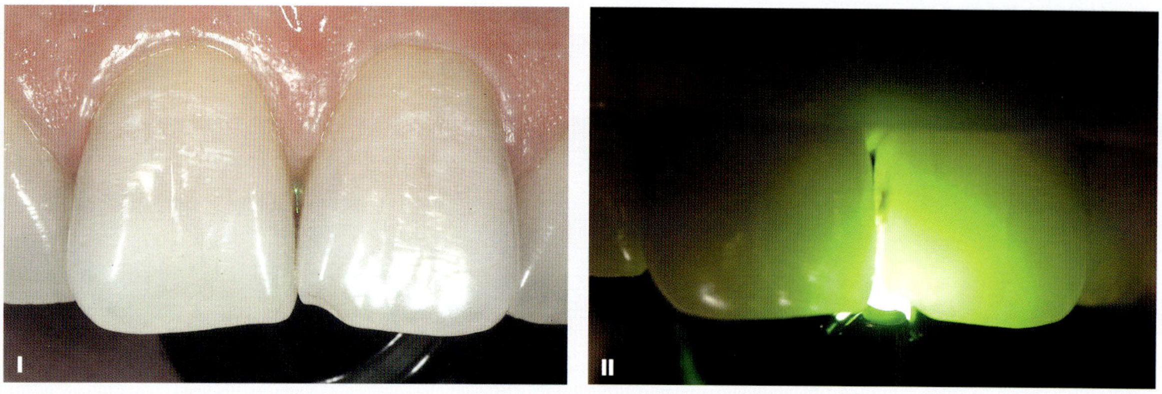

Fig 23 Transillumination. An interproximal caries lesion is revealed as a dark area.

that these state-of-the-art technologies could play a significant role in longitudinal evaluation and in monitoring the type of activity and the patient's risk of caries, although they are unable to replace conventional examinations.[7,8]

The new diagnostic instruments employ technologies that make use of laser emissions, electrical conductance, and ultrasound. Some of these should be considered to be still at the experimental stage, while others are already available for clinical use.[9]

Reports in the literature agree that the easiest technique to use is laser fluorescence, which is important for the early diagnosis of caries lesions and demineralization, particularly occlusal.

This principle is based on light activation of a laser diode on the surface to be examined and consequent evaluation of fluorescence generated in the diseased tooth tissue. This phenomenon is detected by the instrument and then processed and converted to a digital parameter that can be read off a display with the aid of a photoconductor and an electronic evaluation device[4,10] (Fig 24).

Laser fluorescence has proved particularly useful in the evaluation of occlusal grooves and in the diagnosis of hidden caries, where the enamel is apparently intact, but the underlying dentin has already been affected by the process of decay. This type of insidious caries lesion can be identified in 10% to 50% of adolescents.[4]

To conclude, a summary table can be drawn up of the potential applications of diagnostic methods based on the type of surface to be analyzed.

	Interproximal surfaces	Smooth surfaces	Occlusal surfaces	Root surfaces
Visual examination	–*	++	+	+
Tactile examination with probe	–	–	–	–
Laser fluorescence	+	+	++	+
Transillumination	+	–	–	–
Radiography	++	–	+	–

+, usable; –, unusable; ++ method of choice. *Usable after interdental separation.

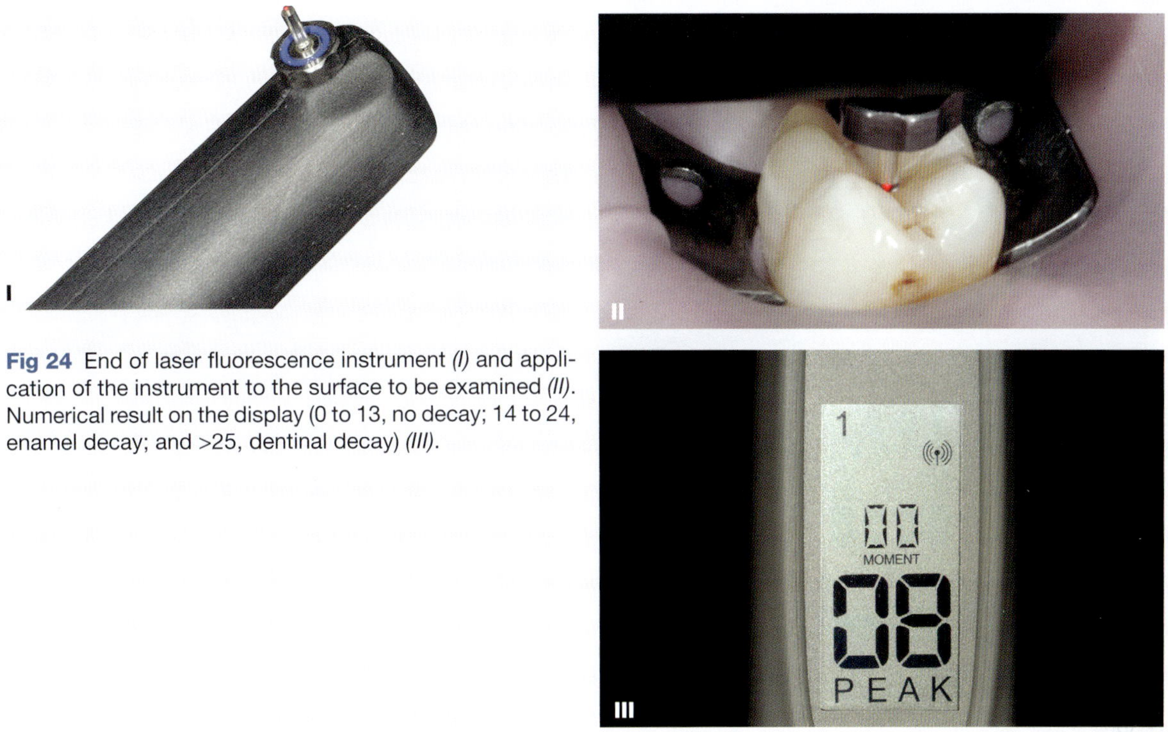

Fig 24 End of laser fluorescence instrument *(I)* and application of the instrument to the surface to be examined *(II)*. Numerical result on the display (0 to 13, no decay; 14 to 24, enamel decay; and >25, dentinal decay) *(III)*.

Diagnosis of activity

Caries lesion activity is diagnosed mainly by evaluating tissue color, location, and consistency.

In active and progressive lesions, the enamel is generally opaque, porous, chalky, and irregular in appearance, and these areas occur more commonly in places where bacterial plaque builds up, ie, at the gingival margin or in interproximal regions (Fig 25).

Arrested or regressive lesions, on the other hand, are characterized by enamel with a smooth, shiny, hard, and intact surface, sometimes pigmented, that may be assessed by gently rubbing with a probe.[11,12]

At the dentinal level, a pale color and soft consistency combined with a certain level of sensitivity indicates an active lesion, while the presence of darker, firm, and less sensitive tissue could suggest reduced or arrested progression.[1,2]

At root level, some authors believe that dentinal coloration is less important than surface consistency, and the presence of soft tissue certainly indicates an active lesion.[4]

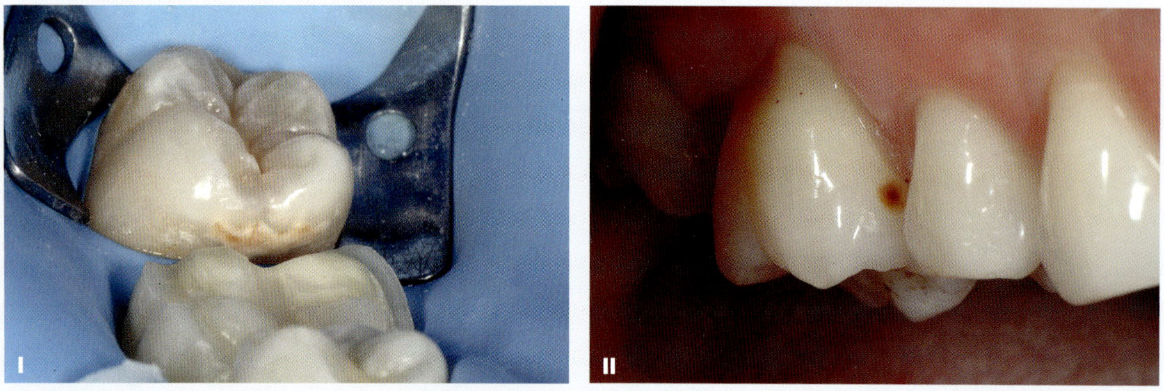

Fig 25 Opaque, porous, and chalky appearance of an active caries lesion *(I)*. Image of a slowly developing caries lesion *(II)*.

Diagnosis of risk

The risk of caries is defined as the probability of caries arising over a certain period. A potential change in the size and activity of existing caries lesions must also be considered.[13]

The main parameters for evaluating risk of caries are as follows[14]:

- Number of teeth decayed, missing, or filled (DMF score)
- Age and state of oral health
- Microbiologic tests
- Salivary flow and buffer potential
- Fluoridation
- Oral hygiene
- Diet and eating habits

The main factors affecting risk of caries onset may therefore be identified as a predisposition on the part of the host (hygiene, saliva, fluoride, and family history), presence of acidogenic bacteria, and type of diet (particularly carbohydrates).
According to some authors, the three main stages of risk assessment concern medical history, clinical examination, and microbiologic saliva tests.[15]
High-risk patients are therefore considered to be those with predisposing systemic diseases, receiving drug treatment interfering with saliva flow, with reduced salivary flow and buffering capacity, with poor oral hygiene who frequently consume carbohydrates, who have high levels of *Streptococcus mutans*, not receiving preventive fluoride treatment, and who have recent cavitated lesions and caries on low-risk surfaces. This defines the risk categories into which different patients may be classified.
The American Dental Association distinguishes three risk categories: low, moderate, and high. It considers adult patients at high risk to be those with three or more caries lesions in the last 3 years or two or more

of the following conditions: deep grooves and fissures with previous episodes of significant or numerous caries, frequent exposure to sugars, reduced salivary flow, inadequate oral hygiene and fluoridation, and irregular checkups.[16]

An evaluation of the risk of caries seems to be fundamental to the management of a proper treatment plan considering that the elimination and control of risk factors should always precede any restorative therapy.[15]

Based on these considerations, a modern conservative approach should always indicate the necessary preventive measures for high-risk patients and identify patients with low risk to limit the placement of restorations and avoid unnecessary interventions.[17]

The importance of early diagnosis and prevention should then be further emphasized since these are the cornerstones of a minimally invasive approach adopted with the aim of being able to "prevent or delay the execution of a restoration."[18,19]

Silver amalgam

Back in the 1980s, when the author had the great fortune to study at the University of Geneva under Professor Holz, to whom, needless to say, he owes a debt of gratitude, amalgam was the most commonly used material in posterior tooth restorations (Fig 26). As 30 years have gone by, great strides have been and continue to be made in research and technology, and one is entitled to wonder whether amalgam restorations have any place in today's clinical practice. Younger colleagues often say, almost as a boast, that there is no longer any trace of amalgam in their practices (Fig 27). Without wishing to go into the debate over the toxicity of the material, its ease of use, and the very long-term results it allows, the author will borrow Dr Monari's words and say that the correct use of amalgam certainly brought more benefits than documented risks for many decades. These pages, however, will discuss replacing amalgam with present-day resins, and it may appear counterintuitive to praise amalgam when the option of higher-performing nanohybrids is available. The author nevertheless finds that there are specific indications for the use of amalgam, even today. The most important is the management of root caries lesions (Figs 28 to 30), where it is impossible to isolate the surgical field properly with rubber dam. The second indication is for clinical situations involving patients who are difficult to motivate, show poor hygiene, have no cosmetic needs, fail to attend checkups, cannot tolerate rubber dam, or do not present for treatment until they are in pain. The third indication is for patients who request treatment for a caries lesion in a tooth that is covered with plaque and tartar, where

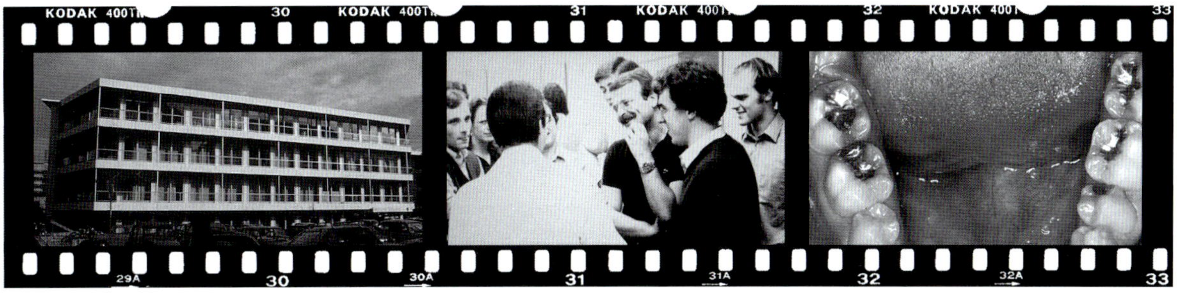

Fig 26 Arch with amalgam restorations *(far right)* performed at the University of Geneva (1979–1982) *(far left and center)*.

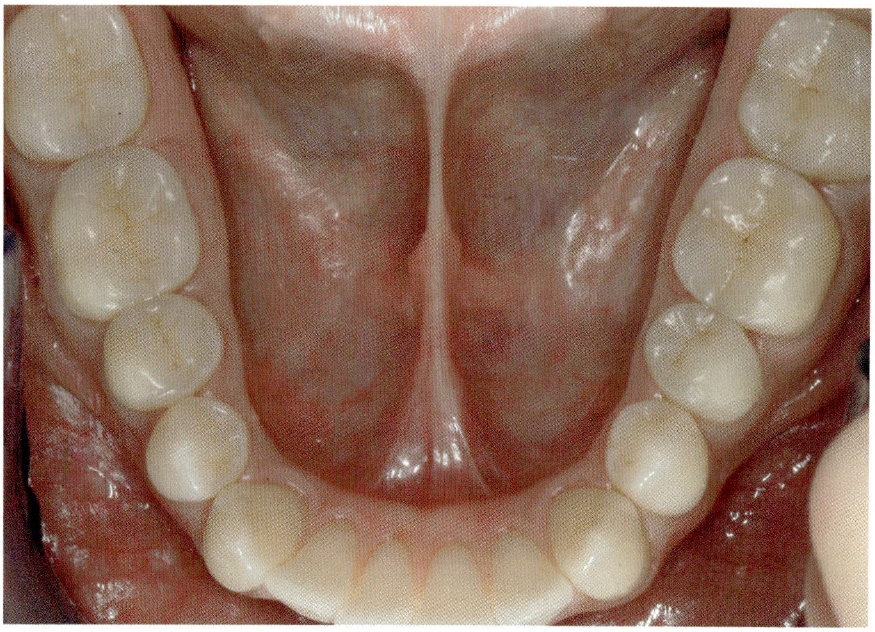

Fig 27 Cosmetic requirements, peer pressure, and the properties of new materials work in favor of dentists' acceptance of composite resins.

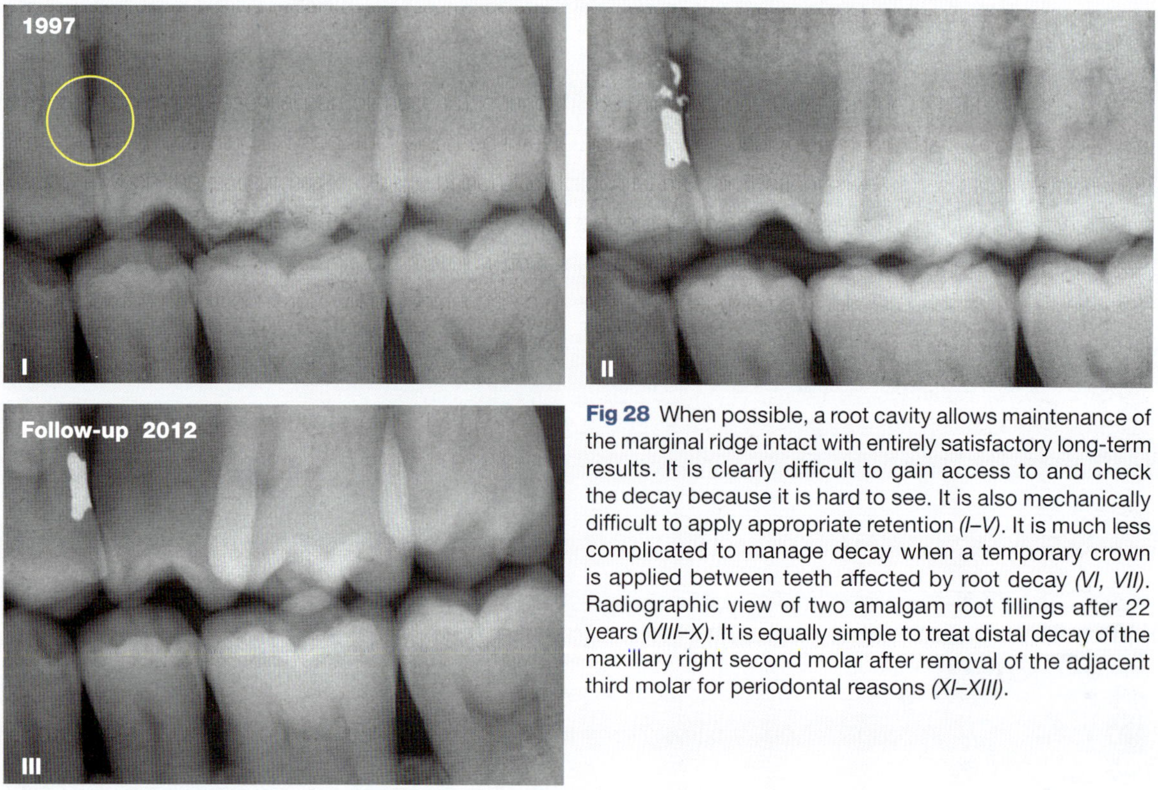

Fig 28 When possible, a root cavity allows maintenance of the marginal ridge intact with entirely satisfactory long-term results. It is clearly difficult to gain access to and check the decay because it is hard to see. It is also mechanically difficult to apply appropriate retention *(I–V)*. It is much less complicated to manage decay when a temporary crown is applied between teeth affected by root decay *(VI, VII)*. Radiographic view of two amalgam root fillings after 22 years *(VIII–X)*. It is equally simple to treat distal decay of the maxillary right second molar after removal of the adjacent third molar for periodontal reasons *(XI–XIII)*.

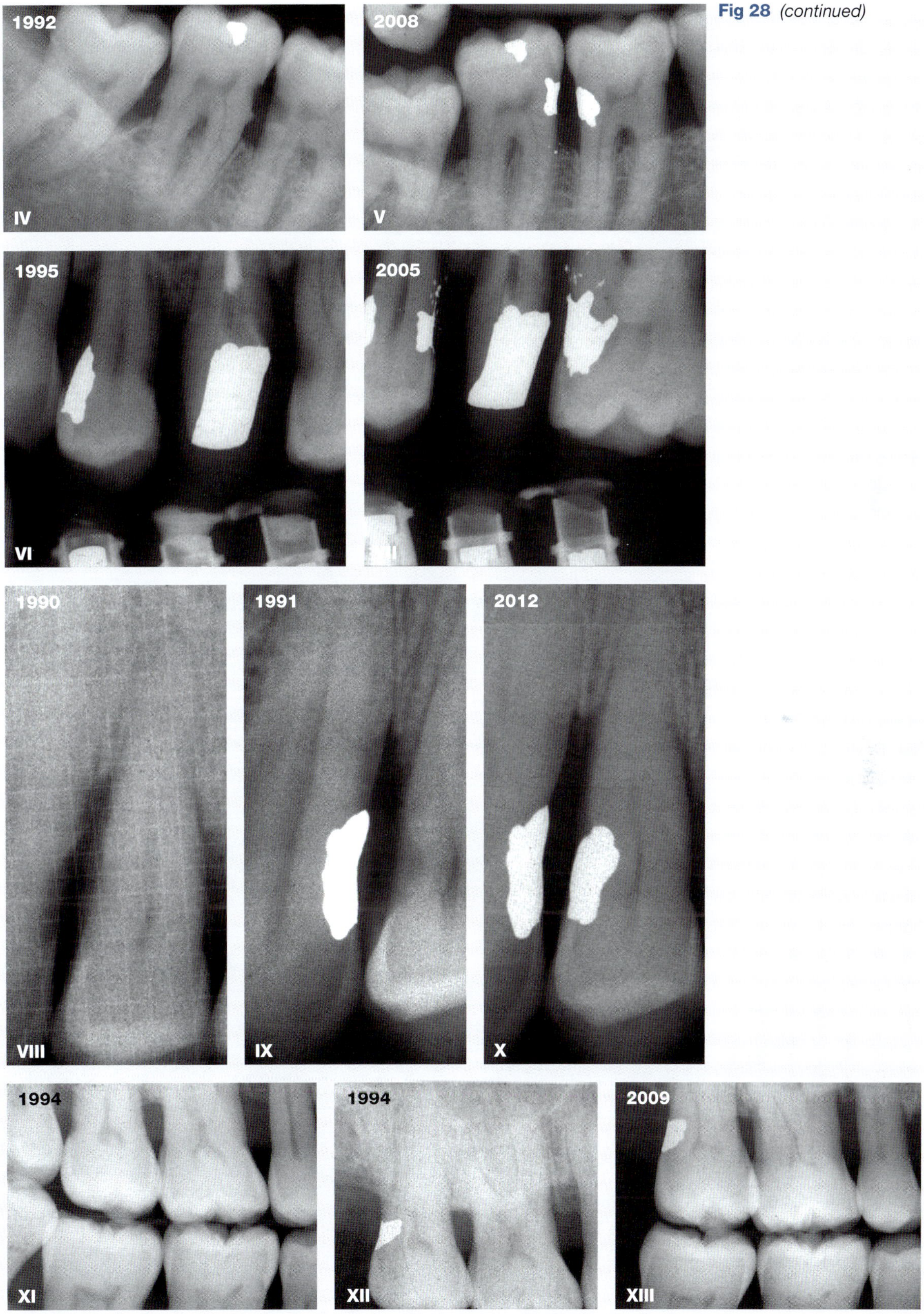

Fig 28 *(continued)*

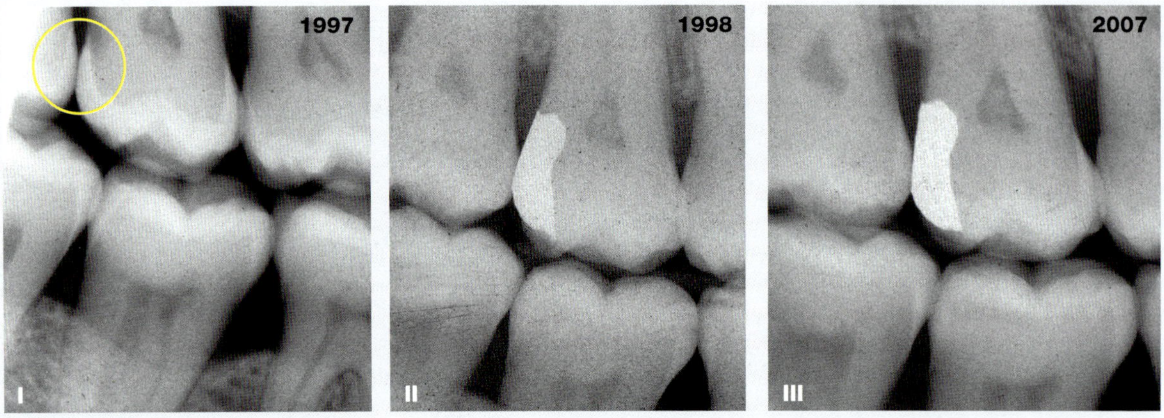

Fig 29 When it is not operationally possible to create a root cavity, a Class 2 restoration that is as conservative as possible is indicated.

Fig 30 Sometimes an unsuccessful root cavity, in this case due to detachment of the amalgam, leads to severe tissue loss. The only consolation is very long-term stability.

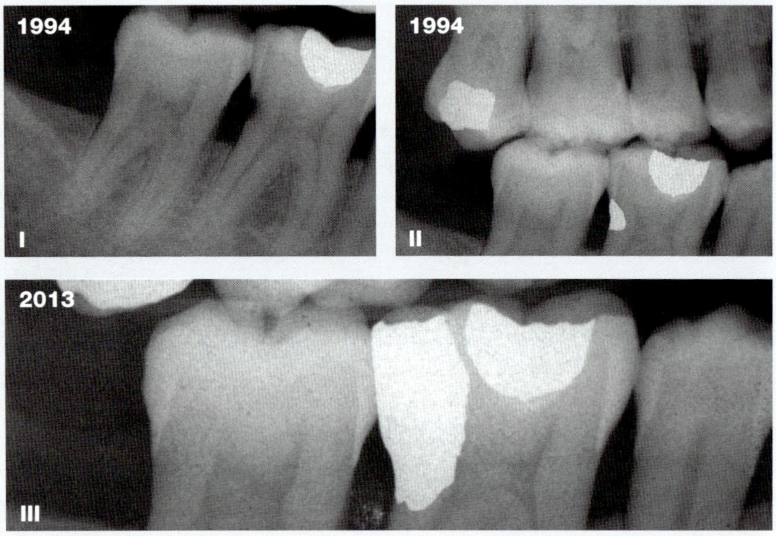

the absolute requirement is that the treatment should be as fast and economical as possible. Instead of turning away such patients, the dentist can perform an amalgam restoration that gives excellent results over time and, naturally, attempt to motivate them (Figs 31 to 36).

It is much more difficult to salvage the situation when the indication is to remove old metal restorations that are not causing any problems: one typical example is the innumerable fracture lines, sometimes horizontal but often vertical, that are routinely found whenever infiltrated restorations are removed due to recurrence of caries because the patient says, *"When I chew I feel a twinge."* Is it ethically correct to replace amalgam restorations that have been working well for so long as a matter of routine practice?

There are plenty of reasons, of course, such as the undeniable benefits of returning to a correct modulus of elasticity instead of one that is so different from the modulus of dentin as well as the low resistance to fracture.[20]

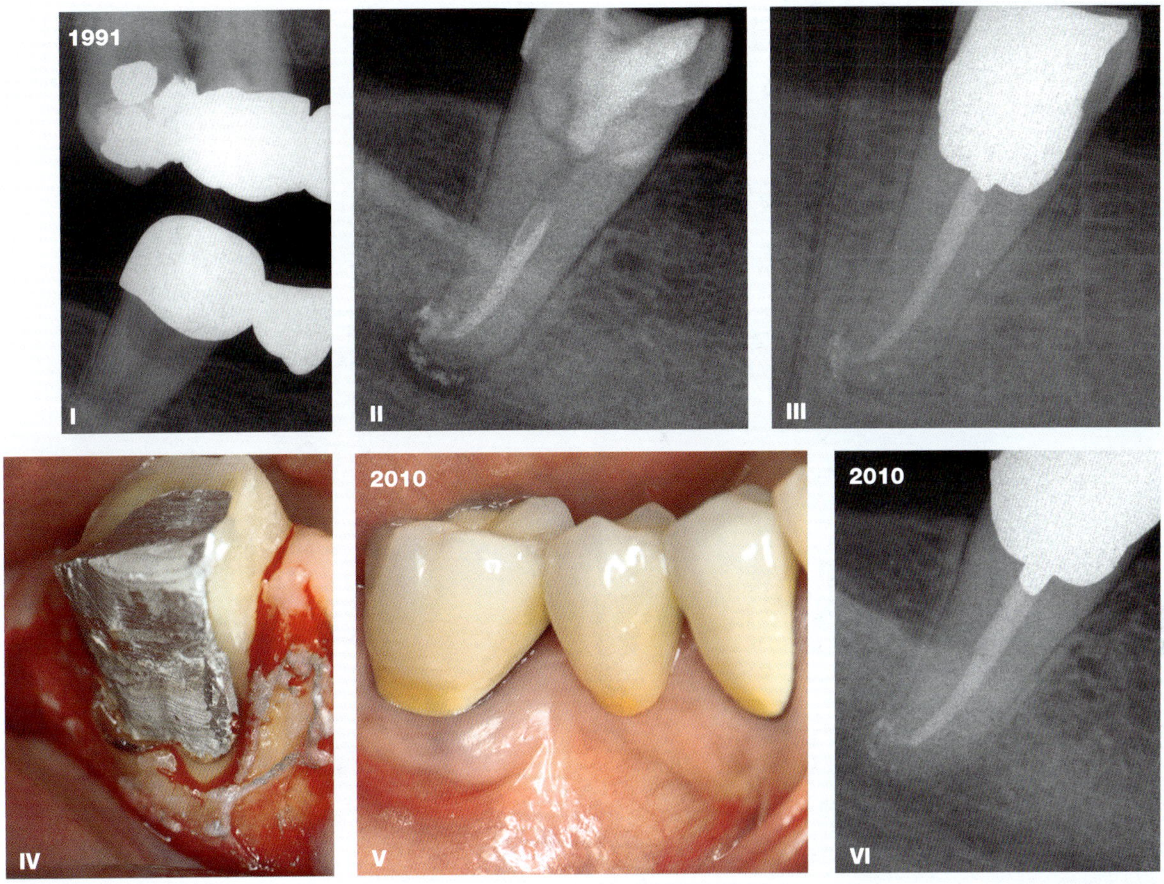

Fig 31 After endodontic treatment for penetrating decay *(I, II)*, a tooth acting as an abutment for a partial denture was reconstructed with amalgam after periodontal surgery *(III, IV)*. After polishing and preparation of the abutments, a new partial denture was made. Clinical and radiographic follow-up of the multidisciplinary treatment after 19 years *(V, VI)*.

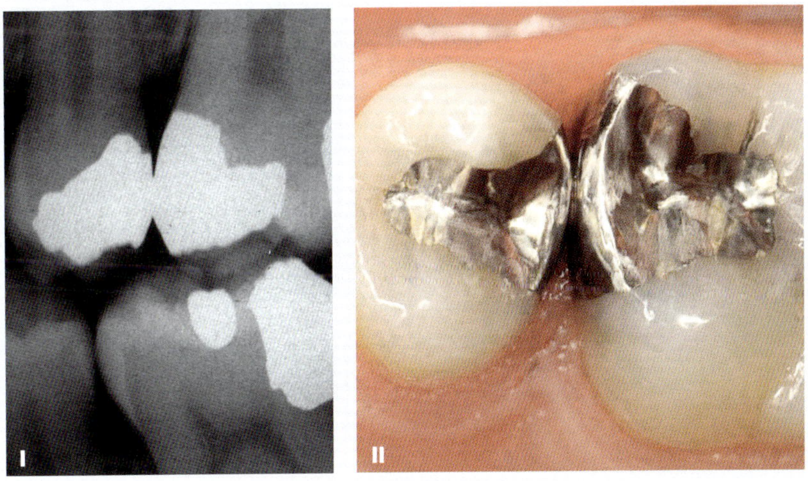

Fig 32 Follow-up of two amalgam restorations after 16 years. Marginal seal and emergence profiles may be seen radiographically, while a clinical view shows very satisfactory interproximal contacts and anatomical modeling.

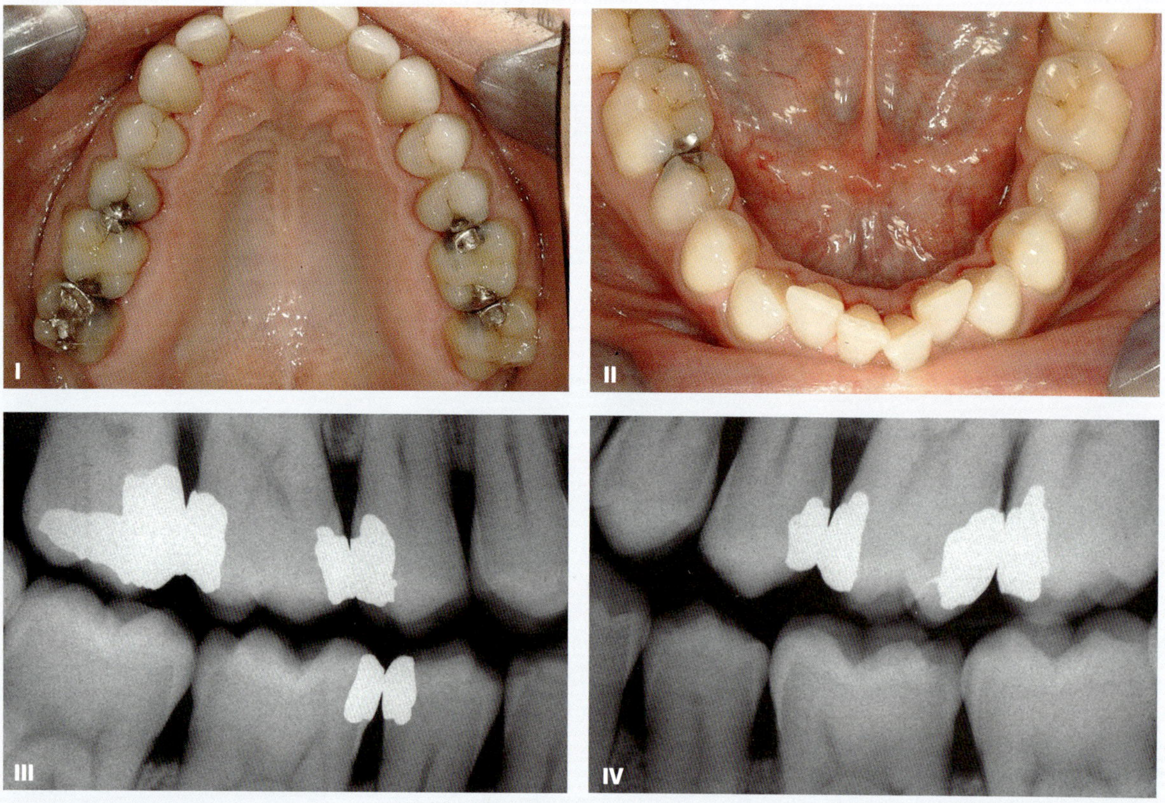

Fig 33 Clinical and radiographic follow-up of amalgam restorations after 19 years. The patient attends regular hygienist appointments and reports no discomfort. Maintenance treatment was therefore performed to the author's and the patient's satisfaction.

Fig 34 Intact margins after 10 years. The amalgam restorations were re-polished over time to prevent plaque buildup.

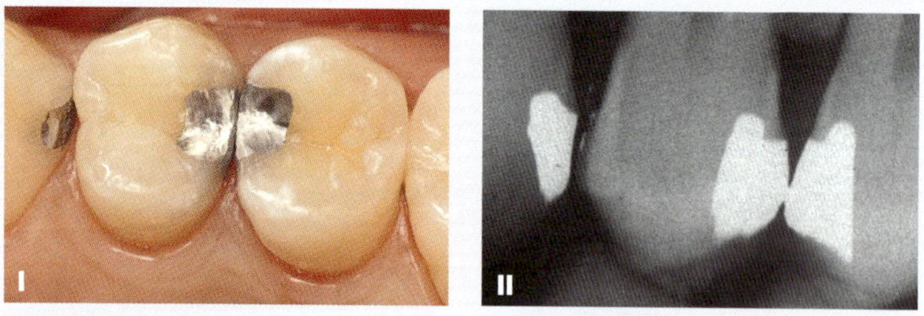

Fig 35 Excellent condition of an amalgam restoration on the mesial aspect of the maxillary right first premolar when checked after 15 years. The metal restorations are consistently re-polished every 4 to 5 years so that decay does not recur on the smooth surface.

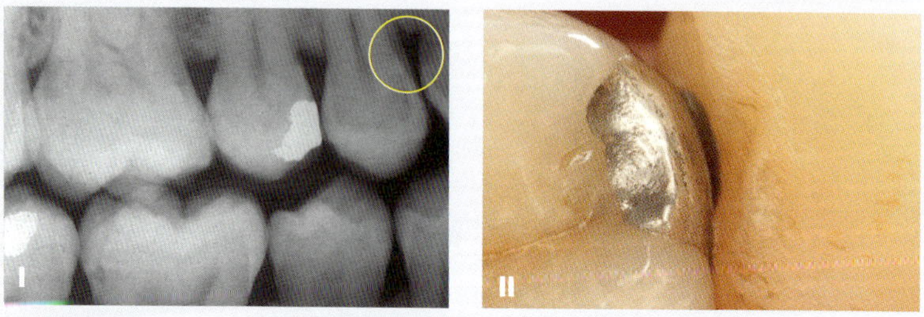

Fig 36 Small amalgam restorations attest to an early diagnosis.

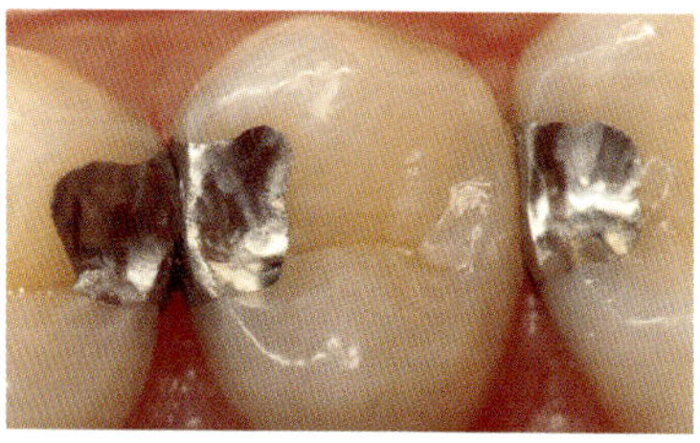

The author believes that the current insistent request for composite restorations is, apart from anything else, simply a great desire for a result with good esthetics (Figs 37 and 38).

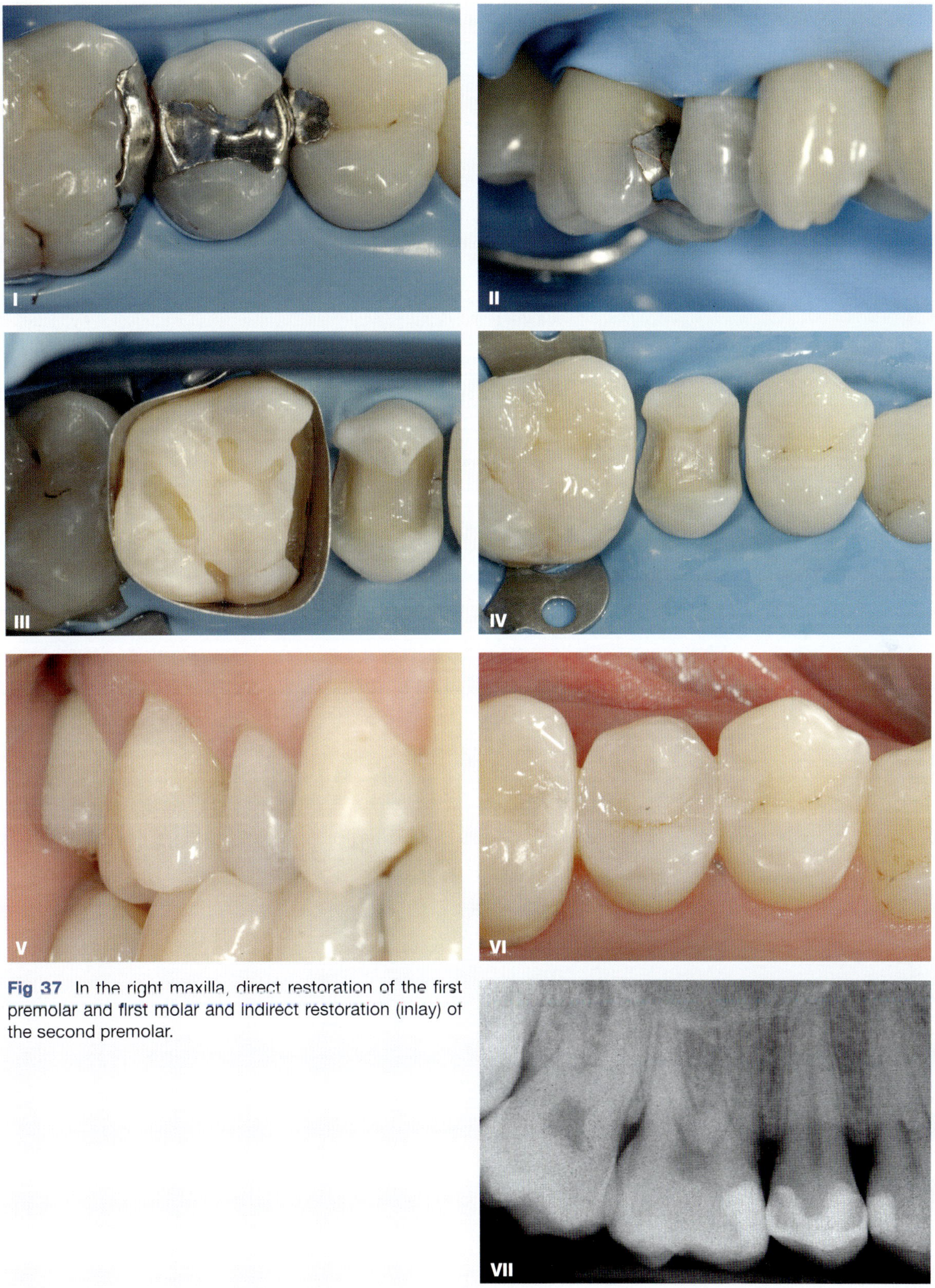

Fig 37 In the right maxilla, direct restoration of the first premolar and first molar and indirect restoration (inlay) of the second premolar.

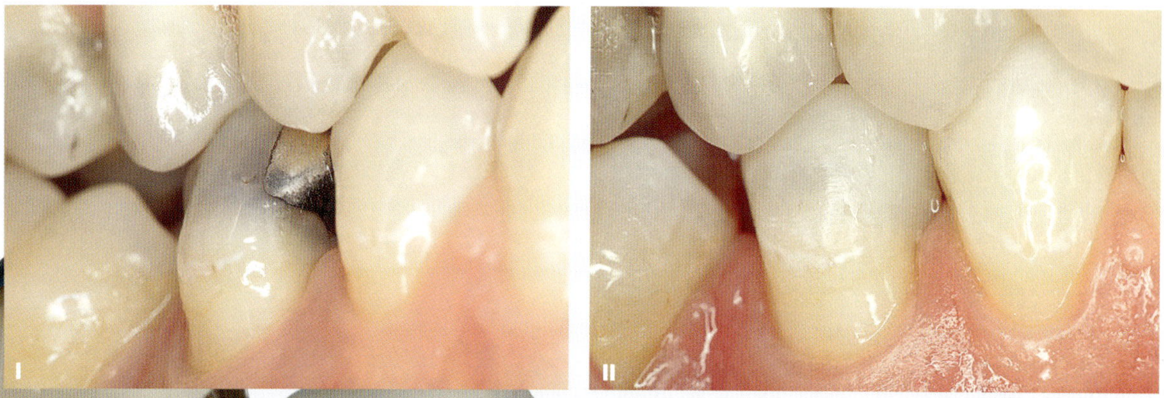

Fig 38 Much more satisfactory esthetics after replacing the amalgam fillings with composite resins at the patient's request.

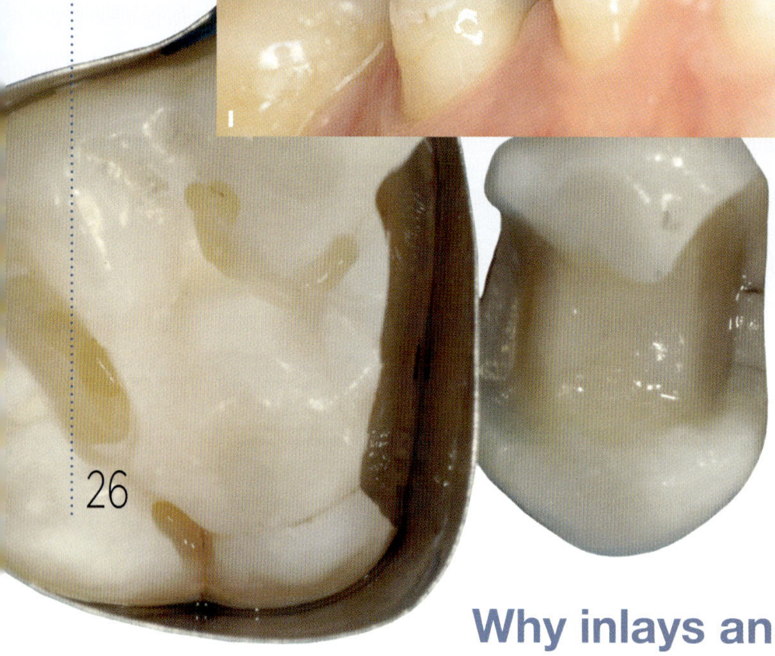

Why inlays and onlays?

Saving healthy tooth tissue during the stages of any dental preparation must represent the best choice in a treatment plan where biology assumes a significant role (Fig 39).

I would therefore be glad to see conservative dentistry being interpreted not as a branch of dentistry concerned with fillings but as an overall philosophy, ie, a therapeutic strategy of conserving as regards restoration, endodontic treatment, or periodontal and surgical treatment rather than as a general step-by-step reconstructive procedure (Fig 40).

The clinician must focus on the problem presented by the patient and, based on an accurate diagnosis, draw up a multidisciplinary treatment plan aimed at achieving an excellent result at the lowest biologic cost.

This is illustrated by a clinical example of a young patient who presented to the author's practice with defective resin restorations and caries lesions. After removing the old restorations and cleaning decay from the cavity, the mandibular right second molar showed a specific indication for a direct restoration, which the author carried out using the stratification technique. The first molar, on the other hand, had re-

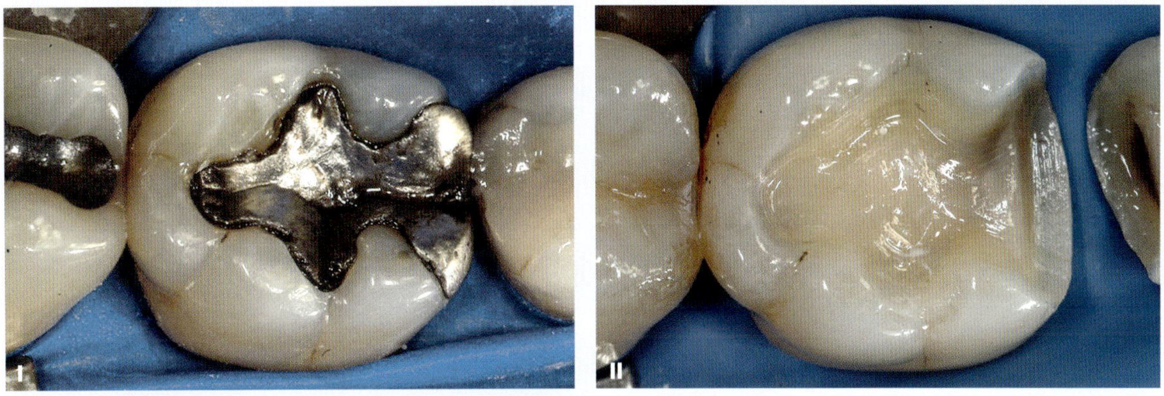

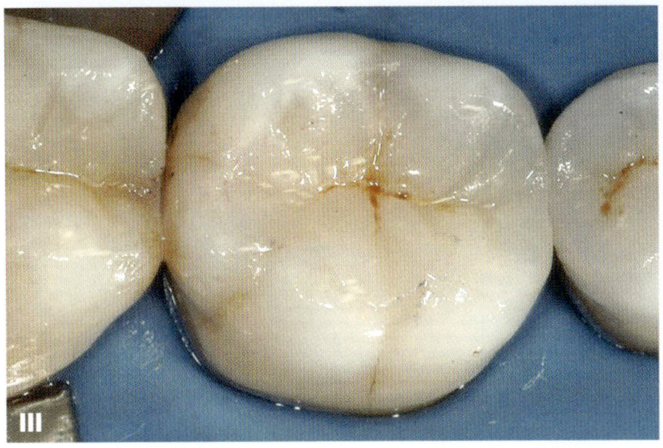

Fig 39 Example of a conservative cavity to replace a leaking amalgam restoration with a composite inlay.

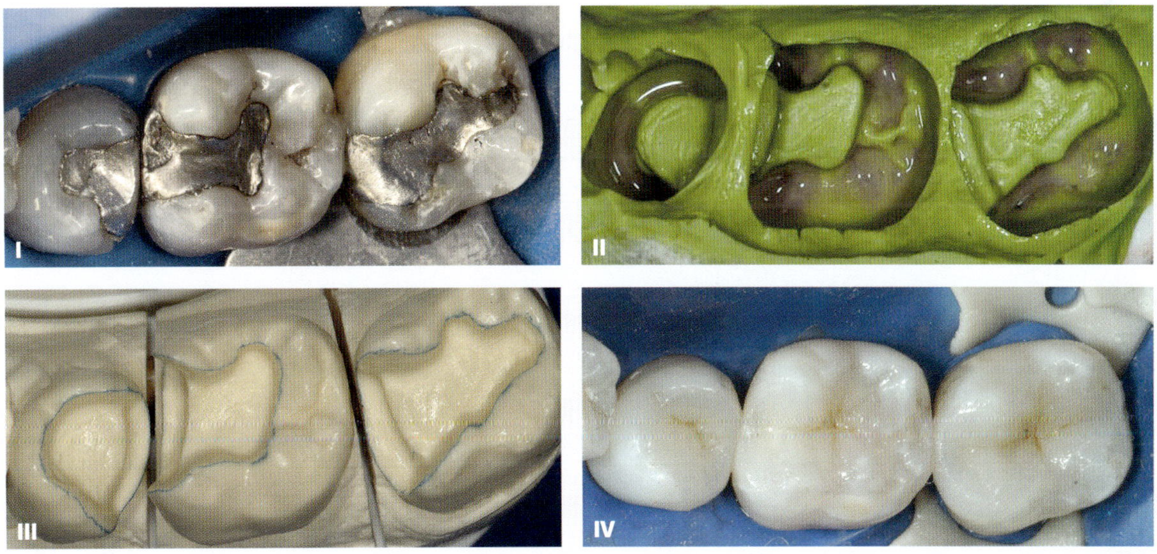

Fig 40 Quadrant with defective restorations. Images of impressions and working casts of the third quadrant, showing conservative preparations and margins that are easy to manage after clinical crown lengthening, cemented inlays, and full-arch direct (mandibular right second molar) and indirect restorations (mandibular left second premolar and first and second molars) *(I–IV)*. Clinical and radiographic follow-up of the mandible after 7 years and of the maxilla after 2 years *(V–VIII)*.

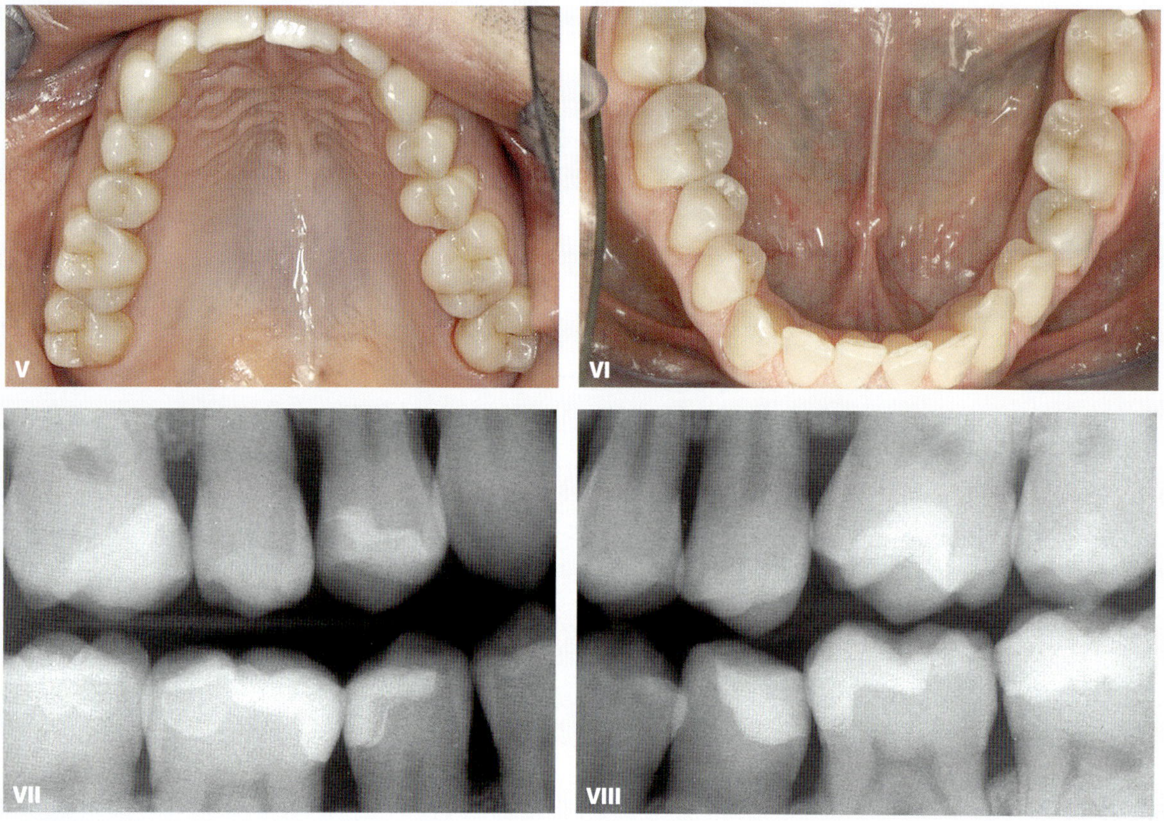

Fig 40 *(continued)*

sidual enamel walls unsupported by dentin, and the treatment plan included preparation of an overlay. The cast constructed in the laboratory showed the supragingival position of all preparation margins and, after cementation, good contact surfaces in both the buccolingual and apicocoronal directions. In the first quadrant, after analyzing the residual dental matter, the author's treatment team opted to add an onlay to the maxillary right first premolar and a direct restoration to the maxillary right second molar. The second quadrant showed multiple caries lesions with subgingival margins and caries lesions located at the cervical level. Periodontal surgery to lengthen the clinical crown was followed by inlays, onlays, and Class 5 restorations. One onlay and one direct restoration were applied to the first and second molars, respectively, of the third quadrant.

As the radiographic images show, none of the teeth were treated endodontically, and the marginal seals and emergence profiles are accurate. Clinical and follow-up radiographs of the restorations were carried out after 4 years (Fig 41).

Over the past decade, the proceedings of various congresses have included reports discussing restorations in posterior sectors where cosmetic appearance took precedence over physiologic aspect. In this case it is legitimate to wonder how physiologic a composite inlay or onlay can be. This opens a debate over the difference in elastic modulus between amalgam and composite, the fragility of ceramic and composite, the different thicknesses required of ceramic and composite material, the drastic reduction in endodontic treatment that arises as a result of partial as opposed to total preparations, the ability to respect biologic parameters by routinely positioning margins in a supragingival position, the quantity of healthy tooth structure that remains after a total or partial preparation, the condition of the pulp and dentin complex after a total or partial procedure carried out under rubber dam, and the length of working times.

The message the author wishes to convey is that by means of a simple but rigorous operating protocol clinicians can respect tooth structure, pulp vitality, and periodontal structures through partial coronal restorations characterized by part of the clinical crown remaining intact, maintenance of pulp vitality, and a supragingival margin position (Figs 42 to 44).

The possibility of correcting an indirect restoration in composite before cementation (Figs 45 and 46) and the potential for re-treatment at a later stage after cementation (Figs 47 and 48) are other essential characteristics of this therapeutic option.

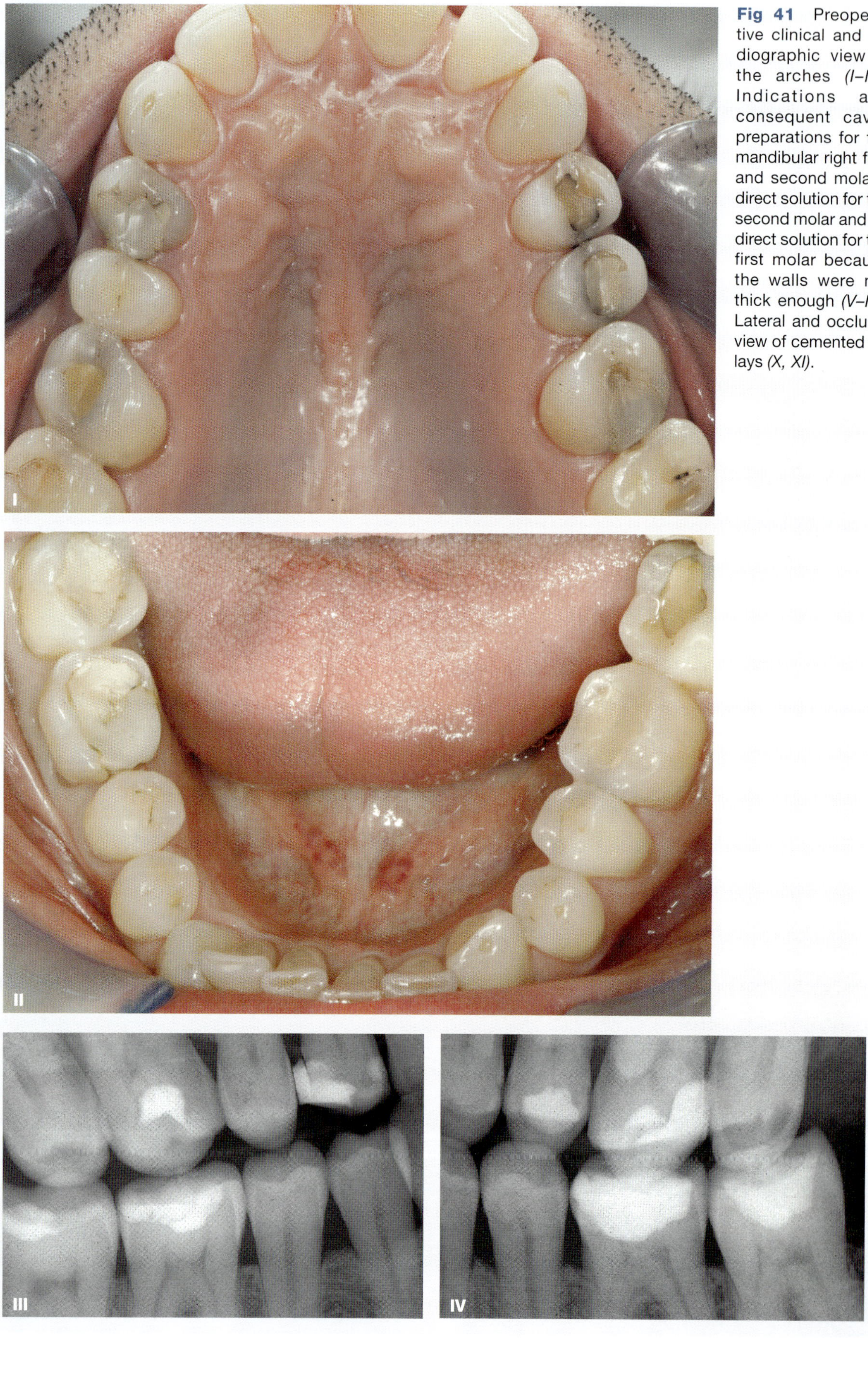

Fig 41 Preoperative clinical and radiographic view of the arches *(I–IV)*. Indications and consequent cavity preparations for the mandibular right first and second molars: direct solution for the second molar and indirect solution for the first molar because the walls were not thick enough *(V–IX)*. Lateral and occlusal view of cemented inlays *(X, XI)*.

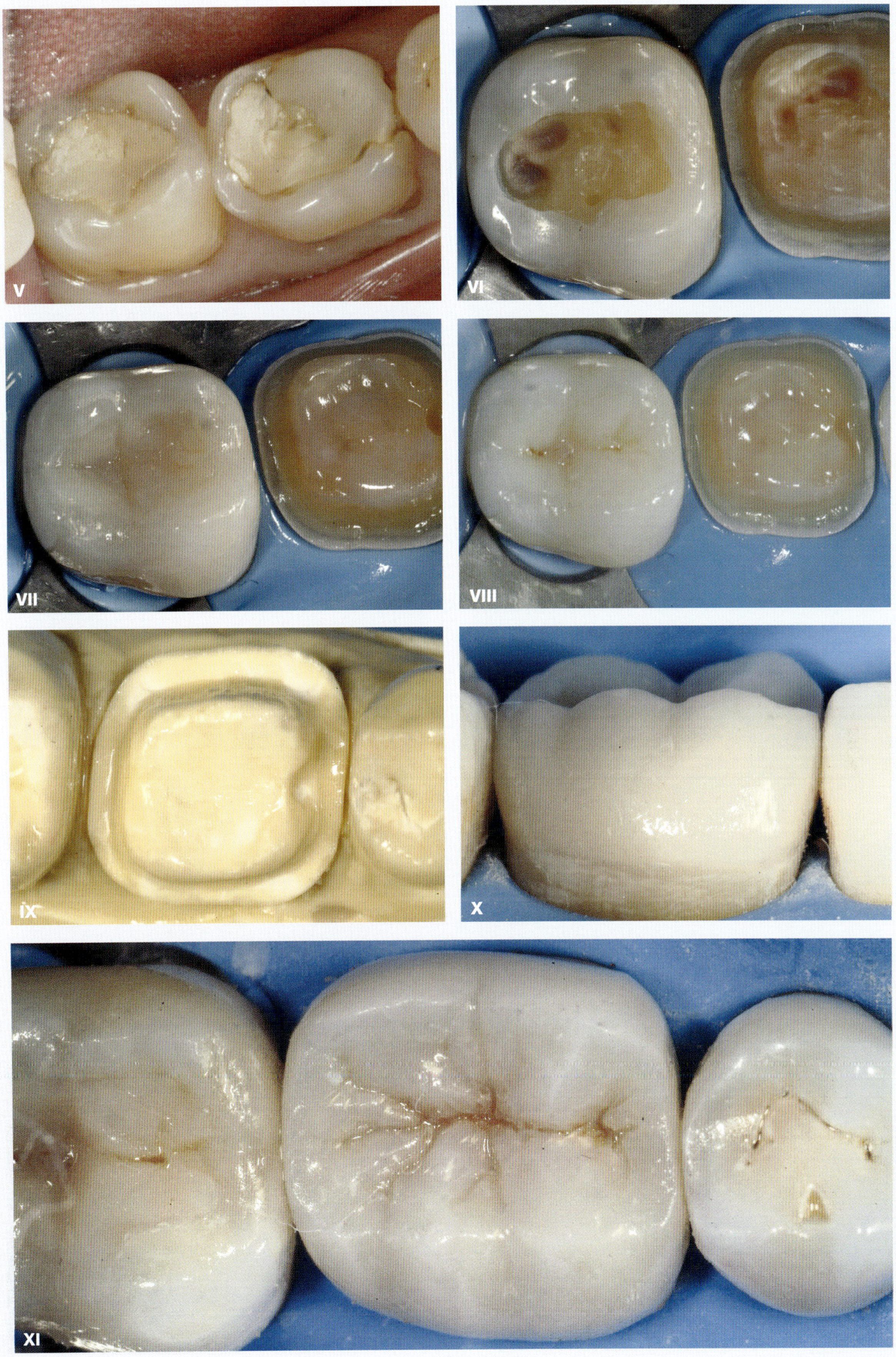
V
VI
VII
VIII
IX
X
XI

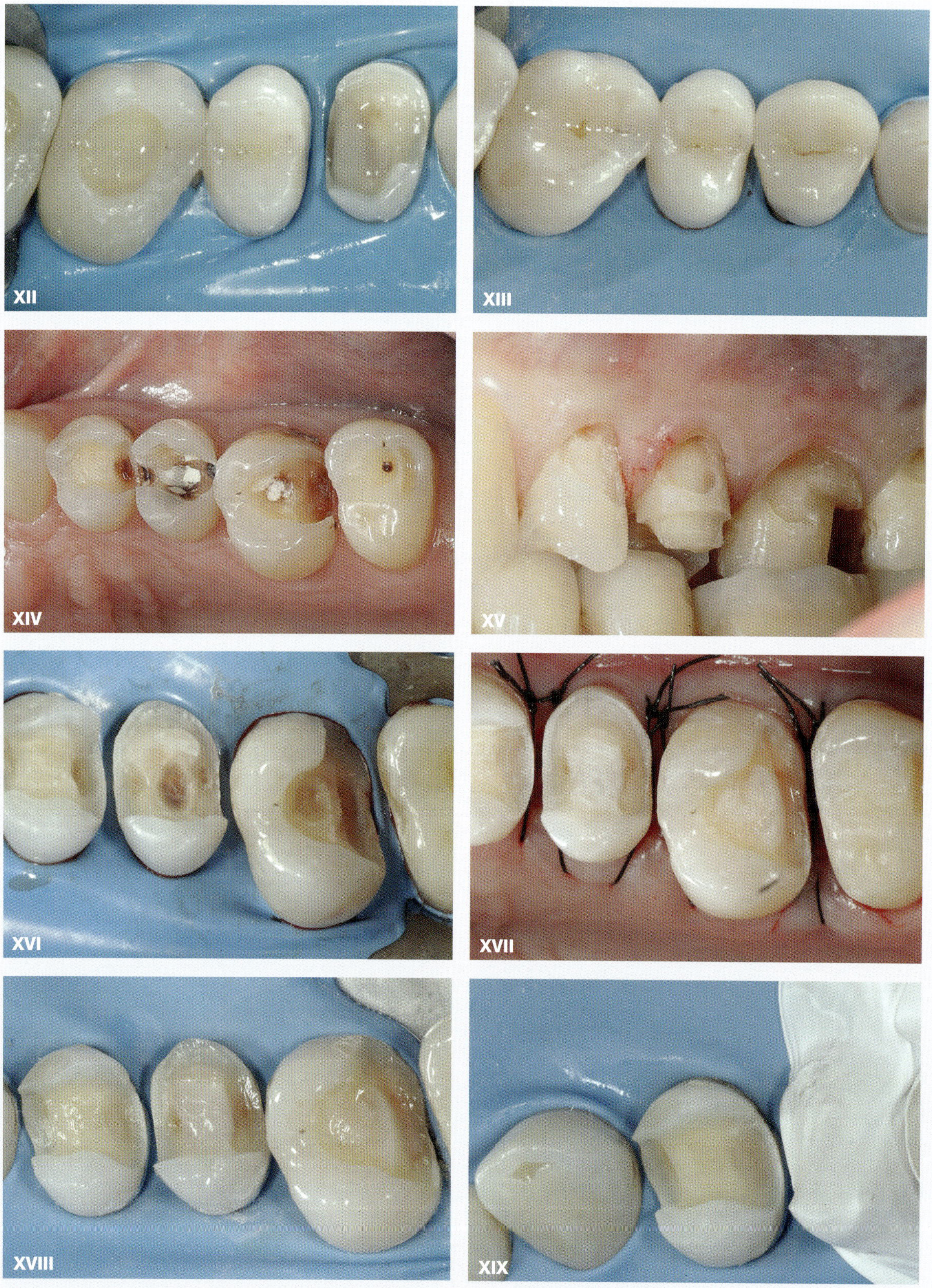

Fig 41 *(continued)* Management of the maxillary right quadrant with direct restoration of the first molar and indirect restoration of the first premolar *(XII, XIII)*. Multiple Class 2 and buccal caries lesions affecting the maxillary left quadrant *(XIV, XV)*. After removal of the decayed tissue and surgical lengthening of the clinical crowns, the healthy remaining tooth tissue indicated the type of preparation to be used *(XVI, XVII)*.

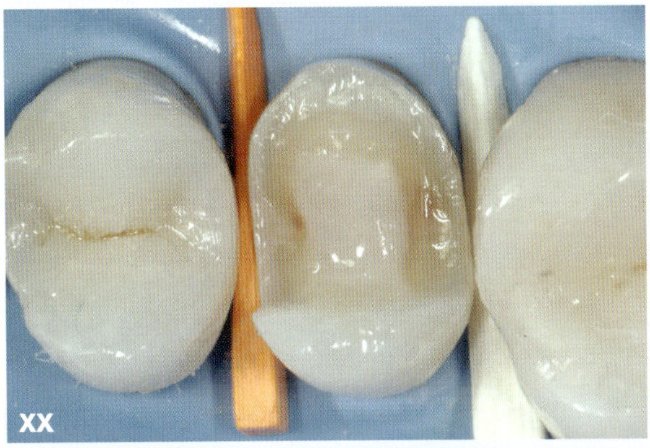
XX

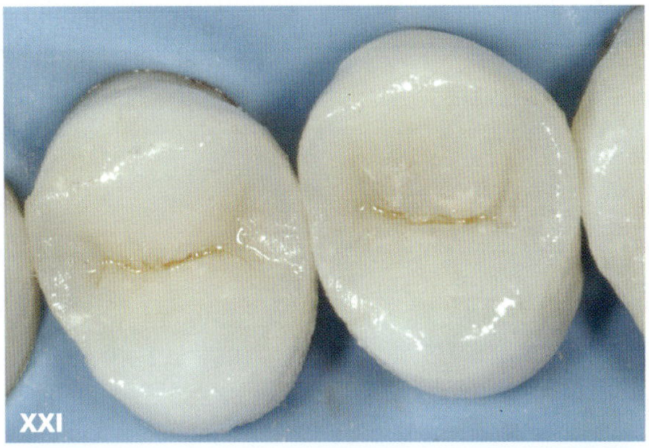
XXI

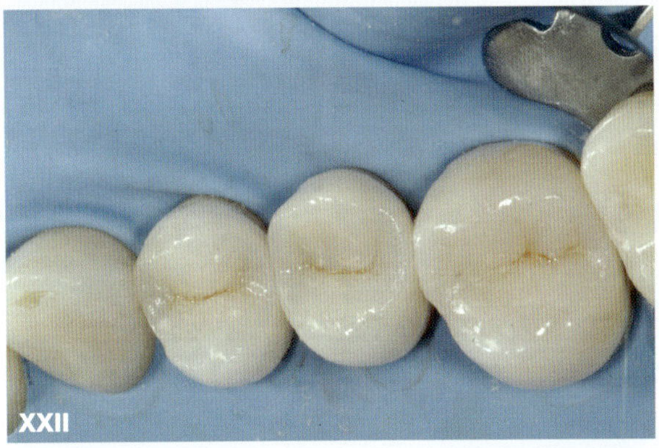
XXII

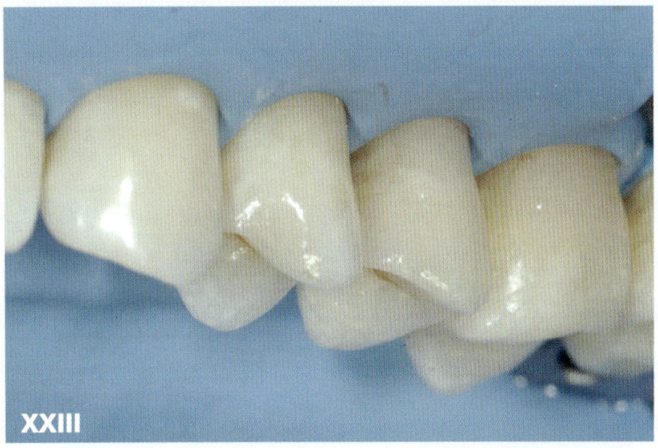
XXIII

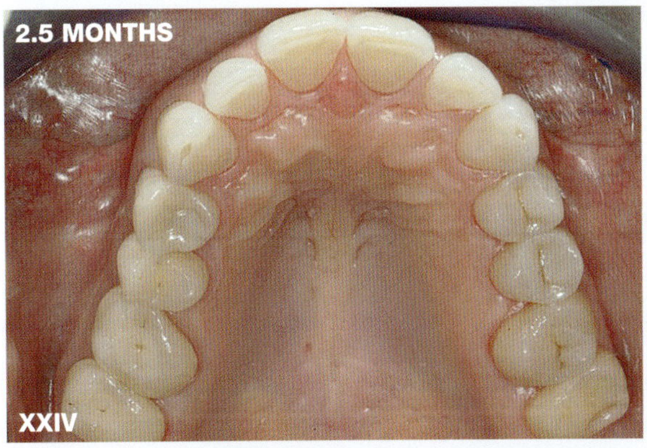

XXIV

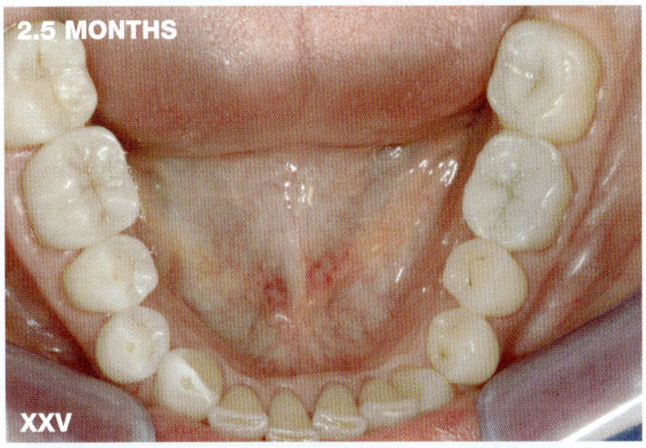

XXV

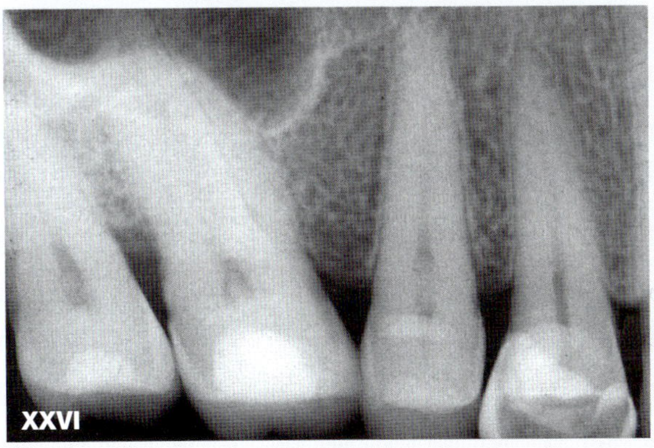
XXVI

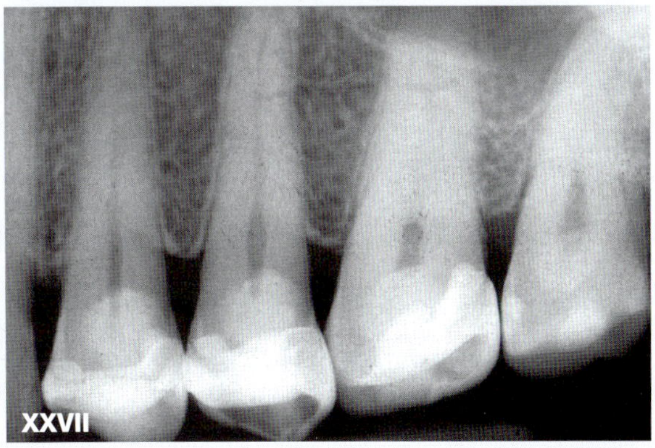
XXVII

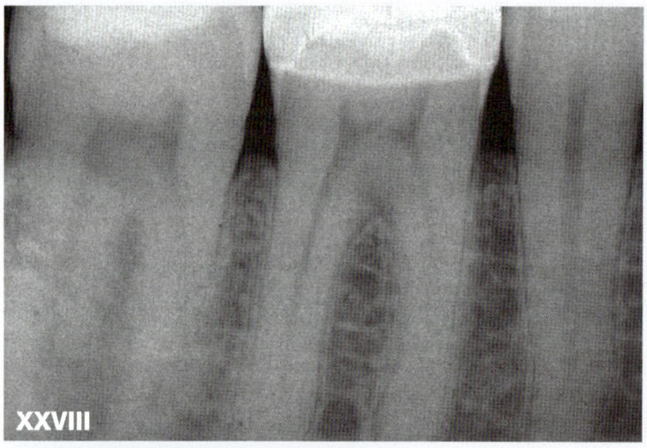

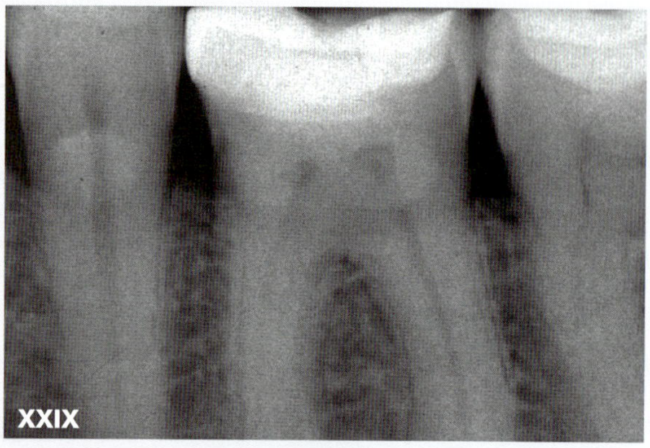

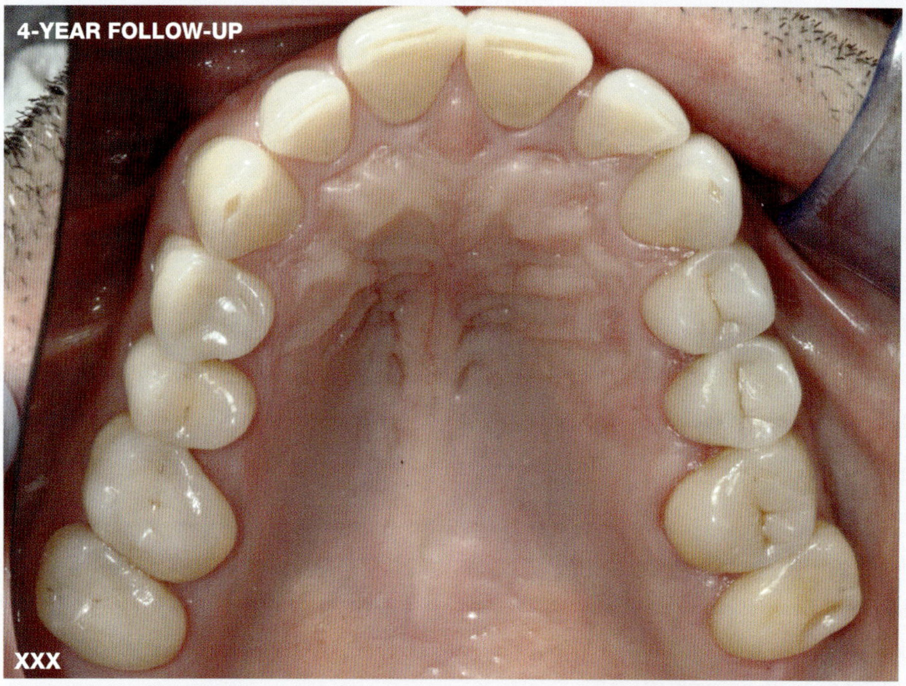

Fig 41 *(continued)* Stages of cementation and view of completed restorations *(XVIII–XXIII)*. Clinical and radiographic follow-up after 2.5 months *(XXIV–XXIX)*. Clinical follow-up after 4 years and associated radiographic status *(XXX–XXXII)*.

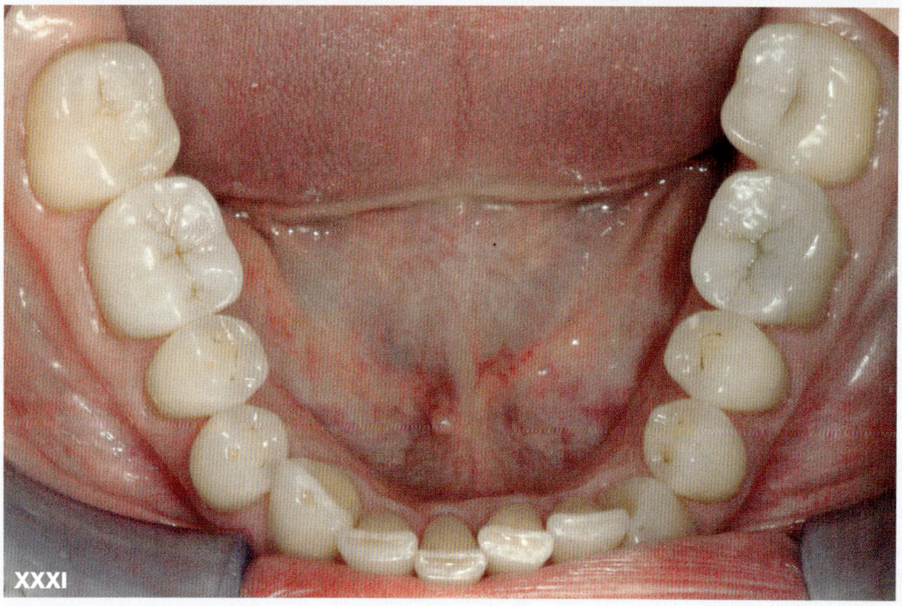

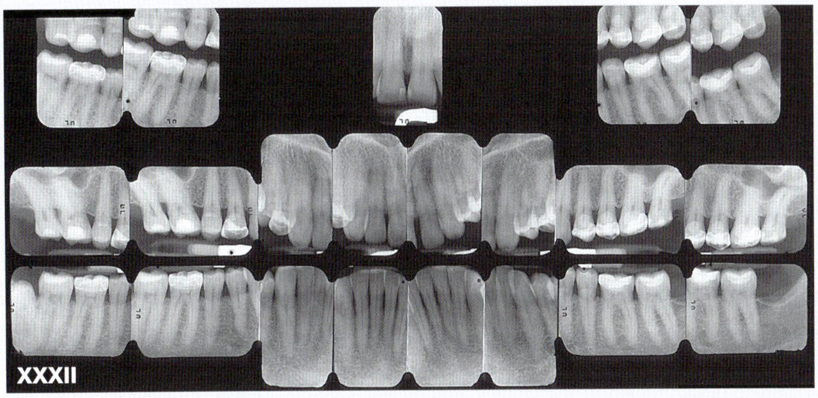

Fig 41 *(continued)*

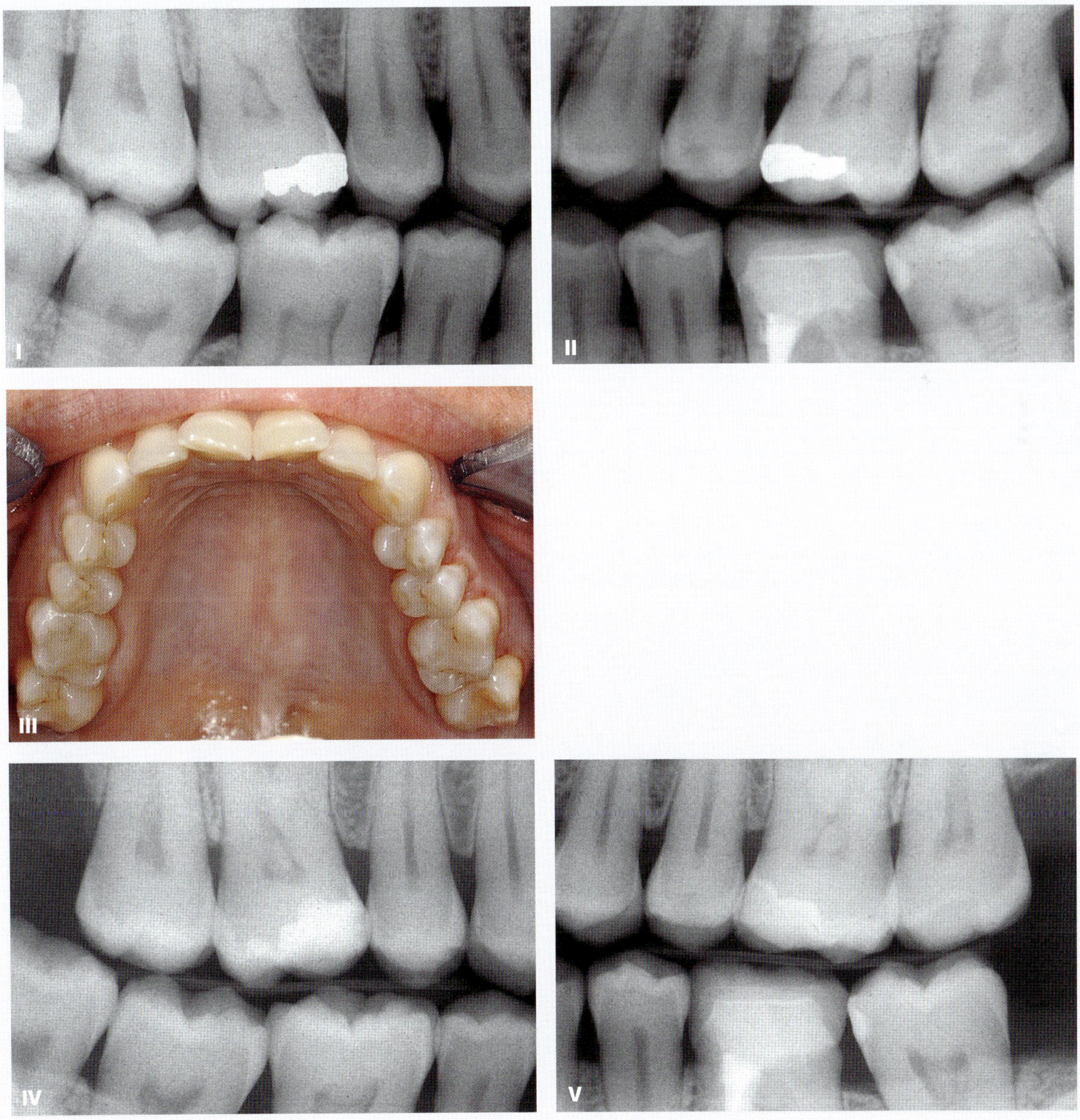

Fig 42 Replacement of old restorations due to the patient's cosmetic requirements.

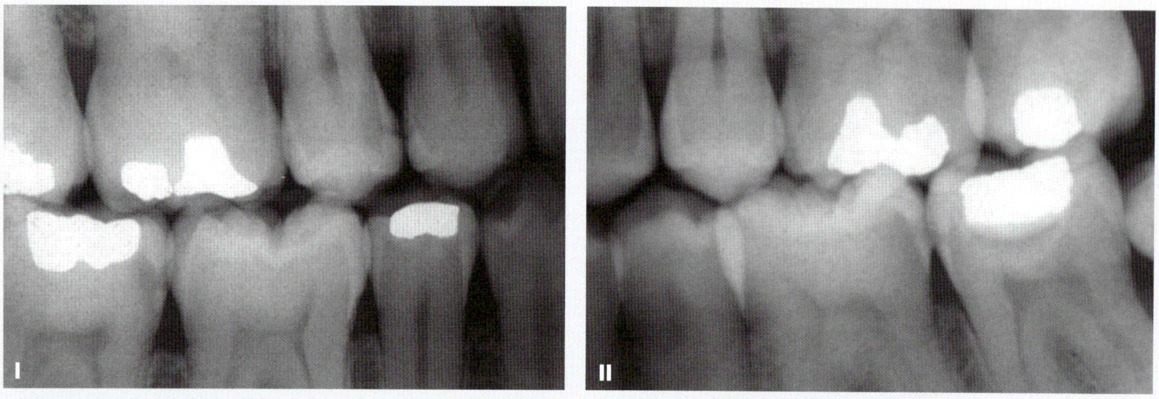

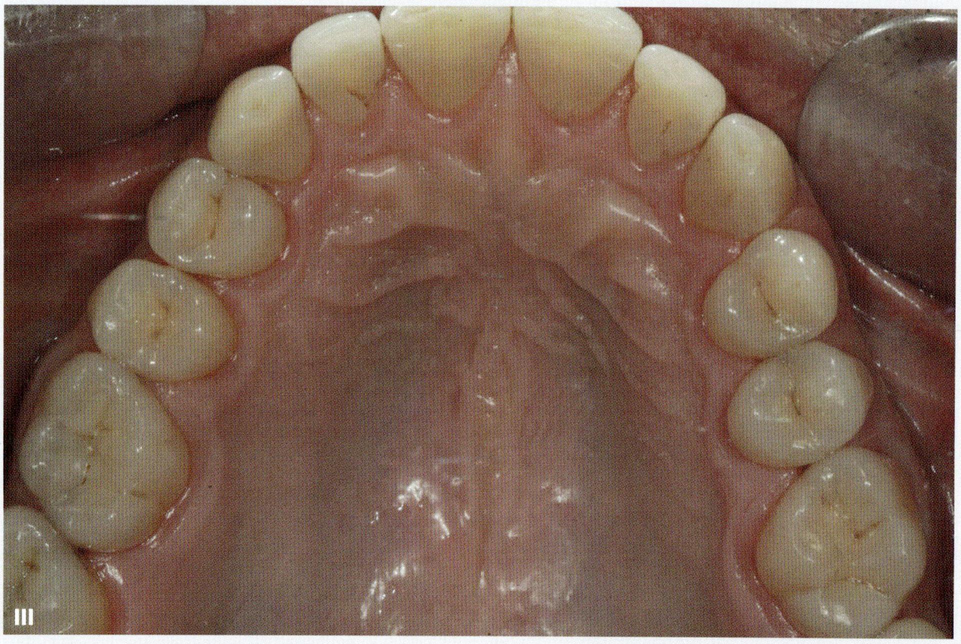

Fig 43 Multiple caries lesions involving molars and premolars on both arches *(I, II)* managed by means of direct and indirect restorations *(III, IV)*. Notably, pulp vitality was maintained in the mandibular left first and second molars at follow-ups after 3 *(V–VIII)* and 5 years *(IX–XI)*.

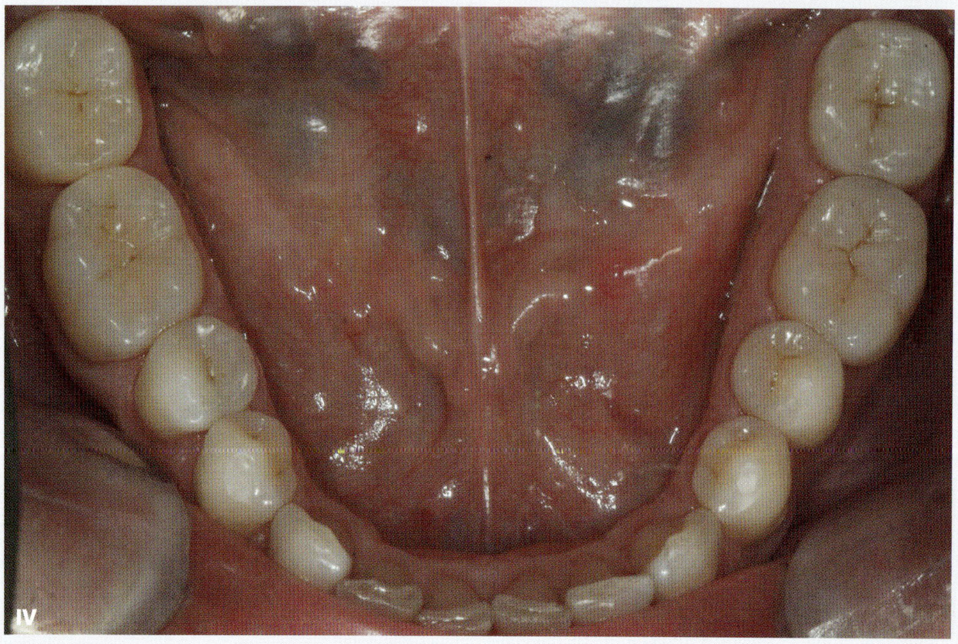

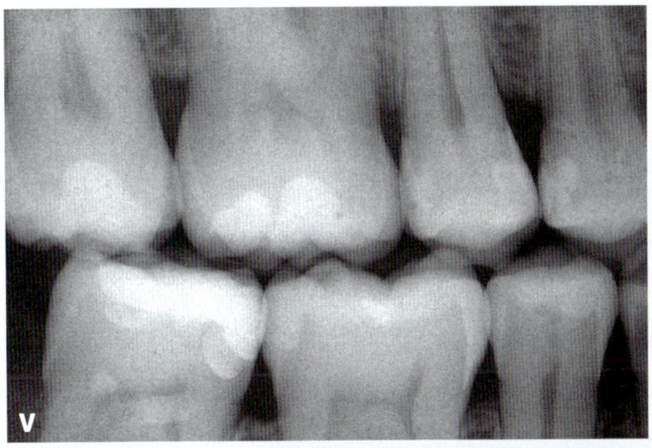
V

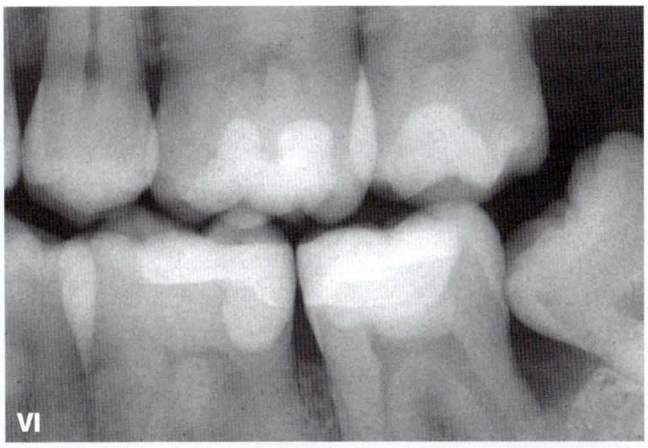
VI

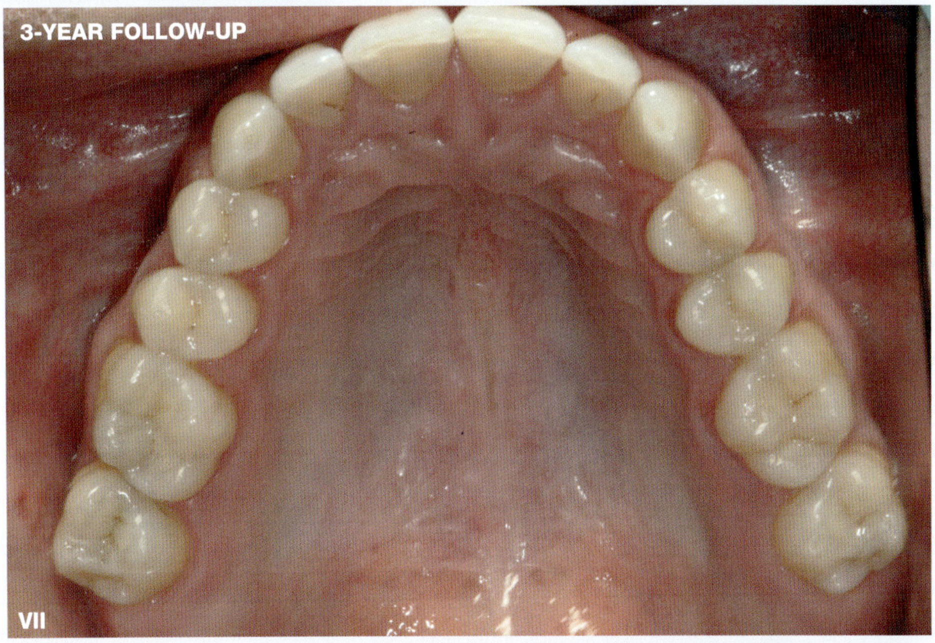
3-YEAR FOLLOW-UP
VII

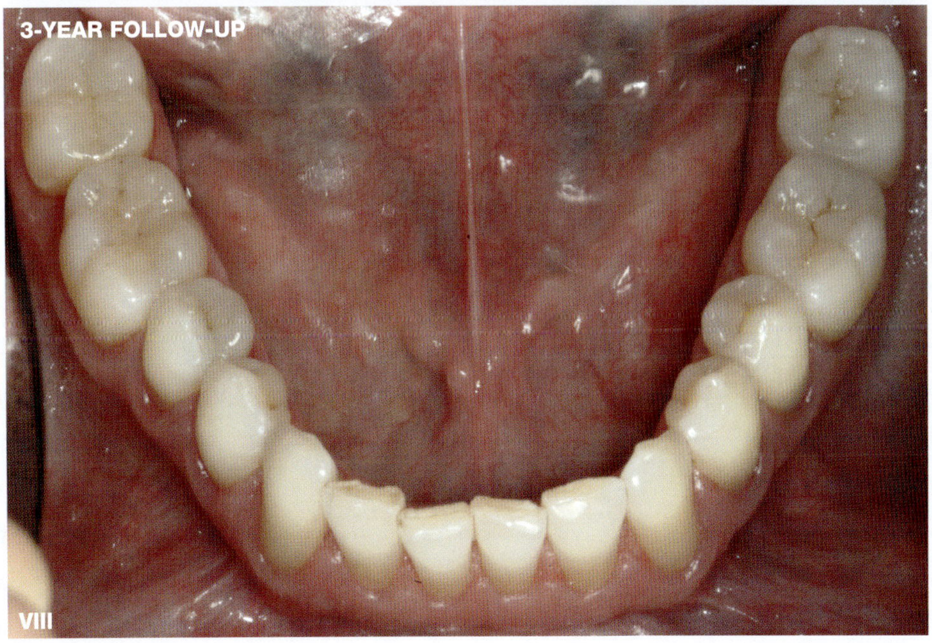
3-YEAR FOLLOW-UP
VIII

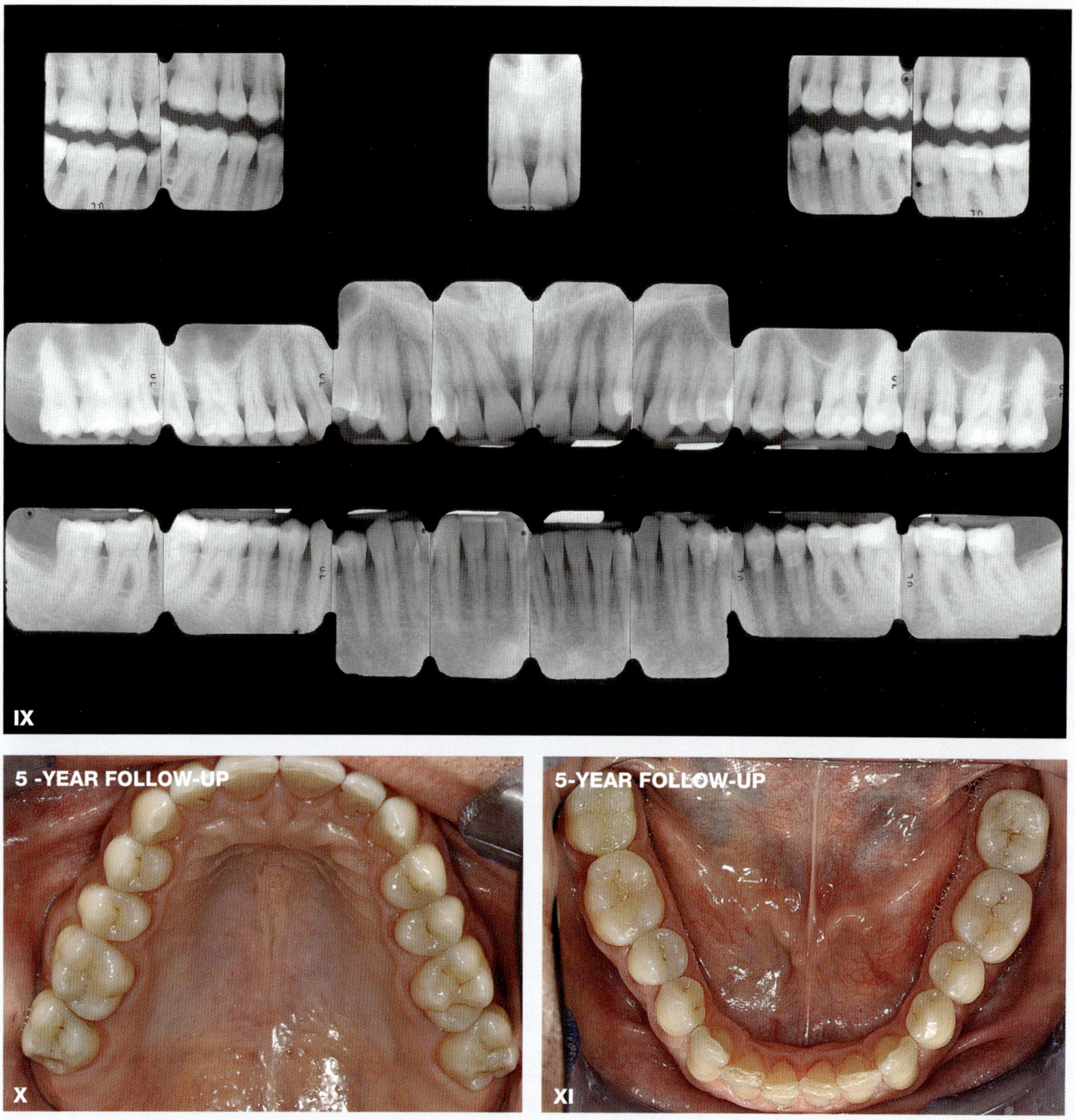

Fig 43 (*continued*) The radiographic status reveals removal of the mandibular left third molar due to periodontal problems *(IX)*. Clinical follow-up after 5 years *(X, XI)*.

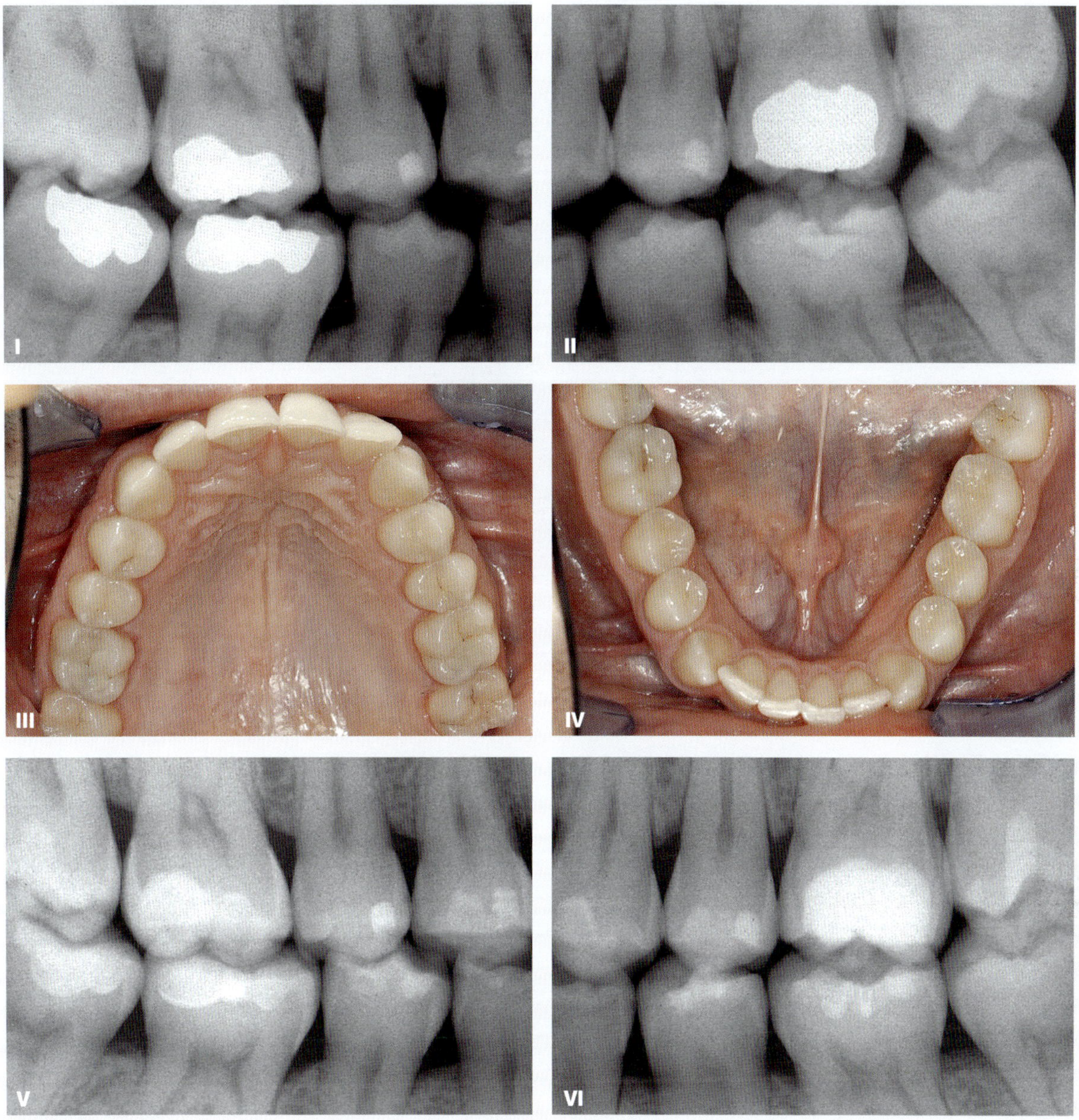

Fig 44 Replacement of old defective restorations with direct fillings due to pain on chewing. Despite the restoration depth, all the teeth are free of endodontic treatment because pulp vitality was maintained.

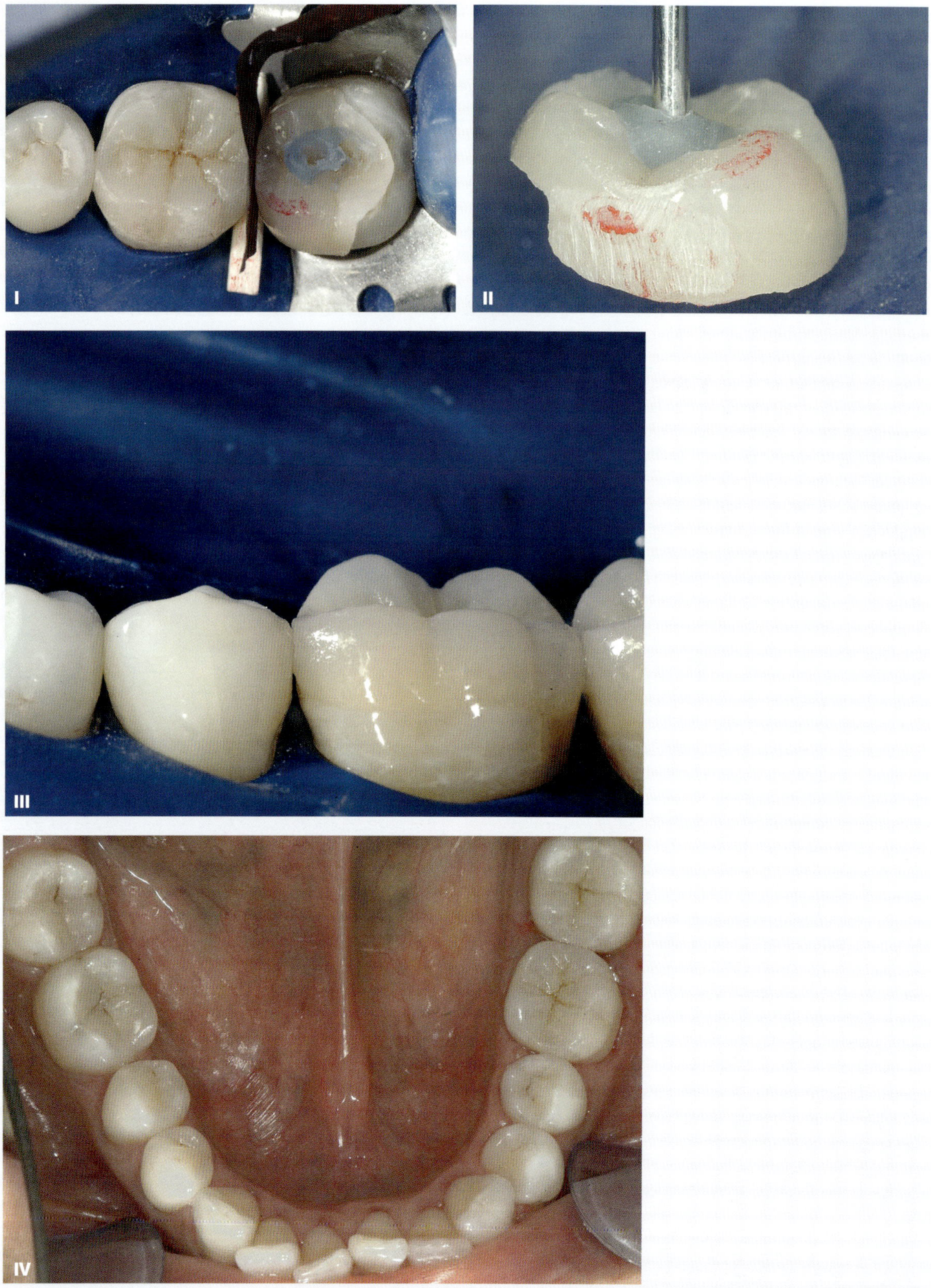

Fig 45 Trying the inlay and correction prior to cementation *(I, II)*, view of interproximal contacts *(III)*, and occlusal view of arch *(IV)*.

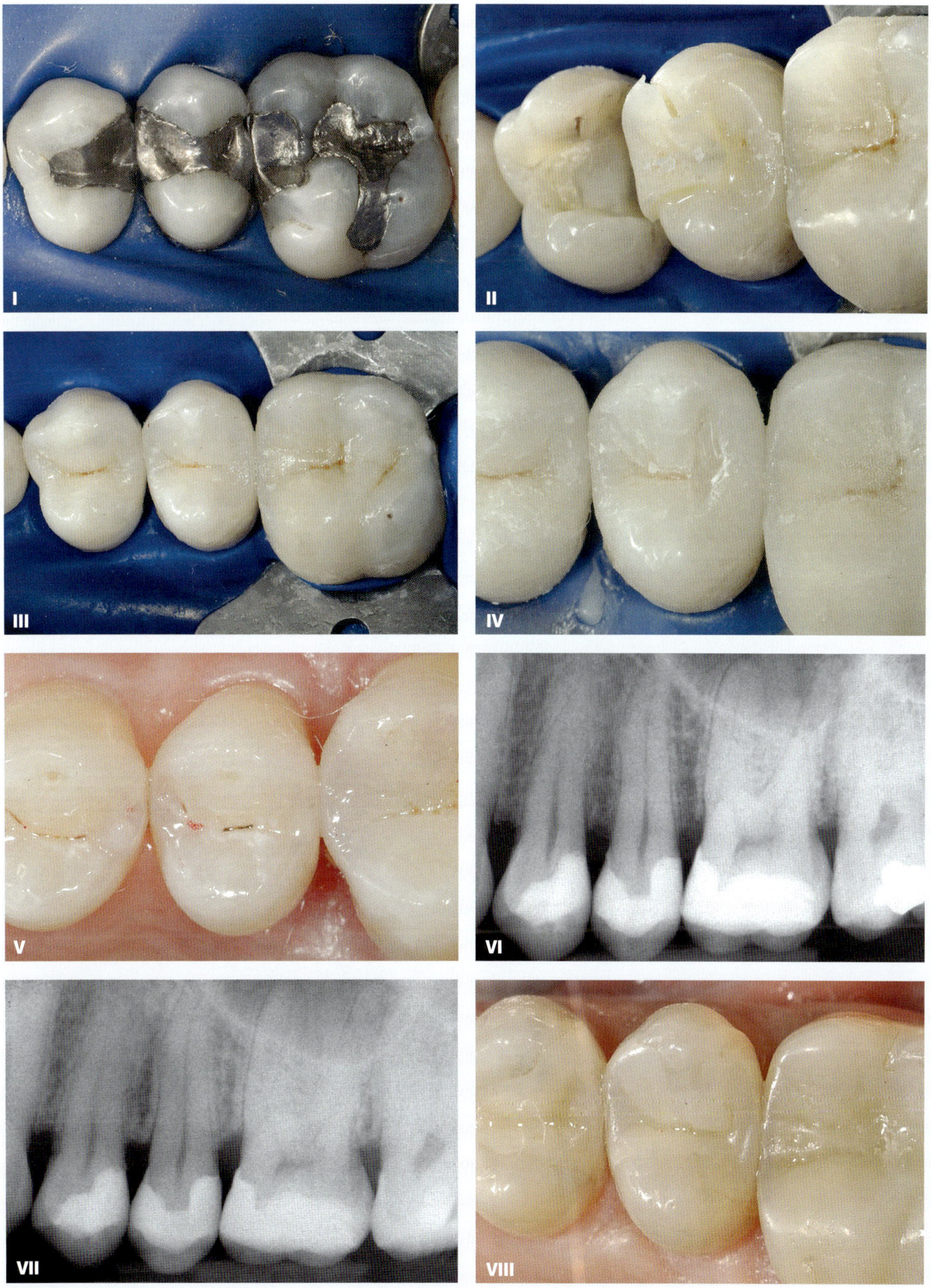

Fig 46 Fracture of inlay during cementation *(I, II)*. Because the buildup, cement, and inlay were made of the same composite material, both fragments were cemented together, and then the compactness of the joined material was checked *(III–VI)*. Radiographic and clinical follow-up after 5 years *(VII, VIII)*.

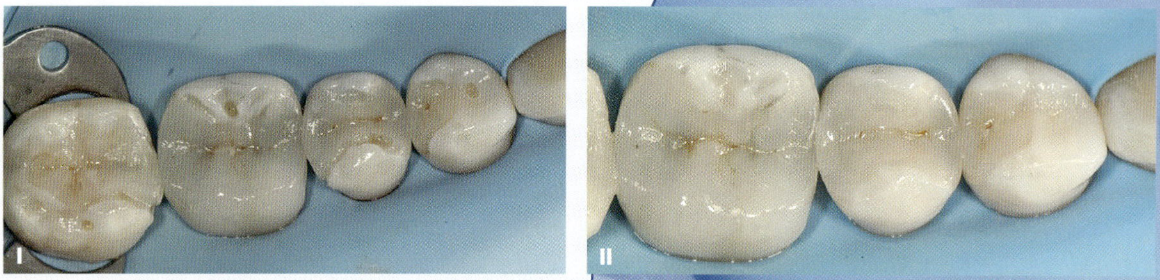

Fig 47 Clinical view of restoration of marginal integrity years after cementation.

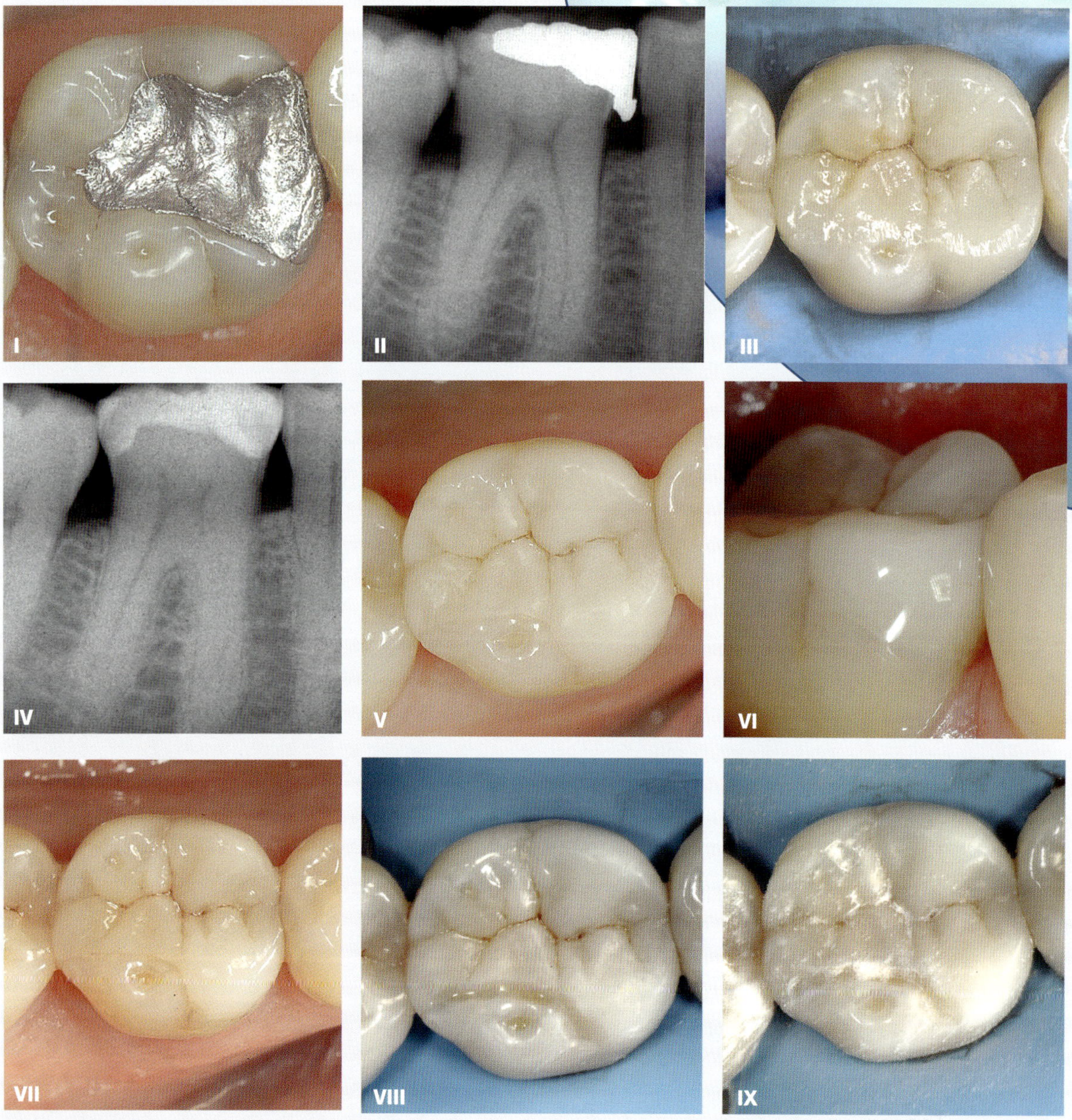

Fig 48 Step-by-step restoration of an inlay after 10 years: after making a minimal cavity in the now defective margin, sanding, acid etching of the enamel, application of the bonding agent, curing, and filling of the cavity with composite, the characteristics of the restoration return to their original form.

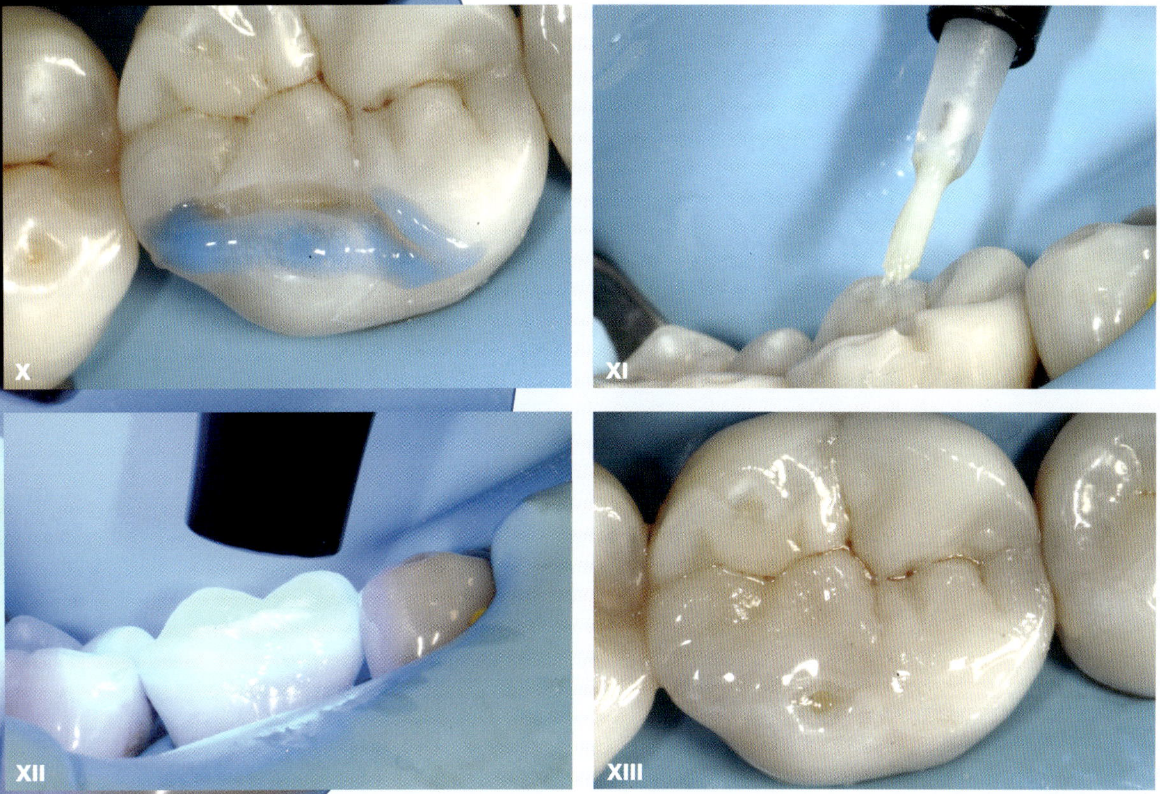

Fig 48 *(continued)*

Why composite?

For the following reasons, the choice of material to be used for the restoration of the posterior teeth inevitably falls on composites.

Microhybrid or nanoparticle composites represent the material of choice for direct and indirect restorations because:

- Their elastic modulus is very close to that of dentin. The elastic moduli of enamel and dentin are 84.1 and 18.3 GPa, respectively[21]; it is clear that the modulus of a composite under masticatory stress must be between these values. When a restoration material with an appropriate modulus of elasticity is inserted in a tooth, the result is a homogenous mechanical response without areas of high rigidity, where the concentrations of force would inevitably result in structural yield.
- They offer excellent physical and mechanical properties because they are highly filled.
- They are very tough and radiopaque.

- The duration of the adhesive bond is high in three-step etch-and-rinse adhesive systems and two-step self-etch systems.
- Their resistance to wear is 10 to 30 μm/year, and new material developments have resulted in the availability of composites with extremely high mechanical performance due to the high filling percentage, with considerably improved wear resistance due to the smaller particle size of the filler.

Pintado and Douglas[22] identified enamel wear of approximately 10 μm per year, Leinfelder et al[23] identified average wear of 13.2 μm per year, and the University of Manitoba identified wear of 39 μm overall for Z100 (3M Espe).
The wear resistance of modern composites is not only due to material technology but is also proportional to the polymer conversion level.
Ferracane et al[24] showed that the wear resistance of composite increases with increasing exposure time (Figs 49 to 52).
One negative characteristic of composite materials is stress caused by shrinkage due to polymerization. This problem can easily be resolved if the relatively narrow range of indications for direct restorations is observed. Shrinkage is avoided altogether in indirect techniques, where only the fine film of composite used for cementation contracts (Figs 53 and 54).

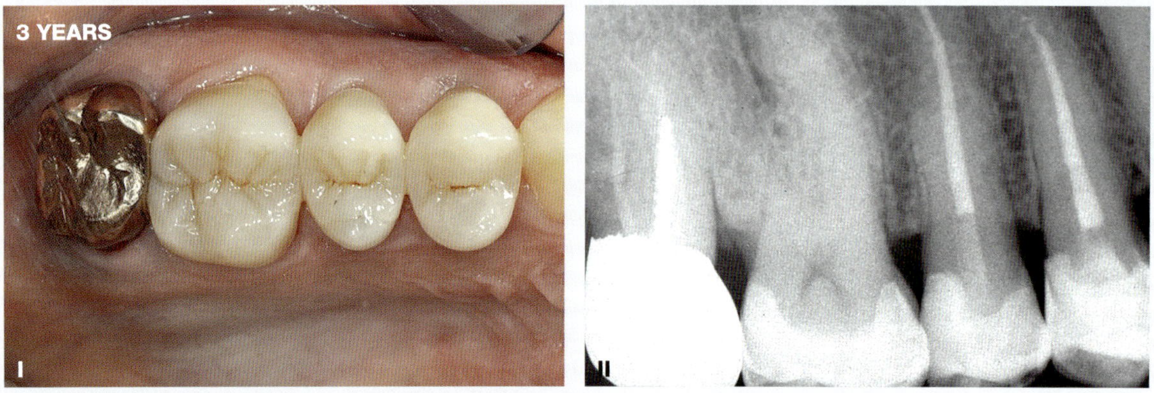

Fig 49 Clinical and radiographic follow-ups of indirect composite restorations after 3 years.

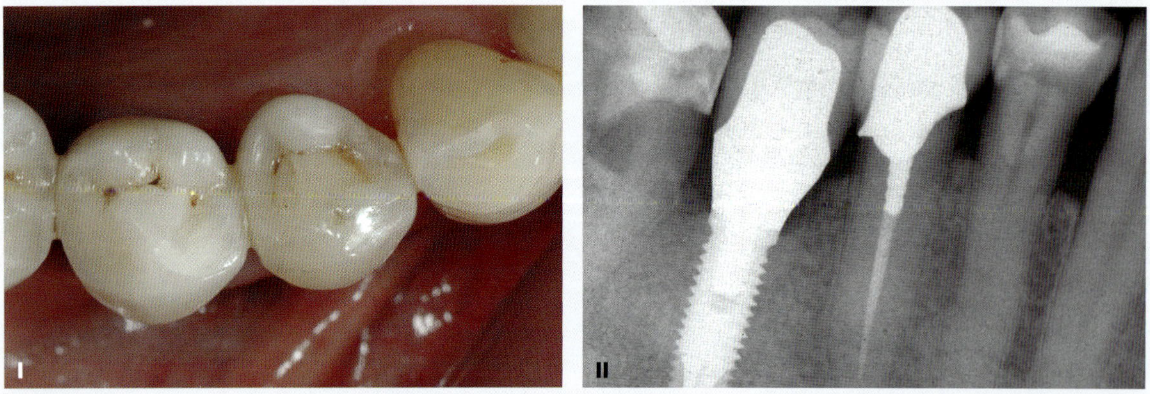

Fig 50 Clinical and radiographic follow-ups of wear in an indirect composite restoration of a mandibular right first premolar 6 years after cementation.

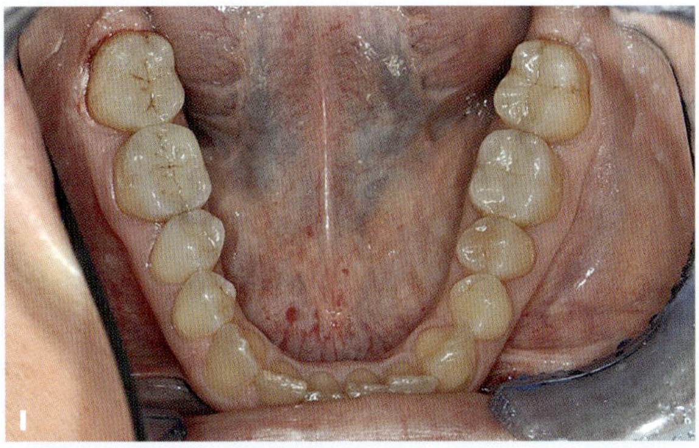

Fig 51 Wear on the four molars is acceptable 5 years after placement of restorations.

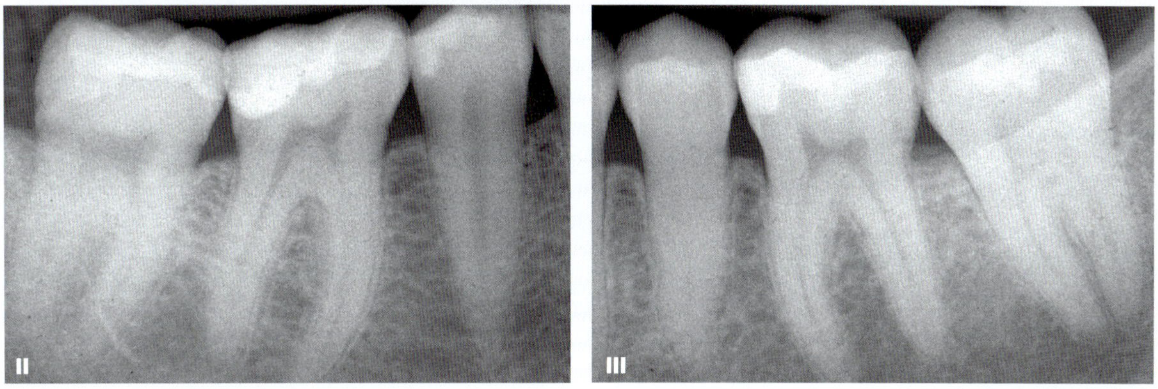

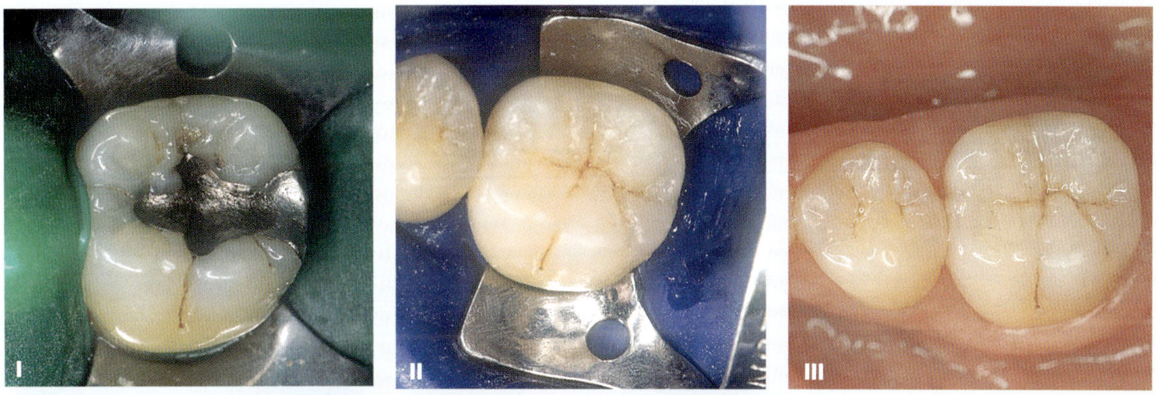

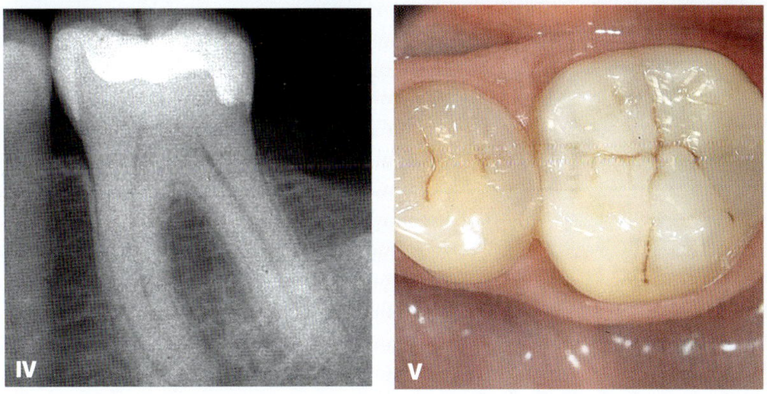

Fig 52 The mandibular left first molar is still structurally intact after 8 years despite being subject to all the masticatory stress because the adjacent second molar is missing.

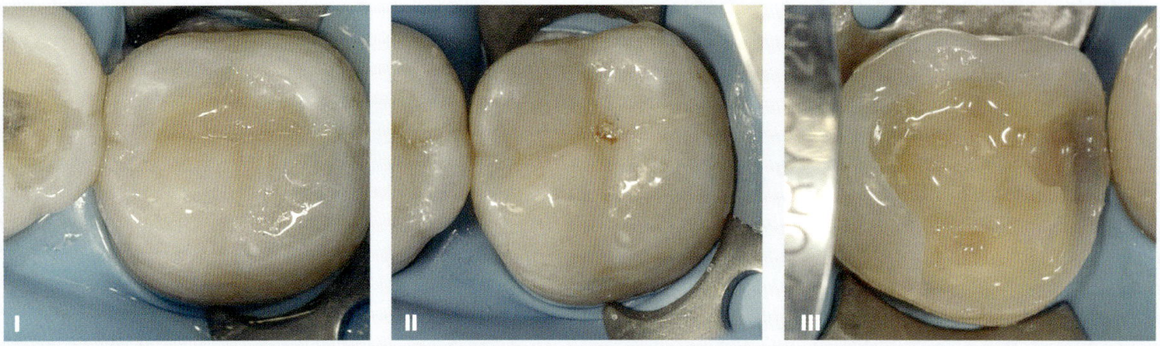

Fig 53 Example of stratification of a direct composite restoration *(I, II)*. A flexible intermediate layer (flowable composite) reduces stress due to shrinkage caused by polymerization by 20% to 50%[25] *(III)*.

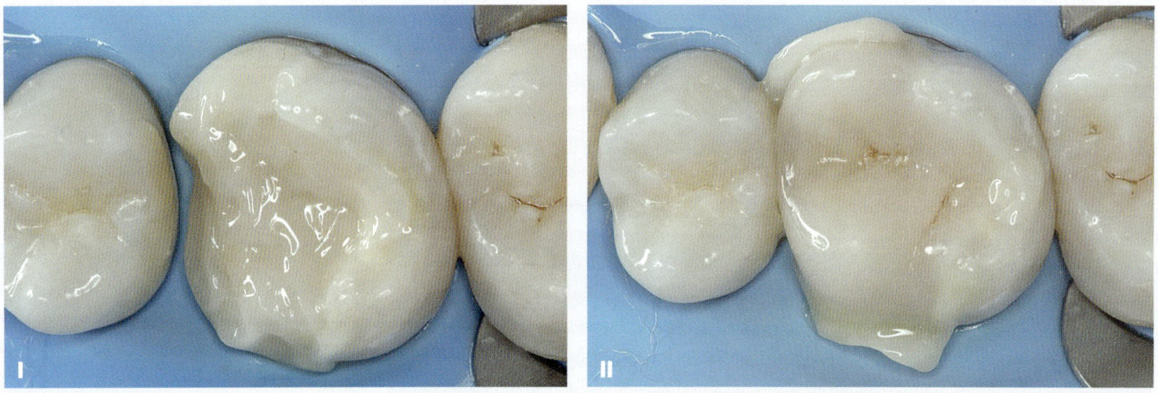

Fig 54 Only the composite used as cement in indirect techniques is subject to stress caused by shrinkage due to polymerization.

It goes without saying that the stratification technique assumes a fundamental role when performing restorations in medium to large cavities (Fig 55).
As far as adhesive systems are concerned, after using a three-step system for 8 years with excellent medium- and long-term clinical results, the author has noticed practically no difference over the past 3 years of using a two-step self-etch system, except that the latter is much easier to use.

As already stated, composite is a better choice than ceramic when restoring posterior sectors because composite is correctable at the cementation stage of the indirect restoration and above all repairable following cementation without any change in the mechanical and physical properties (Figs 56 to 58).

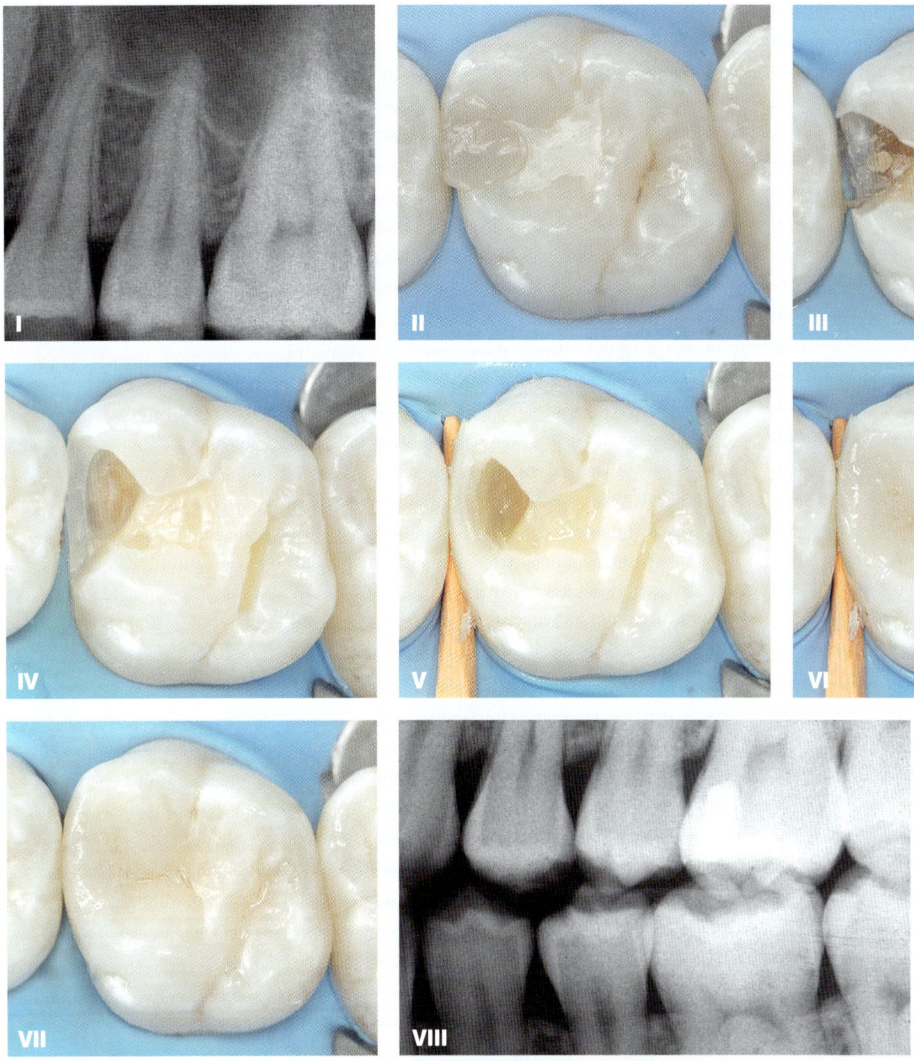

Fig 55 Step-by-step images of a direct restoration. Removal of the decayed tissue, recreation of the marginal ridge, filling of occlusal surface, and postoperative radiography. (Courtesy of Dr Lavinia Landi.)

Fig 56 Maxillary ceramic restorations.

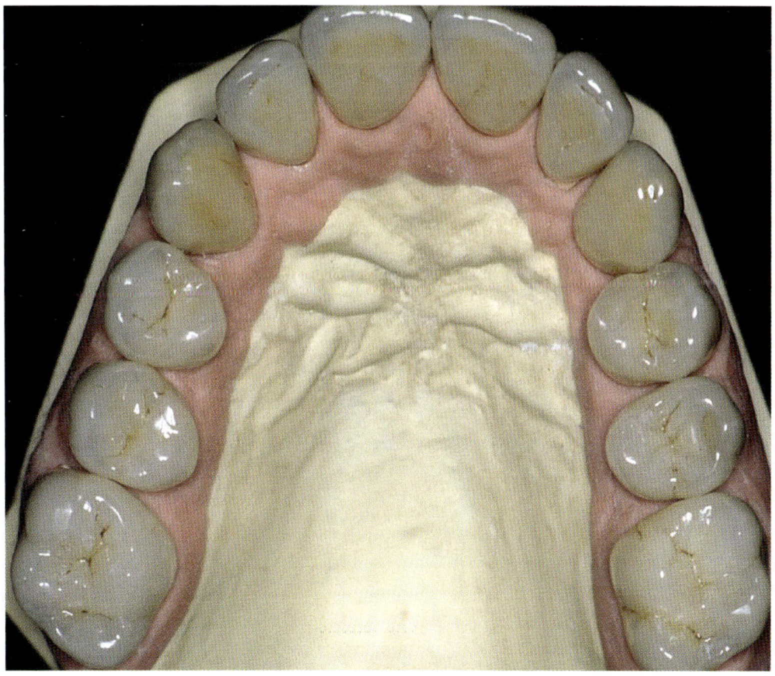

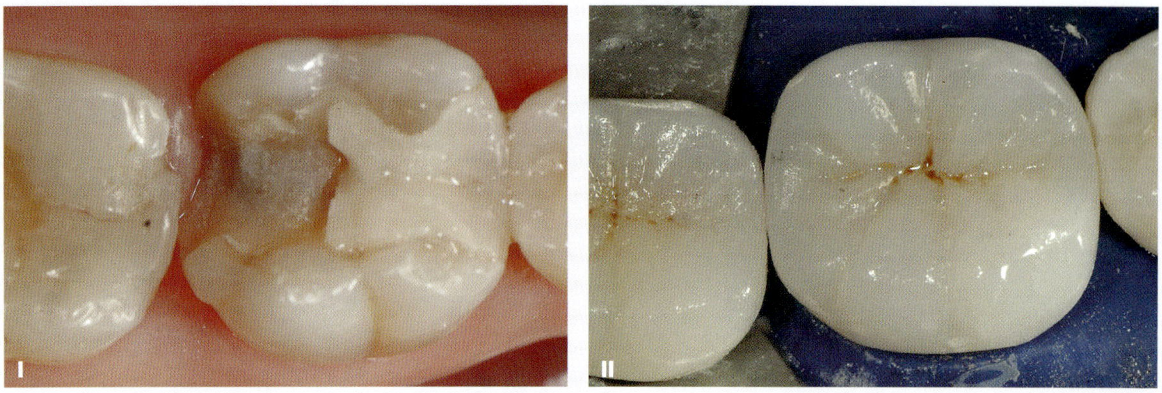

Fig 57 Fracture of two ceramic molars in a patient with parafunctions and their reconstruction using composite material.

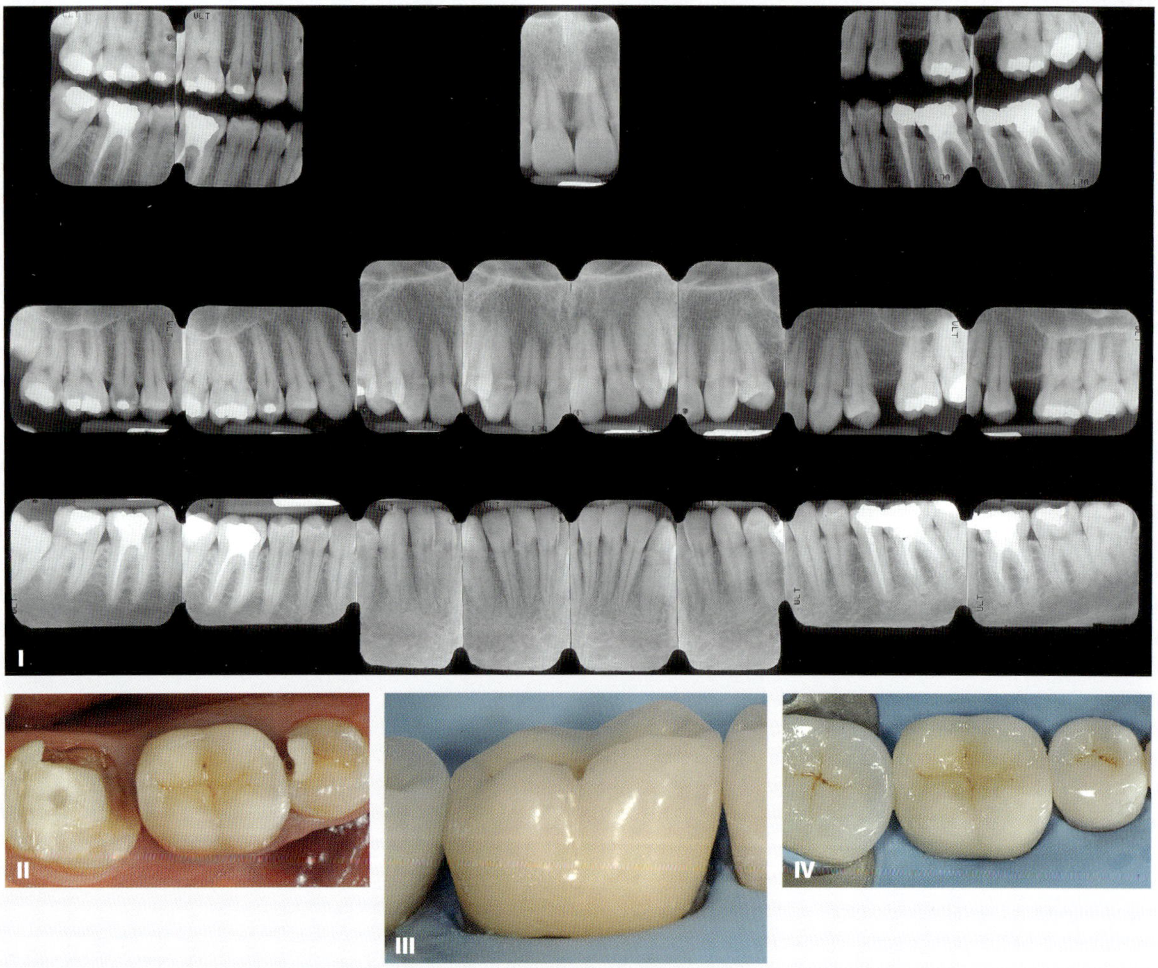

Fig 58 Fractured teeth in a patient suffering from bruxism *(I, II)*. Restorations were made in composite, and the patient was strongly advised to wear a protective mouthguard. Views of contact surfaces *(III–VIII)*. Radiographic follow-up *(IX)*.

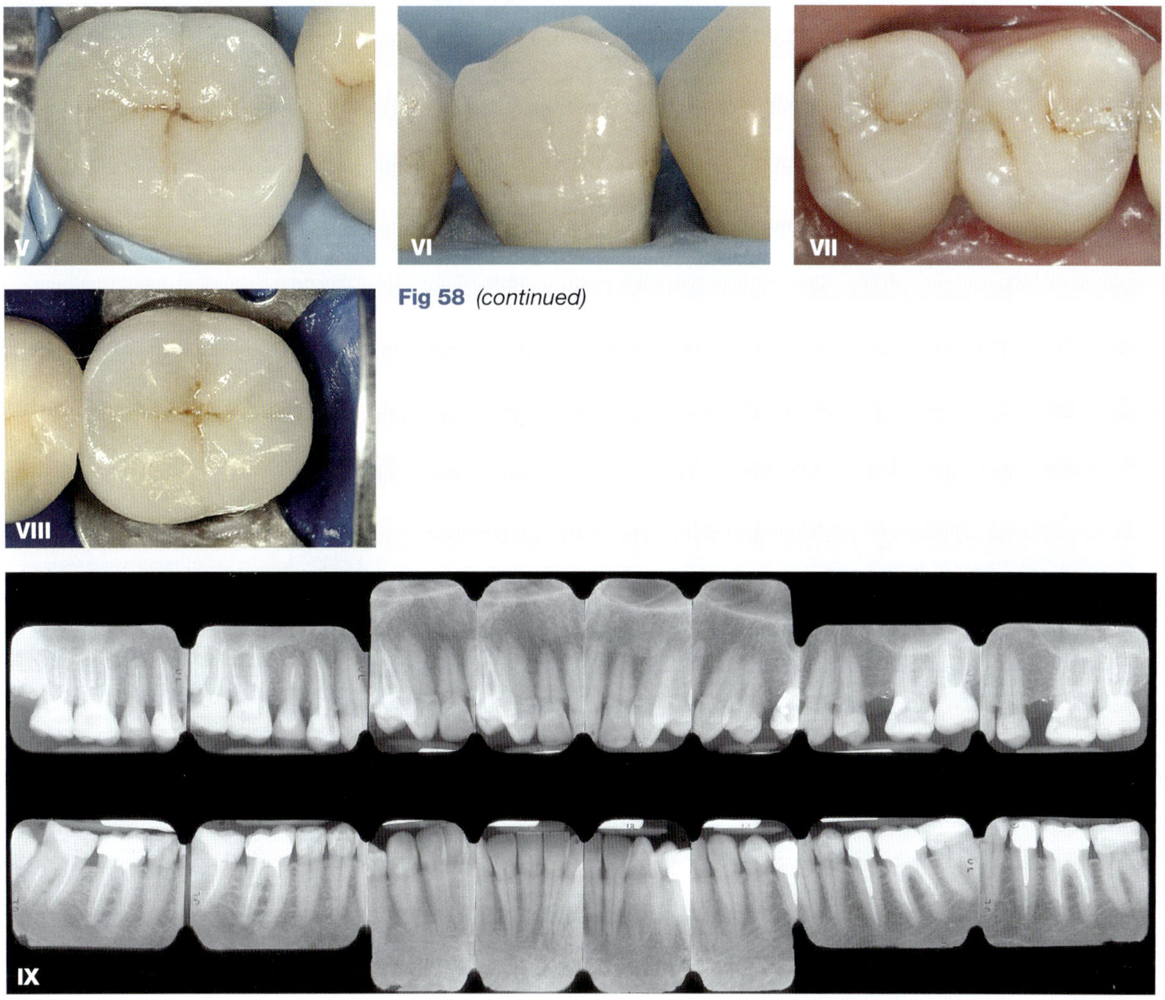

Fig 58 *(continued)*

For the sake of completeness, the author is bound to emphasize the marvelous performance of gold. Even today, it remains the ideal solution for patients with significant dysfunction, but it is hardly ever requested by the patients themselves.

Returning to the selection of composite or ceramic for the posterior sectors, the author is bound to add some comments after a review of the international scientific literature:

- The marginal discrepancy of ceramic inlays and onlays is significantly greater than that of composite.[26]
- Ceramic inlays and onlays show a significantly lower resistance to fracture than those made of composite.[27]

There is much more that could be said; however, although the author has the greatest respect for the scientific literature, he feels that stressing the clinical evidence is a form of intellectual honesty toward his colleagues. The international scientific literature also provides reassuring evidence of the strength added to dental structures through the use of partial restorations in composite[28] (Figs 59 to 105).

CLINICAL EXAMPLES OF REINFORCING DENTAL STRUCTURES WITH PARTIAL-COVERAGE COMPOSITE RESTORATIONS

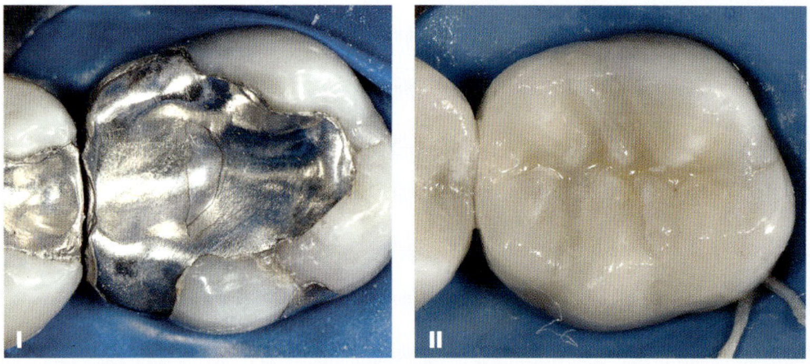

Fig 59

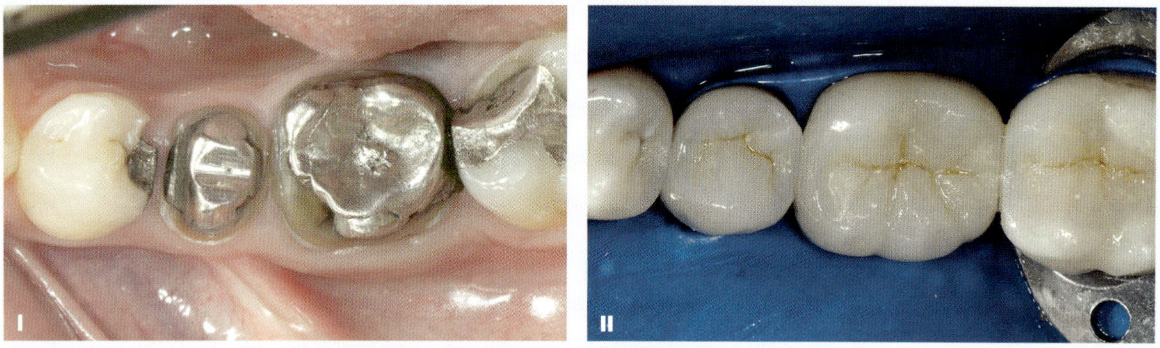

Fig 60

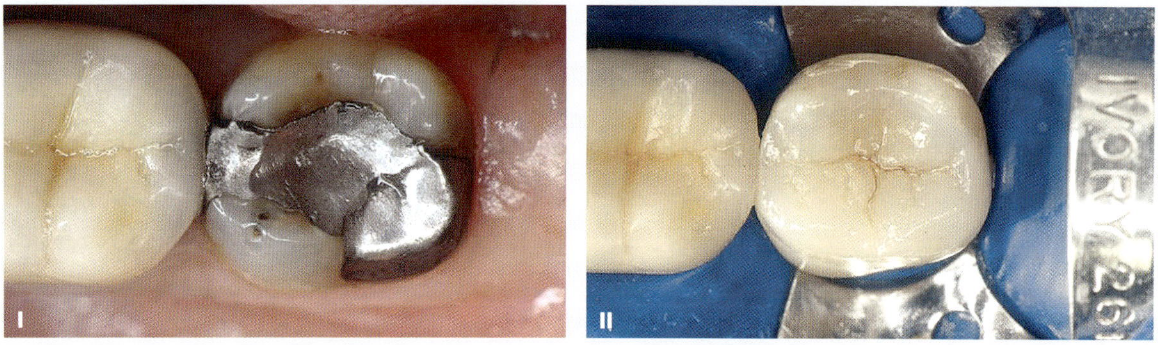

Fig 61

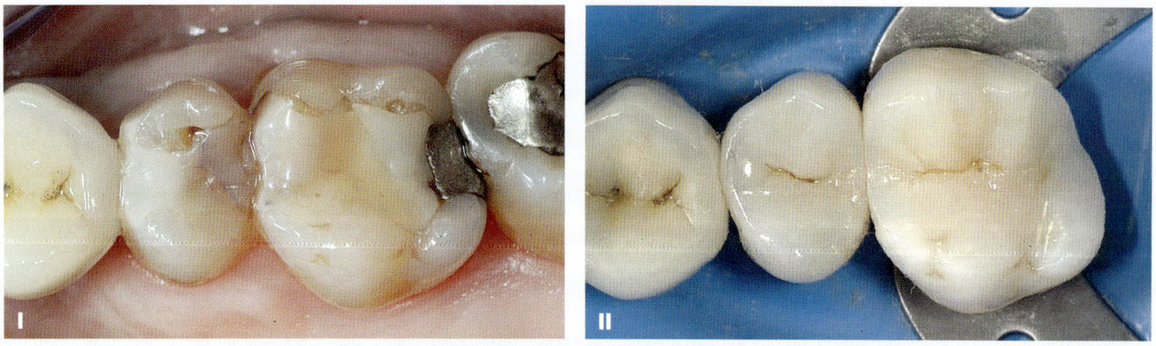

Fig 62

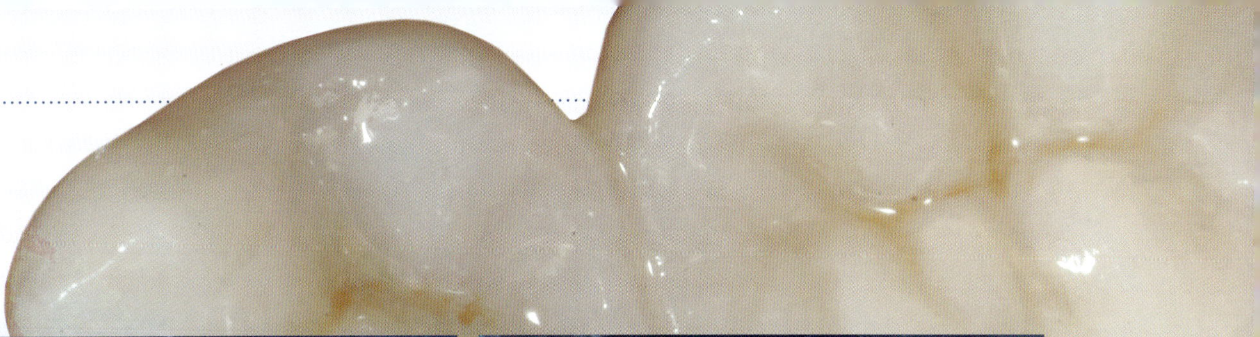

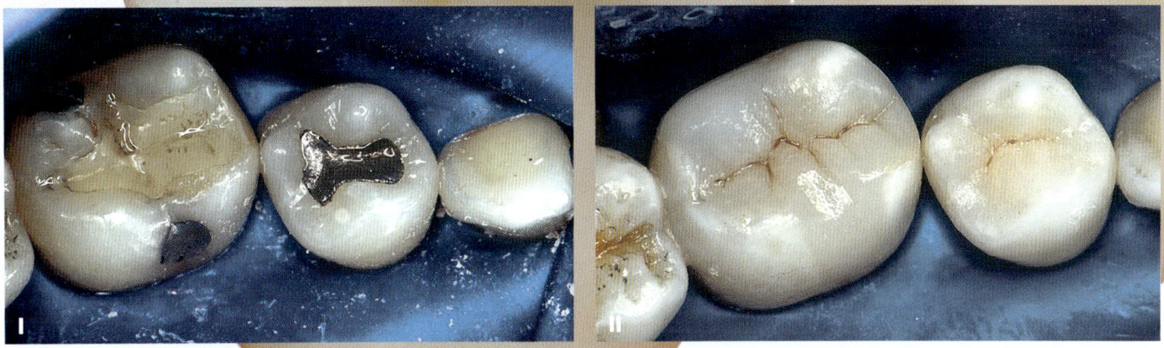

Fig 63

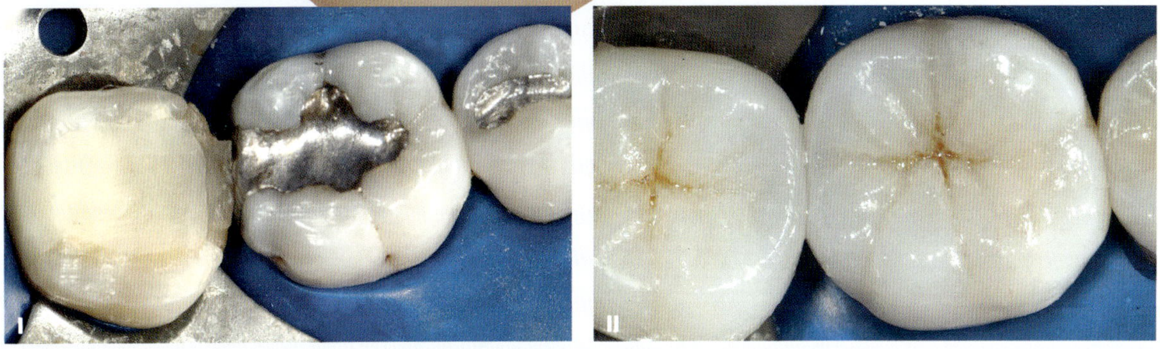

Fig 64

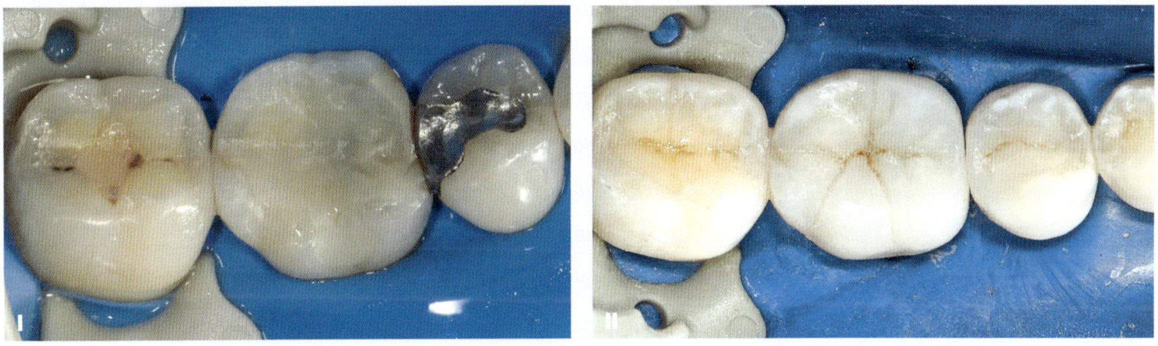

Fig 65

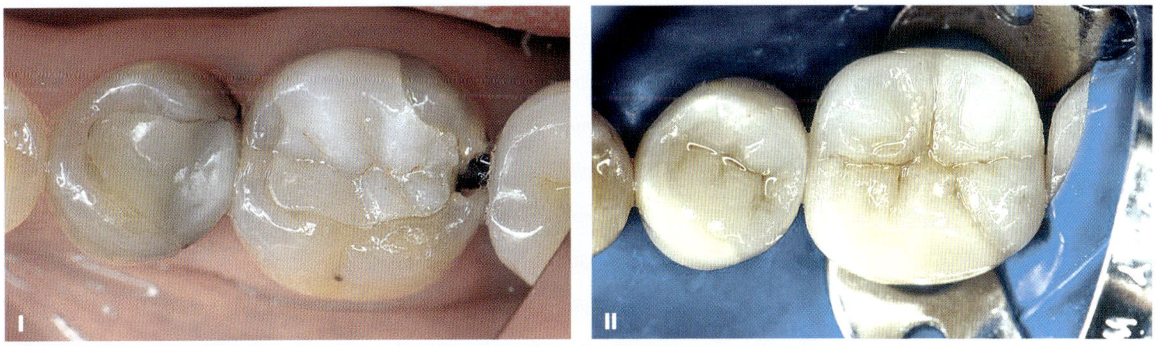

Fig 66

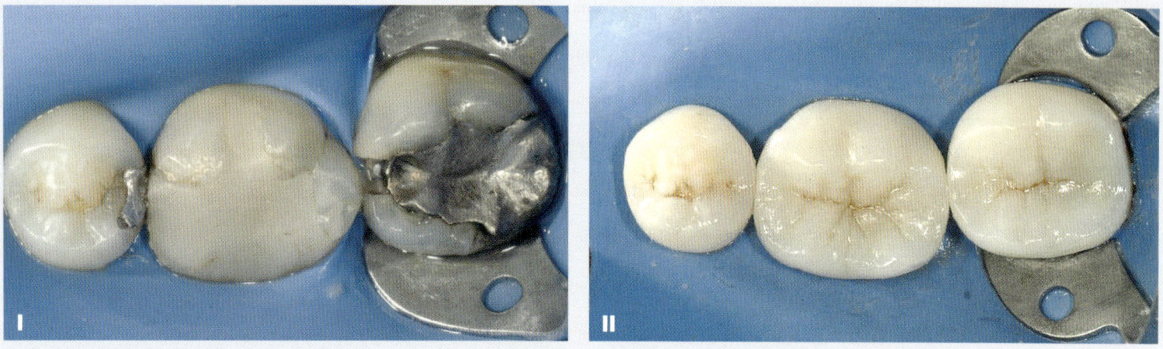

Fig 67

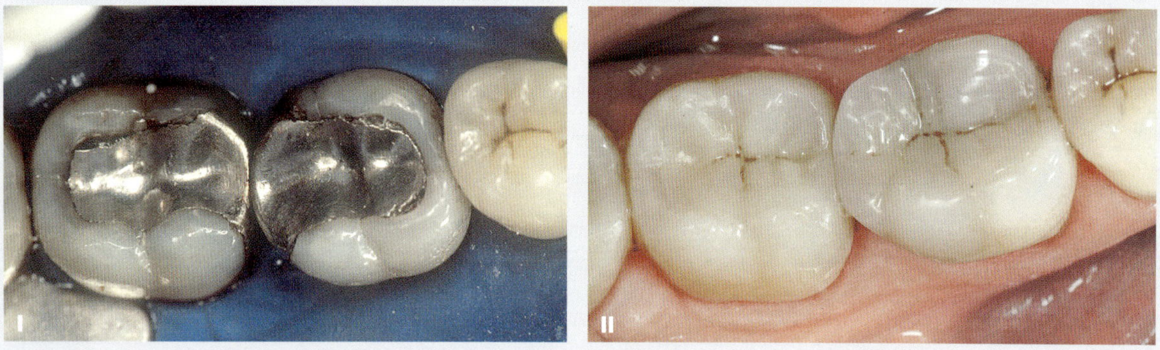

Fig 68

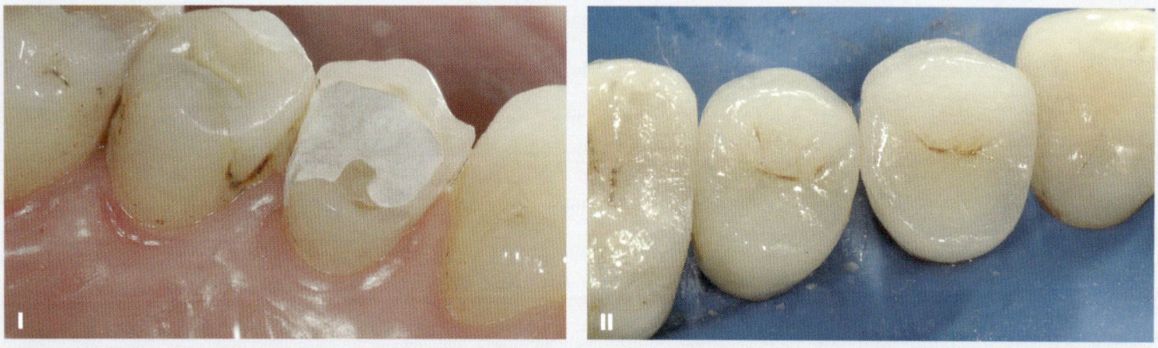

Fig 69

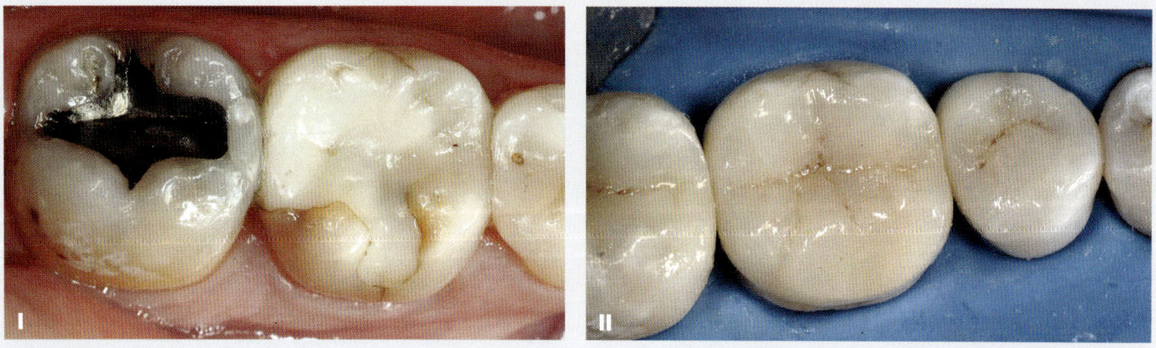

Fig 70

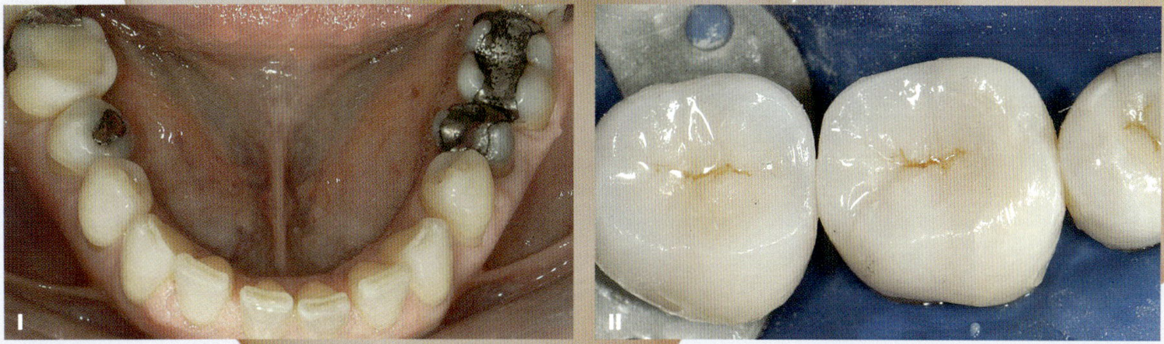

Fig 71

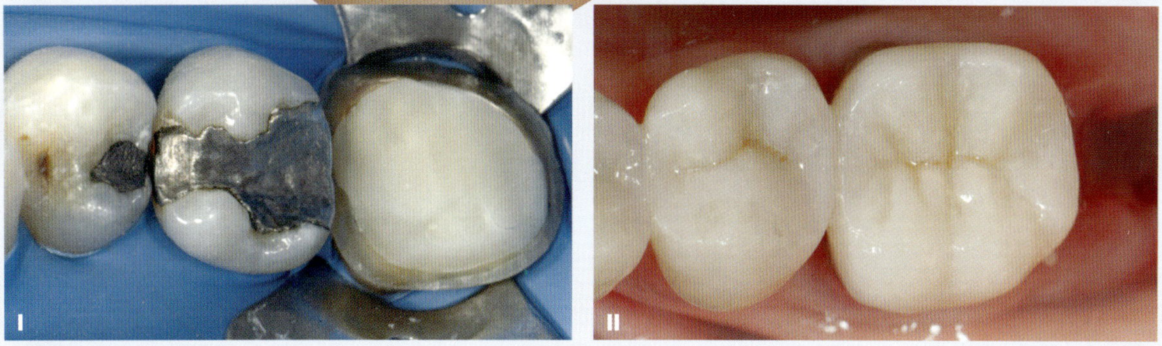

Fig 72

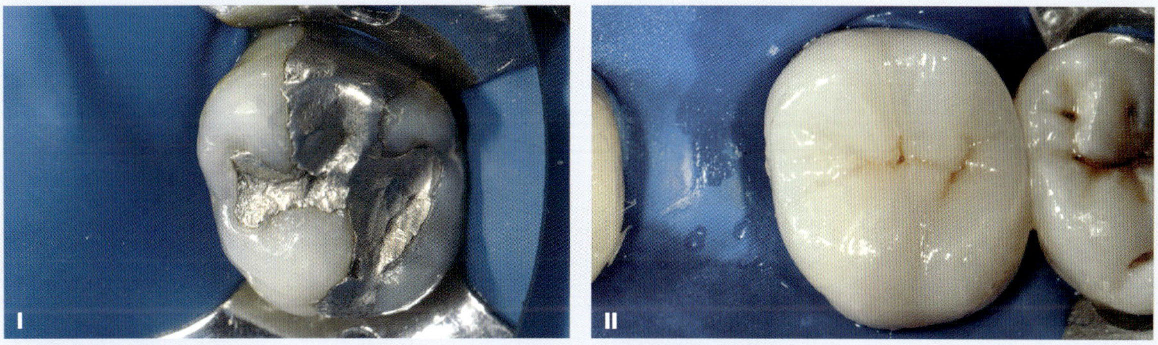

Fig 73

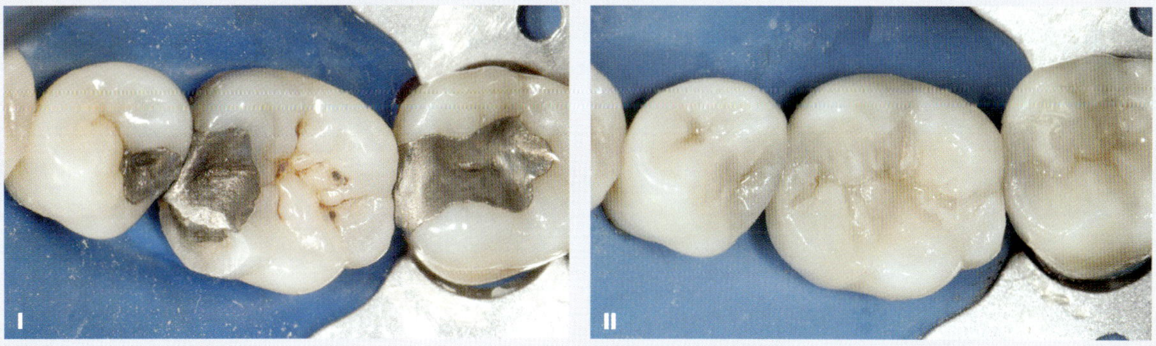

Fig 74

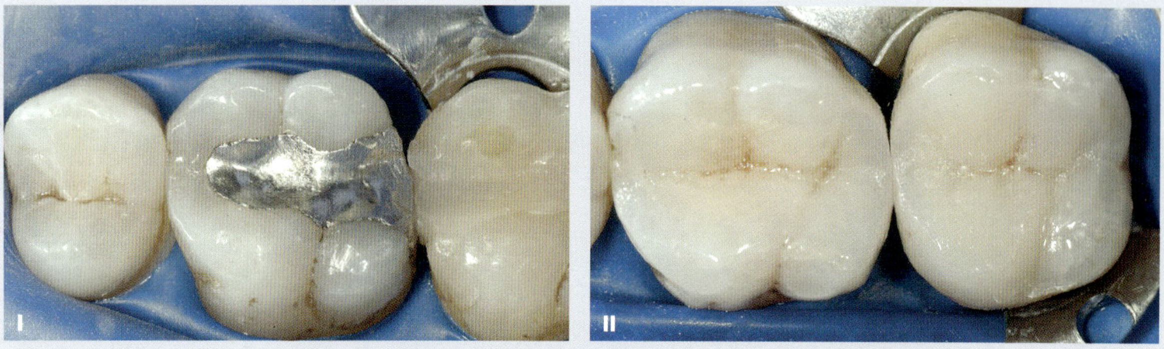

Fig 75

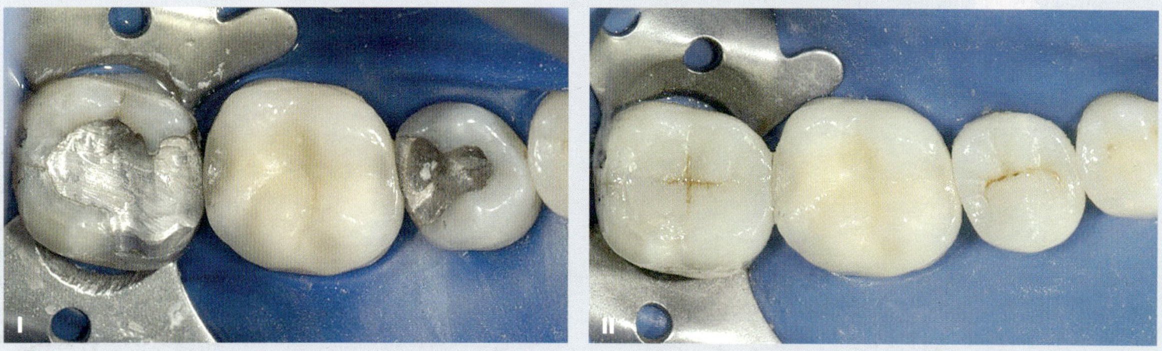

Fig 76

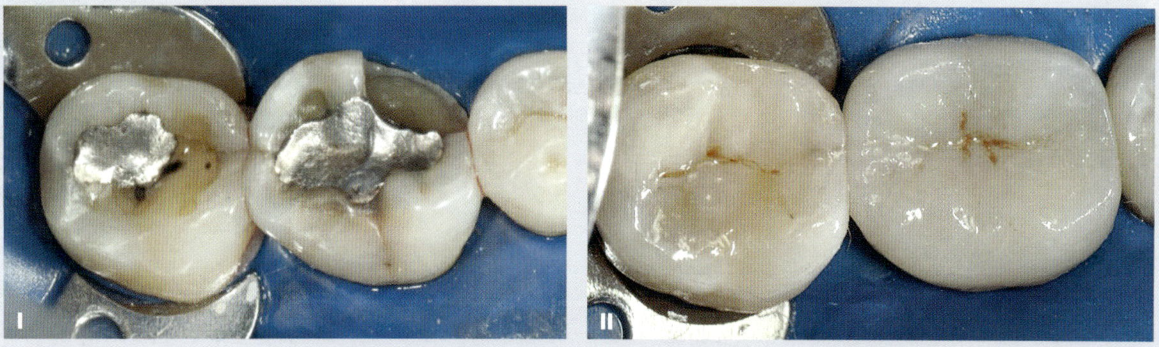

Fig 77

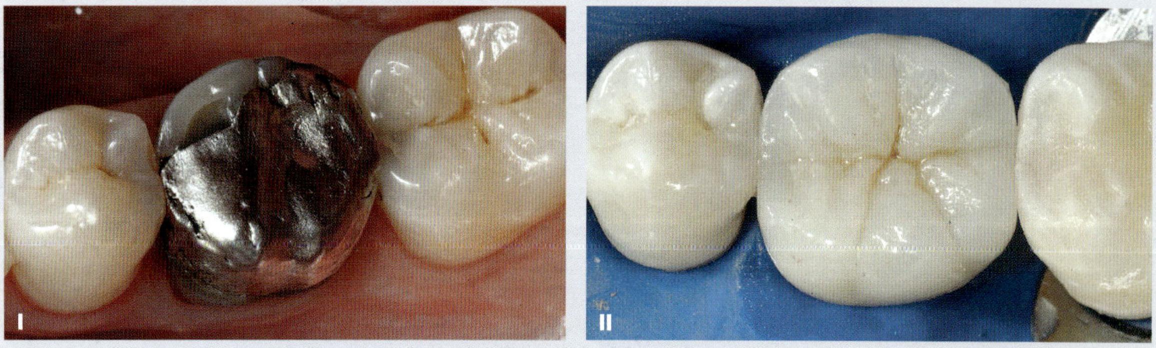

Fig 78

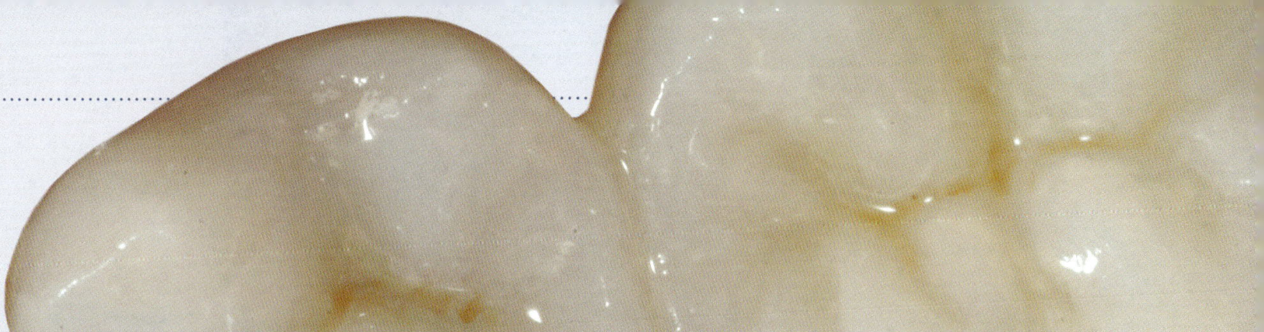

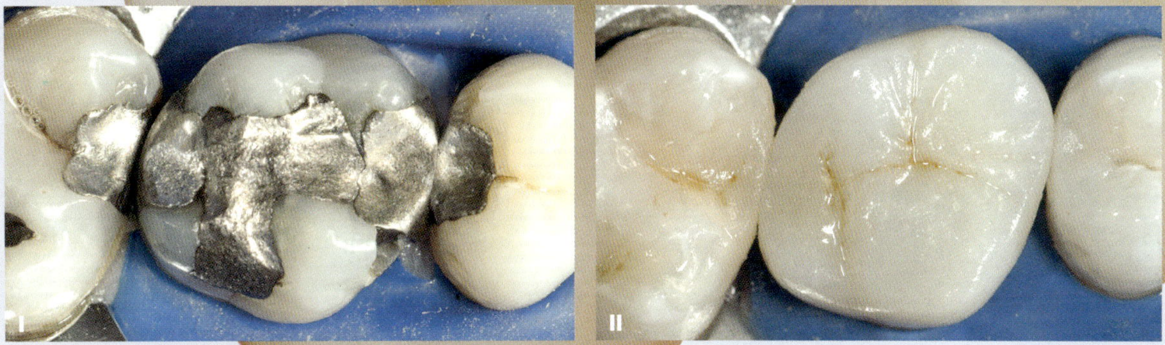

Fig 79

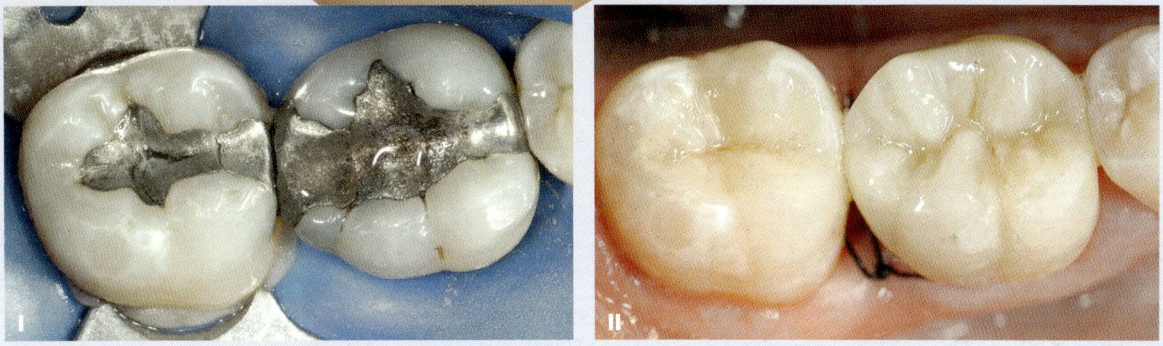

Fig 80

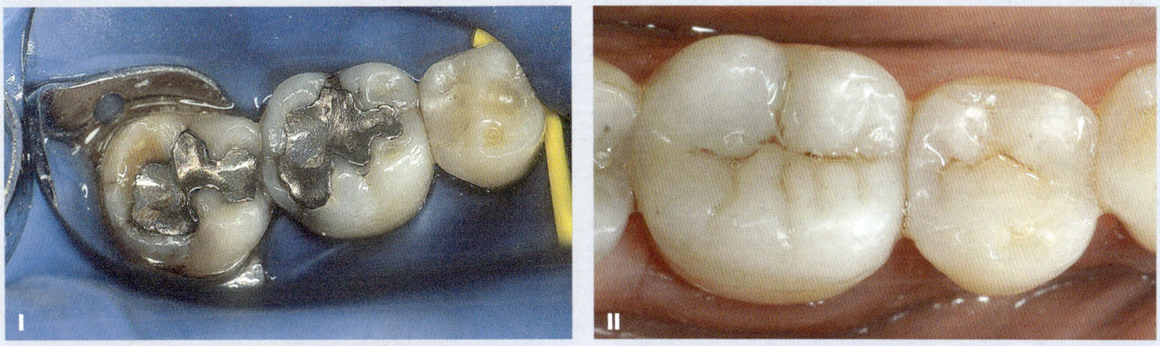

Fig 81

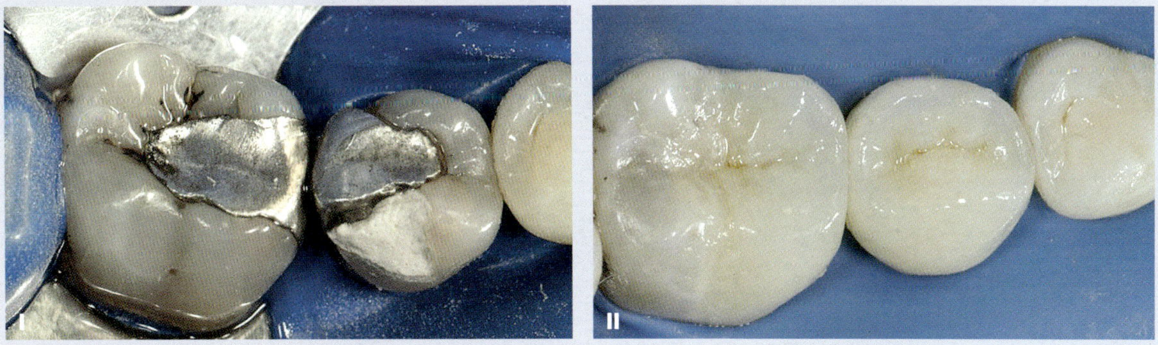

Fig 82

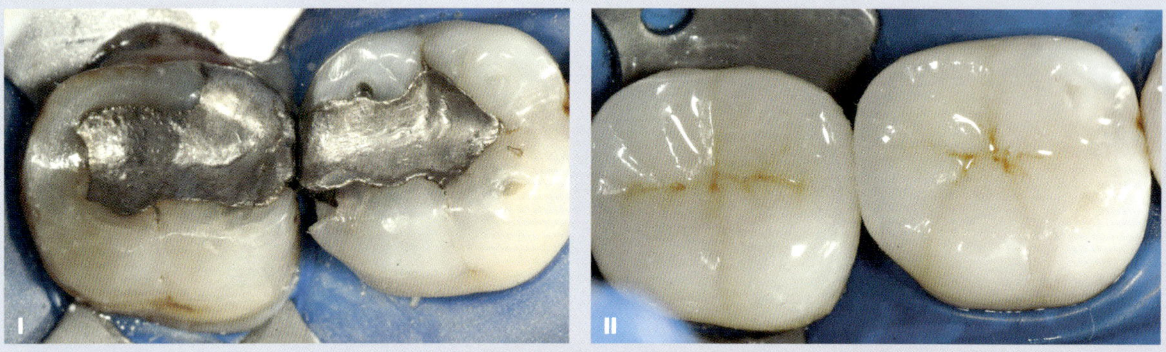

Fig 83

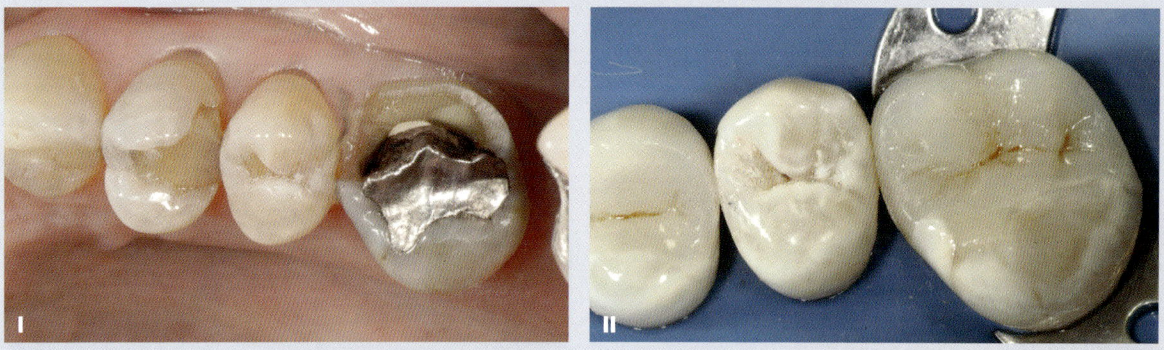

Fig 84

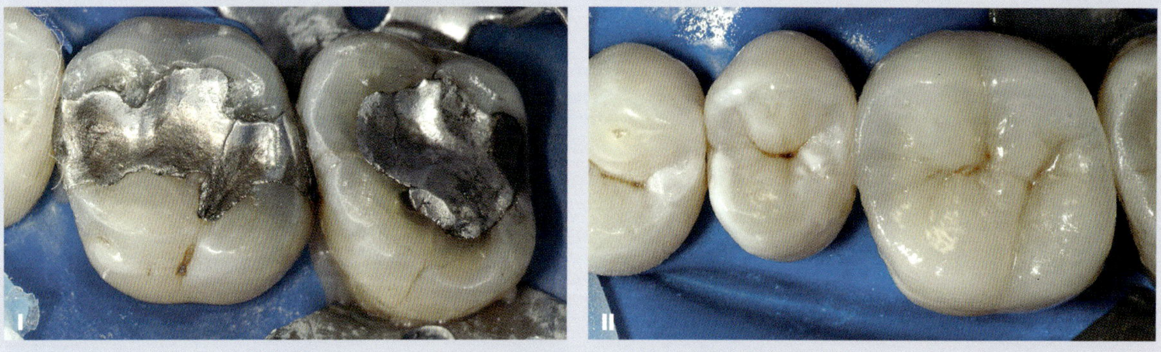

Fig 85

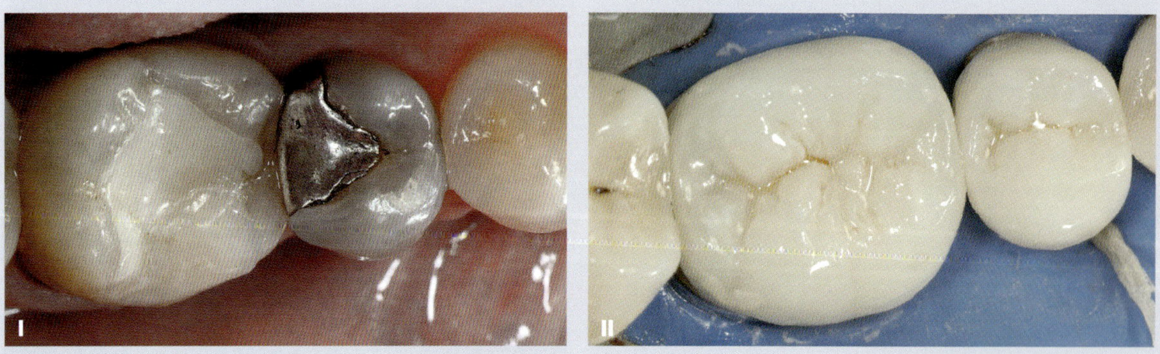

Fig 86

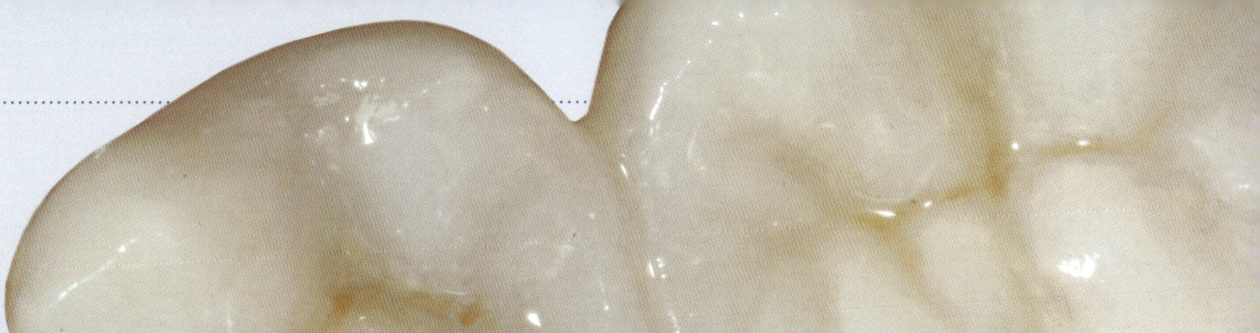

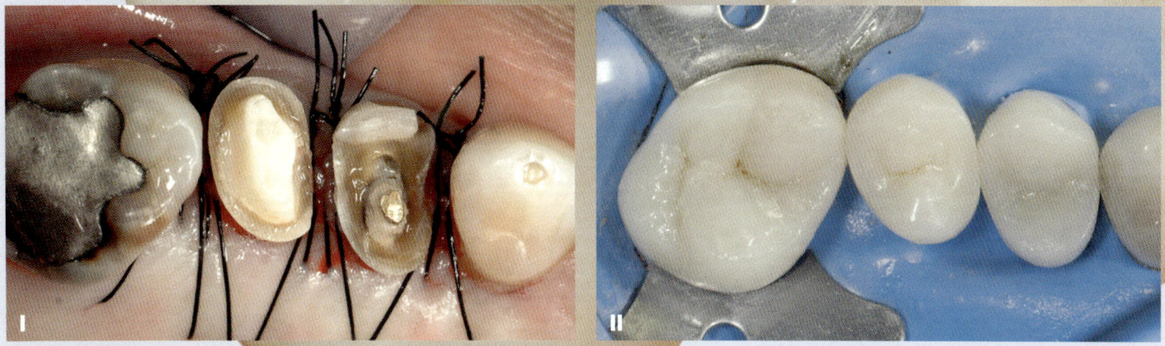

Fig 87

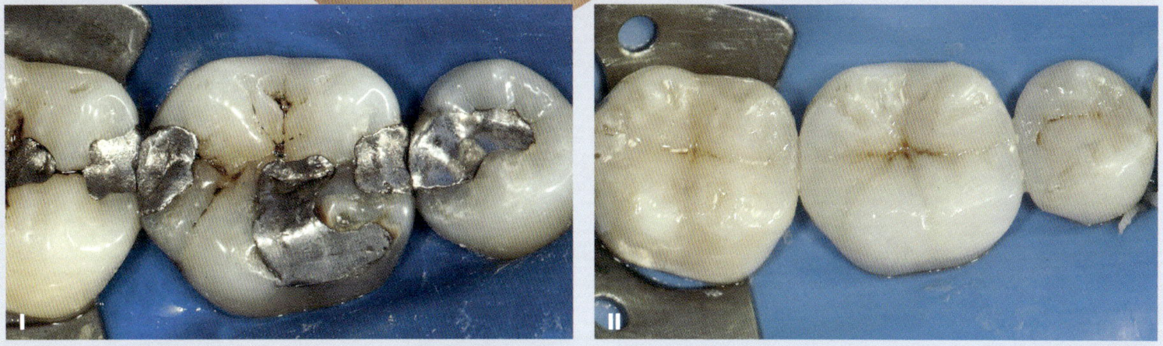

Fig 88

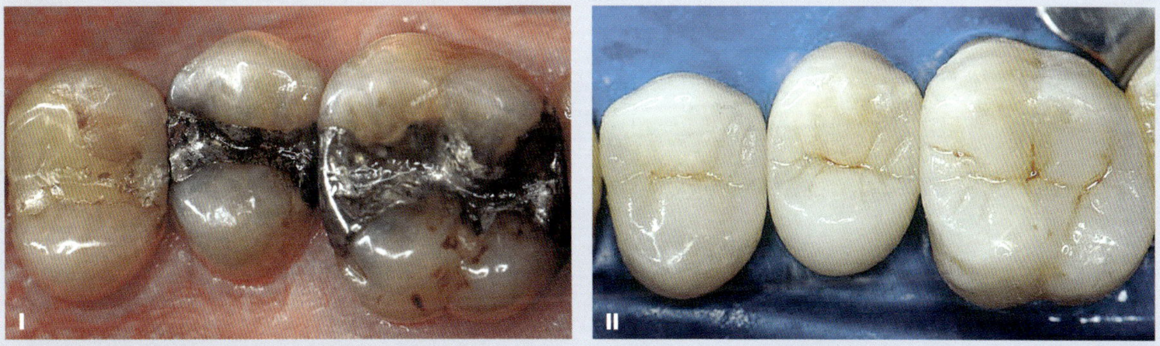

Fig 89

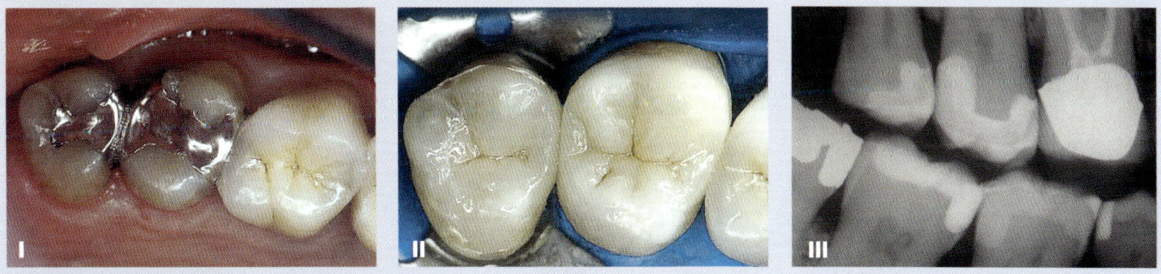

Fig 90

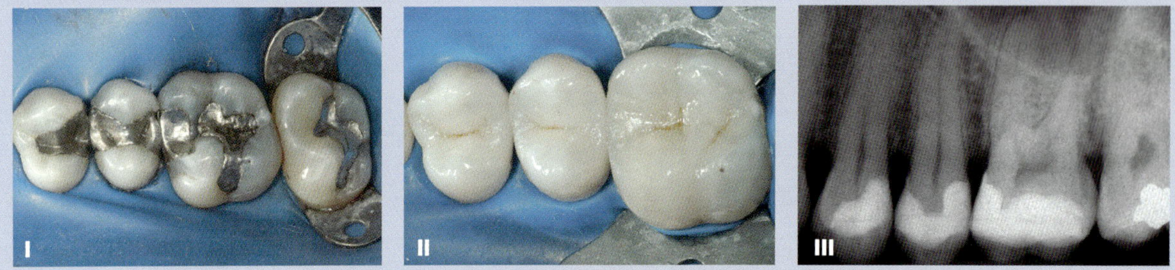

Fig 91

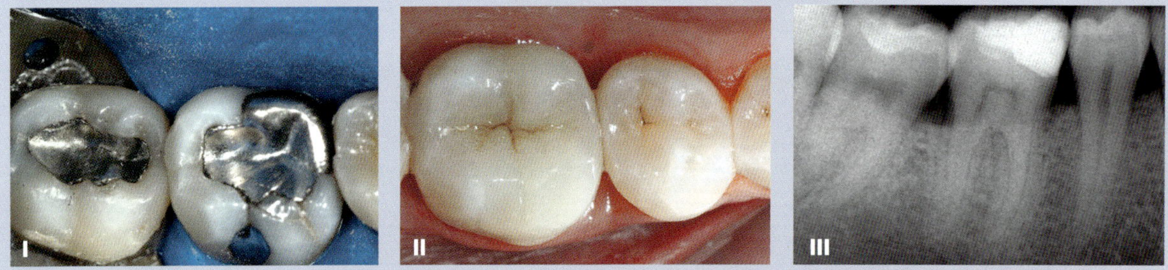

Fig 92

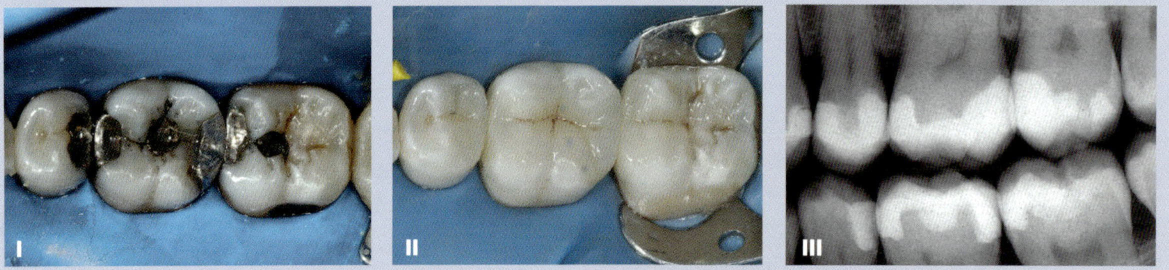

Fig 93

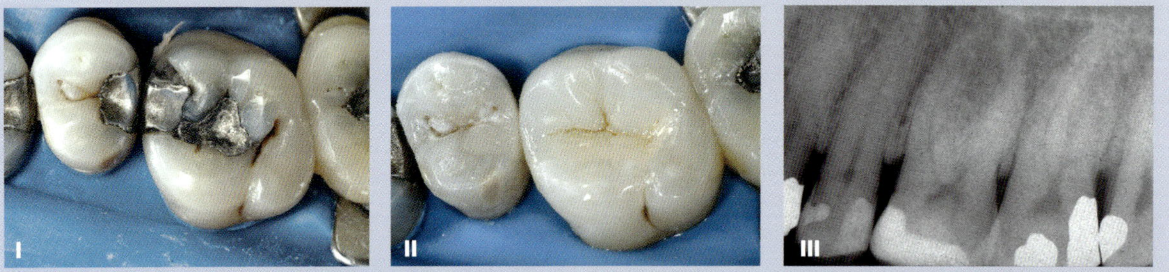

Fig 94

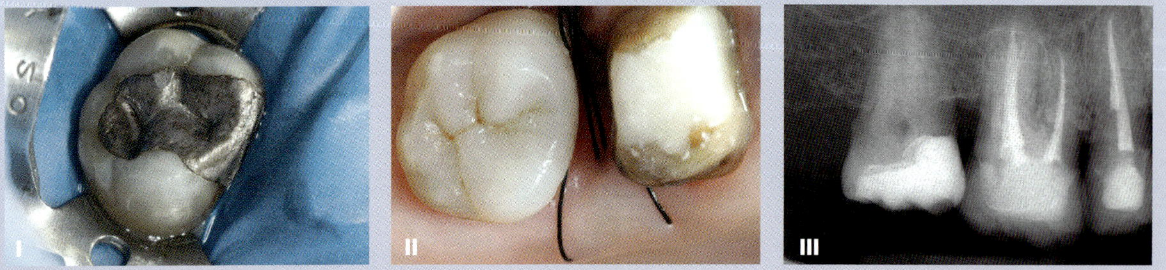

Fig 95

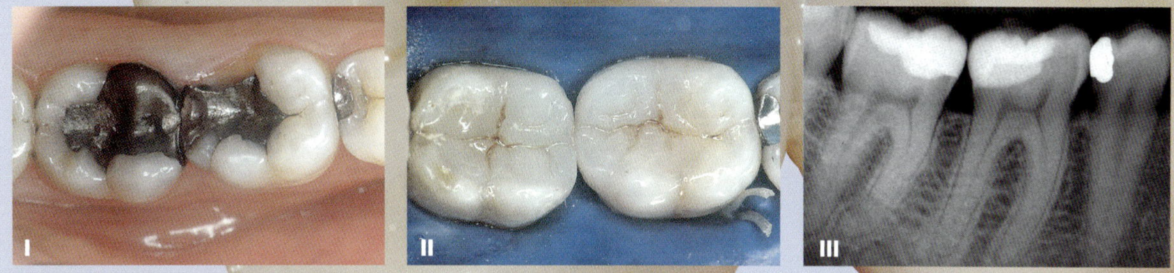

Fig 96

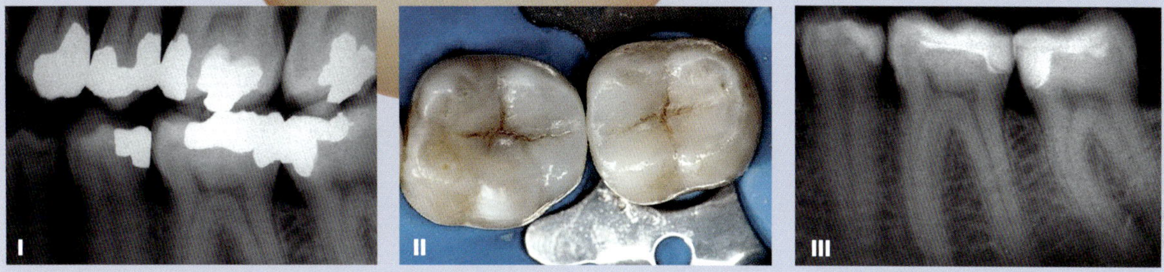

Fig 97

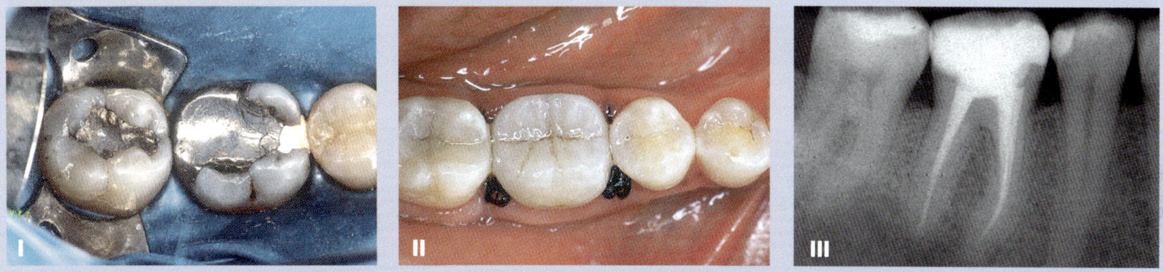

Fig 98

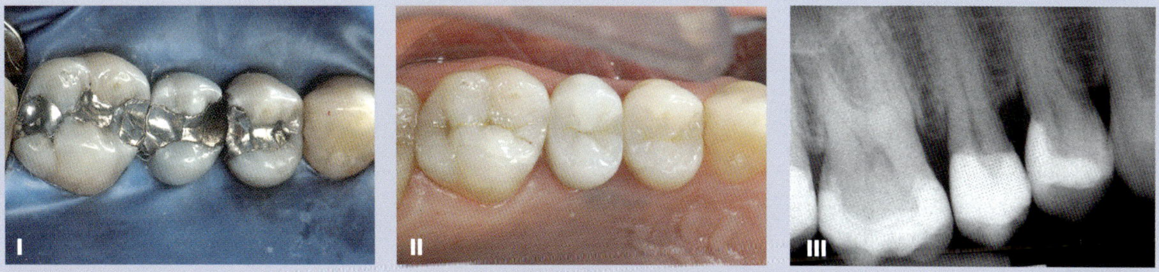

Fig 99

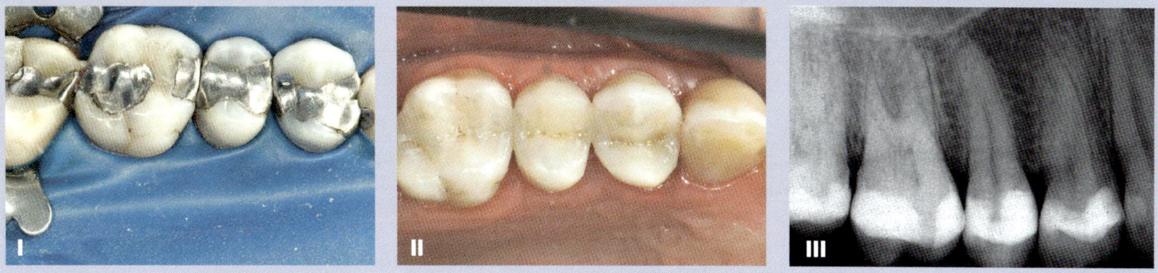

Fig 100

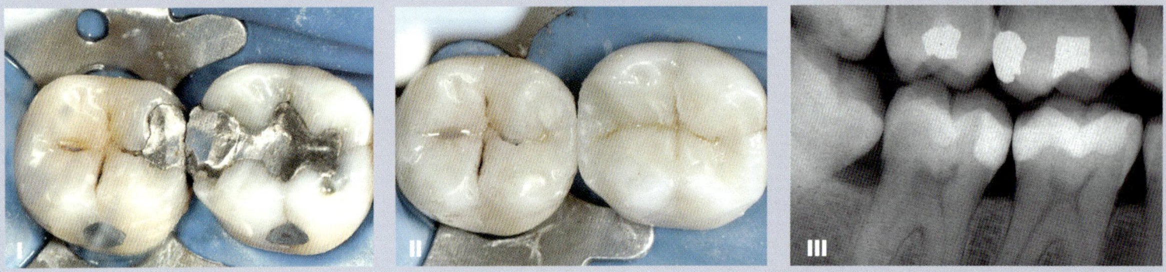

Fig 101

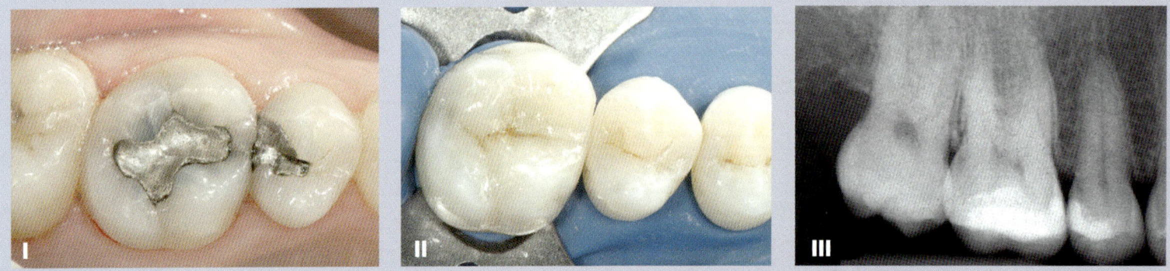

Fig 102

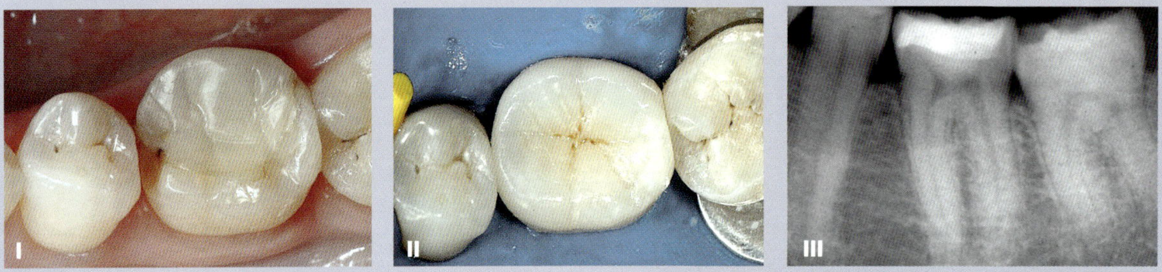

Fig 103

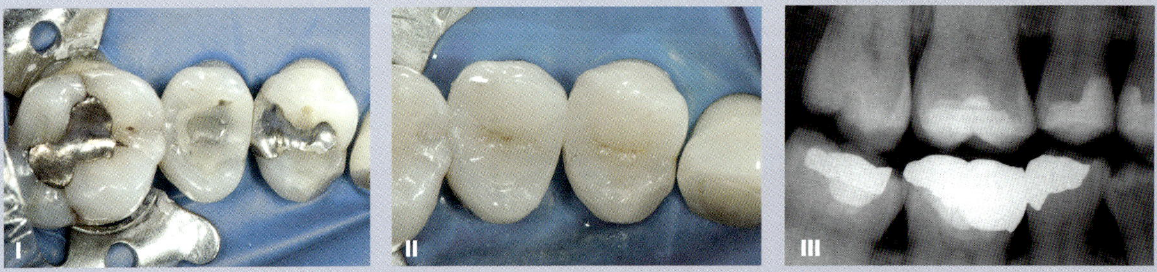

Fig 104

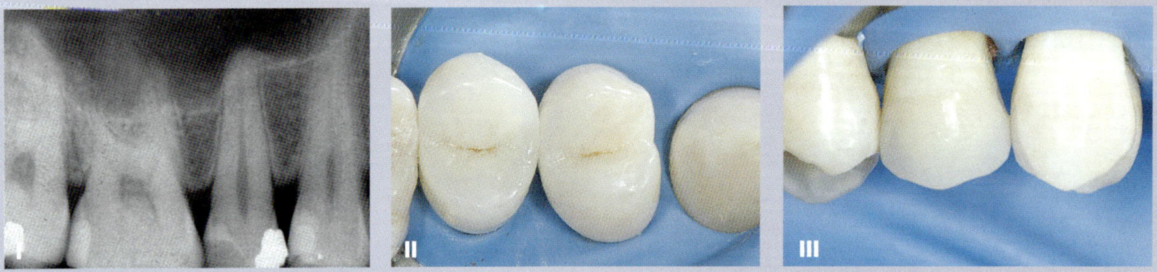

Fig 105

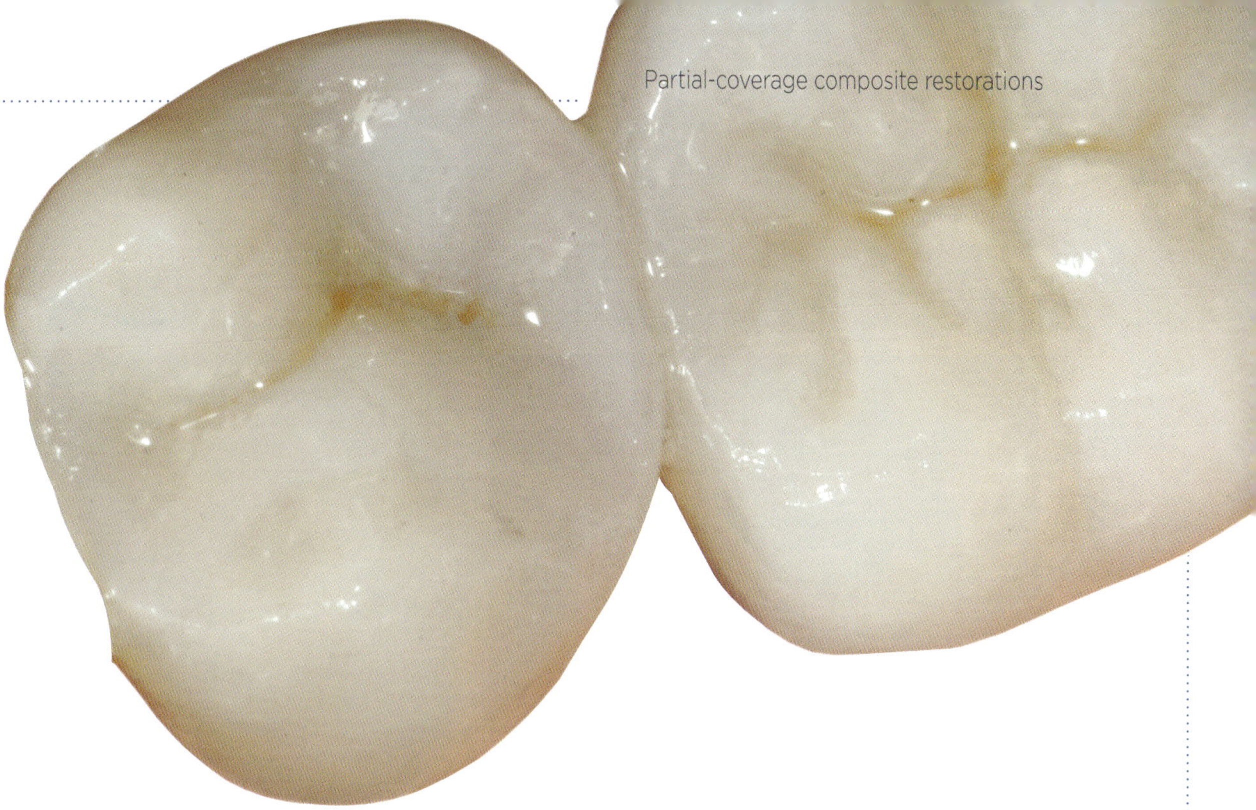

The main characteristics of partial-coverage restorations are great conservation of tooth structure, preservation of pulp vitality in most cases, and supragingival location of preparation margins. These have had a radical effect on treatment plans, rendering them conservative and minimally invasive (Figs 106 and 107). The reconstruction of endodontically treated teeth with partial-coverage restorations in composite also employs this philosophy of saving the teeth, which is borne out by observing the healthy remaining tissue, including maximally preserved root structures and strict use of intraradicular anchorage, ensuring very impressive medium- and long-term results (Figs 108 and 109).

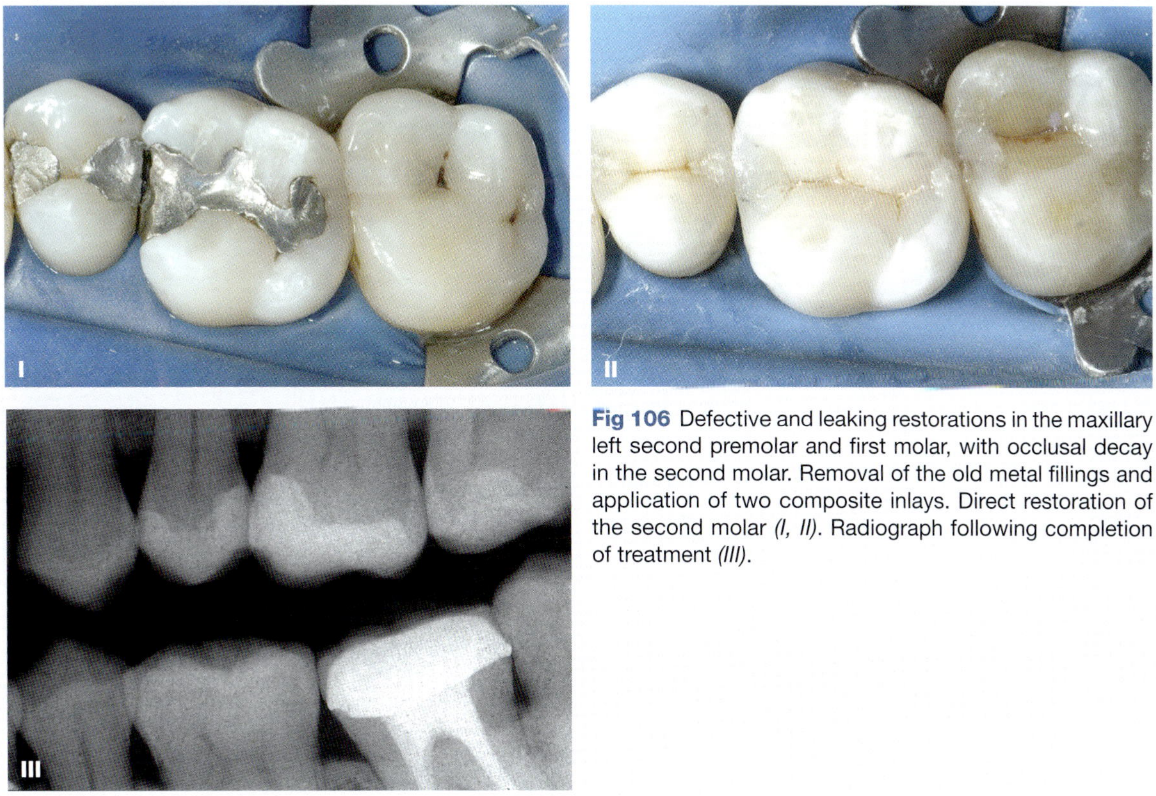

Fig 106 Defective and leaking restorations in the maxillary left second premolar and first molar, with occlusal decay in the second molar. Removal of the old metal fillings and application of two composite inlays. Direct restoration of the second molar *(I, II)*. Radiograph following completion of treatment *(III)*.

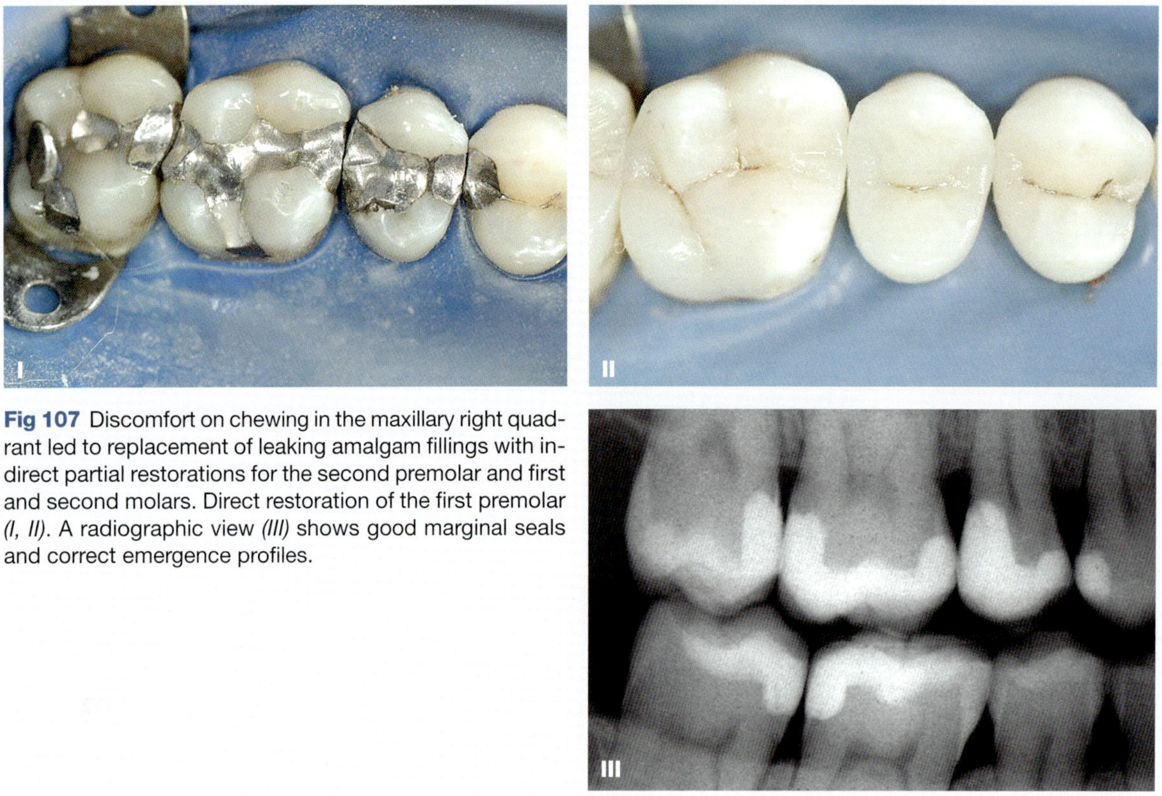

Fig 107 Discomfort on chewing in the maxillary right quadrant led to replacement of leaking amalgam fillings with indirect partial restorations for the second premolar and first and second molars. Direct restoration of the first premolar *(I, II)*. A radiographic view *(III)* shows good marginal seals and correct emergence profiles.

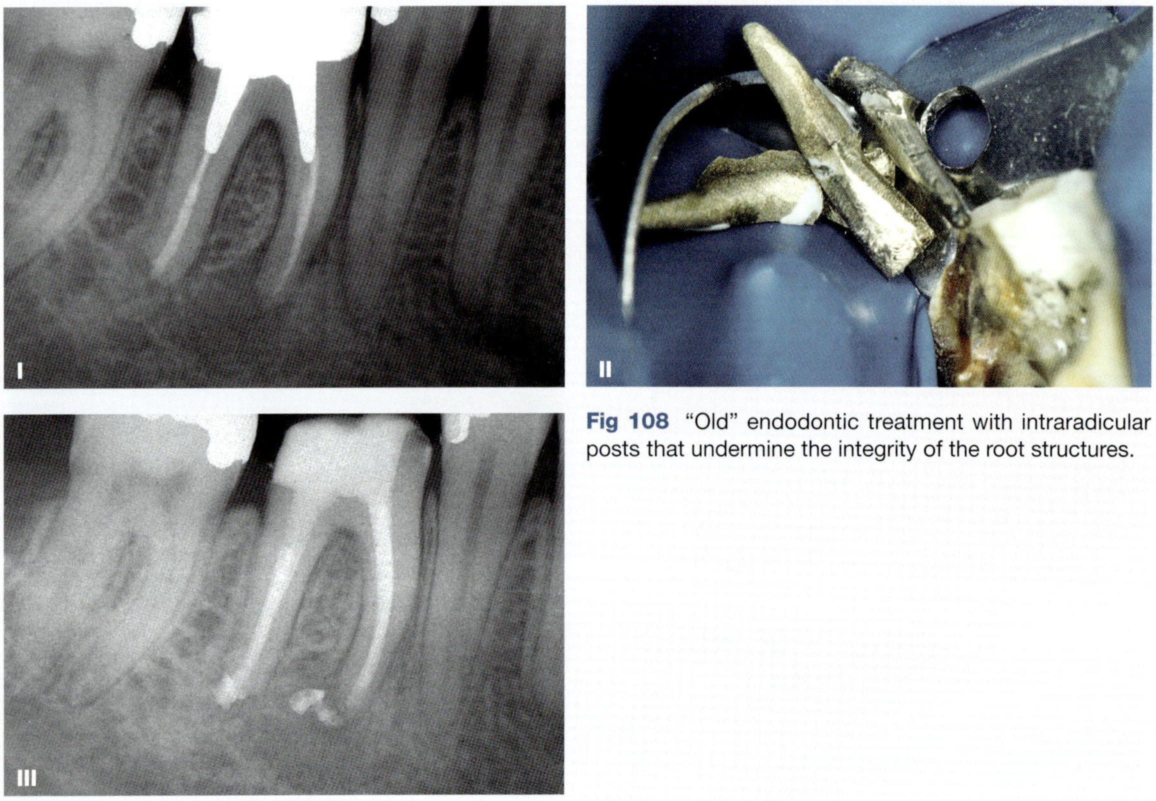

Fig 108 "Old" endodontic treatment with intraradicular posts that undermine the integrity of the root structures.

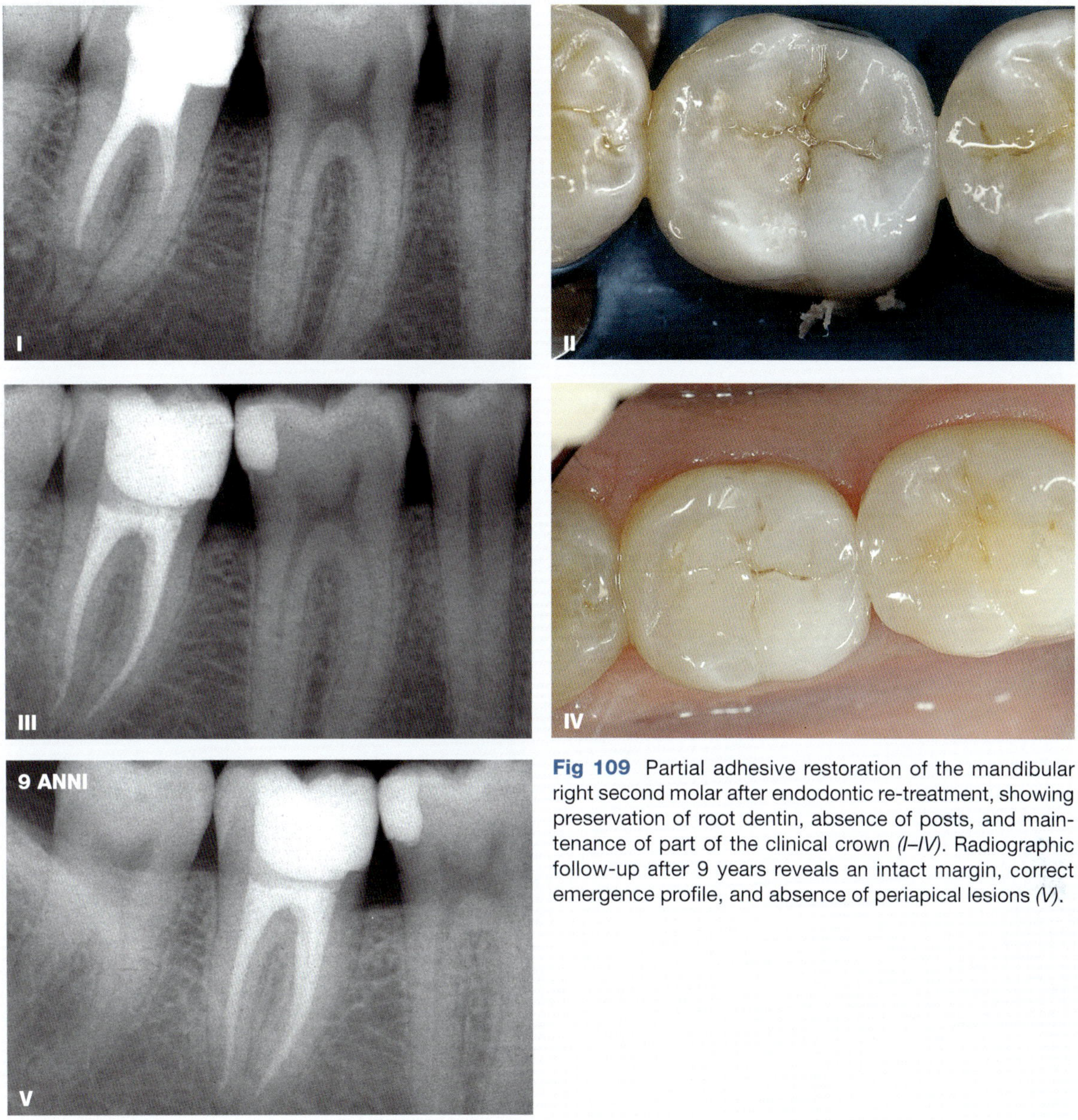

Fig 109 Partial adhesive restoration of the mandibular right second molar after endodontic re-treatment, showing preservation of root dentin, absence of posts, and maintenance of part of the clinical crown *(I–IV)*. Radiographic follow-up after 9 years reveals an intact margin, correct emergence profile, and absence of periapical lesions *(V)*.

Does this mean treatment plans are changing? Yes, or rather they have already changed.

Last but not least, one final consideration is the timing of adhesive techniques. Entire quadrants may routinely be reconstructed within a very short time frame, even within 24 to 48 hours.

The fact that practically all stages of this process require the use of rubber dam as an absolutely essential condition demonstrates how well this technique protects the dentin-pulp complex, which is a particularly delicate structure, against bacterial attack in the oral cavity (Fig 110).

Once the learning process has been completed, with the most difficult stage being the cementing of partial-coverage restorations, the practitioner will find great satisfaction in the results achieved using this technique. It is no wonder that authors such as Roulet and Degrange[29] called this technique a "silent revolution." This is illustrated by the photographs of the composite inlay produced by Dr Landi after only 2 years of experience (Figs 111 and 112).

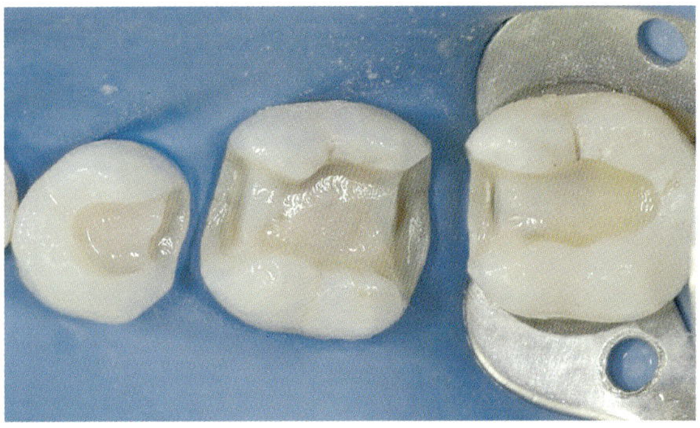

Fig 110 Preparations with rubber dam in place.

From a strictly clinical viewpoint, since this book is about clinical practice, the results of applying partial adhesive techniques allow achievement of the final outcome of arches without caries lesions, increasingly fewer endodontic treatments, and total periodontal tissue health, as is illustrated by the two arches that the author treated during his early days of performing adhesive techniques (Fig 113).

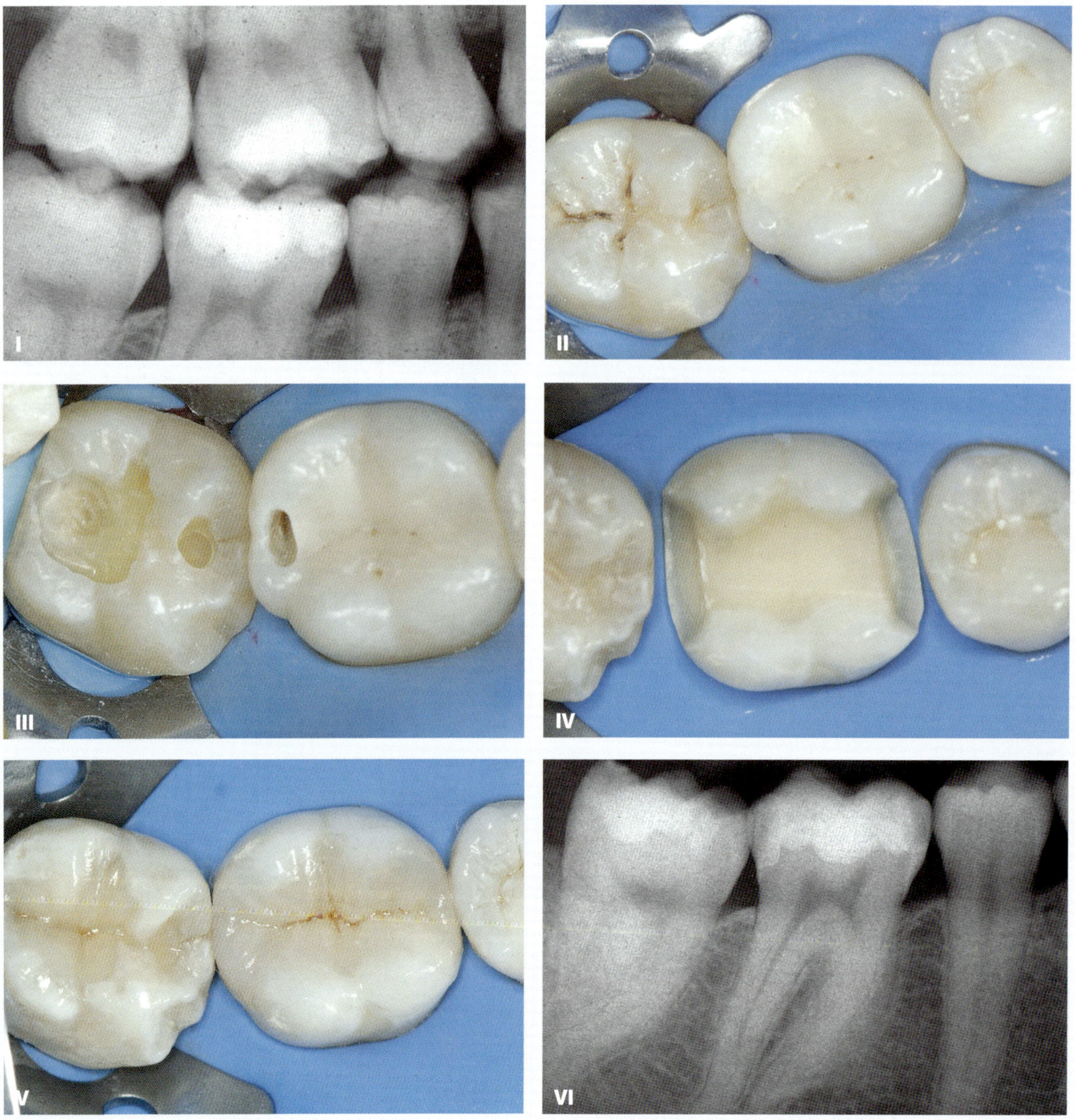

Fig 111 Construction of a mesio-occlusodistal inlay by Dr Lavinia Landi after 2 years of experience.

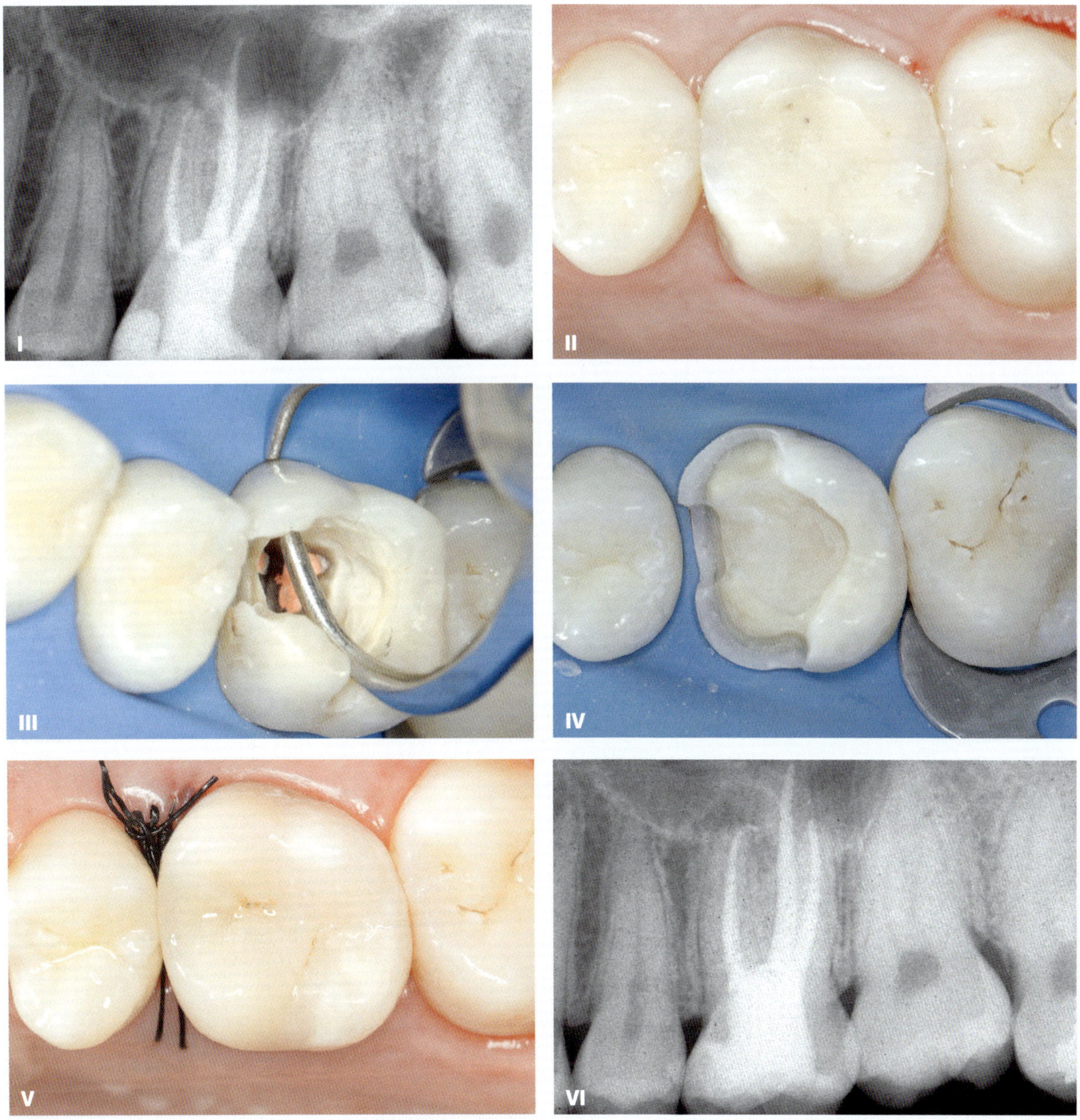

Fig 112 Creation of a mesio-occlusal onlay for reconstruction of an endodontically treated tooth. (Courtesy of Dr Lavinia Landi.)

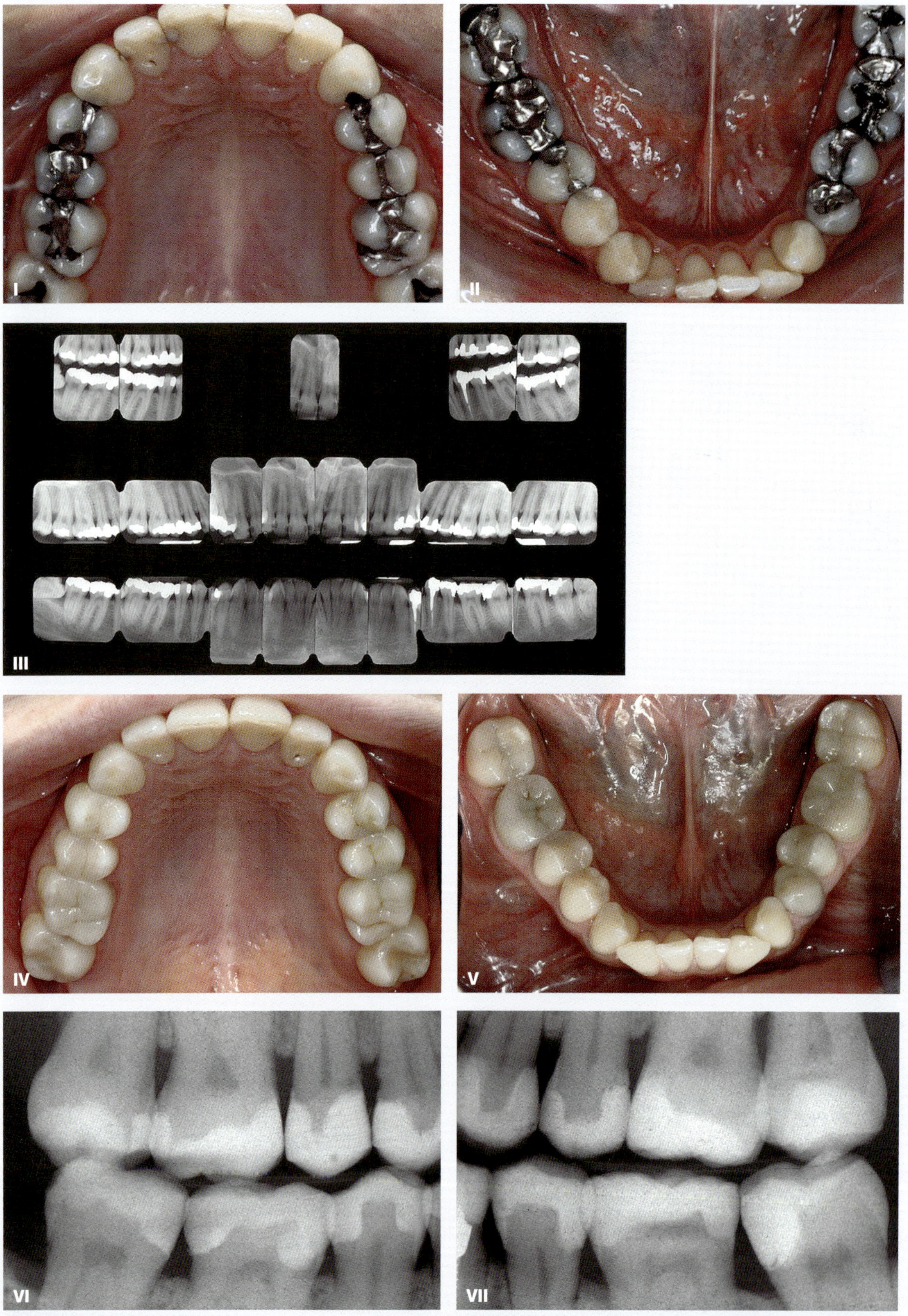

Fig 113 Preoperative view of two arches with caries lesions and defective restorations and the associated radiographic status *(I–III)*. Eight-year follow-up views of arches restored using direct and indirect techniques and follow-up radiographs *(IV–XI)*.

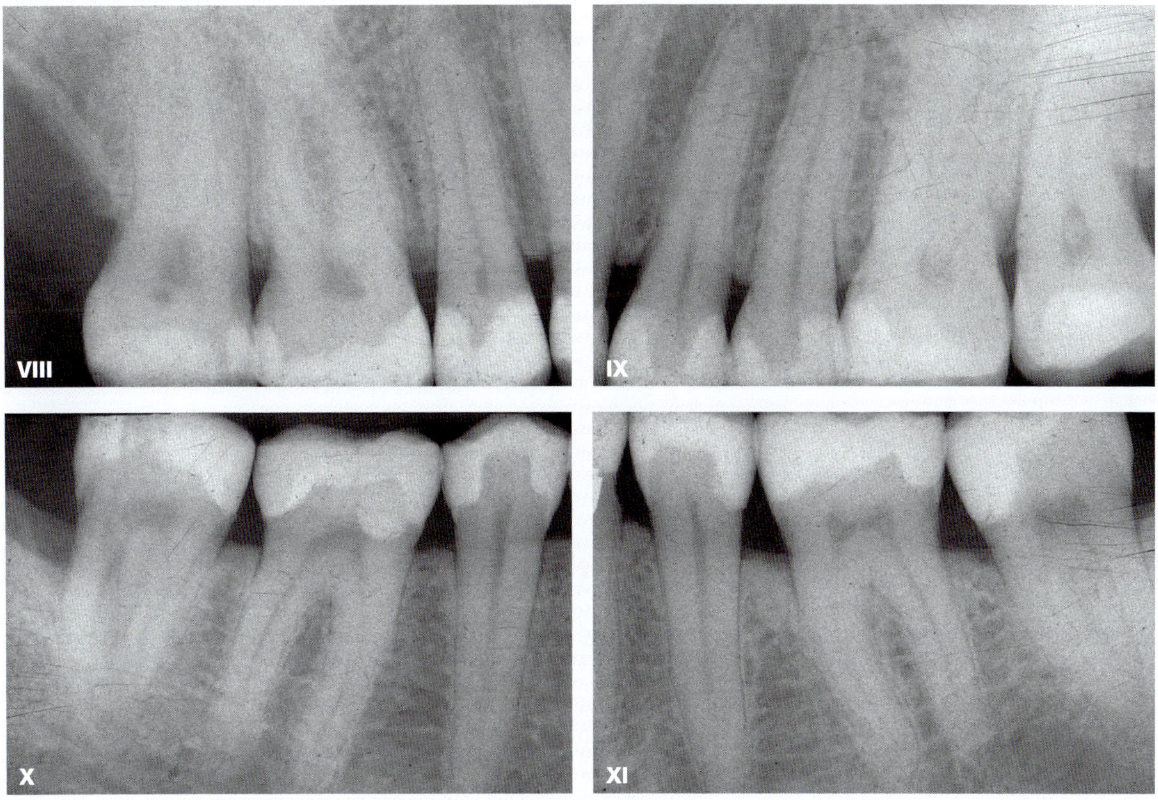

Fig 113 *(continued)*

Medium- and long-term clinical and follow-up radiographs are absolutely satisfactory, and meanwhile if any problem should arise (eg, minor fractures, defective contact surfaces), the clinician can proceed with complete peace of mind because the material used is repairable.

The author likes to talk about the "manageability" of restructured arches and to say that the arches have undergone a "reset" to eliminate the inconsistencies present prior to the intervention.

Even in severely compromised clinical situations, these new arches will satisfy biologic needs, functional stability, and, last but not least, the increasing esthetic demands of patients; however, the latter should not be the primary consideration in the treatment plan (Fig 114). The radiographic appearance is all-important in this protocol; in fact, the author jokingly threatened the four people who have been good enough to put up with his arguments over the years that "anyone who fails to take radiographs will go straight to hell!" Of course, there is no real risk of such severe punishment, but it goes without saying that however good the restoration, if it is performed without a radiographic follow-up at the end of treatment and radiographic checkups over the years, it will lack any credibility at all (Figs 115 and 116).

It is impossible to choose between color and black and white images for esthetic dentistry purposes; they are both important and reveal clinical accuracy and also perhaps a certain ethical approach that is all too often forgotten because today clinicians can ensure that biology, esthetics, function, and stability are all typical features of partial-coverage composite restorations (Figs 117 and 118).

Clinicians perform their work to ensure that the final result performs consistently over time and their patients do not have to keep returning for more treatment. Careful monitoring, including hygiene appointments with clinical and radiographic checkups, allows them to address any problems in the early stages, which makes them much easier to resolve.

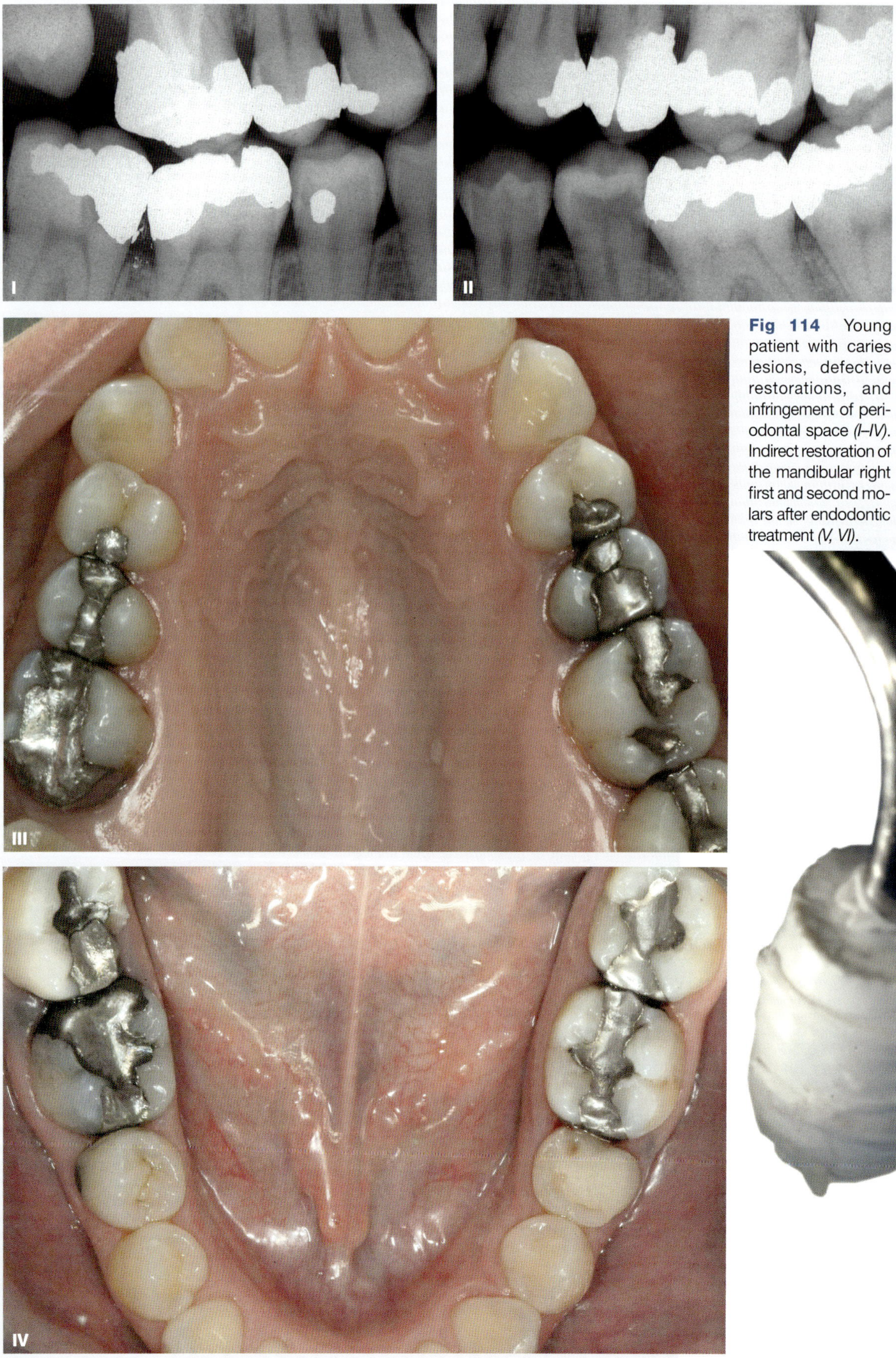

Fig 114 Young patient with caries lesions, defective restorations, and infringement of periodontal space *(I–IV)*. Indirect restoration of the mandibular right first and second molars after endodontic treatment *(V, VI)*.

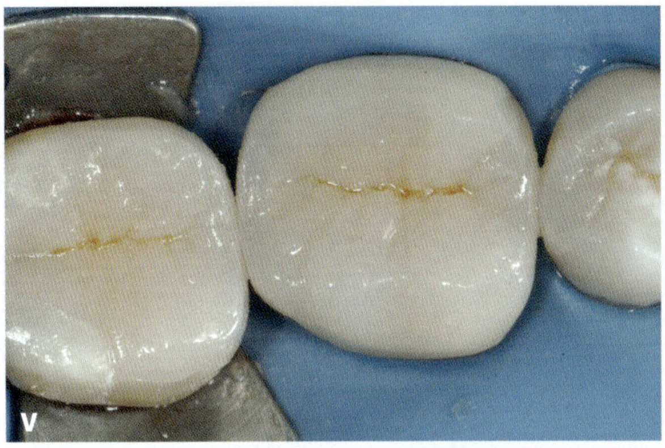

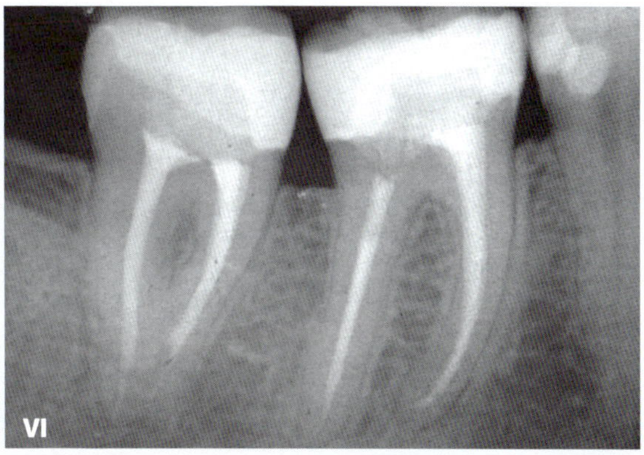

Fig 114 *(continued)* Restorations in the mandibular left quadrant following periodontal surgery *(VII)* and checkup after 3 months *(VIII)*. Intraoperative stages in the maxilla *(IX–XVII)* and the successful result of interdisciplinary treatment *(XVIII)*. Radiographic follow-up showing status at the end of treatment *(XIX)*.

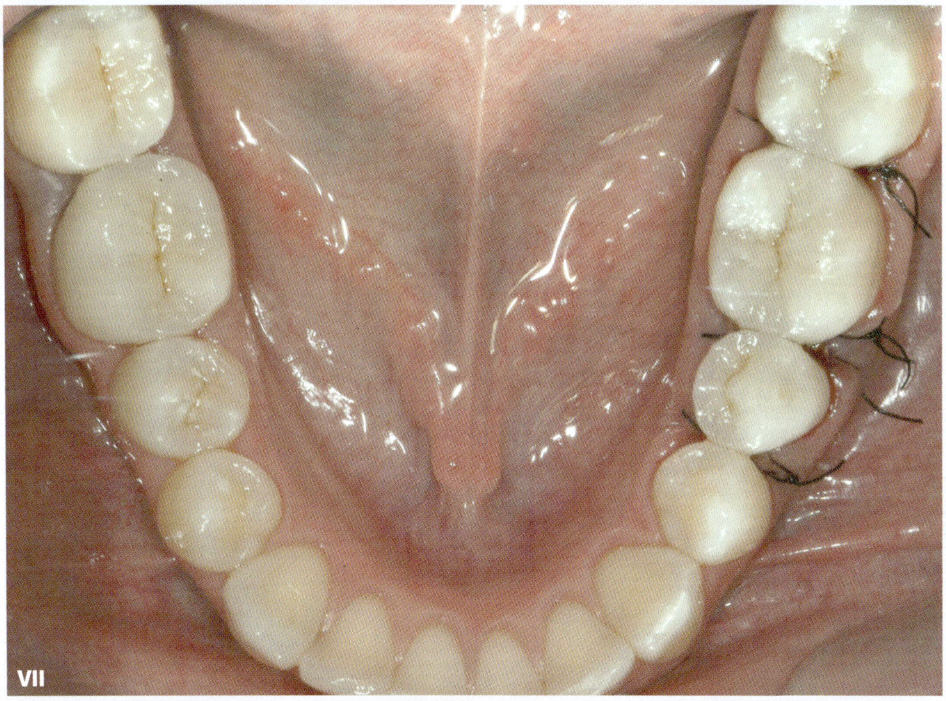

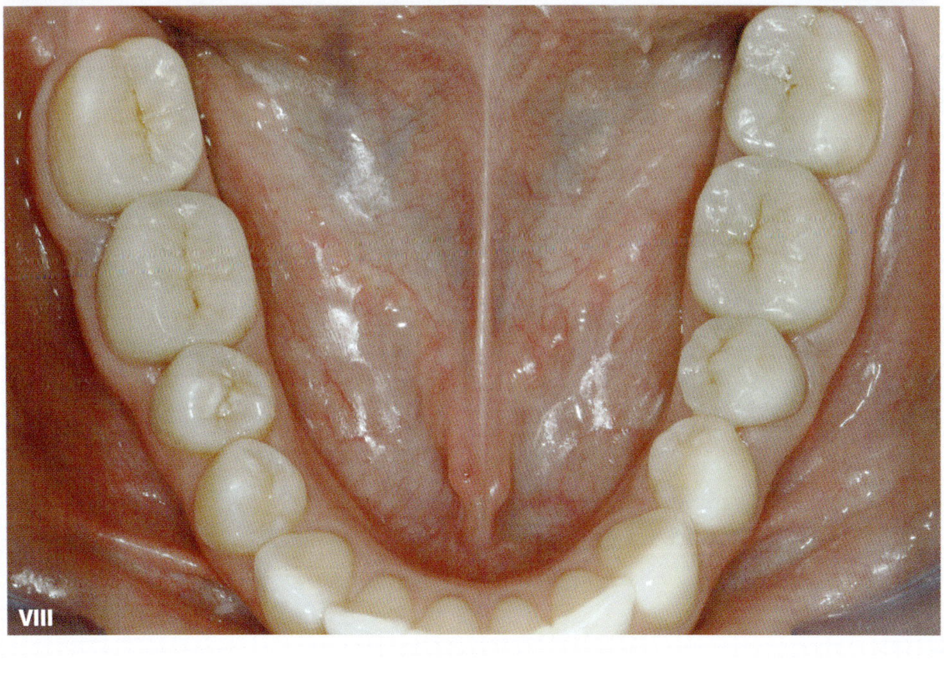

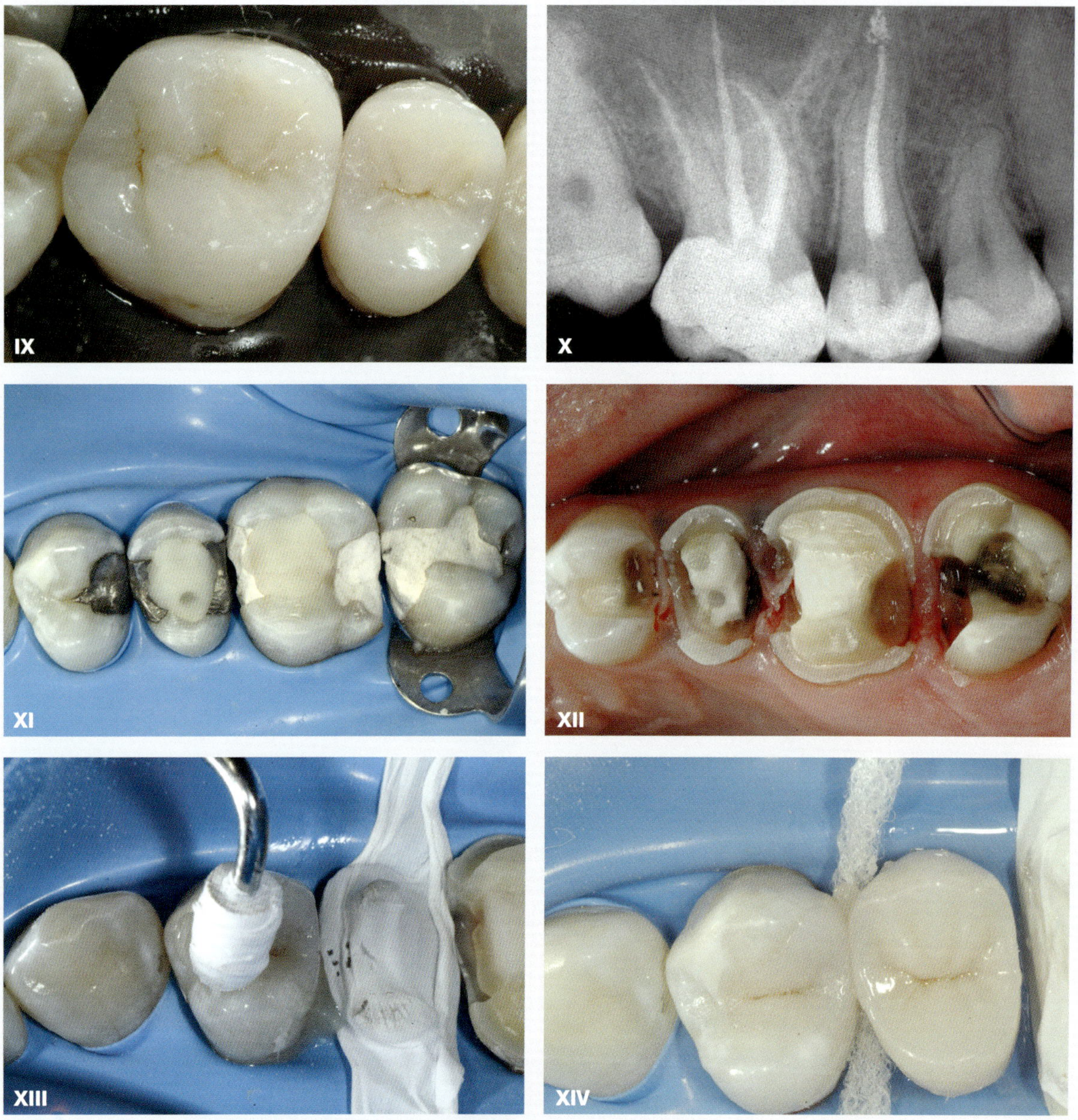

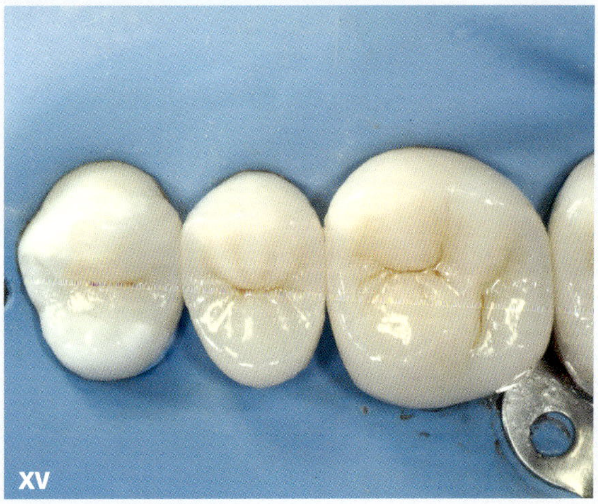

Fig 114 *(continued)*

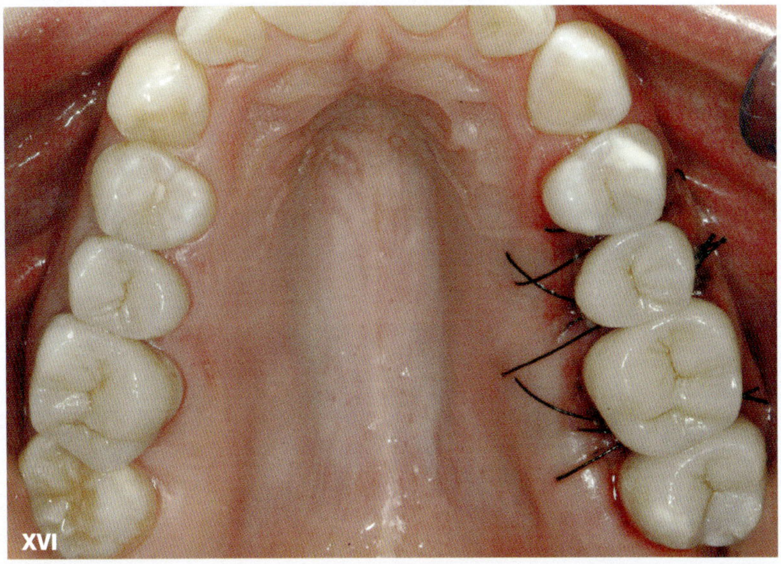

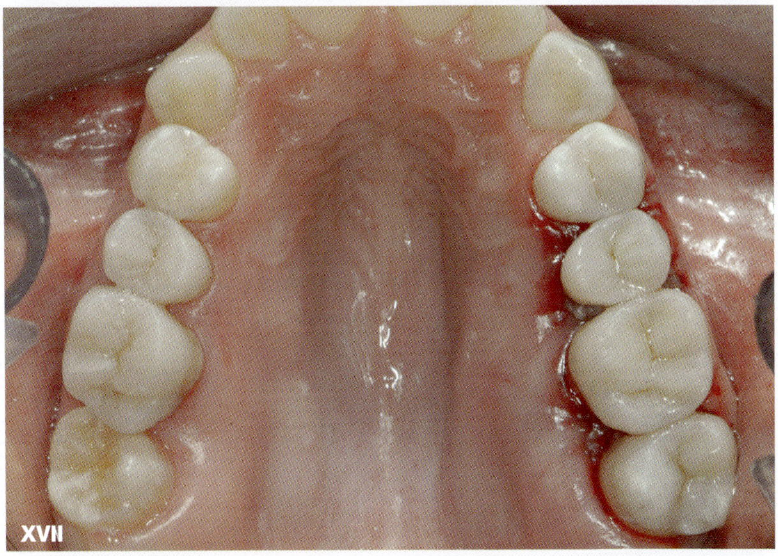

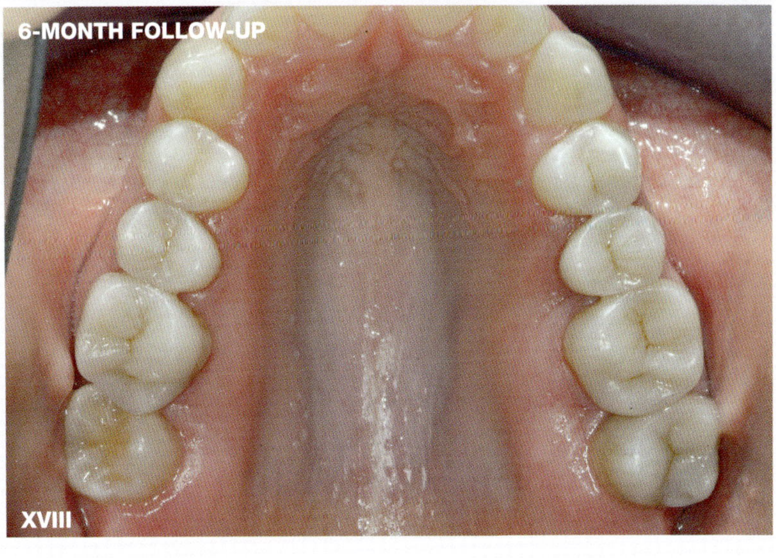

Fig 114 *(continued)*

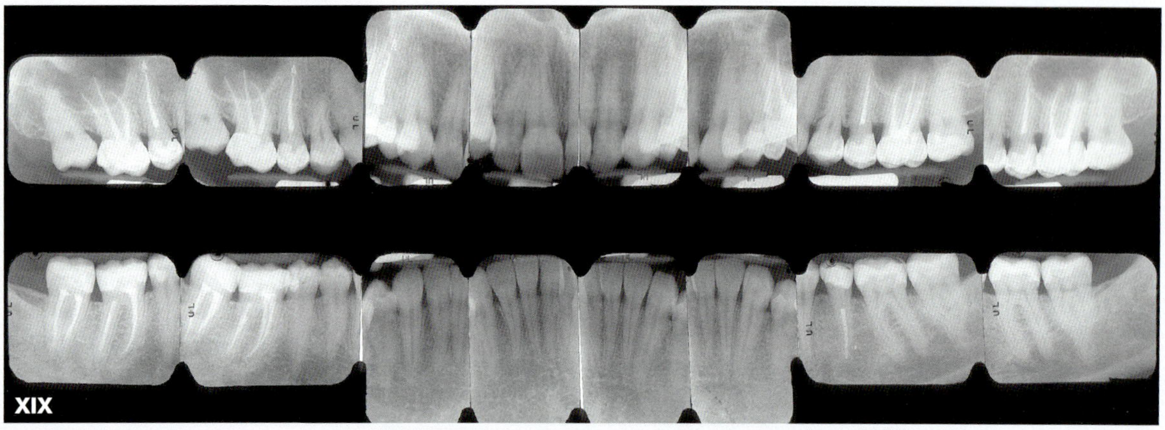

Fig 114 *(continued)*

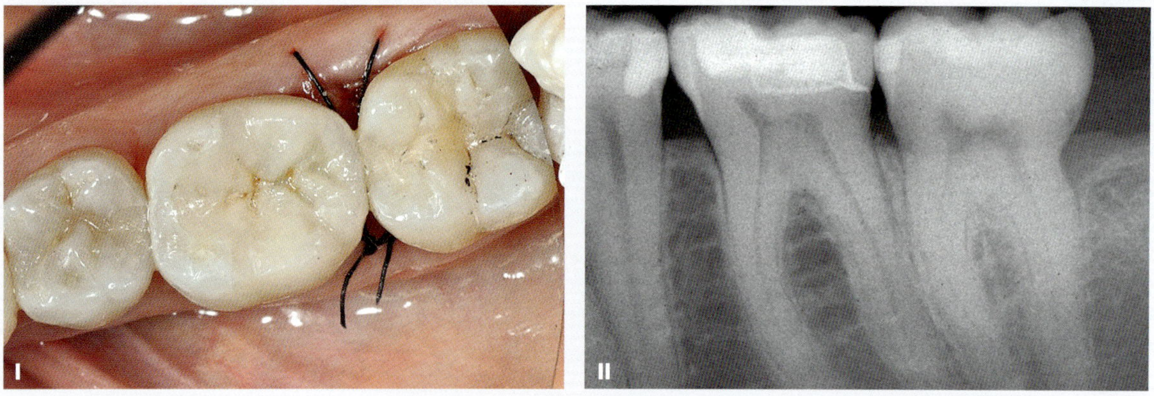

Fig 115 Important post-cementation radiographic checkup, showing correct marginal seal and emergence profile.

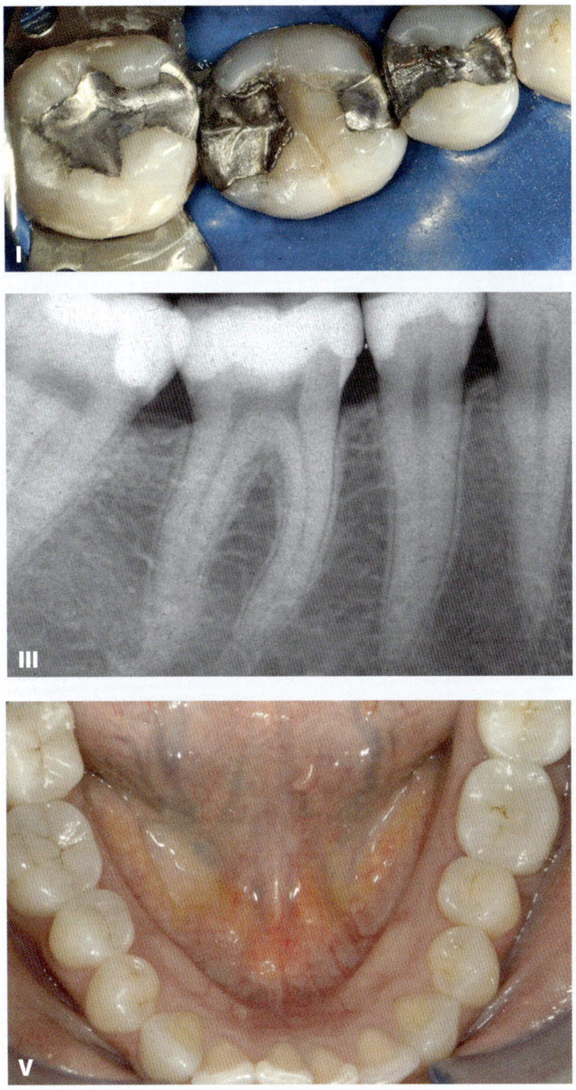

Fig 116 Control radiographs immediately after indirect restoration treatment *(I–IV)* and 7-year clinical follow-up *(V)*.

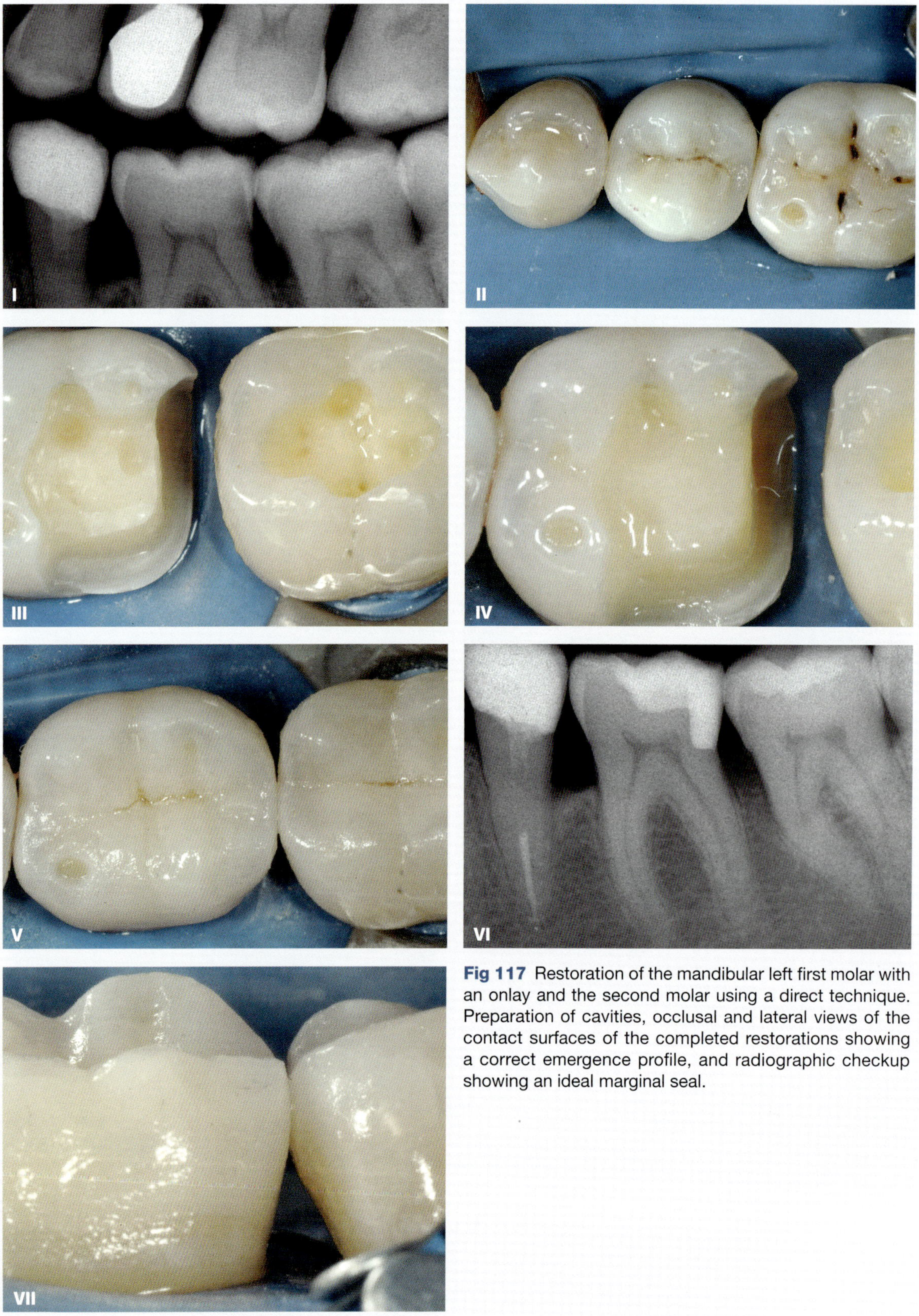

Fig 117 Restoration of the mandibular left first molar with an onlay and the second molar using a direct technique. Preparation of cavities, occlusal and lateral views of the contact surfaces of the completed restorations showing a correct emergence profile, and radiographic checkup showing an ideal marginal seal.

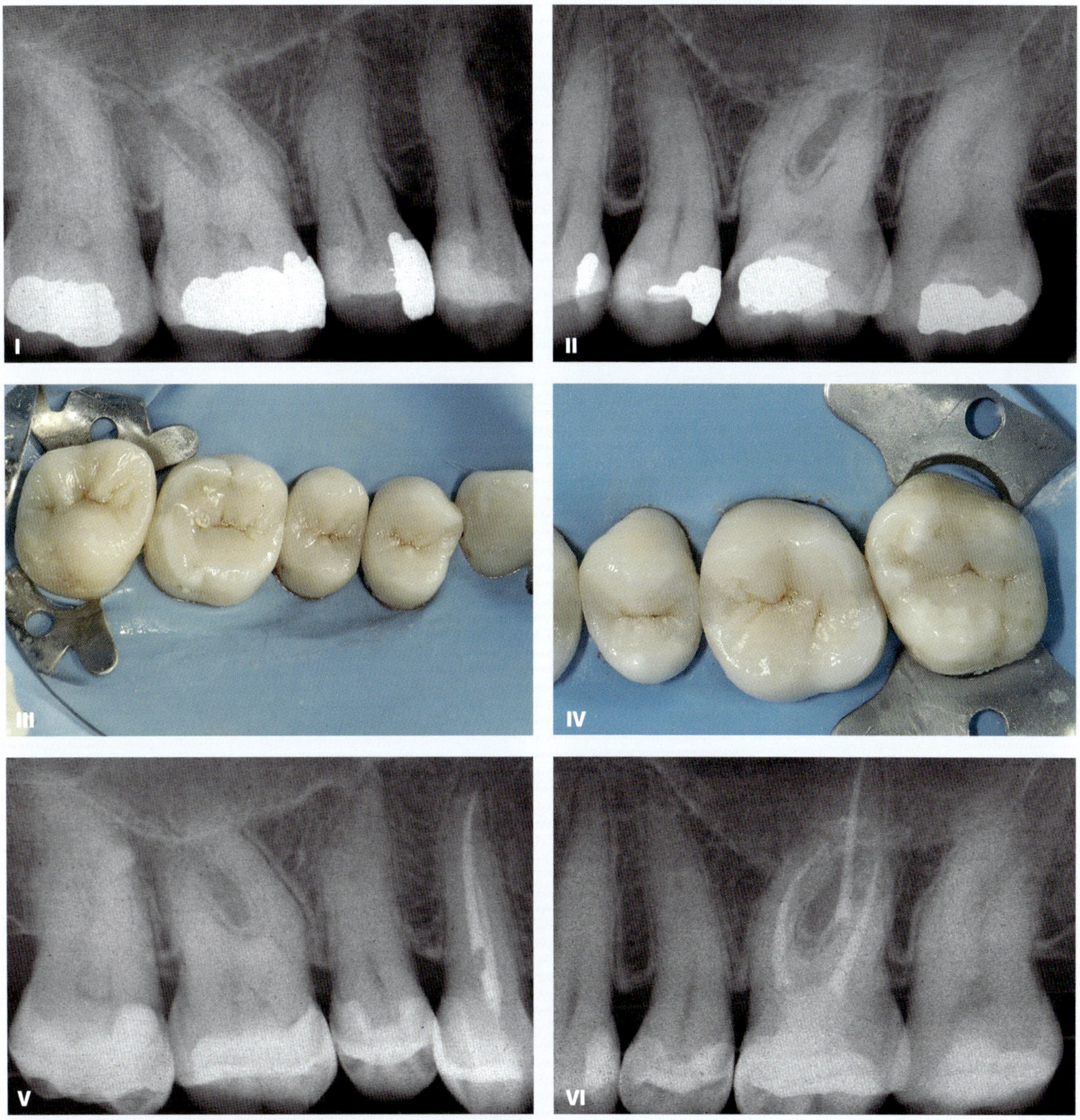

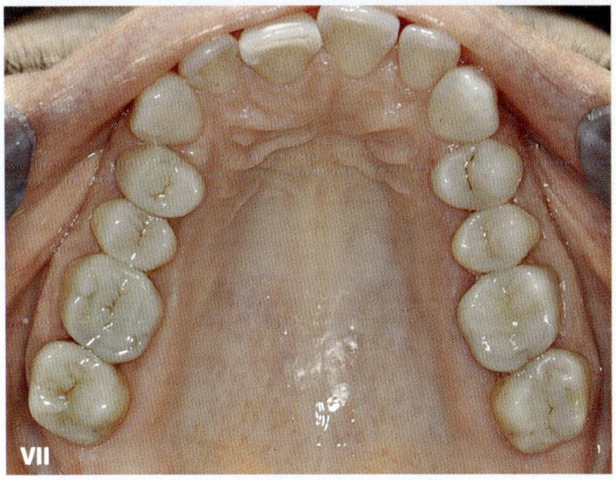

Fig 118 Maxillary direct and indirect restorations *(I–IV)* and 2-year follow-up *(V–VII)*.

Respecting dental structure

When carrying out a treatment plan, clinicians are often faced with a dilemma that the author has referred to as "the big misunderstanding."

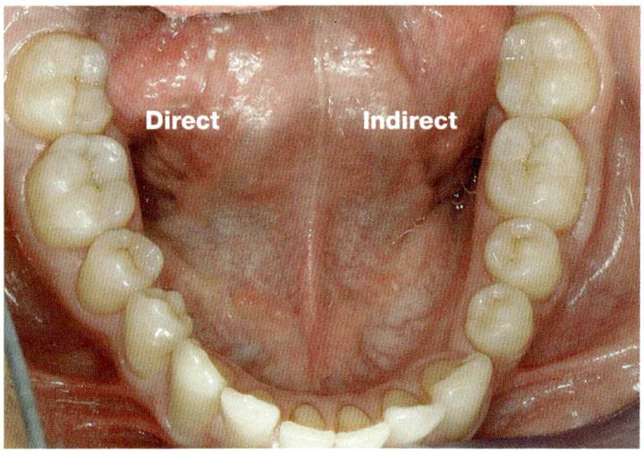

Fig 119 Direct restorations in the right mandible and indirect restorations in the left mandible.

When faced with a defective restoration that needs to be replaced, clinicians often wonder whether to perform a direct or indirect restoration. The misunderstanding lies in the fact that there are very specific guidelines for resolving this dilemma because there are indications for direct restorations and indications for indirect restorations (Fig 119).

An indirect or partial-coverage restoration is simply an alternative to a prosthetic crown or a restoration offering full coverage. Naturally one of the most important indications for the use of composite is restoration of the anterior teeth (Figs 120 to 127).

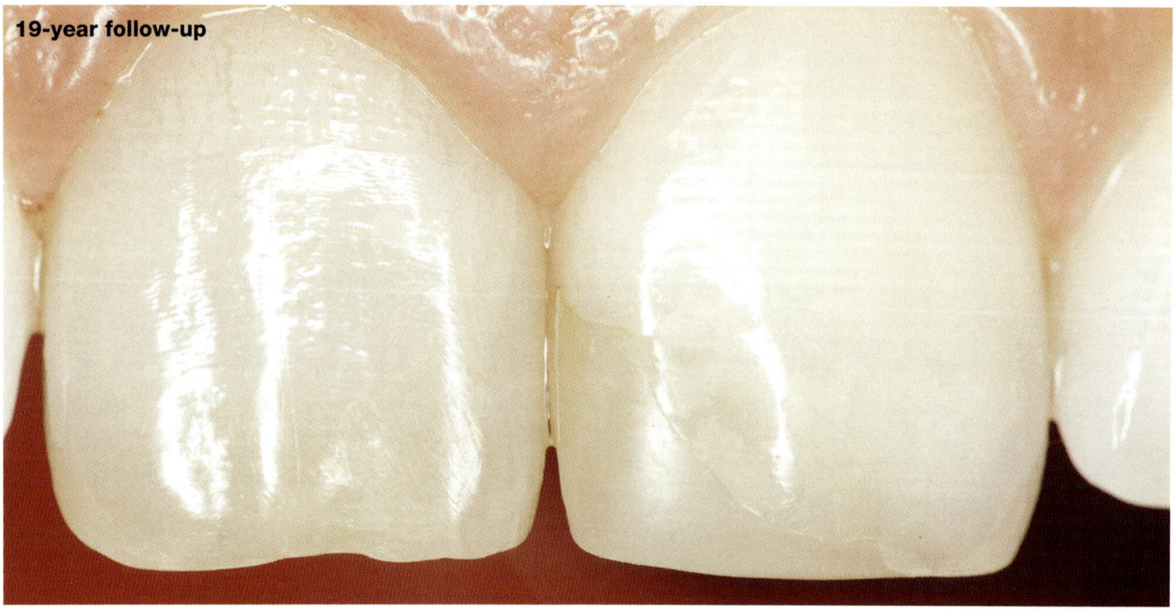

Fig 120 Direct composite restorations for the anterior teeth

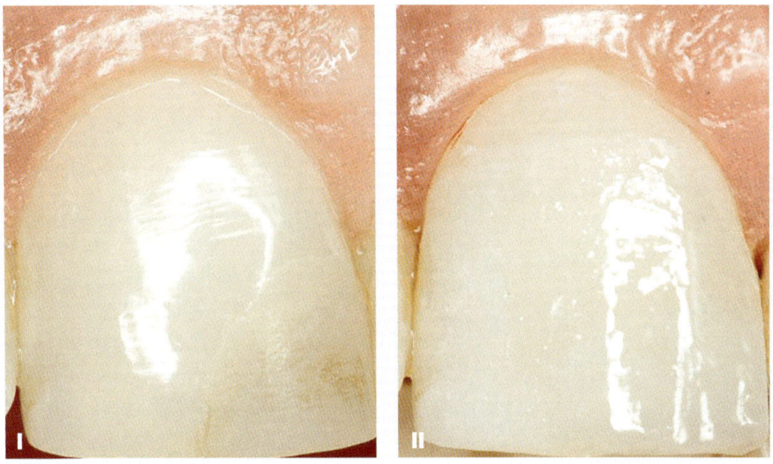

Fig 121 Direct composite restorations for the anterior teeth.

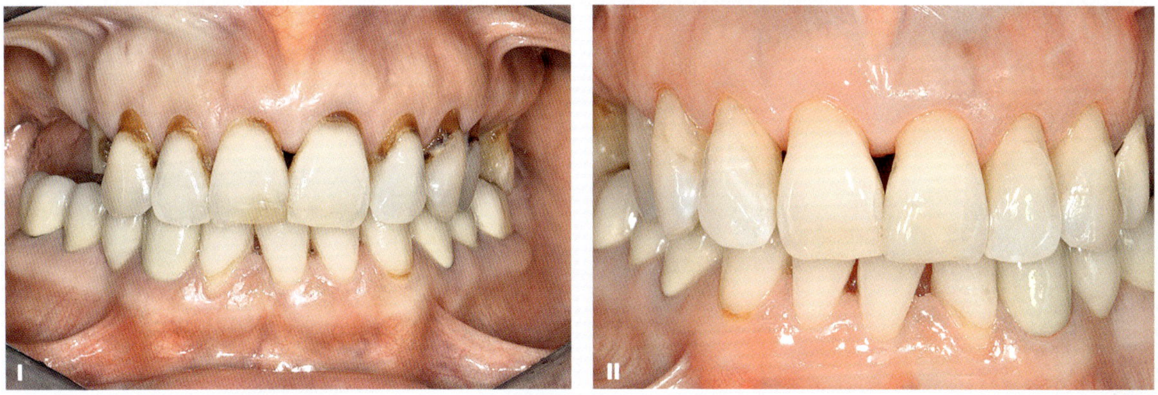

Fig 122 Direct composite restorations for the anterior teeth.

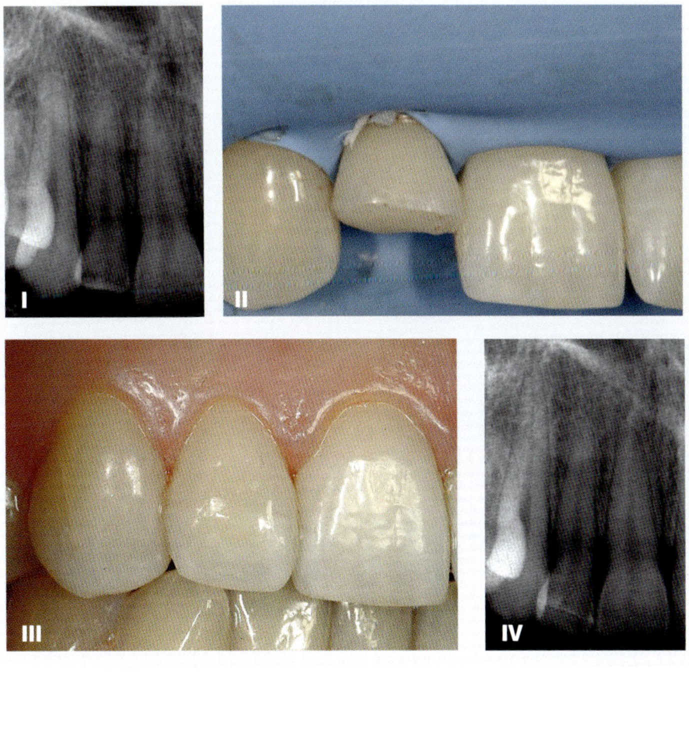

Fig 123 Direct composite restorations for the anterior teeth.

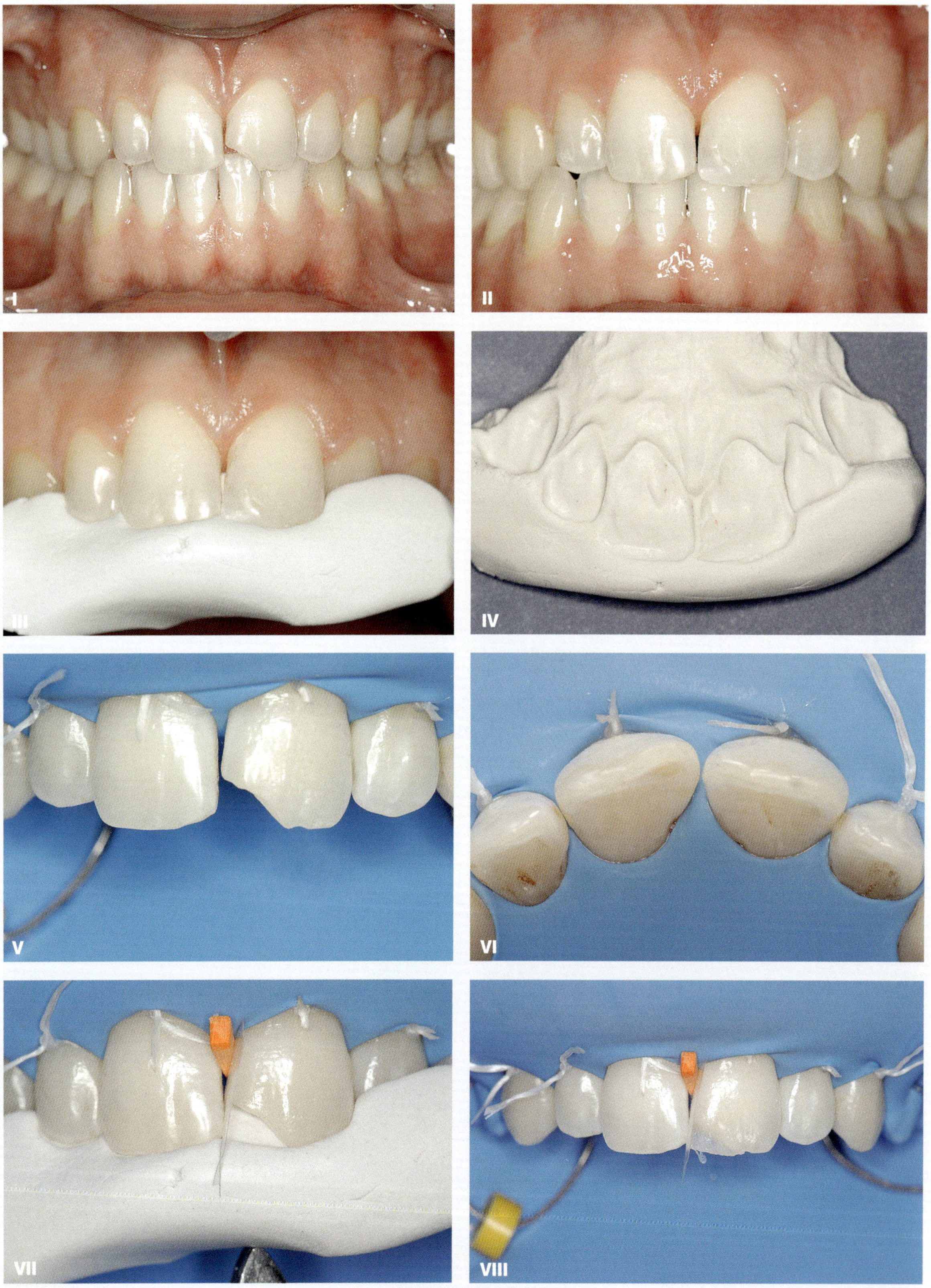

Fig 124 Direct composite restorations for the anterior teeth. (Courtesy of Dr Lavinia Landi.)

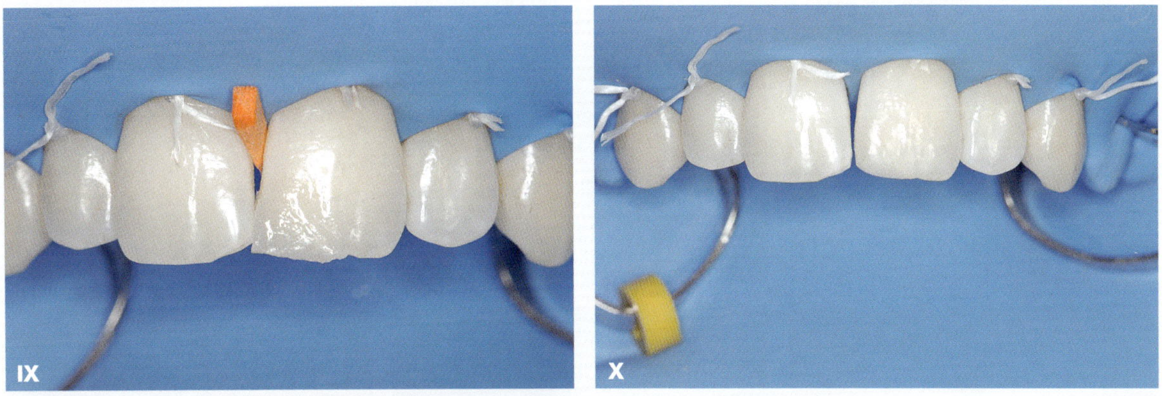

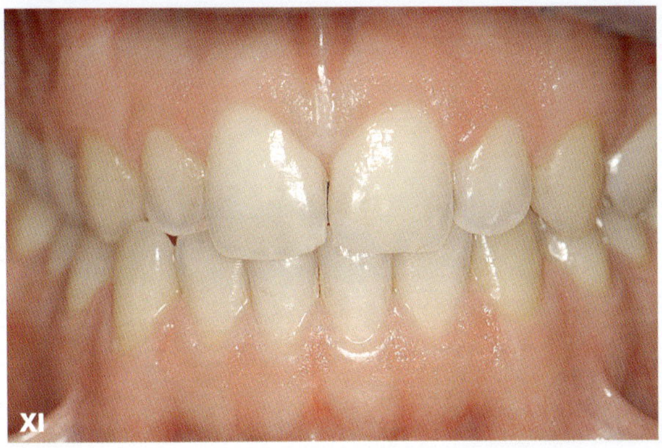

Fig 124 *(continued)*

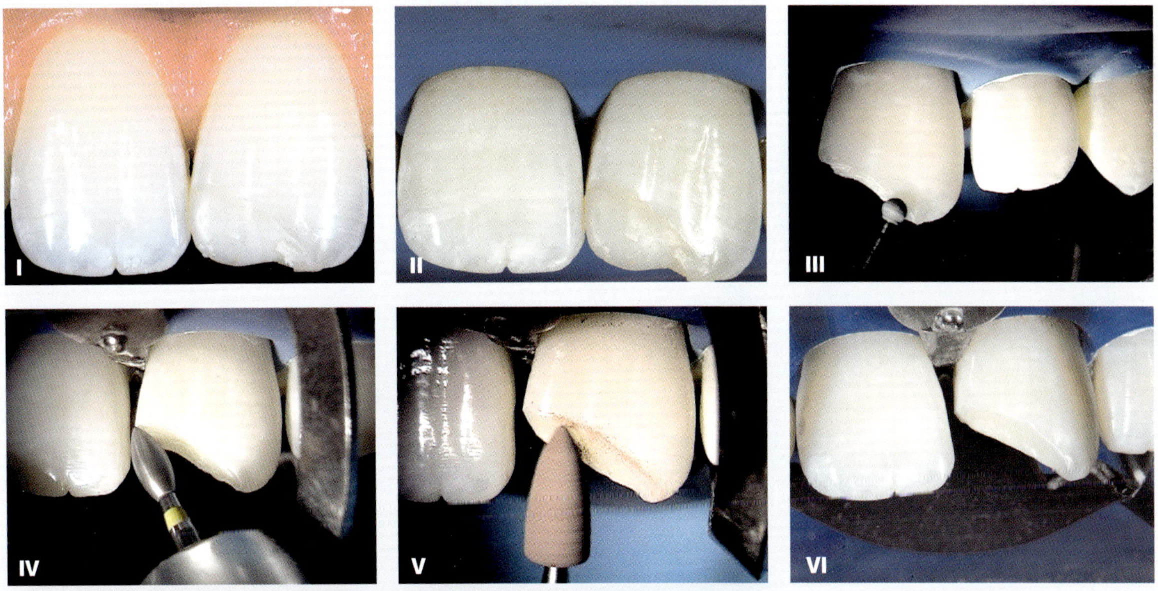

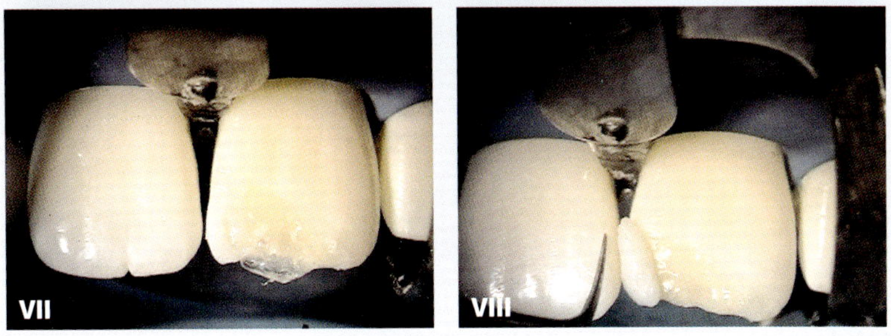

Fig 125 Direct composite restorations for the anterior teeth. (Courtesy of Dr Enzo Lamorgese.)

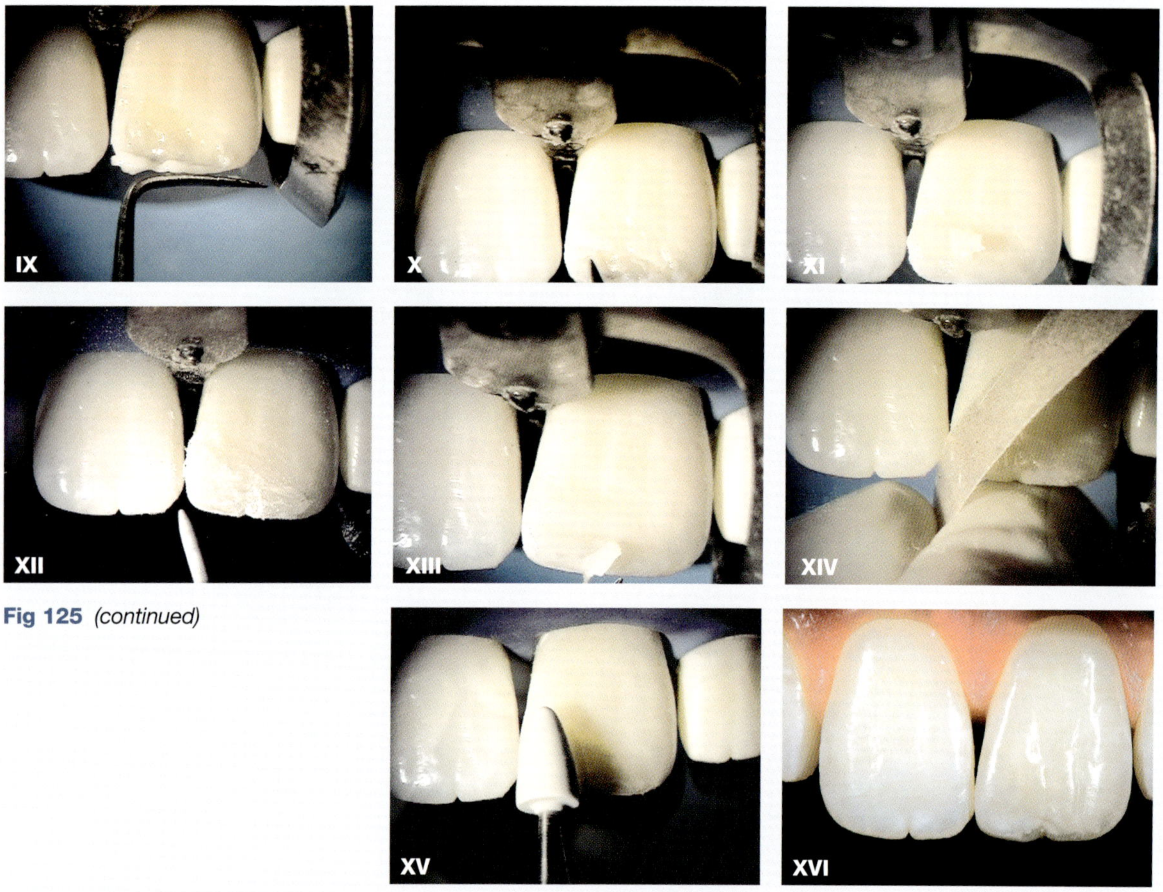

Fig 125 *(continued)*

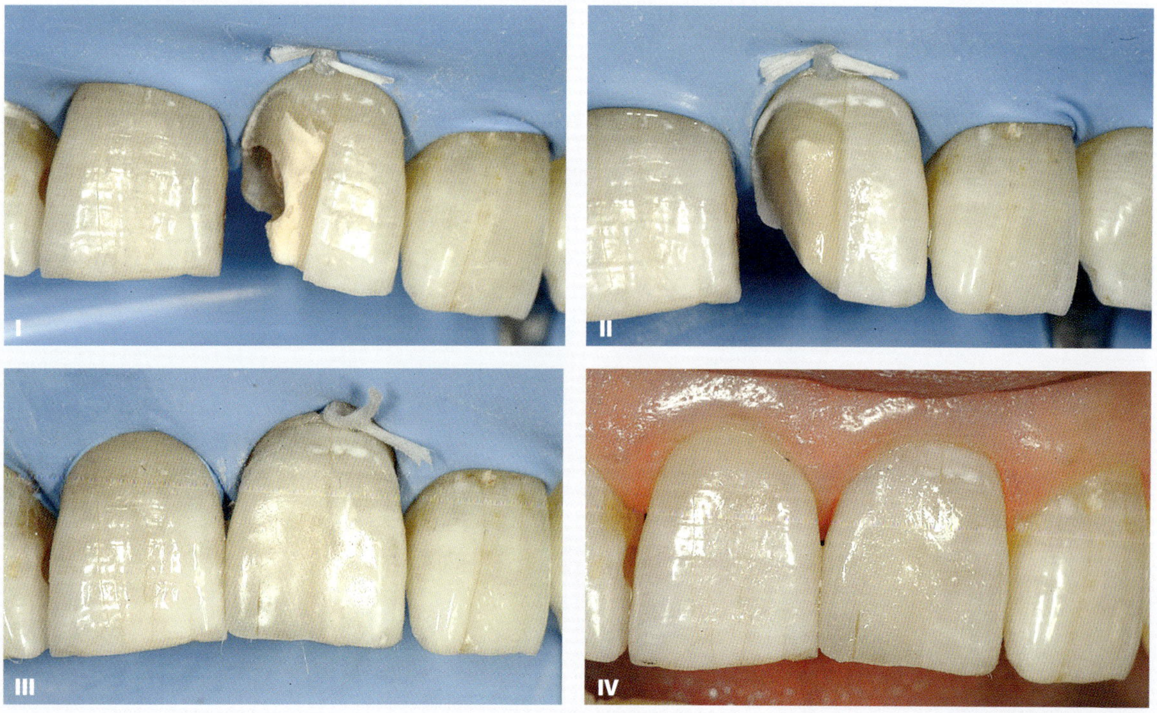

Fig 126 Indirect composite restoration of the maxillary left central incisor.

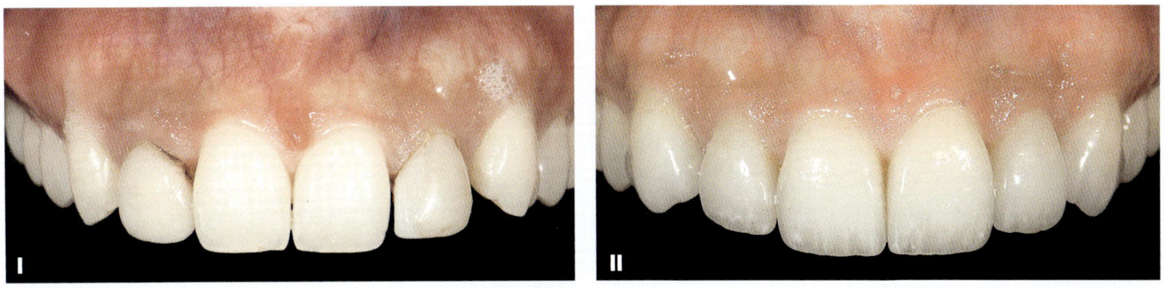

Fig 127 Indirect ceramic restorations of the maxillary anterior teeth. (Courtesy of Dr Marco Nicastro.)

Returning to the posterior teeth, direct techniques are indicated for sealing and for small- and medium-sized Class 1 and 2 cavities (Figs 128 to 144).
Indirect techniques are indicated for the restoration of large cavities, particularly if one or more cusps are missing, and for medium-sized and multiple cavities in the same quadrant (Figs 145 to 158).
The confusion arises when indications are on the borderline between direct and indirect restorations. Aside from anything else, the literature shows that indirect techniques have less risk of infiltration with a better seal of the tooth-restoration interface.[30,31]

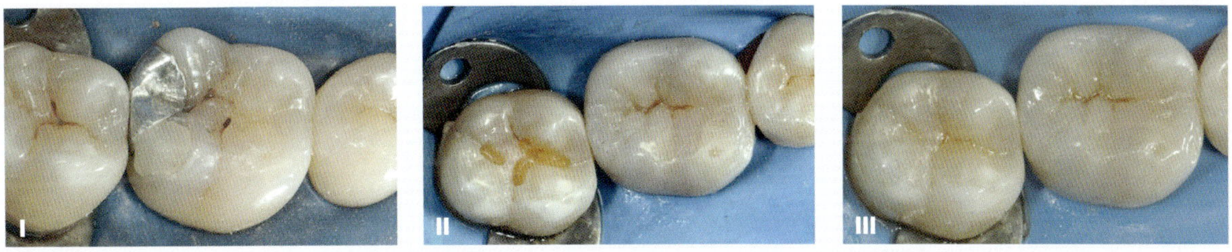

Fig 128 Indication for direct restoration of the mandibular right second molar and indirect restoration of the first molar.

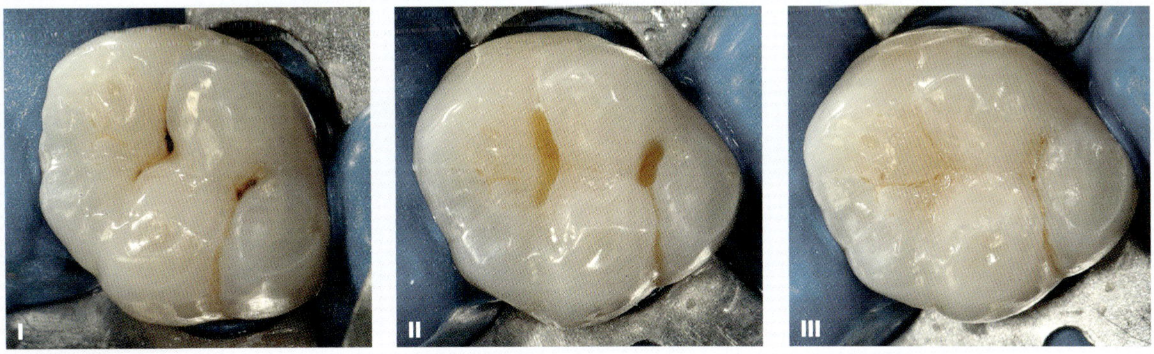

Fig 129 Indication for a very small Class 1 cavity: sealing.

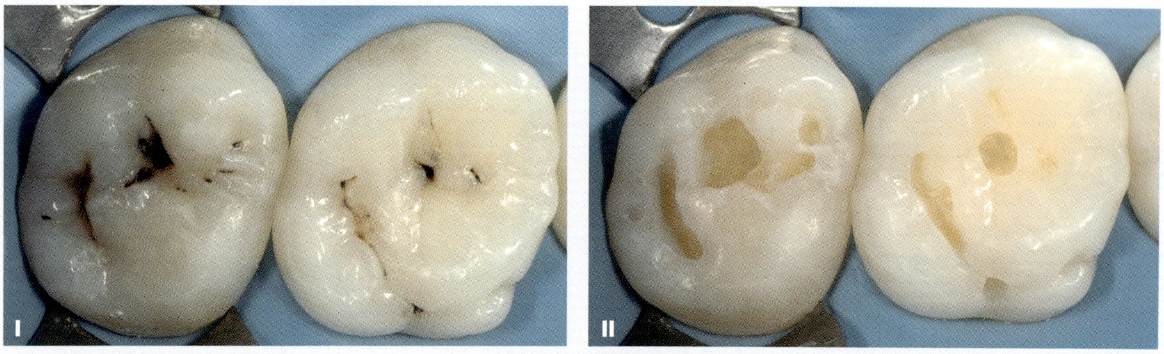

Fig 130 Application of two Class 1 direct restorations: the photographs clearly show the caries lesions *(I)*, complete cleaning of the cavities *(II)*, and anatomically perfect fillings in composite *(III)*. (Courtesy of Dr Paolo Ferrari.)

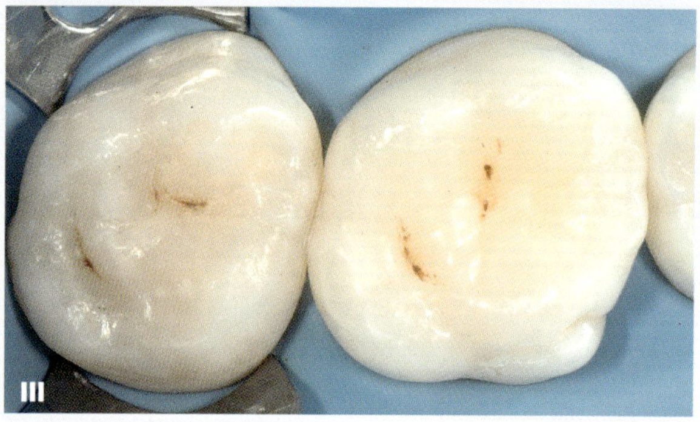

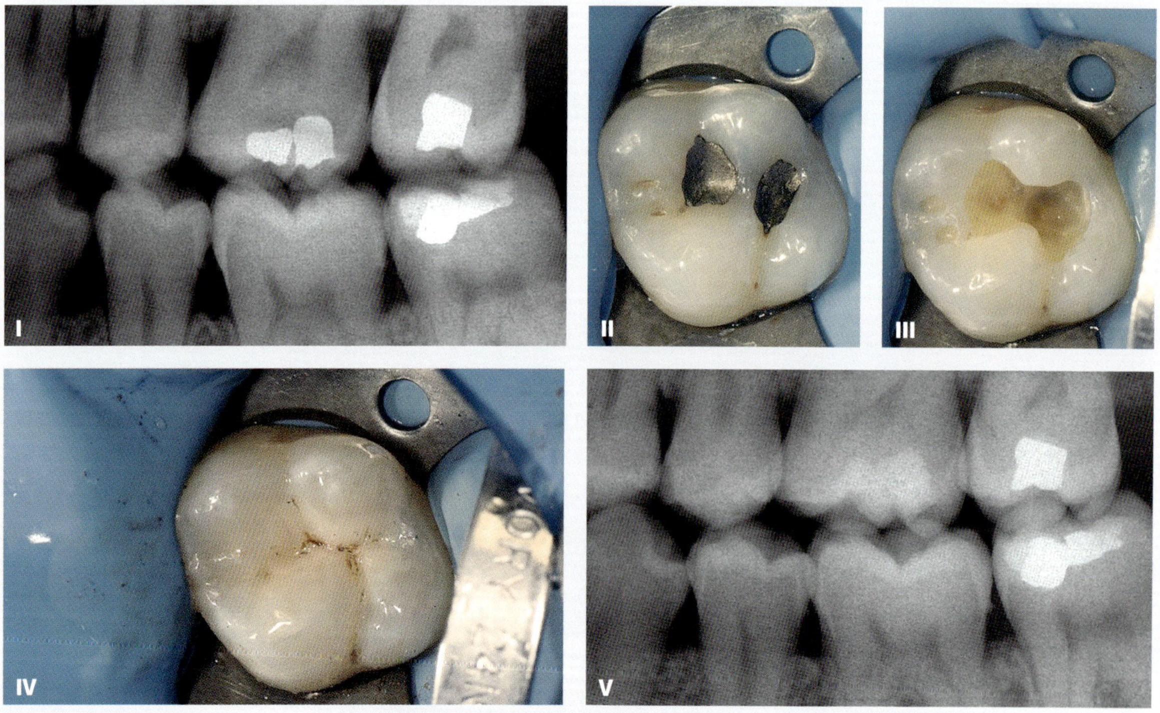

Fig 131 This clinical case also shows ideal anatomical modeling of the composite for a Class 1 restoration. (Courtesy of Dr Paolo Ferrari.)

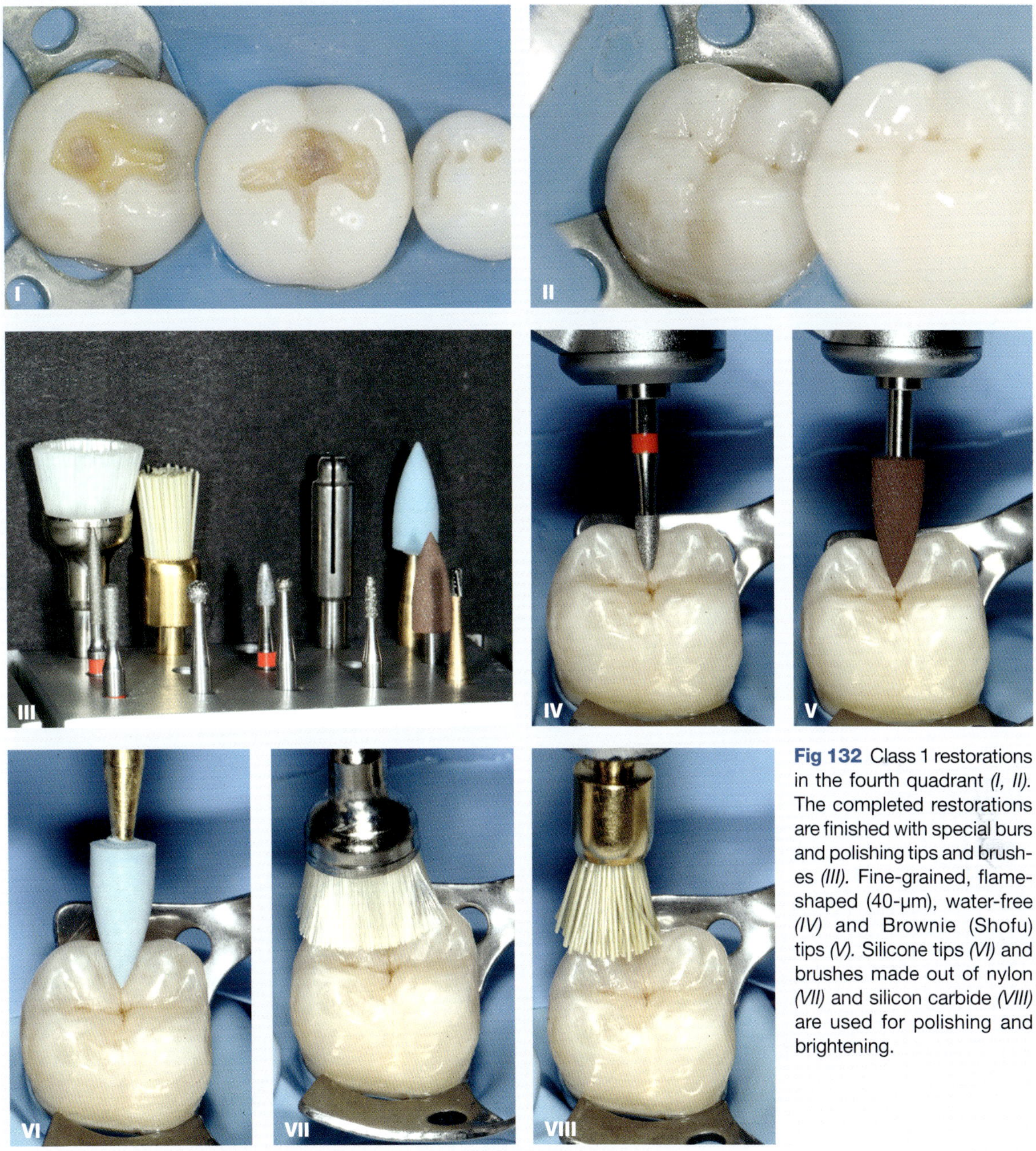

Fig 132 Class 1 restorations in the fourth quadrant *(I, II)*. The completed restorations are finished with special burs and polishing tips and brushes *(III)*. Fine-grained, flame-shaped (40-µm), water-free *(IV)* and Brownie (Shofu) tips *(V)*. Silicone tips *(VI)* and brushes made out of nylon *(VII)* and silicon carbide *(VIII)* are used for polishing and brightening.

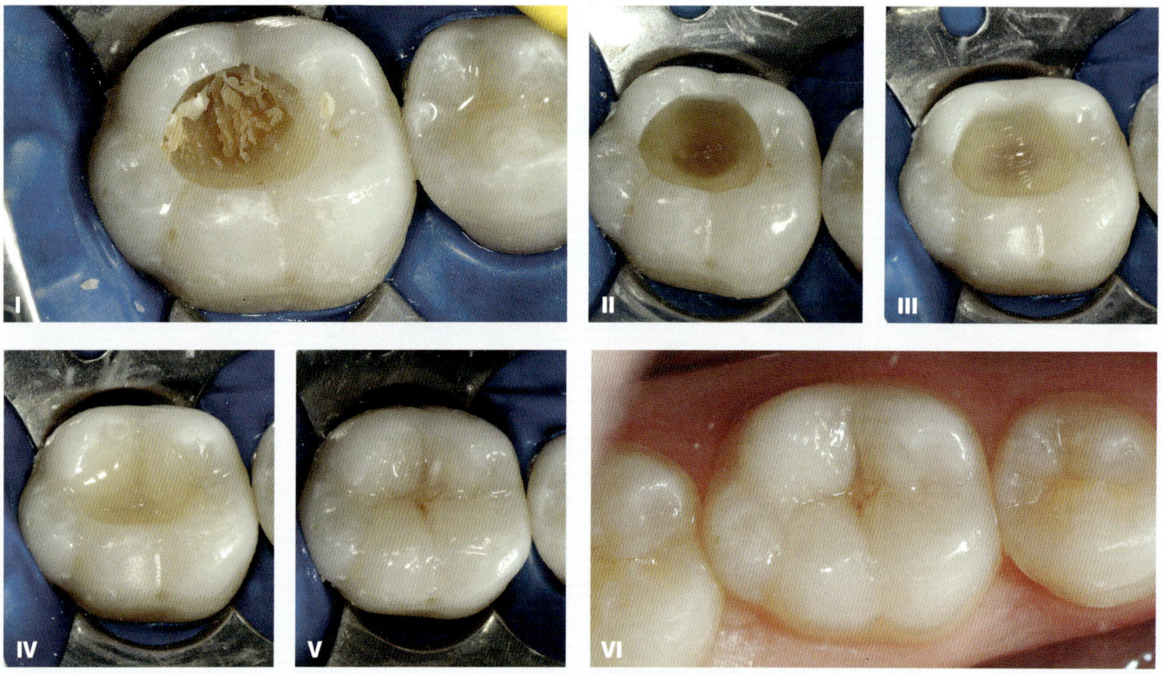

Fig 133 Removal of very deep decayed tissue *(I)*, cavity ready for the restoration *(II)*, application of a fine layer of flowable composite *(III)*, stratification of composite *(IV)*, and completed anatomical modeling *(V, VI)*.

Fig 134 Pain on chewing led to the replacement of a metal restoration with a composite restoration created using a direct technique. The painful symptoms disappeared after a few days.

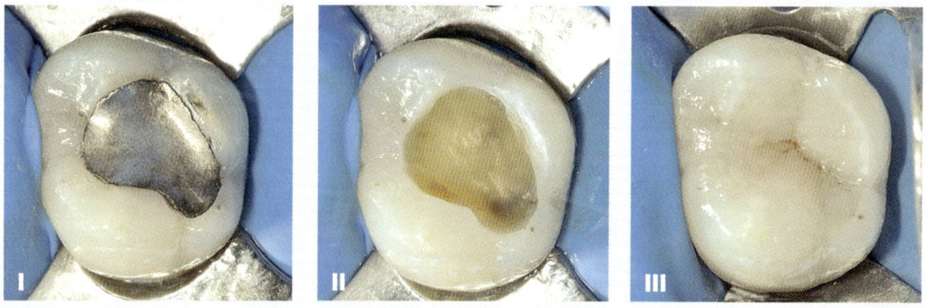

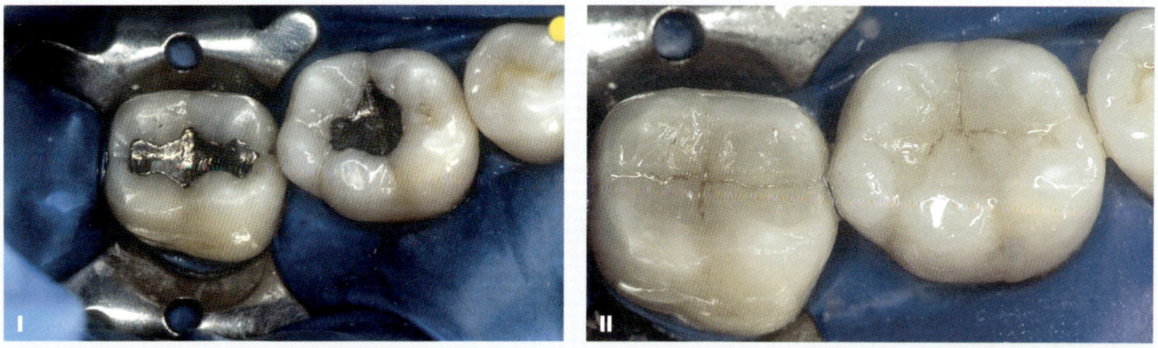

Fig 135 Clinical view showing replacement of metal restorations with composite restorations in Class 1 situations: the cosmetic aspect plays an entirely secondary role because the true indication for the replacement is determined by the difference between the elastic moduli of both materials.

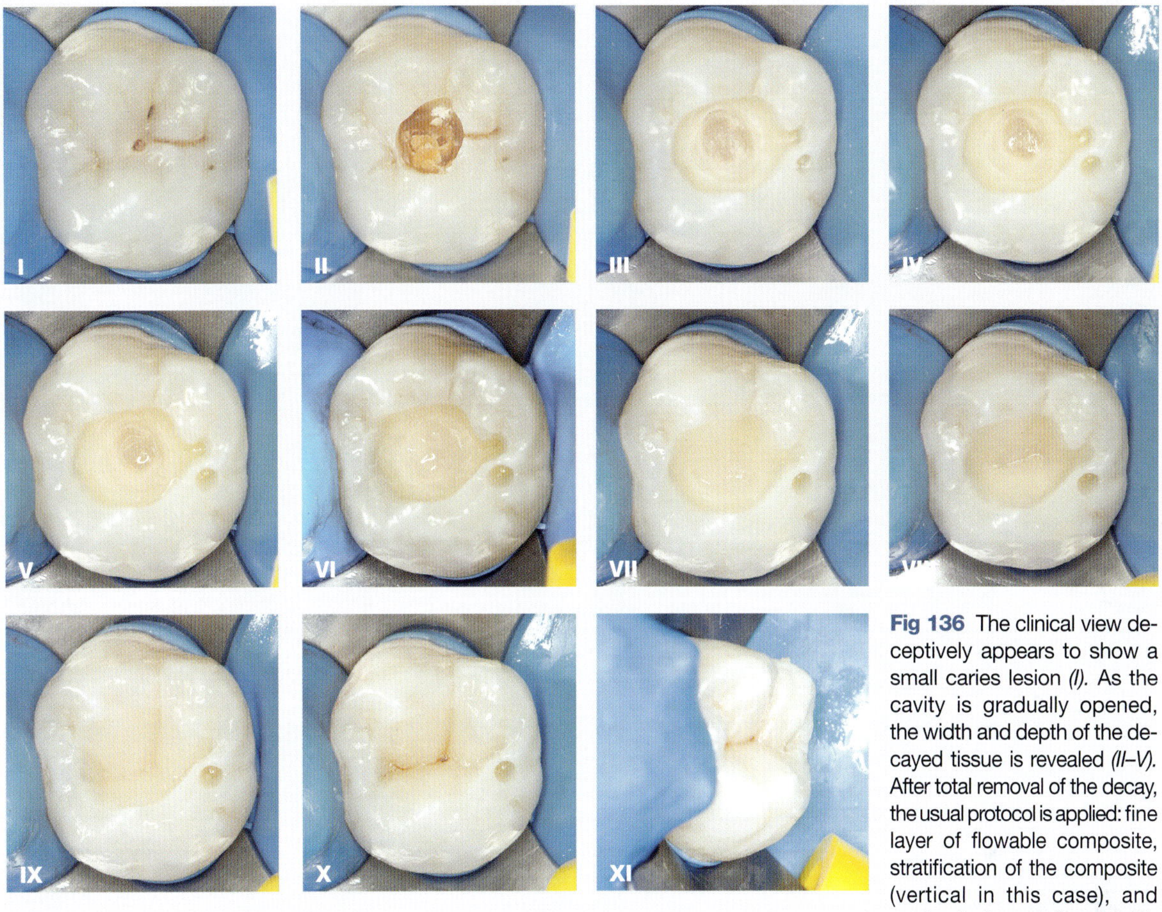

Fig 136 The clinical view deceptively appears to show a small caries lesion *(I)*. As the cavity is gradually opened, the width and depth of the decayed tissue is revealed *(II–V)*. After total removal of the decay, the usual protocol is applied: fine layer of flowable composite, stratification of the composite (vertical in this case), and anatomical modeling *(VI–XI)*. (Courtesy of Dr Lavinia Landi.)

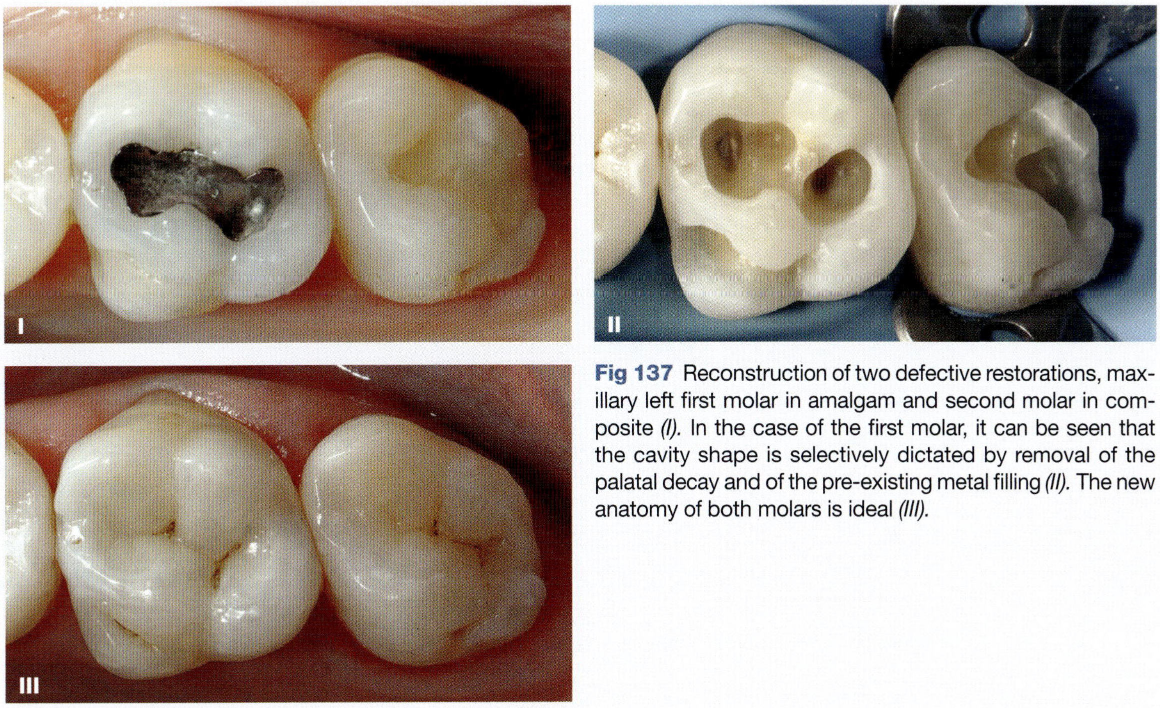

Fig 137 Reconstruction of two defective restorations, maxillary left first molar in amalgam and second molar in composite *(I)*. In the case of the first molar, it can be seen that the cavity shape is selectively dictated by removal of the palatal decay and of the pre-existing metal filling *(II)*. The new anatomy of both molars is ideal *(III)*.

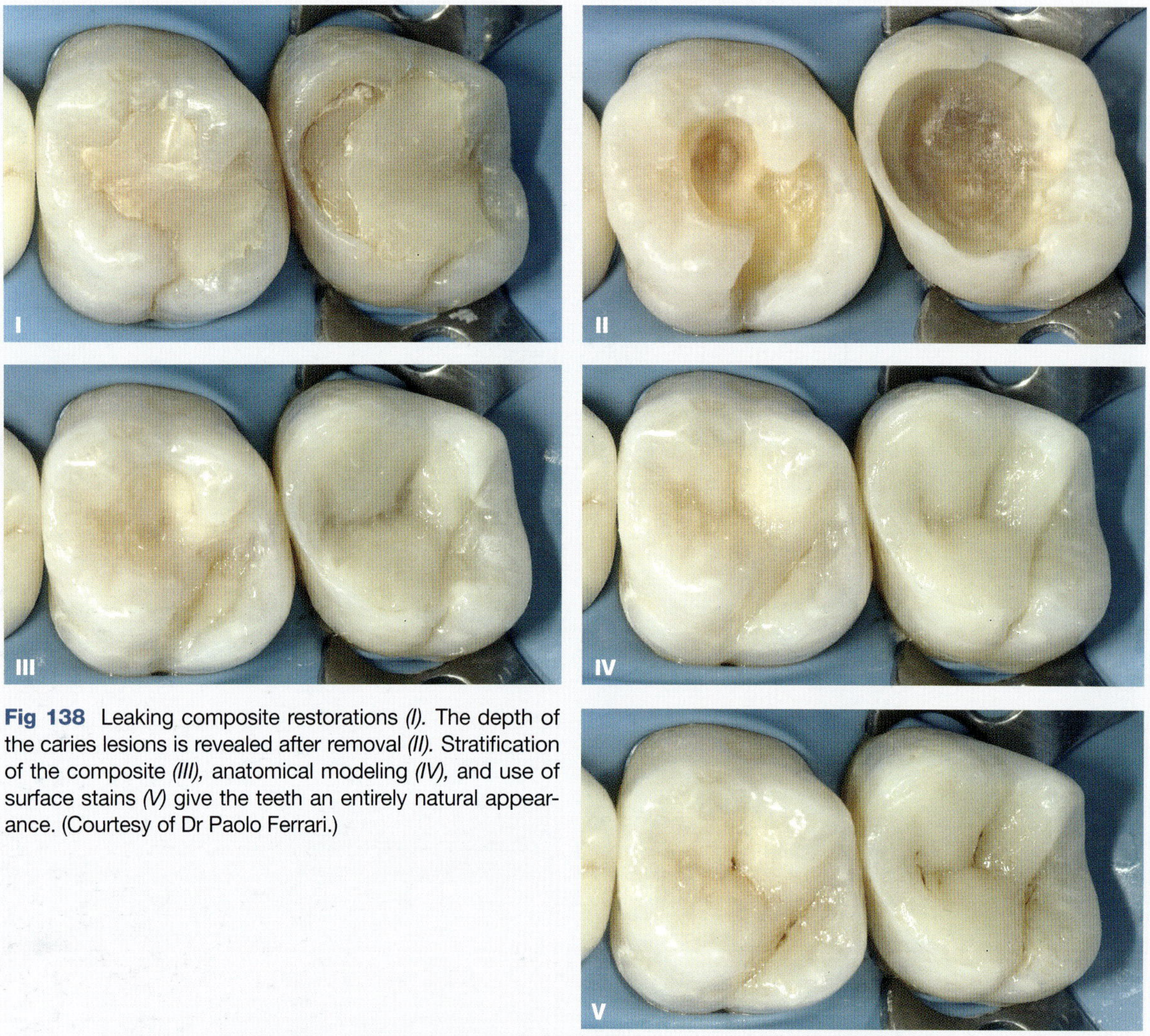

Fig 138 Leaking composite restorations *(I)*. The depth of the caries lesions is revealed after removal *(II)*. Stratification of the composite *(III)*, anatomical modeling *(IV)*, and use of surface stains *(V)* give the teeth an entirely natural appearance. (Courtesy of Dr Paolo Ferrari.)

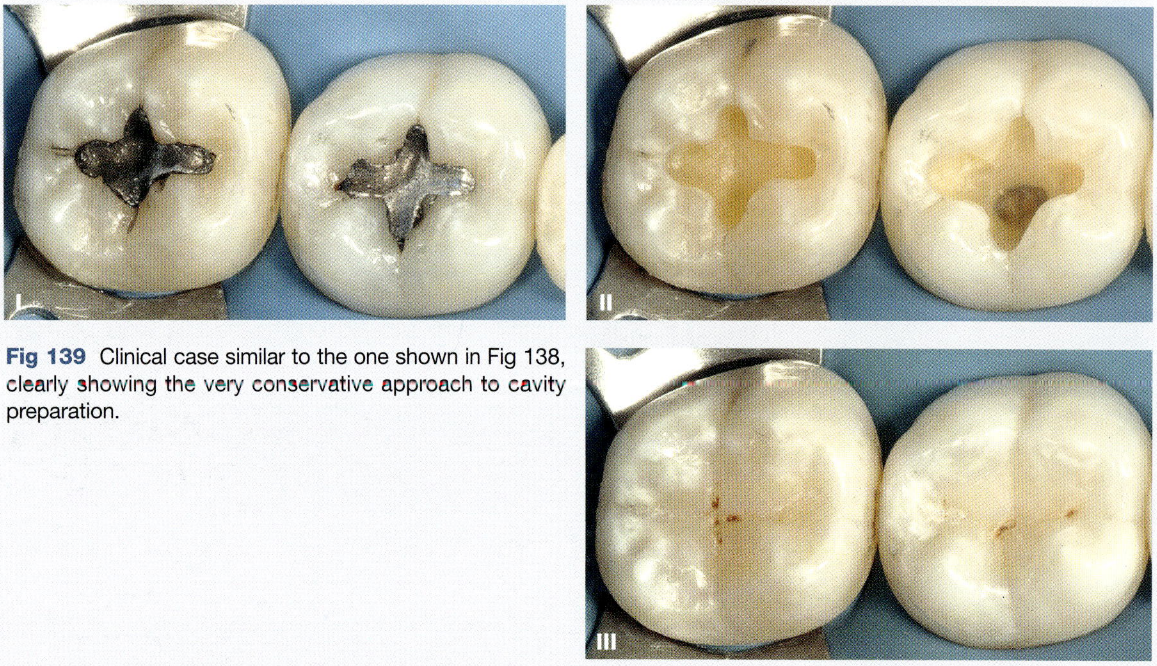

Fig 139 Clinical case similar to the one shown in Fig 138, clearly showing the very conservative approach to cavity preparation.

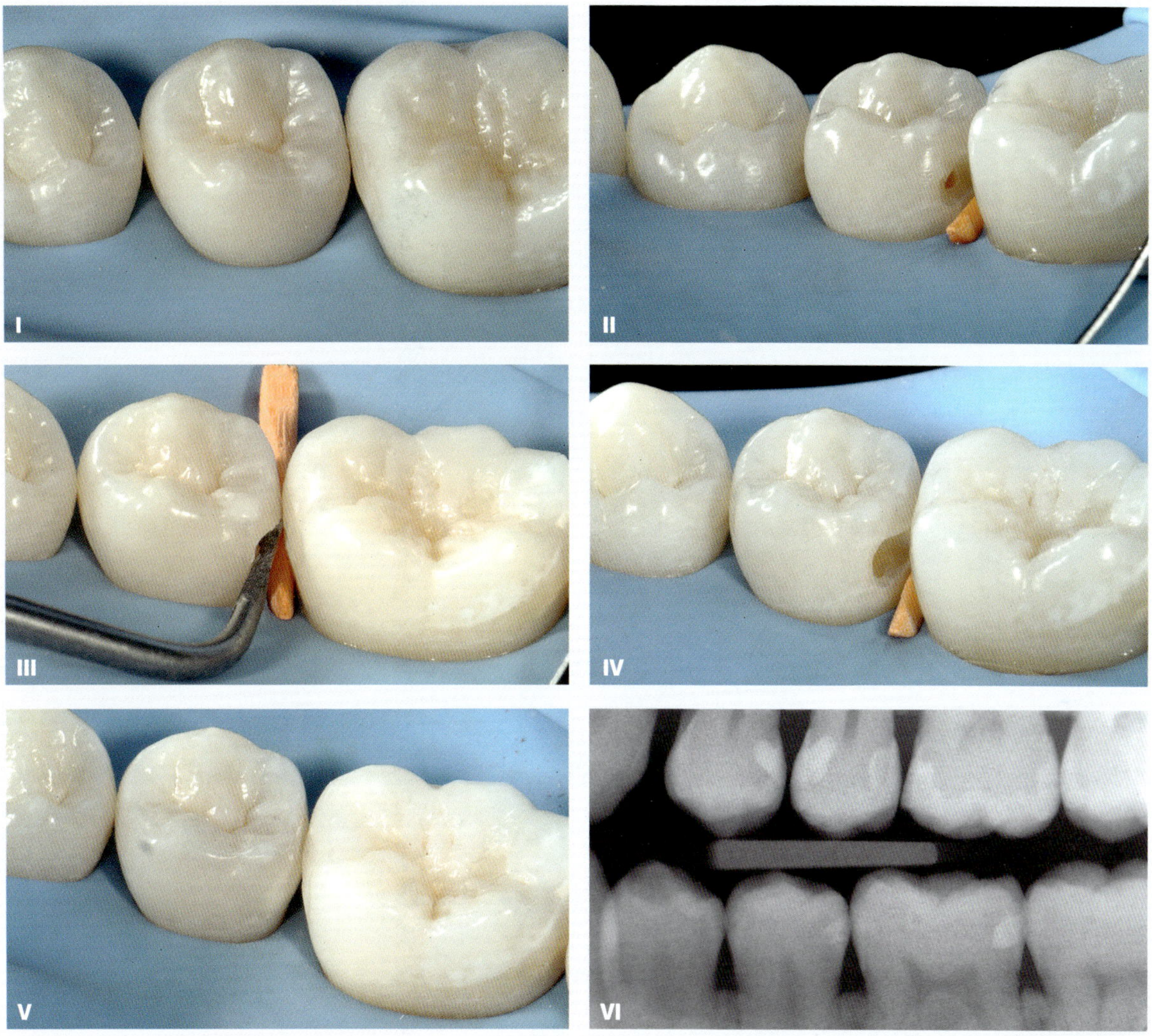

Fig 140 Distal caries lesion and creation of a tunnel cavity to maintain the marginal ridge intact. (Courtesy of Dr Paolo Ferrari.)

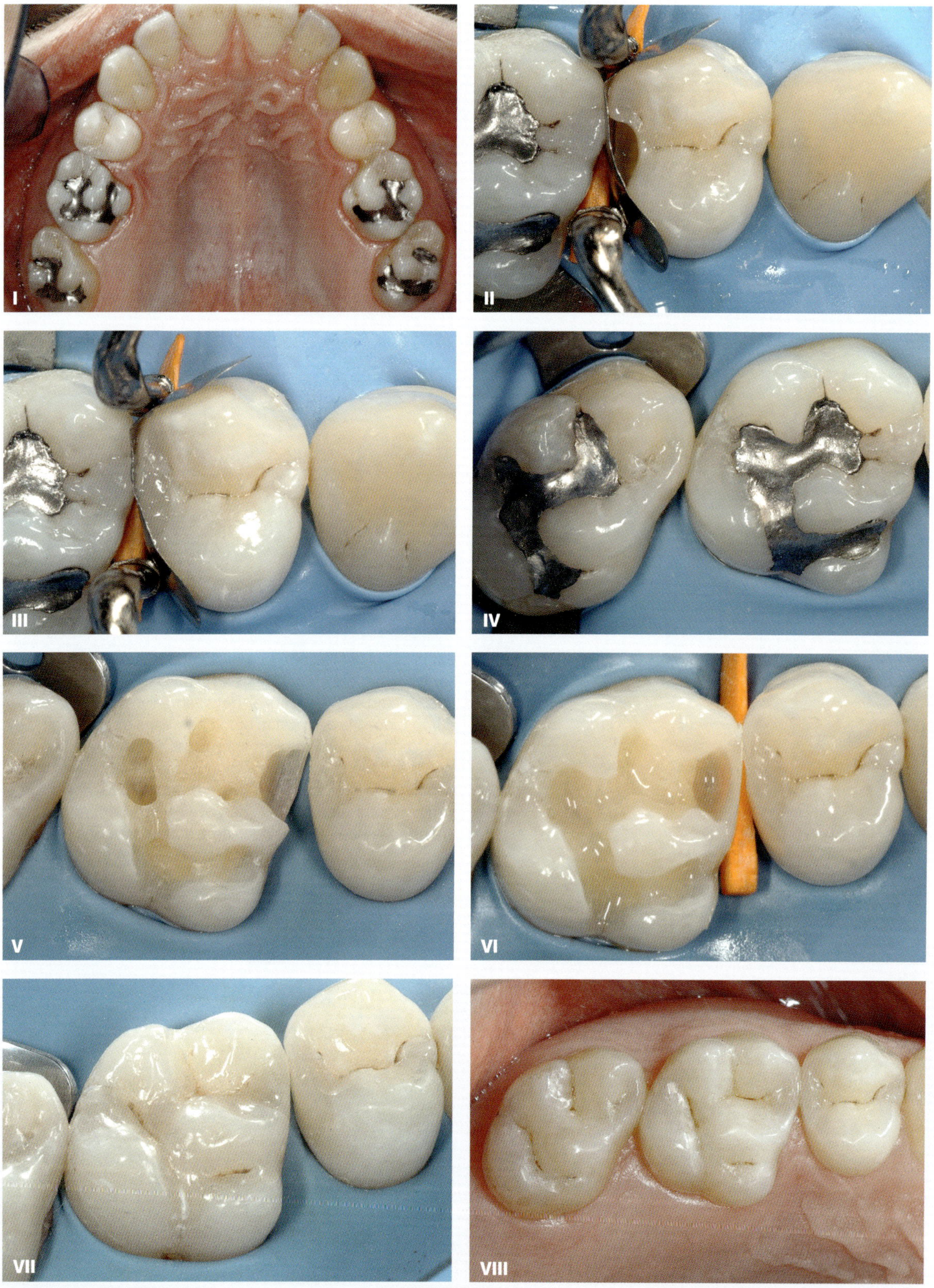

Fig 141 Clinical case involving rebuilding of defective restorations with new direct composite restorations *(I)*. In the right maxilla, positioning of sectional matrices and interdental wedge *(II)* was followed by complete removal of the decayed tissue *(III–V)*. Following the creation of the marginal ridge by means of a direct technique *(VI)*, the accuracy of the anatomical appearance is clearly evident *(VII, VIII)*. Same clinical approach for rebuilding of maxillary left molars using a direct technique *(IX–XIII)*. Occlusal view of the maxilla at the end of treatment *(XIV)* and follow-up bitewing radiographs *(XV, XVI)*. (Courtesy of Dr Paolo Ferrari.)

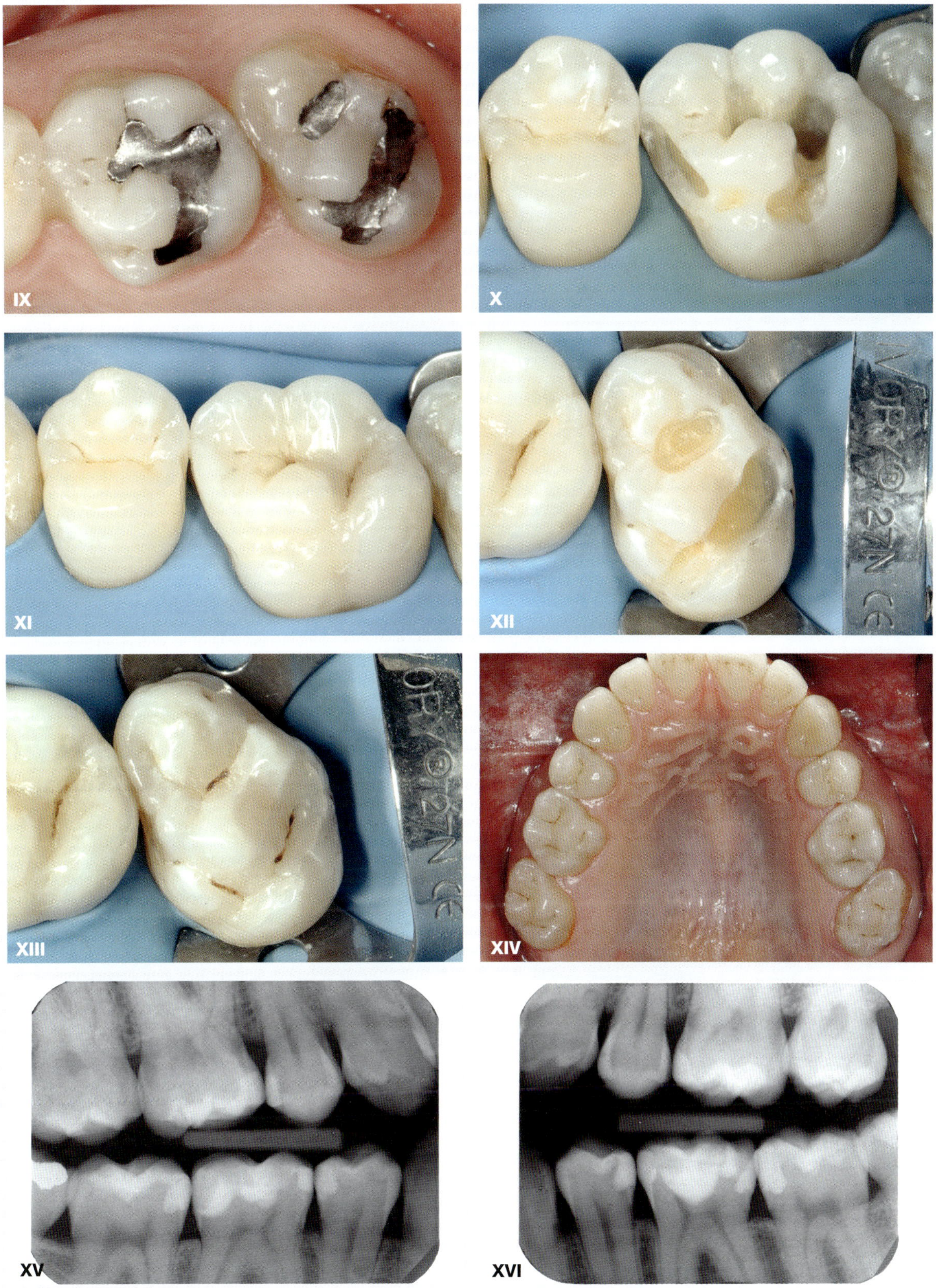

Fig 141 *(continued)*

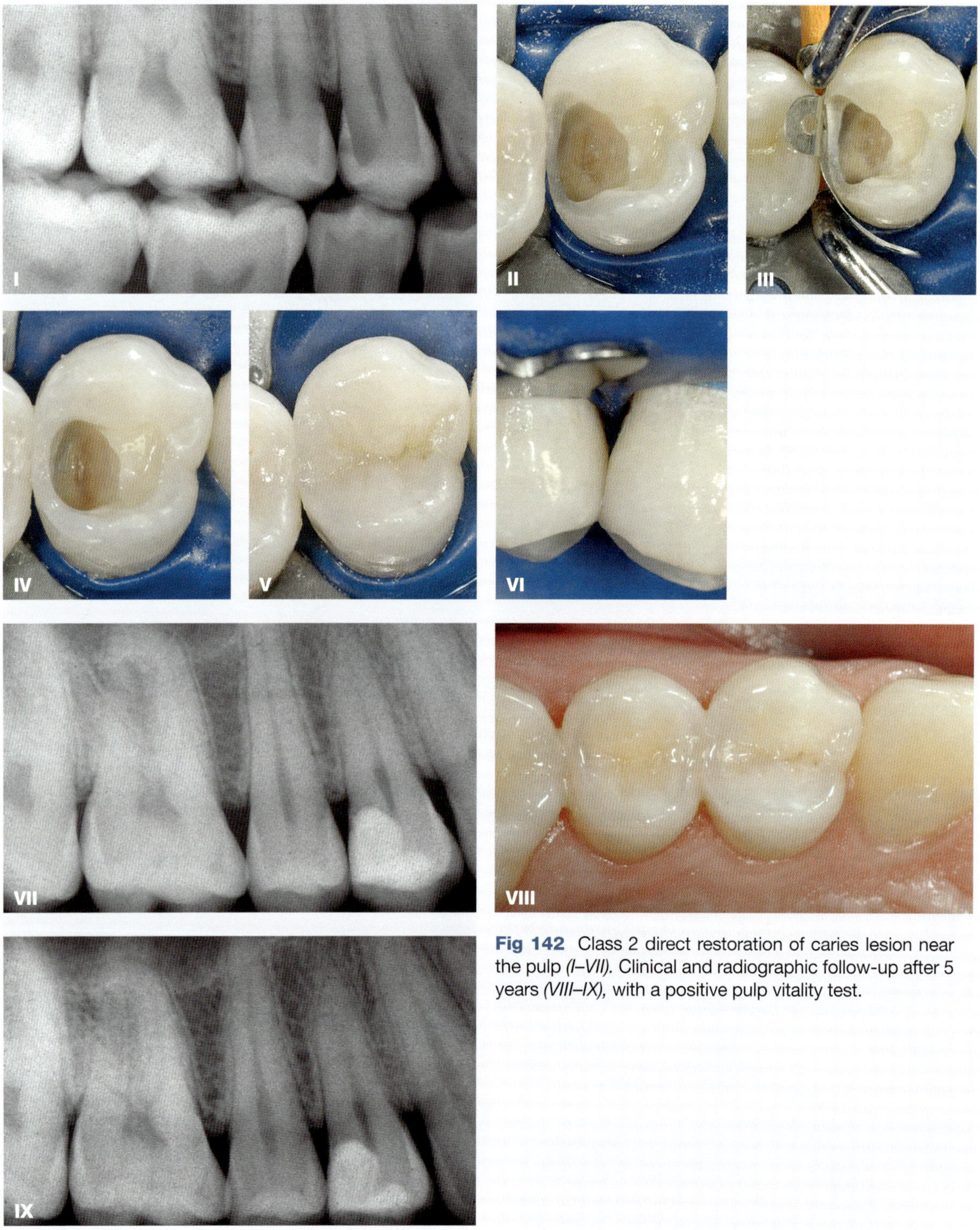

Fig 142 Class 2 direct restoration of caries lesion near the pulp *(I–VII)*. Clinical and radiographic follow-up after 5 years *(VIII–IX)*, with a positive pulp vitality test.

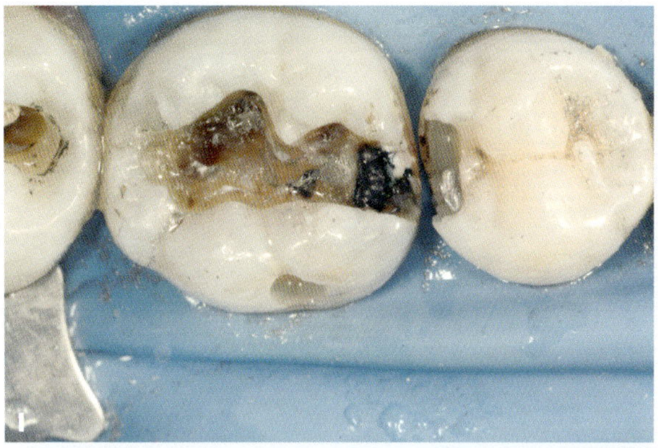

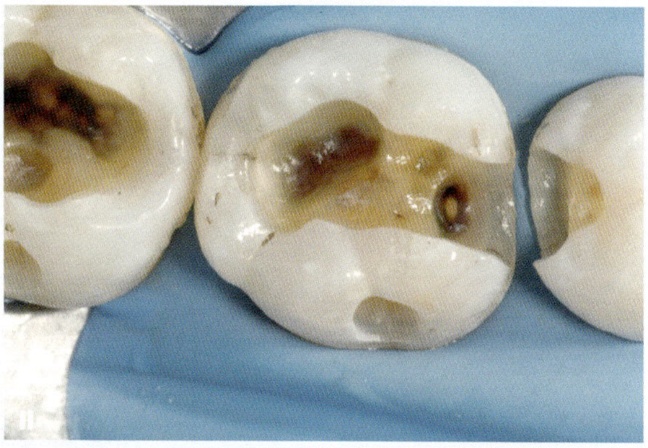

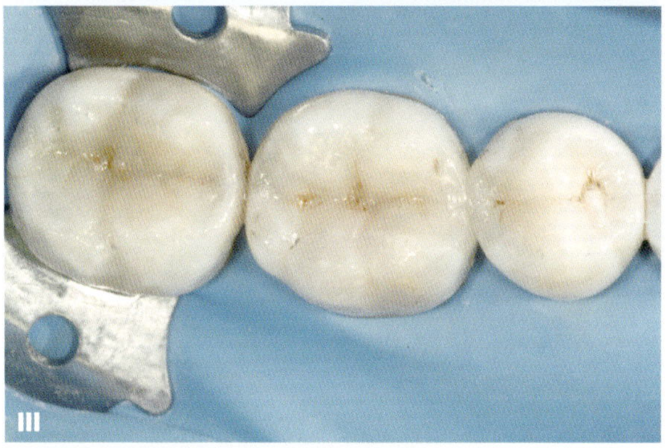

Fig 143 Clinical view of three mandibular right teeth with Class 1 and 2 cavities *(I)*. Note the depth of the cavity following removal of the decayed tissue in both molars *(II)*. The teeth have been restored using a direct technique *(III)*.

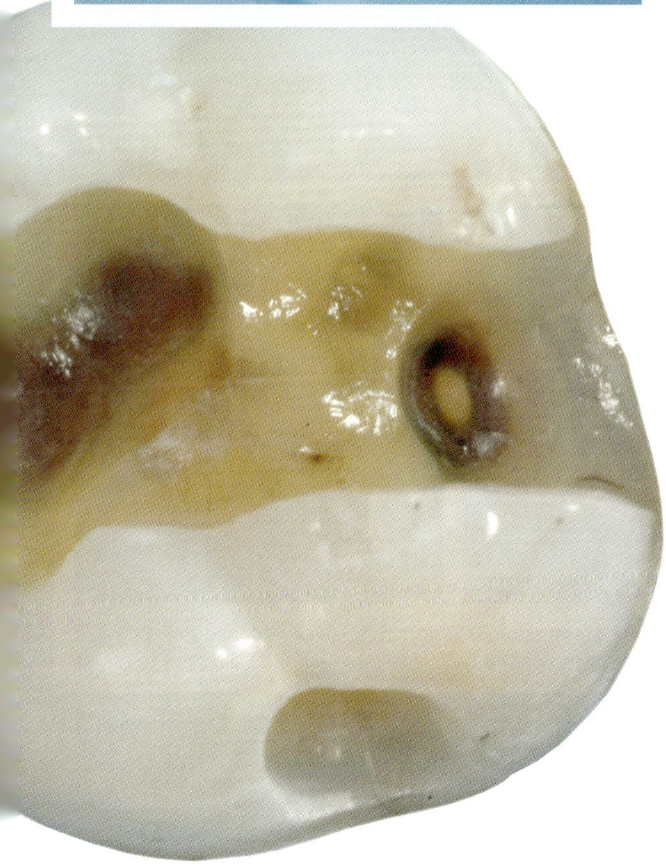

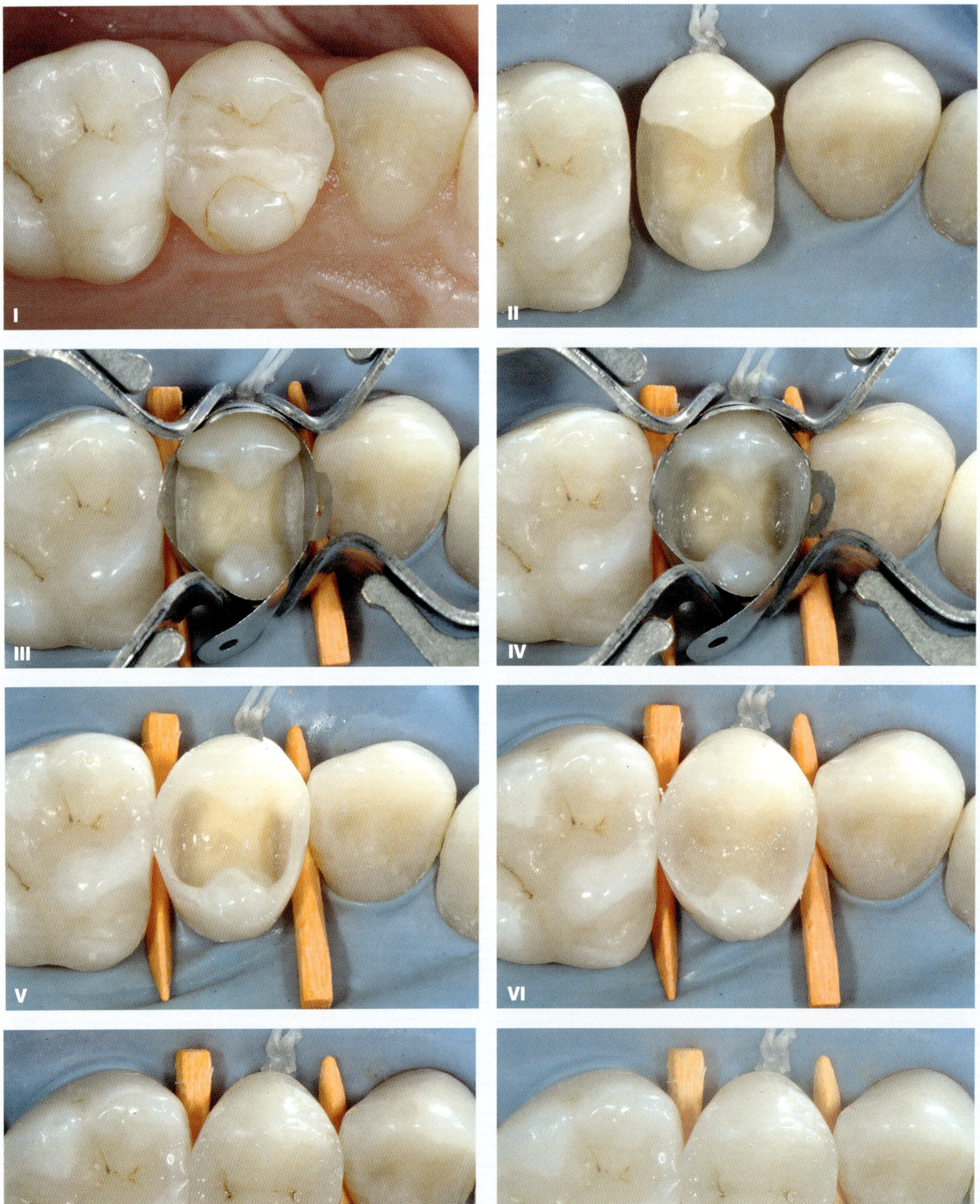

Fig 144 Following removal of a defective restoration *(I, II)*, the author believed that on balance the appearance of the healthy residual tooth structure indicated an indirect restoration. His friend and colleague Paolo Ferrari nevertheless tackled the problem by simultaneously positioning two sectional matrices and two interdental wedges to reconstruct the marginal ridges *(III–V)* and complete a direct restoration *(VI–X)*. Follow-up radiograph at the end of treatment *(XI)*.

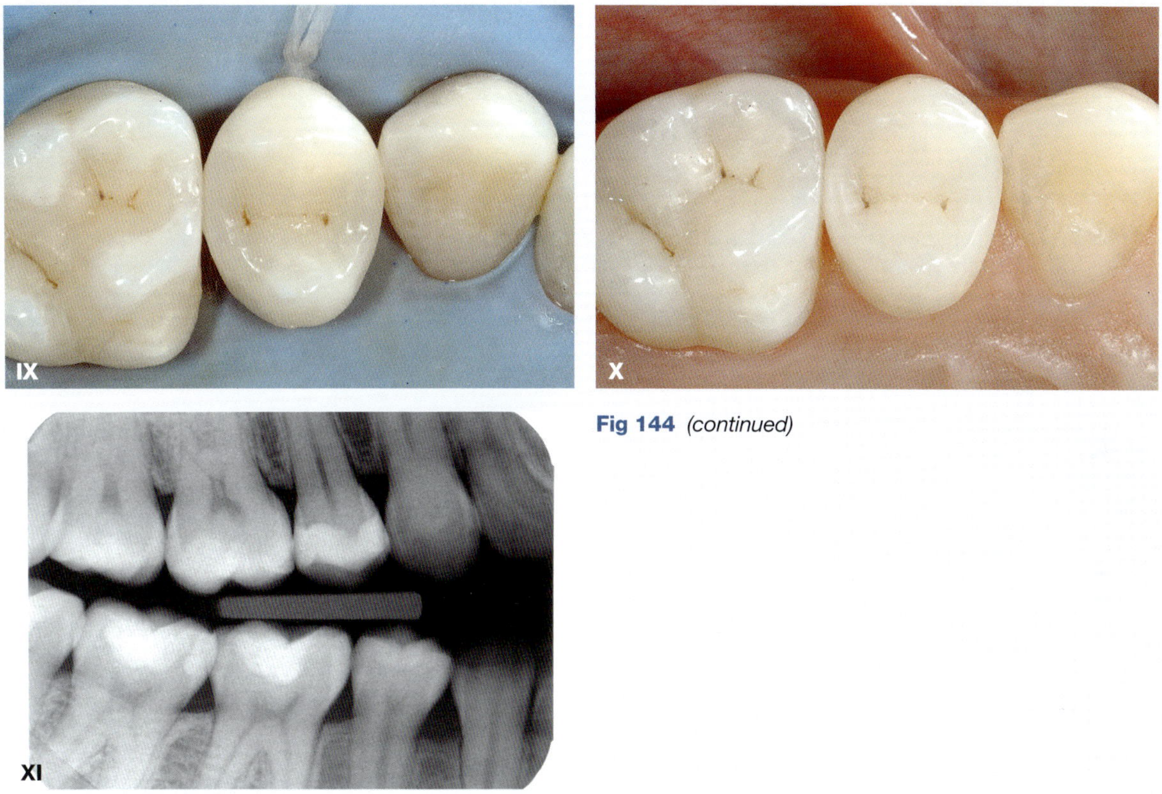

Fig 144 *(continued)*

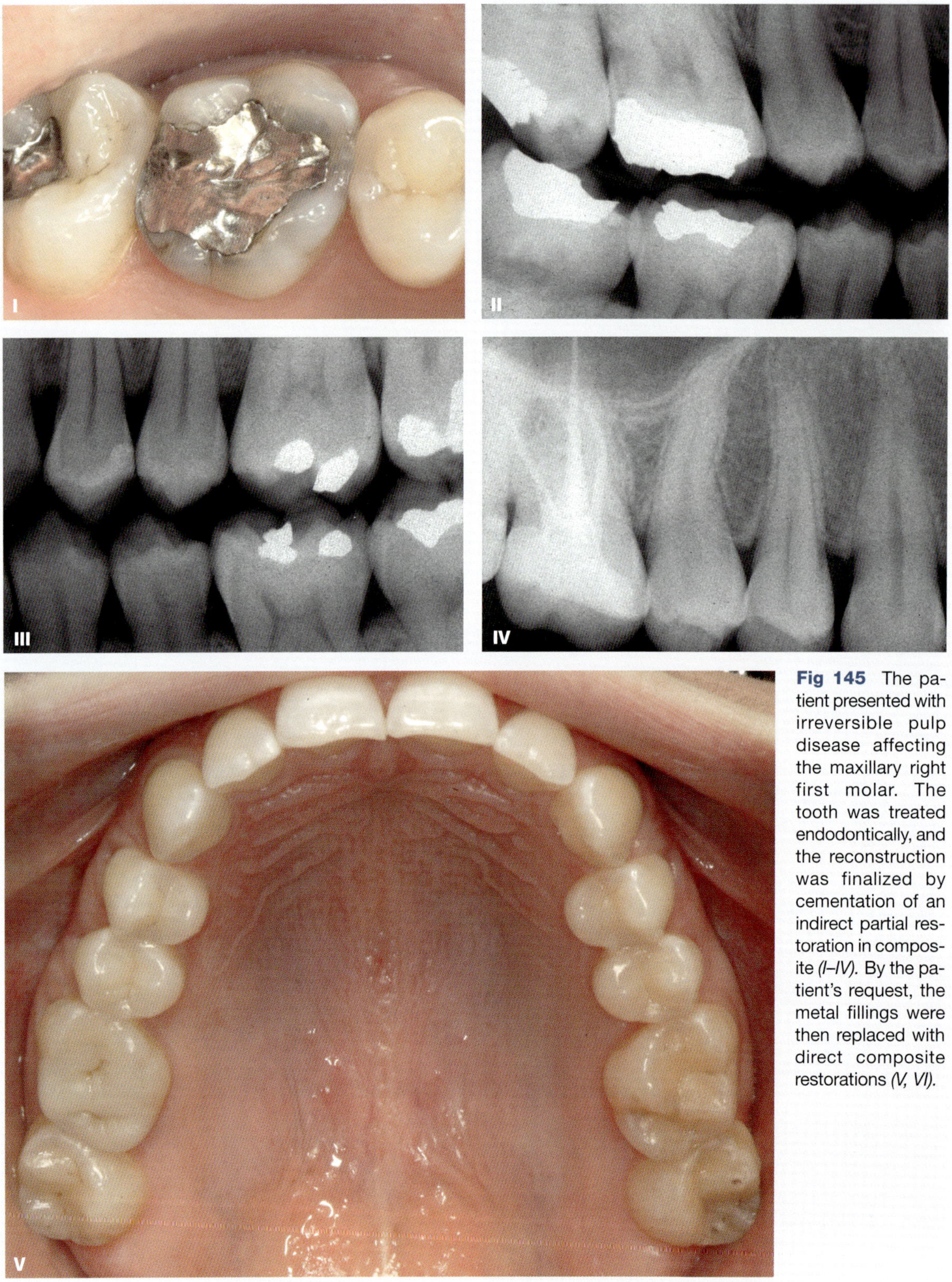

Fig 145 The patient presented with irreversible pulp disease affecting the maxillary right first molar. The tooth was treated endodontically, and the reconstruction was finalized by cementation of an indirect partial restoration in composite *(I–IV)*. By the patient's request, the metal fillings were then replaced with direct composite restorations *(V, VI)*.

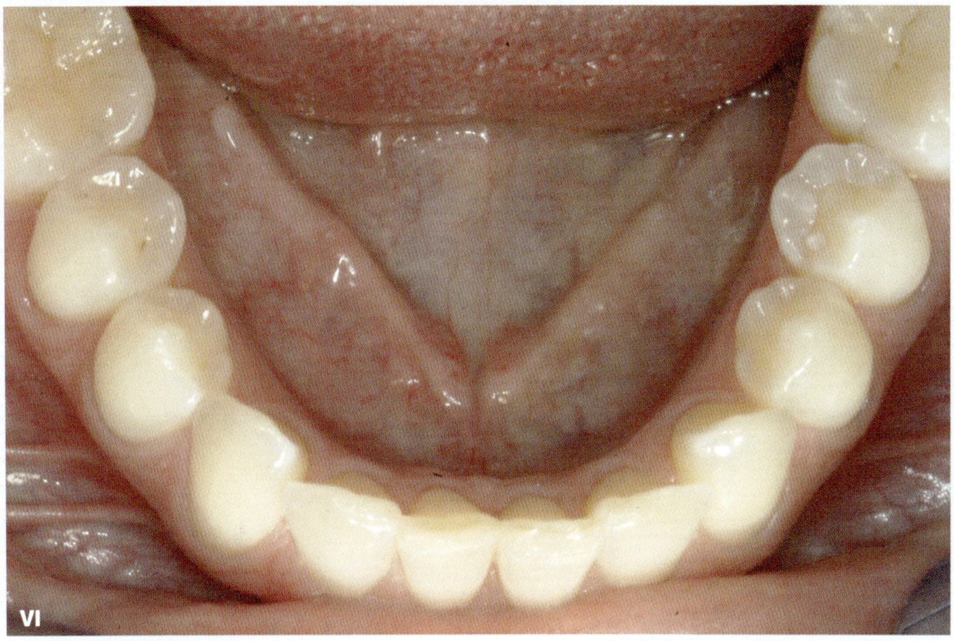

Fig 145 *(continued)*

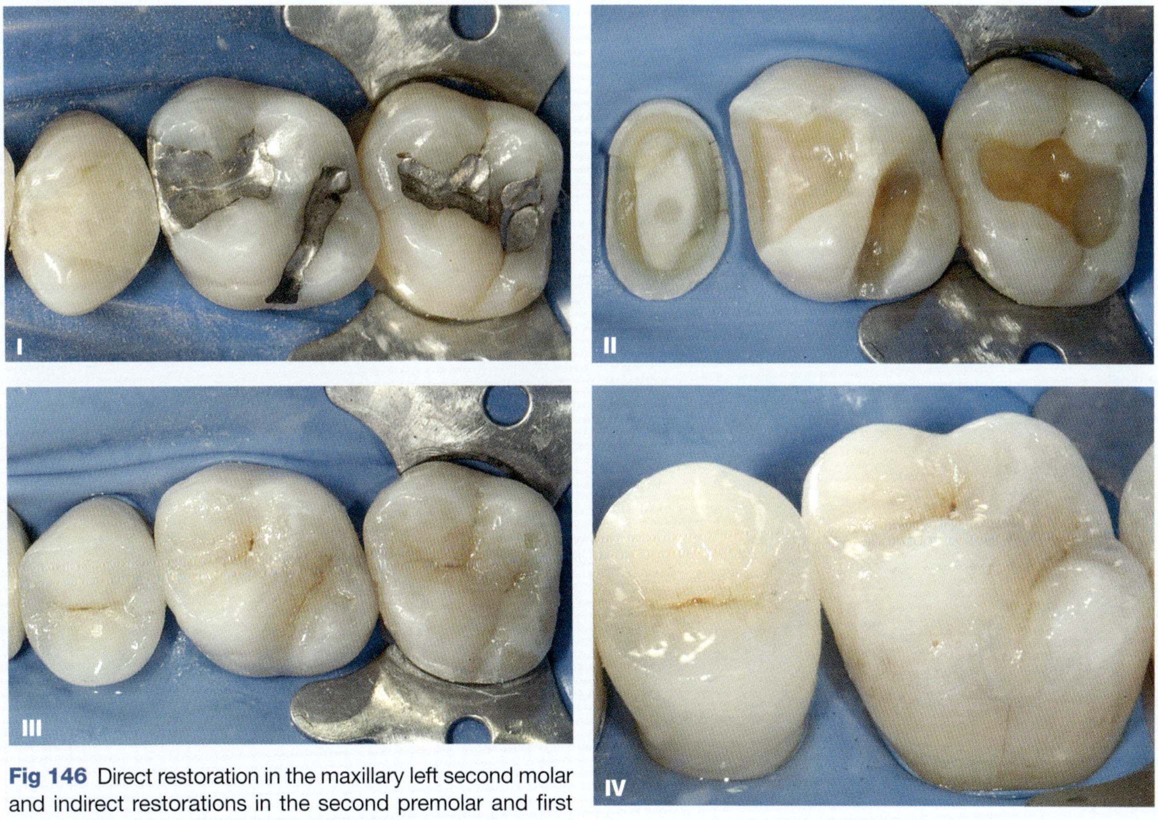

Fig 146 Direct restoration in the maxillary left second molar and indirect restorations in the second premolar and first molar *(I–III)*, with a close-up view of the interproximal contact and emergence profiles of the indirect restorations *(IV)*.

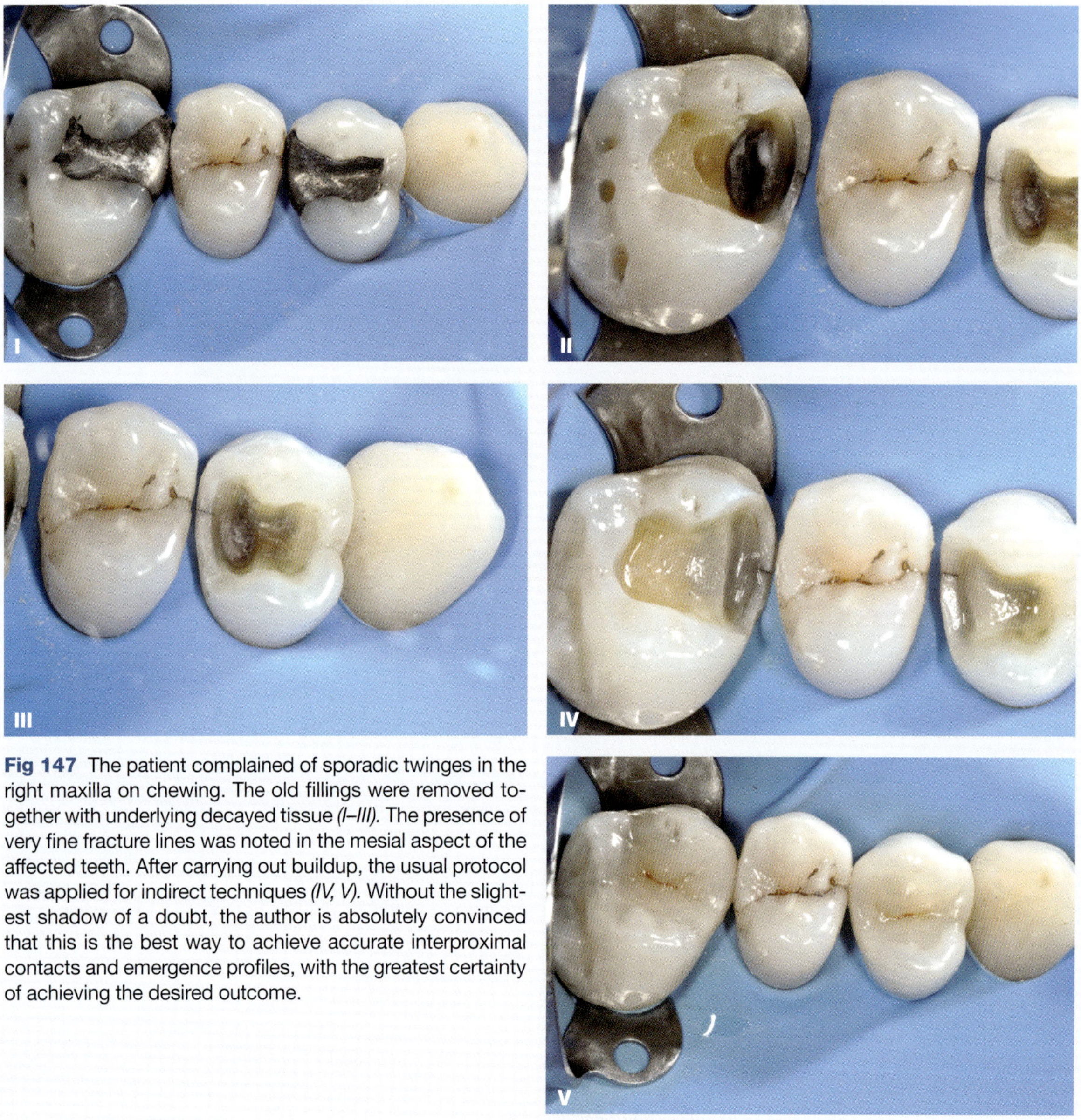

Fig 147 The patient complained of sporadic twinges in the right maxilla on chewing. The old fillings were removed together with underlying decayed tissue *(I–III)*. The presence of very fine fracture lines was noted in the mesial aspect of the affected teeth. After carrying out buildup, the usual protocol was applied for indirect techniques *(IV, V)*. Without the slightest shadow of a doubt, the author is absolutely convinced that this is the best way to achieve accurate interproximal contacts and emergence profiles, with the greatest certainty of achieving the desired outcome.

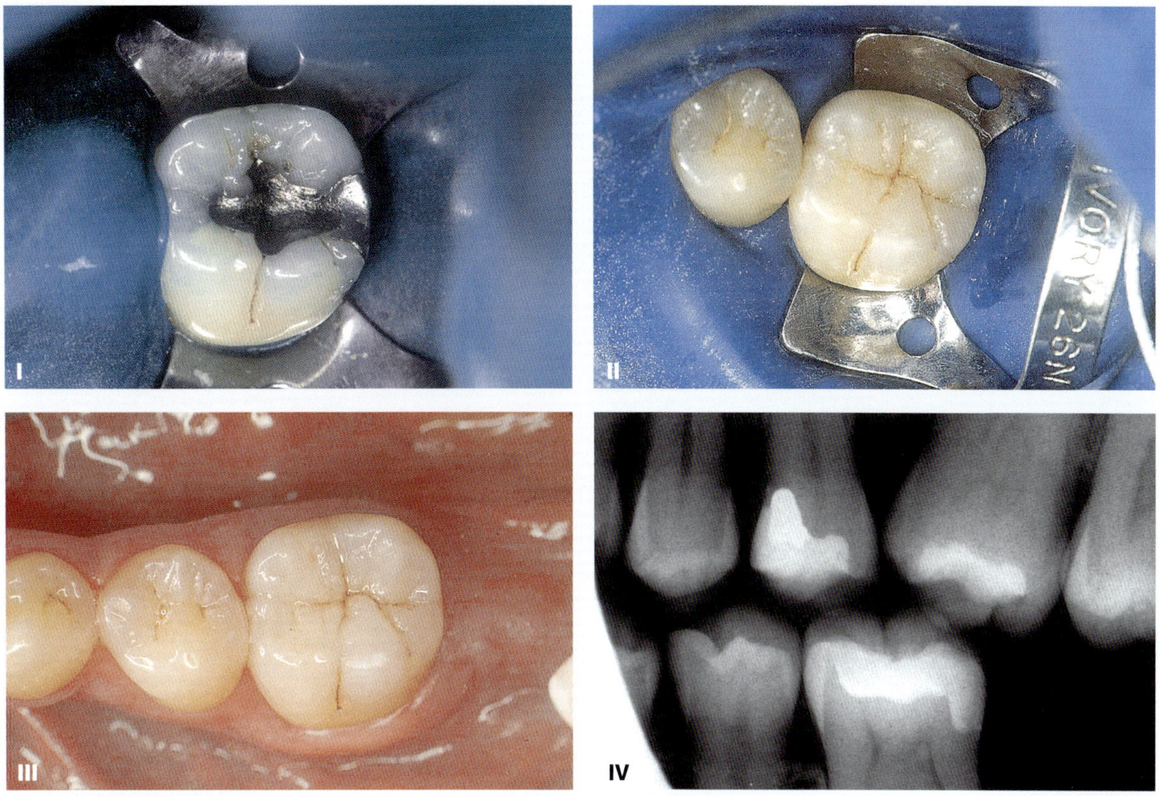

Fig 148 Inlay of a mandibular left first molar *(I, II)*, with clinical and radiographic views of 8-year follow-up *(III, IV)*. Because the mandibular left second molar is missing, the first molar had to support the entire load.

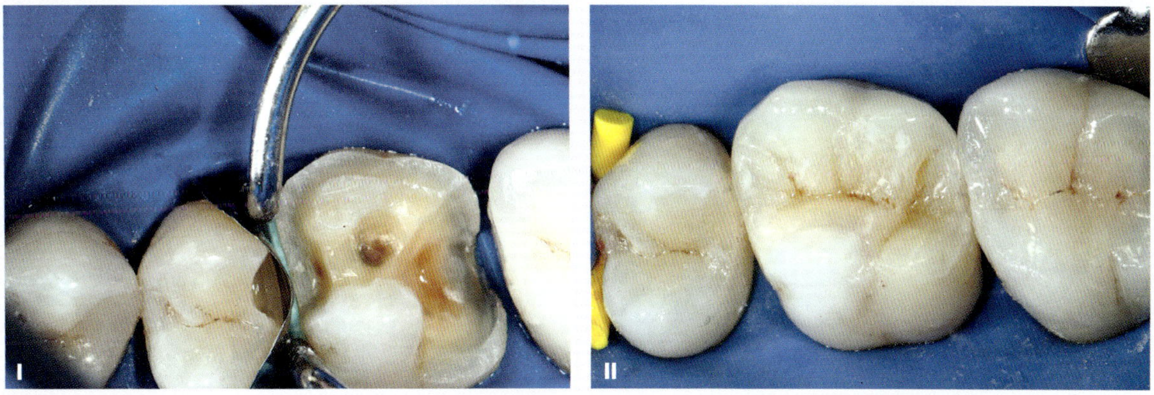

Fig 149 Small Class 2 cavity *(I)* close to a prepared tooth, managed using a direct technique *(II)*.

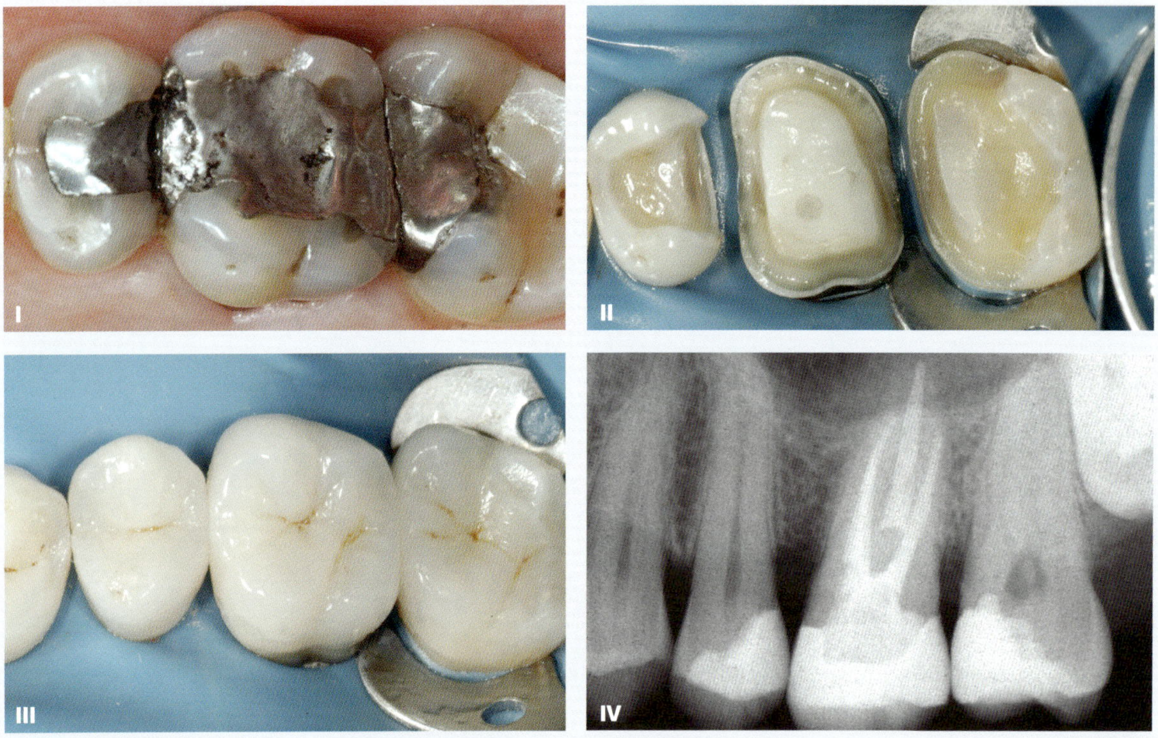

Fig 150 Pulpitis of the maxillary left first molar with old mesio-occlusodistal amalgam restoration required endodontic treatment. For reconstruction of the relevant tooth, after assessing the healthy residual structure, a full-coverage restoration was constructed with supragingival margins. After repeating the all-important analysis of the residual tooth structure, the premolar was finalized with a simple inlay, while for the second molar it was necessary to remove the walls adjacent to the missing marginal ridge and consequently prepare an onlay *(I, II)*. Clinical view of the inlays after cementation *(III)* and radiograph *(IV)* taken at the end of treatment, revealing accuracy of the marginal seals and emergence profiles.

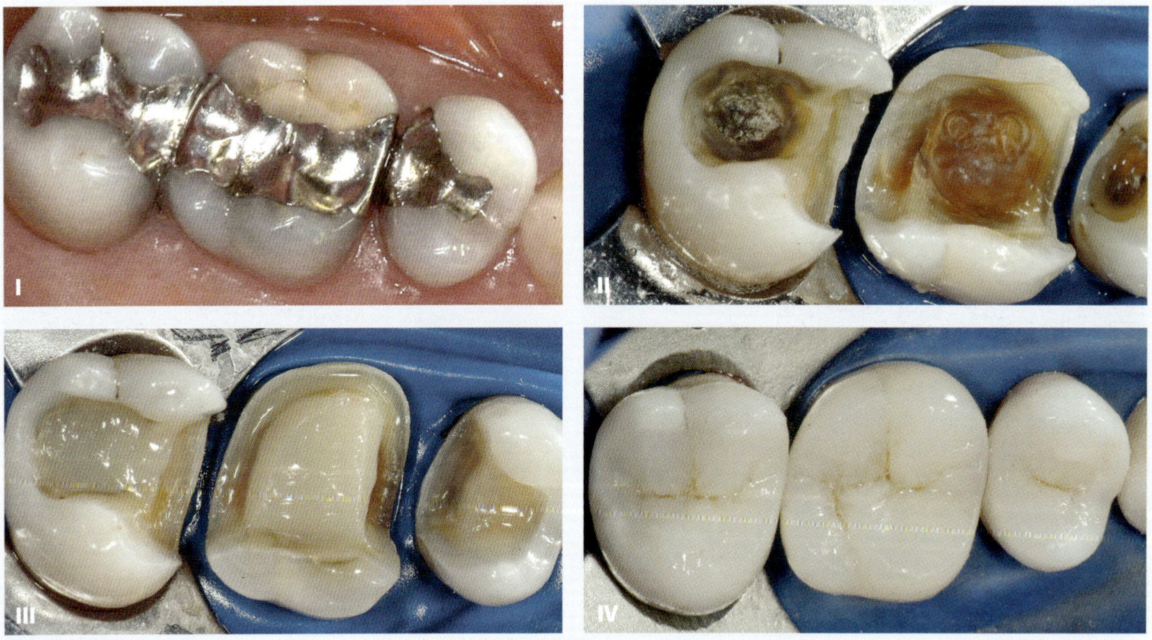

Fig 151 Analysis of the healthy tooth structure remaining after removal of a defective restoration on the maxillary right first molar *(I, II)* led to preparation with removal of the walls and consequent coverage of all cusps *(III)*. A 90-degree shoulder preparation was carried out on the buccal and interproximal aspects, with a shoulder finish line on the palatal aspect. Clinical view of the inlays following cementation *(IV)*.

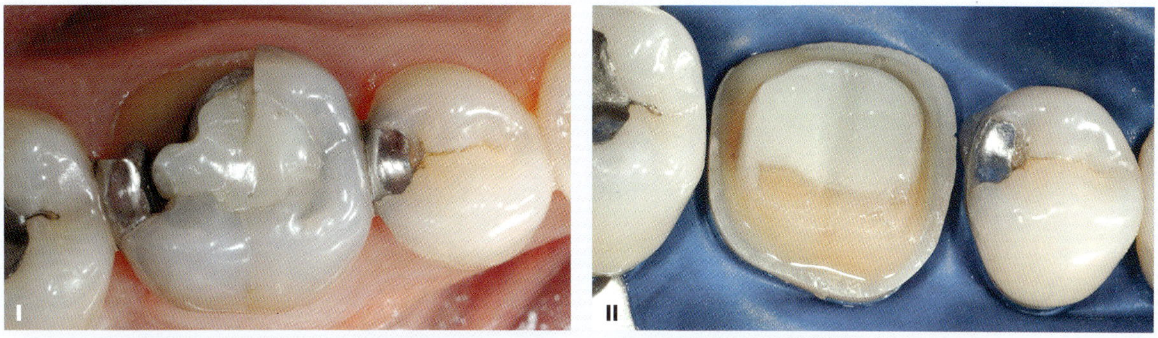

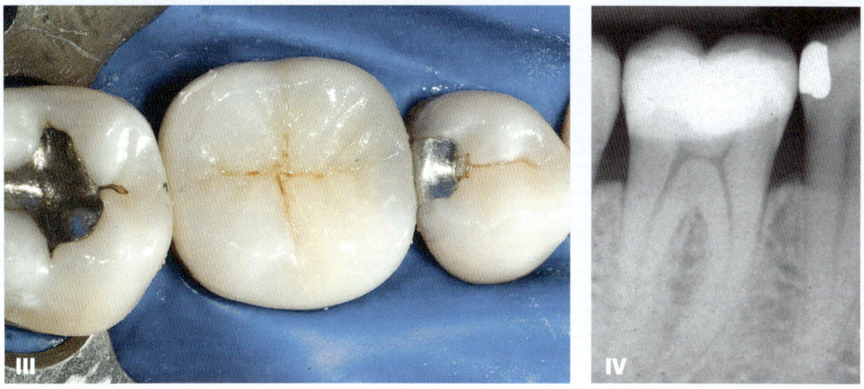

Fig 152 Overlay of the mandibular right first molar *(I–III)* and follow-up after 6 years *(IV)*, showing the marginal seals and emergence profiles.

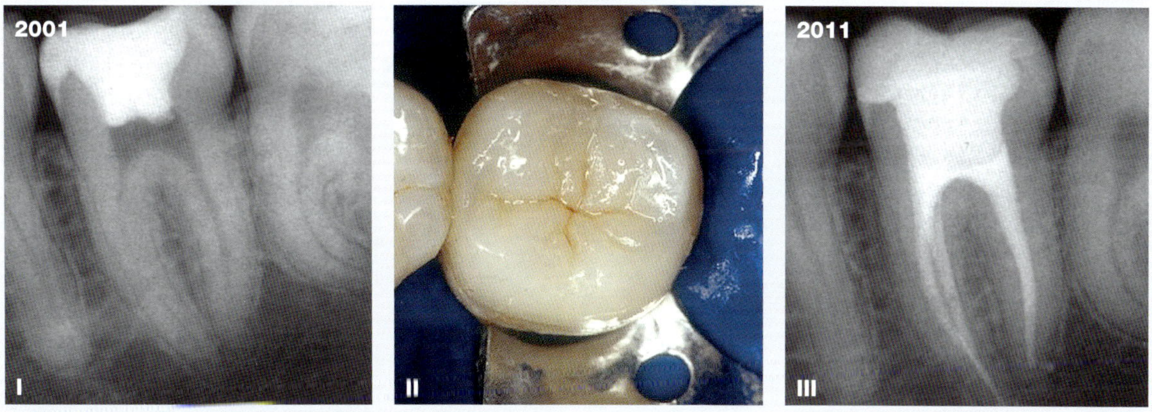

Fig 153 Ten-year follow-up of mandibular molar treated endodontically and reconstructed with a composite onlay. The depth of the pulp chamber was exploited as the only retention.

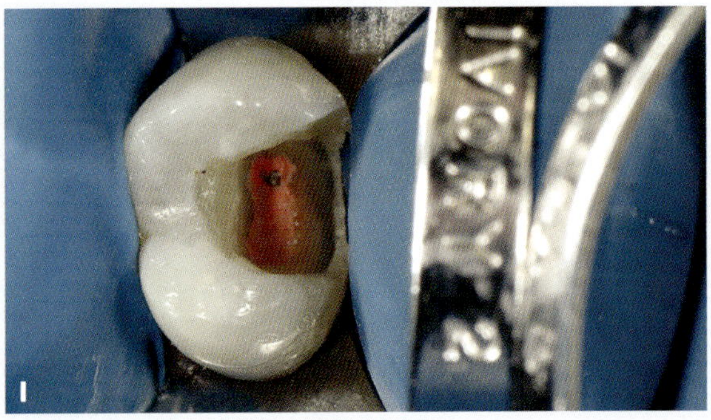
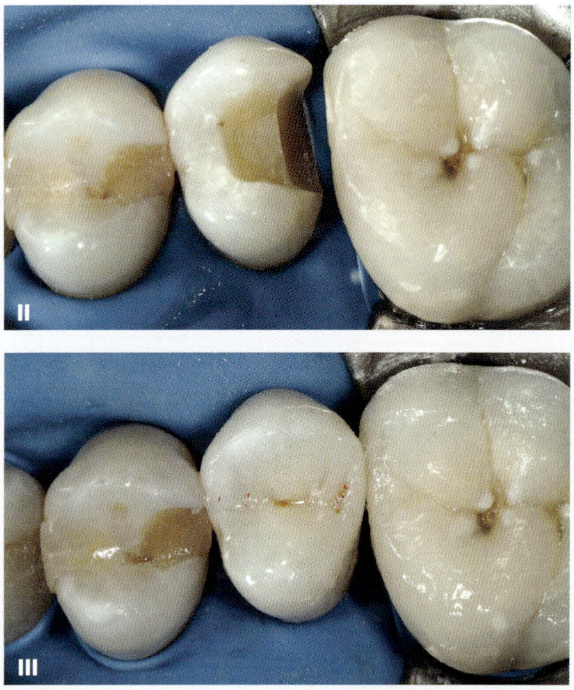

Fig 154 Substantial thickness at the base of the cusps allows a simple inlay for reconstruction of an endodontically treated maxillary premolar.

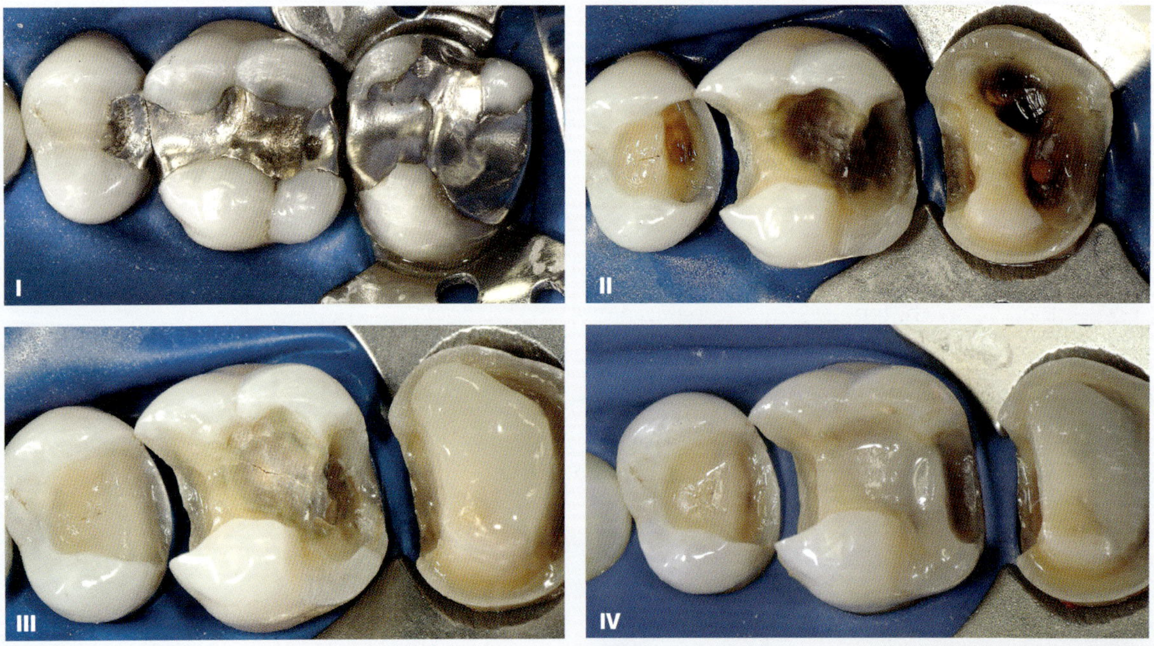
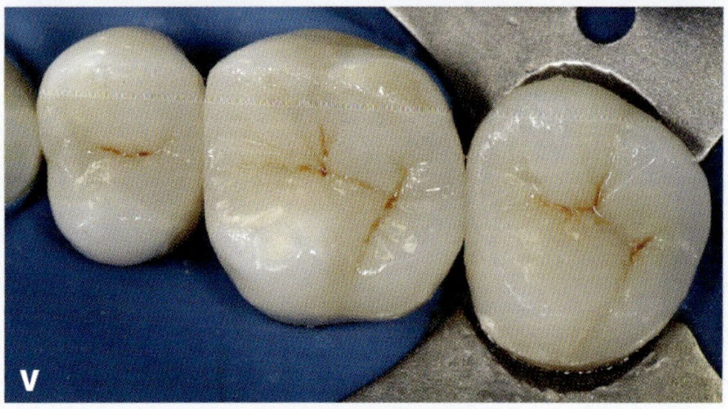

Fig 155 Fracture line in a molar with previous mesio-occlusodistal restoration in amalgam. After cleaning of the fracture line, internal reconstruction was performed with an adhesive technique, flowable composite, and traditional composite, followed by indirect restoration for finalization.

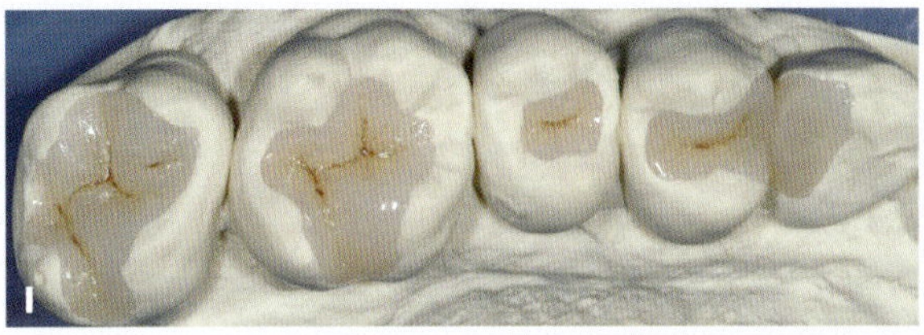

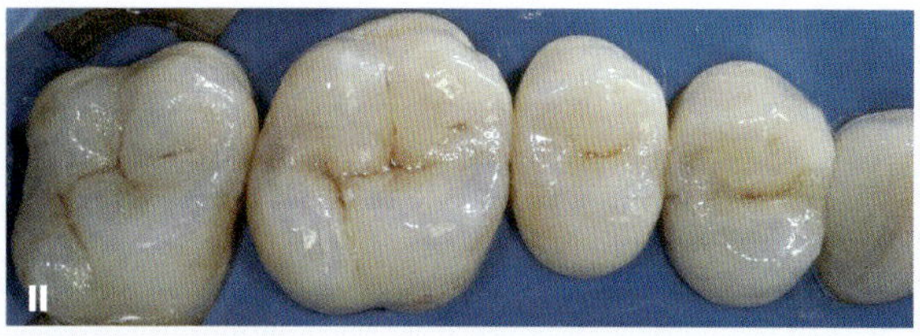

Fig 156 Quadrant restored using an indirect technique: the cavity in the maxillary right second premolar is obviously the result of a direct technique, but this was a trick played on the author's friend Andrea, his very fine dental technician!

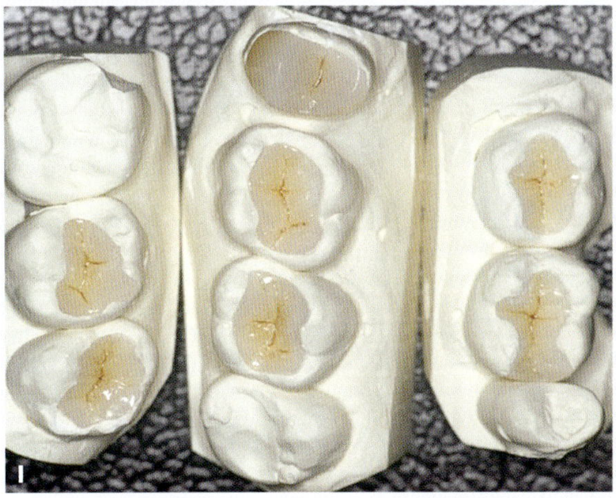

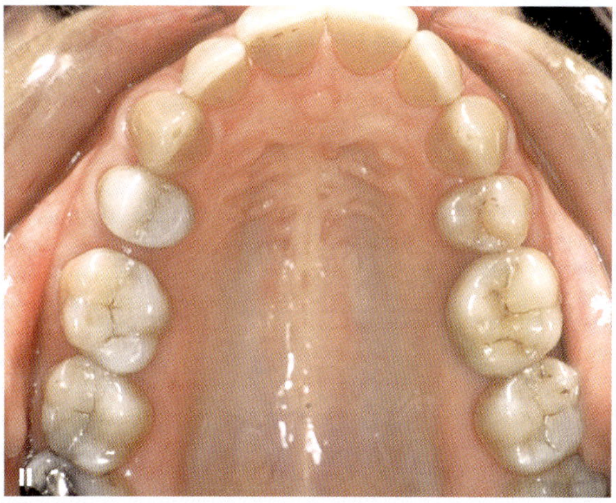

Fig 157 Single session for preparation of Class 1 inlays and onlays *(I)*, followed by another session for cementation. Clinical follow-up after 8 years *(II)*.

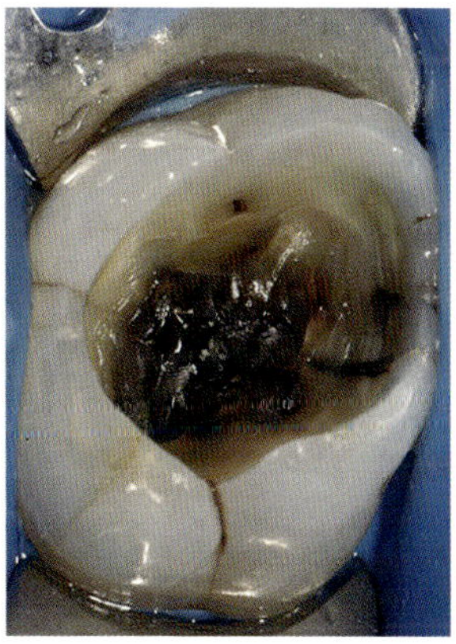

Fig 158 Very deep cavity with significant fracture lines. To prevent stress caused by polymerization shrinkage, which is inevitable and dangerous in such clinical situations, it was decided to perform an indirect restoration, where shrinkage only occurred in the very small amount of composite used for cementation.

When restoring a tooth, the goals are to remove decayed tissue, protect the dentin-pulp complex, and ensure the preparation is minimally invasive as well as to achieve an anatomically correct and impeccable marginal seal, satisfactory internal filling, an accurate emergence profile, and contact surfaces that are consistent both from a clinical and radiographic viewpoint (Figs 159 and 160).

On the subject of contact surfaces, many years ago Marmasse[32] asserted the incontestable superiority of a proximal inlay over fillings: "This is the only solution that can be corrected, adjusted, and hand-finished after tests that make it possible to add to, reduce, replace, and shape the contact point until the required shape, location, and intensity are achieved."

"It offers the unparalleled benefit of making it possible at one stroke to prevent food building up between teeth, injury to the gingival papilla, and secondary decay of the neighboring tooth."

The author is in full agreement with the fact that it is difficult to clean the proximal surface of fillings carried out in situ; as far as he is concerned, this is the main argument in favor of an inlay in this type of reconstruction.

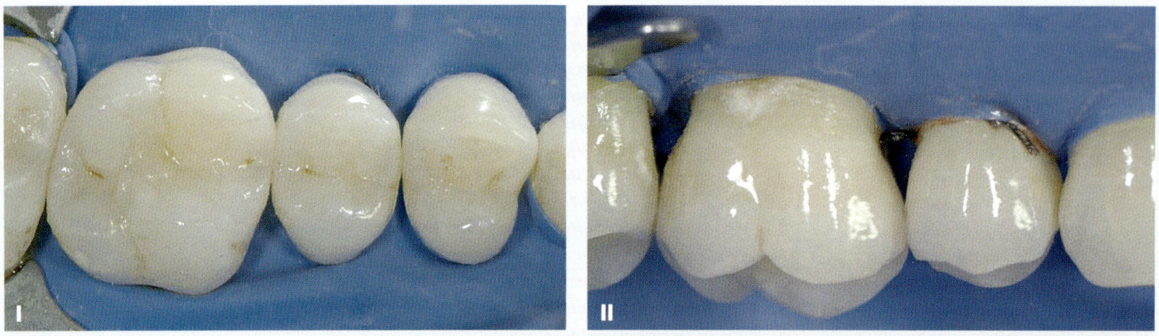

Fig 159 Occlusal and lateral clinical views of three inlays performed on a cavity with a long buccopalatal extension. The accurate contacts and emergence profiles are evident *(I, II)*. Following use of abrasive strips under rubber dam, a suture thread and blood can be observed. Radiographic follow-up *(III)*.

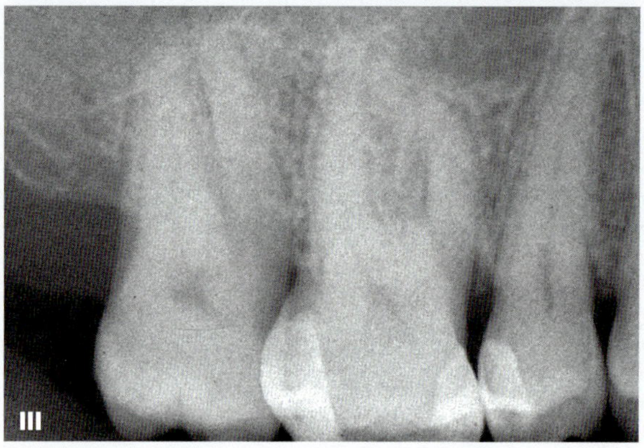

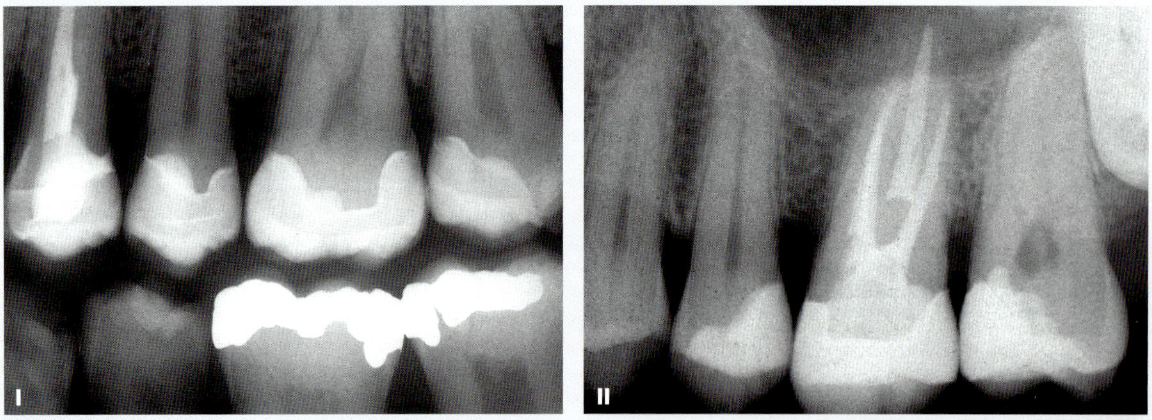

Fig 160 Radiographic views for checking marginal seals and emergence profiles.

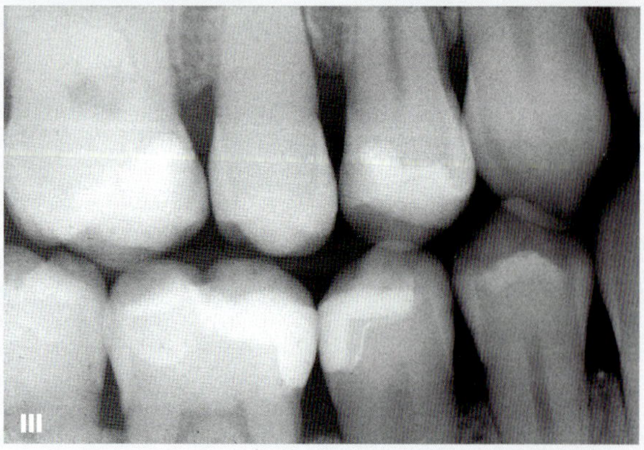

The answer to the question of whether such considerations are still applicable today is a resounding yes (Figs 161 and 162).

It is therefore entirely justified to attempt to establish the best approach for respecting all of these parameters, which is the purpose of the present discussion.

The author believes that clinical and radiographic evidence, combined with medium- and long-term follow-up, is essential in establishing an approach, which naturally must also take into account the literature.

The literature provides valuable information about the properties and applications of the materials clinicians use, but the work is ultimately carried out by the practitioners, who are solely responsible for the success or failure of the techniques that they use in specific situations.

One example that illustrates this situation is the difficulty the author finds in routinely creating restorations with satisfactory contact surfaces and an accurate emergence profile in Class 2 medium-large cavities using a direct technique; the result is inevitably dependent on the practitioner's skill (Figs 163 to 165).

Many reputable colleagues believe that direct composite restorations can match the clinical results achieved with indirect composite restorations in posterior sectors, provided the choice of materials and the application of restoration and curing techniques are extremely intelligent and effective, above all allowing each practitioner to make the necessary adjustment to working times.

Consideration of strictly clinical aspects inevitably calls to mind the practical difficulty of routinely obtaining extensive and strong contact surfaces and ideal emergence profiles when working with large cavities.

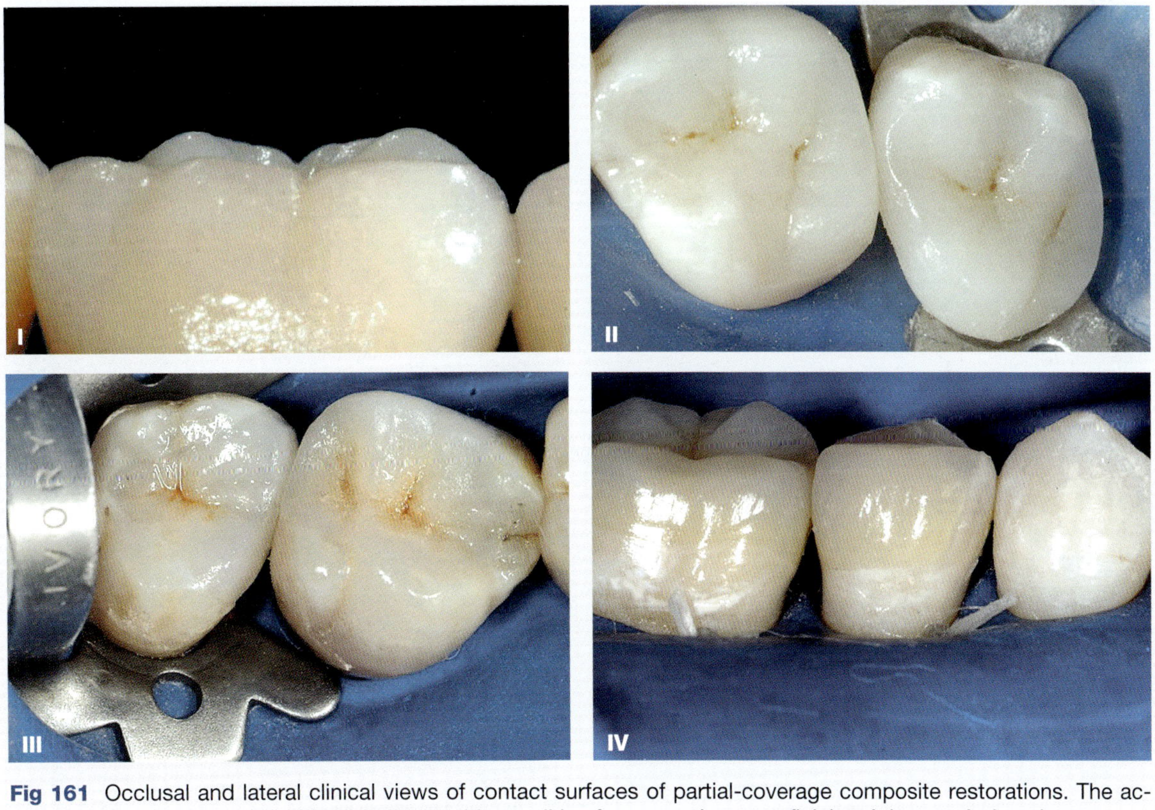

Fig 161 Occlusal and lateral clinical views of contact surfaces of partial-coverage composite restorations. The accuracy of the contact surfaces is an indispensable condition for respecting superficial and deep periodontal structures.

Fig 162 Radiographs of a direct restoration with correct marginal seal and emergence profile.

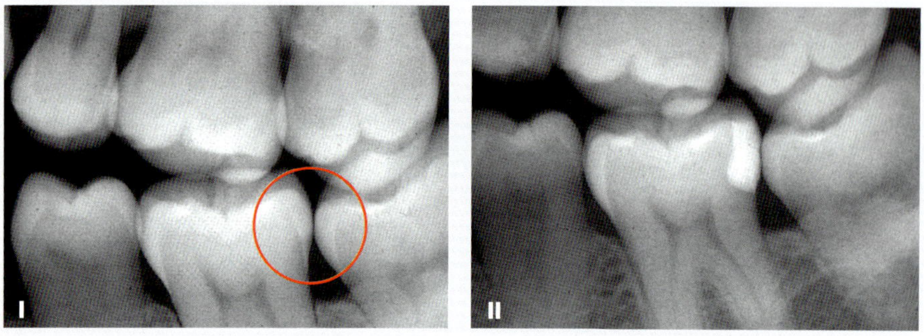

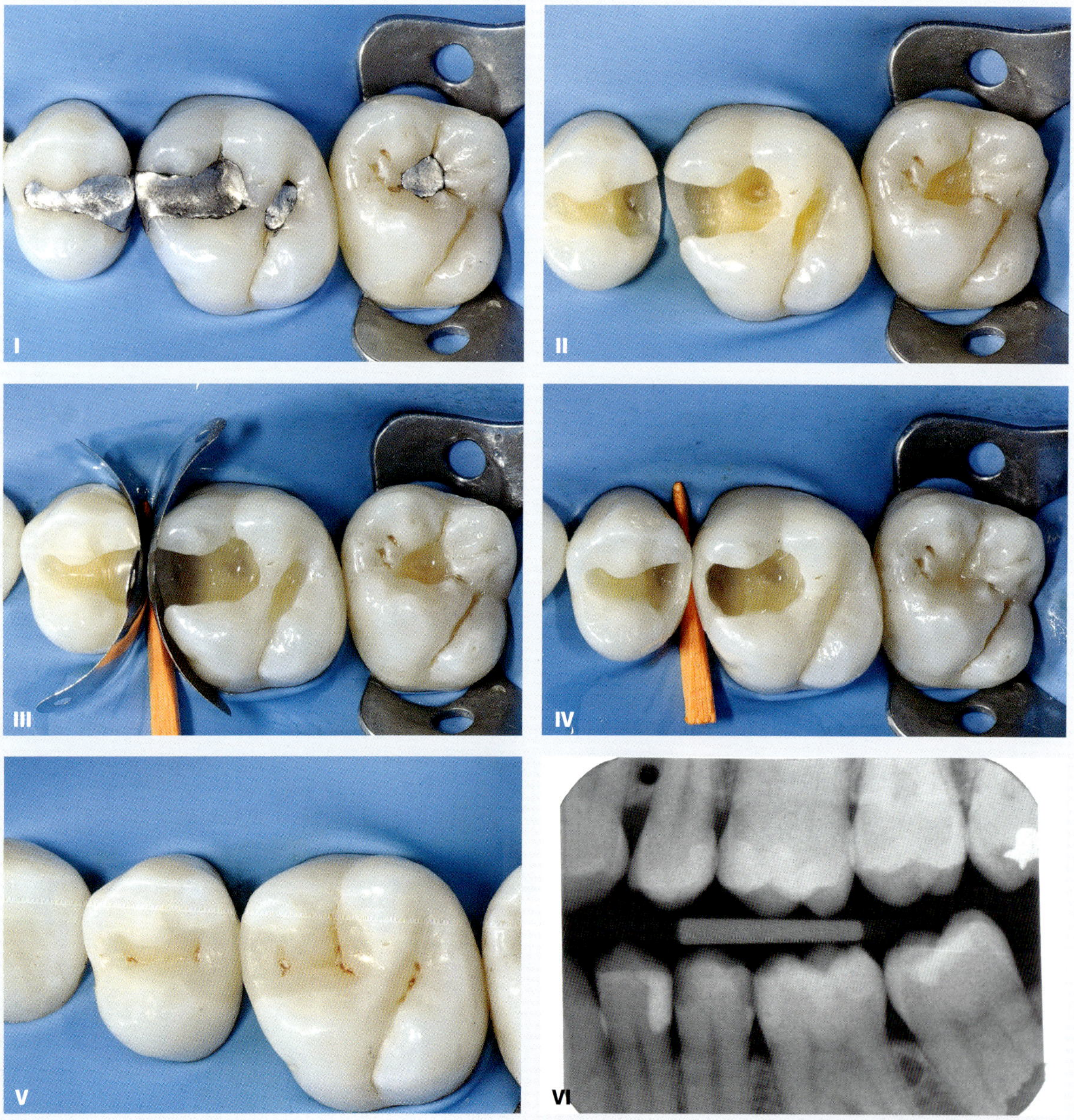

Fig 163 Class 2 cavity treated with a direct restoration, providing effective reproduction of the marginal ridge.

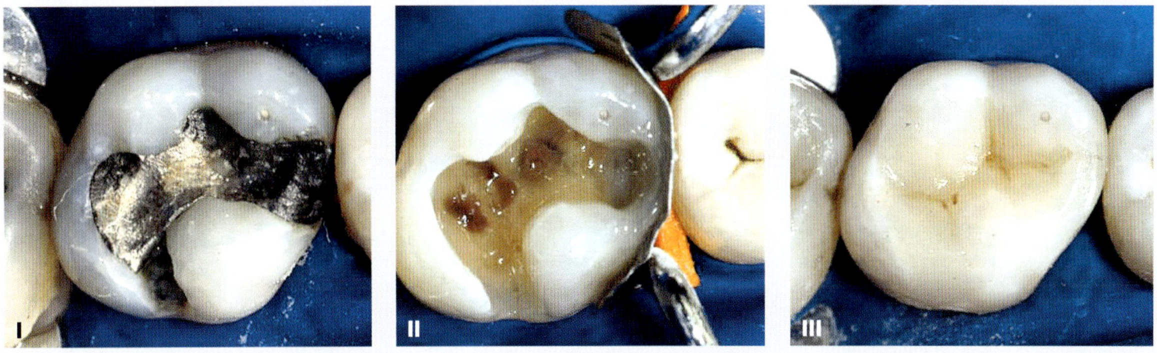

Fig 164 Class 2 cavity treated with a direct restoration, providing effective reproduction of the marginal ridge.

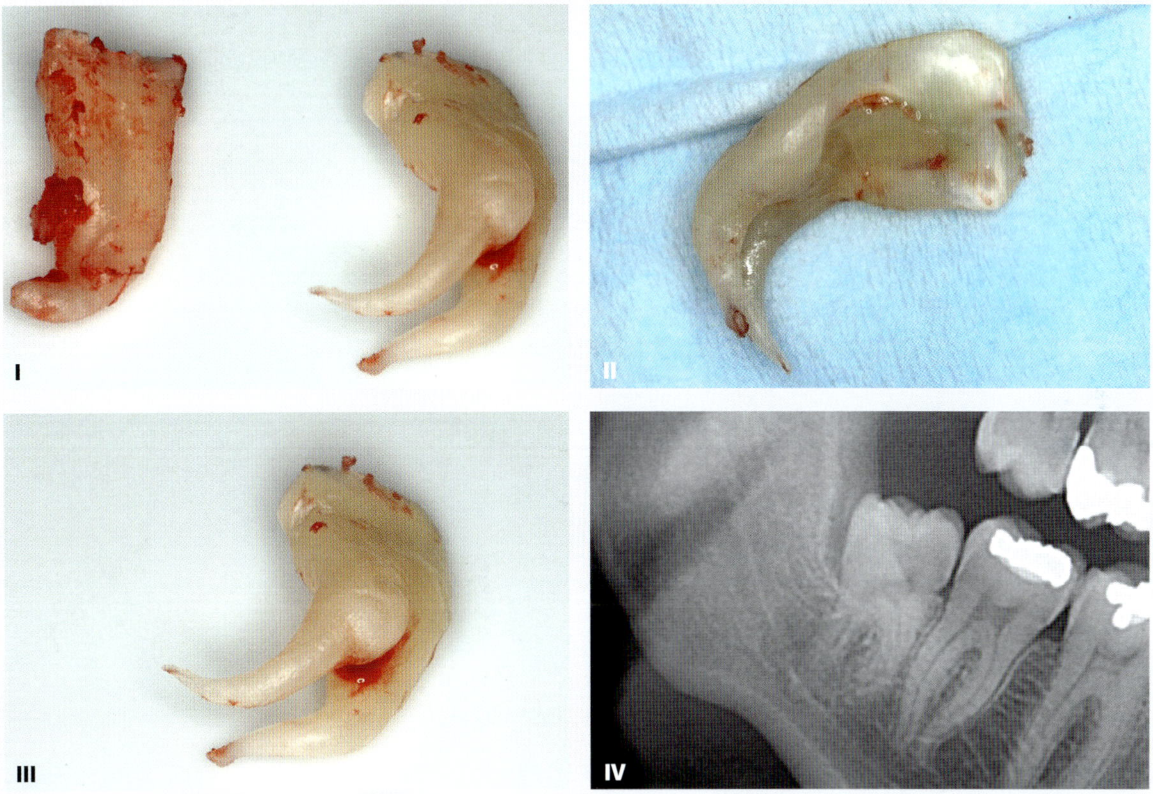

Fig 165 Great manual dexterity was required to remove this impacted third molar. (Courtesy of Dr Stefano Piras.)

The author therefore maintains that each clinical situation must be individually assessed. If a patient's treatment requires a single restoration, even a large mesio-occlusodistal (MOD) restoration, it is fine to go ahead with a direct solution provided the work is performed by the correct practitioner. Otherwise, the author sees no alternative to indirect restorations if the treatment plan involves one or more quadrants in which the replacement of several large defective restorations is required, perhaps with periodontal involvement and subgingival margins.

At lectures and congresses when the author sees quadrants with marvelous MOD restorations carried out using a direct technique, he has to restrain himself from a strong desire to get out his dental floss and personally check the contact surfaces.
A rigorous but simple protocol will aid in the achievement of entirely satisfactory clinical results in most cases in which there is an indication for indirect restorations. As a point of emphasis, the only real problem with such cases remains difficulties encountered during the stage of adhesive cementation (Figs 166 and 167).

Furthermore, when carrying out a restoration with a medium to large Class 2 cavity, certain factors must be considered, based on a knowledge of the literature:

1. The conversion level affects both the physical and mechanical properties of polymers. It increases in direct proportion with the hardness of the matrix, the flexural modulus

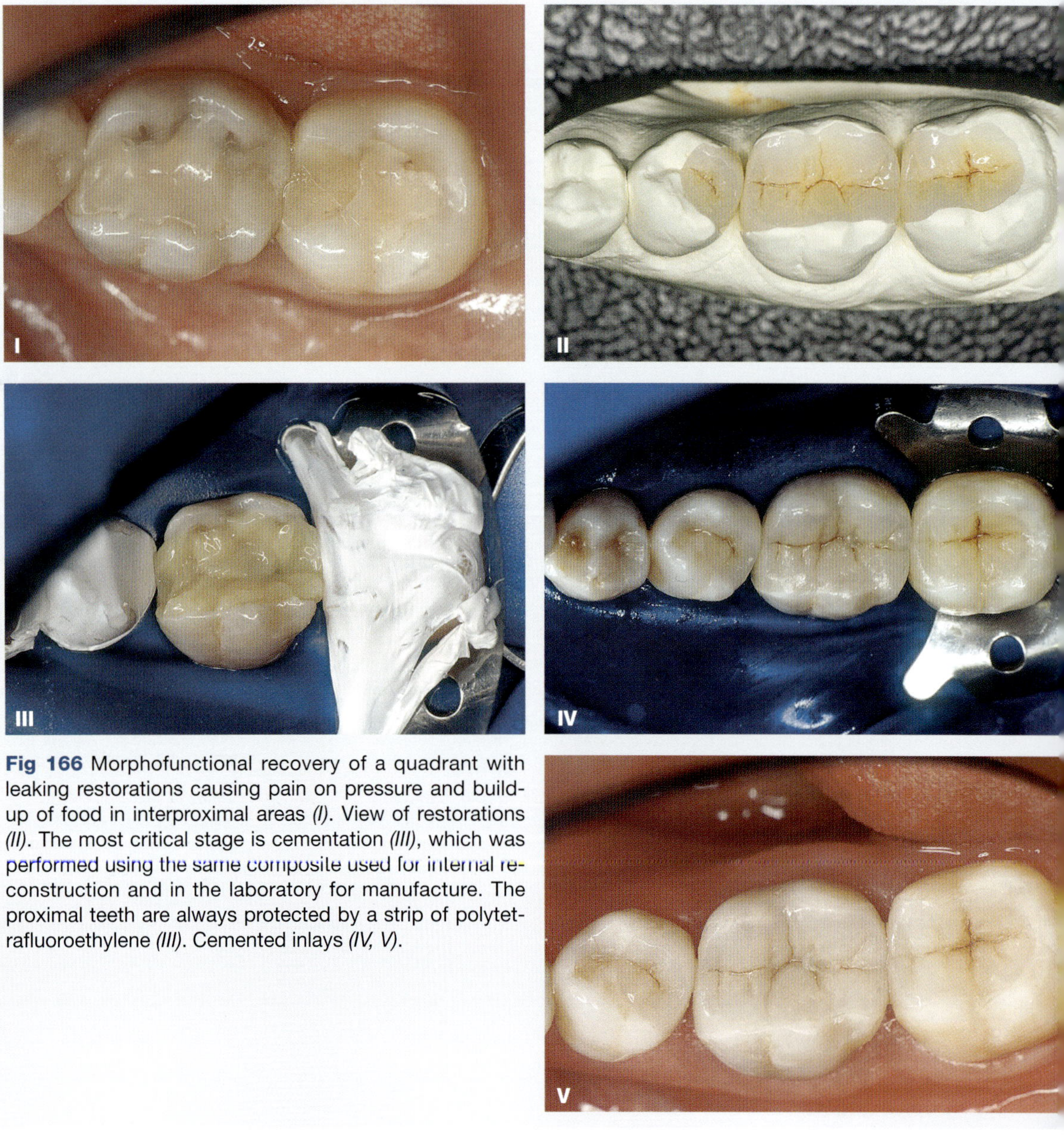

Fig 166 Morphofunctional recovery of a quadrant with leaking restorations causing pain on pressure and build-up of food in interproximal areas *(I)*. View of restorations *(II)*. The most critical stage is cementation *(III)*, which was performed using the same composite used for internal reconstruction and in the laboratory for manufacture. The proximal teeth are always protected by a strip of polytetrafluoroethylene *(III)*. Cemented inlays *(IV, V)*.

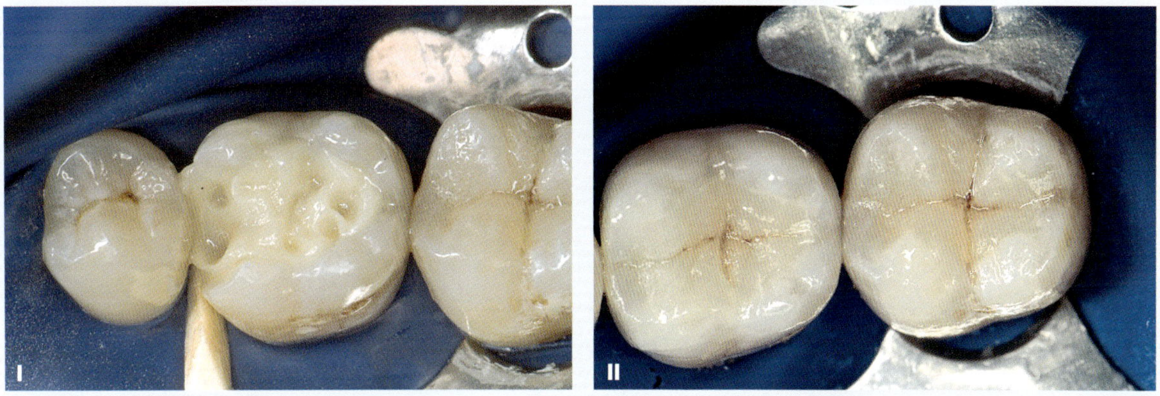

Fig 167 View of one stage of cementation, during which a wooden wedge was inserted to facilitate positioning of the inlay *(I)*. Cemented inlay *(II)*.

and strength, fracture resistance, compressive strength, tensile strength, and wear resistance.[33–37]

2. The conversion level achieved with a curing light is less than that obtained with the light plus heat; indirect techniques allow an increase in the conversion level of the monomer to a polymer due to post-curing, improving the material's mechanical performance.[38,39]
3. Post-curing of the indirect restorations allows a better tooth-restoration interface seal and an outcome with less likelihood of leakage.[30,40] As previously stated, this allows better final physical properties (modulus of elasticity, fragility, coefficient of expansion) and mechanical properties (microhardness, wear resistance) due to the lower conversion level.[41]
4. The indirect technique cancels out stress due to shrinkage,[42] the antagonistic effect between the contraction force of the composite and the adhesion force of the walls (the C-factor, ie, the relationship between free and bonded surfaces). This stress may be expressed by anything from an initial enamel crack to irretrievable fractures (Figs 168 and 169).
5. The stress caused by shrinkage is the force per unit area that develops during the shrinkage and is applied to the walls. It is measured as a percentage.
6. One millimeter of stratification corresponds to 10 MPa of shrinkage.
7. Where there is an indication for a direct restoration, the stress caused by shrinkage is canceled out or at least reduced by stratification of the composite, application of an intermediate elastic layer between the substrate (dentin) and composite, and slow curing. Although the stress is reduced, the shrinkage, which is an inevitable chemical and physical phenomenon, cannot be prevented and ranges from 1.67% to 5.68%.[43,44]
8. Reduction in the activation intensity slows the conversion level of the composite and reduces stress caused by shrinkage.[45,46]
9. Slow and gradual light curing significantly improves the marginal seal.[47]

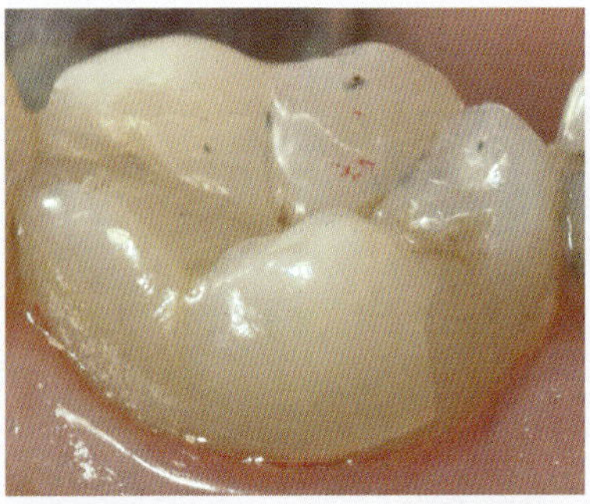

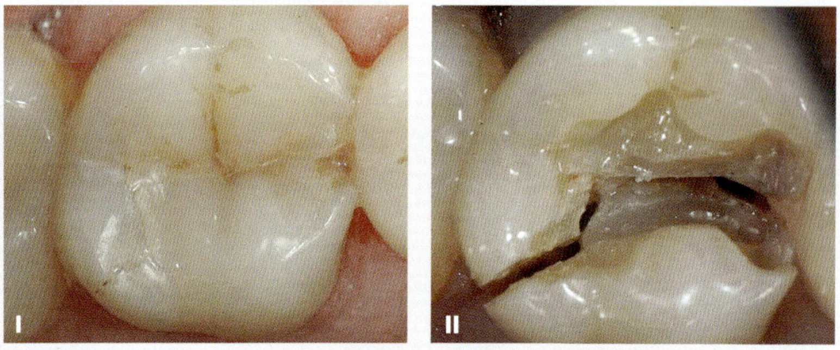

Fig 168 A palatal fracture line in a large composite restoration created using a direct technique, probably caused by excessive stress due to shrinkage during polymerization.

Fig 169 Deep fracture in a large restoration placed using a direct technique that could unfortunately only be resolved by removing the tooth.

Having said this, when treating medium-large and large cavities, inlays and onlays really come into their own in the competition between partial preparation versus total preparation.

The conservation of tooth structure is related to the difference between the healthy tooth structure remaining after a partial preparation and that remaining after a total preparation, ie, to the difference between a preparation for an inlay or onlay and that for a prosthetic crown.

The literature teaches us that:

- The tooth structure removed for a full crown ranges from 67% to 75%, and that figure drops to 38% for a partial crown, 34% for an onlay, and 16% for an inlay.[48,49]
- The reduction in tooth strength following conservative procedures and endodontic treatment is 5% in an endodontically treated maxillary premolar with its two marginal ridges left intact.[50]

In the same tooth, with the loss of a single marginal ridge (ie, a mesio-occlusal or occlusodistal preparation) and vital pulp, the reduction in strength is 35%, rising to 55% in an MOD preparation with loss of vital pulp.[50]

The cusps of a loaded posterior tooth deform differently according to whether a marginal ridge is present or absent: teeth with a missing ridge deform much more than those with an intact ridge.[51–53]

Knowledge of these parameters is of fundamental importance in extremely conservative preparation of a cavity, both when the pulp in the tooth is vital and when the tooth has been treated endodontically.

In the past, there was a general opinion that endodontically treated posterior teeth required the use of an intracanal post and a full crown; however, biomechanical analysis of the residual tooth tissue as well as the proven reliability of adhesive techniques and restoration materials led to a review of this treatment plan[49] (Figs 170 to 172).

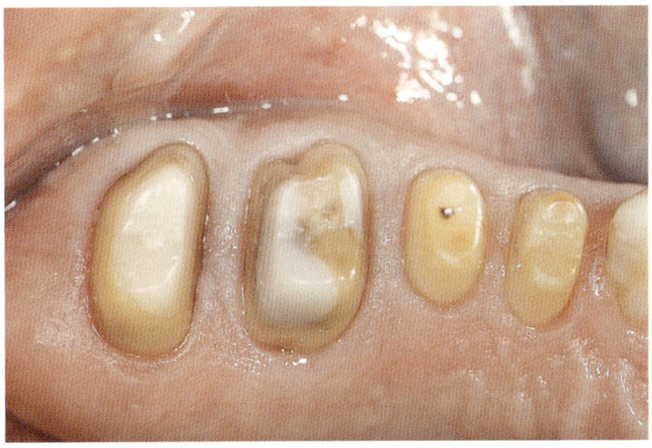

Fig 170 Classic example of accurate prosthetic preparations clearly showing the amount of tooth structure removed. (Courtesy of Dr Marco Nicastro).

Clinicians should undoubtedly opt for alternative treatments over full crowns to observe the principle of saving as much healthy residual tooth tissue as possible.[54]

Much research confirms that the main factor determining resistance to occlusal and masticatory stress is the quantity of HEALTHY RESIDUAL TOOTH TISSUE.[55,56]

These concepts are revisited and examined in greater depth in the chapter on cavity preparation (chapter 3).

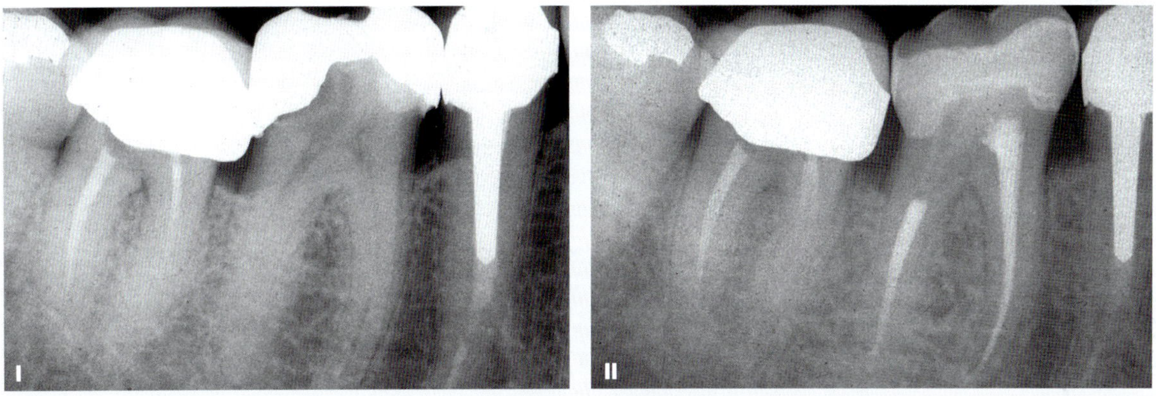

Fig 171 Radiographic view of a mandibular right first molar treated endodontically for pulpitis and reconstructed by means of indirect composite restoration (an overlay replacing the old crown): fiber post, marginal seals, and emergence profile can be observed. The patient was strongly advised to carry out interdisciplinary intervention on the adjacent second molar as well in order to finalize the treatment plan in a streamlined manner, but he refused. Luckily this rarely happens, but it is certainly not pleasant having to work while knowing that the outcome is bound to be a compromise.

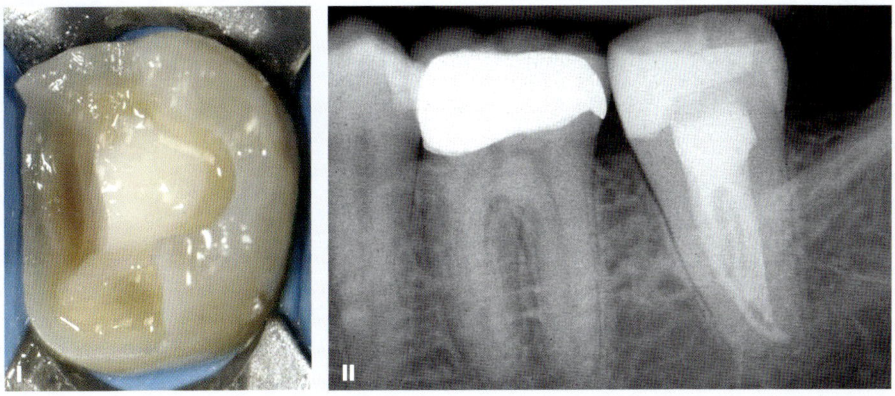

Fig 172 A significant amount of healthy residual tooth structure was maintained to reconstruct an endodontically treated tooth. This is a perfect example of conservative dentistry with maintenance of a distal marginal ridge, adjacent cusps, and supragingival tooth-restoration margins.

Clinical cases

When rehabilitating one or more quadrants, the therapeutic approach often requires techniques for which a multidisciplinary team is of fundamental importance: in the first clinical case (Fig 173), radiographic examination suggested endodontic, periodontal, and restorative treatments of the mandibular arch using indirect techniques, while the caries lesions in the maxilla were treated using direct techniques.

In the mandibular right (fourth) quadrant, endodontic treatment had been carried out on the first molar with previous biopulpotomy, causing persistent painful symptoms that led the patient to consult the author's team. After removing the deep decayed tissue in the second premolar and second molar, the healthy margins of the cavity were found to be subgingival, and it was therefore necessary to lengthen the clinical crown throughout the entire quadrant.

Clinical case 1

Fig 173 Young patient with caries lesions in all four quadrants (see the text for a description of the case).

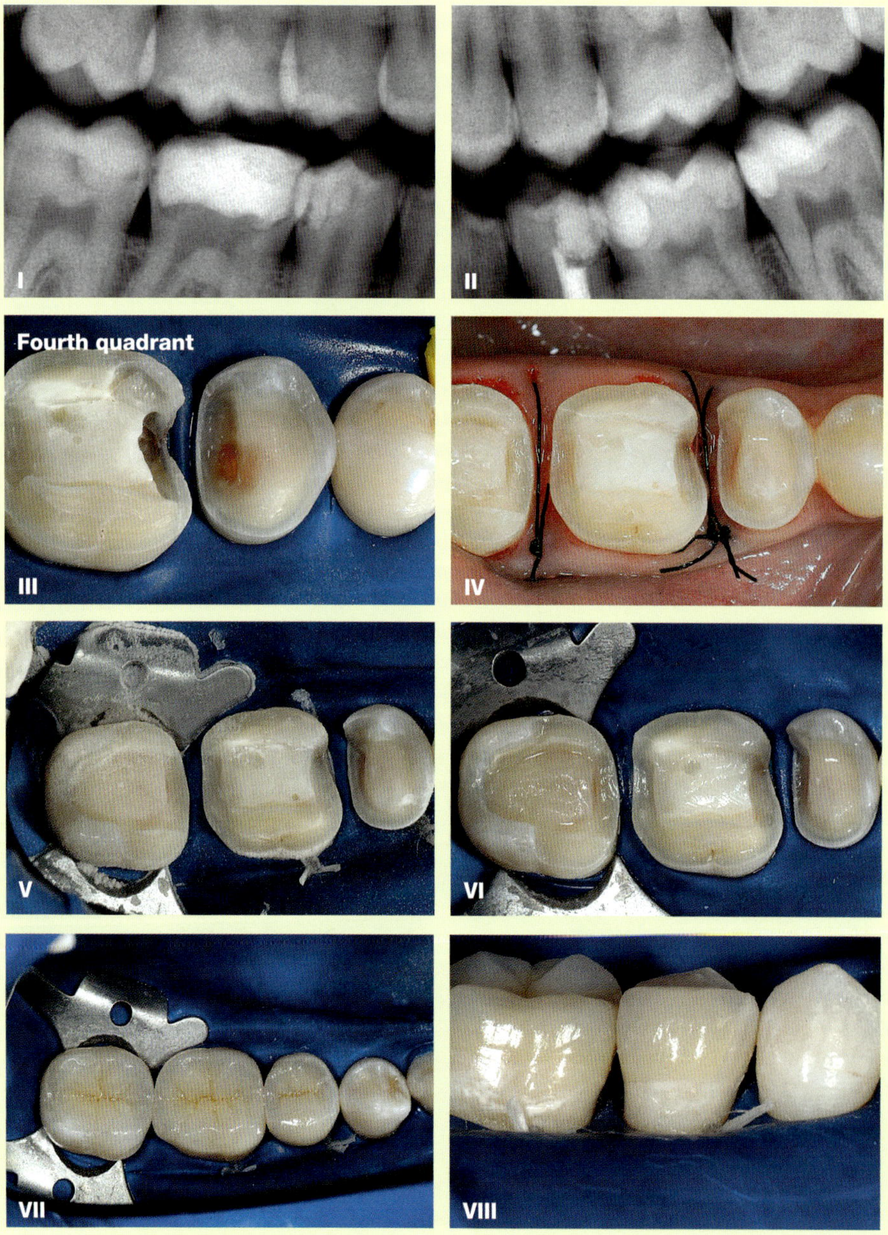

After performing the adhesive protocol, the teeth were built up using composite, a cavity was prepared, an impression was taken, and a provisional filling was positioned. A few days later, the adhesive partial restorations were cemented in accordance with the protocol described in the chapters on adhesion and cavity preparation (chapters 2 and 3). Figures 173 VII and VIII show the occlusal and interproximal aspects of the inlays, revealing good contact surfaces and emergence profiles.
In the mandibular left (third) quadrant, it was significant that the preparations and of course the cementation could be conducted in full surgical isolation with the use of rubber dam. These procedures were followed by clinical and radiographic checkups showing intact marginal seals, maintenance of pulp vitality, and a very satisfactory level of wear.
Additional clinical cases are presented in Figs 174 to 184.

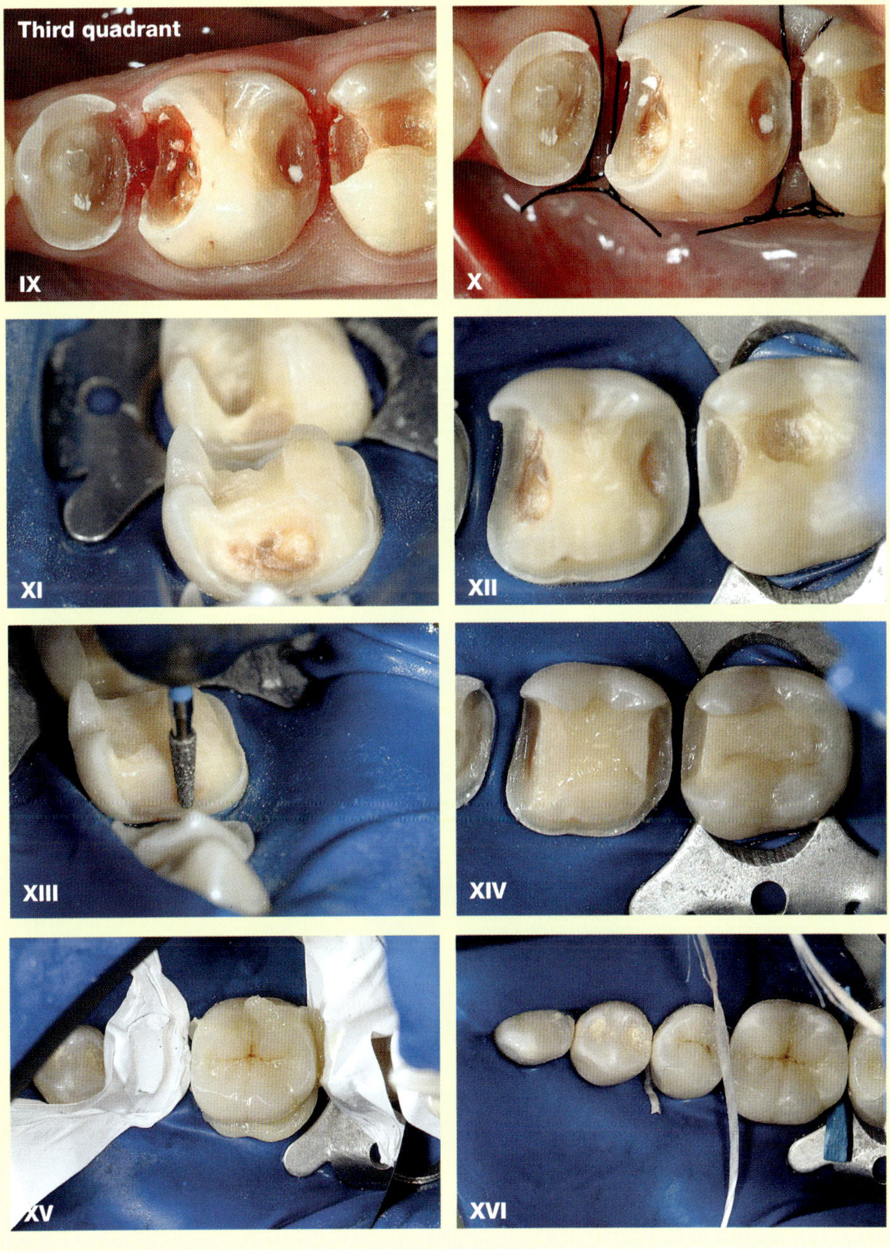

Fig 173 *(continued)*

Fig 173 *(continued)*

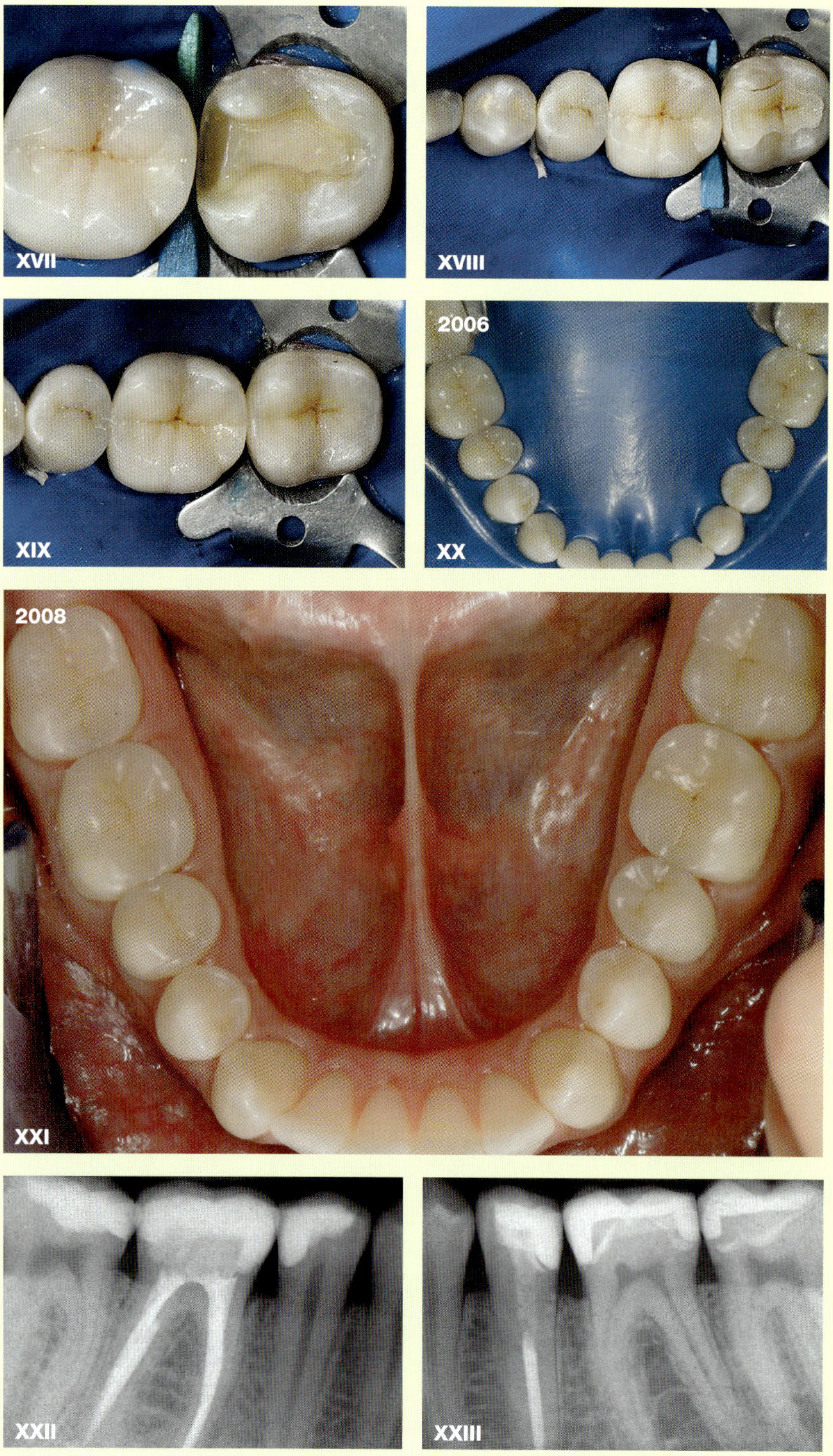

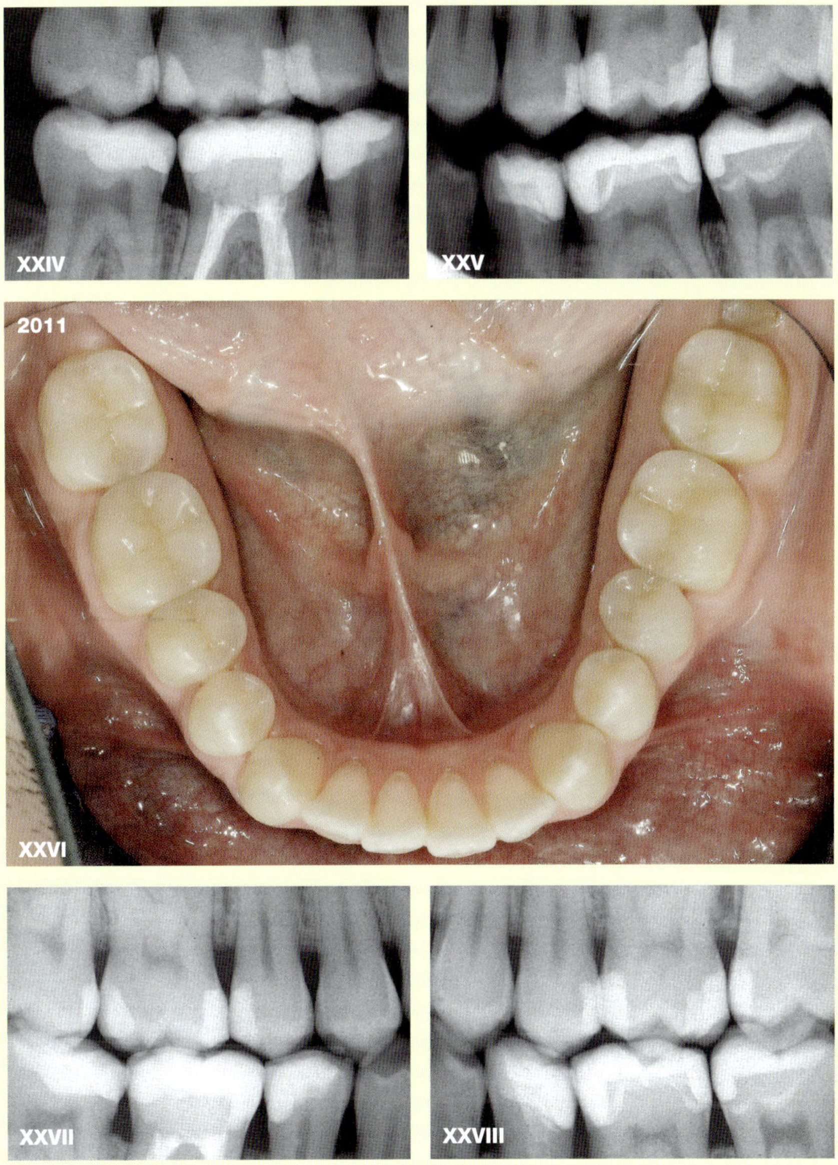

Fig 173 *(continued)*

Clinical case 2

Fig 174 Preoperative bitewing radiograph in a young patient who presented because of pains of pulpal origin in the mandibular left quadrant. Note the defective restorations and multiple, deep caries lesions *(I, II)*. Cementation stage of an inlay in the maxillary left quadrant and view of the inlay after cementing indirect restorations on both premolars and the first and second molars *(III, IV)*. Occlusal views of arches and radiographic status at the end of treatment *(V–VII)*. Clinical follow-up after 3 years *(VIII, IX)*.

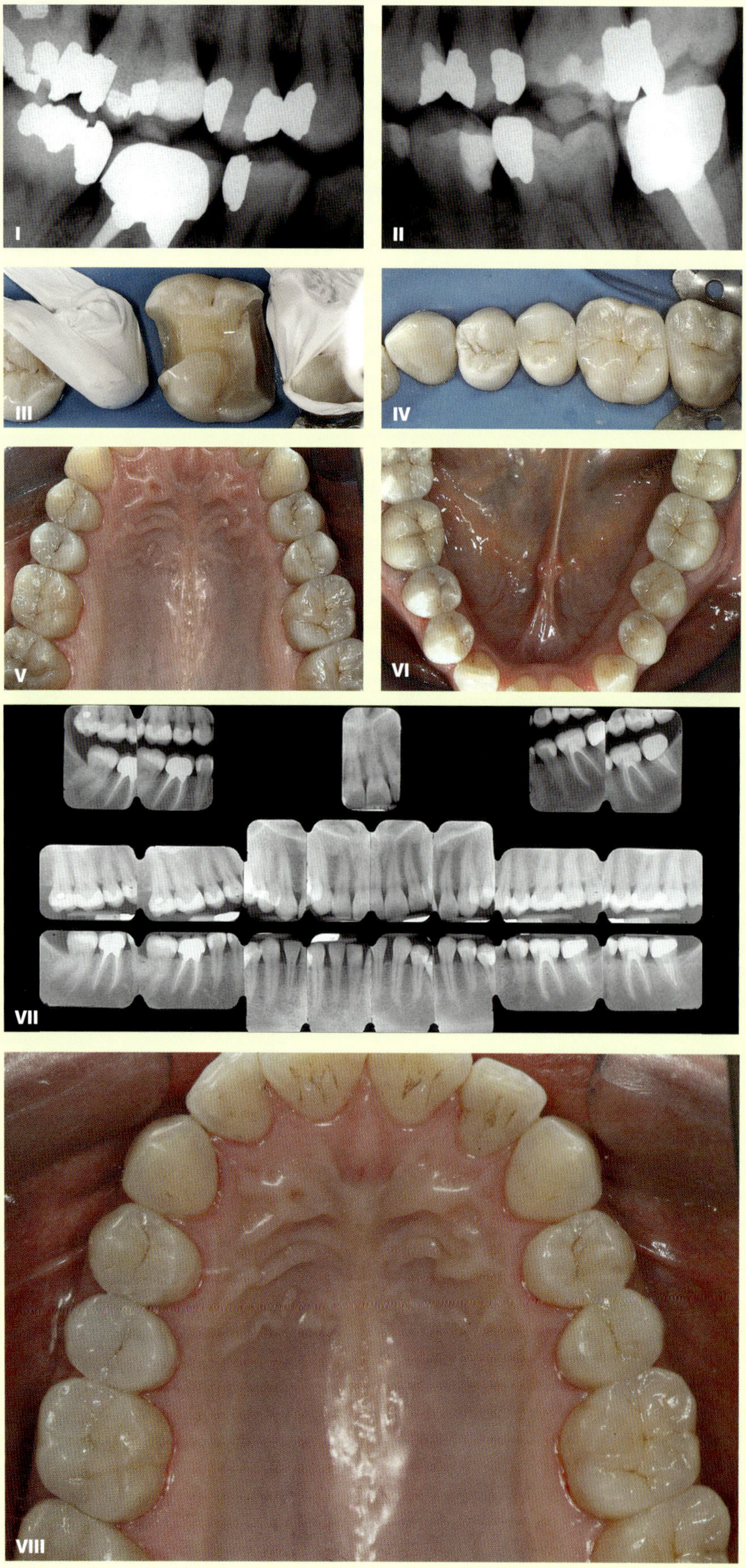

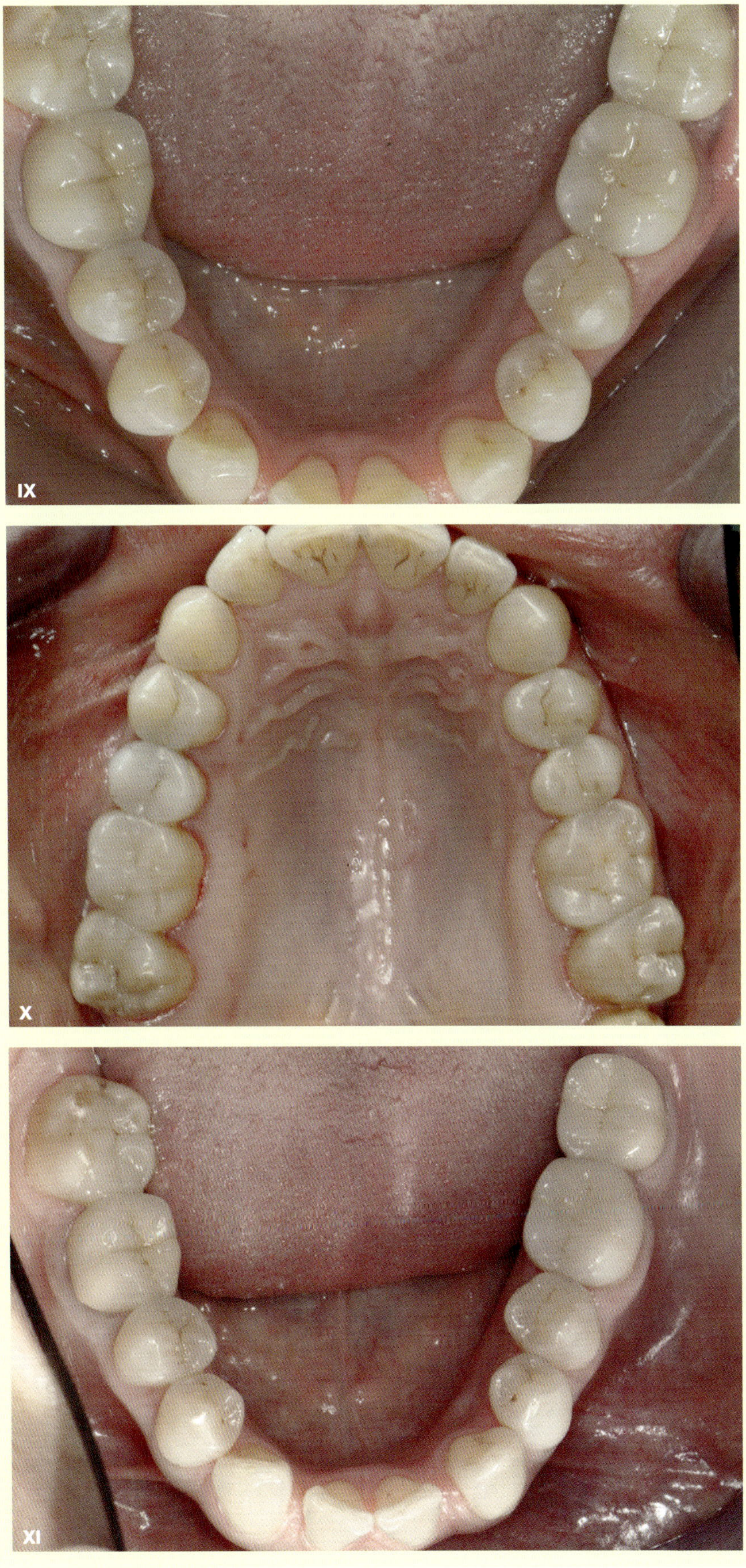

Fig 174 *(continued)* Follow-up views of the maxilla after 5 years *(X)* and the mandible after 4 years *(XI)*.

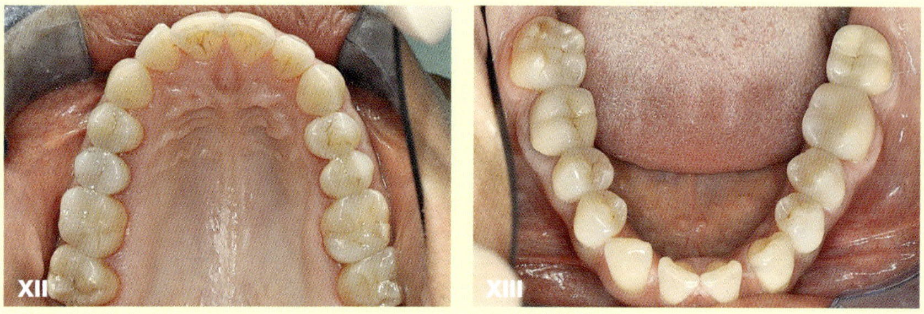

Fig 174 *(continued)* Follow-up views of the maxilla after 8 years *(XII)* and the mandible after 10 years *(XIII)*.

Clinical case 3

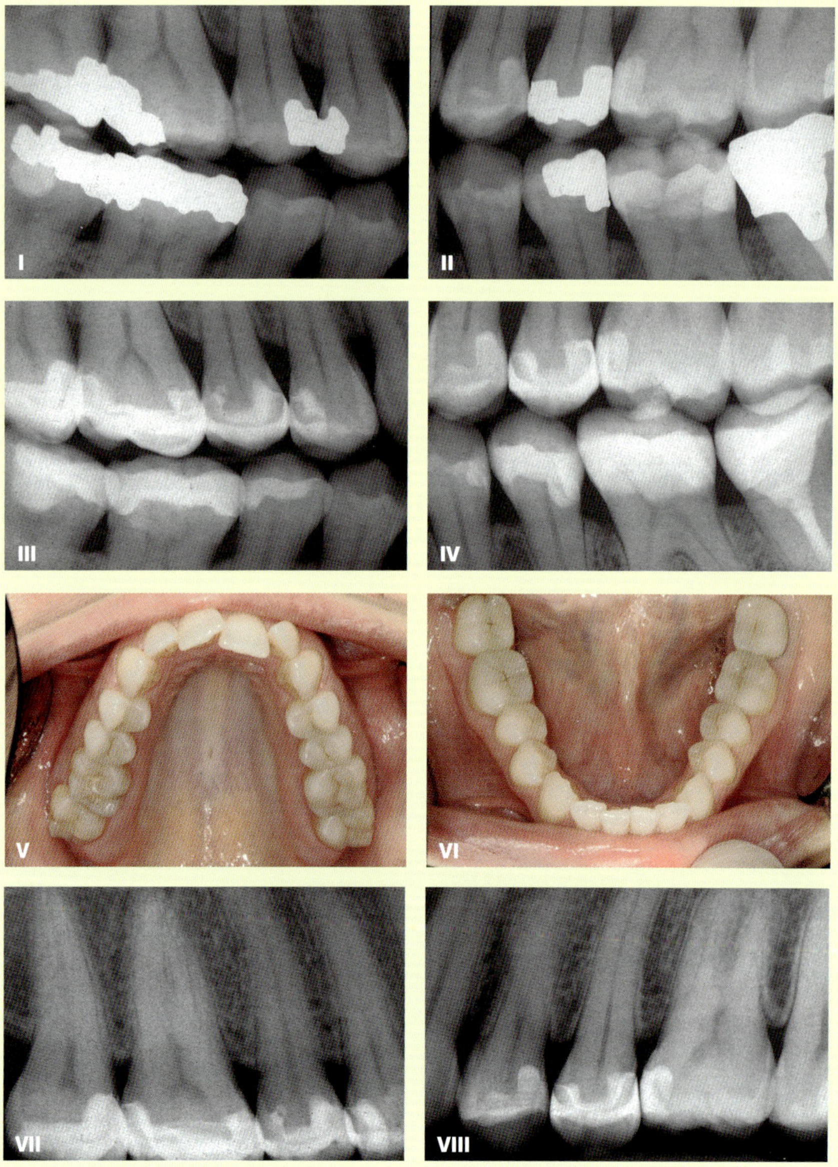

Fig 175 Pre- and postoperative bitewing radiographs of indirect restorations on a young patient *(I–IV)*. Clinical and radiographic follow-up after 2 years *(V–X)*. Clinical follow-ups after 3 *(XI, XII)* and 4 years *(XIII, XIV)*.

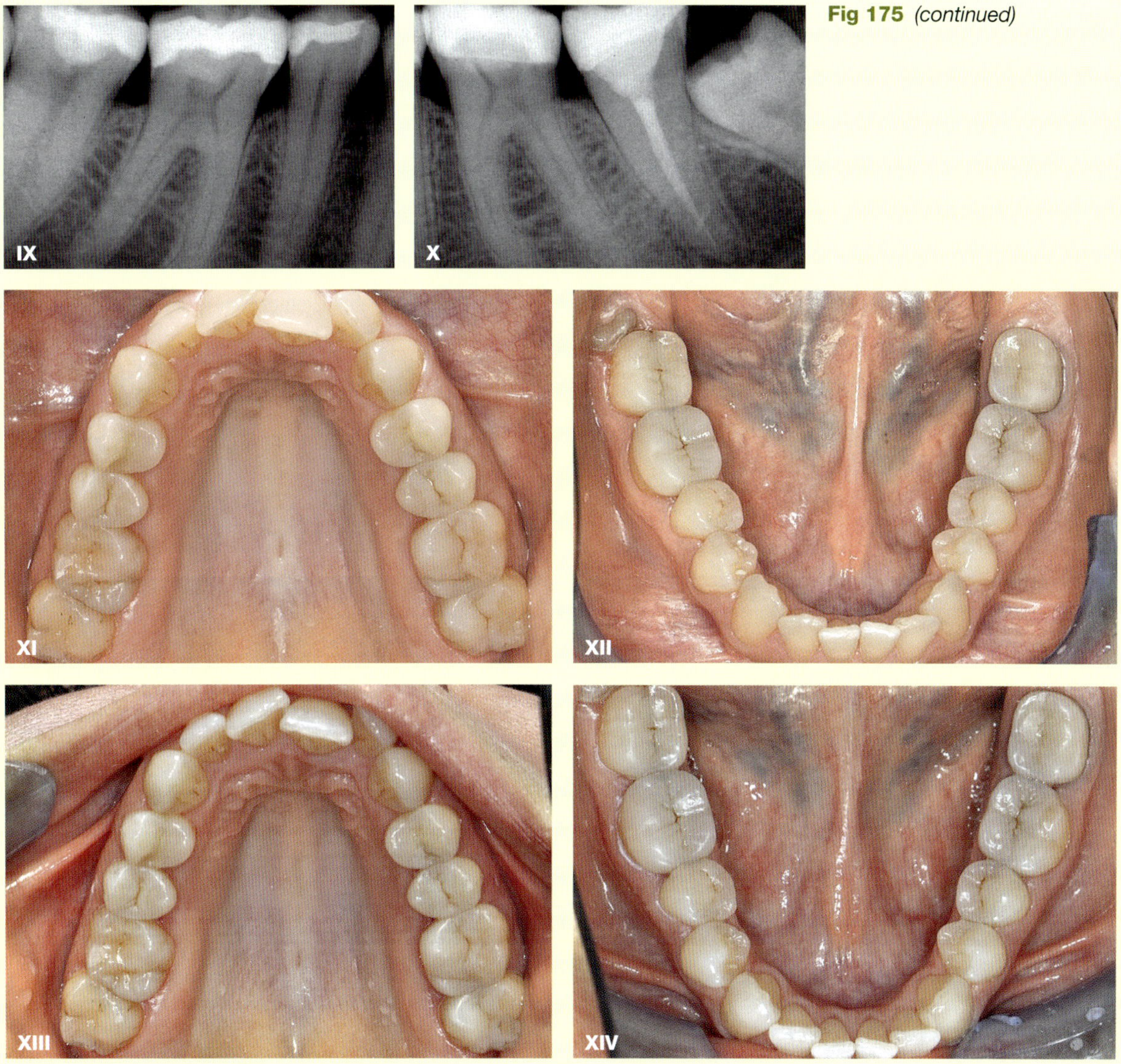

Fig 175 *(continued)*

Clinical case 4

Fig 176 Preoperative bitewing radiographs and occlusal and lateral views of arches after cementation of restorations *(I–VI)*. The sutures were removed during the same session after cementation, which was no more than 1 week after the preparations.

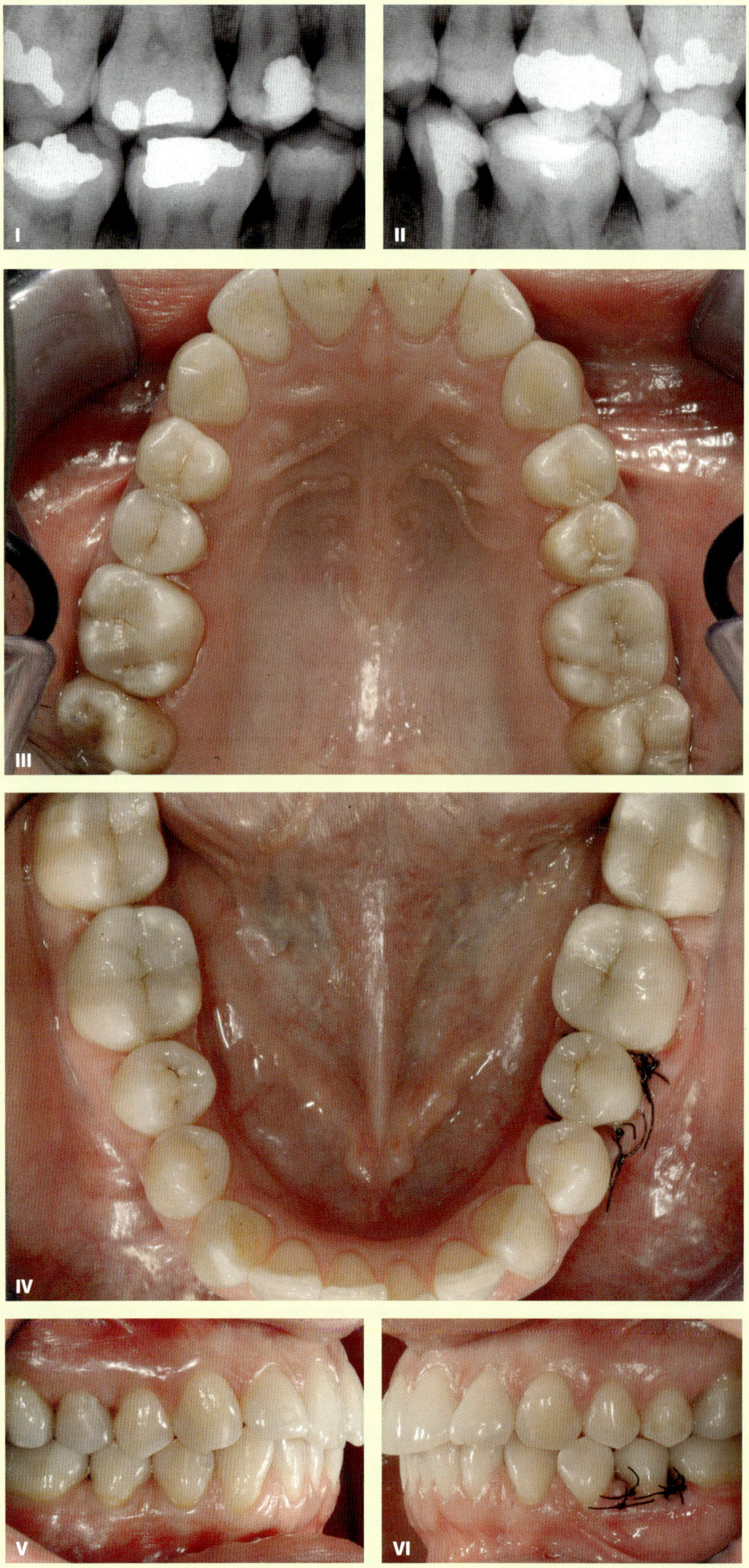

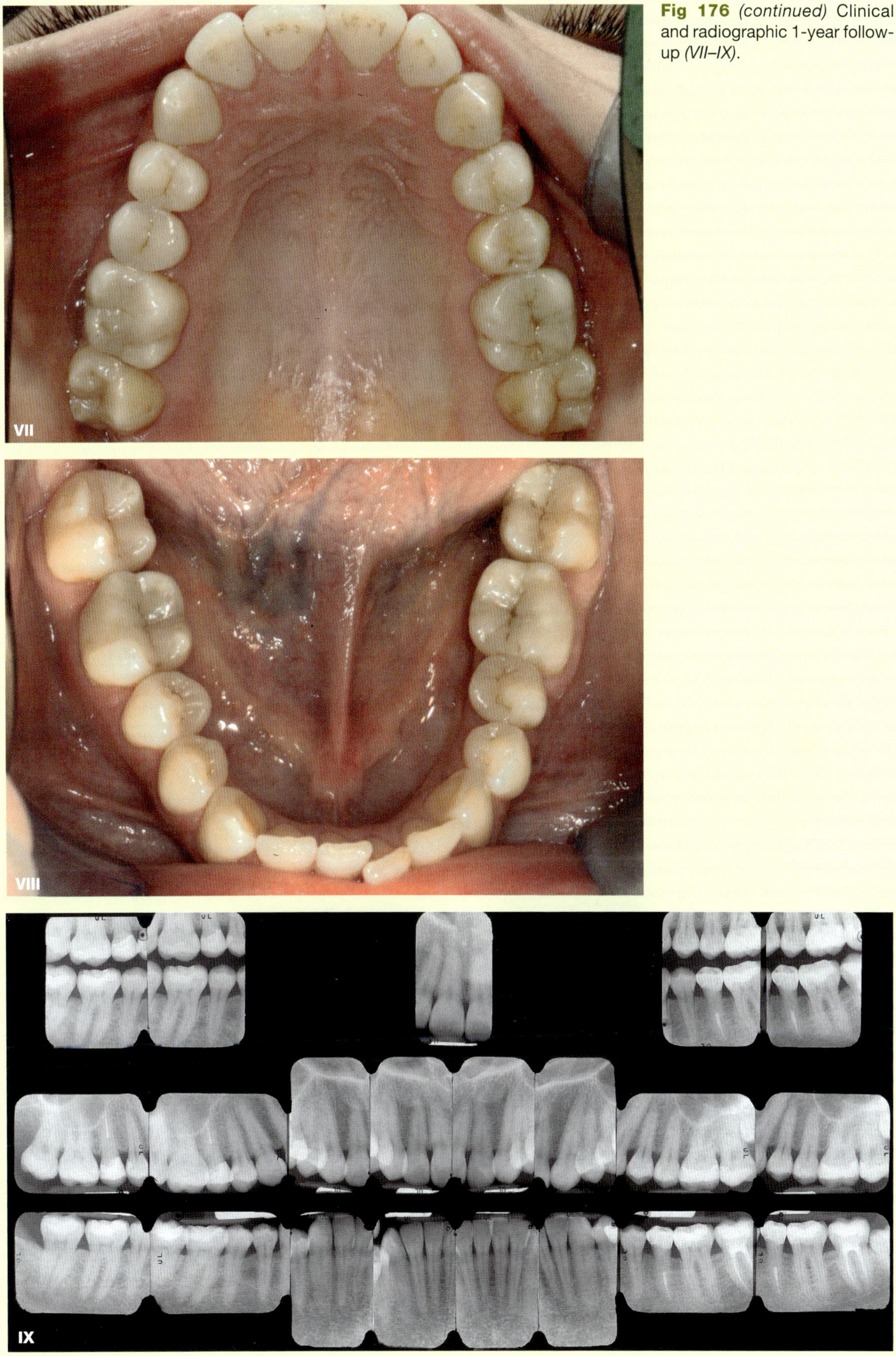

Fig 176 *(continued)* Clinical and radiographic 1-year follow-up *(VII–IX)*.

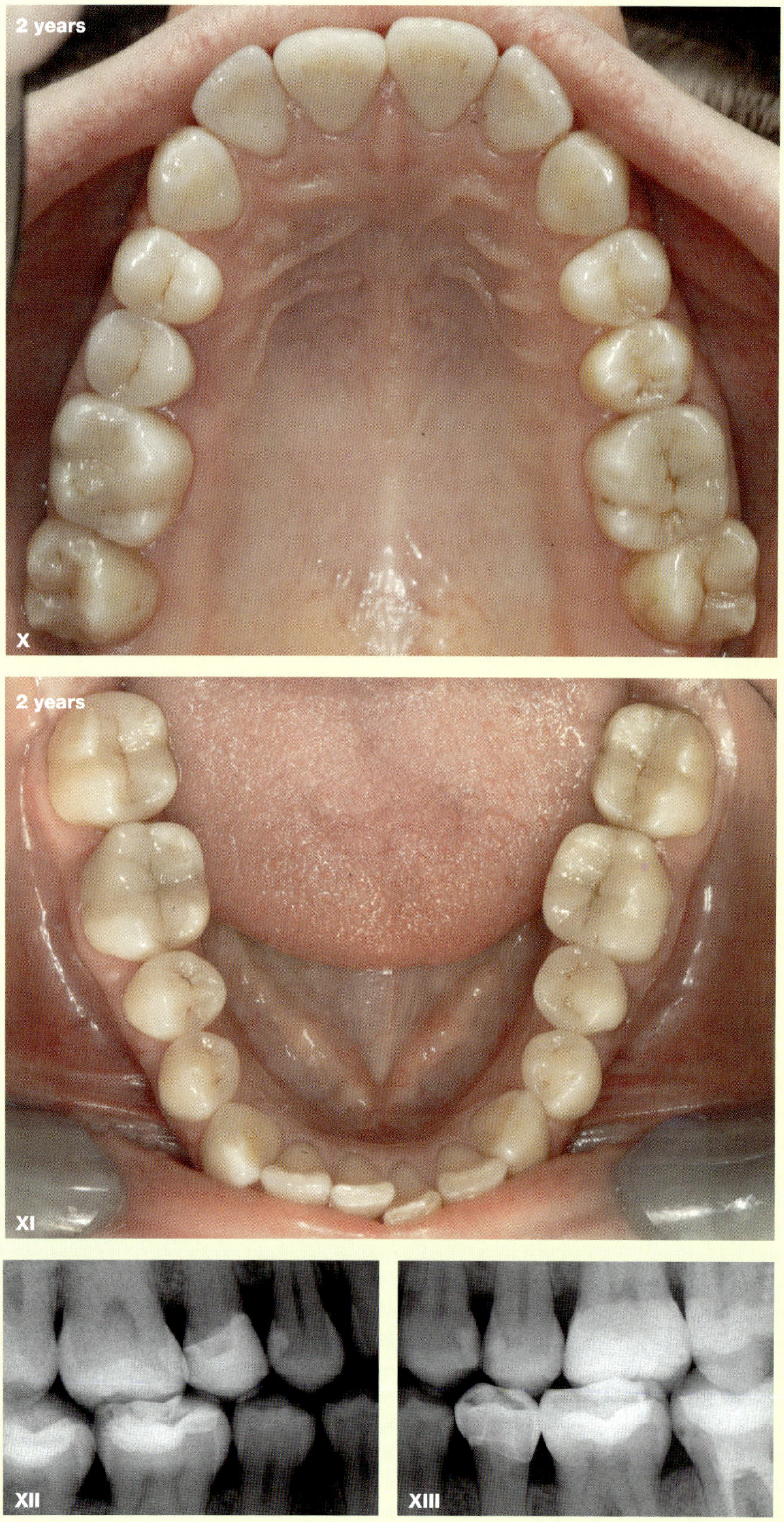

Fig 176 *(continued)* Follow-up after 2 years *(X–XIII)*. Clinical and radiographic 5-year follow-up *(XIV–XVII)*.

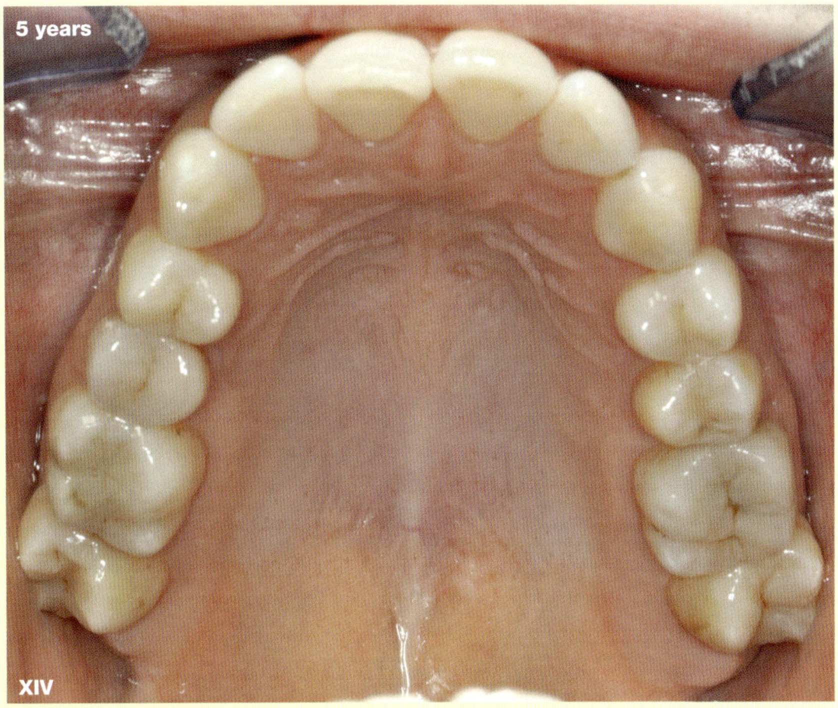

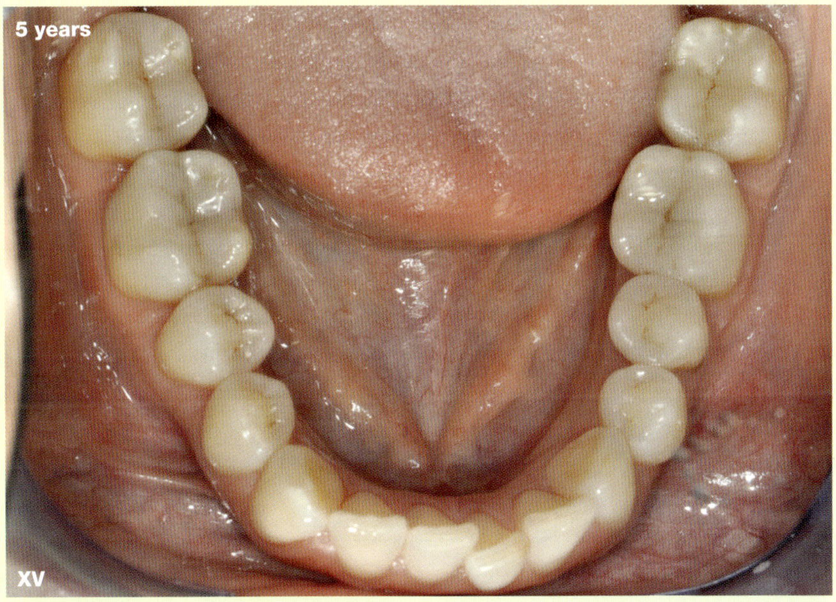

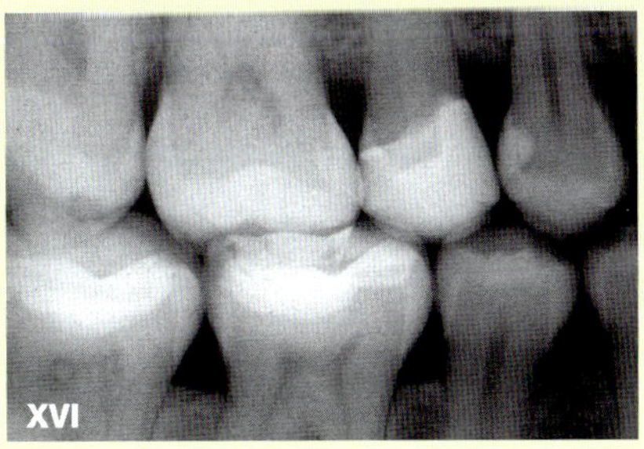

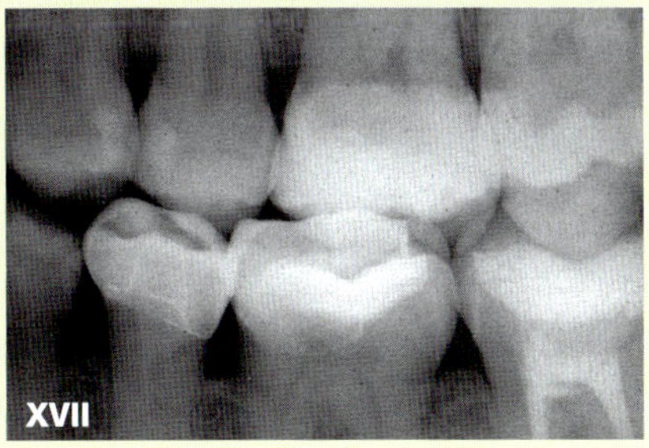

Fig 176 *(continued)*

Clinical case 5

Fig 177 Preoperative radiographs and views of the arches *(I–IV)*. Intraoperative stages in the maxillary left (second) quadrant; cementation of the first molar restoration was extremely difficult *(V–VII)*.

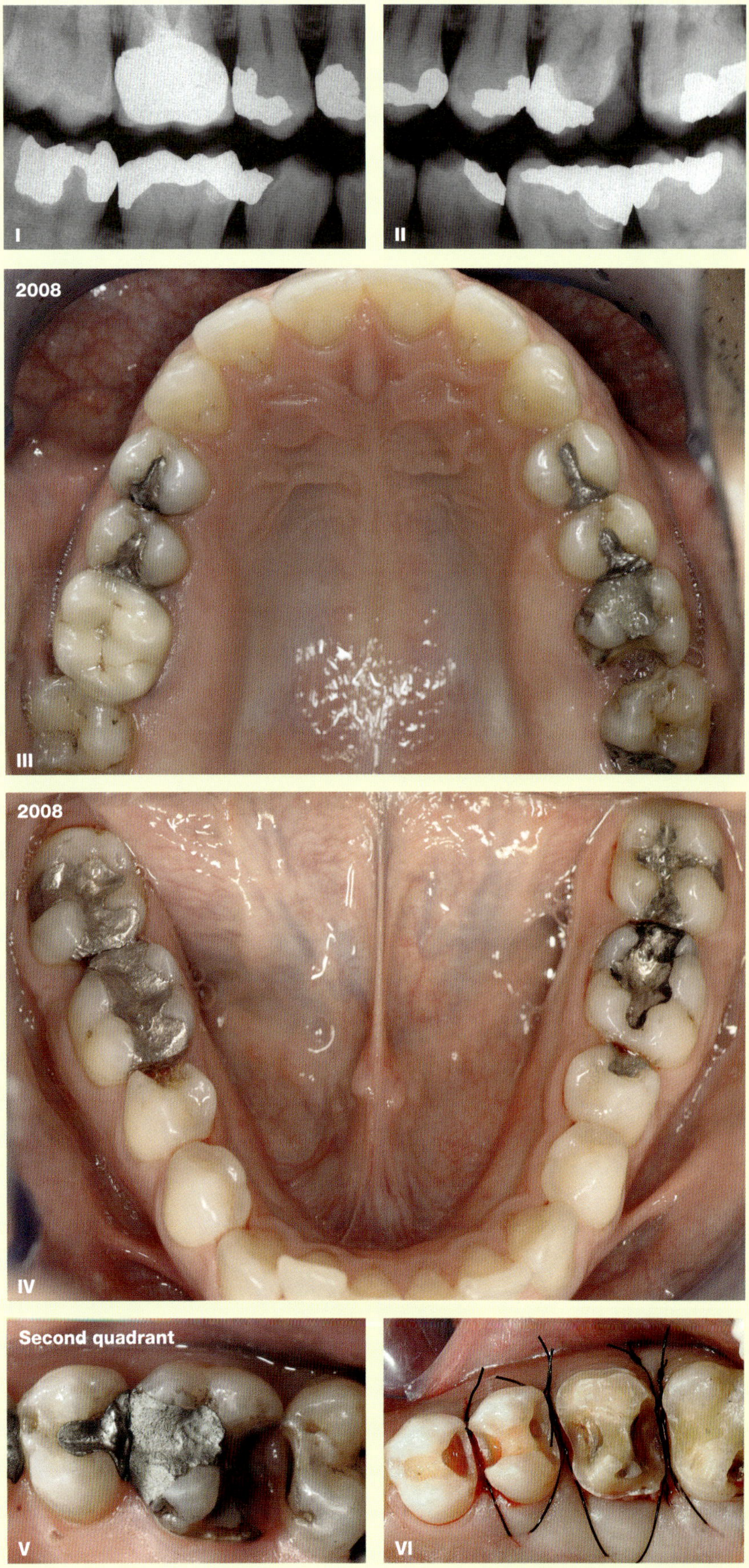

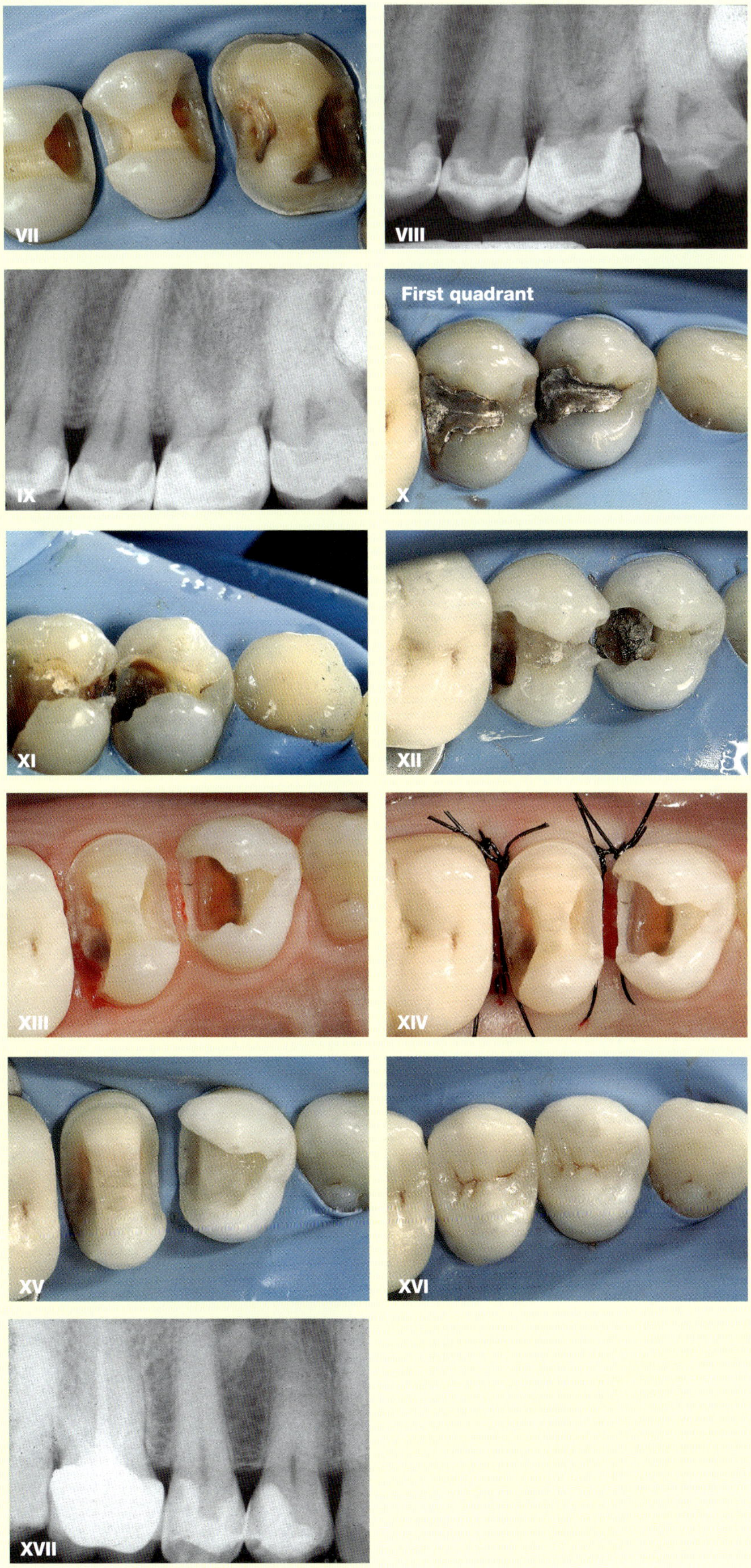

Fig 177 *(continued)* An intraoperative radiograph *(VIII)*, obviously taken prior to curing, showed an unacceptable distal margin seal. It was therefore necessary to remove the inlay and the composite used as cement and then clean the preparation in order to repeat the cementation *(IX)*. Intraoperative and postoperative views of the maxillary right (first) quadrant, where an old prosthetic crown was replaced by an overlay with supragingival margins *(X–XIX)*.

Fig 177 *(continued)* Maxilla after cementation of inlays *(XX)*. Finalization of the mandibular right (fourth) quadrant and radiographic follow-up *(XXI–XXVI)*.

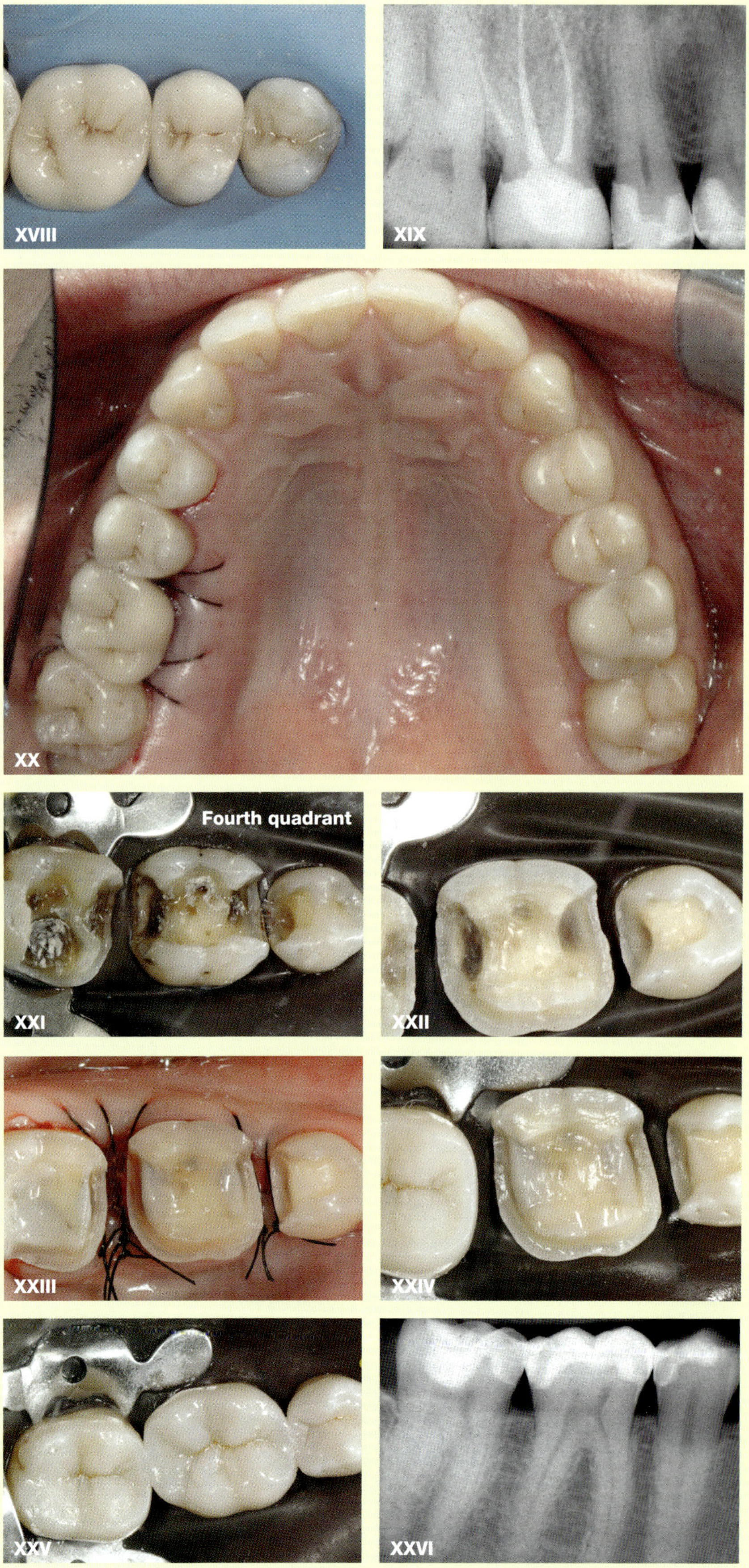

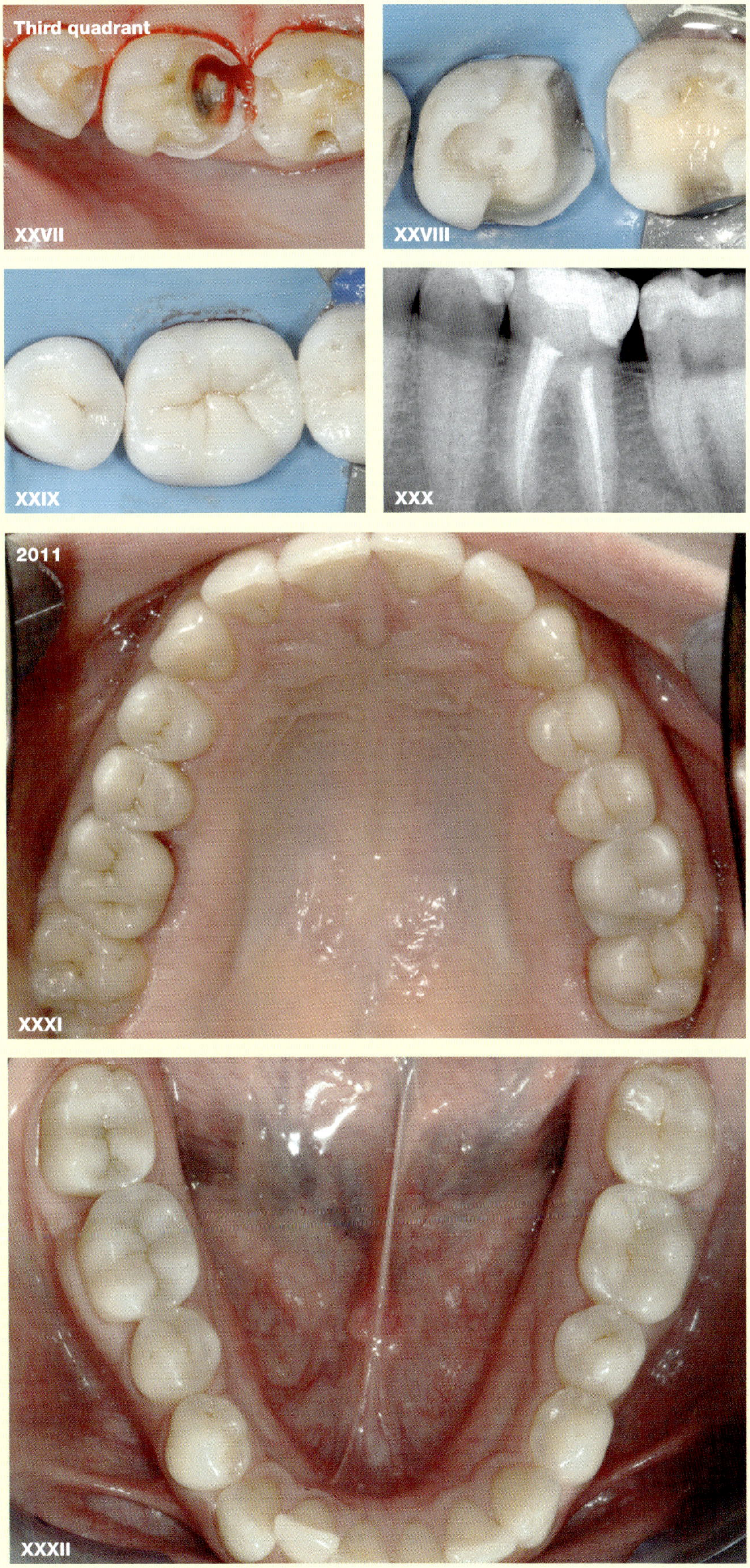

Fig 177 *(continued)* Difficulty in positioning rubber dam in order to isolate the surgical field properly in the mandibular left (third) quadrant, despite clinical lengthening of the crown and follow-up radiographs *(XX–VII–XXX)*.

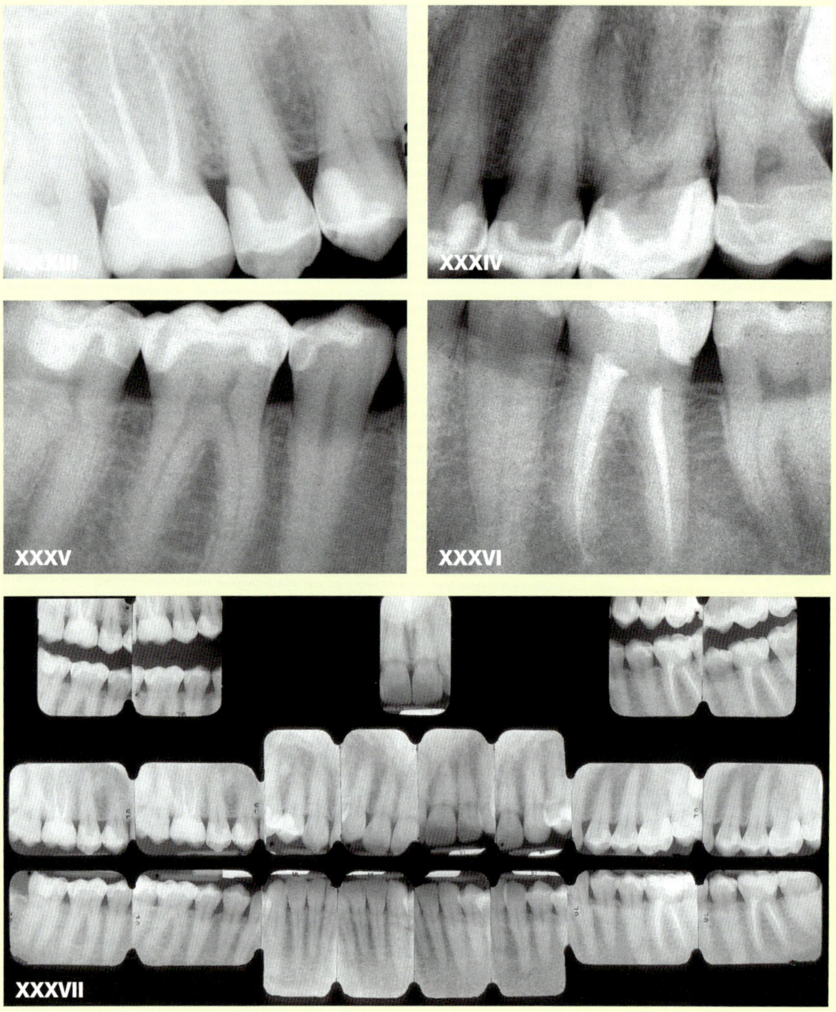

Fig 177 (*continued*) Clinical and radiographic follow-up after 3 years *(XXXI–XXXVII)*.

Clinical case 6

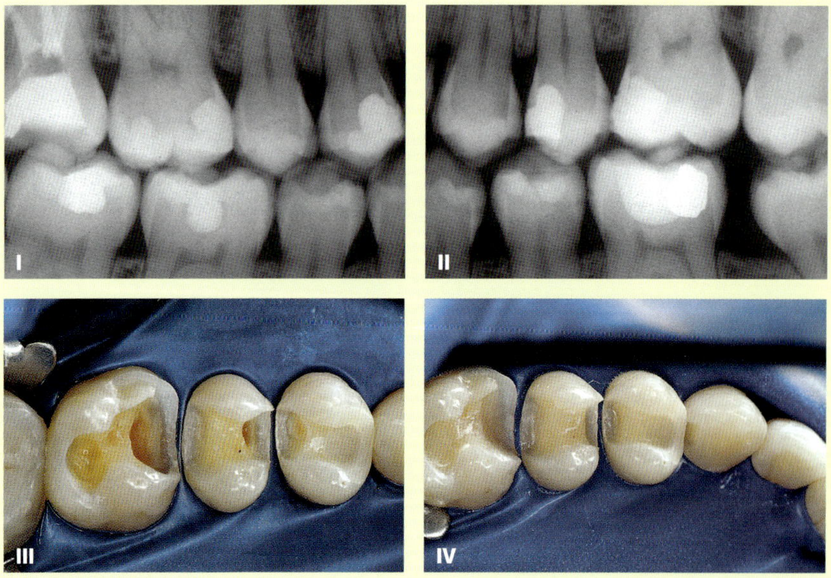

Fig 178 Preoperative bitewing radiographs *(I, II)*. Cemented preparations and inlays in maxillary right quadrant *(III–V)*.

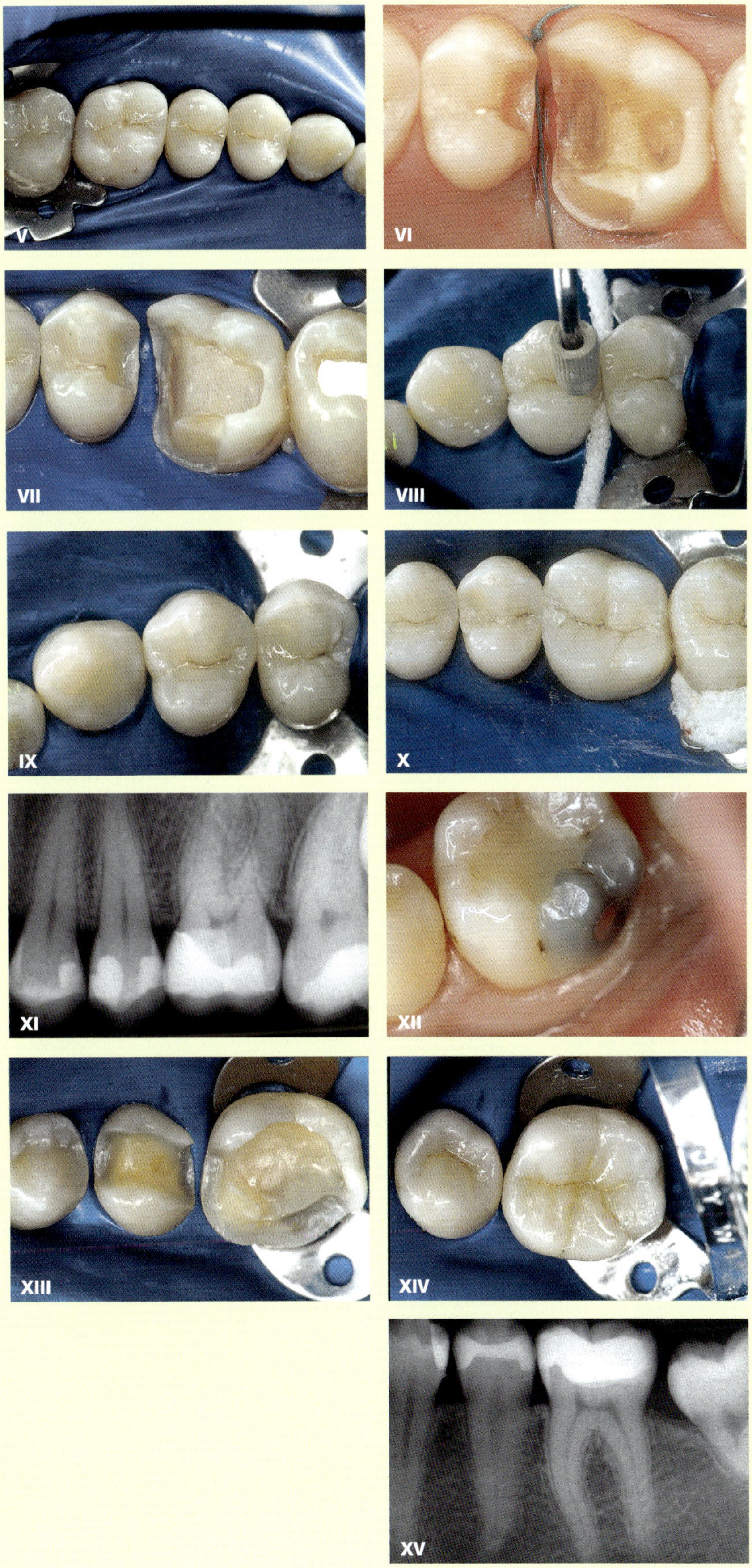

Fig 178 *(continued)* Periodontal surgery, preparations, cementation, and radiographic follow-up in the maxillary left quadrant *(VI–XI)*. Preparations, cemented inlays, and radiographic follow-up of the mandibular left quadrant *(XII–XV)*.

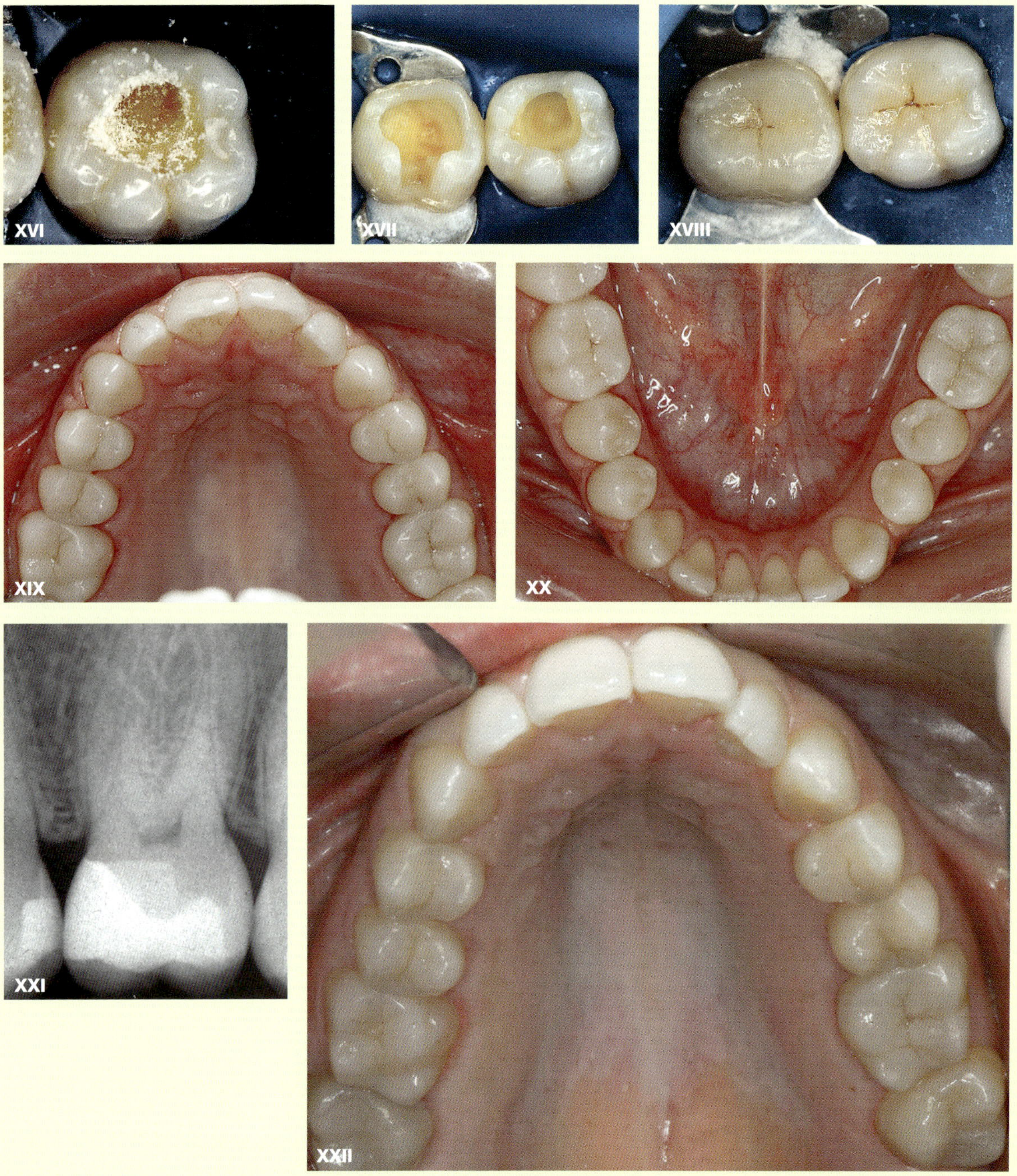

Fig 178 *(continued)* Restorations in the mandibular right quadrant *(XVI–XVIII)*. Follow-up after 2.5 years without any hygienist appointments as a result of problems in the patient's personal life *(XIX–XXI)*.

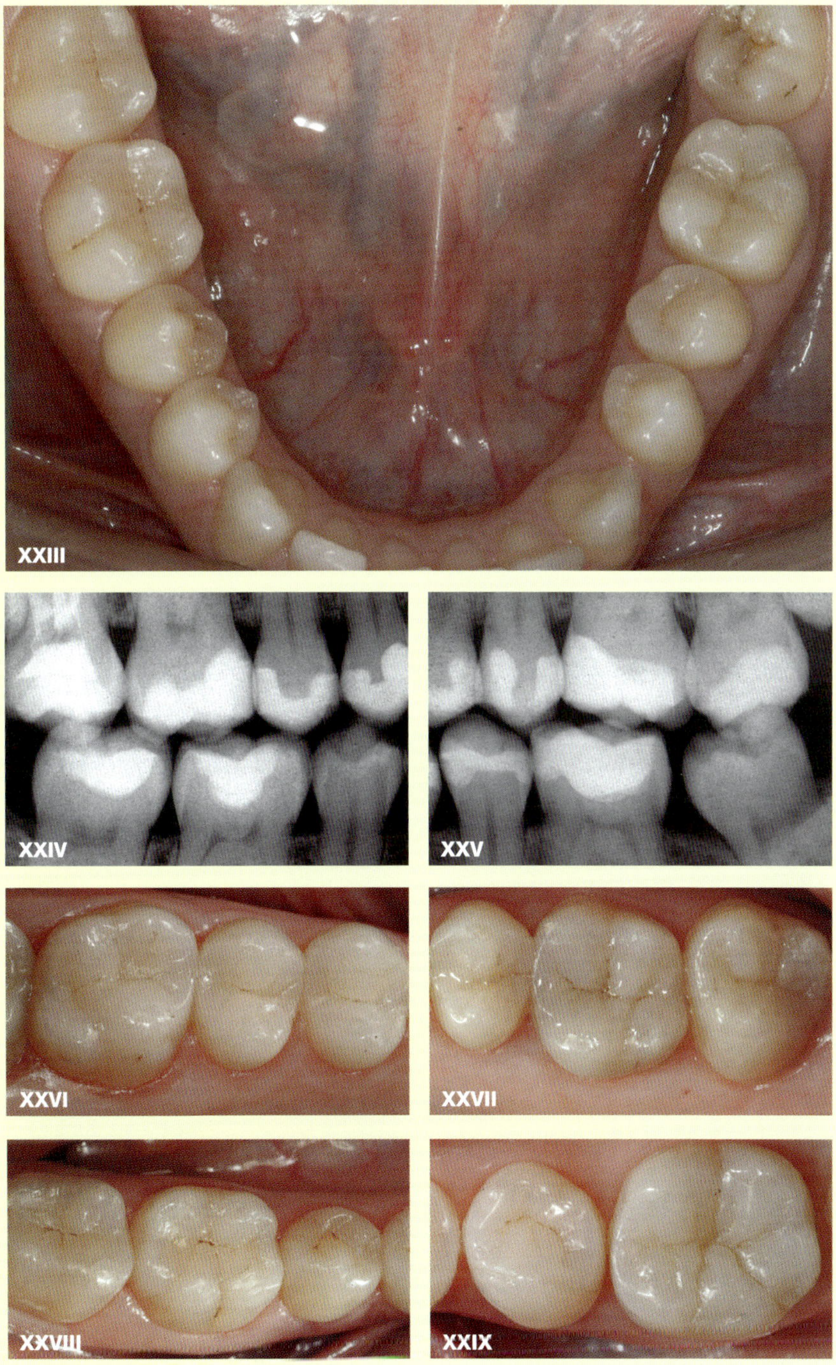

Fig 178 *(continued)* Clinical and radiographic follow-up after 5 years, showing excellent maintenance of the restorations *(XXII–XXIX)*.

Fig 178 *(continued)* Clinical and radiographic follow-up after 7 years *(XXX–XXXIII)*.

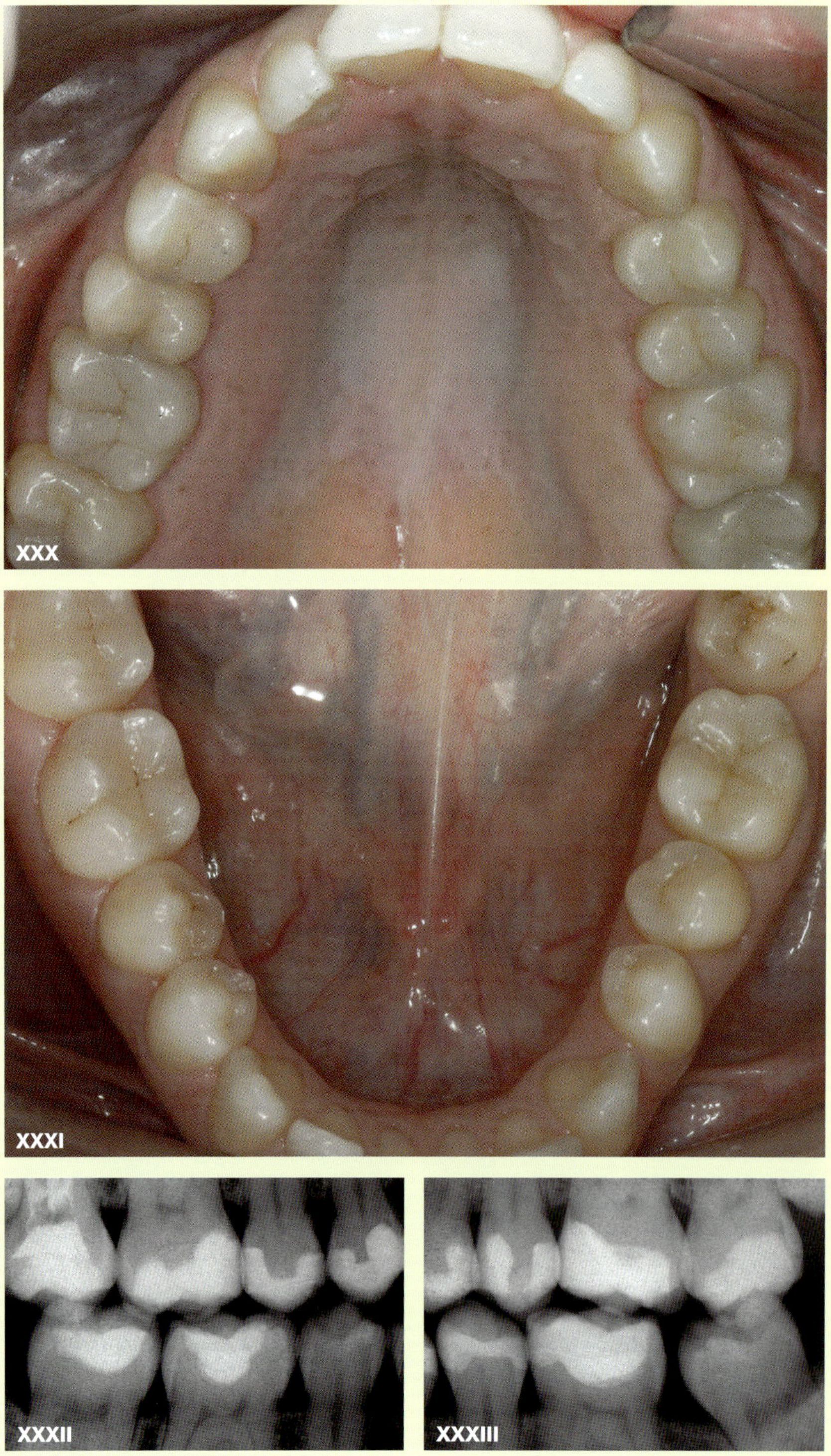

Clinical case 7

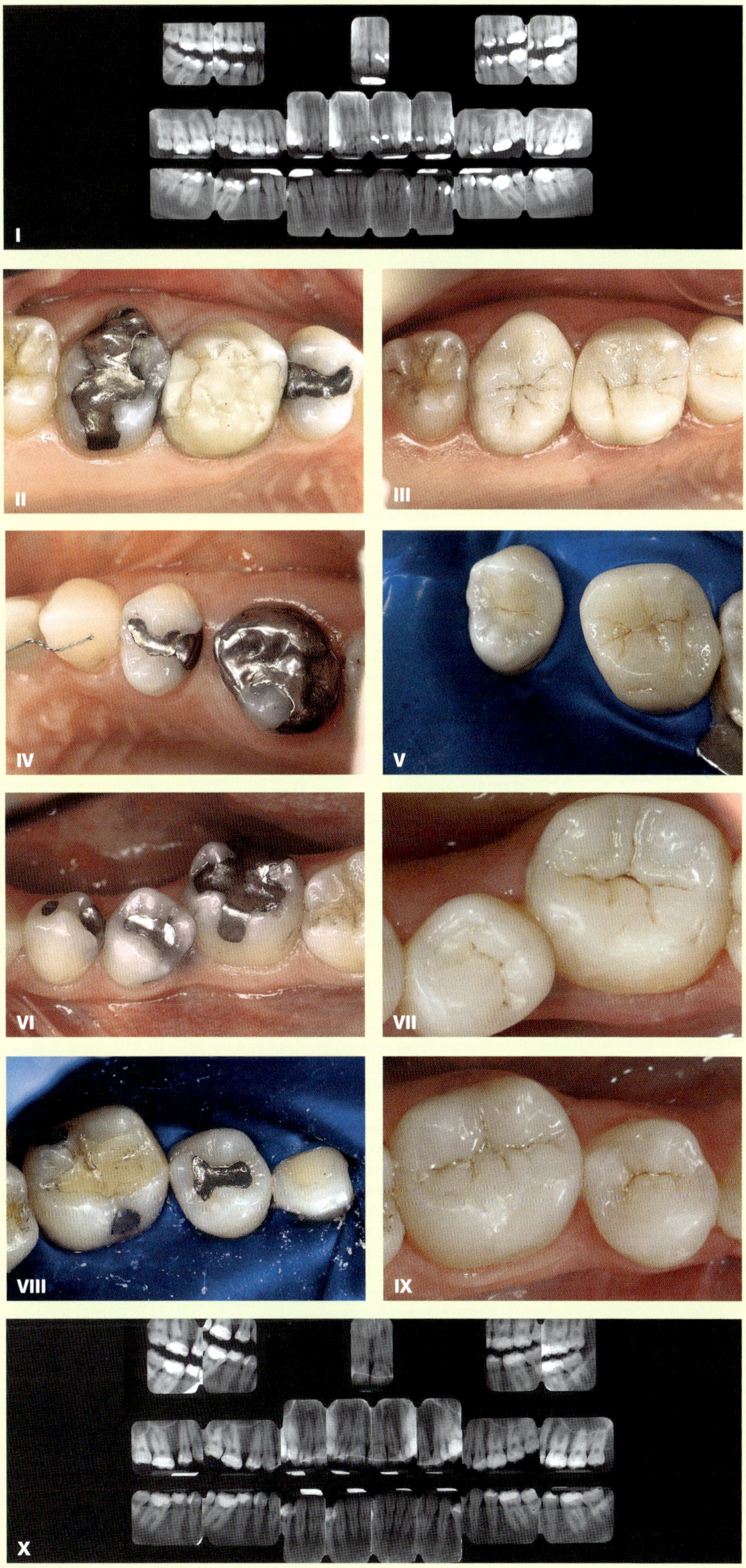

Fig 179 Preoperative radiographic status: amalgam fillings in the anterior teeth, large defective restorations in the posterior teeth, and compromised maxillary left second premolar *(I)*. The patient refused orthodontic treatment. Replacement of the old restorations with composite inlays *(II–IX)*. Radiographic follow-up after 3 years: none of the teeth were endodontically treated *(X)*.

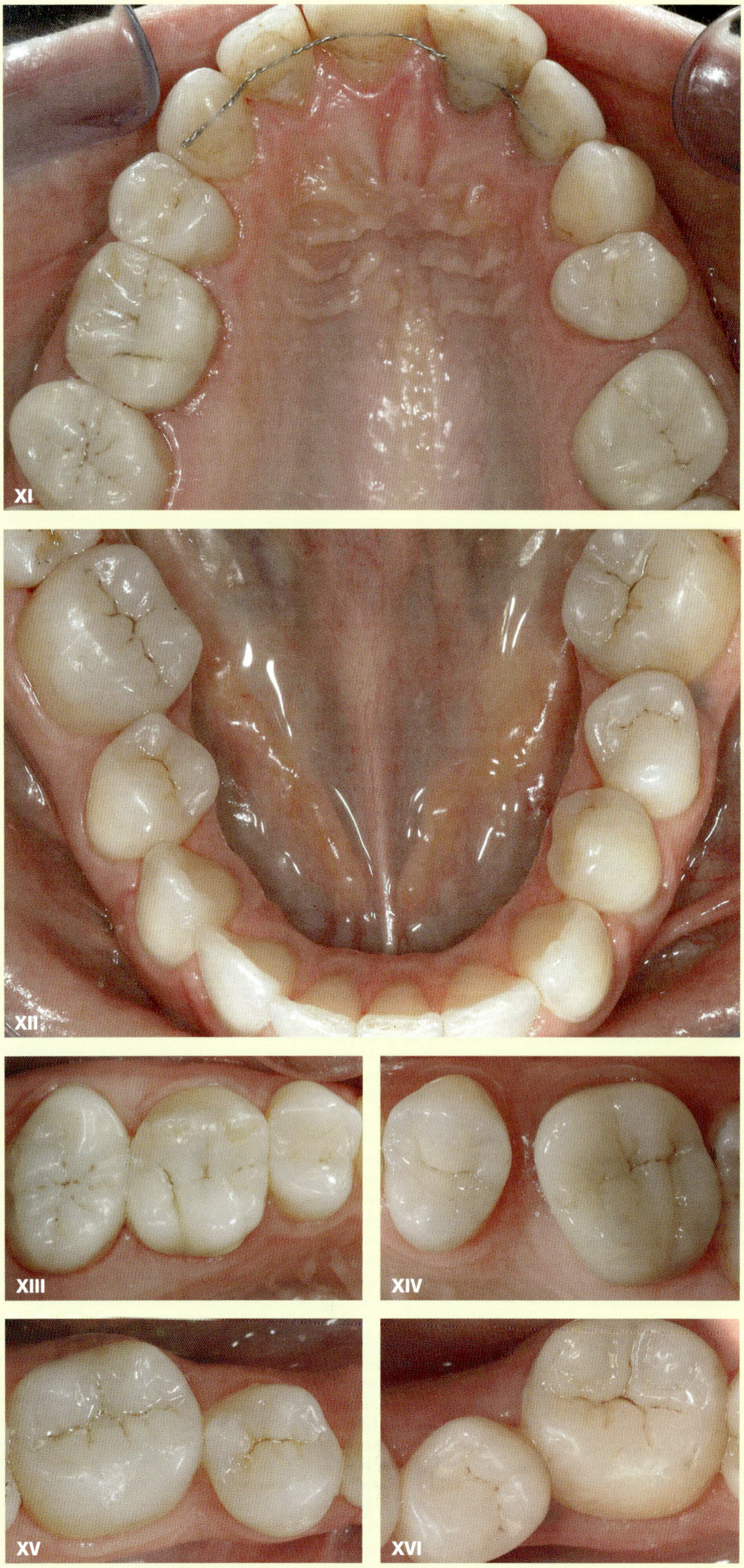

Fig 179 *(continued)* Clinical follow-up after 5 and 6 years: all the treated teeth responded positively to electric and heat tests *(XI–XVI)*.

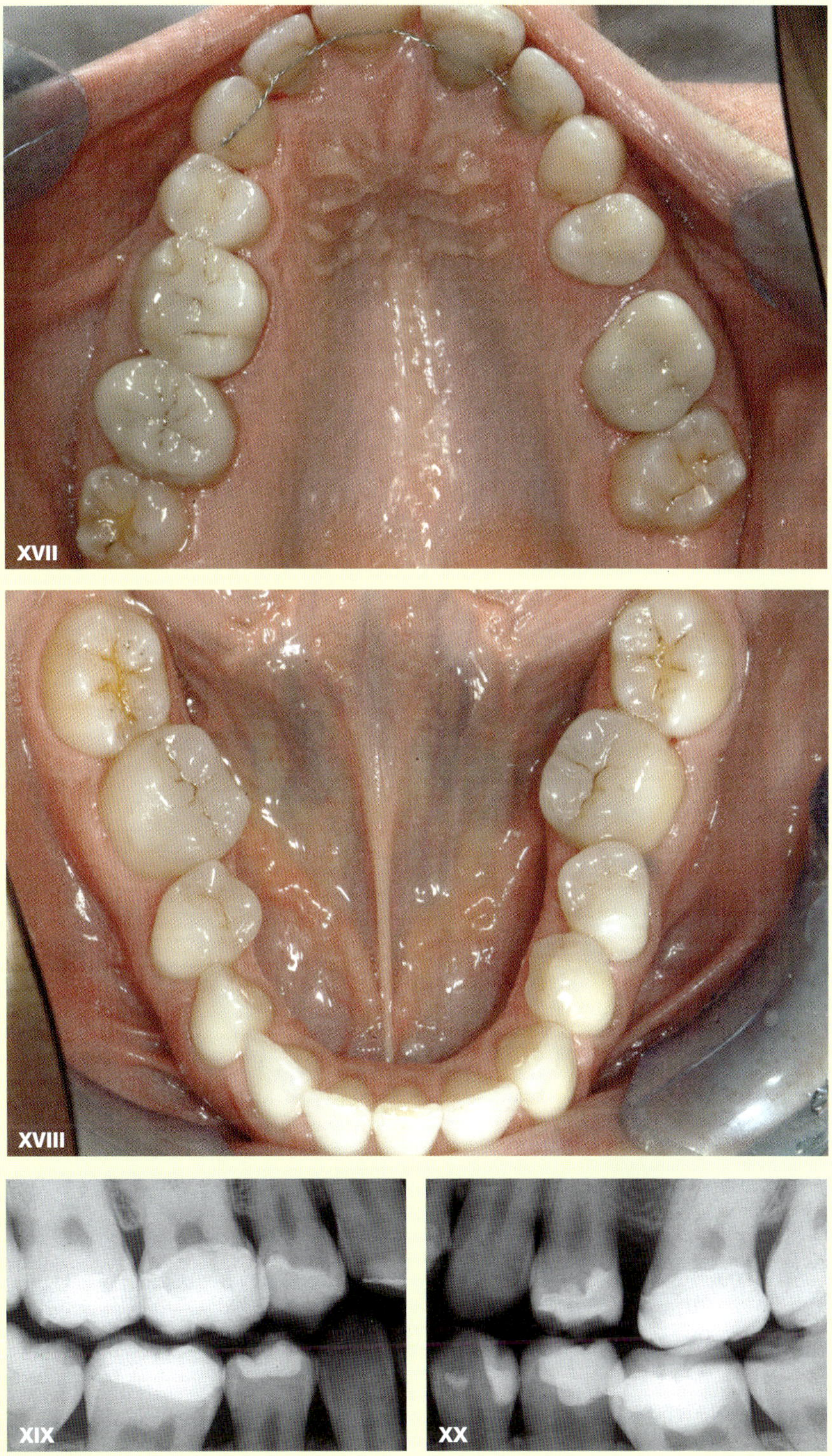

Fig 179 *(continued)* Clinical and radiographic follow-up after 8 and 9 years *(XVII–XX)*.

Fig 179 *(continued)* The patient's clinical record. After the delivery of the inlays in 2003, the patient only underwent hygienist visits and clinical and radiographic checkups for 8 years *(XXI, XXII)*.

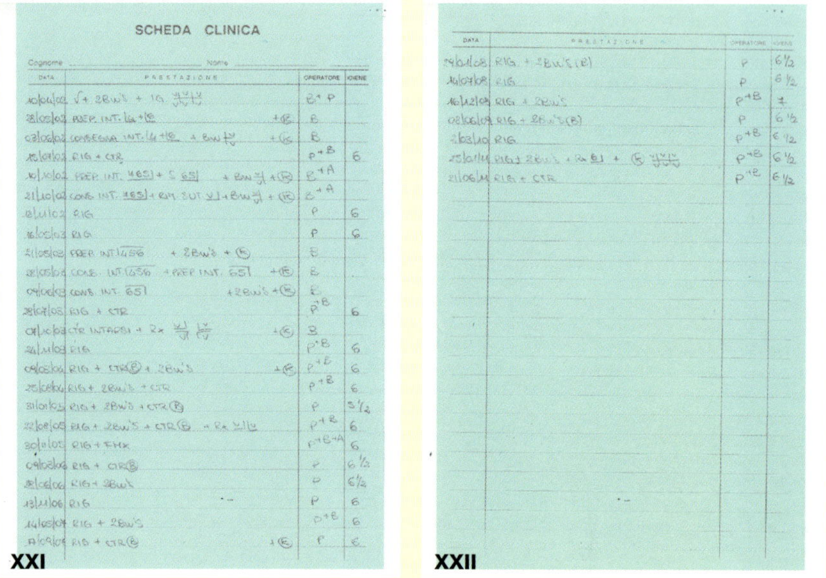

Clinical case 8

Fig 180 Preoperative bitewing radiograph of a 20-year-old patient who presented after noticing a "black spot" on the mandibular right second molar *(I, II)*. Clinical appearance of the completely asymptomatic caries lesion and restorations of the first and second molars *(III–VII)*.

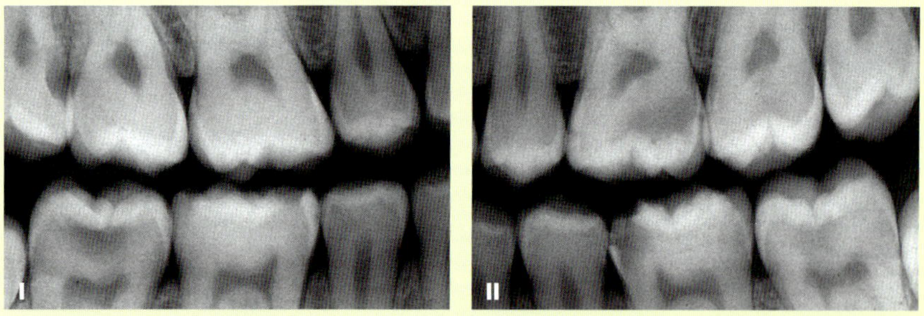

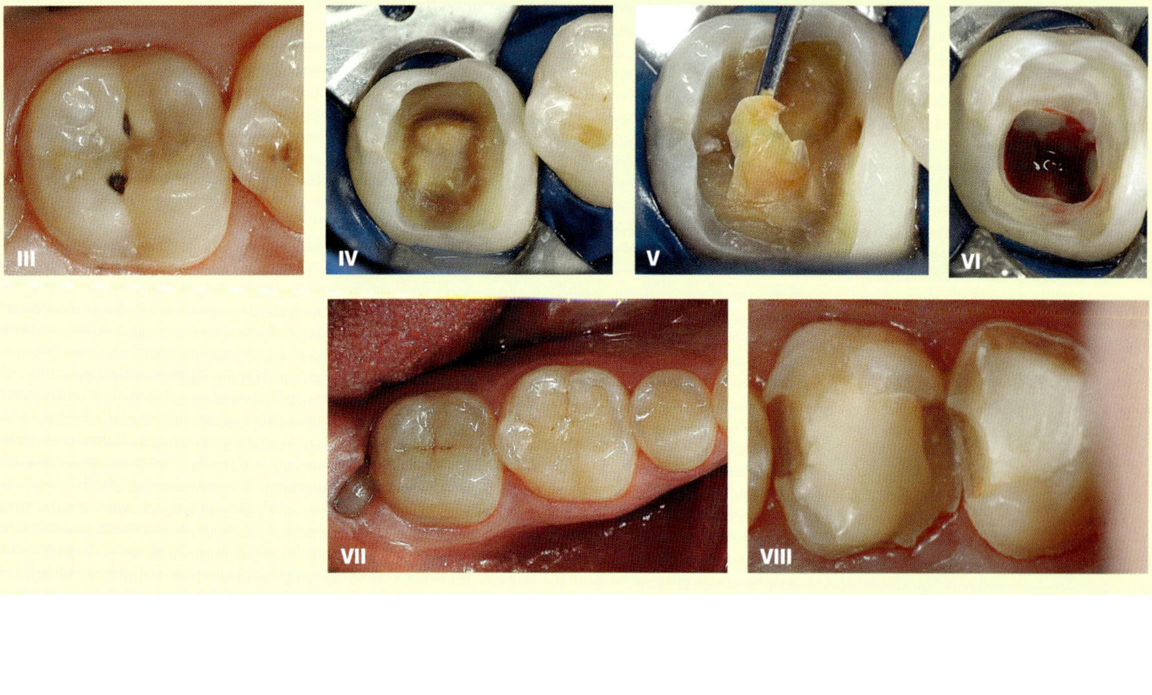

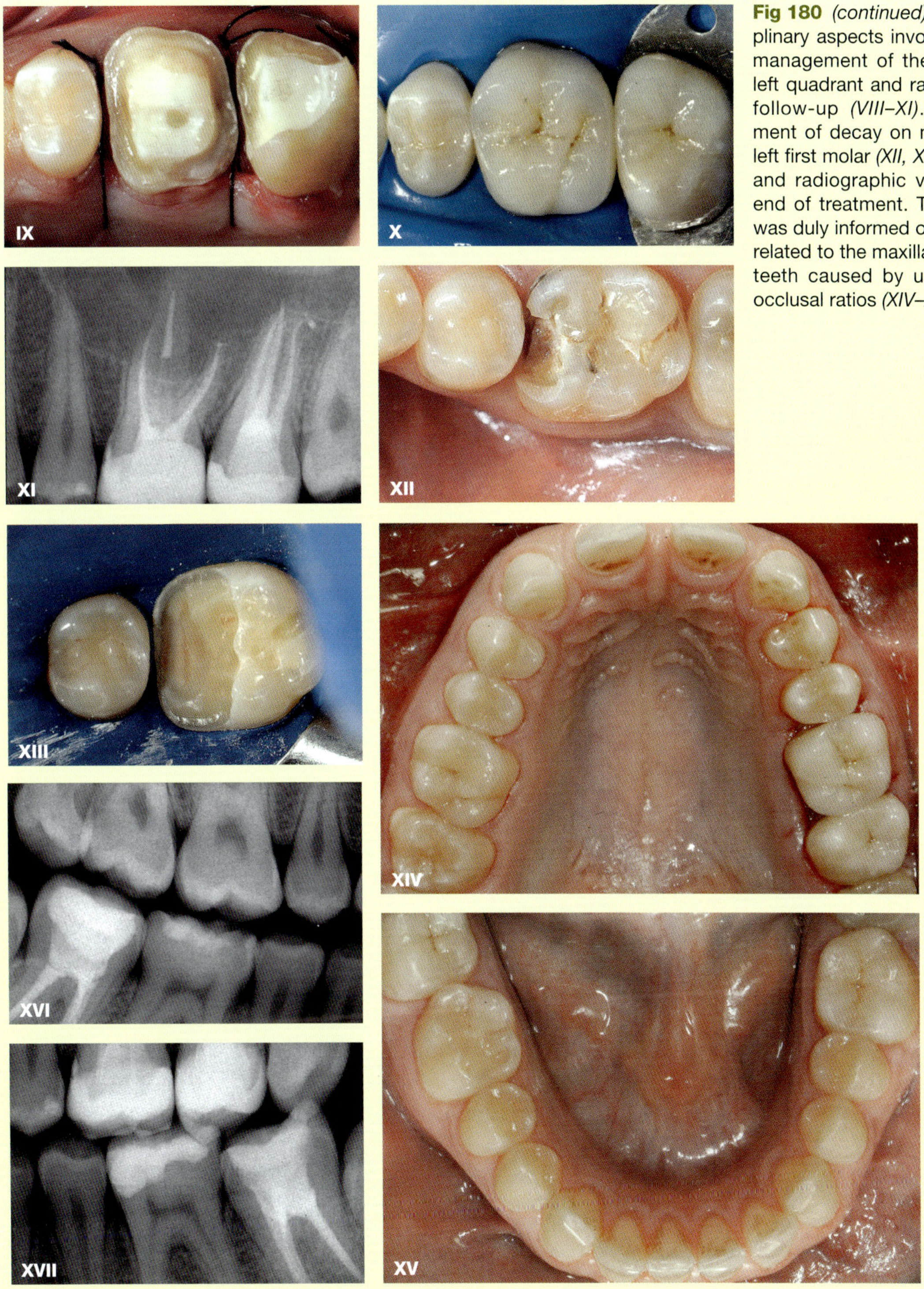

Fig 180 *(continued)* Interdisciplinary aspects involved in the management of the maxillary left quadrant and radiographic follow-up *(VIII–XI)*. Management of decay on mandibular left first molar *(XII, XIII)*. Clinical and radiographic view at the end of treatment. The patient was duly informed of problems related to the maxillary anterior teeth caused by unfavorable occlusal ratios *(XIV–XVII)*.

Clinical case 9

Fig 181 Preoperative bitewing radiographs *(I, II)* and clinical and radiographic follow-up after 6 years *(III–VI)*.

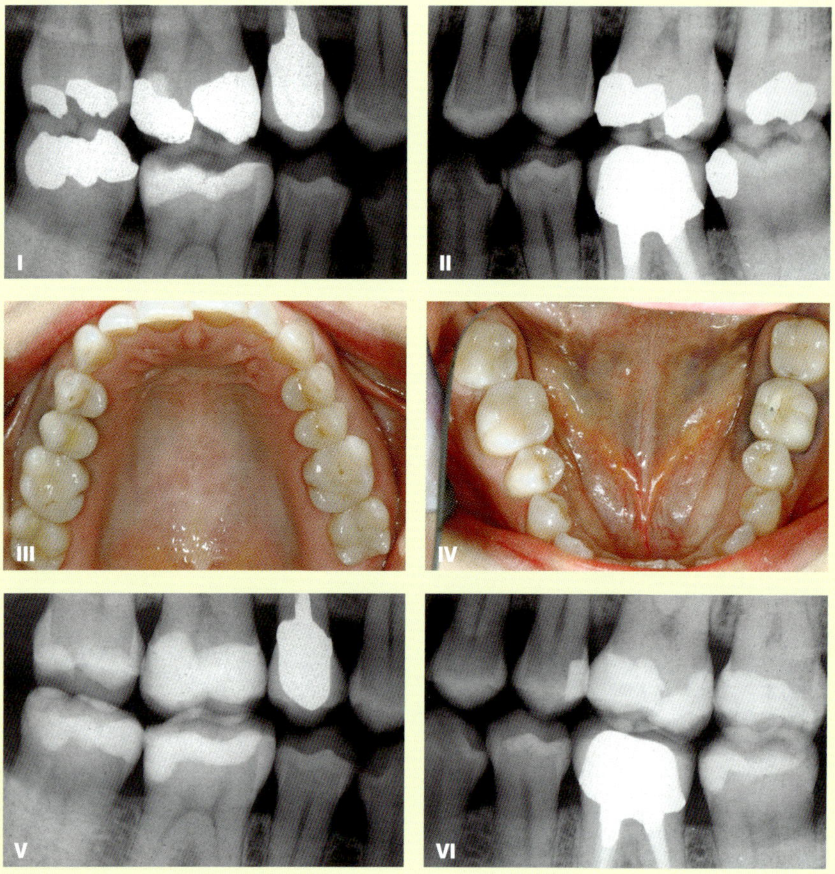

Clinical case 10

Fig 182 Preoperative bitewing radiographs *(I, II)*. Procedural stages in the management of the mandibular right (fourth) quadrant *(III–VII)*.

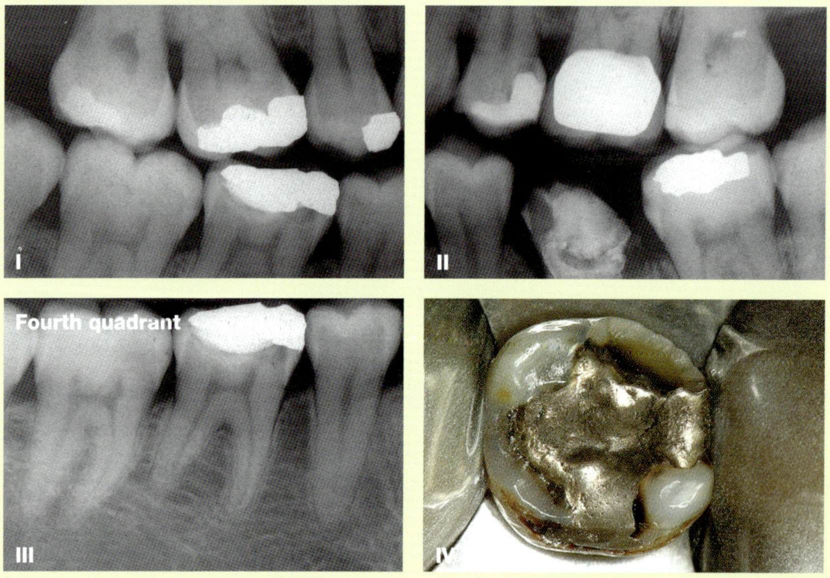

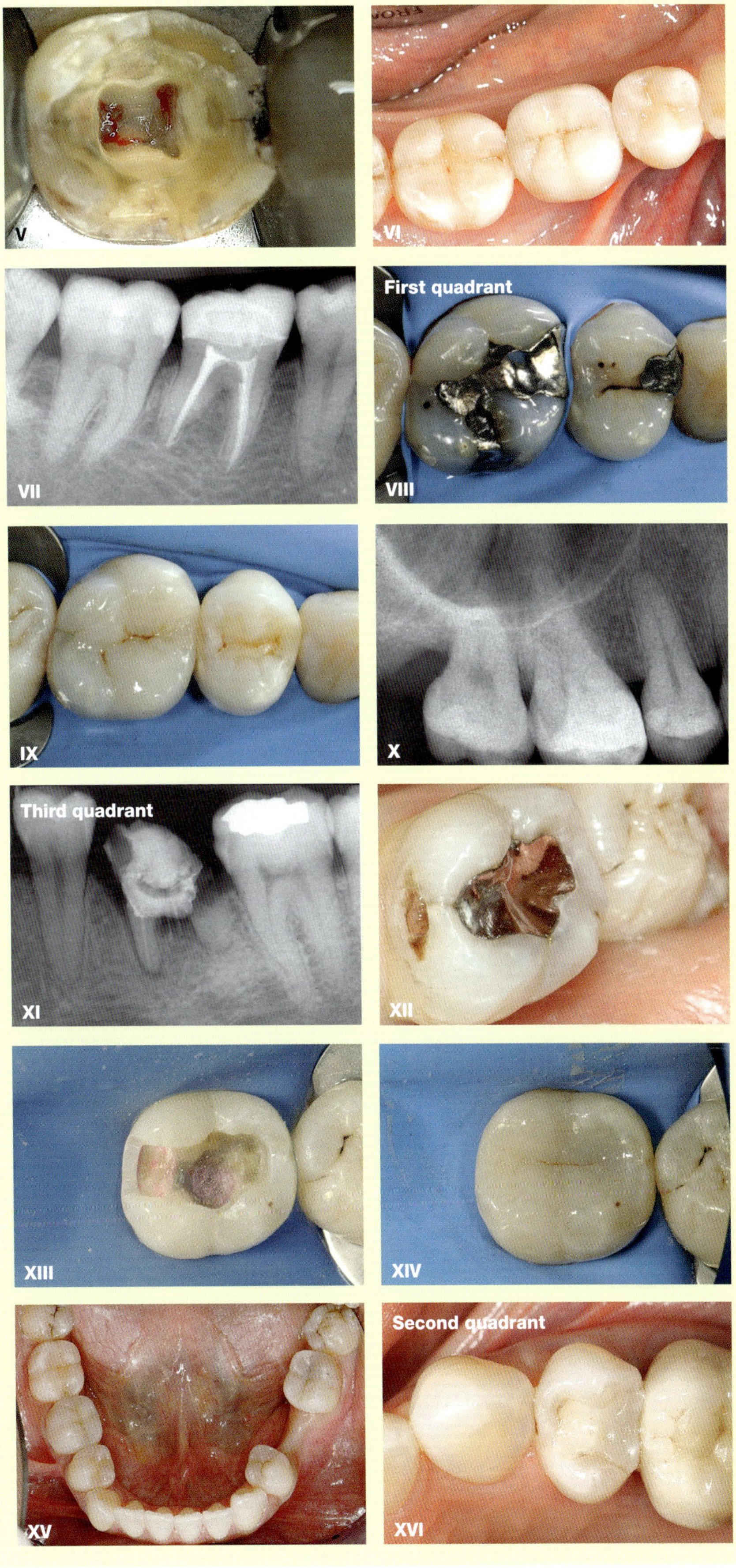

Fig 182 *(continued)* Treatment of the maxillary right (first) quadrant with an inlay on the second molar and post-cementation radiography *(VIII–X)*. In the mandibular left (third) quadrant, deep decay of the first molar and use of a dental decay detector *(XI–XIV)*. View of restorations in the mandible *(XV)*. In the maxillary left (second) quadrant, preparation and view of the second premolar after cementation *(XVI–XX)*.

Fig 182 *(continued)* Contact surfaces between the maxillary left first and second molars *(XXI, XXII)*. Occlusal view of maxilla before suture removal *(XXIII)*.

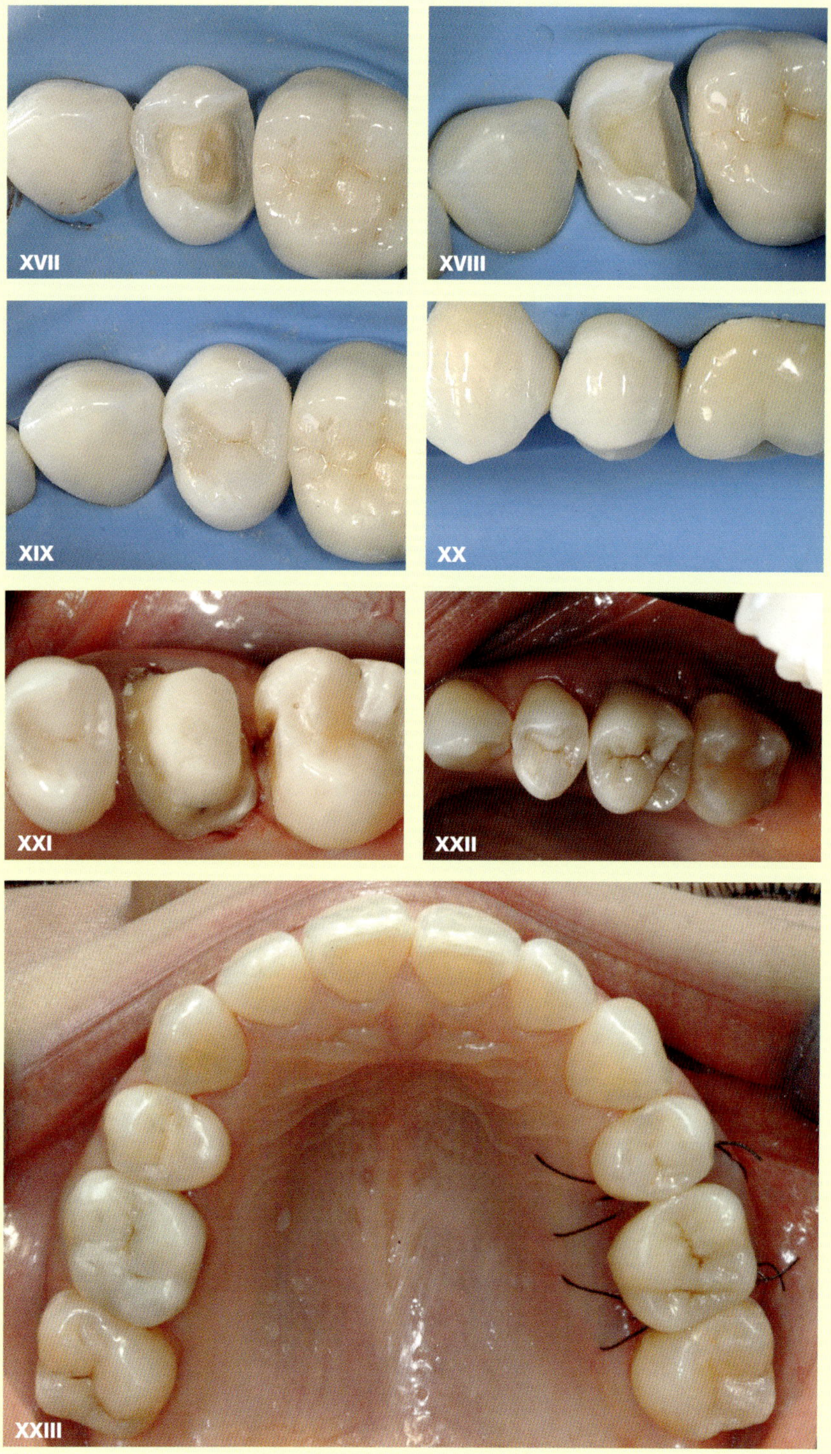

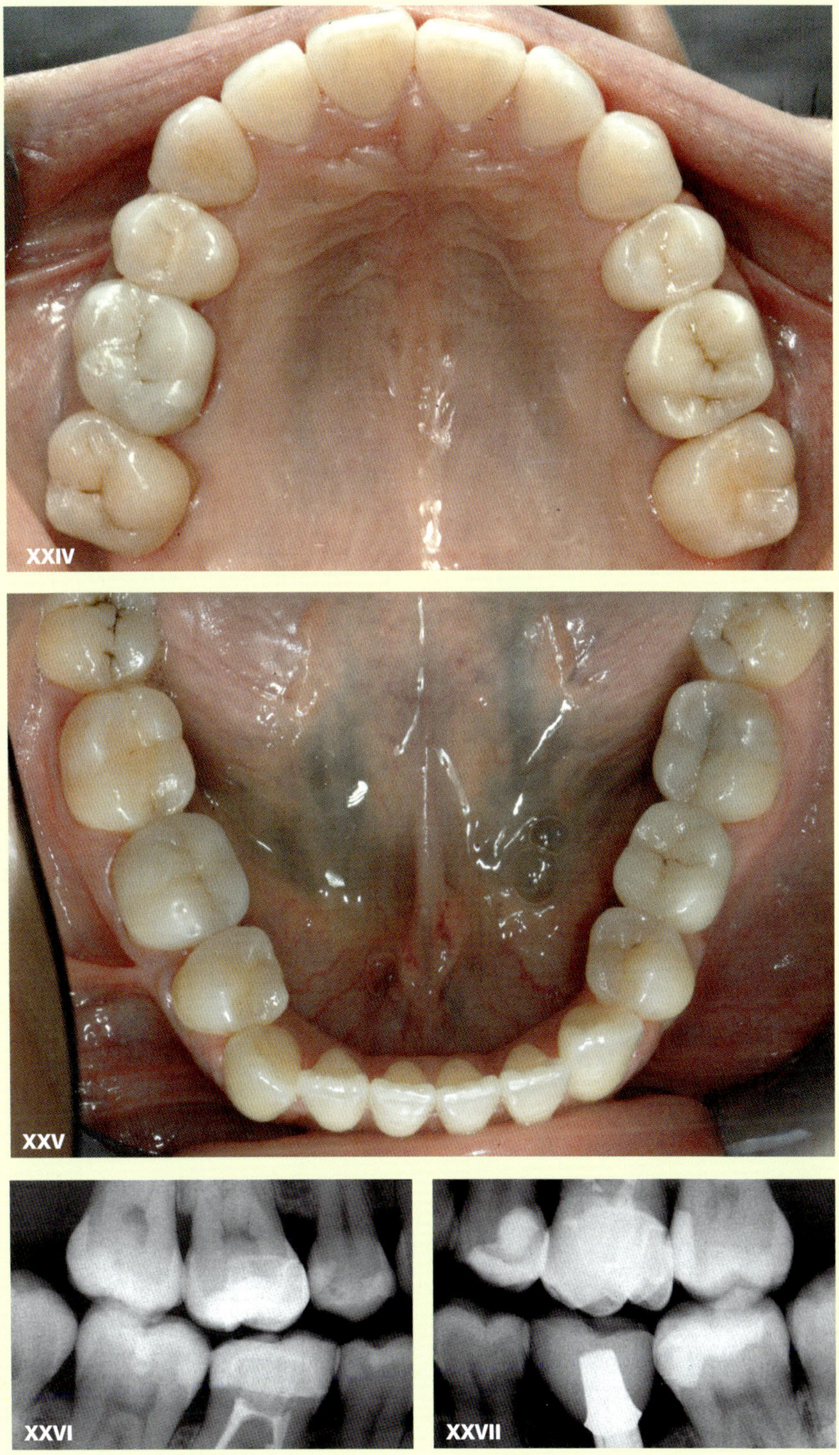

Fig 182 *(continued)* Clinical and radiographic 2-year follow-up *(XXIV–XXVII)*.

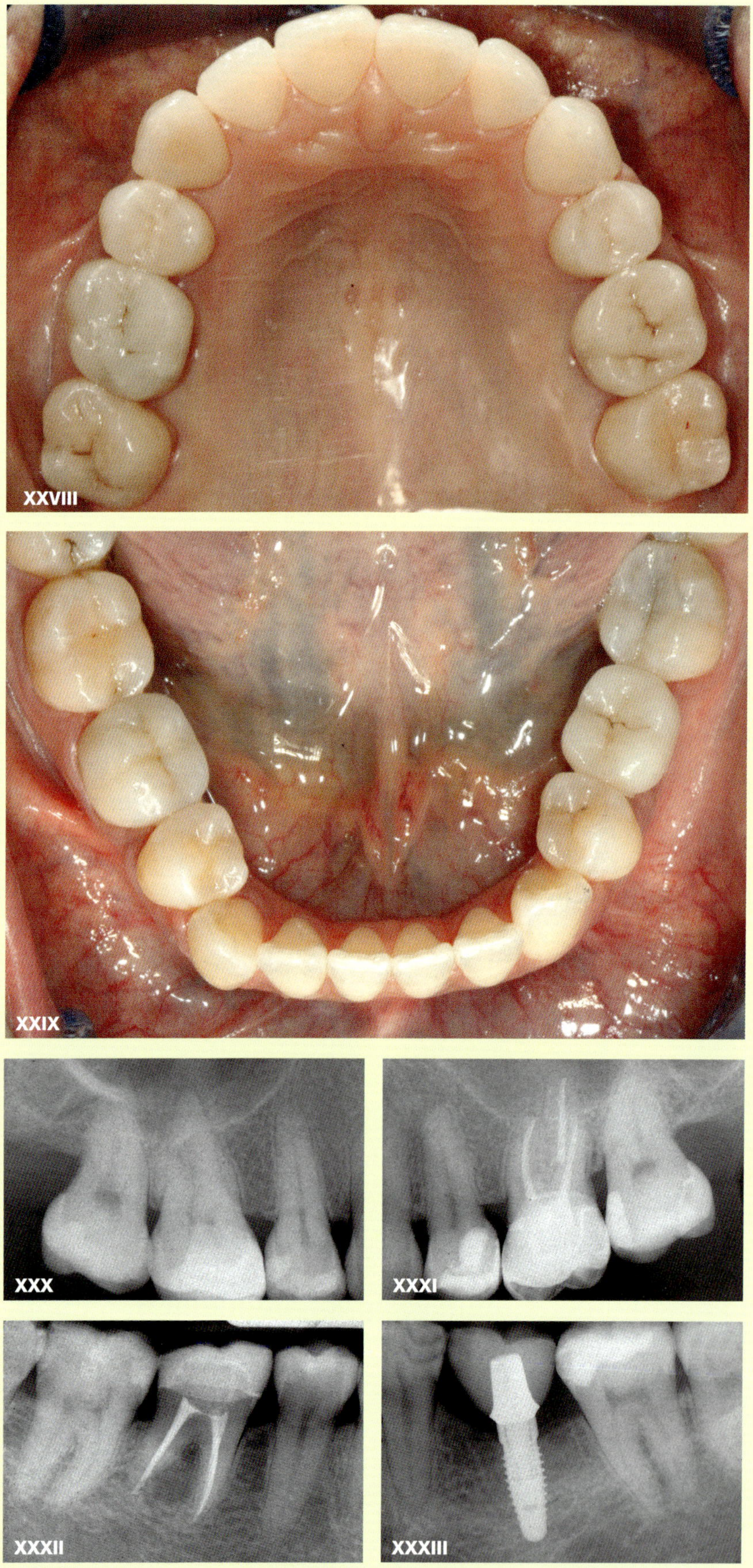

Fig 182 *(continued)* Clinical and periapical radiographic 4-year follow-up *(XXVIII–XXXIII)*.

Clinical case II

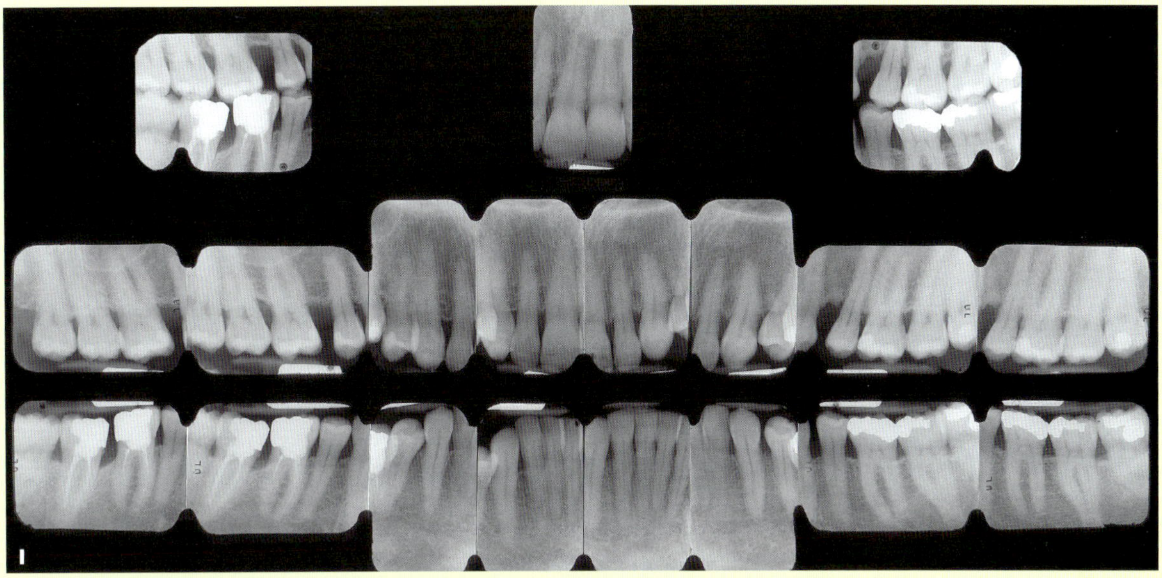

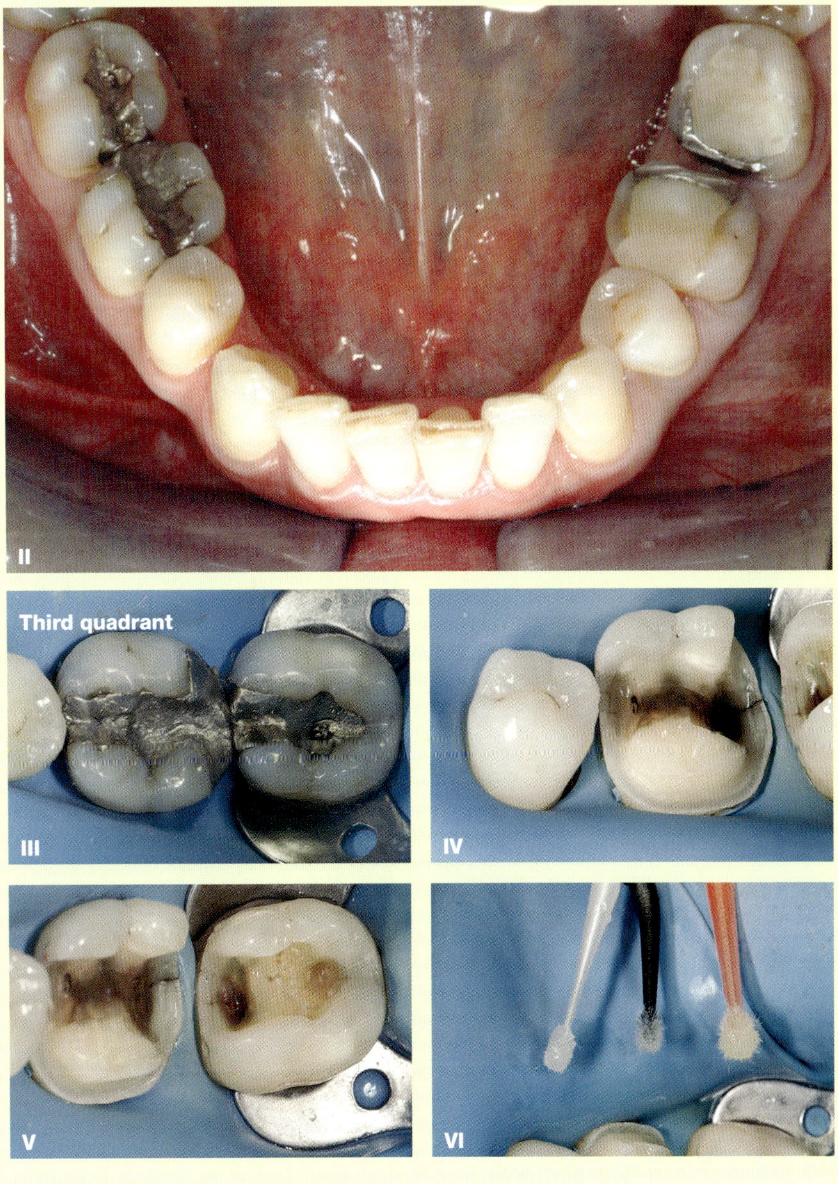

Fig 183 Preoperative radiographic and clinical views *(I, II)*. Intraoperative stages in the mandibular left (third) quadrant: removal of defective restorations, removal of decayed tissue, bonding, buildup with flowable composite and traditional composite, preparation under rubber dam with rotary and ultrasonic instruments, impression, and cementation of inlays *(III–XII)*.

Fig 183 (*continued*) Pre- and postoperative views of the mandibular right (fourth) quadrant (*XIII–XVI*). Full arch (*XVII*). Clinical follow-up after 1 year (*XVIII*).

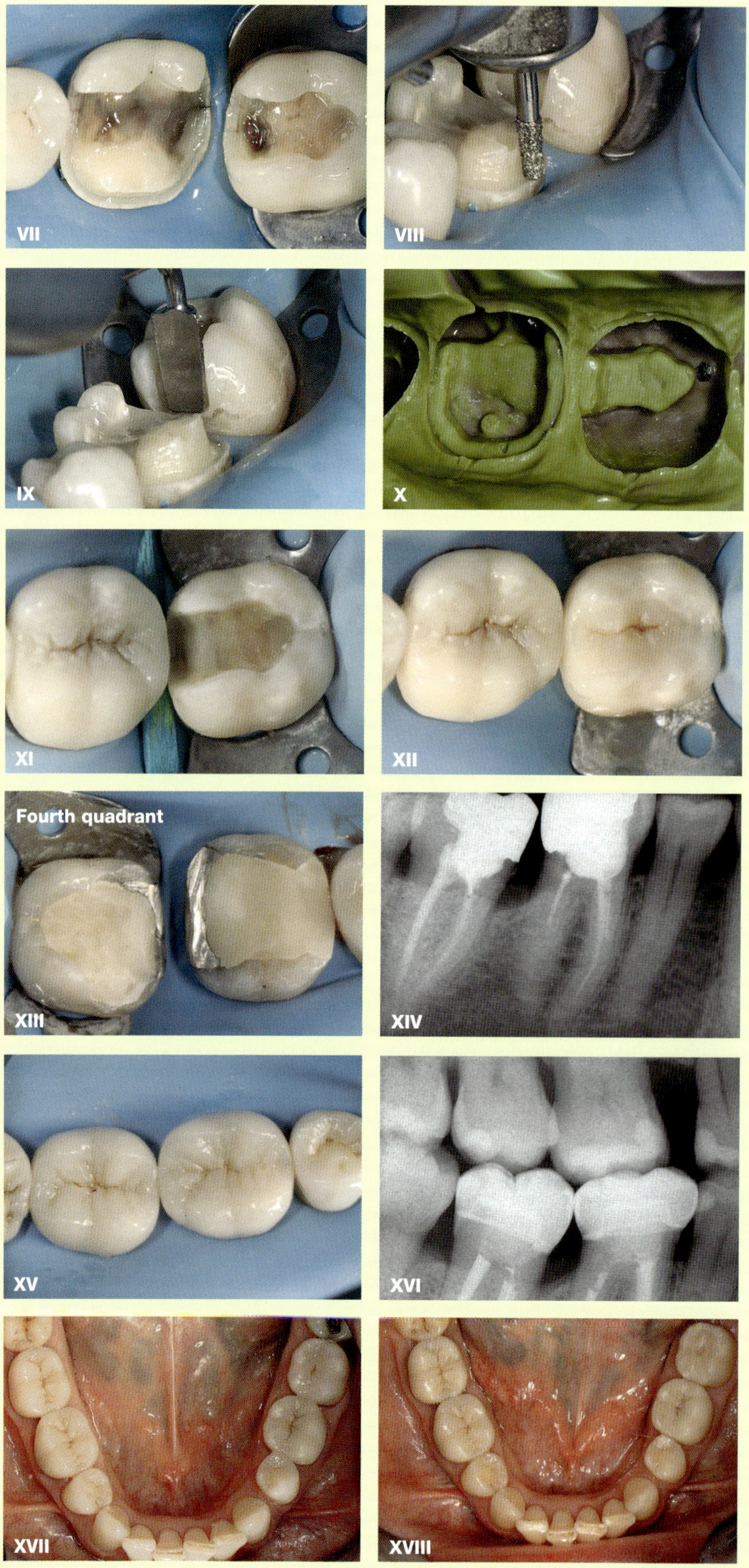

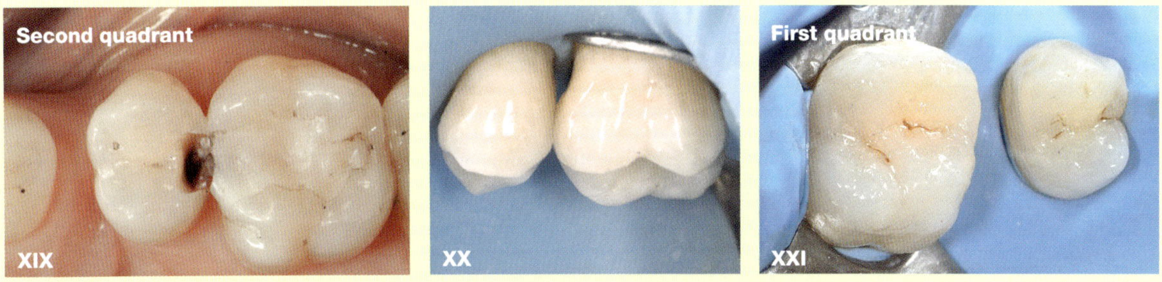

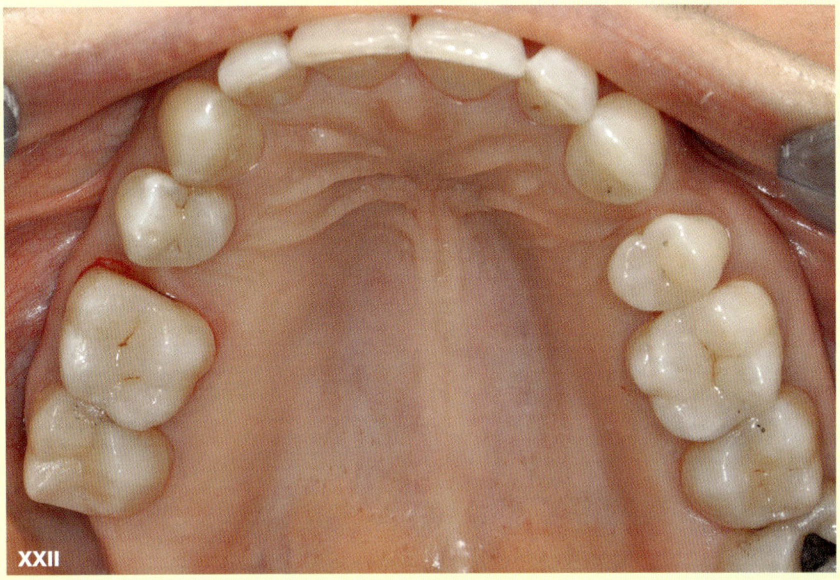

Fig 183 *(continued)* In the maxillary left (second) quadrant, management of the second premolar and first molar: view of interproximal contact surfaces *(XIX, XX)*. Inlays cemented in the maxillary right (first) quadrant *(XXI)*. Occlusal view of maxilla and end-of-treatment radiographs *(XXII, XXIII)*.

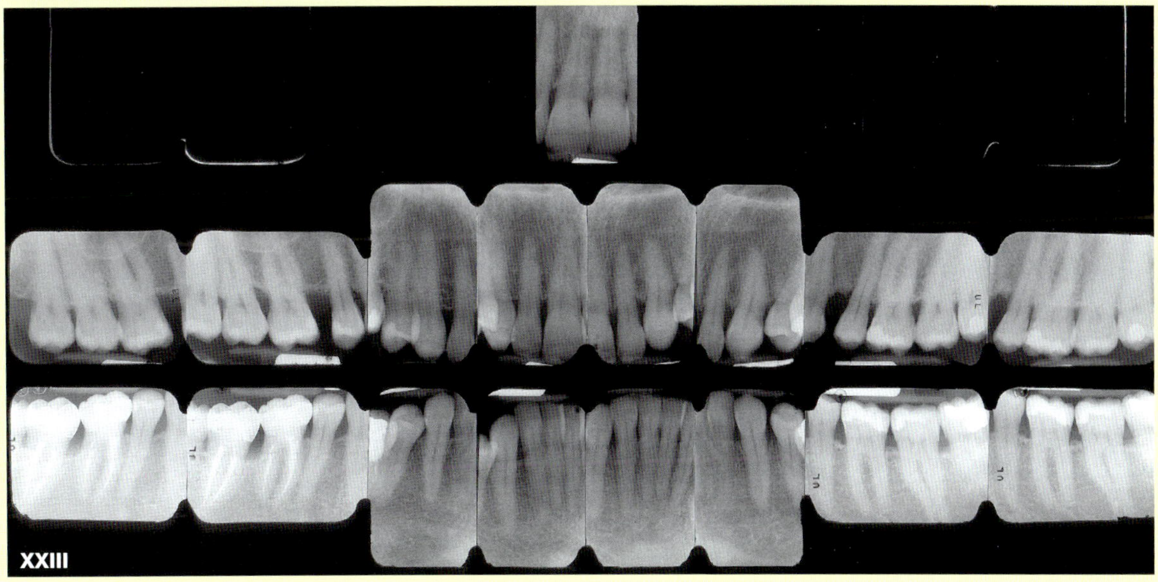

Clinical case 12

Fig 184 Occlusal view of maxilla and preoperative bitewing radiographs *(I–III)*. Direct and indirect restorations in the maxillary right (first) quadrant and radiographic follow-up *(IV–VI)*. Maxillary left (second) quadrant preparations, cementation, and radiographic follow-up *(VII–X)*.

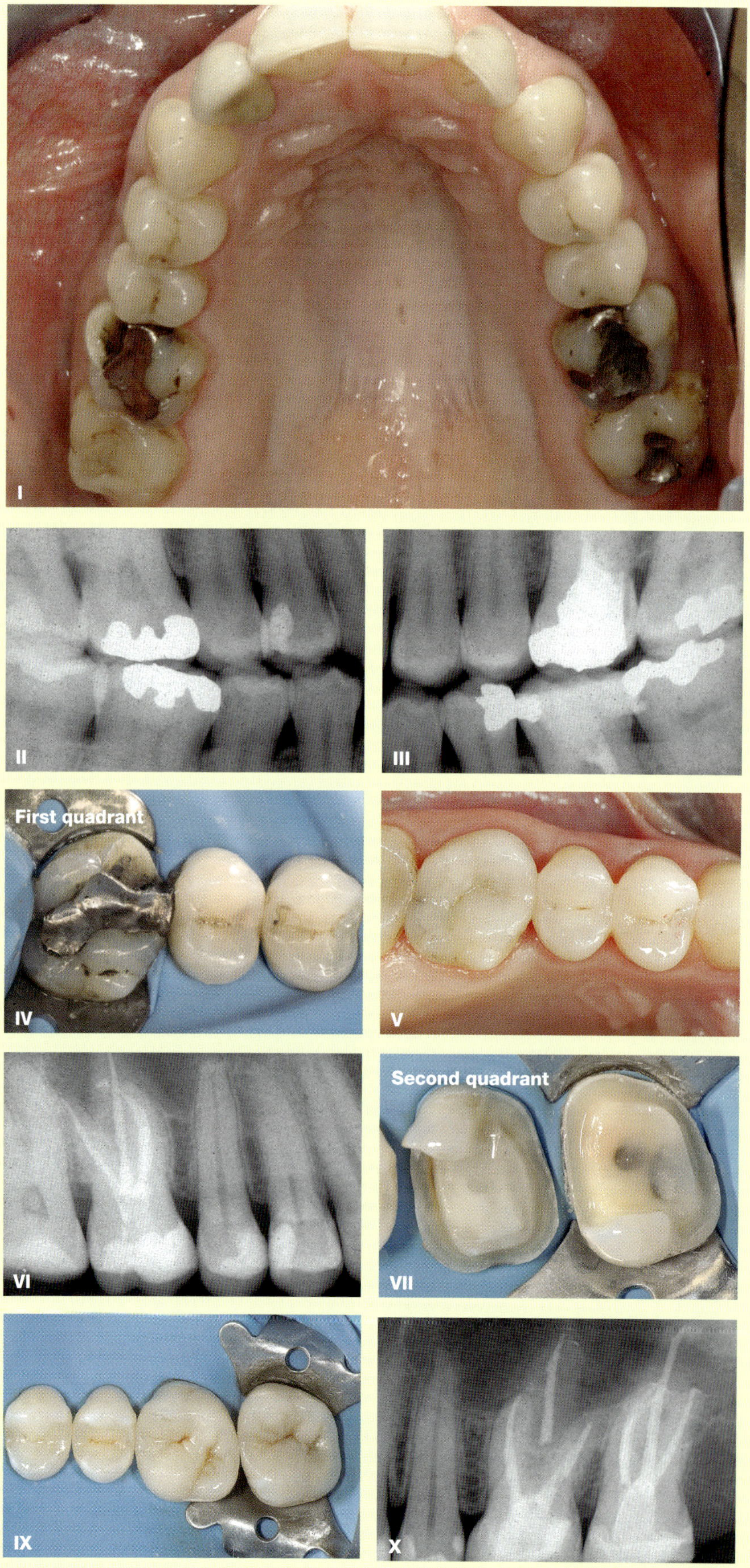

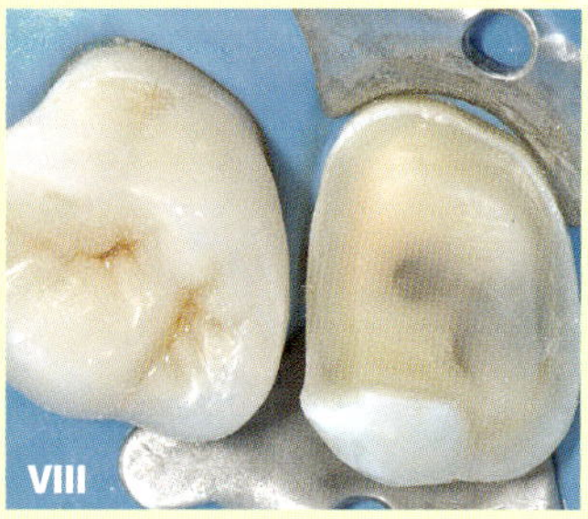

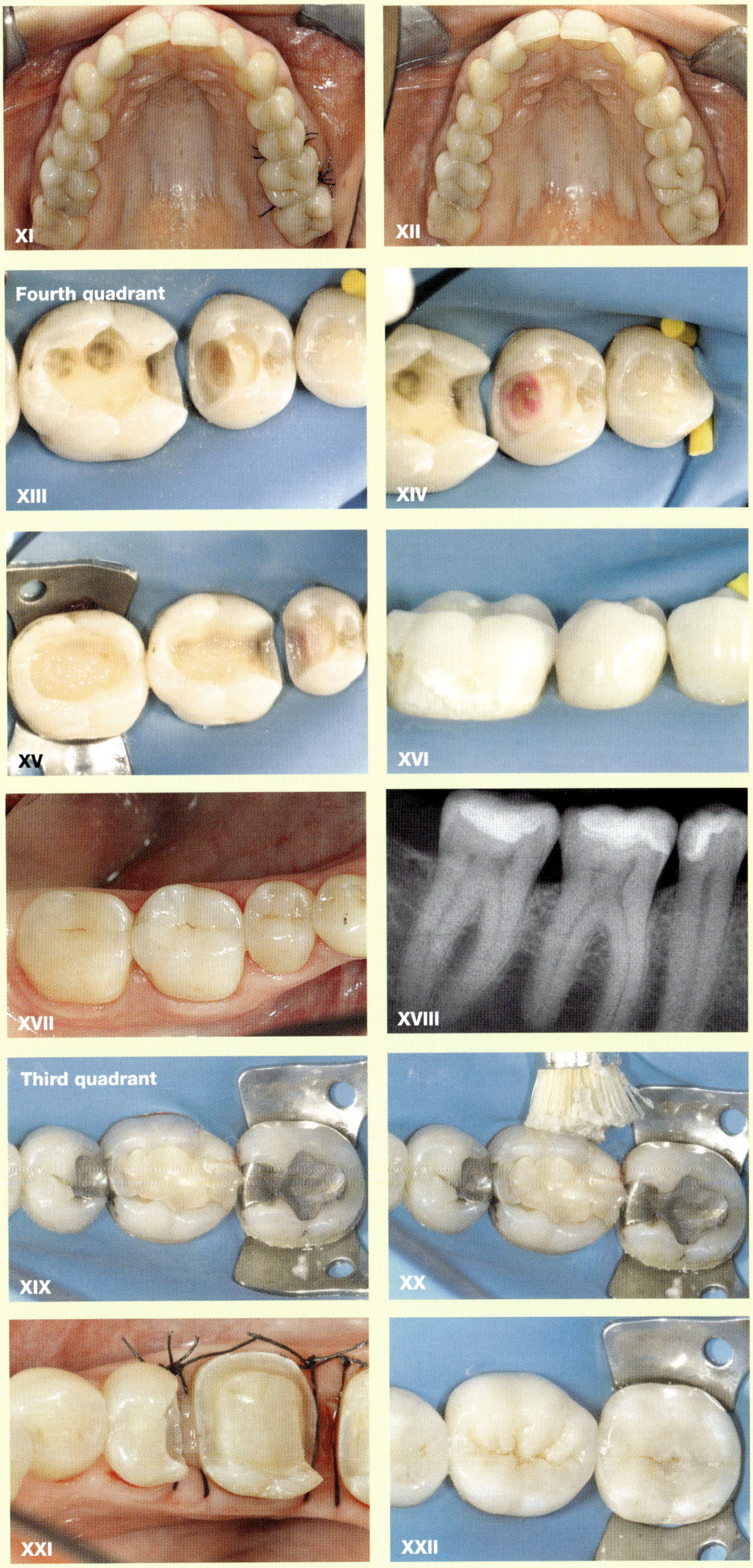

Fig 184 *(continued)* Views of the maxilla before and after suture removal *(XI, XII)*. Management of the mandibular right (fourth) quadrant *(XIII–XVIII)*. Indirect restorations of the mandibular left (third) quadrant: well-performed sutures routinely allow excellent isolation of the surgical field in order to perform inlay cementation effectively *(XIX–XXII)*.

Fig 184 *(continued)* View of the mandible with sutures in situ and 3 weeks after their removal *(XXIII, XXIV)*. Follow-up radiograph of the mandibular left quadrant *(XXV)*.

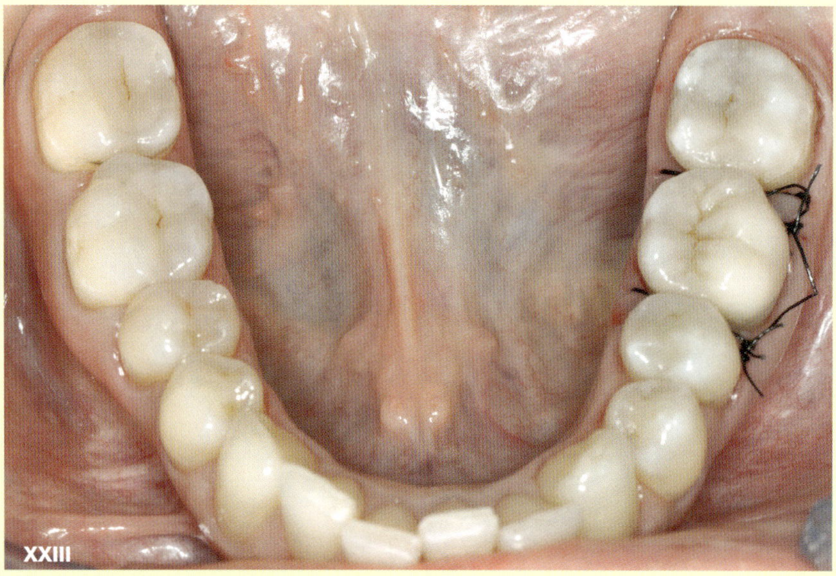

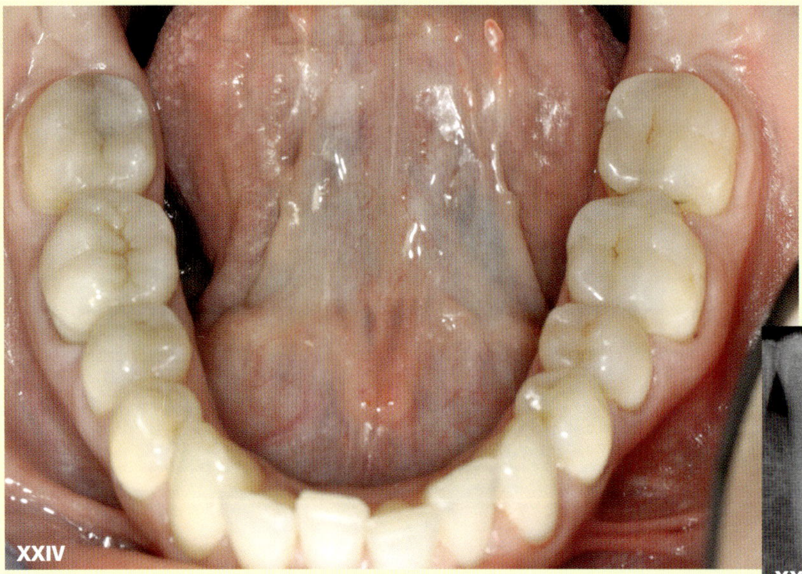

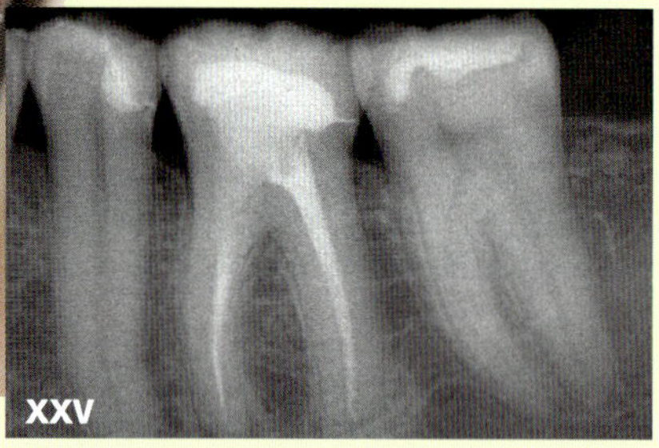

Respecting pulp vitality

Maintenance of pulp vitality must be a primary aim when preparing teeth using partial- and total-coverage techniques (Fig 185).

This goal is achieved by removing all decay (Fig 186); avoiding overheating, dehydration, mechanical trauma, and excessive pressure; and using rotary instruments with effective cutting capacity under a constant water jet.

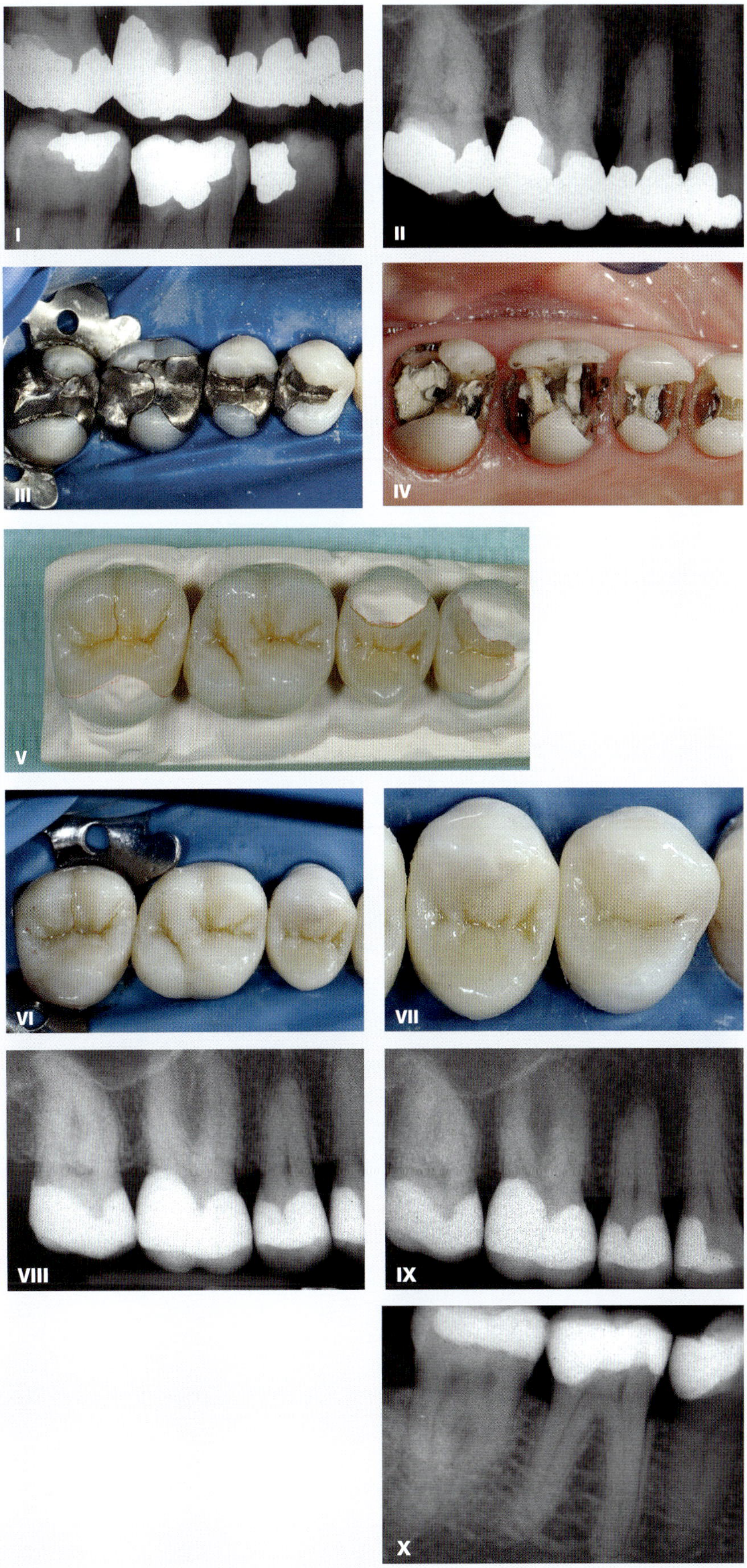

Fig 185 Bitewing radiographs showing large amalgam restorations near the pulp *(I)*. After taking periapical radiographs to check for any lesions at the apices *(II)* and performing pulp vitality tests, the restorations were removed, and the cavities were cleaned. These images clearly show the difficulty in cleaning the cavities *(III, IV)*. Preparation of inlays in the laboratory *(V)*. Views of inlays and periapical radiography *(VI–VIII)*. After 6 years, radiographic follow-up found no apical lesions, and vitality tests were positive; the intact marginal seals and accurate emergence profiles were also of considerable significance *(IX, X)*.

The pulp complex is afforded maximum protection during preparation by simply using rubber dam (Fig 187). During tooth preparation for a prosthetic crown all the tubules are opened, and the closer the preparation comes to the pulp, the greater the risk of pulp damage because of the increased number and diameter of dentinal tubules that remain at the mercy of bacteria in the oral cavity for longer.[57]

Pulp inflammation is caused by the presence of these bacteria, but if they are removed they will no longer be a danger.

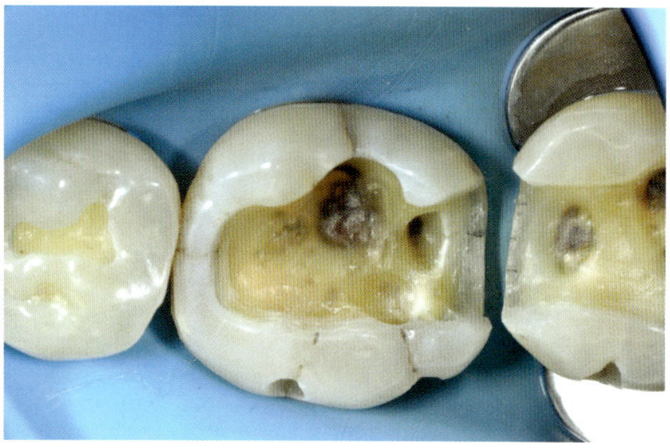

Fig 186 Cavity after removal of decayed tissue.

The use of rubber dam is in accordance with protocol in adhesive techniques for cavity preparation and subsequent buildup and does not need any further recommendations (Fig 188).

When replacing large defective restorations with prosthetic crowns, the preparation work will inevitably remove all the walls; therefore, intraradicular anchorage often becomes essential for the reconstruction.

In such cases one sees the consequences of preprosthetic endodontic treatments that do not fulfill the goal of an all-round conservative approach and above all subvert the real indication for endodontic treatment: irreversible pulp inflammation (Figs 189 to 191).

Fig 187 Important factors in safeguarding pulp vitality include the use of rubber dam, new burs that minimize the pressure exerted during preparation, and a constant jet of water to avoid overheating the pulp.

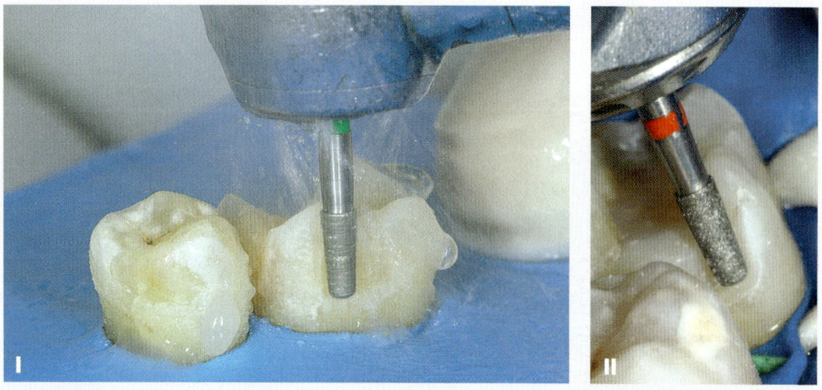

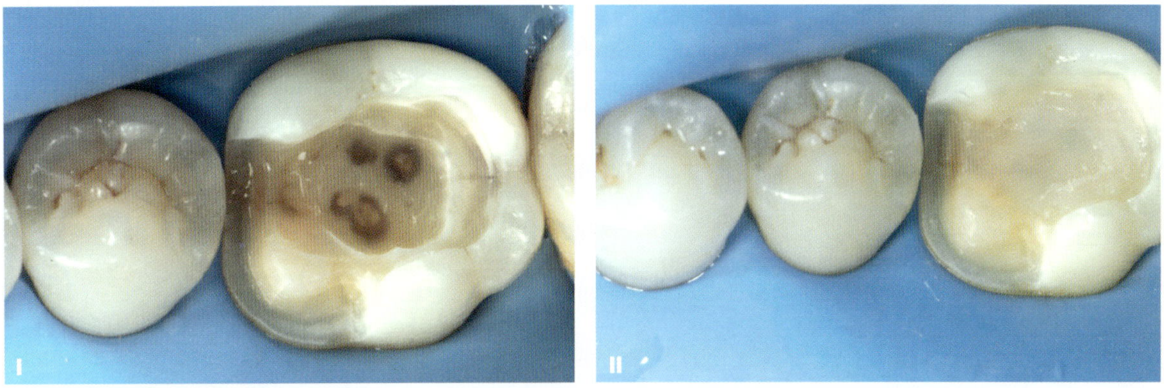

Fig 188 Classic clinical example of the ease of internal preparation and subsequent reconstruction if the tooth is protected by rubber dam, which also serves the important function of ensuring that bacteria in the oral cavity cannot penetrate into the dentinal tubules.

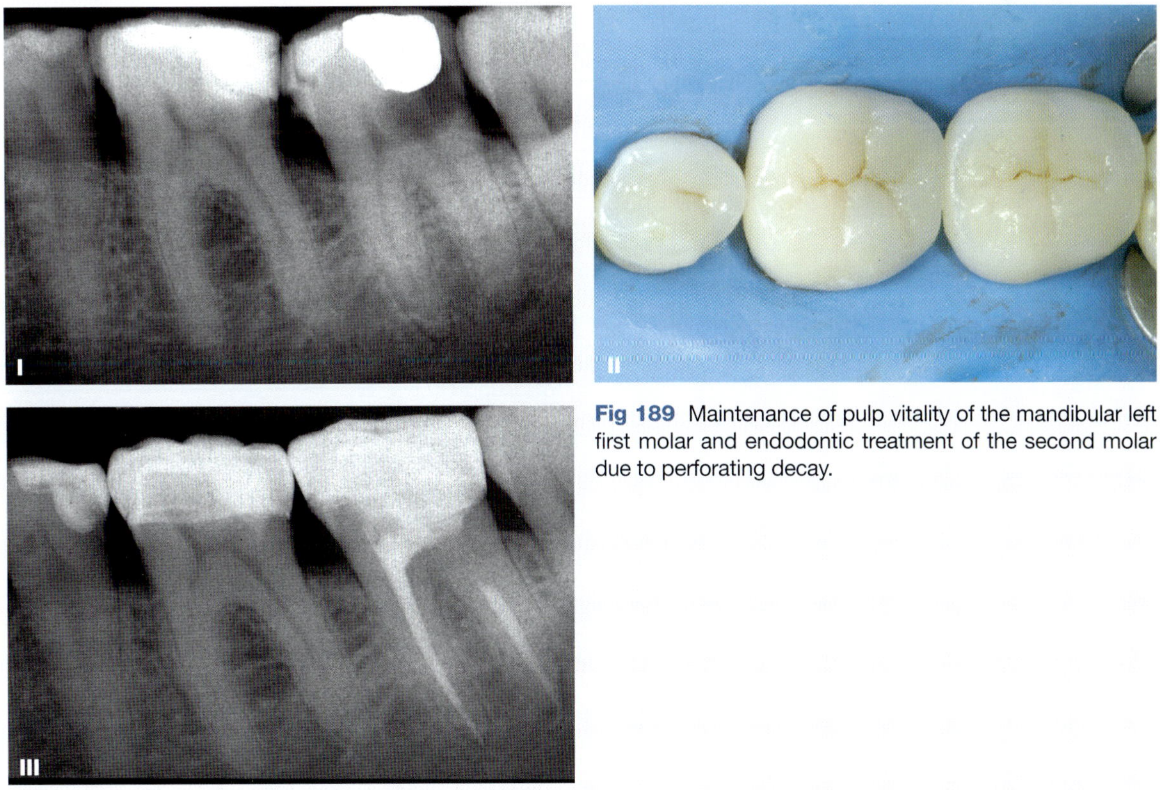

Fig 189 Maintenance of pulp vitality of the mandibular left first molar and endodontic treatment of the second molar due to perforating decay.

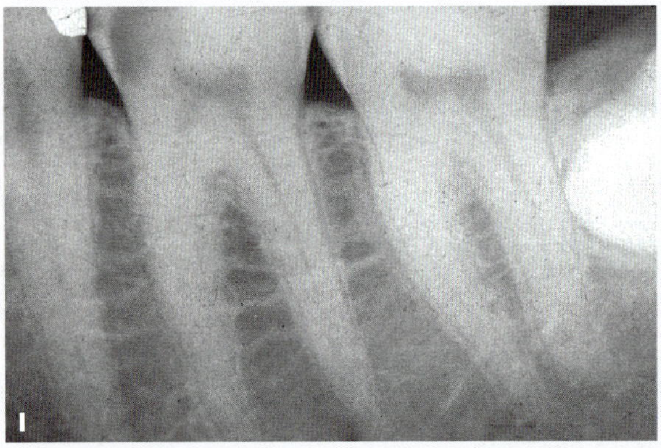

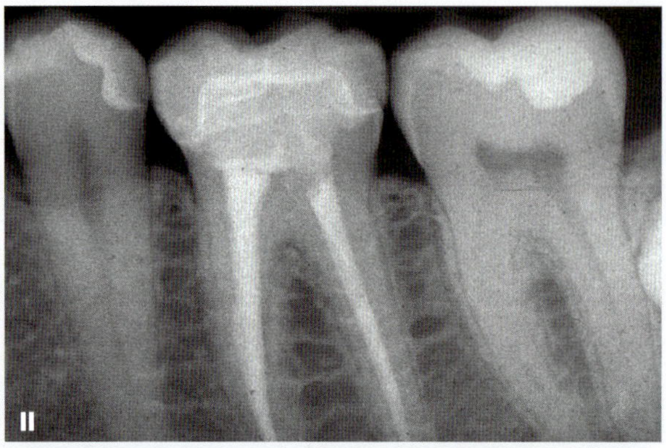

Fig 190 The patient presented with great pain in the third quadrant. The painful symptoms radiated to the maxilla and ear. A radiograph showed deep decay involving the mesial area of the first molar and a caries lesion of moderate size in the distal region. The tooth in question was therefore endodontically treated and then reconstructed with an indirect restoration in composite.

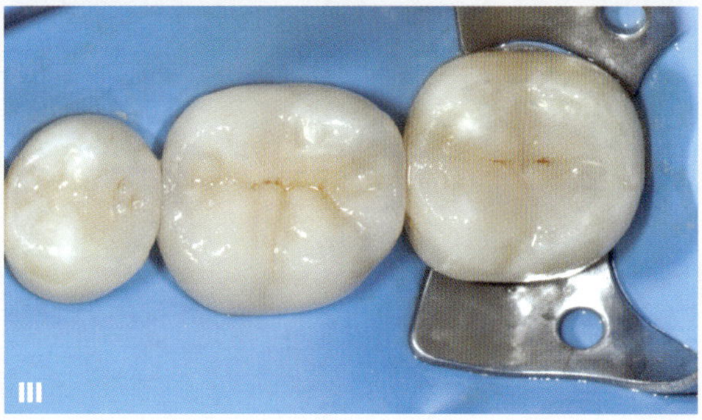

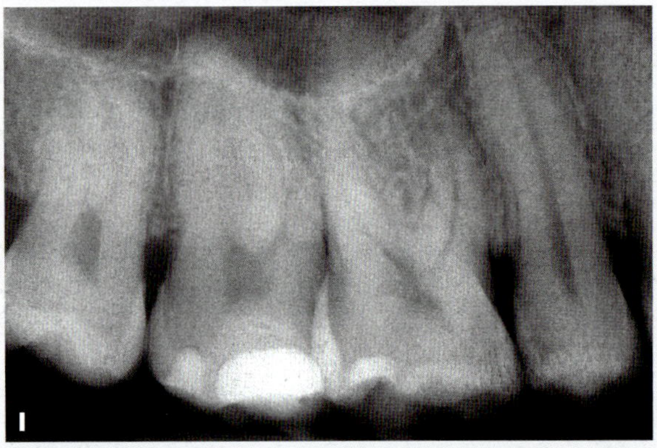

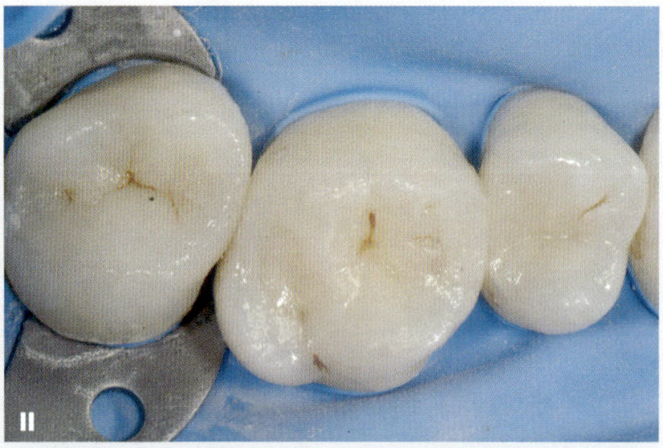

Fig 191 Diagnosis of pulpitis in the maxillary right second molar, which indicated endodontic treatment of the tooth and its subsequent reconstruction by means of a composite onlay. Direct techniques were used for treatment of caries lesions in the second premolar and first molar.

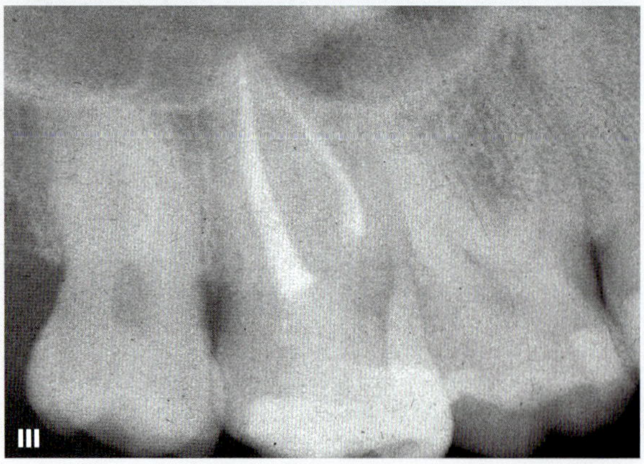

Teeth with previous large restorations near the pulp do not allow the presence of any form of pulp disease to be ruled out with certainty, but there is little point in treating them if they respond positively to vitality tests, they are asymptomatic, and radiographs failed to show the presence of periradicular lesions. To do so would be ignoring the fact that the sole indication for such an invasive intervention is irreversible pulp disease.

Today, adhesive techniques make it possible to reconstruct seriously compromised teeth with great ease while maintaining pulp vitality (Figs 192 to 202).

In any case, if at a later stage the signs and symptoms indicate that endodontic treatment is required, it will simply be necessary to make an access cavity in the inlay, carry out the endodontic treatment, and then seal the cavity by means of a direct technique using the same composite used to make the restoration.

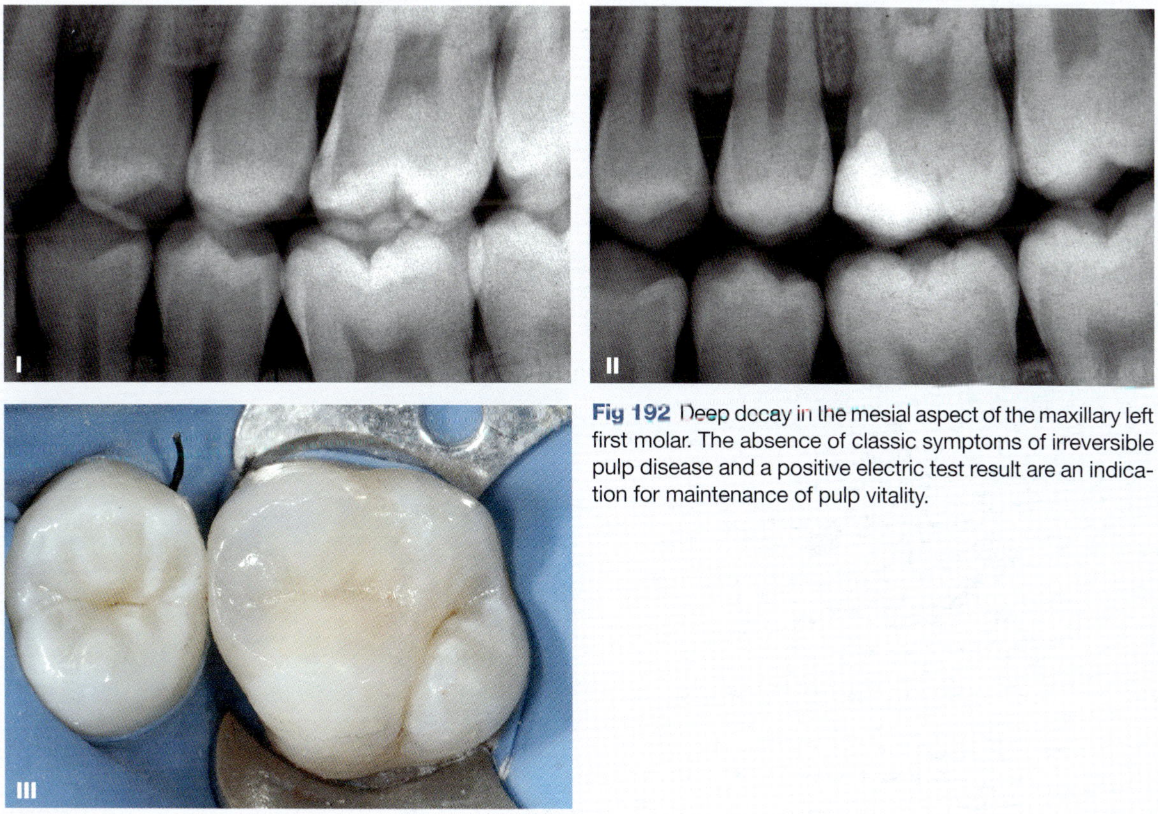

Fig 192 Deep decay in the mesial aspect of the maxillary left first molar. The absence of classic symptoms of irreversible pulp disease and a positive electric test result are an indication for maintenance of pulp vitality.

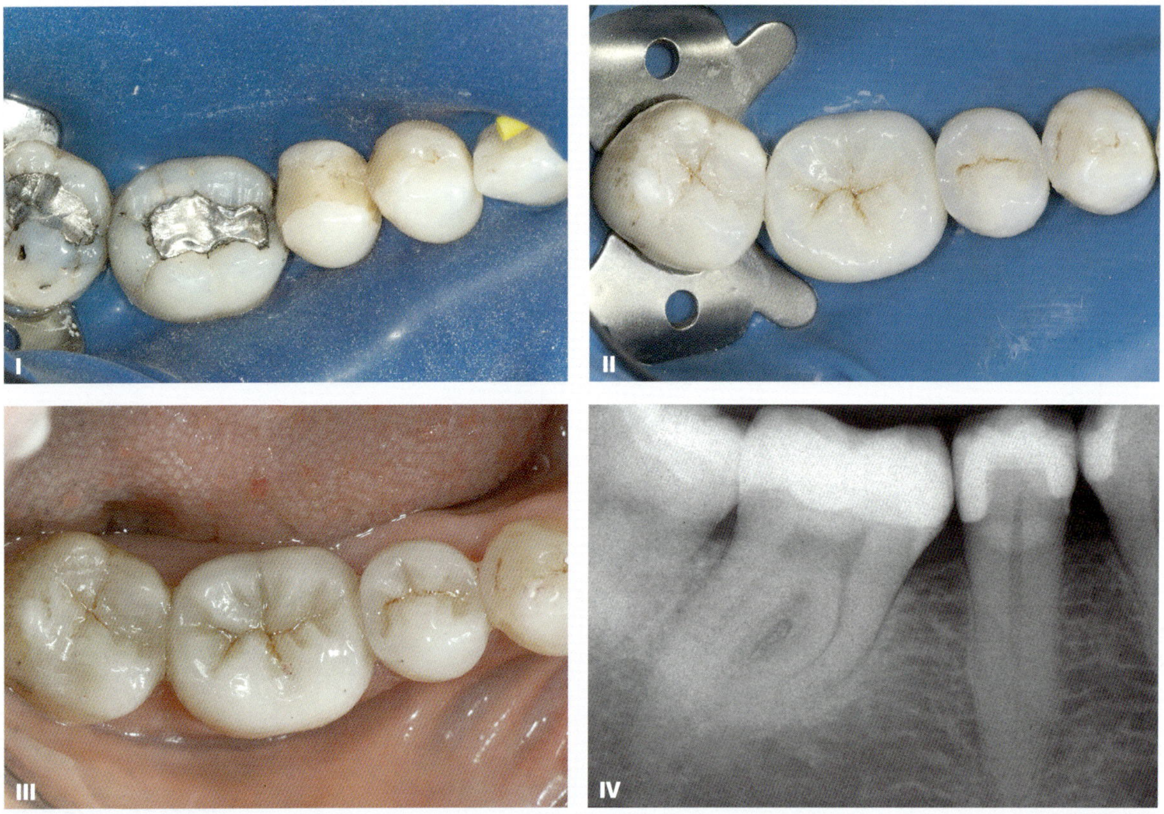

Fig 193 Example of quadrant with defective, deep restorations. Endodontic treatments were avoided in all teeth, which were restored with inlays.

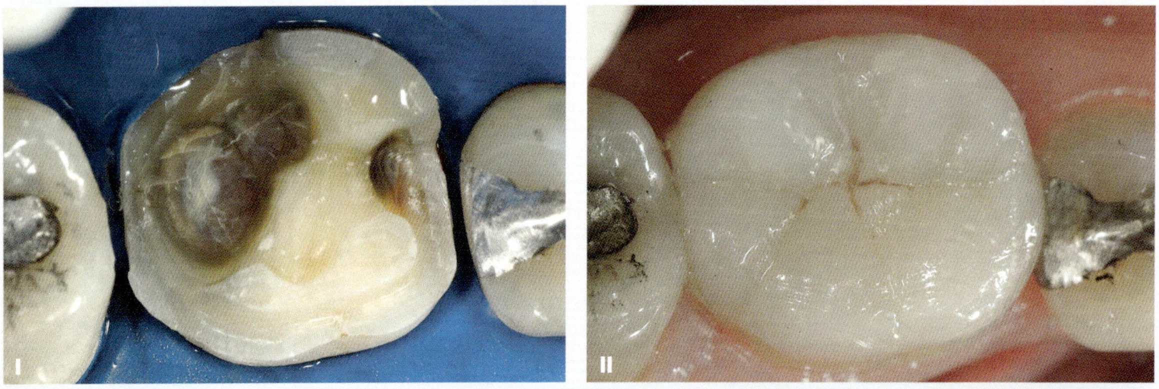

Fig 194 Very deep caries lesion affecting the mandibular right first molar: evident multiple fracture lines, positive vitality test, and subsequent maintenance of pulp vitality.

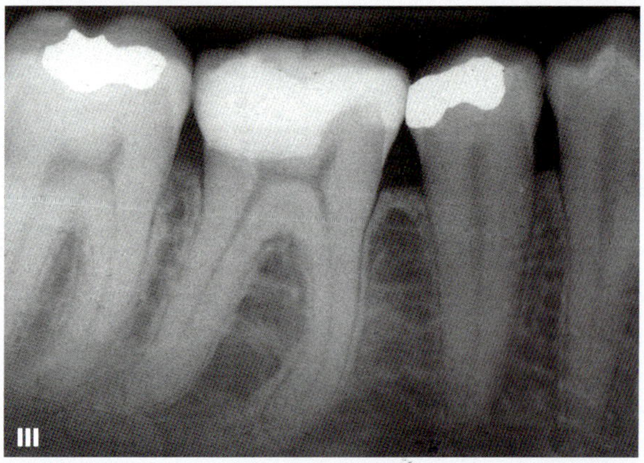

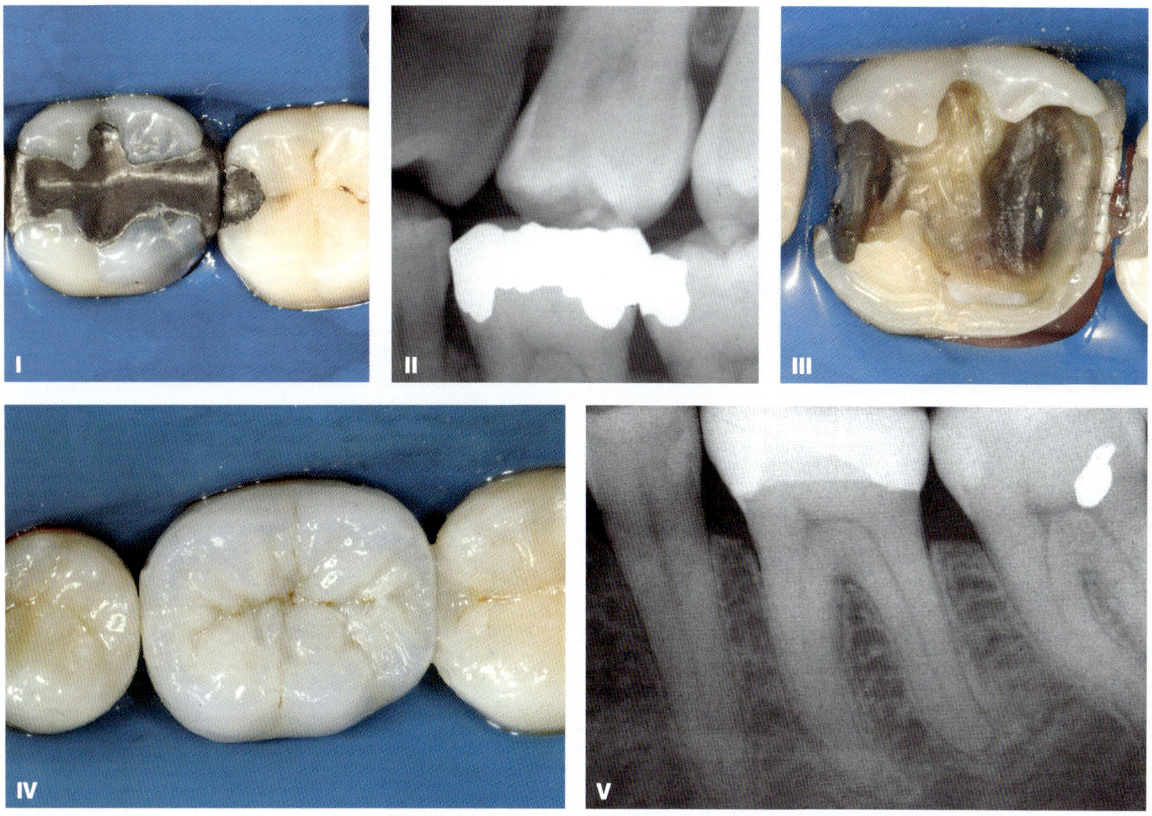

Fig 195 Another caries lesion very close to the pulp. Conservative treatment was carried out with positive long-term pulp vitality tests; marginal seals are extremely consistent.

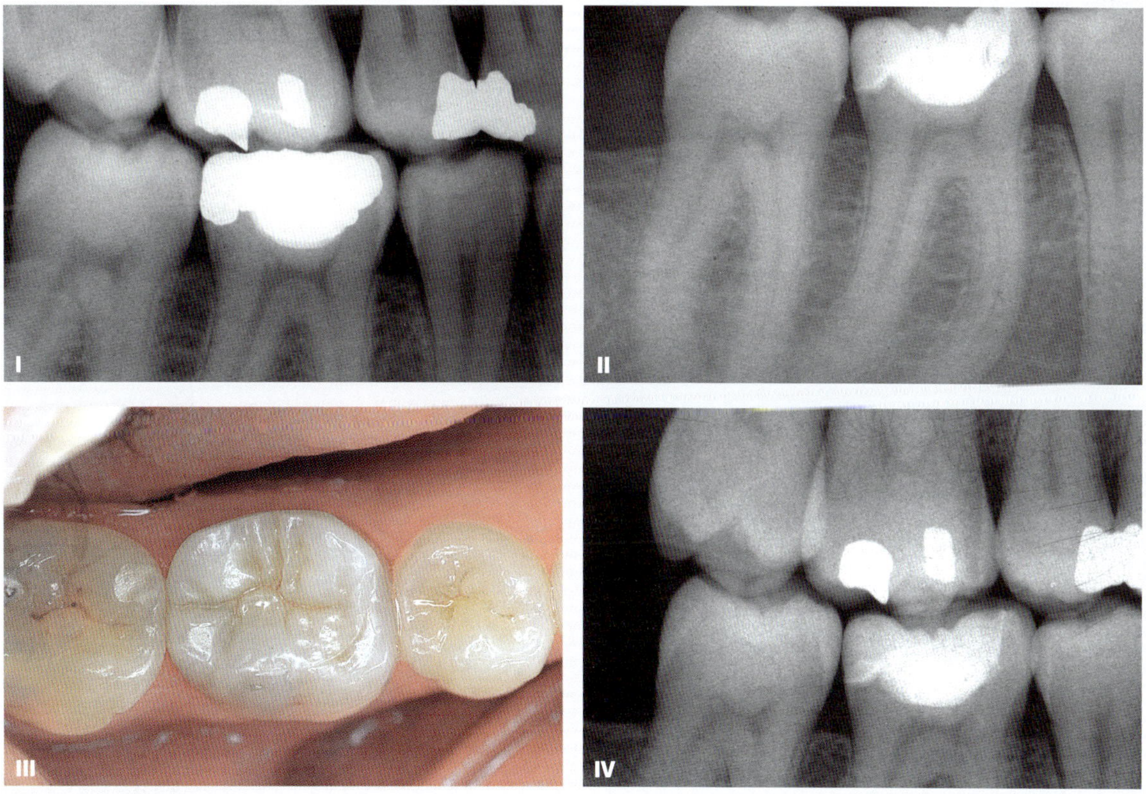

Fig 196 Mandibular right first molar containing a very deep amalgam restoration. After reconstruction using a composite inlay, the pain on chewing that prompted the procedure disappeared.

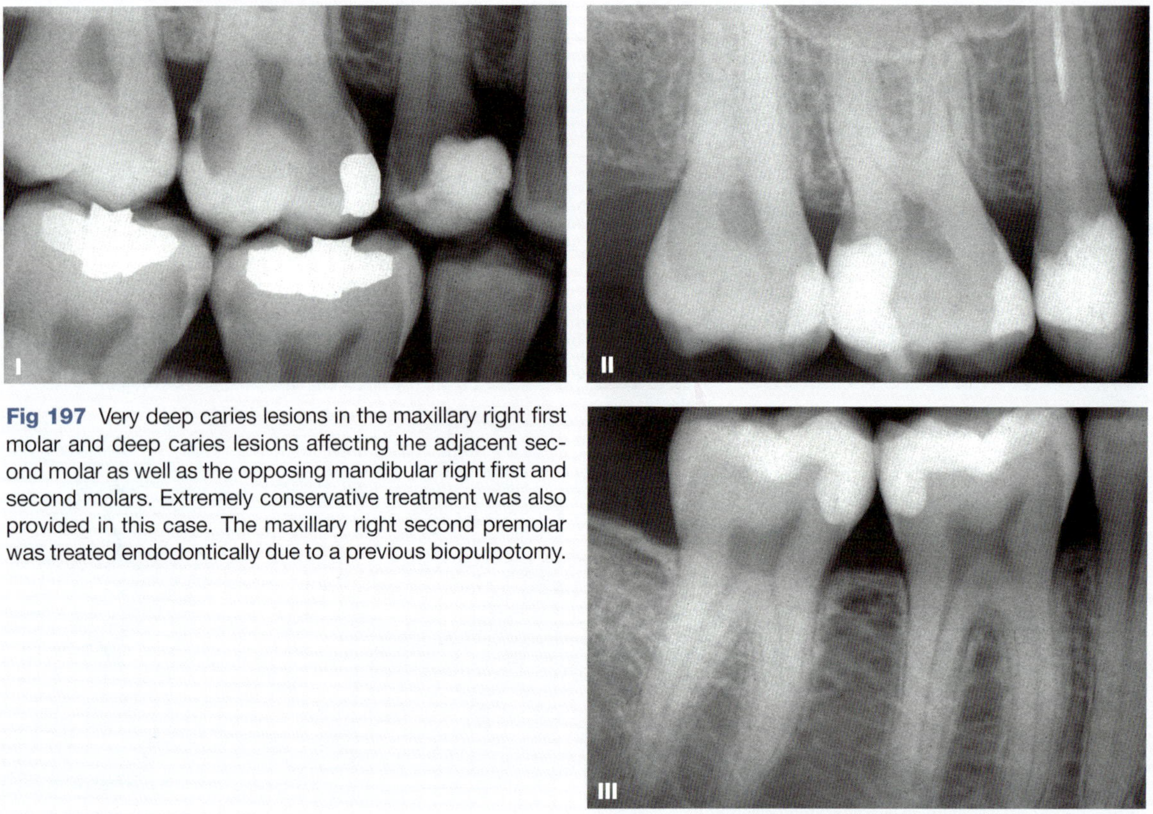

Fig 197 Very deep caries lesions in the maxillary right first molar and deep caries lesions affecting the adjacent second molar as well as the opposing mandibular right first and second molars. Extremely conservative treatment was also provided in this case. The maxillary right second premolar was treated endodontically due to a previous biopulpotomy.

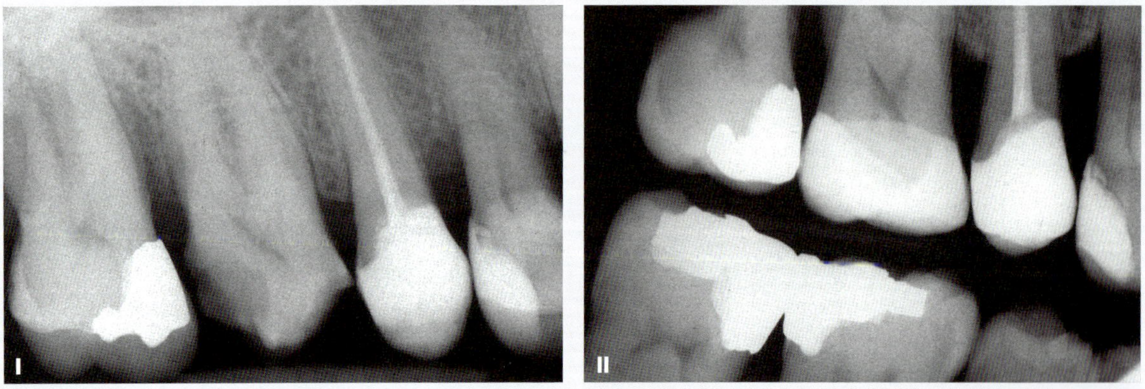

Fig 198 Caries lesion and fracture in the maxillary right first molar: maintenance of pulp vitality and accurate marginal seals.

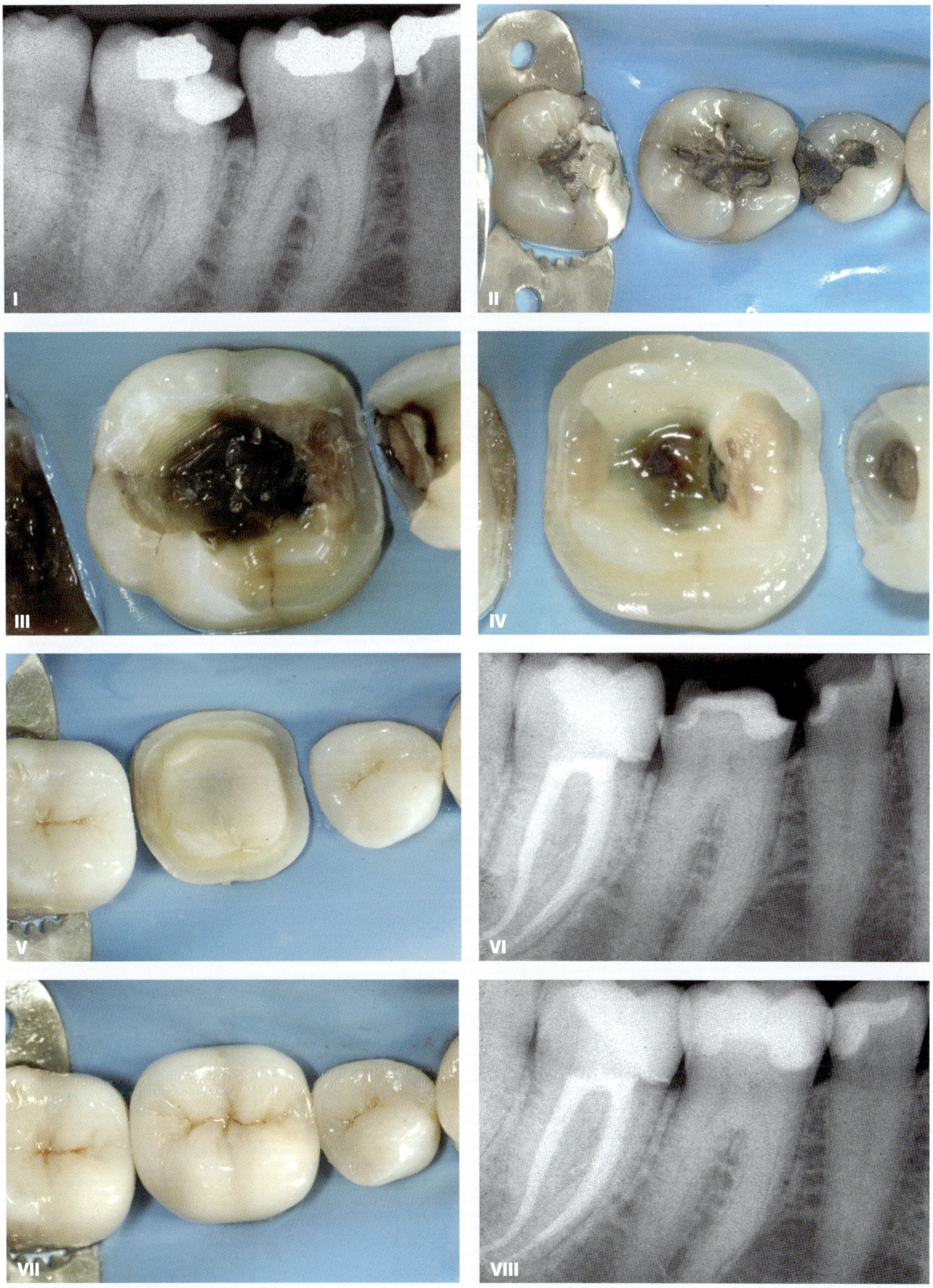

Fig 199 Extreme case of maintenance of pulp vitality: after removing decayed tissue, mesial pulp horns were visible *(I–IV)*. Because they were completely calcified, the author considered it advisable to proceed directly to the stage of buildup using flowable composite and traditional composite and then prepared an overlay *(V–VII)*. The accuracy of the margins and internal filling are evident *(VIII)*. The vitality tests were positive after 2 years, and the patient did not complain of any discomfort.

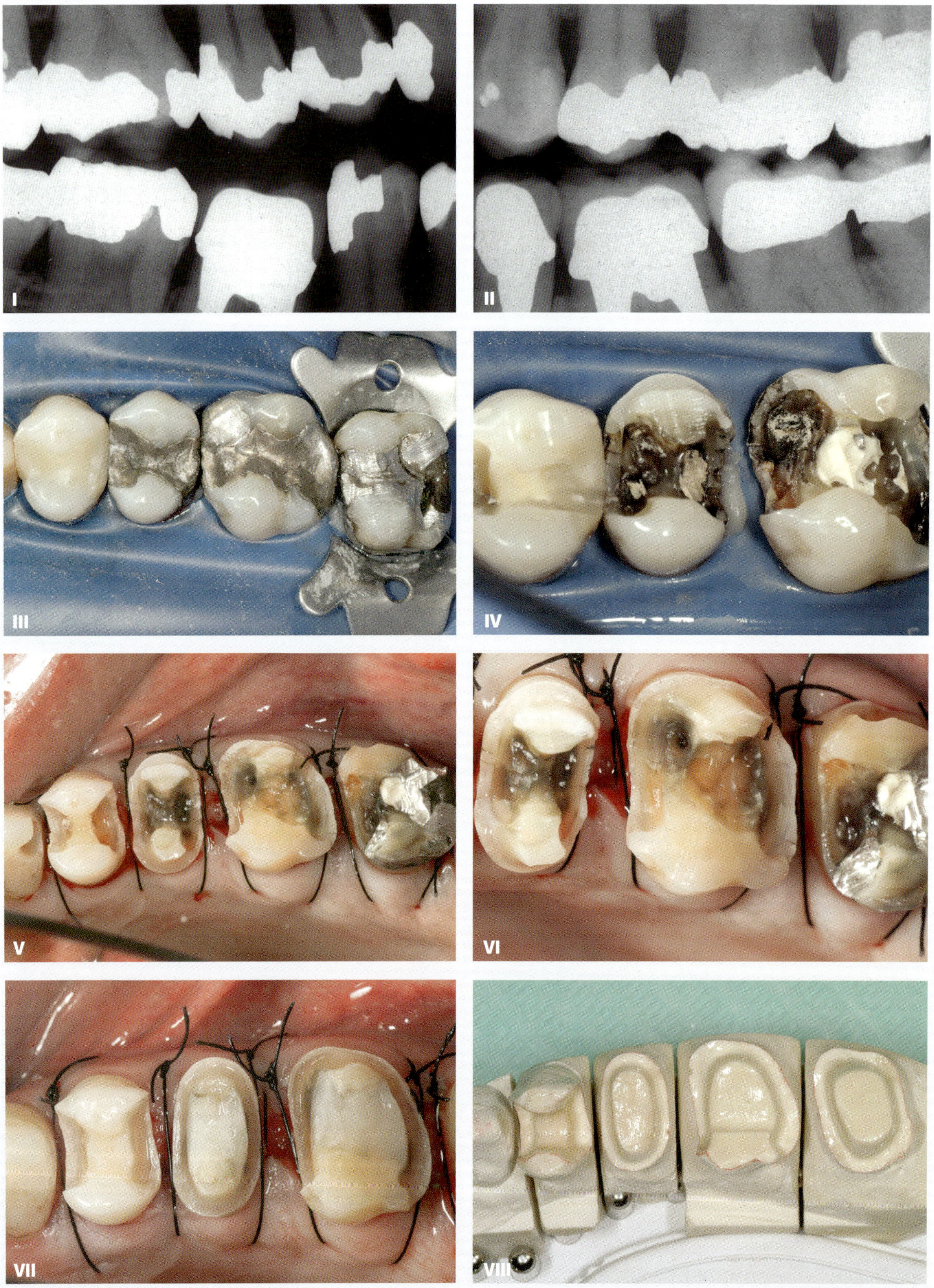

Fig 200 Reconstructing maxillary molars and premolars. After removing defective restorations and cleaning the cavities *(I–IV)*, periodontal surgical lengthening made it possible to achieve supragingival positioning for all margins *(V–X)*. This facilitated preparation of the teeth and the work of the dental technician. The cavity margins are extremely accurate in the follow-up radiograph *(XI)*. View of the maxillary left quadrant 1 week following surgery *(XII)*. The procedures for restoration of the maxillary right quadrant were identical *(XIII–XV)*. Clinical and radiographic follow-ups after 5 *(XVI–XVIII)* and 7 years *(XIX–XXI)*. All the treated teeth achieved positive vitality test results.

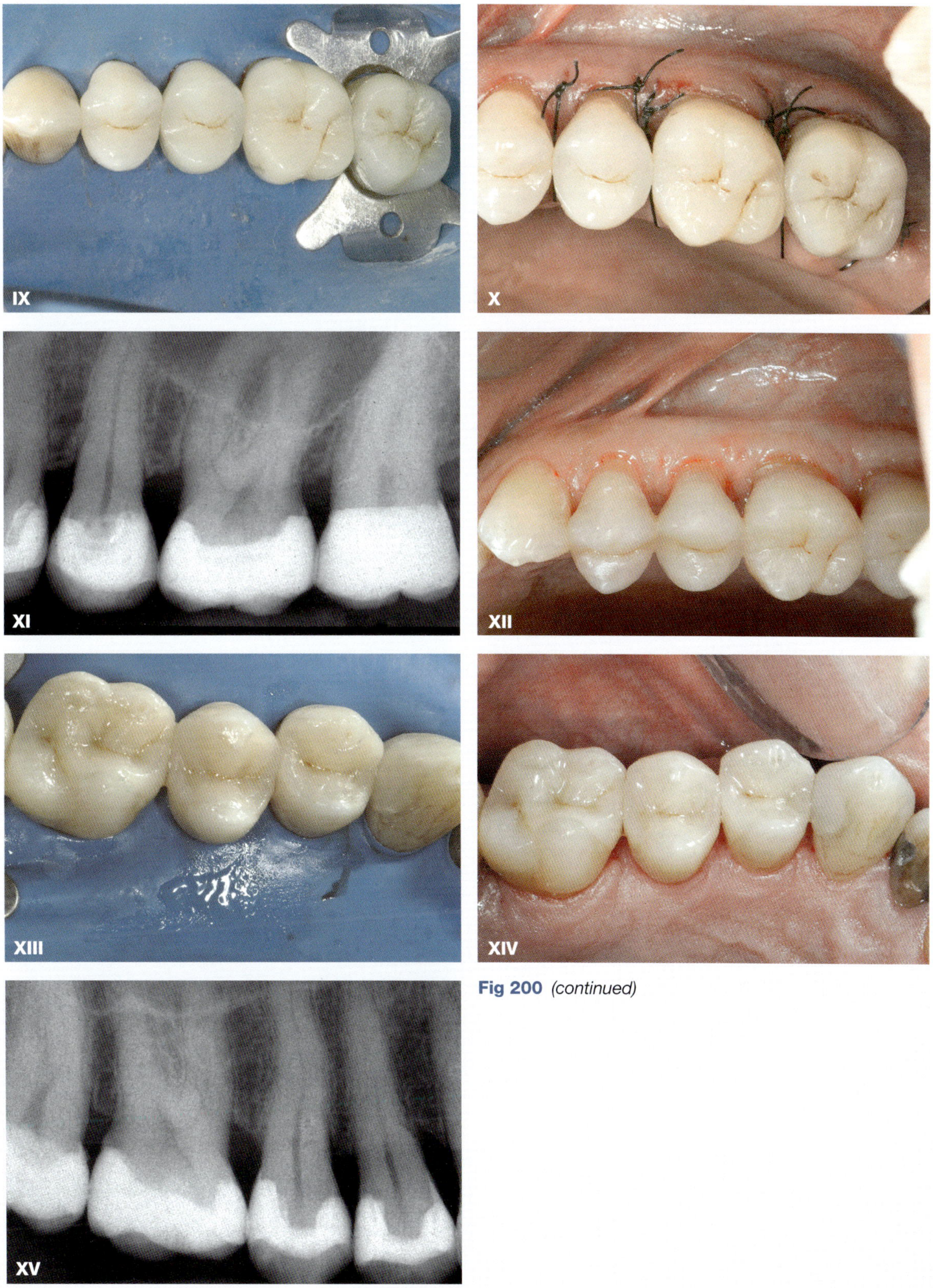

Fig 200 *(continued)*

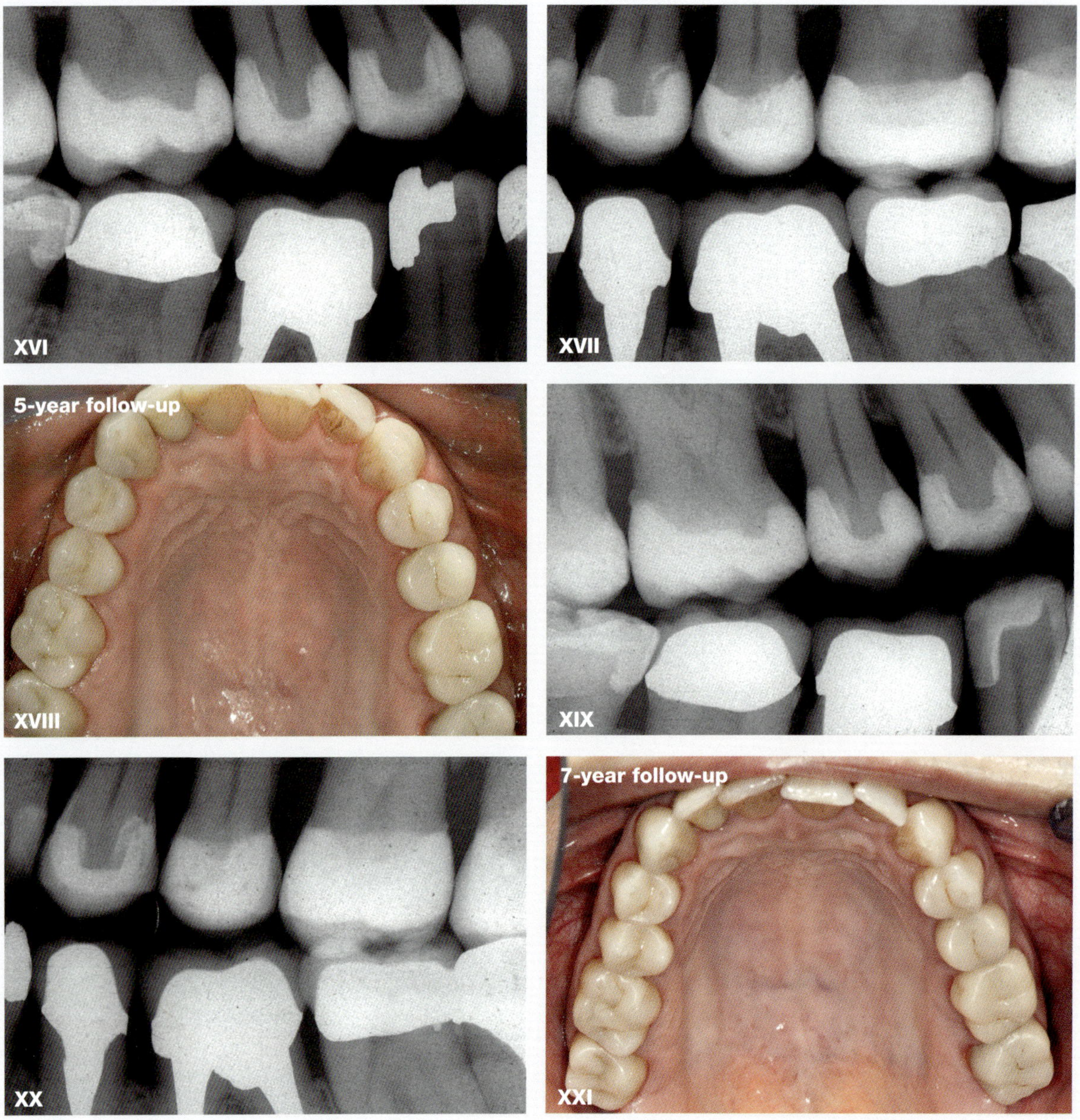

Fig 200 *(continued)*

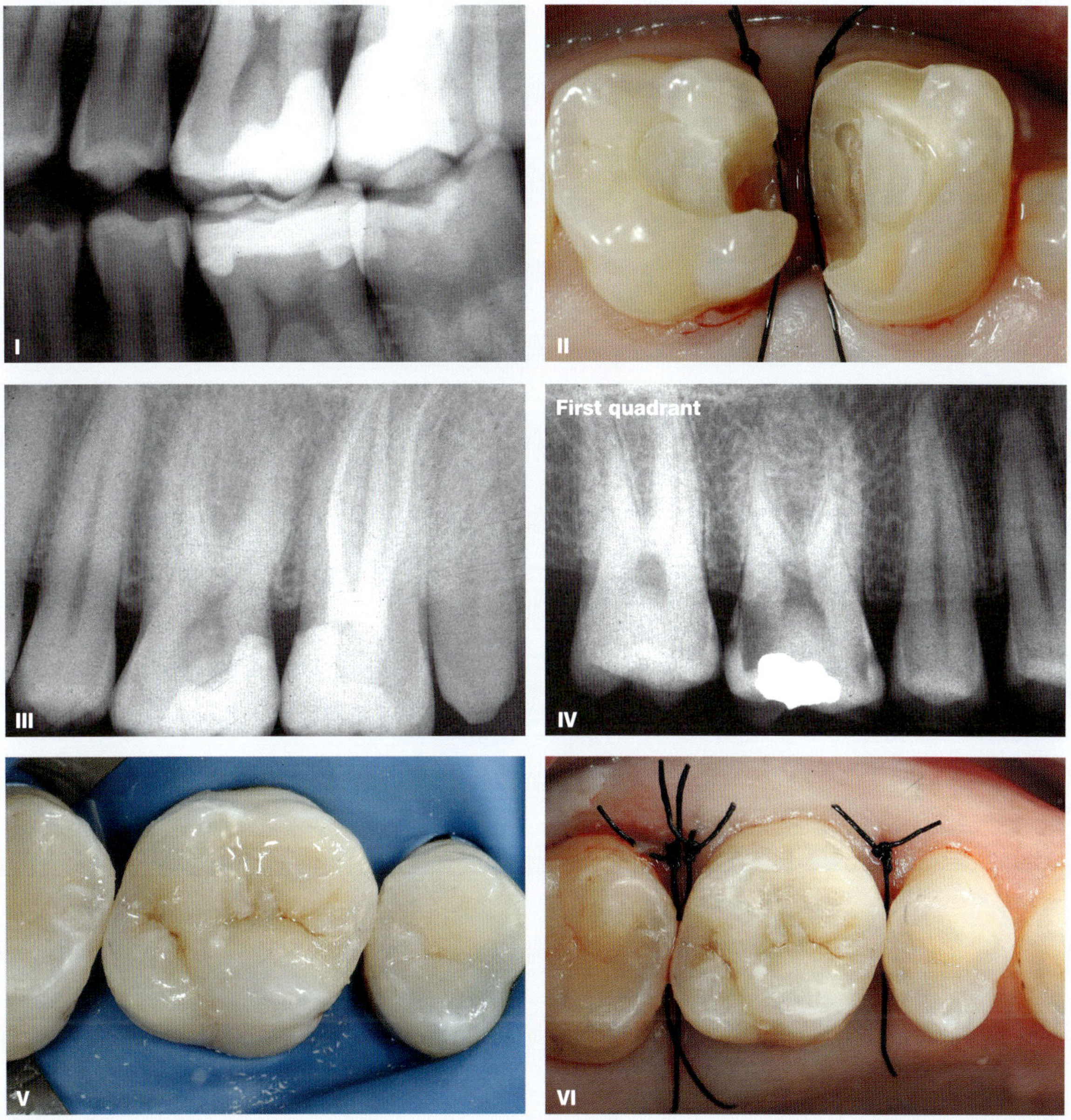

Fig 201 Despite the presence of deep caries lesions, the maxillary right first and second molar and left first molar had a positive pulp test, absence of periapical radiolucency, and absence of painful symptoms, which are very specific indications for not treating teeth endodontically *(I–VII)*. Occlusal view of maxilla following treatment of the aforementioned teeth *(VIII)*.

Fig 201 *(continued)*

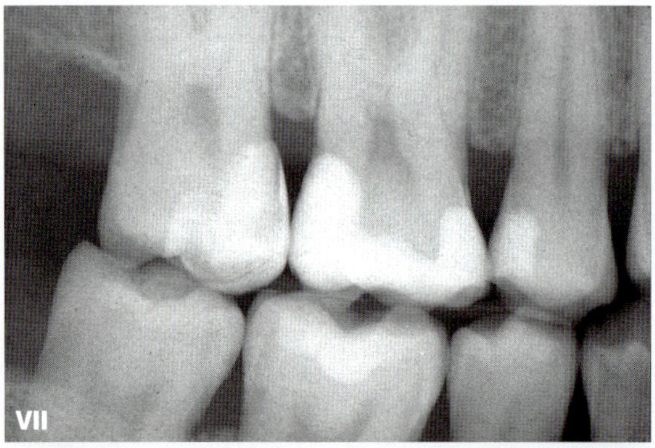

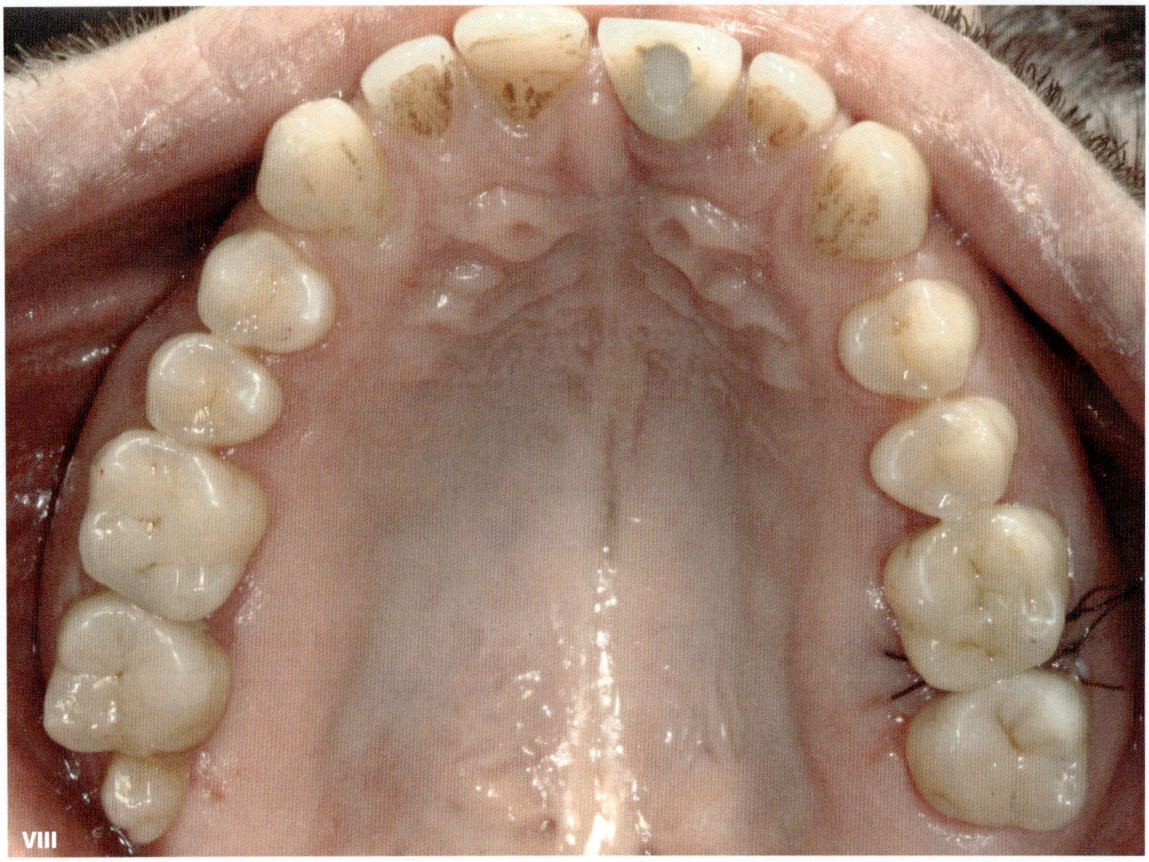

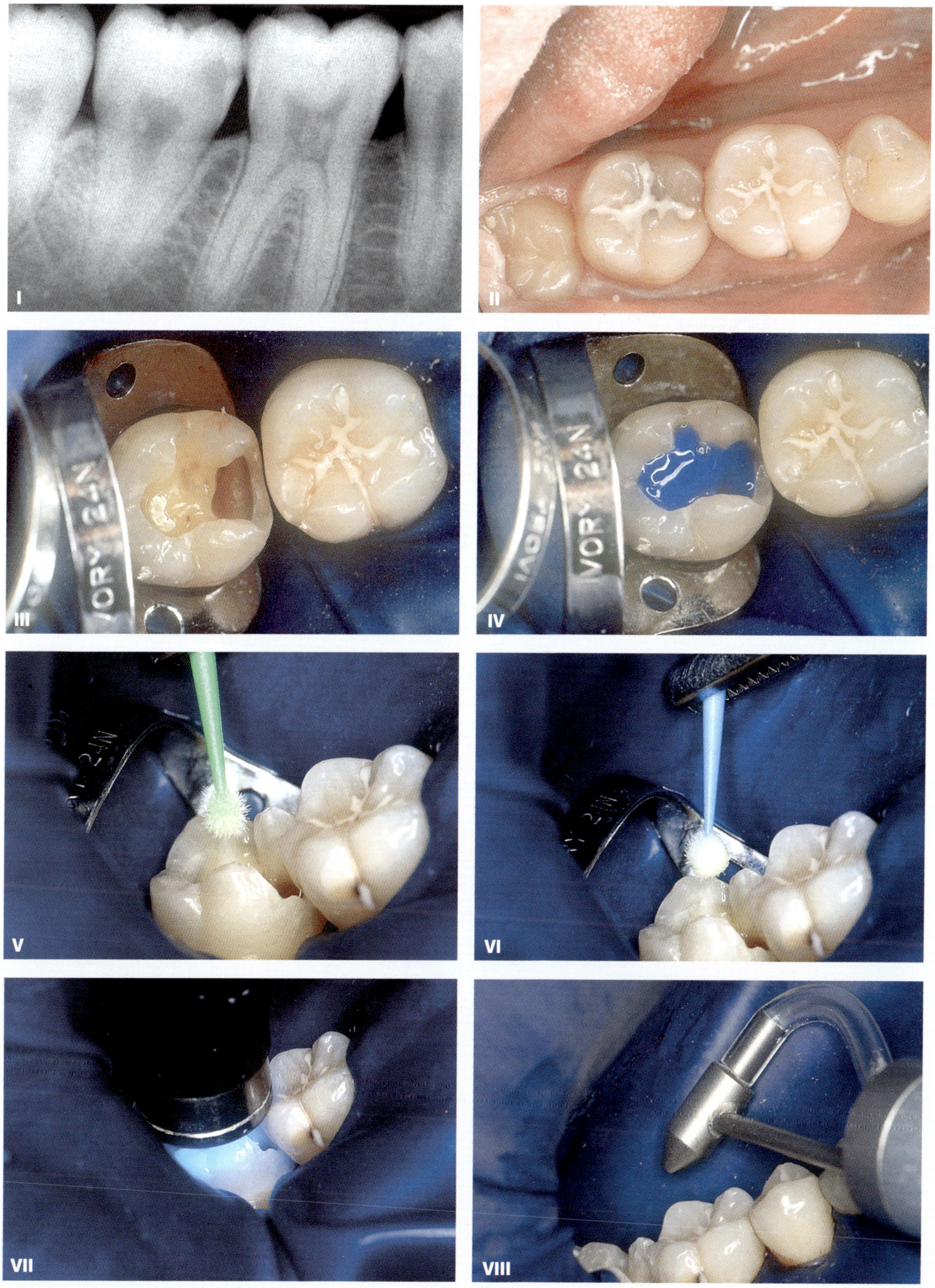

Fig 202 Mandibular right second molar with deep decay: removal of the decay, use of a three-step adhesive system, cementation following restoration, and follow-up radiograph. Conservative treatments were then carried out on the adjacent first molar and the maxillary right second premolar and second molar; the mandibular right third molar was eventually removed.

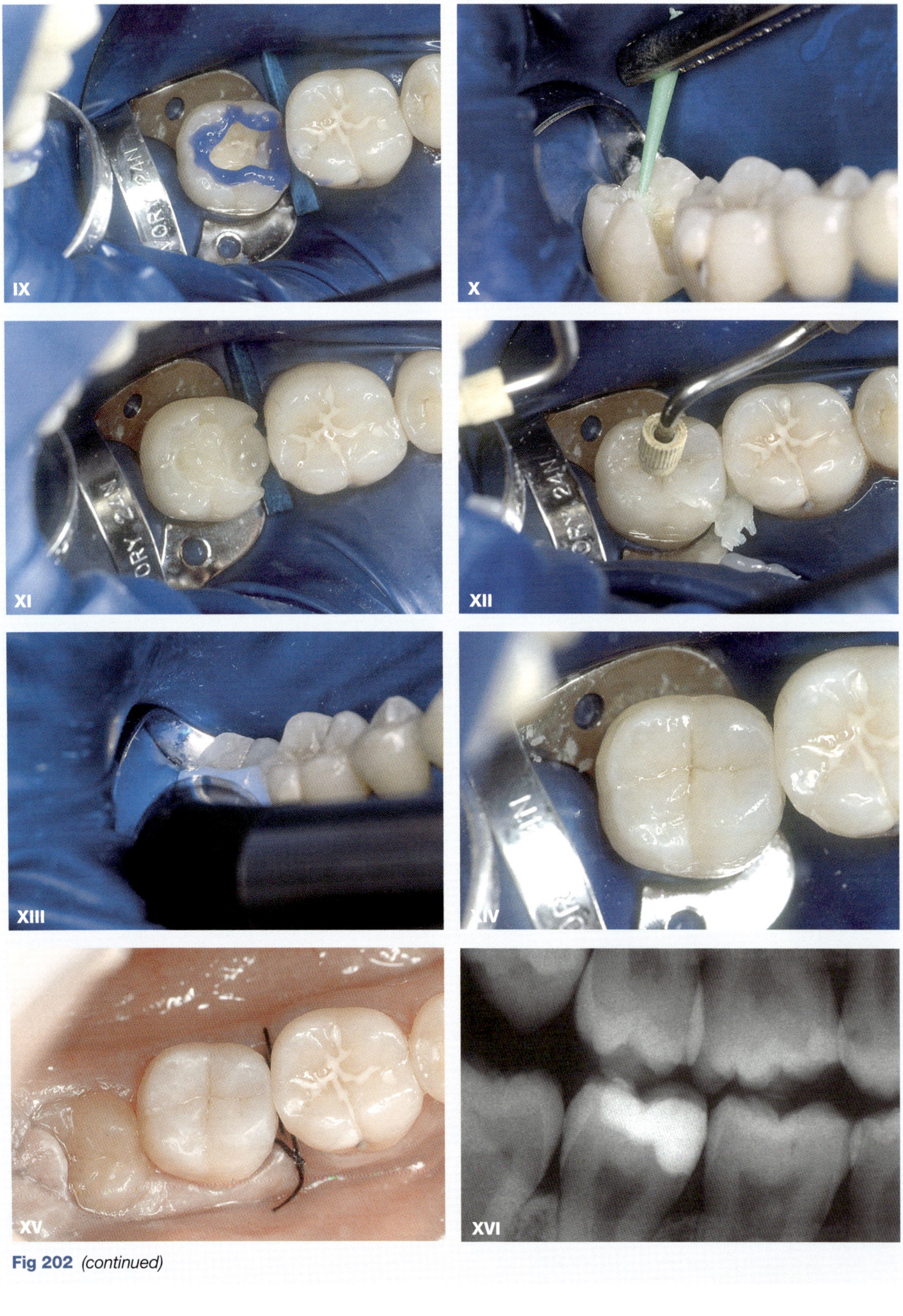

Fig 202 *(continued)*

The author's clinical experience supports this: out of approximately 3,000 restorations, it was only necessary to carry out a subsequent endodontic operation for 2% to 3% of teeth. This figure would very probably have been much higher if full crowns had been applied (Figs 203 and 204).
With regard to the technique of capping the pulp directly, the author is able to claim a 100% success rate, although it is true that his case sample only comprises to two cases (Figs 205 and 206).
Saving healthy tooth tissue makes a significant contribution toward respecting the pulp (Fig 207).

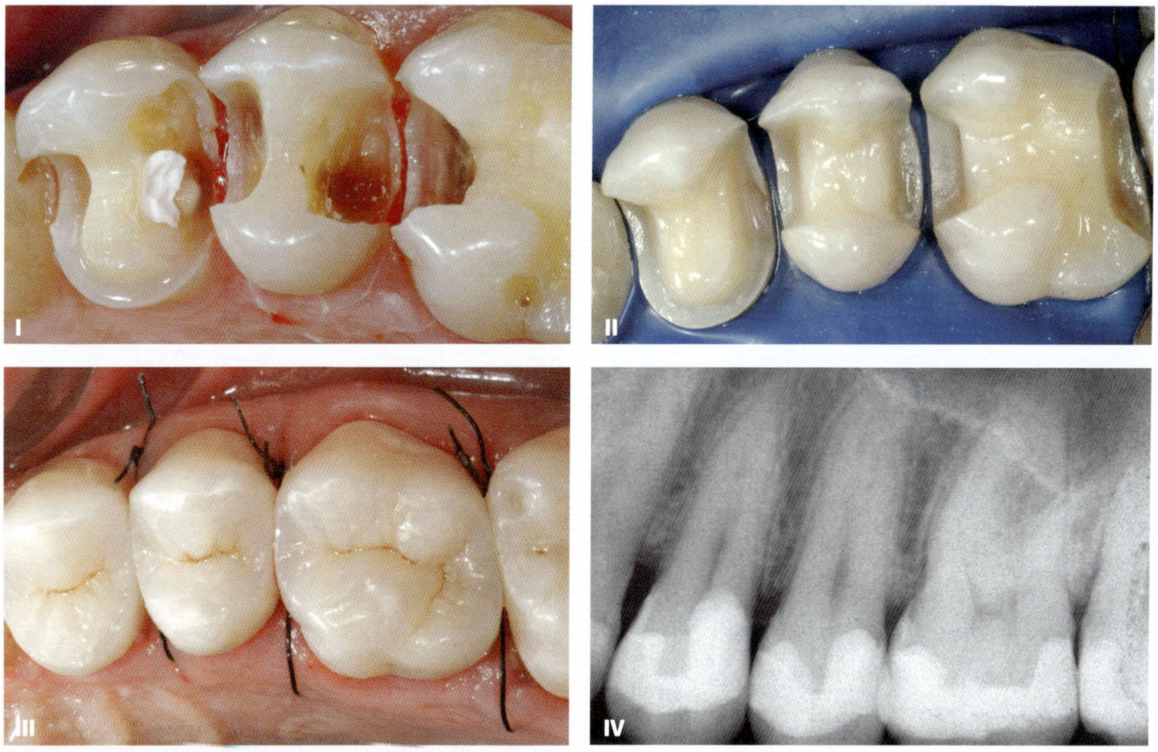

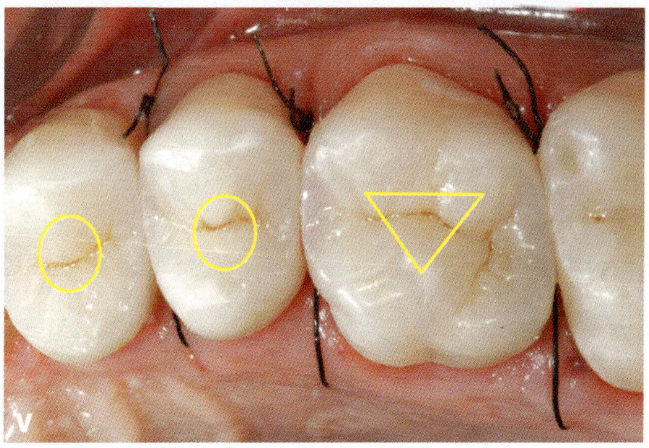

Fig 203 Extreme situation for endodontic treatment: absence of signs and symptoms of irroversible disease involving the pulp (periapical lesions, painful symptoms, pain on pressure, and positive vitality tests) justified preservation of the pulp tissue *(I–IV)*. Illustrations of possible future access cavities for endodontic treatment, to be sealed subsequently by means of an ordinary direct restoration using the same material (composite) used for the inlay, buildup, and cementation *(V)*.

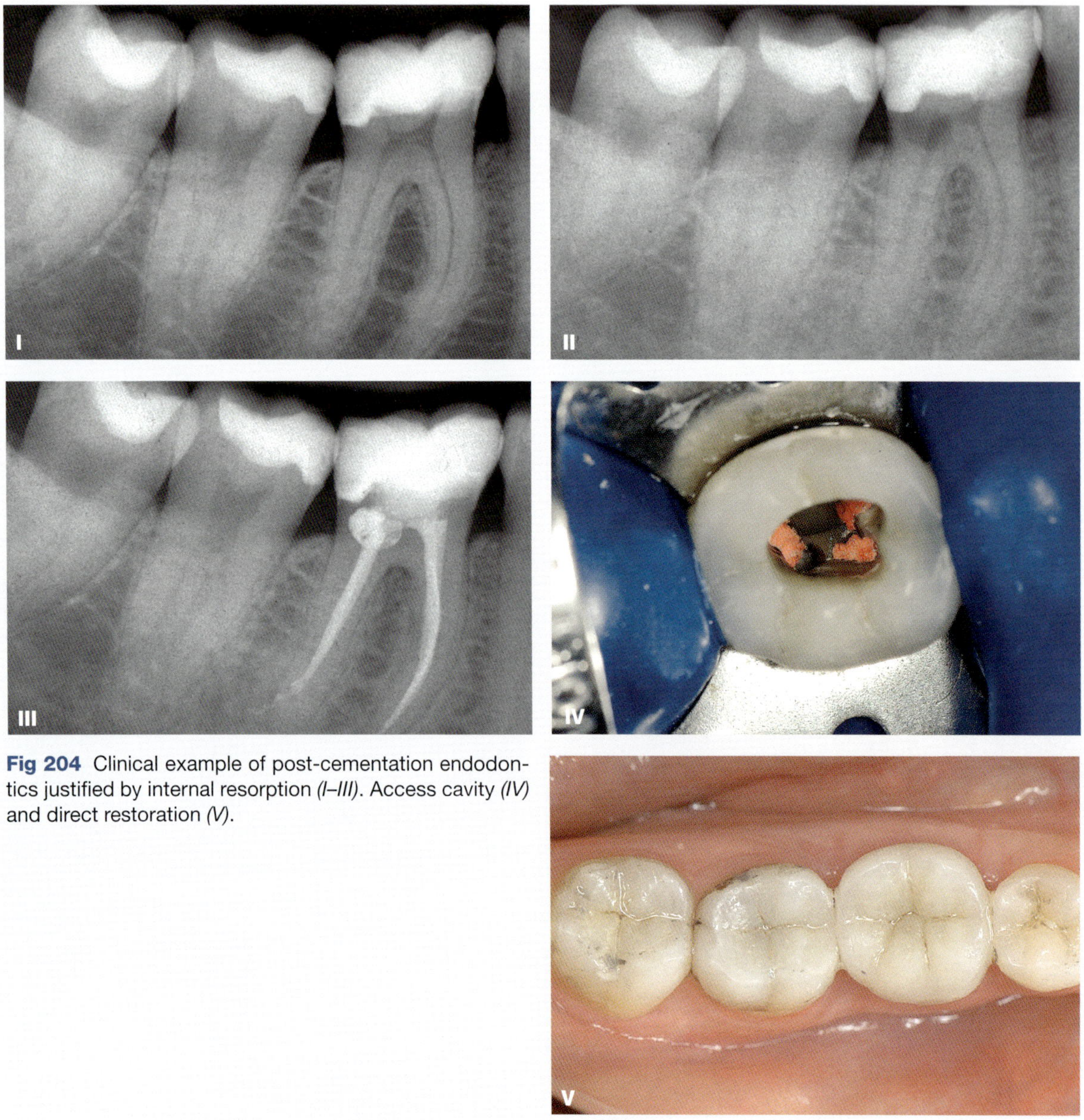

Fig 204 Clinical example of post-cementation endodontics justified by internal resorption *(I–III)*. Access cavity *(IV)* and direct restoration *(V)*.

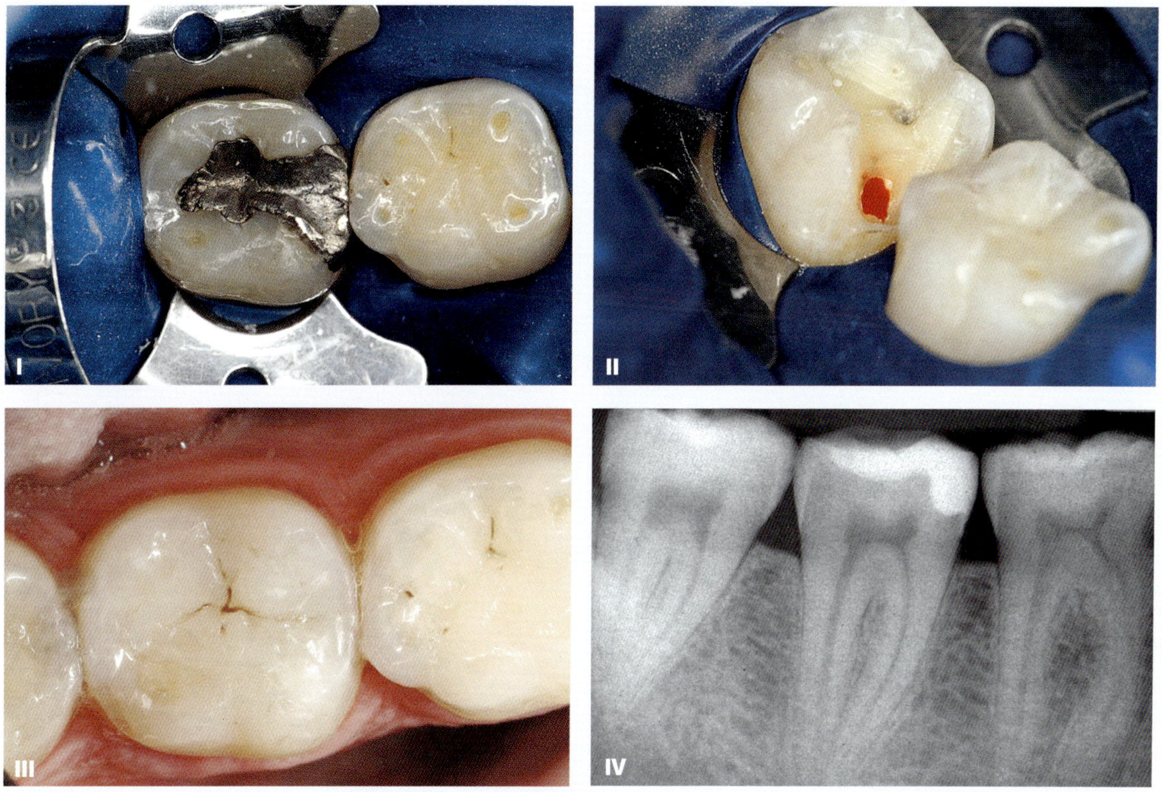

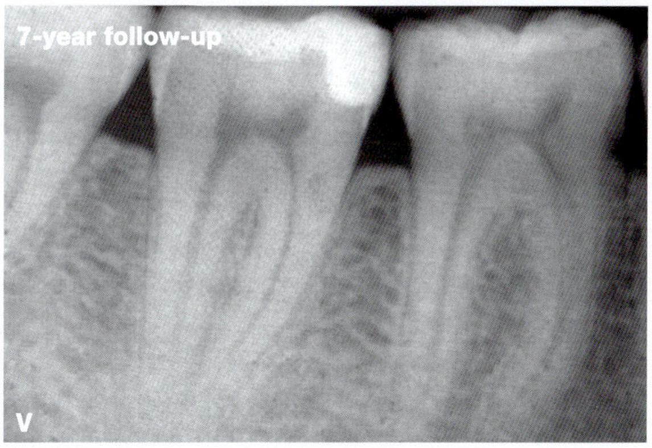

Fig 205 Direct capping of pulp with calcium hydroxide *(I–IV)* and radiographic follow-up after 7 years *(V)*. The vitality test remained positive.

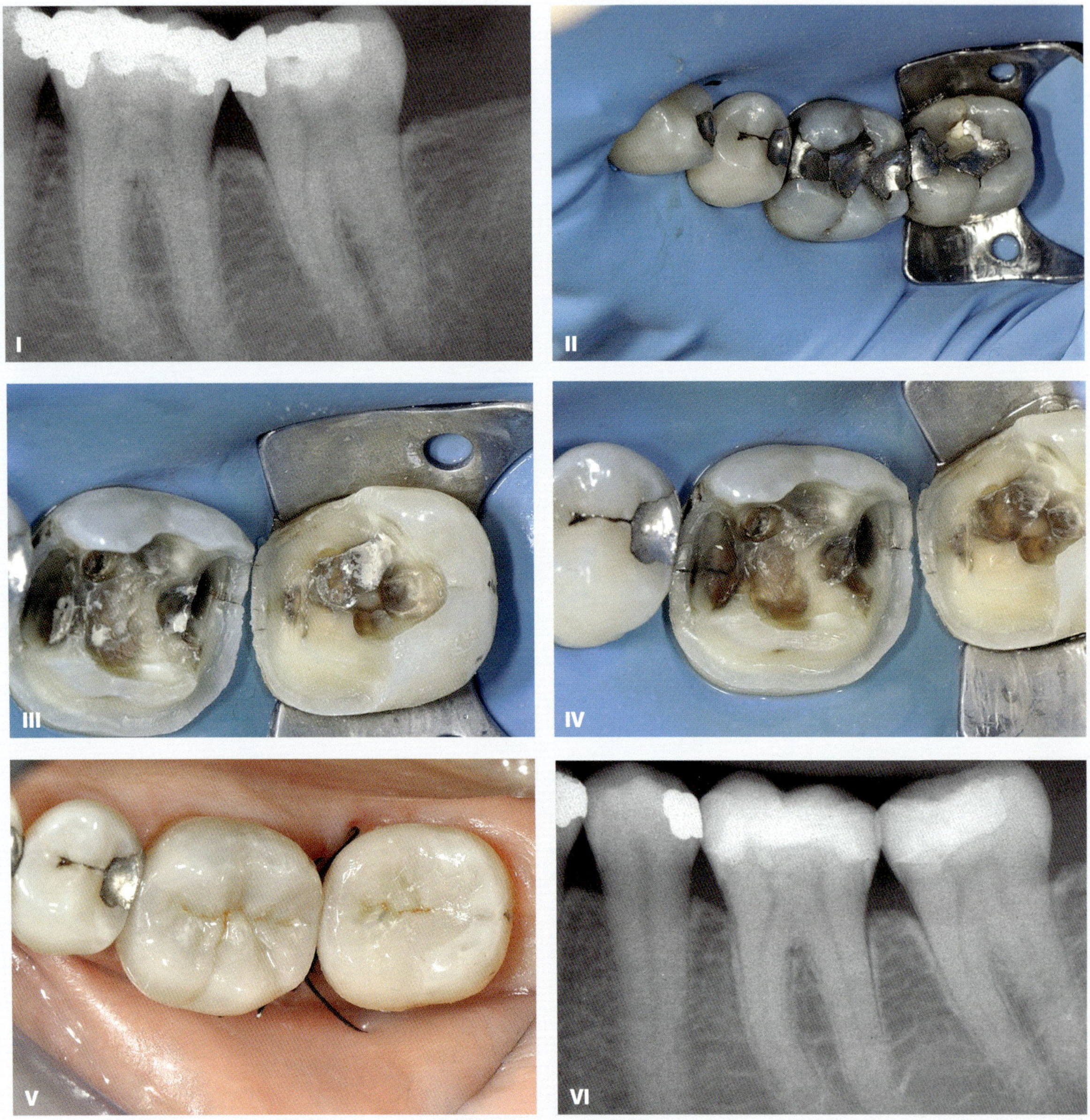

Fig 206 Probable former capping of pulp at point of mesiolingual pulp horn in a mandibular left first molar. The patient was duly notified, and with no signs and symptoms of irreversible disease involving the pulp and the usual positive tests, no endodontic treatment was carried out on the affected tooth.

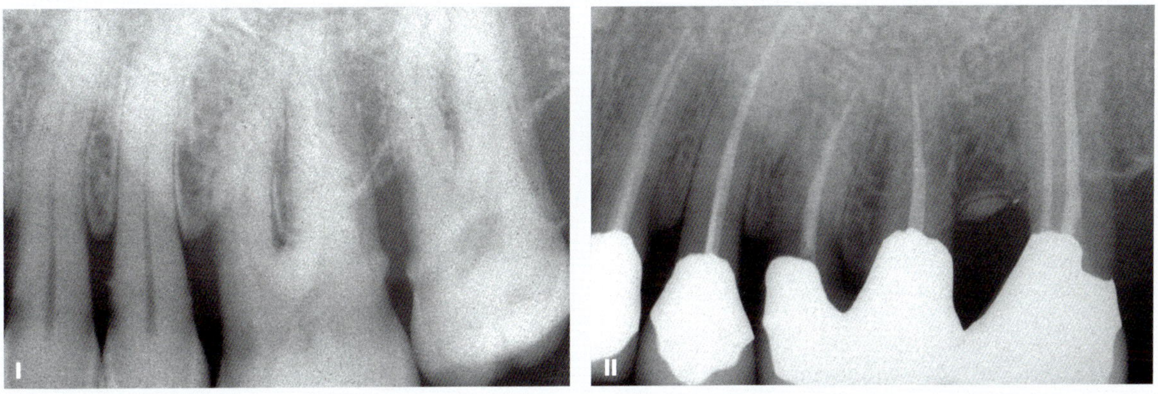

Fig 207 Returning to the topic of conservation, the author prefers not to comment on the treatment plan applied to the caries lesions present in the maxillary left premolars. The 17-year follow-up of the overtreatment was nevertheless encouraging.

When endodontic work is indicated, one should never lose sight of a conservative approach,[58] which in this case involves the root dentin. It is relatively common to see root canals with the coronal and middle thirds indiscriminately widened, almost certainly with the aim of reaching the apex more easily; however, the price paid in terms of reducing the mechanical strength of the treated tooth is very high (Figs 208 to 219). Since the 1980s, the literature has shown that excessive removal of root dentin due to excessive instrumentation and the use of oversized posts considerably compromises the root[49,59,60] (Fig 220).

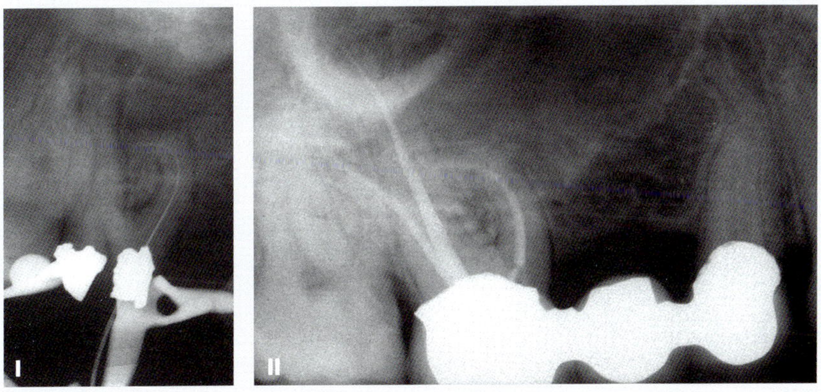

Fig 208 Endodontic treatment of the maxillary right first molar performed using manual instruments *(I)* and radiographic follow-up after 16 years *(II)*.

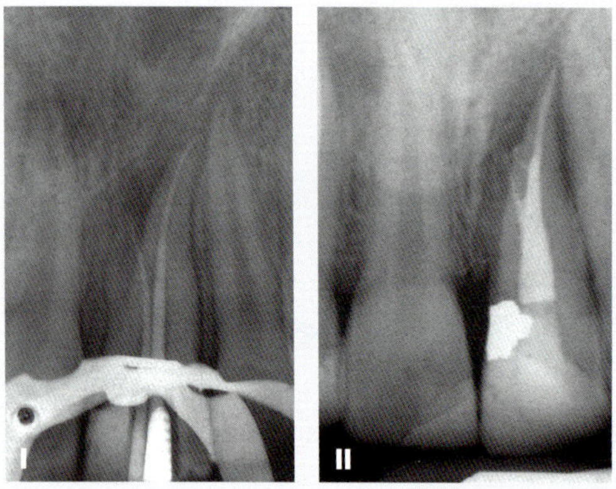

Fig 209 Endodontics and treatment of root decay during the 1990s.

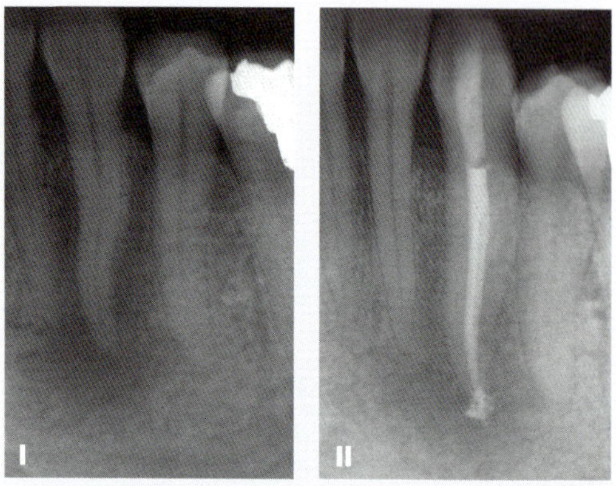

Fig 210 Respect for root dentin in a canine tooth, again using manual instruments.

Fig 211 Endodontic treatment of a pulp lesion with a reconstruction typical of the 1990s: metal post as intraradicular anchorage and amalgam followed by a prosthetic crown.

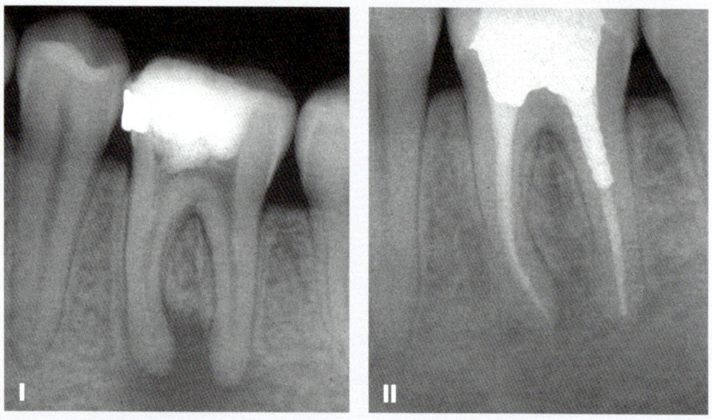

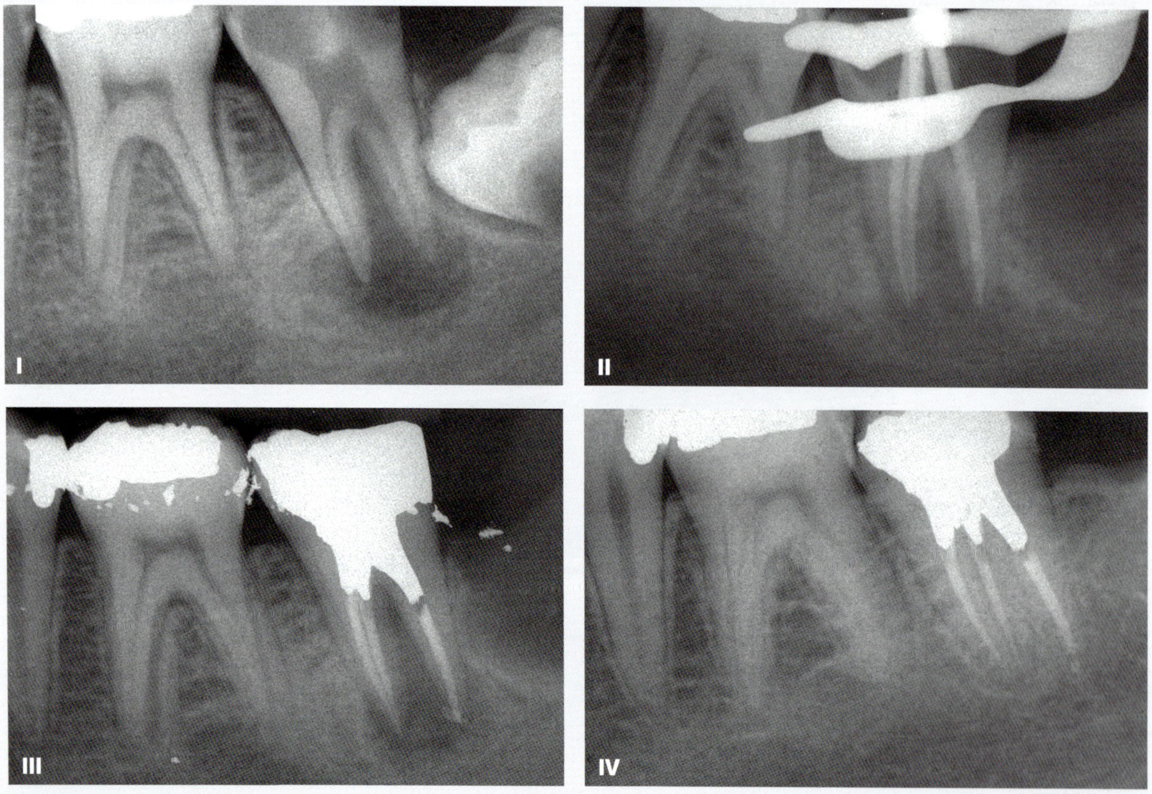

Fig 212 After endodontic treatment, the reconstruction used amalgam intraradicular pins for retention. The removal of these pins in the event of endodontic re-treatment is very difficult and risky.

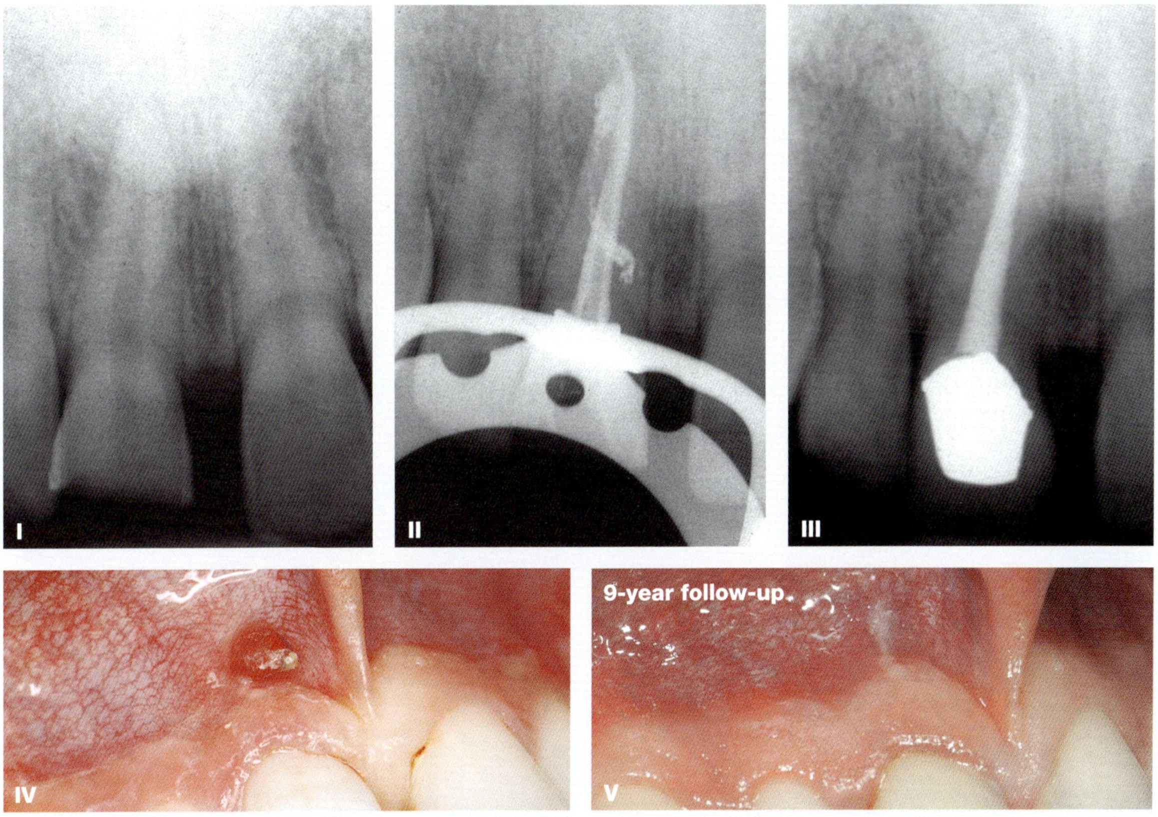

Fig 213 After compaction of warm gutta-percha, it traveled along the length of the fistula *(I, II)* until it appeared in the mucosa *(IV)*. Radiographic follow-up after a few weeks to confirm resolution of the fistula *(III)* and clinical view after 9 years *(V)*.

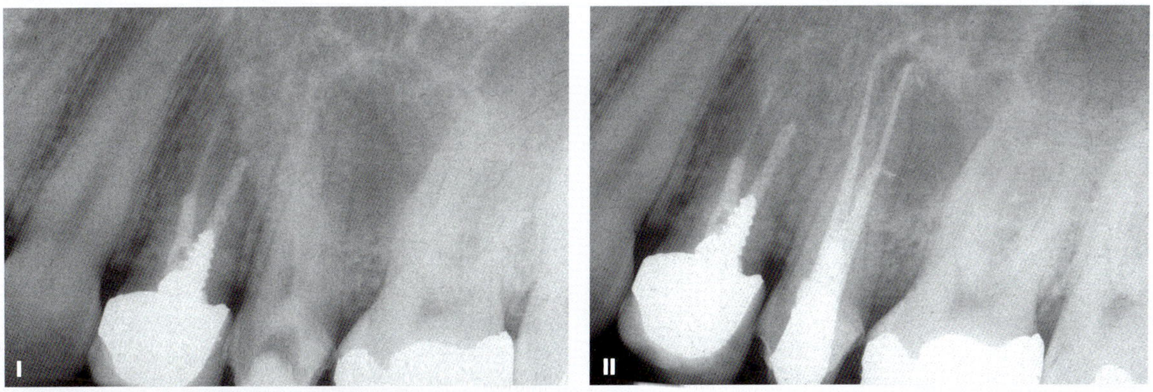

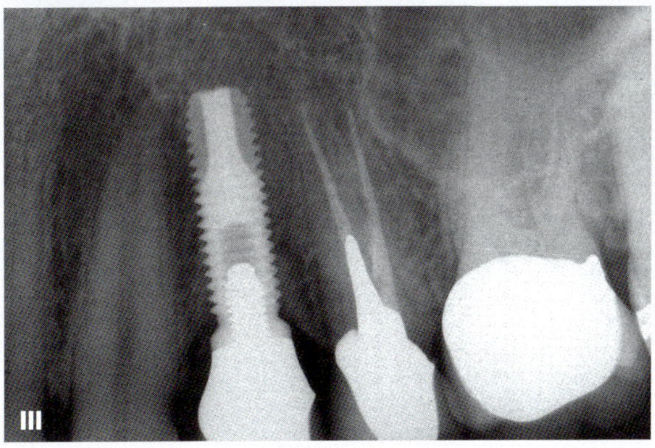

Fig 214 Lateral lesion in the maxillary left second premolar *(I)*. The patient was referred by medical colleagues who could not explain an erythrocyte sedimentation rate (ESR) of 80 following thorough examinations. The author carried out endodontic treatment, and a lateral canal emerging into the lesion site became evident after sealing the endodontic space *(II)*. Complete healing of the lesion was confirmed after a few months with an immediate return of normal ESR values. Radiographic follow-up after 15 years *(III)*.

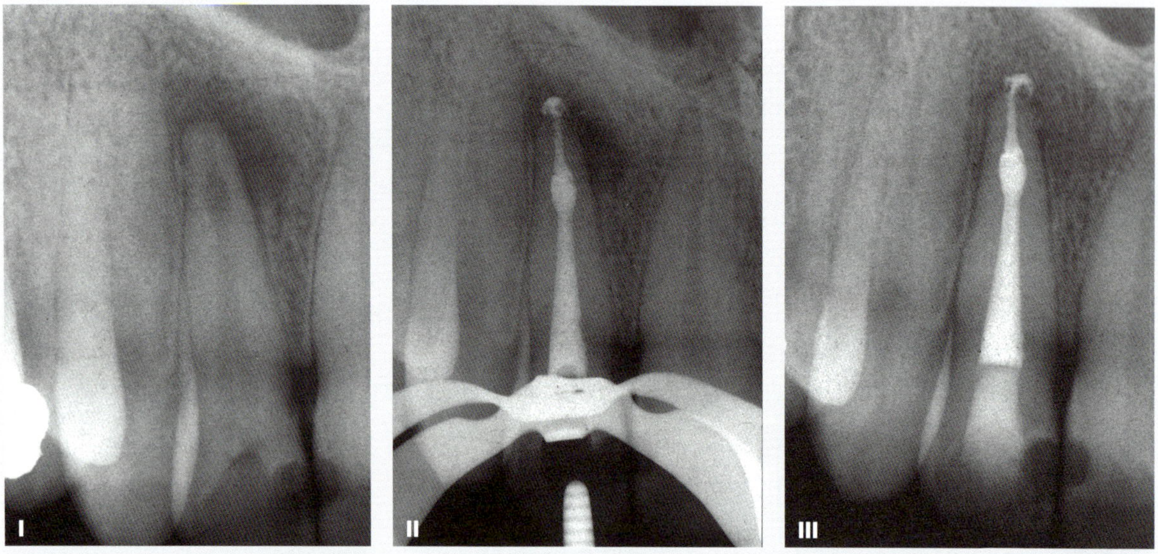

Fig 215 Filling of internal resorption with gutta-percha *(I, II)*. Radiographic follow-up only 9 months later showed a distinct improvement in the lesion *(III)*.

Fig 216 Follow-up 23 years after endodontic treatment was carried out without vertical compaction of warm gutta-percha. The canals were treated with multiple applications of sterile calcium hydroxide.

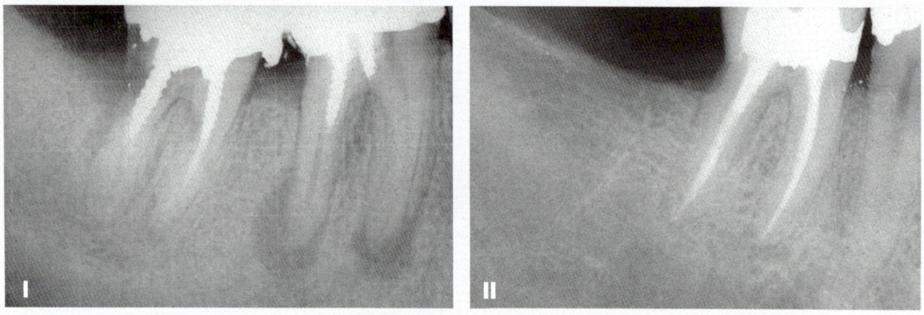

Fig 217 Preoperative radiography shockingly revealed that a channel had been created in the bone using a bur and then filled with material. The periodontologist had to spend many hours cleaning up the bone.

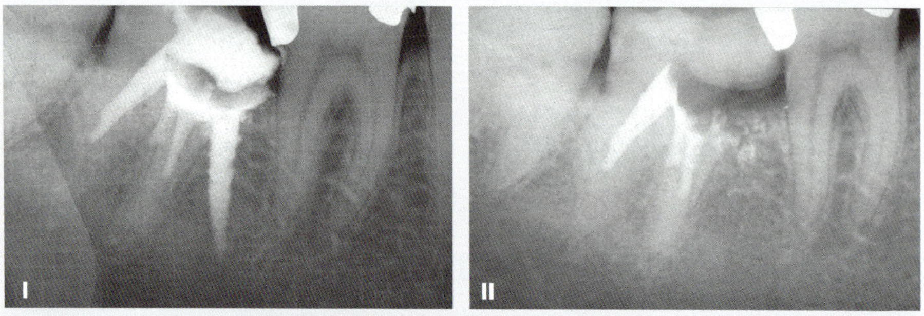

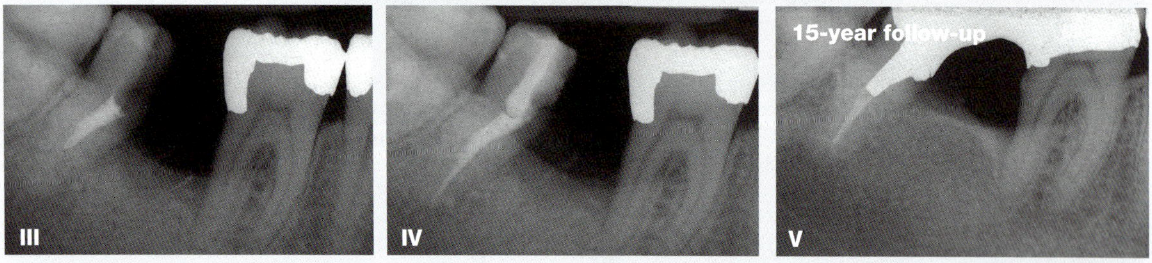

After treating the distal decay in the mandibular right first molar, the mesial root of the second molar was removed because, naturally, it was no longer usable. The distal root was treated endodontically, and a partial denture was constructed using the first molar and the distal root of the second molar as abutments. The patient understandably did not return for 15 years, but a follow-up radiograph taken at that time showed that the treatment had been successful.

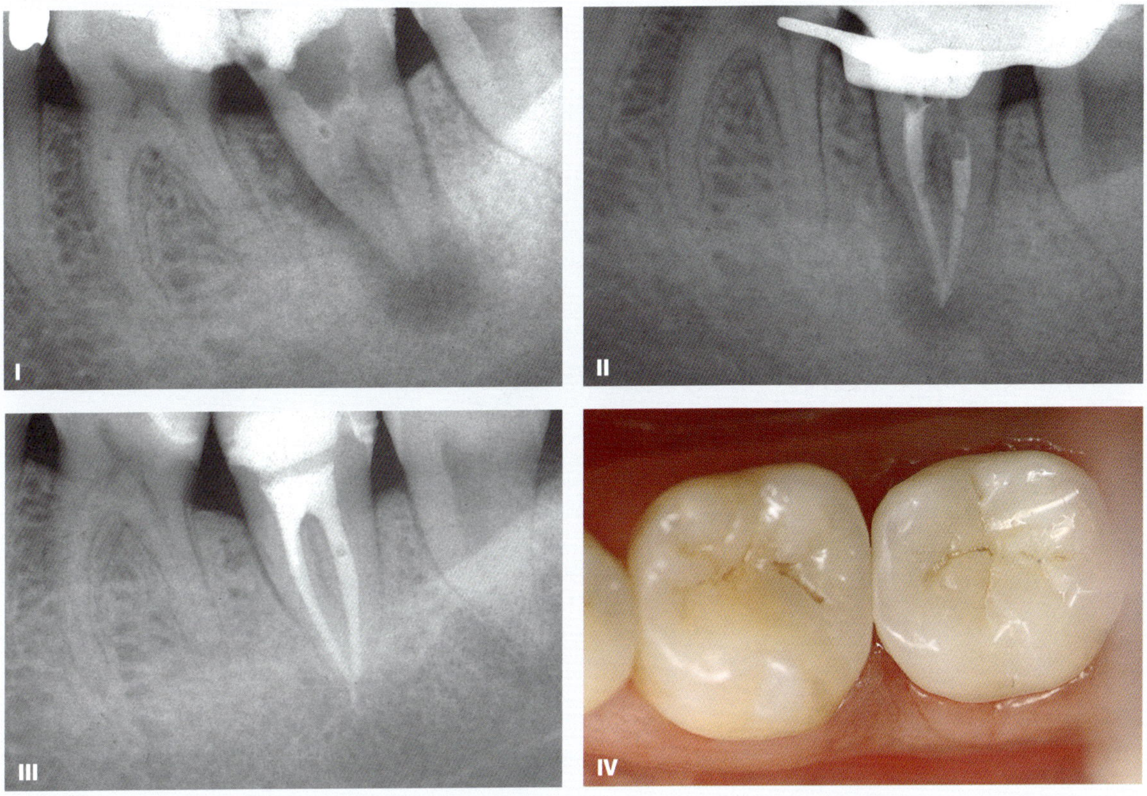

Fig 218 After performing an endodontic-periodontal differential diagnosis, the author treated the tooth endodontically *(I, II)*. The reconstruction was carried out without using posts because of the size of the pulp chamber, and treatment was completed using a composite inlay *(IV)*. Radiographic follow-up after 5 years is shown *(III)*.

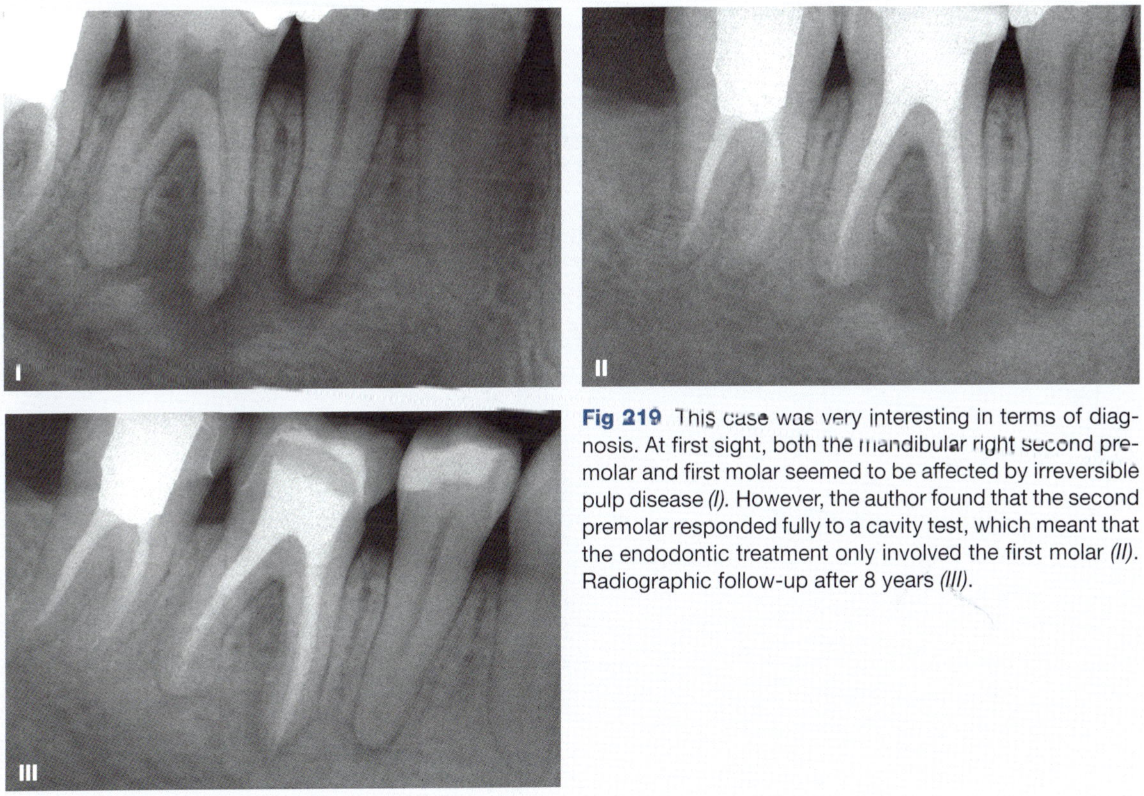

Fig 219 This case was very interesting in terms of diagnosis. At first sight, both the mandibular right second premolar and first molar seemed to be affected by irreversible pulp disease *(I)*. However, the author found that the second premolar responded fully to a cavity test, which meant that the endodontic treatment only involved the first molar *(II)*. Radiographic follow-up after 8 years *(III)*.

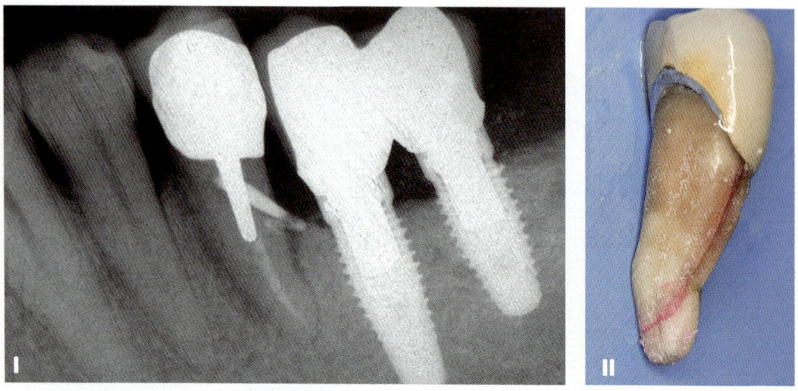

Fig 220 Vertical fracture of a mandibular premolar.

Continuing on the subject of conservative dentistry, the international scientific literature agrees that teeth without posts are stronger than those with posts[49,50,61] (Figs 221 and 222).

The use of a post is indicated in endodontically treated teeth with insufficient residual tooth tissue to support a reconstruction.[55]

Endodontically treated teeth are now reconstructed using adhesive techniques, and the use of fiber posts is indicated, as demonstrated by Fichera et al.[62]

Endodontic procedures have also undergone equally exceptional improvements due to the introduction of nickel-titanium rotary instruments, and endodontic results have been achieved that were once unthinkable in terms of execution times and quality.

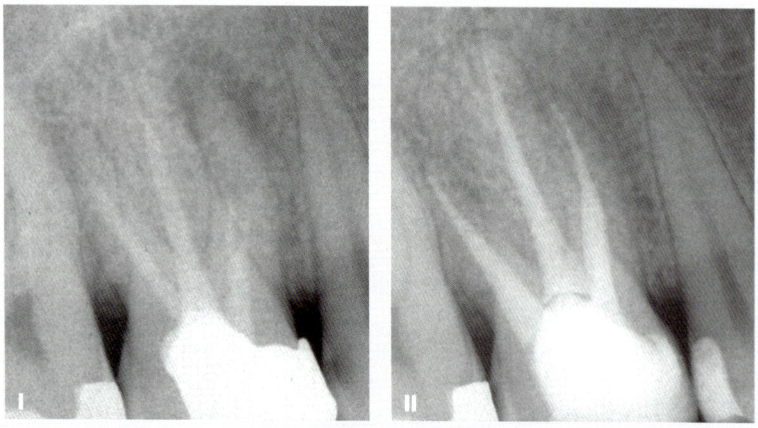

Fig 221 Note the consistent endodontic treatment performed without the use of posts. (Endodontics by Dr Marco Forestali.)

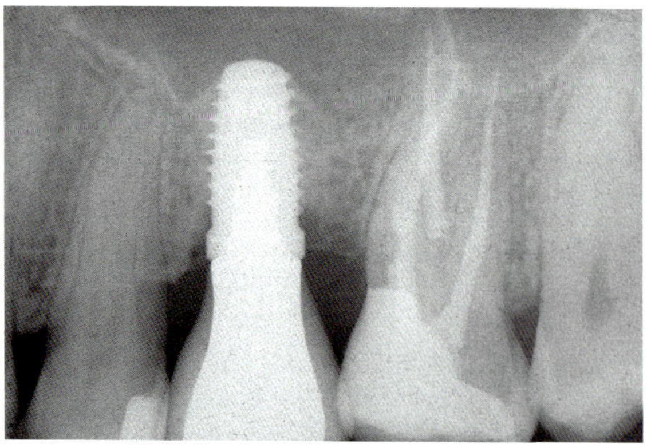

Fig 222 Use of intraradicular anchorage in the reconstruction of endodontically treated teeth showing insufficient healthy residual dental matter.

Until the mid-1990s, endodontically treated teeth in the posterior sectors were often restored using a metal core made up of a cast post buildup or a screw and silver amalgam before being covered with a metal-ceramic crown (Fig 223).

It was believed that the cast post (extending along two-thirds of the root) or a self-tapping prefabricated post cemented using oxyphosphate would reinforce the core-crown complex in teeth with little coronal structure.[63] Clinical evidence has nevertheless revealed numerous root fractures associated with the use of such posts, probably due to a wedge effect.[64,65]

Due to progress in adhesive dentistry and resin cements, dentists have switched to the use of cast or prefabricated passive posts (metal or fiber). Preparation of the post space is limited to removing gutta-percha or endodontic cement to safeguard wall resistance. In this way, the impact of occlusal and masticatory stresses is reduced, partly due to the action of the resin cement, which acts as reinforcement. In endodontically treated teeth to be restored using metal-free materials, epoxy resin posts are used instead, reinforced with fiber and adhesively cemented into the root canal.[66,67]

Clinical experience shows that the use of such posts seems to cancel out or at least significantly reduce the incidence of root fracture associated with active metal posts: the worst that could happen is decementation of the post.[68,69]

Present-day composite materials have achieved outstanding performance even in the indirect restoration of endodontically treated posterior teeth. The Hansen study is a good example of this.[70]

The use of a fiber intracanal post does not reinforce the root but simply acts as an anchorage device in the root-restoration system, above all with the purpose of controlling occlusal stresses with a lateral component.

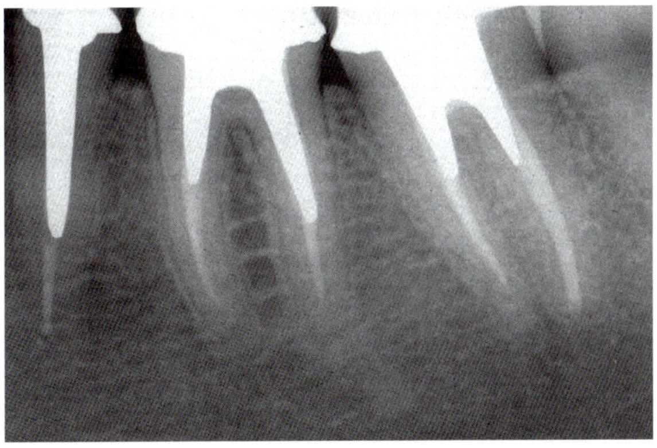

Fig 223 Example of typical restorations placed during the 1980s and 1990s using posts and crowns.

The indication for the use of posts in partial restorations is determined in individual cases by the presence and thickness of the walls present, the presence or absence of marginal ridges, the depths of the pulp chamber (a retaining factor only in molars), the position of the tooth in the arch, and the type of occlusion.

In posterior teeth with four walls, a post is often unnecessary, and a direct restoration is indicated, above all in cases of single restorations without significant fracture lines (Fig 224).

Even when three walls are present, there is often no indication for the use of a post (Figs 225 to 228).

Conversely, severe loss of tooth tissue always requires the positioning of intraradicular retention (Figs 229 to 233).

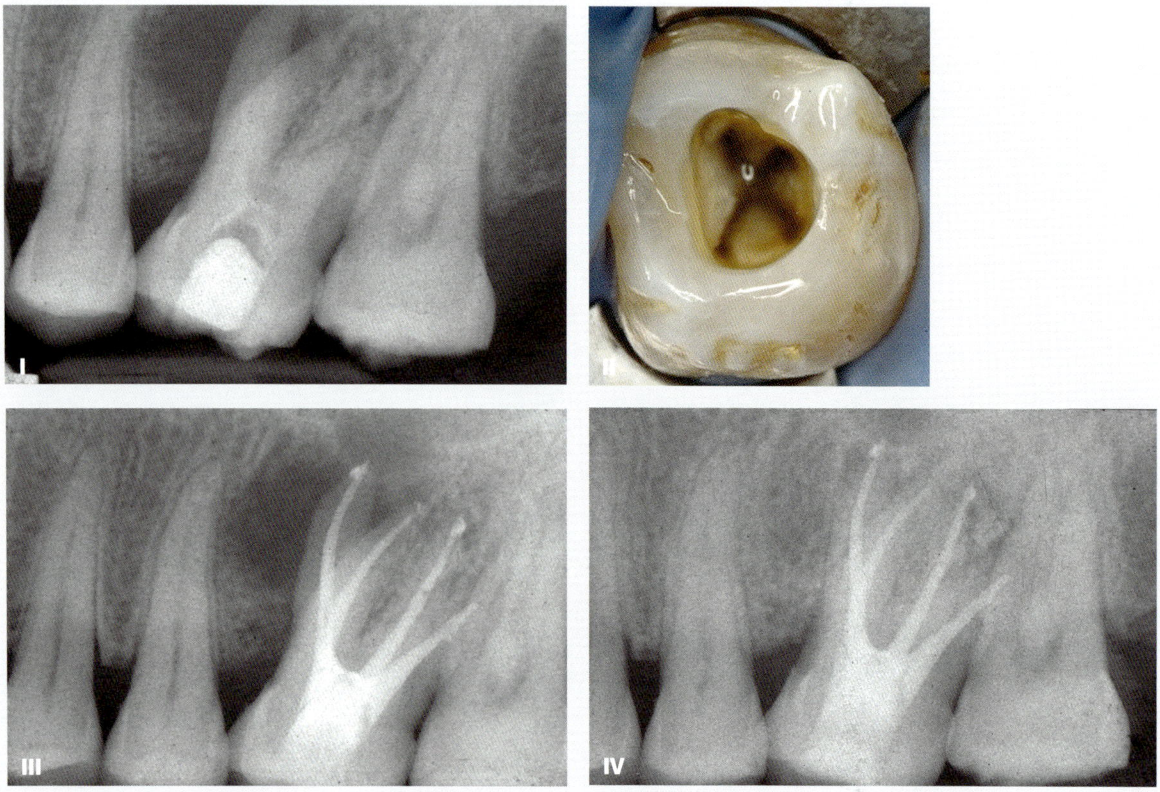

Fig 224 Presence of four walls of sufficient thickness means that the use of posts is not needed.

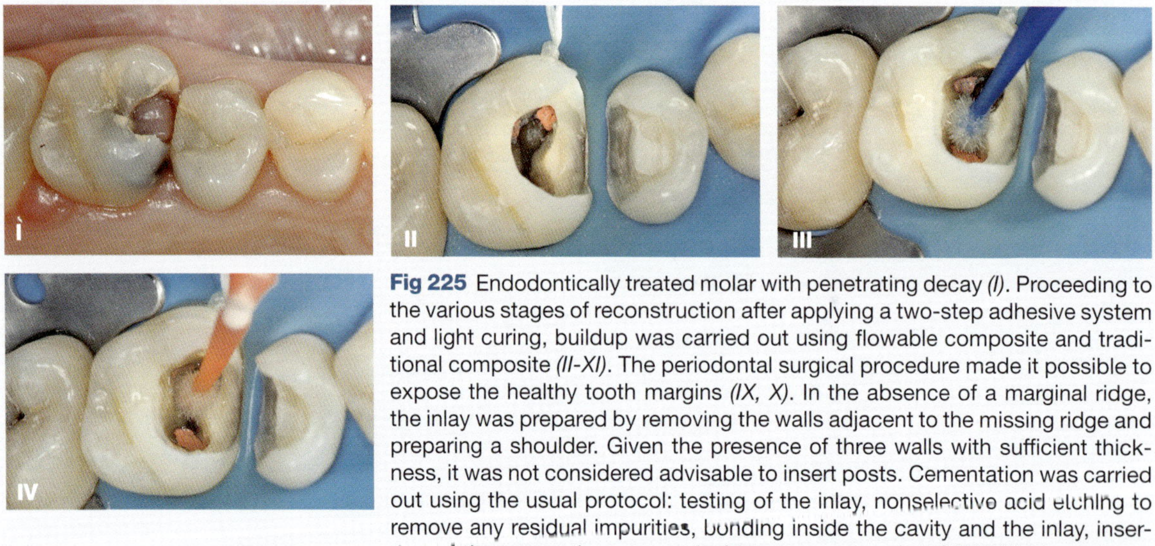

Fig 225 Endodontically treated molar with penetrating decay *(I)*. Proceeding to the various stages of reconstruction after applying a two-step adhesive system and light curing, buildup was carried out using flowable composite and traditional composite *(II-XI)*. The periodontal surgical procedure made it possible to expose the healthy tooth margins *(IX, X)*. In the absence of a marginal ridge, the inlay was prepared by removing the walls adjacent to the missing ridge and preparing a shoulder. Given the presence of three walls with sufficient thickness, it was not considered advisable to insert posts. Cementation was carried out using the usual protocol: testing of the inlay, nonselective acid etching to remove any residual impurities, bonding inside the cavity and the inlay, insertion of the restoration, removal of excess, and curing *(XII-XXX)*. A post was nevertheless positioned in the premolar based on knowledge of the eccentric forces to which these teeth are subject. Once rubber dam had been removed, an occlusal check was carried out.

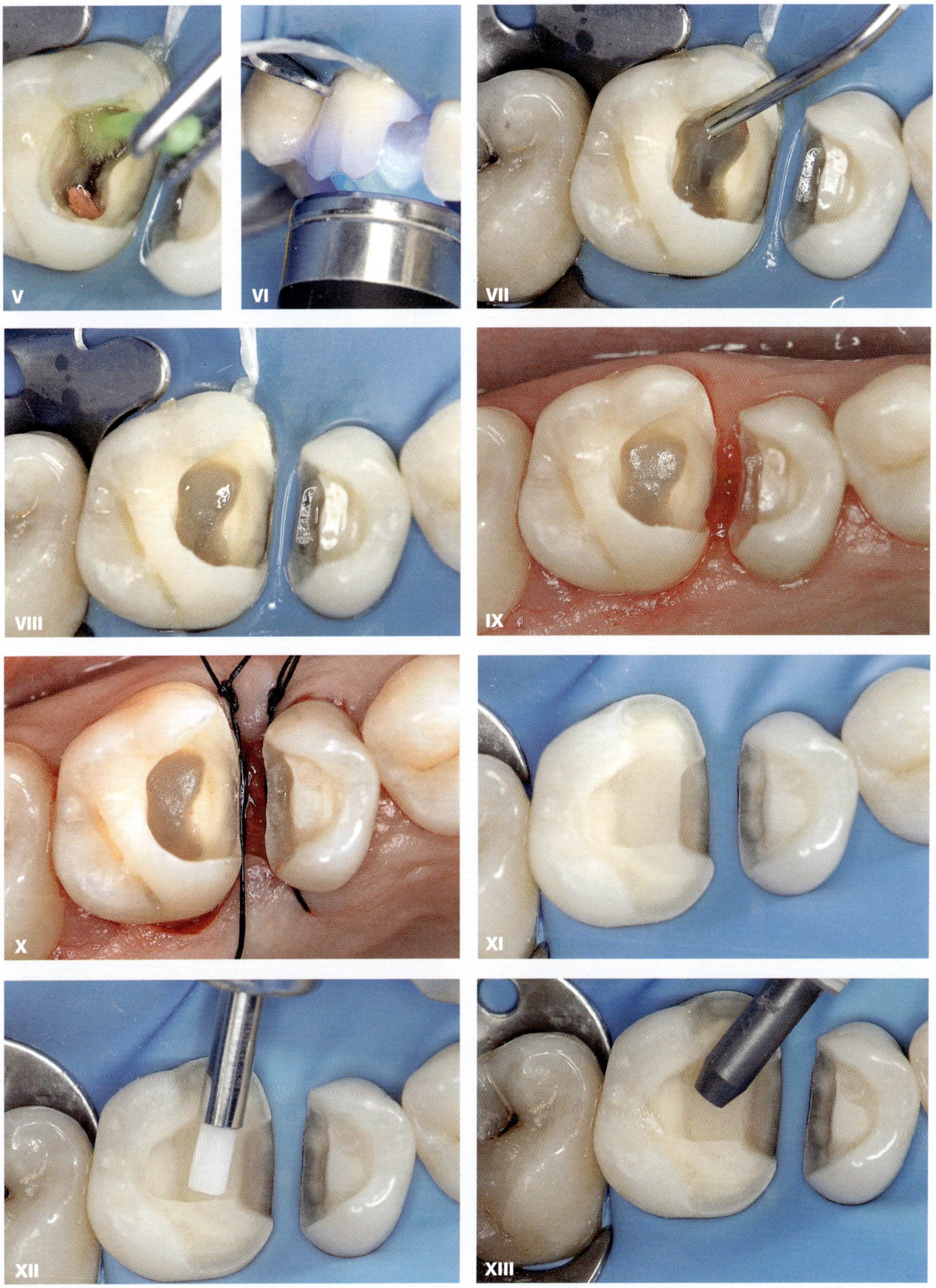

Fig 225 *(continued)*

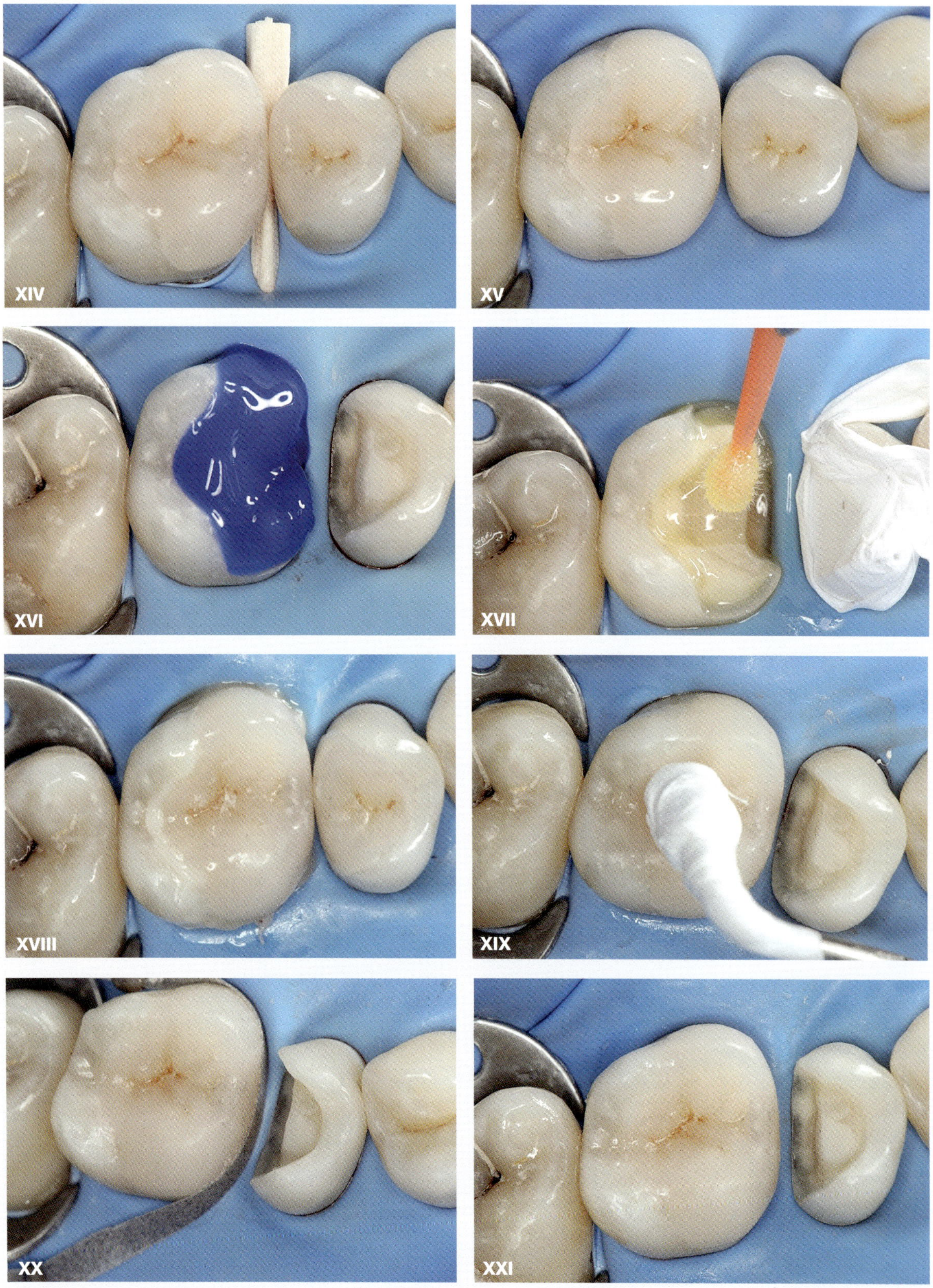

Fig 225 *(continued)*

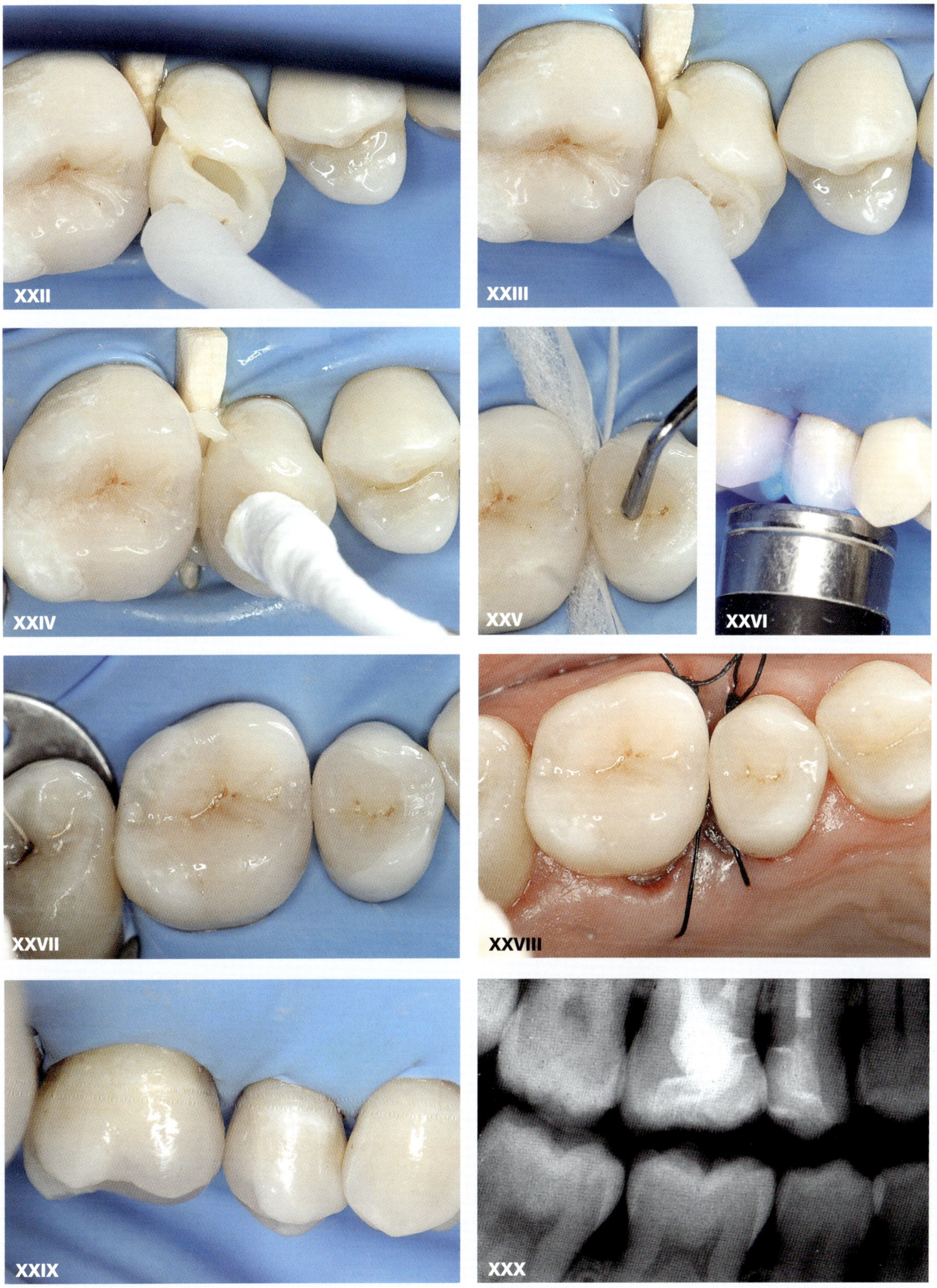

Fig 225 *(continued)*

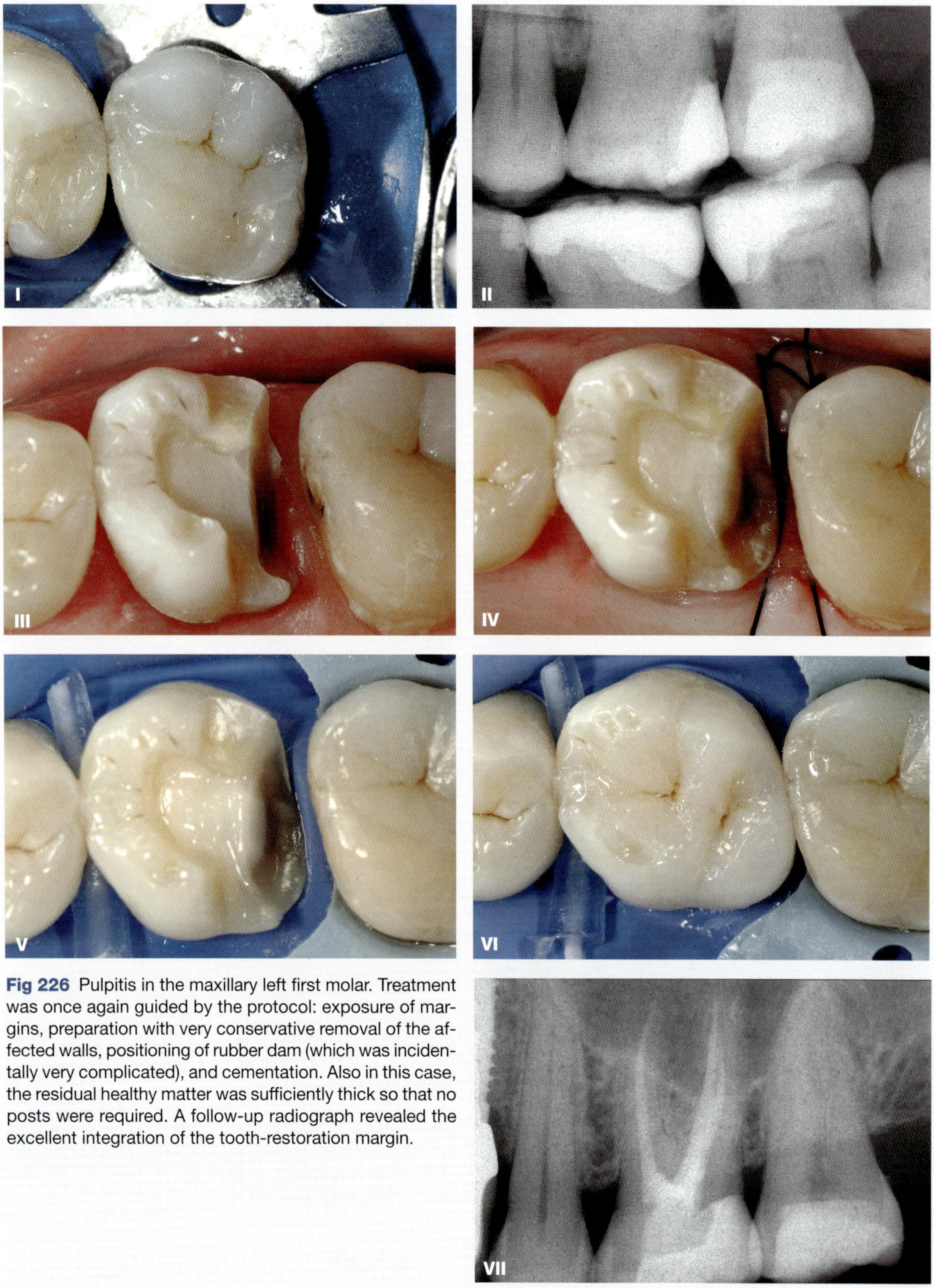

Fig 226 Pulpitis in the maxillary left first molar. Treatment was once again guided by the protocol: exposure of margins, preparation with very conservative removal of the affected walls, positioning of rubber dam (which was incidentally very complicated), and cementation. Also in this case, the residual healthy matter was sufficiently thick so that no posts were required. A follow-up radiograph revealed the excellent integration of the tooth-restoration margin.

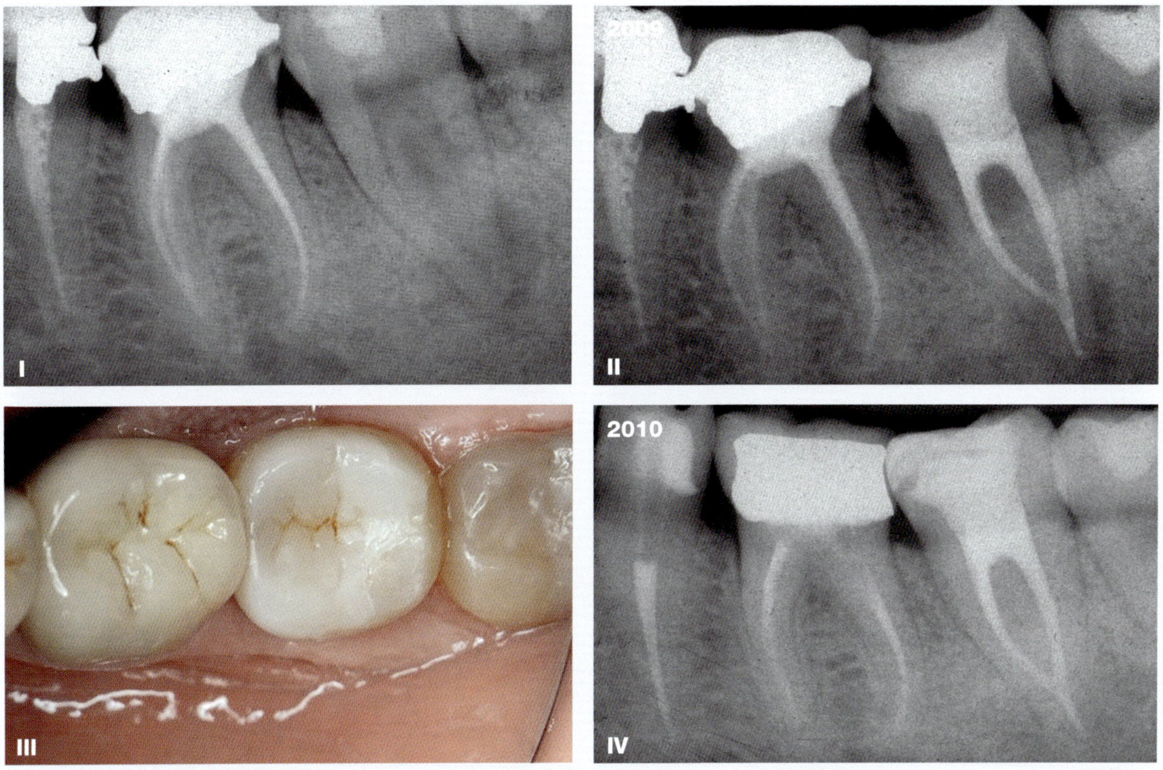

Fig 227 Endodontic treatment of the mandibular left second molar due to a periapical lesion. Because the distal marginal ridge and adjacent walls were present, an onlay was constructed, and no post was inserted. Posts were nevertheless used in the prosthetic crowns applied to the adjacent first molar and second premolar, given that all the walls were missing in these teeth.

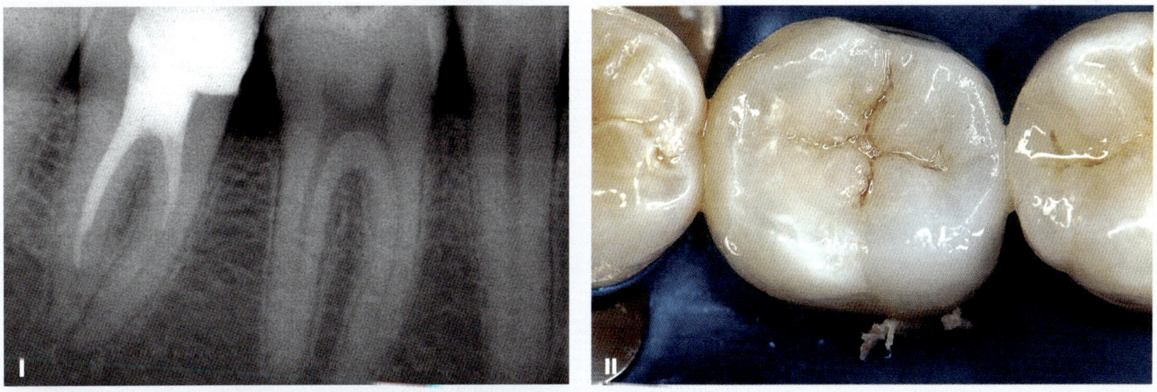

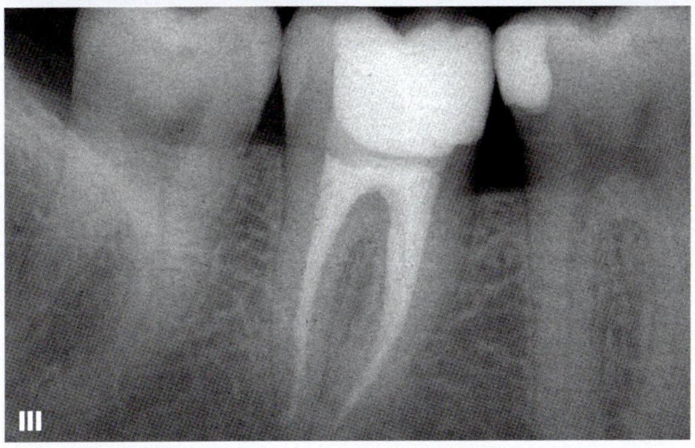

Fig 228 This clinical example is repeated to emphasize the absence of intraradicular anchorage. The author believes that this is the approach to be taken, which is confirmed by the good radiographic follow-up 9 years later.

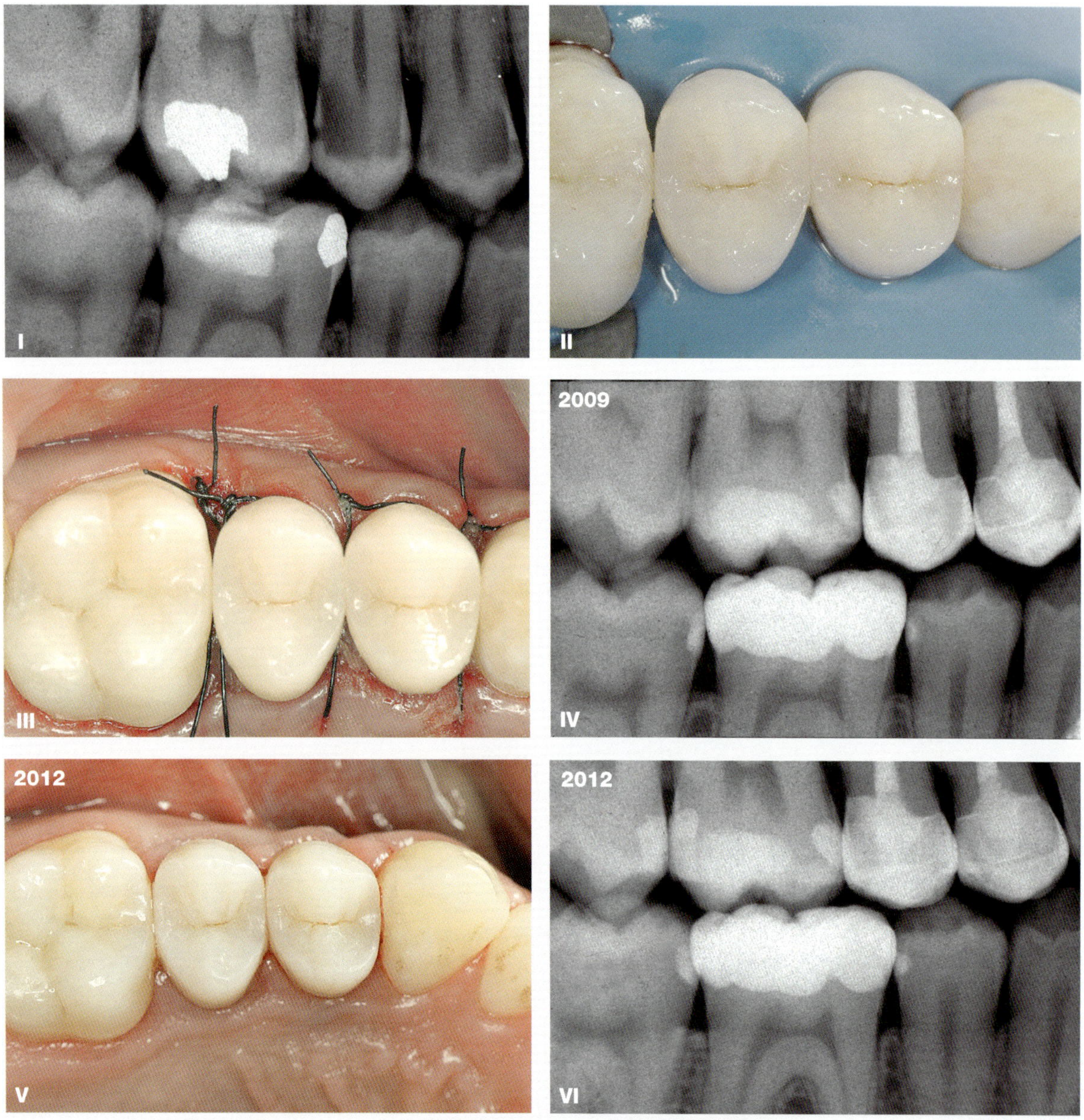

Fig 229 Caries lesions affecting both maxillary right premolars with irreversible pulp disease. Because the preparations were MOD, two overlays were prepared, and two posts were inserted, one for each tooth.

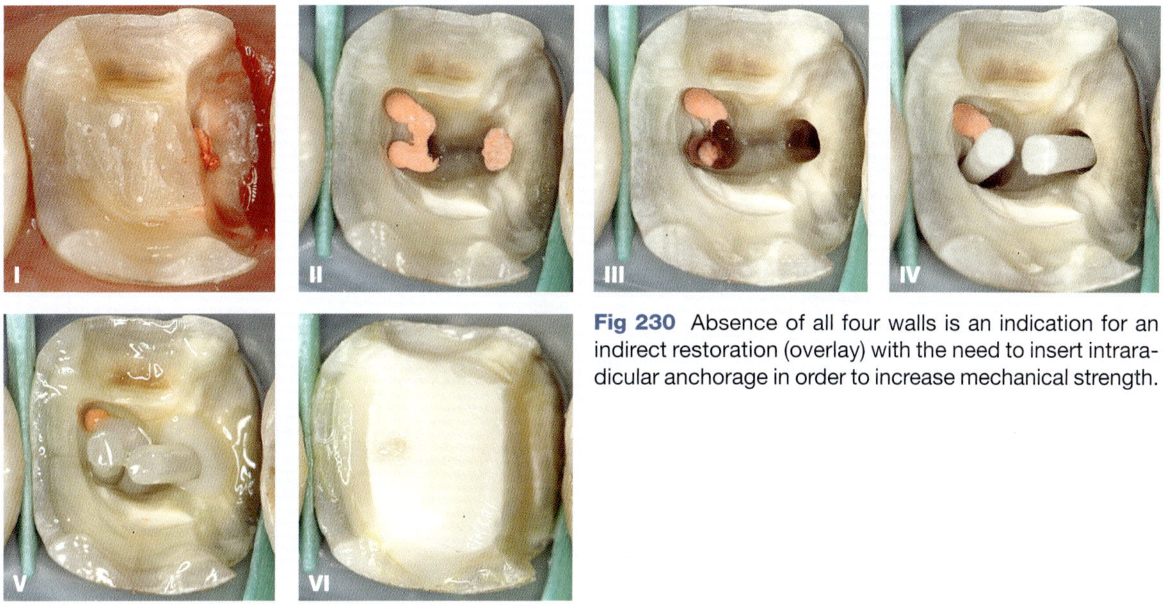

Fig 230 Absence of all four walls is an indication for an indirect restoration (overlay) with the need to insert intraradicular anchorage in order to increase mechanical strength.

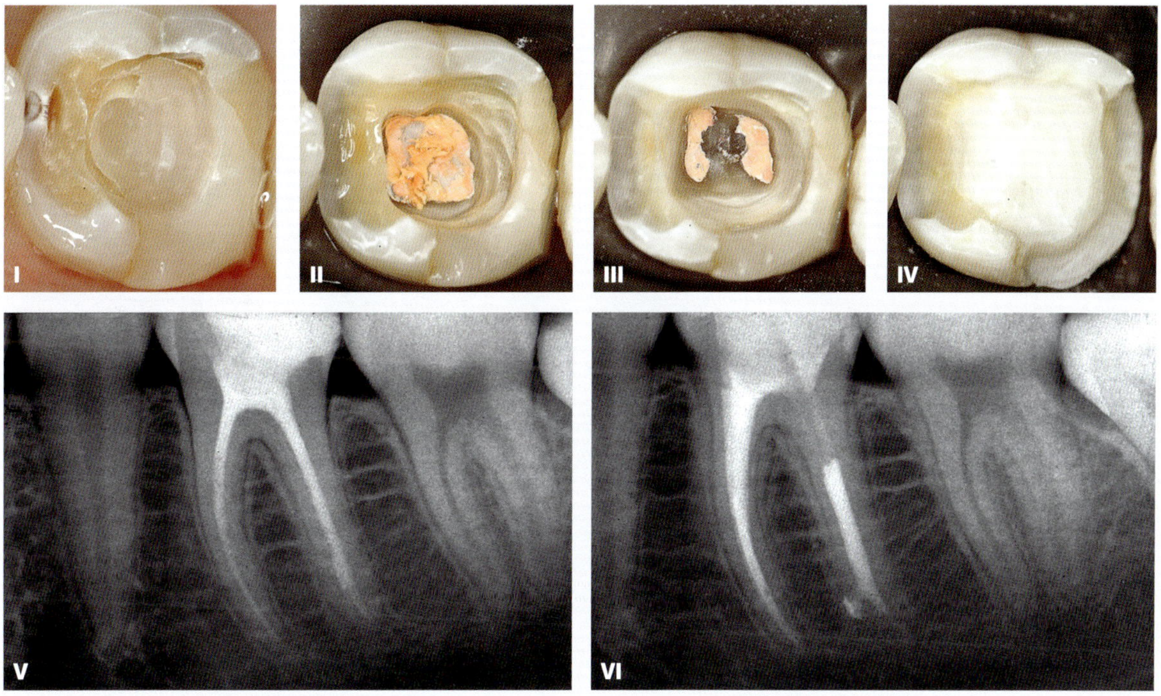

Fig 231 Given the extremely reduced amount of residual dental matter, reconstruction of this tooth required the insertion of two posts.

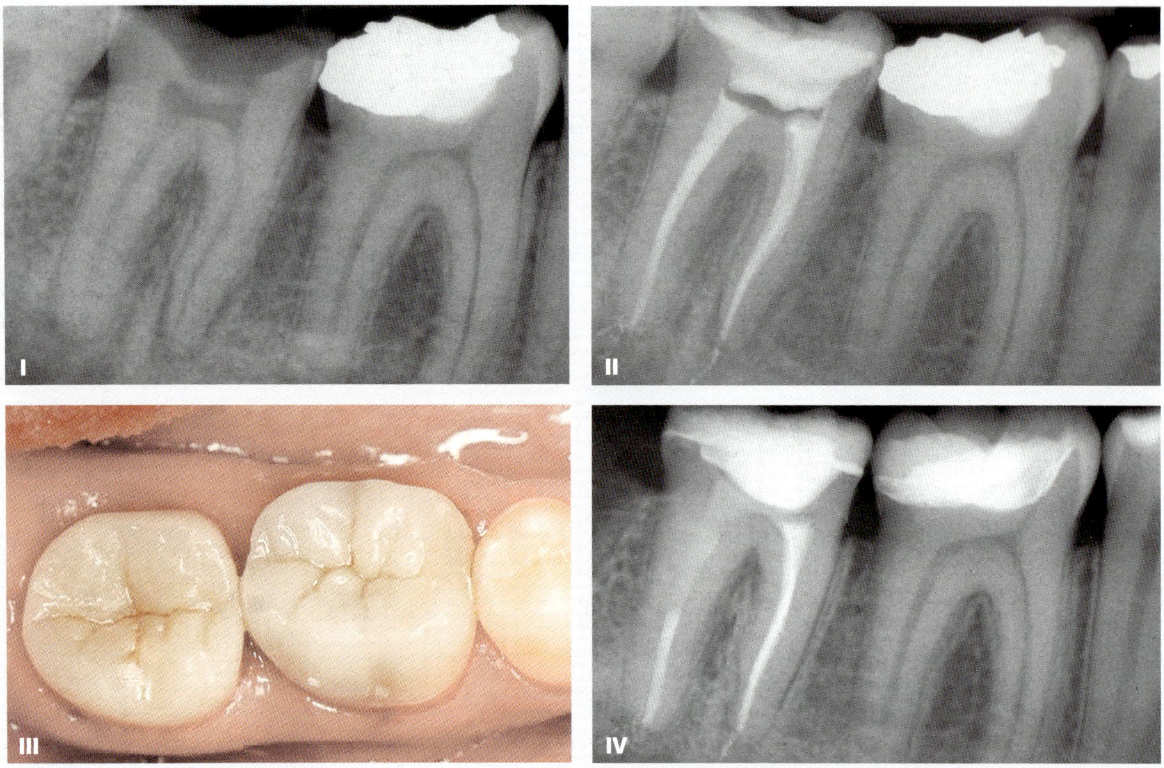

Fig 232 Severely compromised tooth with periapical lesion of the mesial root of the mandibular right second molar. After endodontic treatment and insertion of a post in the distal root, an indirect restoration in composite (overlay) completed the treatment. The absence of painful symptoms and a positive electrical pulp test allowed maintenance of the vitality of the pulp in the adjacent first molar, which was reconstructed by means of an occlusodistal onlay.

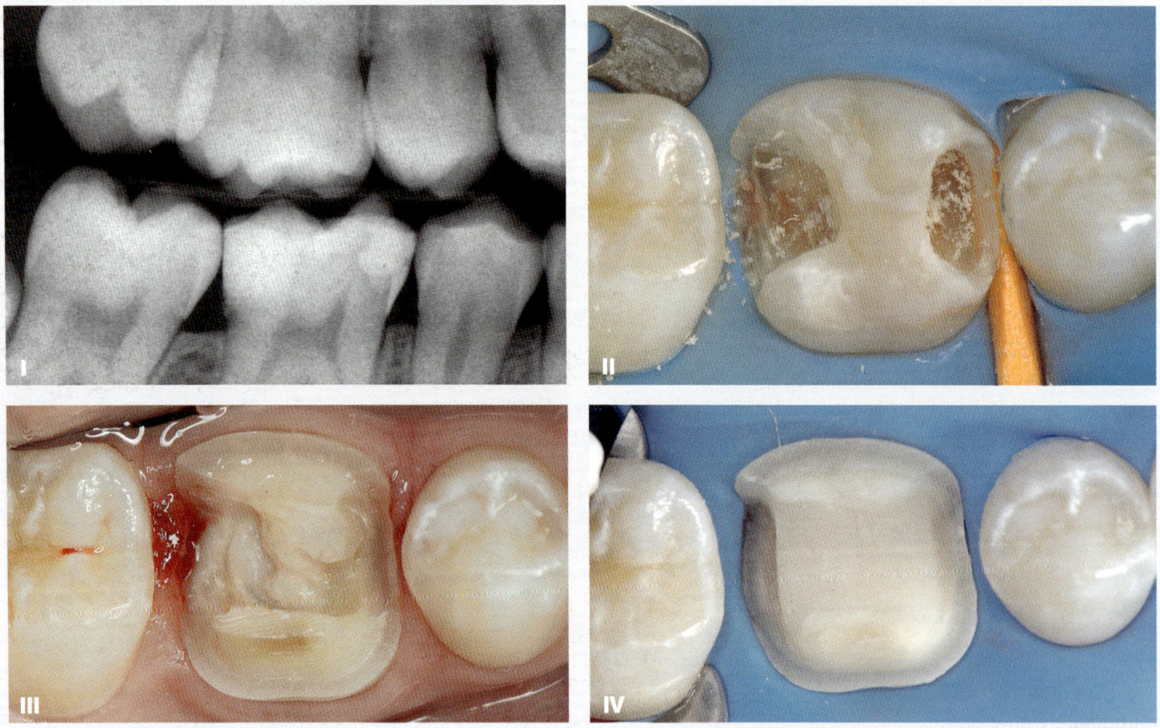

Fig 233 Vital tooth in which the amount of residual dental matter allowed reconstruction without any need for intraradicular anchorage. The fact that the sutures are still in place reveals the extremely short treatment duration, which was a great relief to the patient. (Courtesy of Dr Lavinia Landi.)

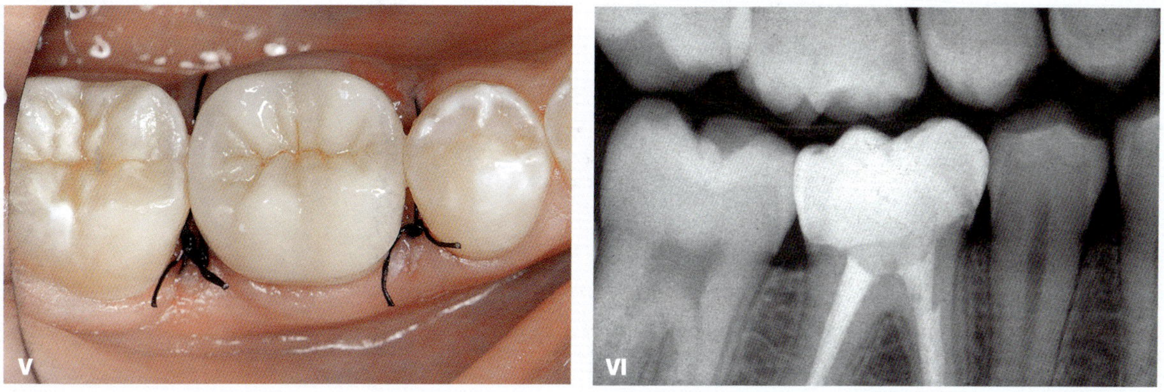

Fig 233 *(continued)*

Respecting periodontal structures

Restoration margins positioned in a supragingival site constitute an indubitable advantage for the health of the superficial and deep periodontium, even though flawless intrasulcular preparations are known to determine long-term periodontal health.

Supragingival margins naturally offer the enormous advantage that they can be optimally managed by the patient, the hygienist, and the practitioner (Fig 234).

In medium- and long-term follow-ups around partial preparations, maintenance of periodontal tissues takes precedence over preservation of natural teeth, a strategy that clearly avoids infringing on biologic width (Fig 235).

Biologic integration of a restoration cannot be achieved if the tooth is treated as a separate entity, divorced from its supporting apparatus, which consists of alveolar bone, periodontal ligament, and gingiva.

If the cavity extends below the gingival margin, the most certain way of safeguarding it against decay, which—to borrow an expression from Dr Valerio—perennially lies in wait, is to surgically lengthen the clinical crown.

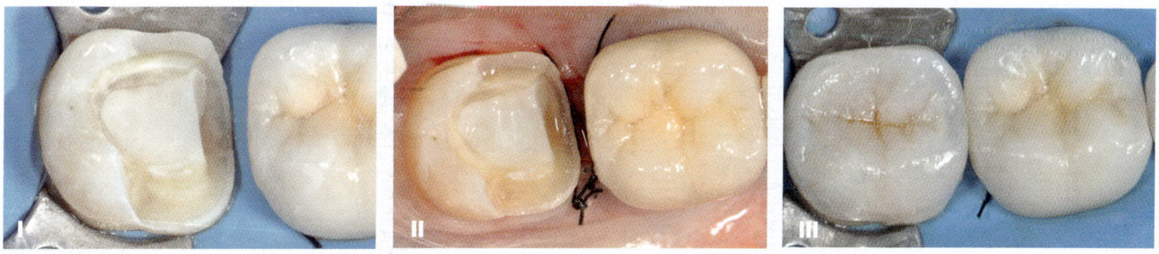

Fig 234 Classic clinical example of buildup and preparations carried out in an effectively isolated surgical field *(I)* immediately after surgical lengthening of the clinical crown *(II)*. View of the cemented restoration *(III)*.

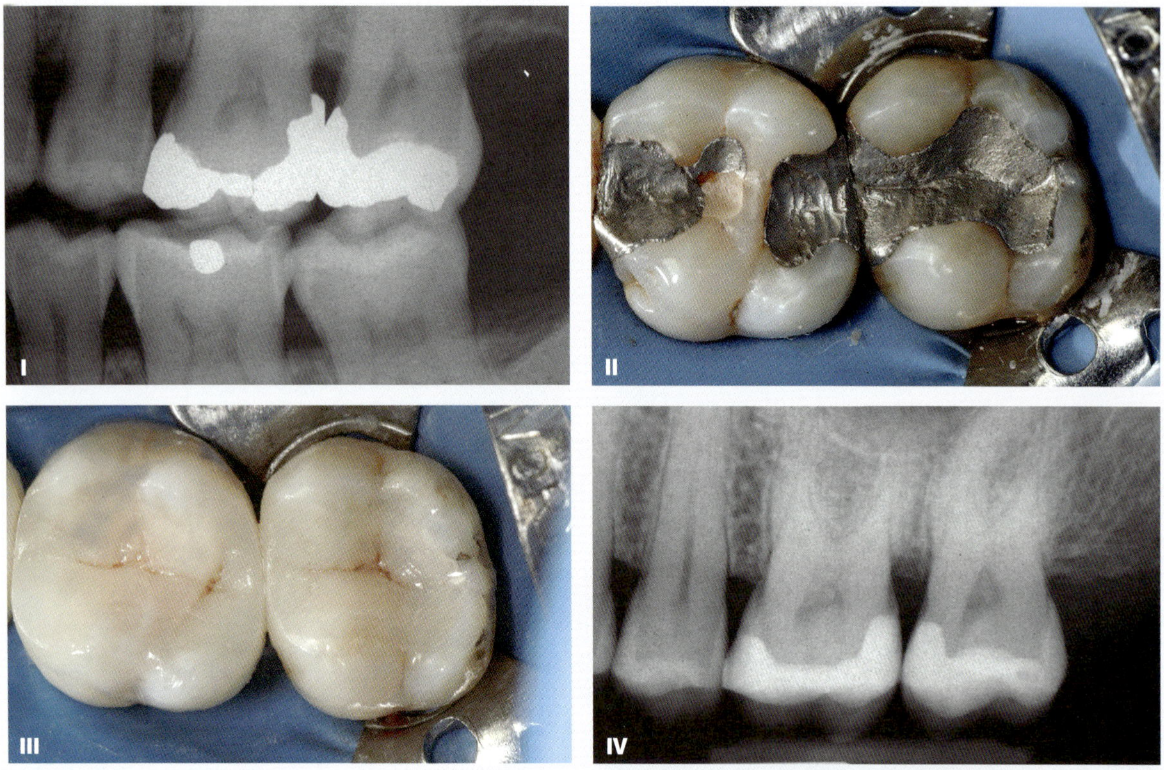

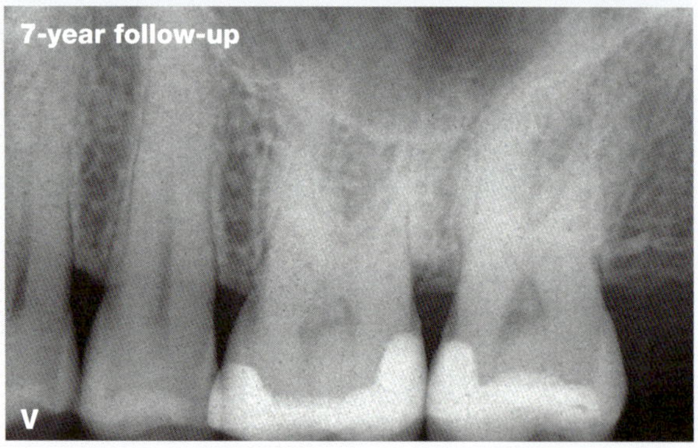

Fig 235 Infringement of periodontal space by defective restorations. Clinical and radiographic situation after reconstruction by means of restorations with proper marginal seals and emergence profiles.

In the proper hands, this procedure is the shortest step in the indirect adhesive restoration protocol, but in the author's opinion it is essential to guarantee success (Fig 236).

Ideal control of cavity preparation and buildup is routinely achieved using this approach. Taking an impression becomes as simple and accurate as could be wished; the "high" margins make all the difference when it comes to the crucial and extremely delicate stage of cementing the adhesive restoration under rubber dam. In addition, the stages of removing excess composite used as cement and those of subsequent margin finishing are greatly simplified (Figs 237 to 239).

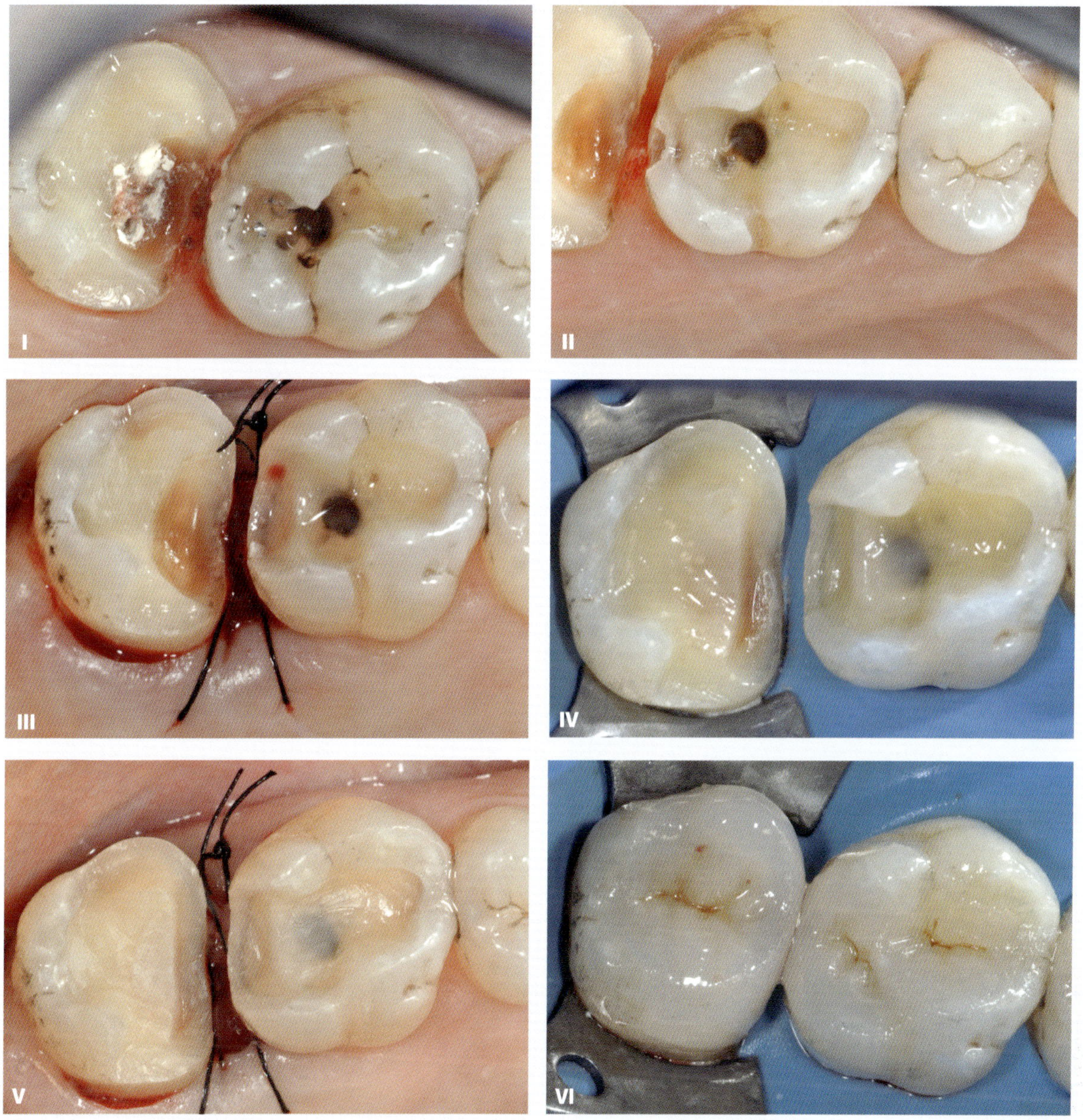

Fig 236 Periodontal procedure to lengthen the clinical crown. The margins, which are now supragingival, make it possible to carry out the reconstruction and cementation stages easily.

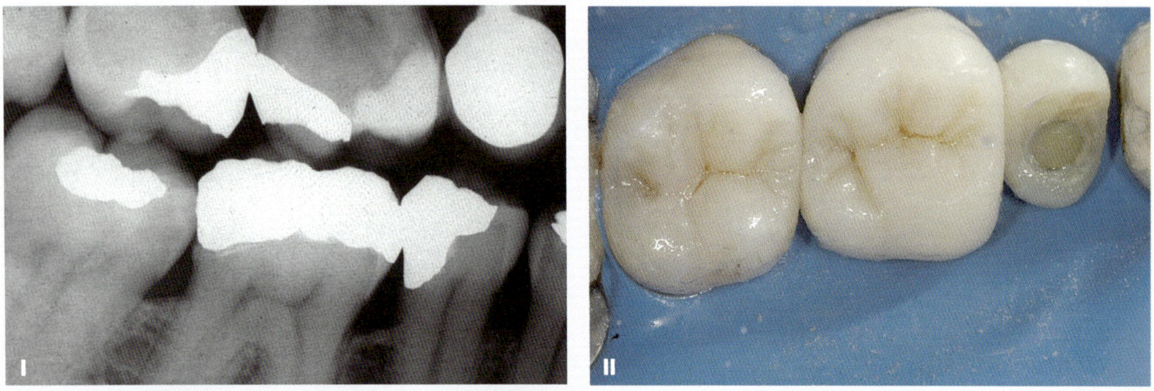

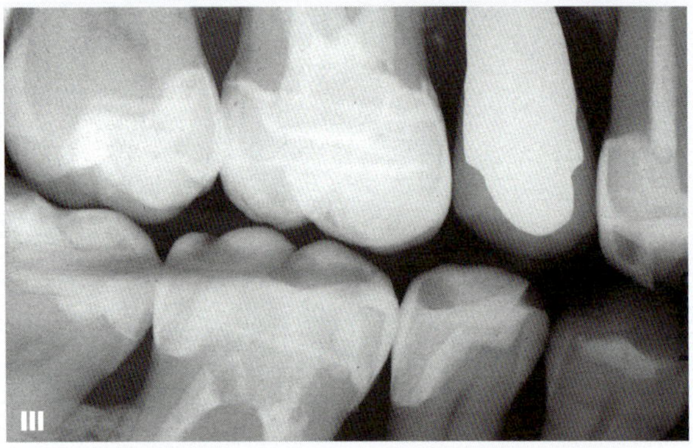

Fig 237 Restorations with ideal margins and contact surfaces after cementation of composite inlays.

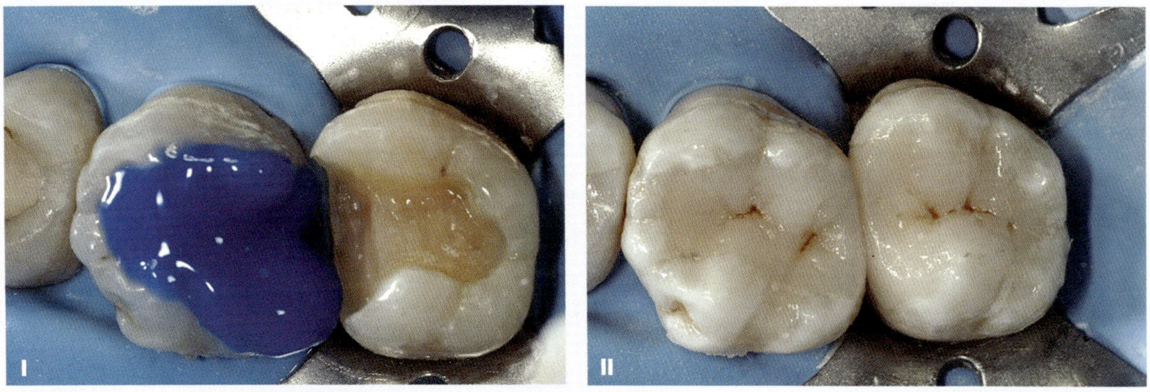

Fig 238 Acid etching of the restoration prior to cementation *(I)* and view of cemented restorations *(II)*. The consistency of the contact surfaces is evident.

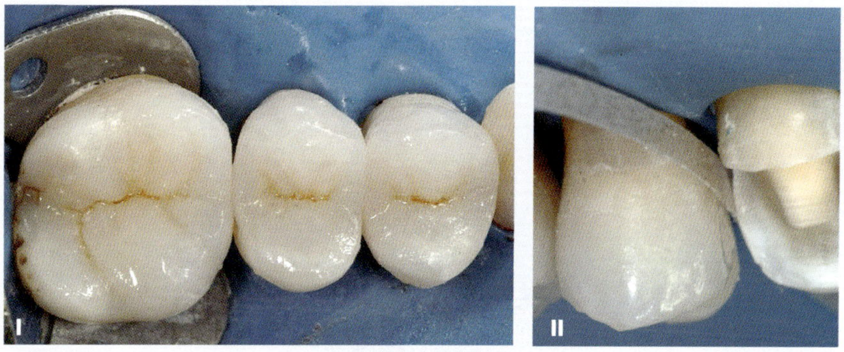

Fig 239 Indications for lengthening of the clinical crown include allowing extremely simplified management of the margin by the practitioner and excellent results. Finishing of the margins, which are in a high position under rubber dam, cannot cause any difficulty to the practitioner. Often it is only necessary to use a simple abrasive strip in order to achieve the inevitable goal: continuity between the margin and restoration.

Where indicated, the use of periodontal surgery for the positioning of margins in a supragingival site plays a fundamental role in correctly determining the emergence profiles, which are crucial to superficial and deep periodontal tissue health. Professor Martignoni always said that patients recover from an acute lesion but can only recover from a defective marginal adaptation or an incorrect emergence profile if the correct contour is restored (Figs 240 to 243).

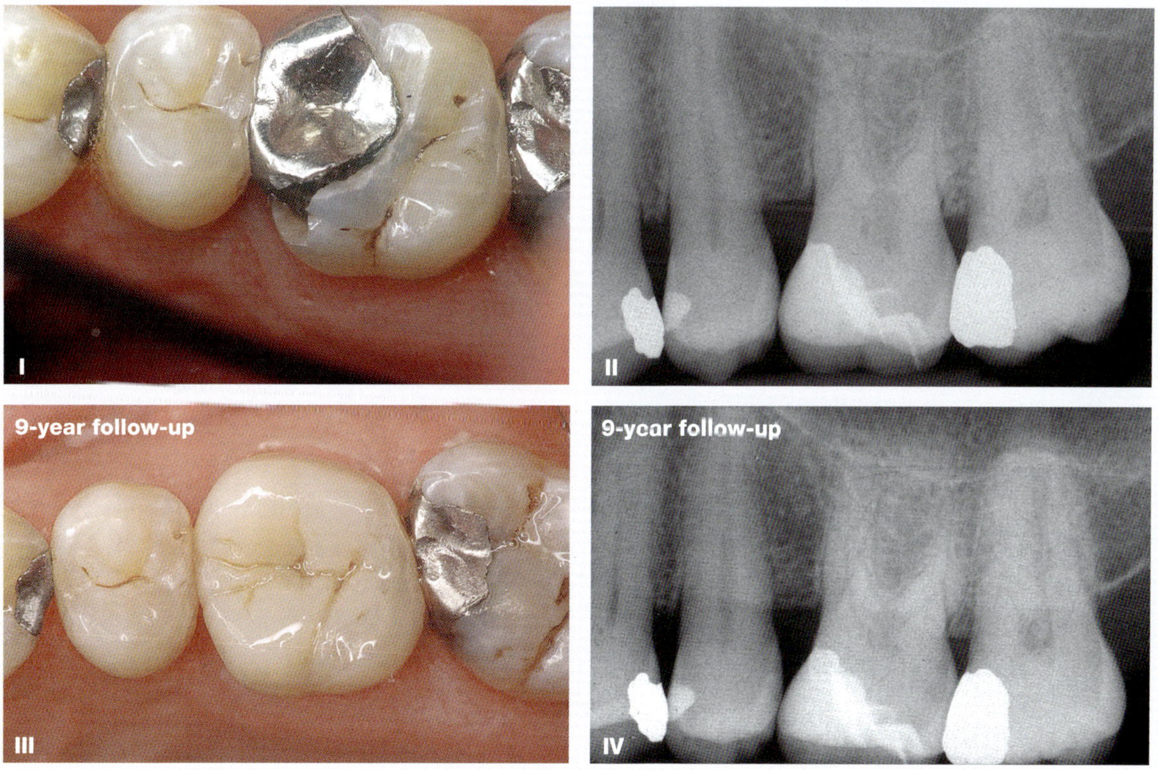

Fig 240 Follow-up revealing accuracy of the relationship between restoration and margin after 9 years.

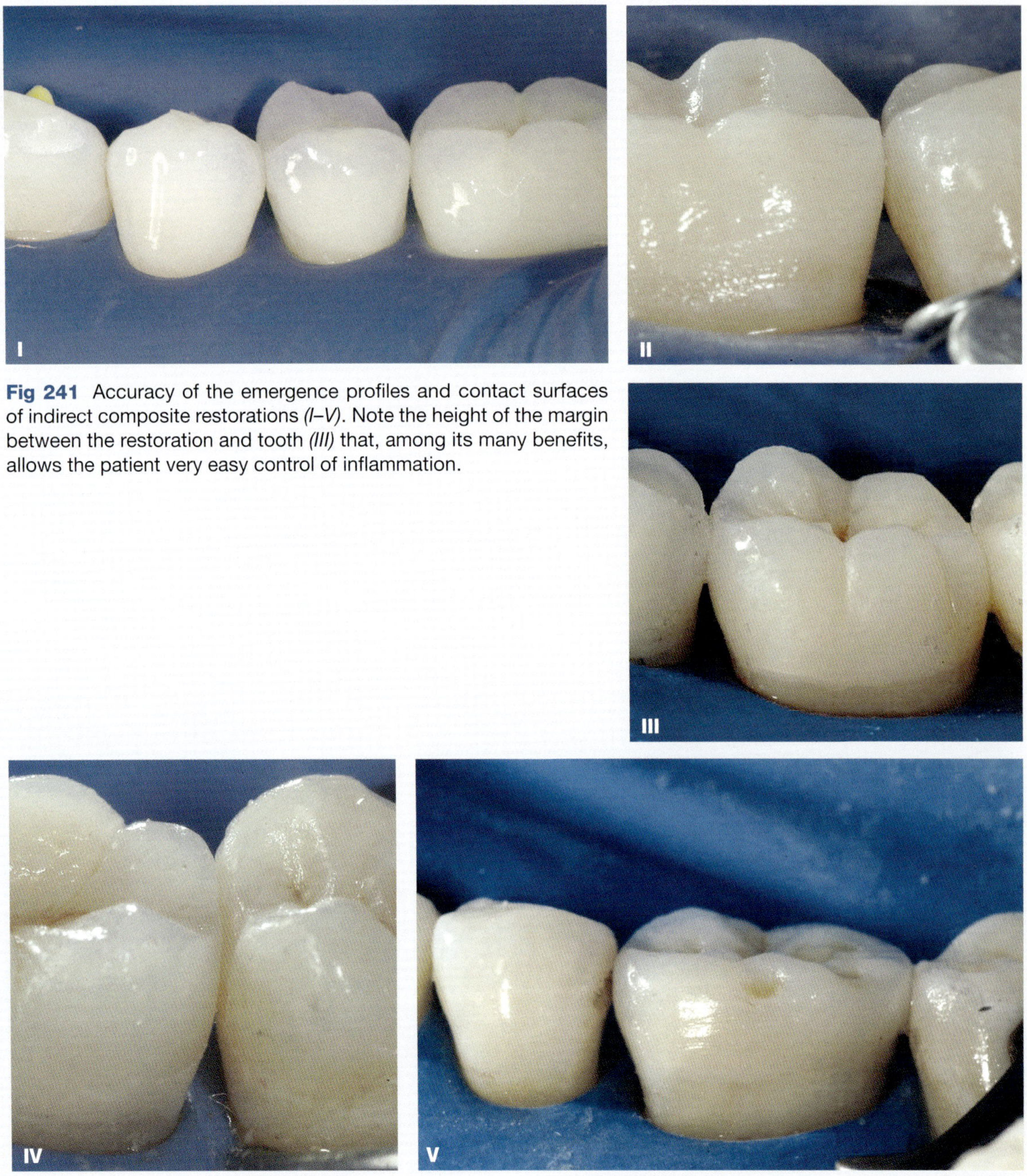

Fig 241 Accuracy of the emergence profiles and contact surfaces of indirect composite restorations *(I–V)*. Note the height of the margin between the restoration and tooth *(III)* that, among its many benefits, allows the patient very easy control of inflammation.

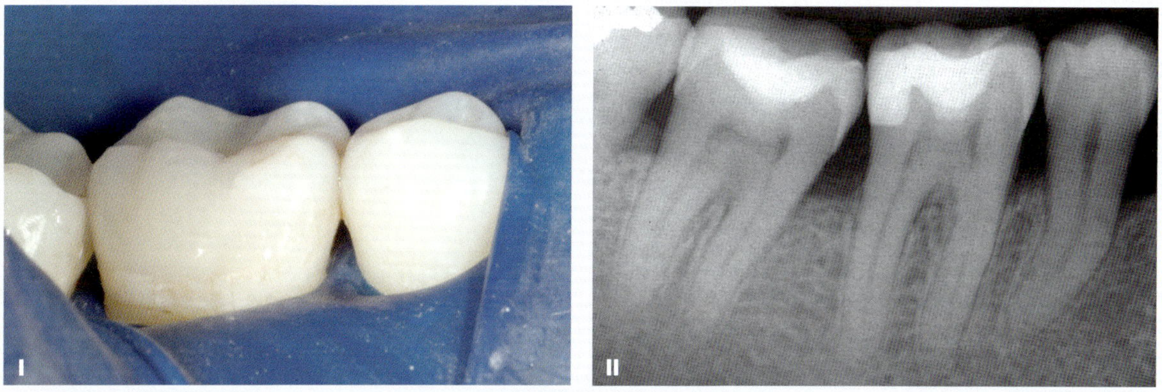

Fig 242 Clinical appearance following treatment *(I)* and 6-year radiographic follow-up *(II)* of the marginal seal of the mandibular right first molar.

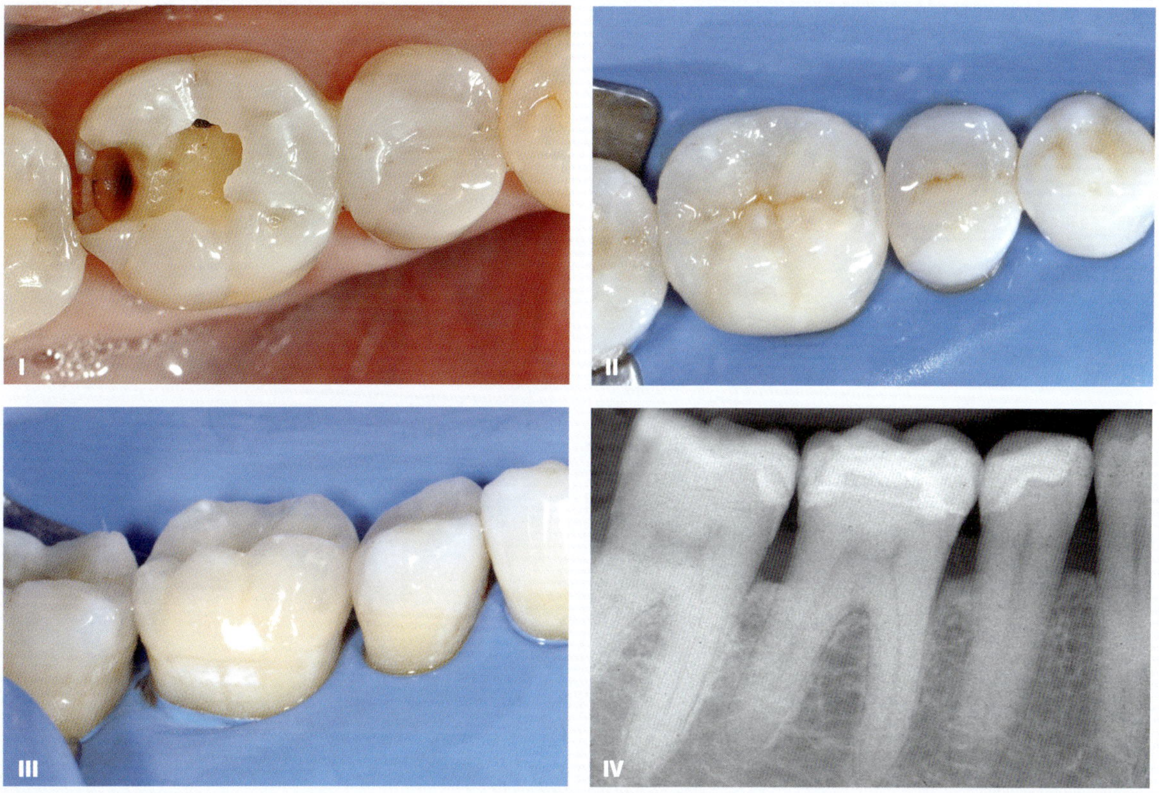

Fig 243 Reconstruction of defective restorations *(I)*, clinical view of the restorations after cementation *(II, III)*, and 9-year radiographic follow-up *(IV)* of the mandibular right second premolar and first and second molars.

Techniques have been proposed for relocating the subgingival margin in a more coronal position by means of small increments of composite instead of using flowable composite techniques. Good results can be achieved using this technique, although the author believes that its merits are debatable, partly due to the difficulty of applying adhesive systems in areas that cannot always be effectively isolated by means of rubber dam (Fig 244).

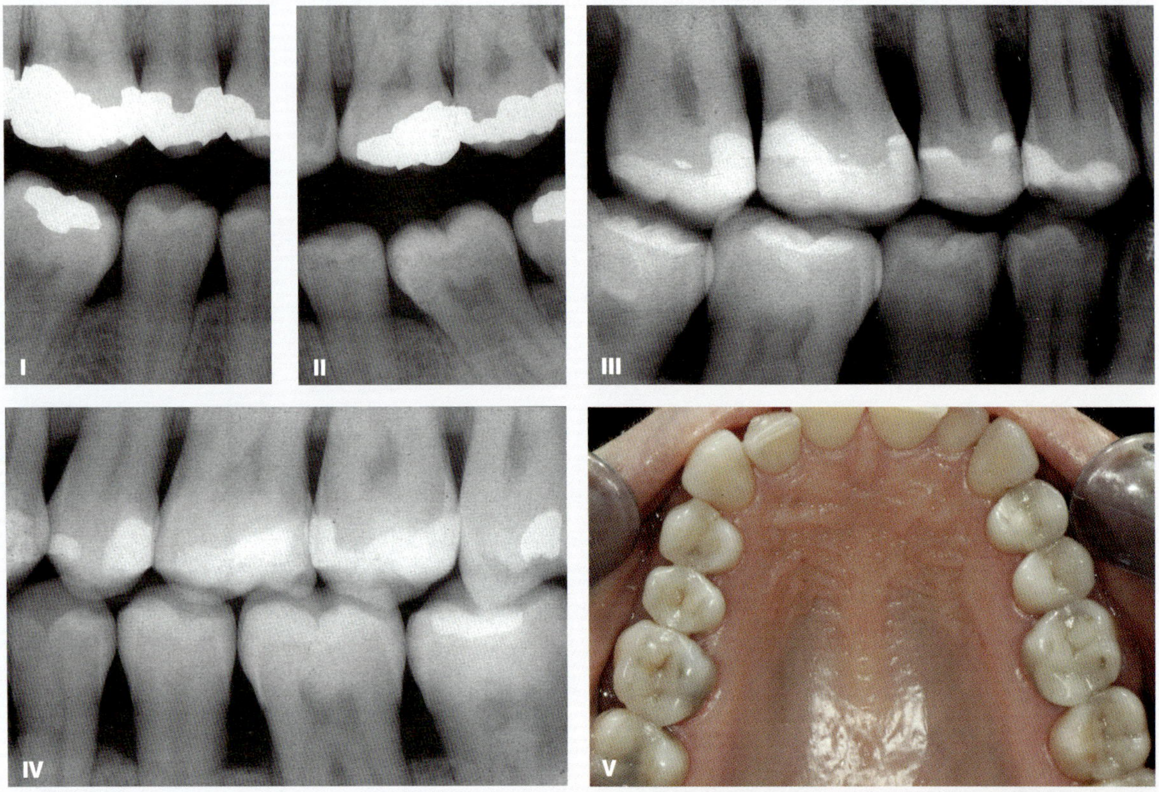

Fig 244 Radiographic and clinical follow-up after 10 years in a patient with parafunction of inlays performed using the technique of incremental application of composite at the cervical margin. The result was acceptable considering that the author performed the treatment while still learning the procedure. The patient reported distinct improvement in the sensitivity that had previously been a problem and cessation of pain on chewing. She was, however, an extremely motivated patient who attended hygienist appointments three to four times a year.

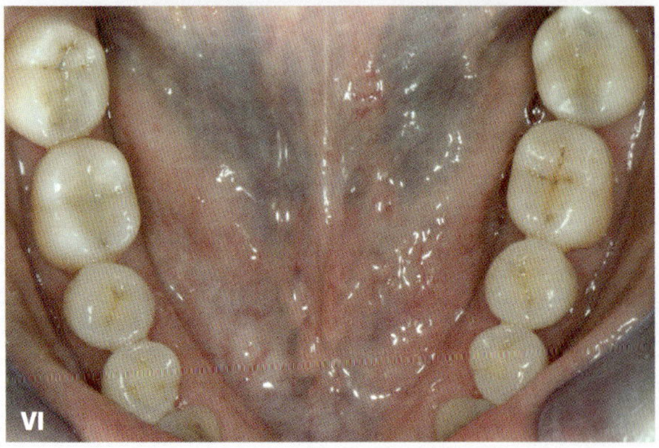

The surest way of achieving predictable results remains the surgical exposure of margins. This technique is simple to implement provided one makes the mental effort to include it routinely in the treatment plan, where indicated.

The protocol results in margins that show proper seals and satisfactory emergence profiles both clinically and radiographically (Figs 245 to 248).

Chapter 4 will examine this important topic.

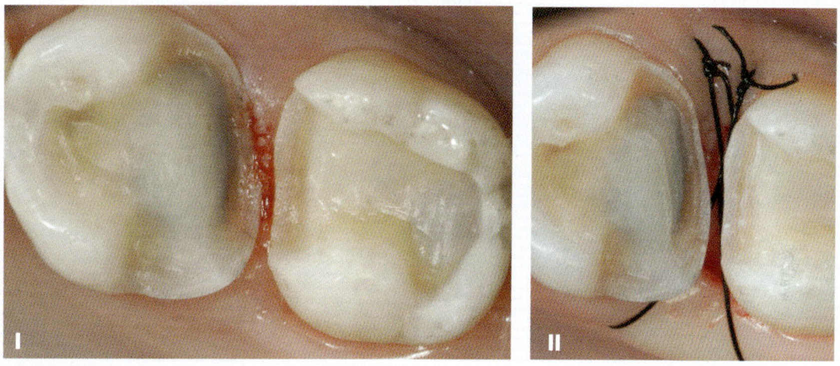

Fig 245 Clinical example of simple surgical exposure of only the affected margin, which makes it possible to routinely optimize future restoration cementation procedures.

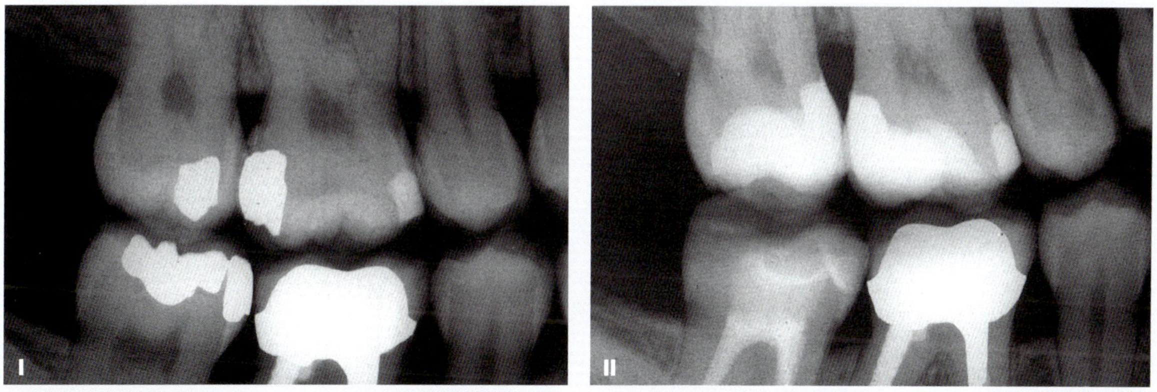

Fig 246 Radiographic follow-up of the mandibular right second molar after 11 years and the maxillary right first and second molars after 6 years.

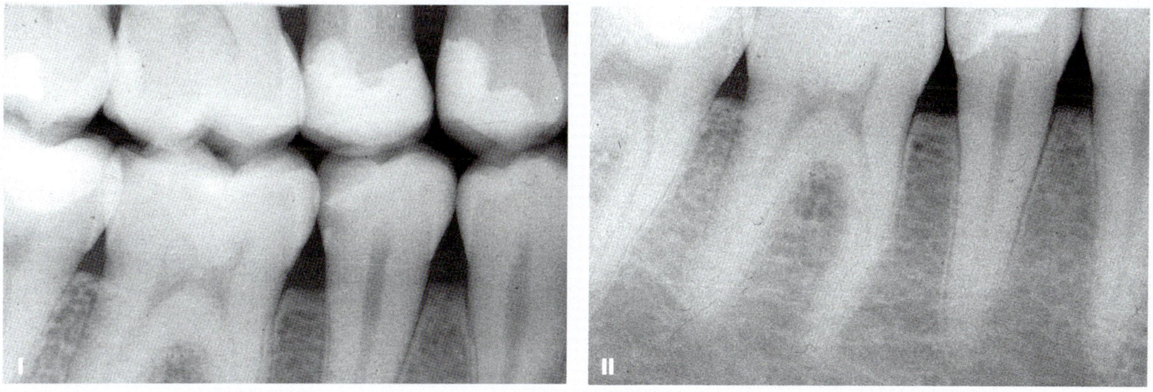

Fig 247 Radiographic follow-up of the mandibular right second premolar after cementation of the inlay.

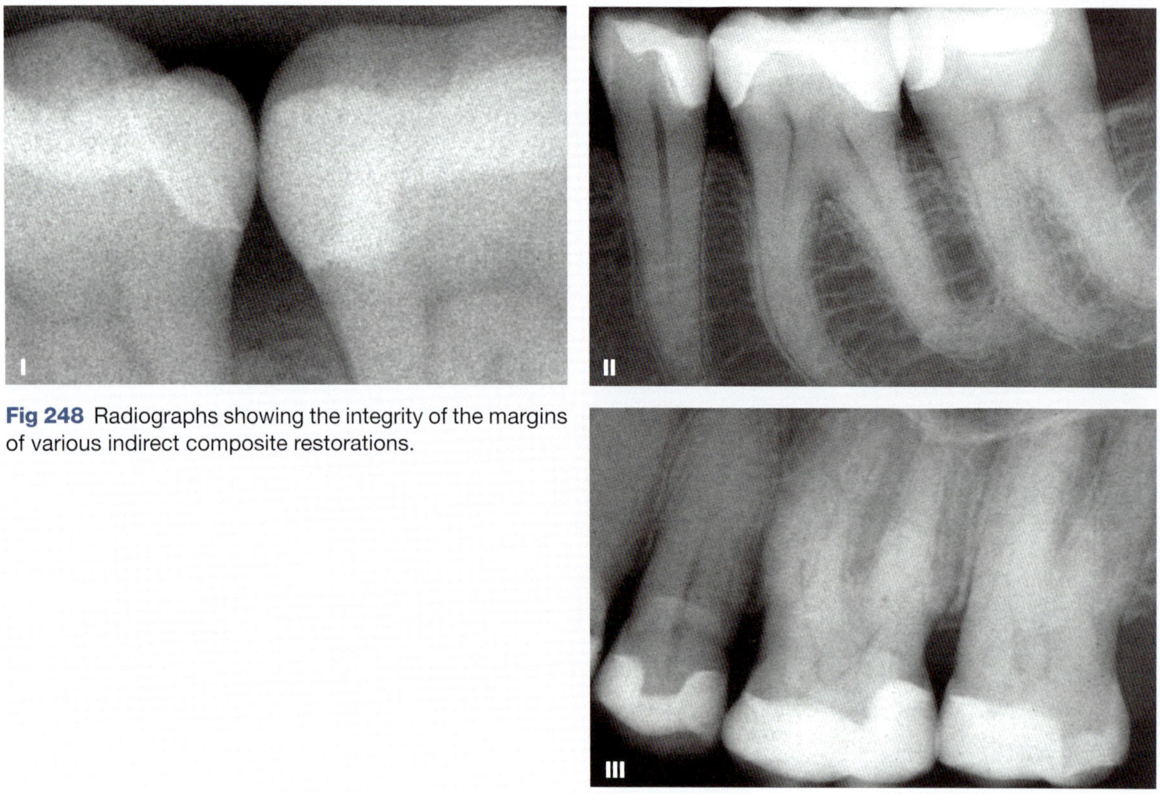

Fig 248 Radiographs showing the integrity of the margins of various indirect composite restorations.

References

1. Toffenetti F. Conservativa, le nuove tendenze. Fatti, possibilità, responsabilità. Dent Cadmos 1992;8:19–46.
2. Anderlini G. Moderni orientamenti per la restaurazione dentale, vol 2. Bologna, Italy: Martina, 1994:441–494.
3. Penning C, van Amerongen JP, Seef RE, ten Cate JM. Validity of probing for fissure caries diagnosis. Caries Res 1992;26:445–449.
4. Lussi A. Methods for caries detection. In: Roulet J-F, Wilson NHF, Fuzzi M (eds). Advances in Operative Dentistry. Vol 2: Challenges of the Future. Chicago: Quintessence, 2001:43–59.
5. Kirkegaard E, Kruidsen WS, Gronbock L. Poulsen E. Comparison of x-ray and clinical caries recording in a nationwide sample of adult Danes. Caries Res 1987;21:187.
6. Galcera Civera V, Almerich Silla JM, Montiel Company JM, Forner Navarro L. Clinical and radiographic diagnosis of approximal and occlusal dental caries in a low risk population. Med Oral Patol Oral Cir Bucal 2007;12:E252–E257.
7. Tam LE, McComb D. Diagnosis of occlusal caries: Part II. Recent diagnostic technologies. J Can Dent Assoc 2001;67:459–463.
8. Tranæus S, Shi XQ, Angmar-Mansson B. Caries risk assessment: Methods available to clinicians for caries detection. Community Dent Oral Epidemiol 2005;33:265–273.
9. Pretty IA. Caries detection and diagnosis: Novel technologies. J Dent 2006;34:727–739.
10. Lussi A, Hellwig E. Performance of a new laser fluorescence device for the detection of occlusal caries in vitro. J Dent 2006;34:467–471.
11. Ekstrand KR, Martignon S, Ricketts DJ, Qvist V. Detection and activity assessment of primary coronal caries lesions: A methodologic study. Oper Dent 2007;32:225–235.
12. Zandoná AF, Zero DT. Diagnostic tools for early caries detection. J Am Dent Assoc 2006;137:1675–1684.
13. Fontana M, Zero DT. Assessing patients' caries risk J Am Dent Assoc 2006;137:1231–1239.
14. Anusavice KJ. Caries risk assessment. Oper Dent 2001;(Suppl 6):19–26.
15. Brambilla E, Garcia-Godoy F, Strohmenger L. Principles of diagnosis and treatment of high-caries-risk subjects. Dent Clin North Am 2000;44:507–540.
16. Caries diagnosis and risk assessment: A review of preventive strategies and management. J Am Dent Assoc 1995;126(Suppl):1S–24S
17. Anusavice K. Clinical decision-making for coronal caries management in the permanent dentition. J Dent Educ 2001;65:1143–1146.
18. Peters MC, McLean ME. Minimally invasive operative care. I. Minimal intervention and concepts for minimally invasive cavity preparations. J Adhes Dent 2001;3:7–16.
19. Ericson D, Kidd E, McComb D, Mjör I, Noack MJ. Minimally invasive dentistry—Concepts and techniques in cariology. Oral Health Prev Dent 2003;1(1):59–72.
20. Bergman M. Side-effects of amalgam and its alternatives: Local, systemic and environmental. Int Dent J 1990;40:4–10.
21. Craig RG (ed). Restorative Dental Materials, ed 9. St Louis: Mosby, 1993.
22. Pintado MR, Douglas WH. Annualized enamel wear rate by volume and depth in young adults. J Dent Res 1996;75:abstract 1198.
23. Leinfelder KF, Beaudreau RW, Mazer RB. An in vitro device for predicting clinical wear. Quintessence Int 1989;20:755–761.
24. Ferracane JL, Mitchem JC, Condon JR, Todd R. Wear and marginal breakdown of composites with various degrees of cure. J Dent Res 1997;76:1508–1516.
25. Kemp Scholte CM, Davidson CL. Marginal integry related to bond strength and strains capacity of composite resin restorative systems. J Prosthet Dent 1990;64:658–664.
26. Soares CJ, Martins LR, Fernandes Neto AJ, Giannini M. Marginal adaptation of indirect composites and ceramic inlay systems. Oper Dent 2003;28:689–694.
27. Soares CJ, Martins LR, Pfeifer JM, Giannini M. Fracture resistance of teeth restored with indirect-composite and ceramic inlay systems. Quintessence Int 2004;35:281–286.
28. Lopes LM, Leitao JG, Douglas WH. Effect of a new resin inlay/onlay restorative material on cuspal reinforcement. Quintessence Int 1991;22:641–645.
29. Degrange M, Roulet JF. Adhesion: The Silent Revolution in Dentistry. Chicago: Quintessence, 2000.
30. Hasegawa EA, Boyer DB, Chan DC. Microleakage of indirect composite inlays. Dent Mater 1989;5:388–391.
31. Soares CJ, Celiberto L, Dechichi P, Fonseca RB, Martins LR. Marginal integrity and microleakage of direct and indirect composite inlays: SEM and stereomicroscopic evaluation. Braz Oral Res 2005;19:295–301.
32. Marmasse A. Dentisterie opératoire, ed 5. Paris: Bailliére, 1974.
33. Caughman WF, Caughman GB, Shiflett RA, Rueggeberg F, Schuster GS. Correlation of cytotoxicity, filler loading and curing time of dental composites. Biomaterials 1991;12:737–740.
34. Kawaguchi M, Takahashi Y, Fukushima T, Habu T. Effect of light-exposure duration on the amount of leachable monomers from light-activated reline material. J Prosthet Dent 1996;75:183–187.
35. Shajii L, Santerre JP. Effect of filler content on the profile of released biodegradation products in micro-filled bis-GMA/TEGDMA dental composite resins. Biomaterials 1999;20:1897–1908.
36. Sideridou I, Tserki V, Papanastasiou G. Effect of chemical structure on degree of conversion in light-cured dimethacrylate-based dental resins. Biomaterials 2002;23:1819–1829.
37. Rueggeberg FA, Craig RG. Correlation of parameters used to estimate monomer conversion in a light-cured composite. J Dent Res 1988;67:932–937.
38. Daronch M, Rueggeberg FA, Hall G, De Goes MF. Effect of composite temperature on in vitro intrapulpal temperature rise. Dent Mater 2007;23:1283–1288.

39. Stansbury JW. Curing dental resins and composites by photopolymerization. J Esthet Dent 2000;12:300–308.
40. Manhart J, Neuerer P, Scheibenbogen-Fuchsbrunner A, Hickel R. Three-year clinical evaluation of direct and indirect composite restorations in posterior teeth. J Prosthet Dent 2000;84:289–296.
41. Park SH. Comparison of degree of conversion for light-cured and additionally heat-cured composites. J Prosthet Dent 1996;76:613–618.
42. Feilzer AJ, De Gee AJ, Davidson CL. Setting stress in composite resin in relation to configuration of the restoration. J Dent Res 1987;66:1636–1639.
43. Van Meerbeek B, Lambrechts P, Inokoshi S, Braem M, Vanherle G. Factors affecting adhesion to mineralized tissues. Oper Dent 1992;(Suppl 5):111–124.
44. Davidson CL, de Gee AJ. Relaxation of polymerization contraction stresses by flow in dental composites. J Dent Res 1984;63:146–148.
45. Uno S, Asmussen E. Marginal adaptation of a restorative resin polymerized at reduced rate. Scand J Dent Res 1991;99:440–444.
46. Sakaguchi RL, Berge HX. Reduced light energy density decreases post-gel contraction while maintaining degree of conversion in composites. J Dent 1998;26:695–700.
47. Mehl A, Hickel R, Kunzelmann KH. Physical properties and gap formation of light-cured composites with and without 'softstart-polymerization'. J Dent 1997;25:321–330.
48. Edelhoff D, Sorensen JA. Tooth structure removal associated with various preparation designs for posterior teeth. Int J Periodontics Restorative Dent 2002;22:241–249.
49. Sorensen JA, Martinoff JT. Intracoronal reinforcement and coronal coverage: A study of endodontically treated teeth. J Prosthet Dent 1984;51:580–584.
50. Reeh ES, Messer HH, Douglas WH. Reduction in tooth stiffness as a result of endodontic and restorative procedures. J Endod 1989;15:512–516.
51. Linn J, Messer HH. Effect of restorative procedures on the strength of endodontically treated molars. J Endod 1994;20:479–485.
52. Sakaguchi RL, Brust EW, Cross M, De-Long R, Douglas WH. Independent movement of cusps during occlusal loading. Dent Mater 1991;7:186–190.
53. Panitvisai P, Messer HH. Cuspal deflection in molars in relation to endodontic and restorative procedures. J Endod 1995;21(2):57–61.
54. Lasfargues JJ, Bukiet F, Tirlet G, Decup F. Bonded partial restorations for endodontically treated teeth. In: Roulet J-F, Wilson NHF, Fuzzi M. Advances in Operative Dentistry. Vol 1: Contemporary Clinical Practice. Chicago: Quintessence, 2001:191–209.
55. Assif D, Gorfil C. Biomechanical considerations in restoring endodontically treated teeth. J Prosthet Dent 1994;71:565–567.
56. Fichera G, Dinapoli C, Dino R. Restauri estetico-adesivi indiretti: modello per diagnosi di configurazione cavitaria. Il Dentista Moderno 2003;2:21–57.
57. Garberoglio R, Brännström M. Scanning electron microscopic investigation of human dentinal tubules. Arch Oral Biol 1976;21:355–362.
58. Ruddle CJ. Endodontic considerations for periodontal prostheses. J Calif Dent Assoc 1989;17(9):41–49.
59. Trope M, Maltz DO, Tronstad L. Resistance to fracture of restored endodontically treated teeth. Endod Dent Traumatol 1985;1:108–111.
60. Robbins JW. Guidelines for the restoration of endodontically treated teeth. J Am Dent Assoc 1990;120:558,560,562.
61. Guzy GE, Nicholls JI. In vitro comparison of intact endodontically treated teeth with and without endo-post reinforcement. J Prosthet Dent 1979;42(1):39–44.
62. Fichera G, Dinapoli C, Ferrari P, Re D. Restaurativa postendodontica con perni in fibra. Indicazioni e tecnica operativa. Il Dentista Moderno 2005;9:23–51.
63. Shillingburg HT Jr, Kessler JC, Wilson EL Jr. Root dimensions and dowel size. CDA J 1982;10(10):43–49.
64. Torbjörner A, Karlsson S, Odman PA. Survival rate and failure characteristics for two post designs. J Prosthet Dent 1995;73:439–444.
65. Mason PN. Contributo sperimentale alla ricerca sul legame Composipost endodonto. Atti simposio Int Odont Adesiva e Ricostruttiva 1997;1:18–24.
66. Duret B, Reynaud M, Duret F. Un nouveau concept de reconstituction Corono-radiculaire: le Composipost (1). Chir Dent Fr 1990;540:131–141.
67. Duret B, Reynaud M, Duret F. Un nouveau concept de reconstituction Corono-radiculaire: le Composipost (2). Chir Dent Fr 1990;542:69–77.
68. Ferrari M, Mannocci F, Vichi A, Cagidiaco MC, Mjör IA. Bonding to root canal: structural characteristics of the substrate. Am J Dent 2000;13:255–260.
69. Martínez-Insua A, da Silva L, Rilo B, Santana U. Comparison of the fracture resistances of pulpless teeth restored with a cast post and core or carbon-fiber post with a composite core. J Prosthet Dent 1998;80:527–532.
70. Hansen EK. In vivo cusp fracture of endodontically treated premolars restored with MOD amalgam or MOD resin fillings. Dent Mater 1988;4:169–173.

Adhesion 2

The use of orthophosphoric acid in 1955 by Buonocore[1] to improve the adhesion of acrylic resins and the development of the monomer bisphenol glycidyl methacrylate (bis-GMA) by Bowen in 1963[2] marked the advent of adhesive dentistry.

Adhesion made reconstructive treatment of teeth easier, quicker, and more practical, revising and sometimes changing the traditional guidelines. Adhesive techniques revolutionized reconstructive treatment of teeth and also brought changes in orthodontic techniques, cementation of fixed prostheses, and fiber intracanal posts.[3]

Despite their ease of use, adhesive systems require a careful protocol based on adequate knowledge of adhesion principles and the substrates on which adhesives act. Each adhesive system should be specifically assessed on a case-by-case basis according to the different substrate and based on the purpose to be achieved.

Principles of adhesion

Adhesion may be defined as a mechanism that joins two substrates in intimate contact with one another through an interface. Adhesion may therefore be quantified as resistance to separation between two materials subject to a mechanical force.[4]

Four different theories have been put forward to explain adhesion phenomena:

1. ***Mechanical theory:*** Once the adhesive has set, it interlocks with the roughness and surface irregularities of the bonded surface to achieve micromechanical retention.
2. ***Adsorption theories:*** All known types of chemical bonds between adhesive and bonded surfaces, including primary (ionic and covalent) and secondary (hydrogen, dipole-dipole, or van der Waals forces) bonds, contribute to achieving adhesion.
3. ***Diffusion theories:*** Adhesion is the result of a bond between moving molecules. The polymers of each interface can move and react with the molecules present on the complementary side.
4. ***Electrostatic theories:*** A double electric gradient forms at the interface between metal and polymer that certainly helps to increase the adhesive force, even though the mode of action is not known as yet.

Whichever type of adhesion is considered, one essential requirement is that the two materials should be as close to one another as possible and free of contamination.

Isolation of the operative field by means of rubber dam is an essential condition for adopting adhesive techniques because saliva, blood, and fluids in general have a negative impact on the quality of the adhesive bond if they contaminate the tooth surface, reducing the bond strength (Fig 1).

To achieve adhesion, it is essential for the surface free energy, a property of the tooth substrate, to be increased by the use of an etching acid. At the same time, the surface tension must be lowered by the use of a bonding agent or primer that allows the adhesive system to adapt properly to the substrate. The adhesive system is defined as an amphiphilic compound, ie, a compound that contains hydrophilic chemicals to ensure a bond to the teeth, as well as chemical groups with hydrophobic properties that enable them to adhere to the composite resin. The adhesion process is therefore performed in successive steps with the aim of making the enamel, dentin, and resin restoration compatible with one another.

Every adhesive system, irrespective of the type of adhesive, contains an etching agent designed to increase the surface free energy, a primer to make the adhesive system more wettable, and a bonding agent for the purposes of infiltrating and constituting the bond.

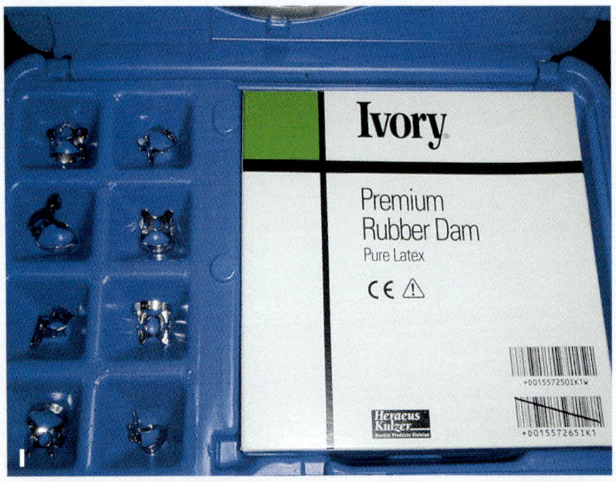

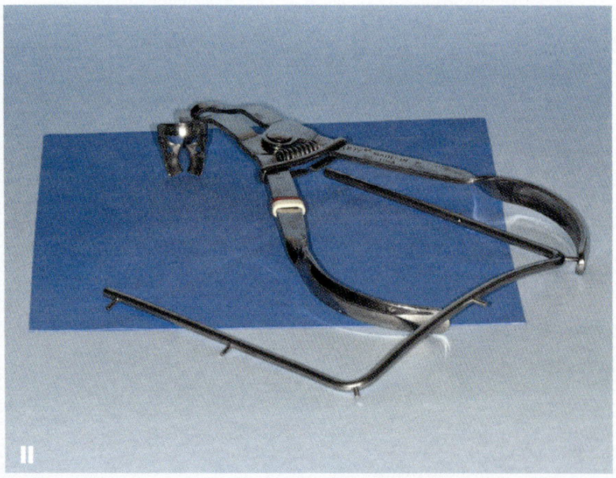

Fig 1 Rubber dam, band, hooks and anti-anxiety patch for patients who feel as though they are suffocating.

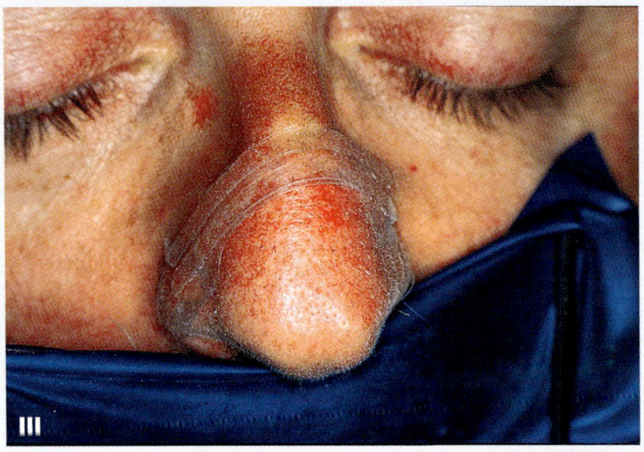

Functions and objectives of adhesive systems

The application of enamel-dentin adhesive is a fundamental procedure in modern dentistry.[5] The adhesive step is a crucial juncture that may be fundamental to the long-term outcome of the restoration.

The main functions to be performed by an adhesive system are as follows:

- Sealing, to allow the restoration to be properly maintained over time
- Distribution of forces, to guarantee proper functional rehabilitation of the tooth
- Resistance to separation, a property that is indispensable to retain the restoration material and overcome shrinkage due to polymerization

The aims of enamel-dentin adhesion described by Lutz et al are as follows[6]:

- Restoration retention and stability
- Countering and absorbing stresses due to contraction
- Perfect marginal adaptation with no cracks and microleaks
- Hermetic seal of the pulp-dentin complex
- Reduction in postoperative sensitivity
- Reinforcement of the residual tooth structure

Enamel and dentin: Chemistry and histology

Enamel and dentin are tissues with different embryologic derivations, chemical and micromorphologic constitutions, and functional and mechanical properties.[7] Enamel is a mineralized secretion, 96% of which is made up of calcium phosphate salts that determine the formation of prisms. These are separated from one another by a fine organic film and interprismatic enamel. The remaining is made up of a protein matrix (amelogenin, enamelin; 1%) and water (3%) (Fig 2).

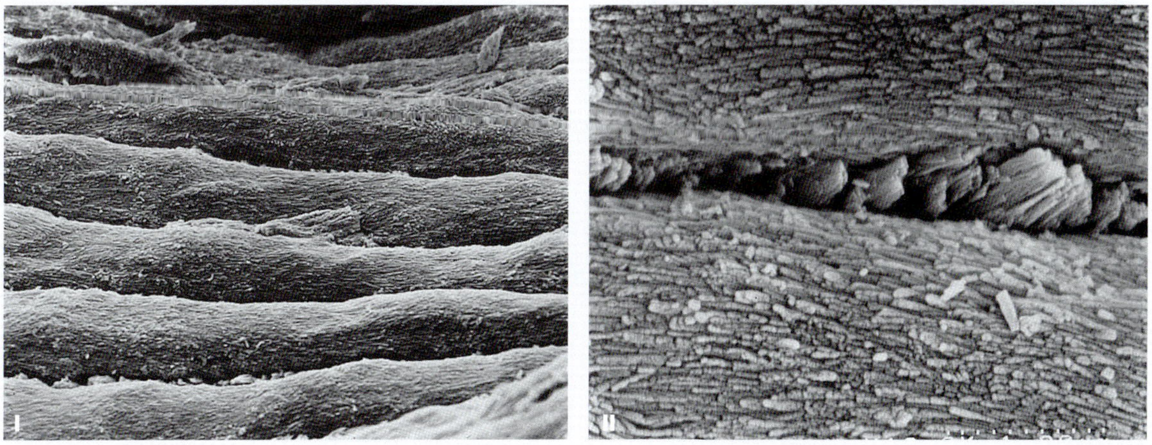

Fig 2 Scanning electron microscopy images of enamel prisms interspersed with interprismatic matter. (Courtesy of Professor Guido Goracci et al.)

The acid etching gives rise to significant morphologic changes in the enamel surface, increasing surface roughness (and therefore the area available for adhesion) and the surface free energy that, in turn, increases the wettability and adhesion capacity. The etched enamel therefore appears to be more receptive to the adhesive resin, with which it will be able to establish a stable and lasting bond (Fig 3).

Dentin is a hydrated biologic complex made up of 70% inorganic matter (hydroxyapatite), 18% organic matrix (type I collagen), and 12% water. It is characterized by the presence of dentinal tubules.[8] Different histologic properties therefore arise according to whether the dentin is considered to be peritubular (with a high water content and low collagen fiber content) or intertubular (with a high collagen content).[9] The odontoblastic tubules are also not parallel to one another but extend in a radial direction (from pulp to periphery). This means that the size of the odontoblastic tubules varies from 0.8 to 2.5 µm, moving from superficial dentin to deep dentin, and the number ranges from 20,000 to 45,000/mm^2 (Fig 4).[10,11]

Given that the number and size of the tubules doubles in deep dentin compared with superficial dentin, there is an inverse ratio between peritubular and intertubular dentin quantity.[12]

Dentin is not a homogenous tissue but dynamic and subject to continuous remodeling, taking different forms: secondary, reparative, or tertiary; sclerotic, subcarious, or hypermineralized.[13] In clinical situations, these forms typically constitute the substrate of most restorations (Fig 5).

In general, these types of dentin are characterized by a high level of mineralization, disorganization of the tubular structure, low permeability, and the presence of crystals blocking the tubule lumen. These major histologic changes determine substantial differences in substrate between superficial and deep dentin and the associated adhesion values.[14]

After the use of any cutting instrument (burs or manual instruments), a sludge made up of organic and inorganic cutting detritus known as a smear layer forms on the dentin. This varies in thickness between 0.5 to 5 µm and 3 to 10 µm. Because it is strongly bonded to the dentin, it prevents the resin from bonding. The cutting operation itself gives rise to the formation of plugs in the tubule openings that are known as smear plugs. These arise due to the entry of detritus during the instrumentation stage[15] (Fig 6).

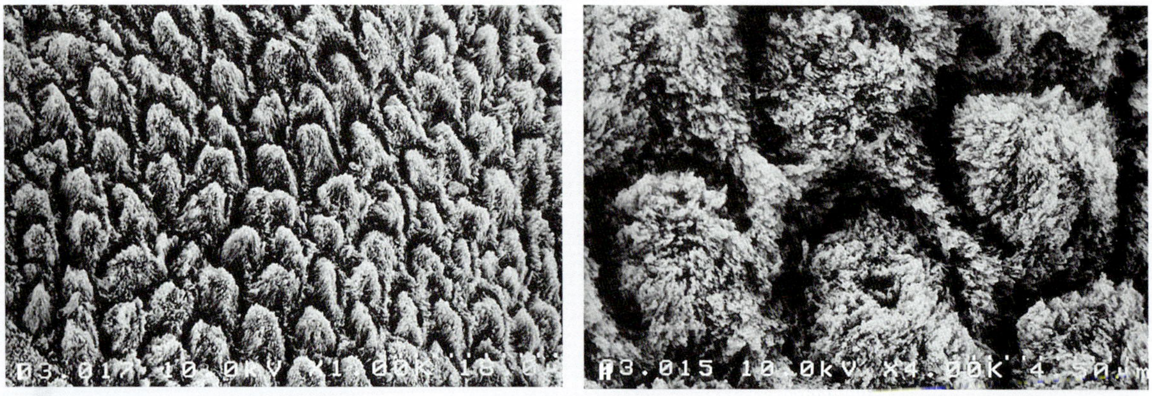

Fig 3 Scanning electron microscopy images of the enamel prisms after acid etching. (Courtesy of Professor Guido Goracci et al.)

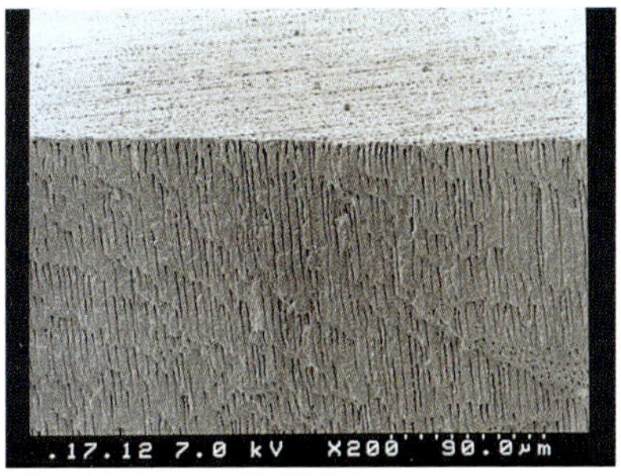

Fig 4 Cross section through dentinal tubules under a scanning electron microscope. (Courtesy of Professor Guido Goracci et al.)

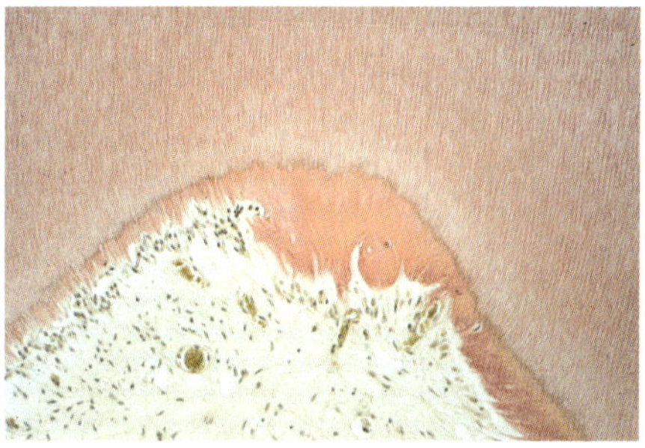

Fig 5 Light microscopy image showing dentinal reaction near a pulp horn. (Courtesy of Professor Guido Goracci et al.)

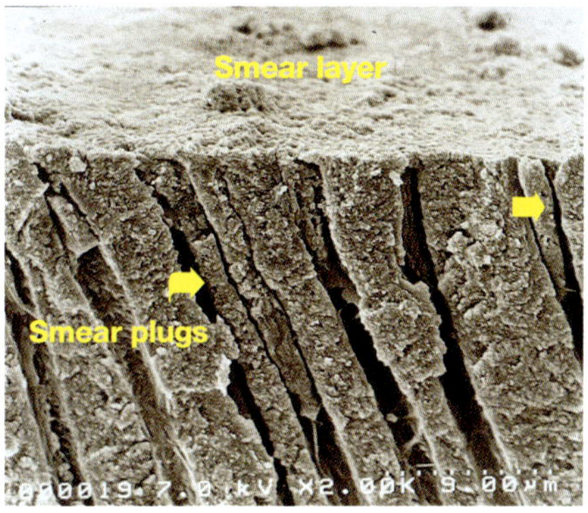

Fig 6 Scanning electron microscopy image of dentin following treatment with rotary instruments that gave rise to the formation of a smear layer on the surface and smear plugs in the tubules. (Courtesy of Professor Guido Goracci et al.)

Classification of present-day adhesives

Present-day adhesive systems may be classified according to different parameters:

1. ***Generation:*** Adhesives are classified based on the time when they appeared on the market.
2. ***Action on the substrate:*** They can be differentiated into two categories, those that remove the smear layer and those that dissolve it.
3. ***Number of steps:*** They may be classified according to the number of clinical steps necessary for correct application.
4. ***Solvent type:*** Adhesives are classified according to the type of solvent that they contain (to improve the fluidity of the resin). This will generally be ethanol, acetone, or water or a combination of these.

Adhesive systems can be subdivided into four groups. Among the many existing classifications, the most significant and most commonly used clinical classification considers the interaction with the substrate and categorizes adhesive systems as etch-and-rinse or self-etch and considers the number of steps required by the system to establish a bond with the tooth substrate.[16,17]

Etch-and-rinse adhesives

Etch-and-rinse adhesives require the application of an etching agent (generally 30% to 40% orthophosphoric acid) to the enamel and dentin followed by rinsing with the aim of removing the acid and salts that are formed by the demineralization process.

The possible formulations are as follows:

- ***Three-step:*** Three classic steps involving the separate application of etching agent, primer, and bonding agent (Fig 7)
- ***Two-step:*** Also known as self-priming adhesives, characterized by an etching stage similar to that of three-step systems, followed by an agent that combines primer and bonding agent within a single product

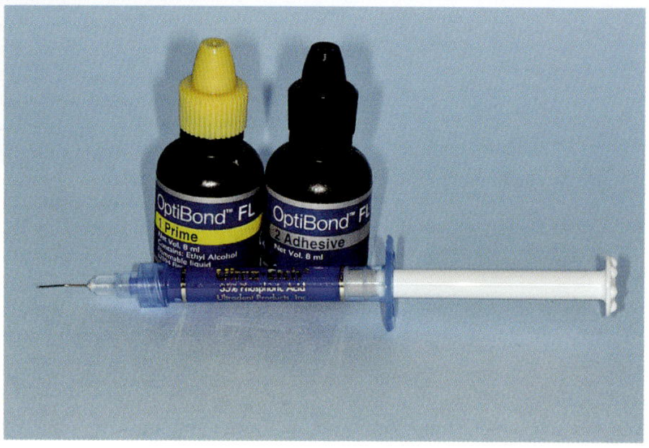

Fig 7 Three-step adhesive system.

Self-etch adhesives

These products, which were also recently termed etch-and-dry, are based on the use of an acid monomer that dissolves the smear layer and simultaneously infiltrates the dentin. They do not need to be rinsed but only dried.

The possible formulations may be:

- ***Two-step:*** These feature an etching agent and primer mixed in a single product that must not be rinsed (in order not to remove the primer), but only dried, followed by a bonding step to be applied and cured (Fig 8).
- ***One-step:*** Adhesives featuring a system that incorporates etching, primer, and bonding all together in a single product.

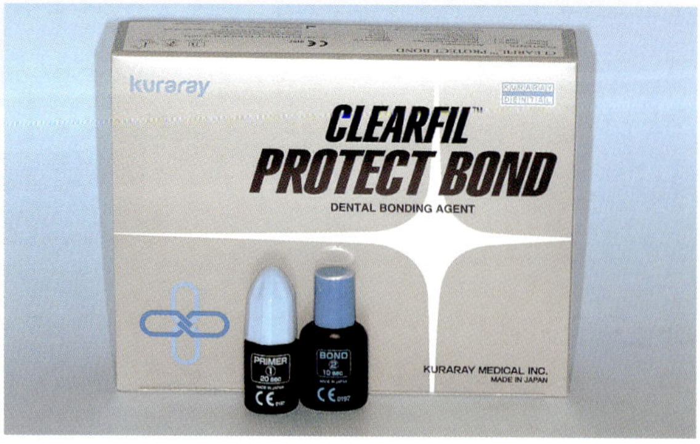

Fig 8 Two-step self-etch adhesive system.

Stability and duration of the adhesive interface

Although the adhesive systems currently on the market have demonstrated adequate short-term adhesion, their long-term stability is nevertheless an unknown factor, particularly for simplified adhesive systems.
The adhesive bond changes and breaks down in time, creating pigmentation and discoloration of the margin, a poor seal, and secondary decay.
This is due to the effects of aging adhesive monomers and collagen fibrils.
These effects also include that of hydrolytic breakdown, ie, breakdown of polymer chains following exposure to water.
The hybrid layer, ie, the area in which the adhesive system resin mechanically interlocks with the dentinal collagen,[18,19] represents a complex entity in which biologic components (collagen-dentin matrix and residual hydroxyapatite crystals) and nonbiologic components (resin monomers and solvents) interact (Fig 9).
Aging effects can exclusively involve, or synergistically break down, both the resin and the tooth components[17] through disorganization of collagen fibers or through hydrolysis of the resin in the interfibrillar spaces.
Hydrolysis is a chemical process that causes the breakdown of the covalent bonds in polymer chains and is considered one of the main contributory causes of a reduction in the adhesive bond over time, particularly in simplified adhesive systems.[20]

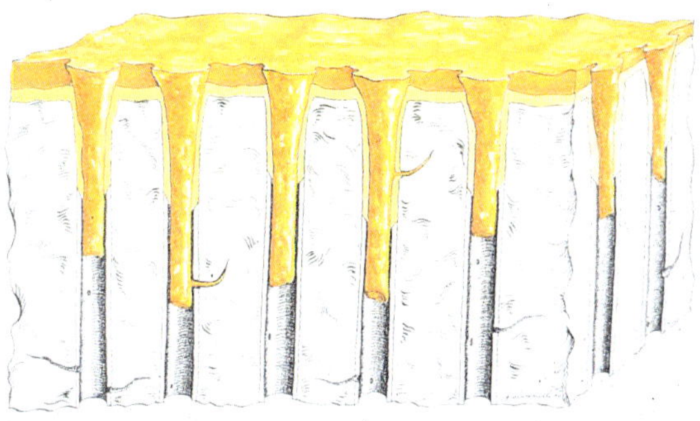

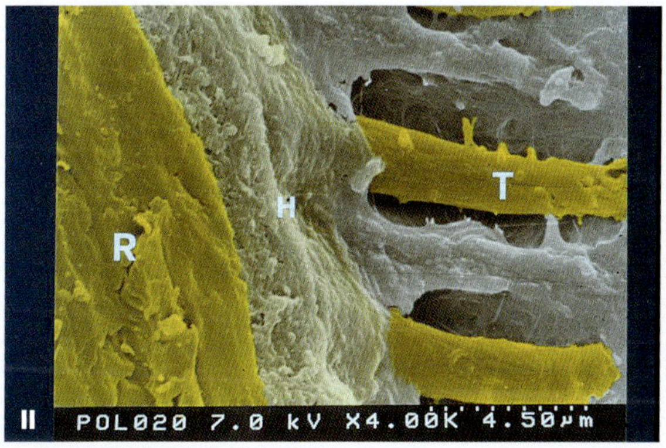

Fig 9 Illustration *(I)* and scanning electron microscopy image *(II)* showing formation of a hybrid layer (H). R, adhesive resin; T, resin tag. (Courtesy of Professor Guido Goracci et al.)

The duration of the adhesive interface is:

- ***Limited:*** One-step self-etch systems
- ***Moderate:*** Two-step etch-and-rinse systems
- ***High:*** Three-step etch-and-rinse and two-step self-etch systems

The combination of hydrophilic monomers in simplified adhesives (two-step etch-and-rinse or one-step self-etch) leads to the formation of a nonhydrophobic hybrid layer that behaves like a semipermeable membrane.[21]

The ultimate aim of adhesive procedures is total infiltration and encapsulation of the collagen fibers by the resin. Incomplete hybridization of the dentinal surface can leave the collagen fibers vulnerable to hydrolytic breakdown due to solvent residues[22] or insufficient water removal.

Recent studies have shown that some autogenic proteins known as metalloproteinases are activated during the adhesion stages and break down the collagen fibers in areas that are incompletely infiltrated by the resin.[11,23] Application of chlorhexidine after etching inhibits their intrinsic breakdown activity, preserving the collagen and the hybrid layer over time[24] (Fig 10).

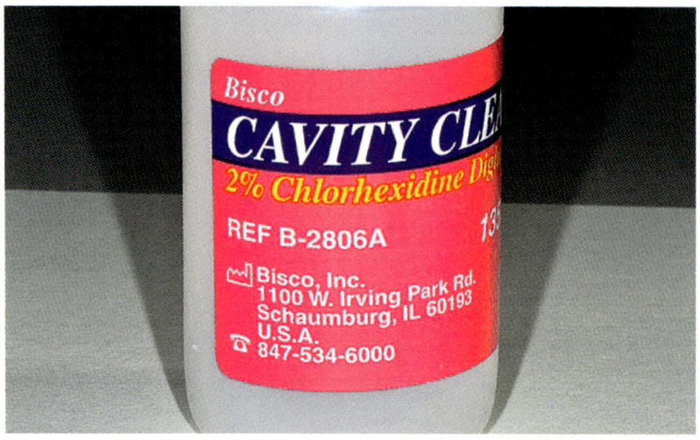

Fig 10 Chlorhexidine.

Different clinical approaches have been proposed for improving the resin infiltration and reducing the level of water absorption and breakdown due to the lysis of collagen.

- ***Using an additional hydrophobic layer:*** Incorporation of hydrophilic monomers in simplified adhesive systems (two-step etch-and-rinse and one-step self-etch) has dramatically reduced the longevity of the bond. The use of a hydrophobic coating layer with a solvent-free adhesive is therefore recommended with the aim of reducing water absorption and stabilizing the hybrid layer over time.[25] (Three-step etch-and-rinse and two-step self-etch systems should therefore take precedence over simplified adhesive systems.)
- ***Increase the curing time:*** Increasing the curing time in simplified adhesive systems beyond that recommended by the manufacturer means improving curing and reducing permeability with a good likelihood of improving the performance of the adhesives.[26]
- ***Using metalloproteinase inhibitors:*** The clinical use of metalloproteinase inhibitors, such as 0.2% or 2% chlorhexidine, as a primer on etched dentin is believed to reduce the breakdown of the adhesive interface over time, inhibiting the activity of the above enzymes present in the dentin that are responsible for the breakdown of collagen fibers.[27]
- ***Improving the impregnation of the adhesive component into the substrate:*** Various methods have recently been suggested with the aim of increasing impregnation of the dentinal substrate, namely prolonged application of the adhesive system, more vigorous mechanical application of the adhesive with a microbrush and, recently, the use of special electrical pulses during adhesive application.[28]

Choosing the system and method of application

ADHESIVE SYSTEM

Small and superficial cavities (prevalently enamel)

Three-step etch-and-rinse (three steps, eg, Optibond FL, Kerr)

Wide and deep cavities (significant amount of dentin)

Two-step self-etch (two steps, eg, Clearfil Protect Bond, Kuraray)

CLINICAL APPLICATION METHOD

Three-step etch-and-rinse

DIRECT RESTORATIONS (Fig 11)

1. *ETCHING*: Apply the etching gel to the enamel surface for 15 seconds and then to the dentin for another 15 seconds. The etched surface is thoroughly rinsed with air-water spray for 15 seconds to remove any acid residue and then gently dried.
2. *CHLORHEXIDINE*: Apply the chlorhexidine in concentrations of 0.12% or 0.2% for 30 seconds.
3. *PRIMER*: Apply the primer generously to the enamel and dentin surfaces in several layers to ensure good wettability of the bonding cavity. This must then be properly dried with the aim of evaporating off the solvent. It may be applied repeatedly if the etched surface is chalky in appearance.
4. *BONDING*: The adhesive then must be applied in cavities to create a homogenous layer and gently blown with the aim of evaporating the solvent.

INDIRECT RESTORATIONS (Fig 12)

In indirect restorations, the only difference is that the enamel is etched only during the inlay/onlay cementation stage.

Two-step self-etch

DIRECT RESTORATIONS (Fig 13)

1. *ETCHING AGENT:* Many studies recommend selective etching of the enamel alone and subsequent application of self-etch agent/primer to the etched enamel and unetched dentin.
2. *CHLORHEXIDINE*: Apply the chlorhexidine in concentrations of 0.12% or 0.2% for 30 seconds.
3. *ETCHING/PRIMER:* The self-etch agent/primer is applied to the enamel and dentin for the time recommended by the manufacturer and then blown to remove excess and stop the demineralization reaction.
4. *BONDING:* The bonding is applied in the same way as the three-step etch-and-rinse bonding, blowing thoroughly with air to create a homogenous layer and promote evaporation of the solvent before curing.

INDIRECT RESTORATIONS (Fig 14)

As already mentioned for three-step etch-and-rinse indirect restorations, the enamel etching is only applied at the time of cementation, even when using two-step self-etch systems.

Five clinical cases are presented, demonstrating the use of different adhesive systems (Figs 15 to 19).

Three-step etch-and-rinse: Direct restorations

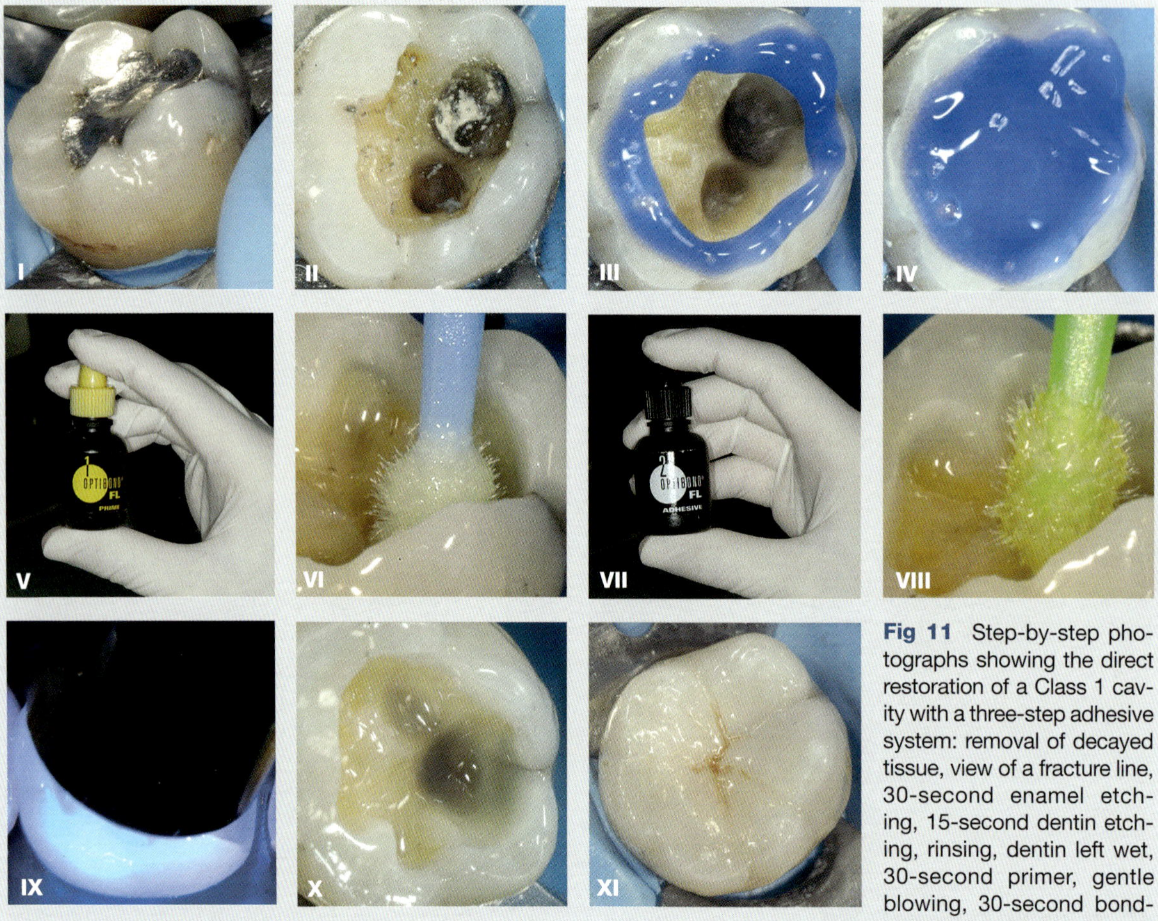

Fig 11 Step-by-step photographs showing the direct restoration of a Class 1 cavity with a three-step adhesive system: removal of decayed tissue, view of a fracture line, 30-second enamel etching, 15-second dentin etching, rinsing, dentin left wet, 30-second primer, gentle blowing, 30-second bonding, blown and cured for 40 seconds, 0.5 mm of flowable composite added to the walls and base of the cavity, cured for 40 seconds, then stratification carried out by adding traditional composite to a maximum thickness of 2 mm at a time, curing each individual layer. The restoration was carried out approximately 8 years ago. Today it is very useful to use chlorhexidine immediately after the etching.

Three-step etch-and-rinse: Indirect restorations

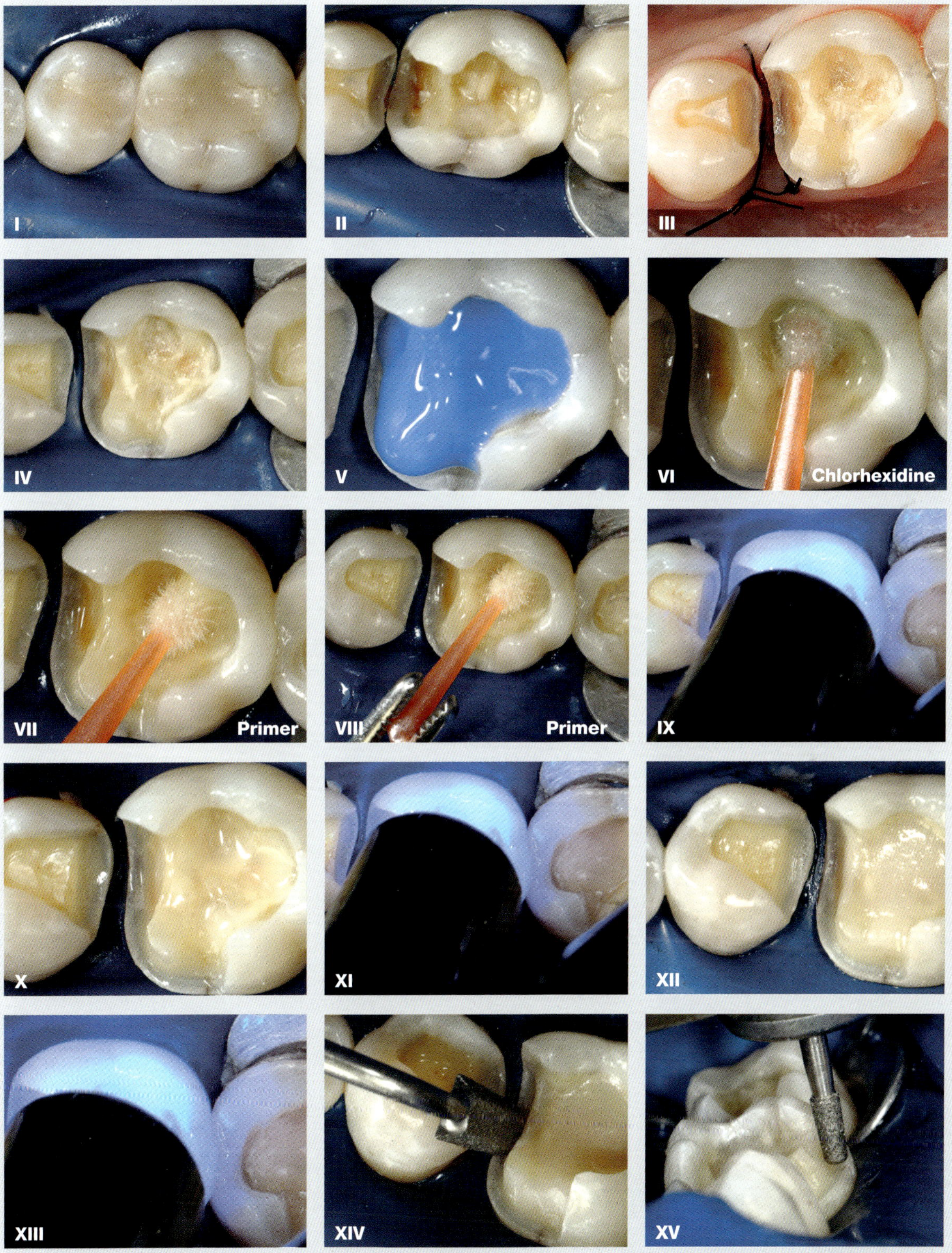

Fig 12 Stages of adhesion and buildup for the preparation of indirect restorations *(I–XIII)*. Completion of preparations with rubber dam and the aid of rotary and subsonic instruments *(XIV–XVI)*.

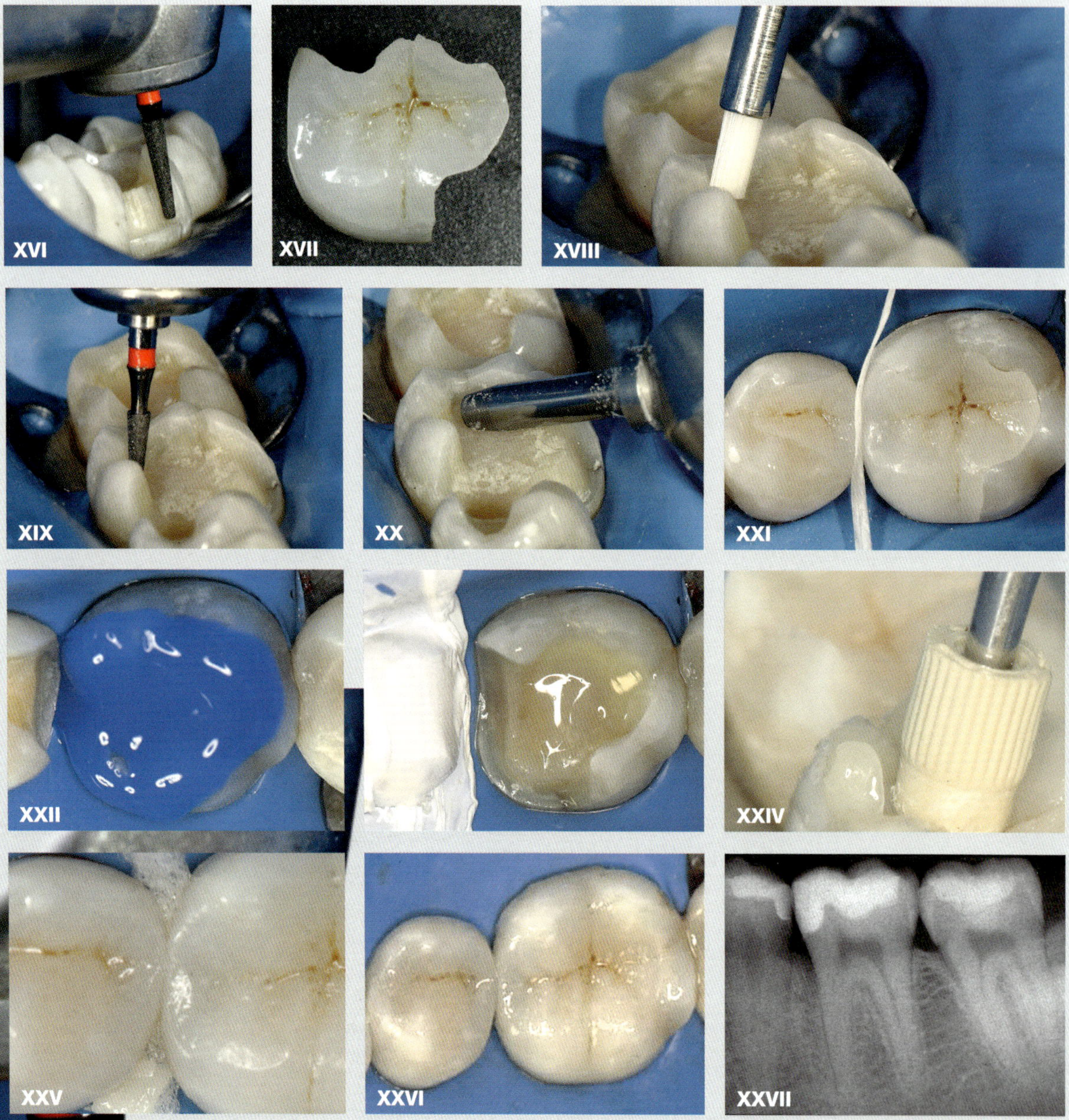

Fig 12 *(continued)* Before cementing the inlay, the cavity was thoroughly cleaned and sanded, and the structure was tested before cementation *(XVII–XXVI)*. Follow-up radiograph *(XXVII)*.

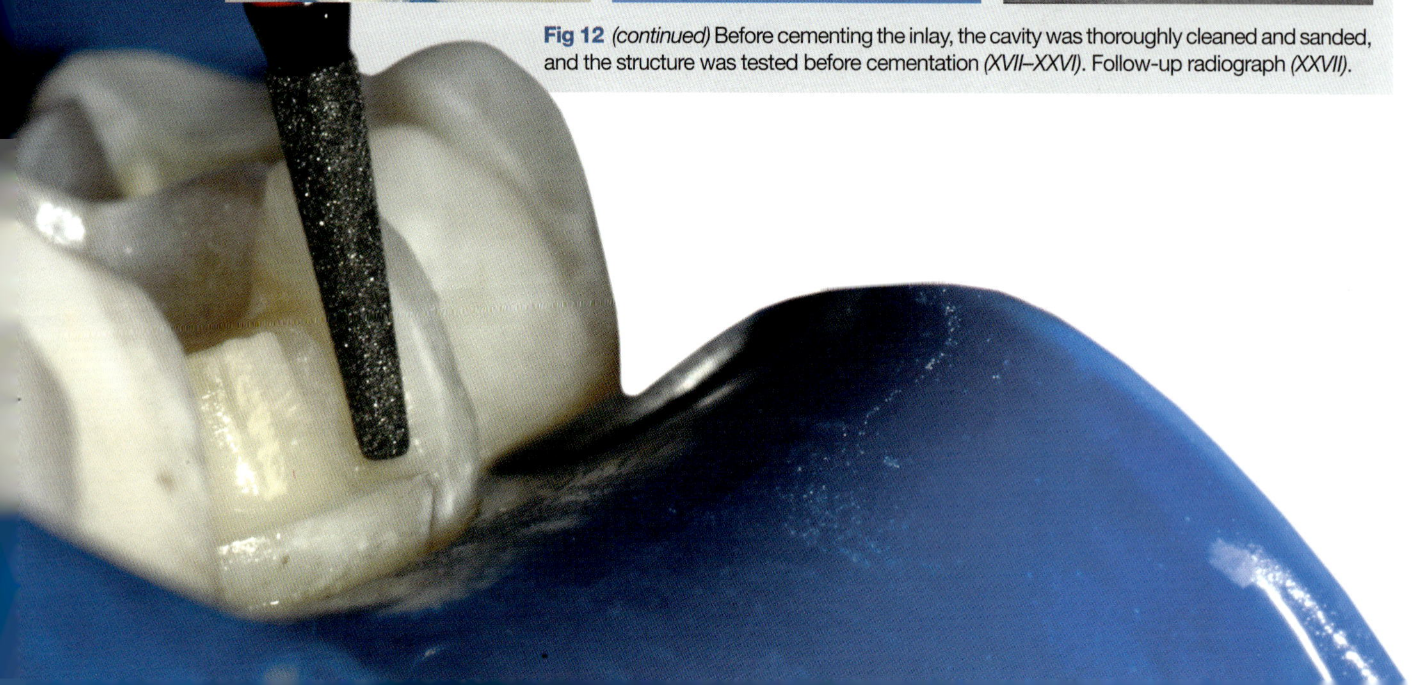

Two-step self-etch: Direct restorations

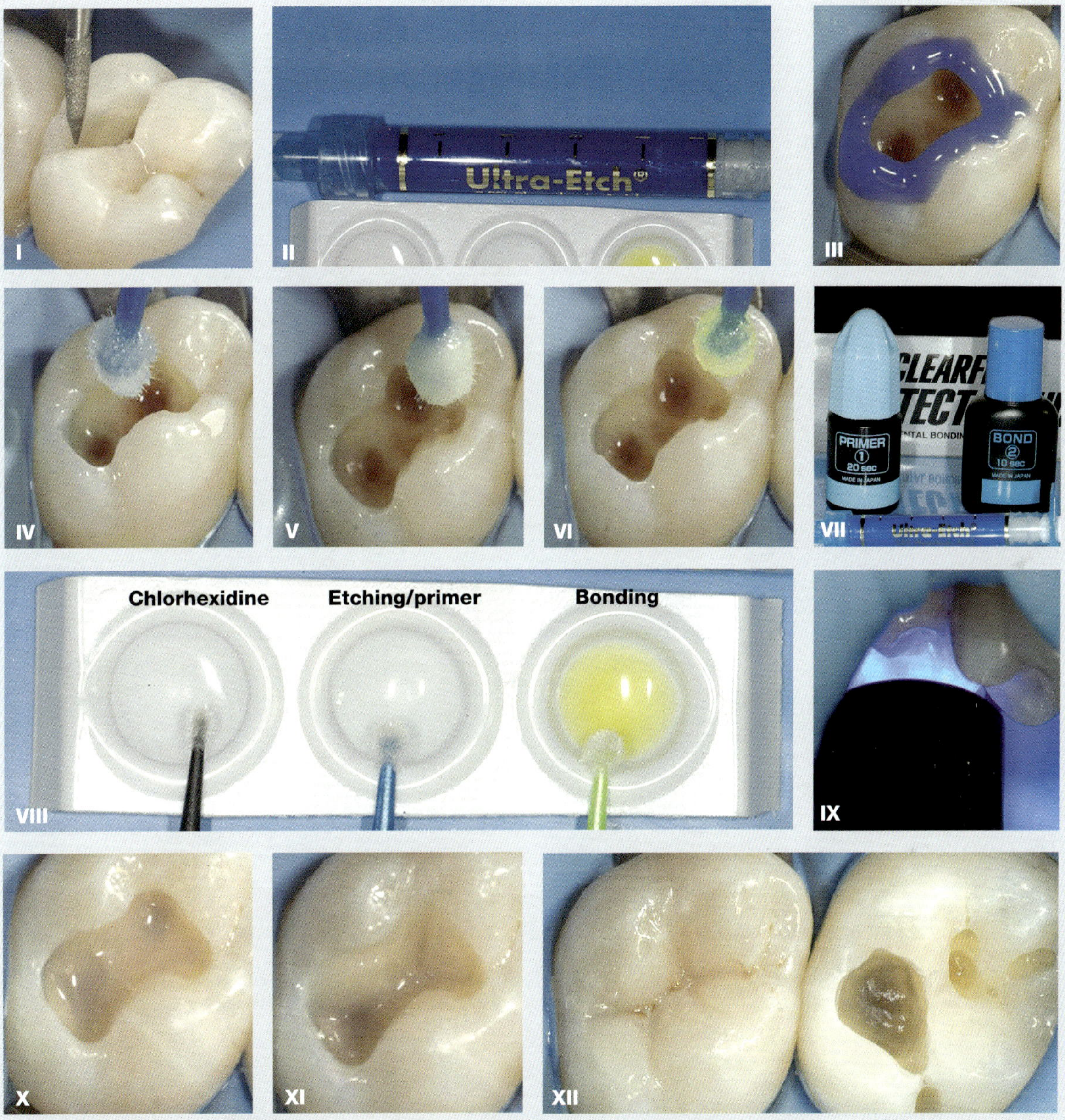

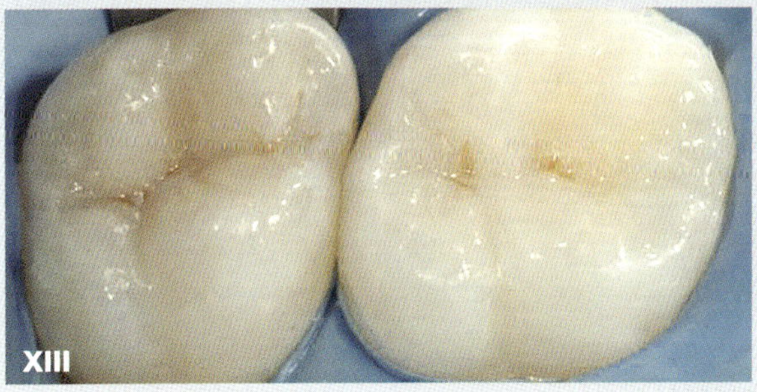

Fig 13 Step-by-step photographs showing a Class 1 cavity treated with a two-step self-etch adhesive system. Finishing of the cavity, selective etching of the enamel for 30 seconds *(I–III)*. Chlorhexidine 30 seconds, dentin primer/etching 30 seconds, blow gently, bonding 30 seconds, blow and cure 40 seconds *(IV–IX)*. Addition of 0.5 mm flowable composite in all cavities, stratification with traditional composite, curing after each layer, anatomical shaping, and completed restorations *(X–XIII)*.

Two-step self-etch: Indirect restorations

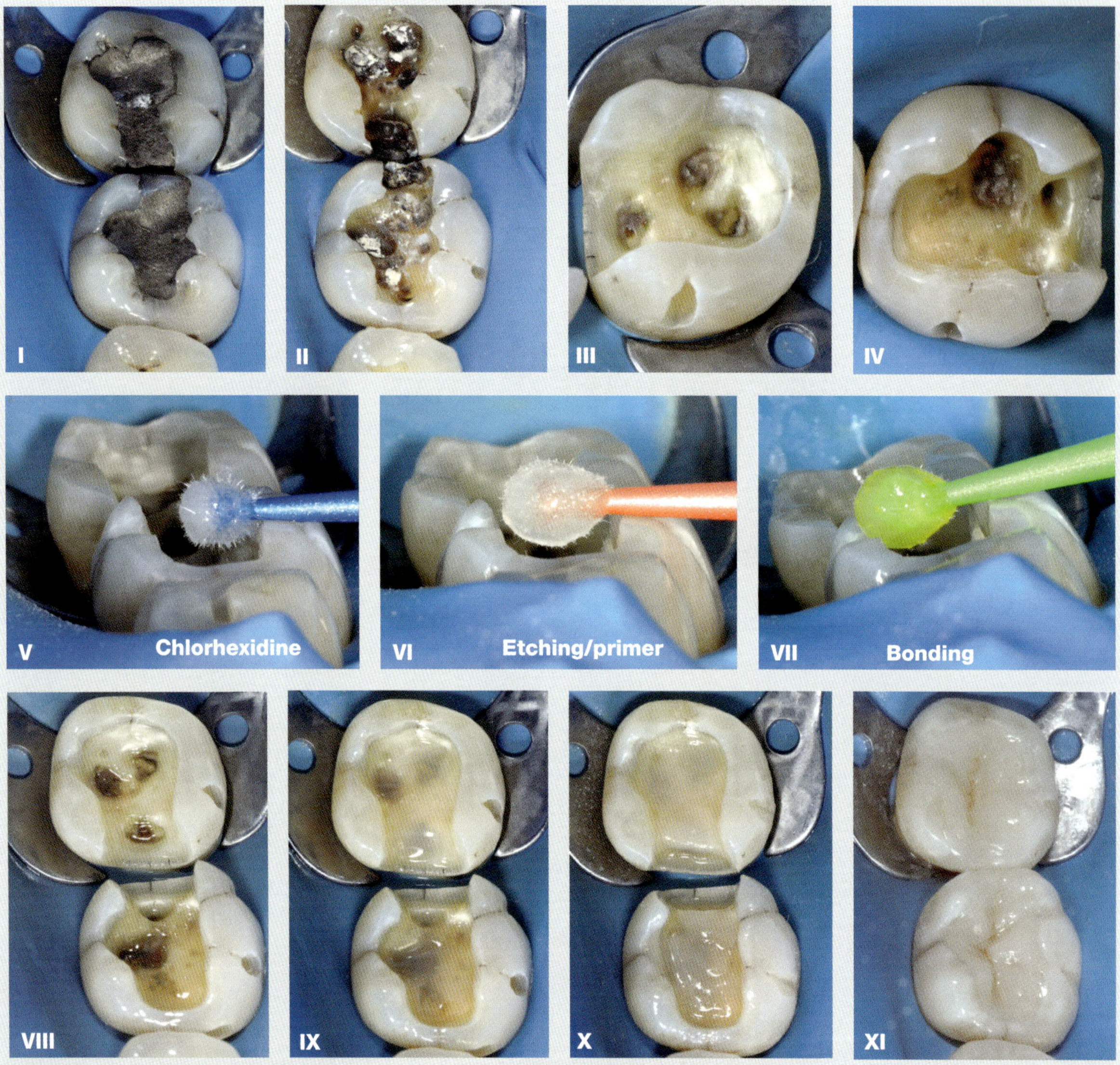

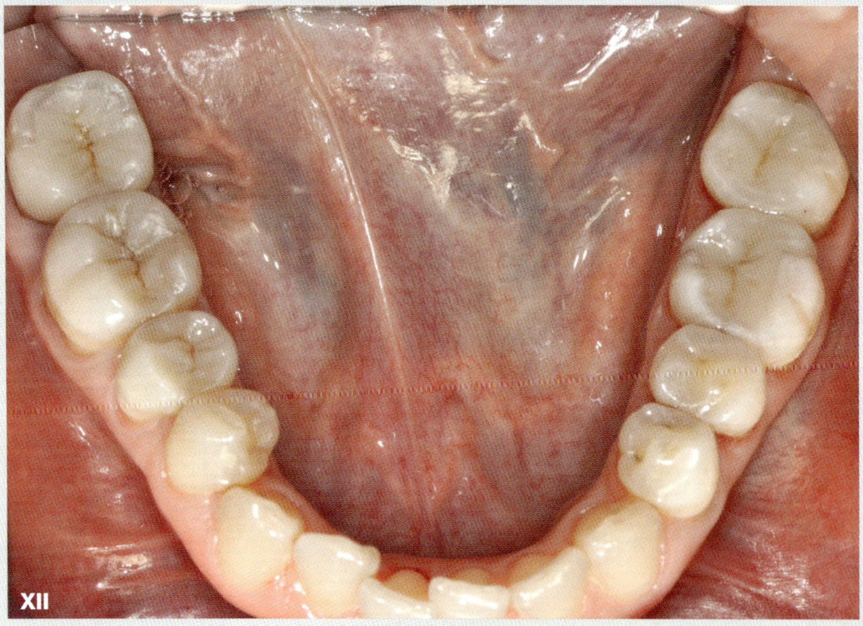

Fig 14 Removal of defective restorations, view of decayed tissue and cavities ready for adhesion *(I–IV)*. Stages of adhesion with chlorhexidine, etching/primer, and bonding *(V–VII)*. Buildup stages *(VIII–X)*. Inlay cemented and view of mandible with inlay cemented bilaterally *(XI, XII)*.

Clinical cases

Clinical case 1

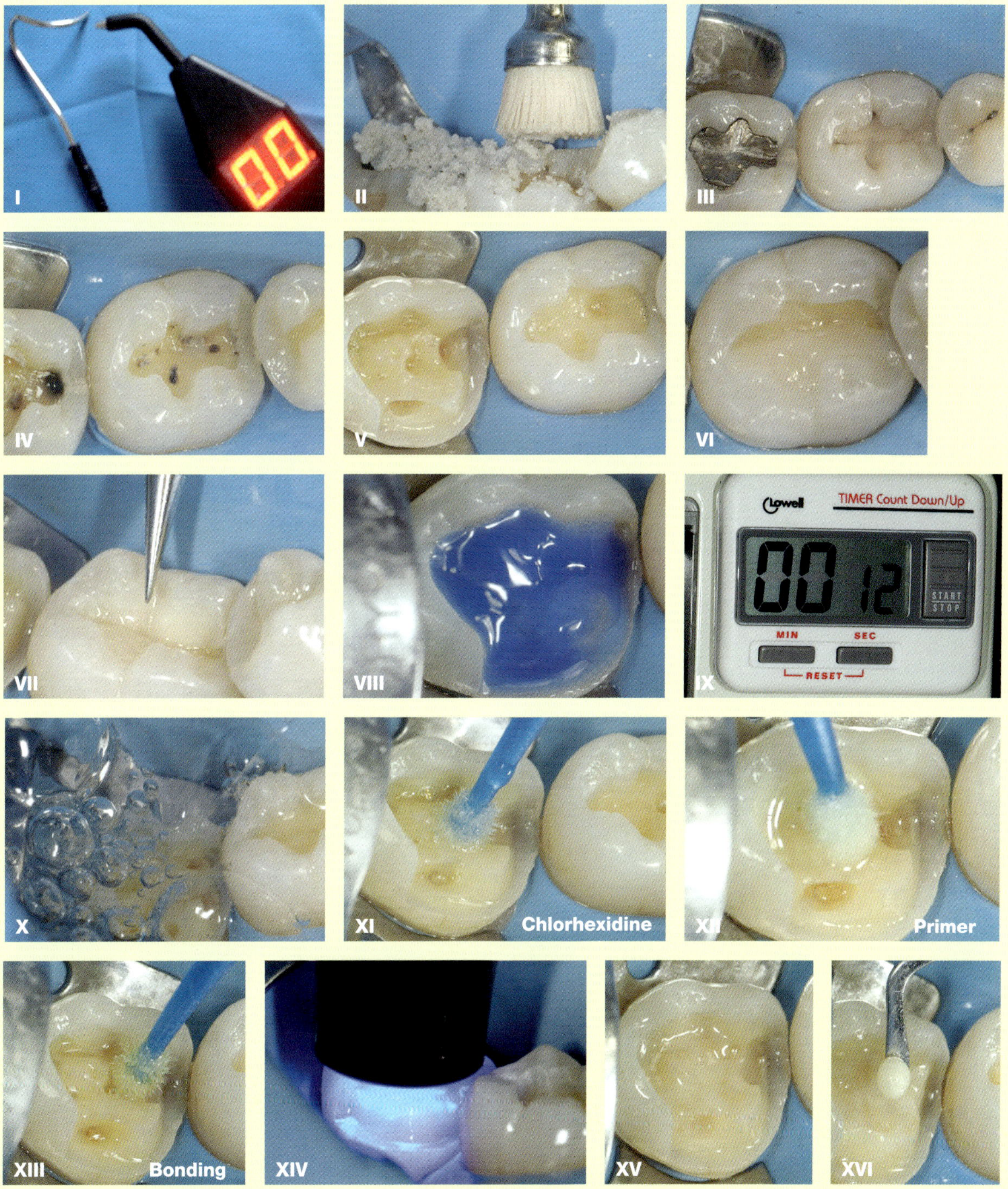

Fig 15 Instrument for vitality test *(I)*. Step-by-step photographs showing treatment of both Class 1 and 2 cavities with a three-step adhesive system. Note the cleanliness of the teeth under rubber dam, removal of the old restorations, cavities free of decay, and indication and execution of a direct restoration for the mandibular right first molar using a stratification technique *(II–VII)*. The indication for the adjacent second molar, on the other hand, is an indirect restoration with coverage of the mesiobuccal cusp (onlay). Selective etching of the dentin is carried out using 37% orthophosphoric acid for 15 seconds with the aim of removing the superficial dentinal smear layer and that plugging the tubules, with exposure of the collagen fibers and increased wettability *(VIII)*. After 15 seconds of etching, timed with a stopwatch *(IX)*, the cavities are thoroughly washed for a long time to prevent the traces of silicone contained in the acid gel from affecting the adhesive process, leaving the dentin slightly wet *(X)*. Adhesion stages: chlorhexidine 30 seconds and blow; primer 30 seconds and blow; bond for 30 seconds, rubbing briskly; repeat the application; then cure for 40 seconds *(XI–XIV)*. Execution of buildup with flowable composite with the aim of achieving a buffering effect to compensate for the mechanical stress caused by polymerization shrinkage. After curing the flowable composite, the buildup is completed with traditional composite that is also cured *(XV, XVI)*.

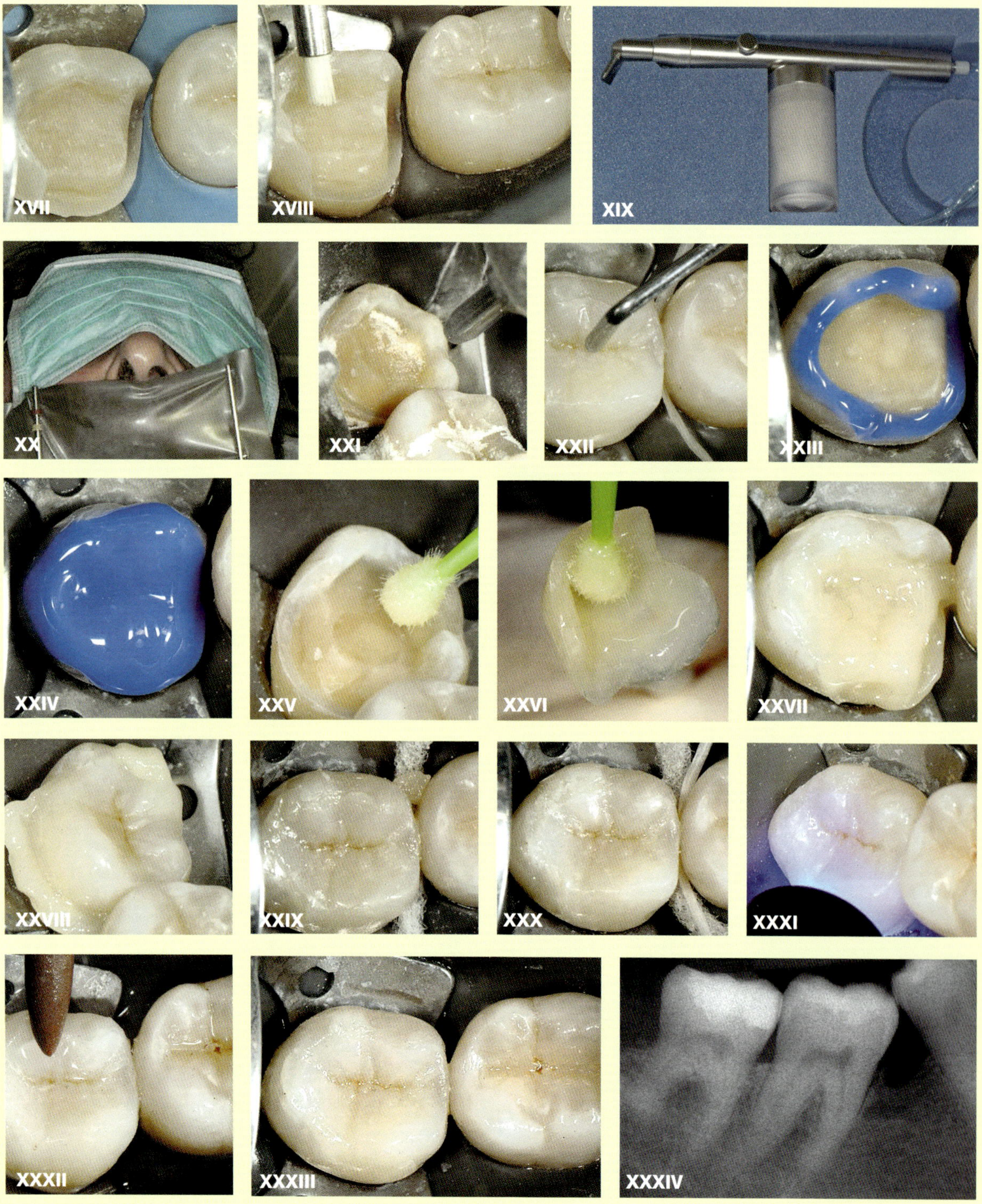

Fig 15 *(continued)* Inlay cementation stages involving cleaning of the tooth after removal of the temporary dressing, sanding in accordance with the recognized procedure, testing of the inlay, acidification of the enamel and buildup to remove any impurities *(XVII–XXIV)*, use of bonding alone *(XXV, XXVI)* in both the internal part of the inlay and in the cavity, filling of the cavity with composite used as cement *(XXVII)*, insertion of the inlay using manual and subsonic instruments, removal of excess and then curing, 1 minute per side *(XXVIII–XXXIV)*. According to D'Arcangelo and Vanini,[29] tooth sanding is a surface treatment carried out with 50-µm aluminum trioxide particles for 10 seconds, at a distance of 5 cm, under a pressure of 2 bars, leading to a significant increase in adhesive strength compared with other methods *(XIX)*.

Clinical case 2

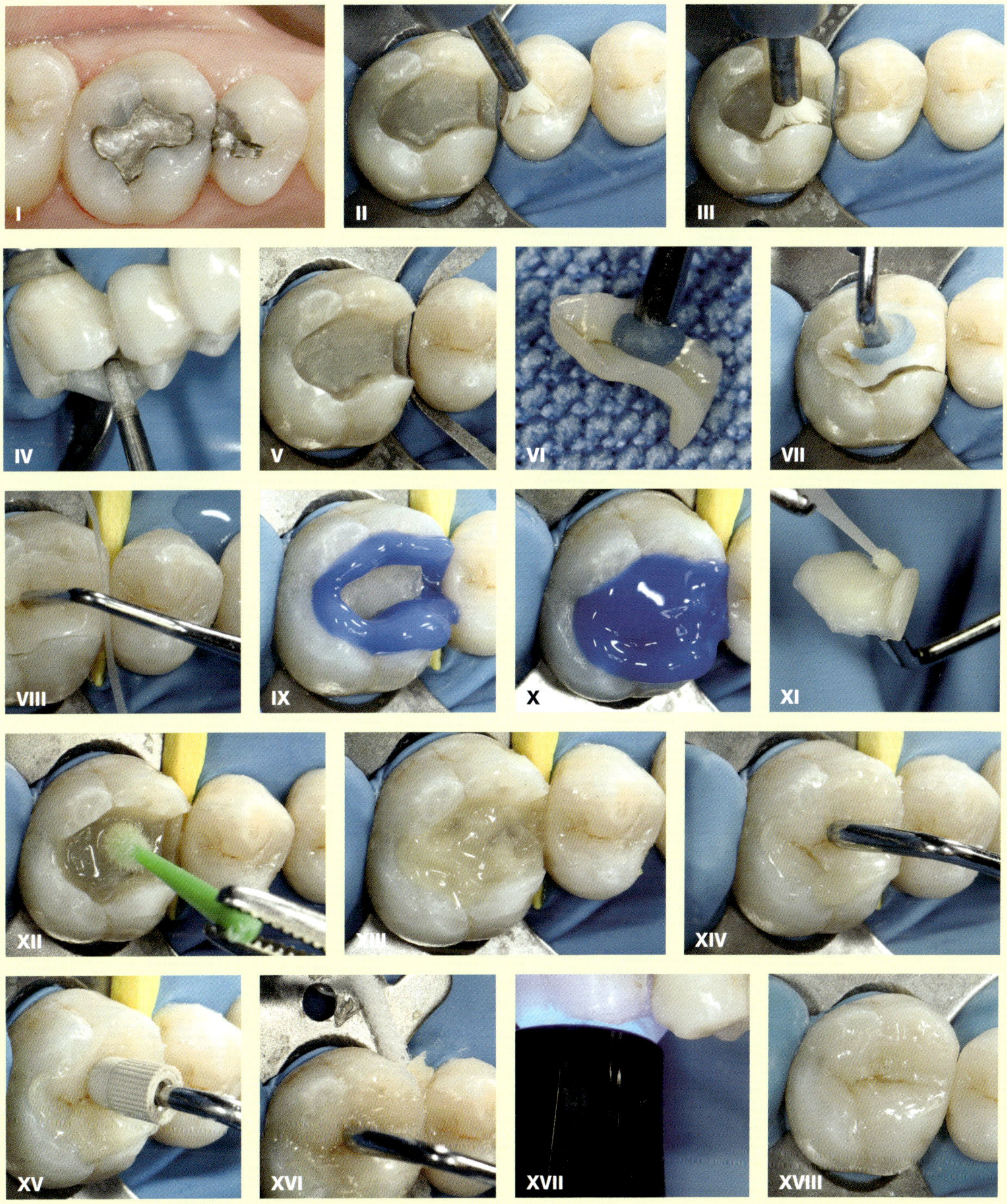

Fig 16 Clinical case showing cementation of two inlays using a three-step adhesive technique.

Clinical case 3

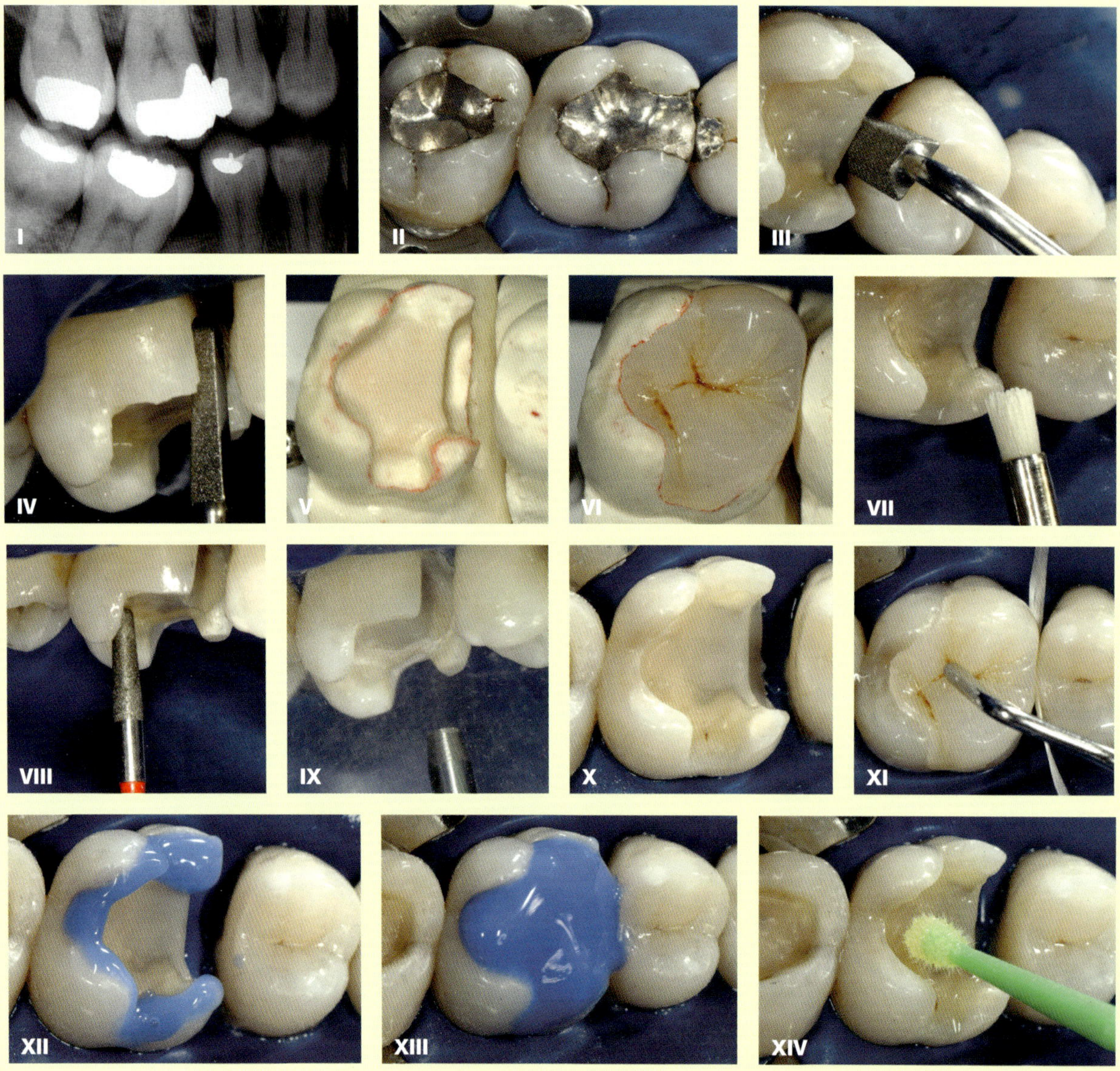

Fig 17 Clinical case showing cementation of an inlay on the maxillary right first molar, involving finishing of the cavity with subsonic burs, carrying out the inlay on a working cast, cleaning of the preparation after removal of the temporary dressing, testing the inlay to check the contact surfaces, adhesion stages (three-step technique) with an additional layer of primer in the cavity and bonding cured to fill in any areas of dentin that have inadvertently been left uncovered (dentin islands) and so on, according to the protocol, before checking the contact surfaces and emergence profiles. These concepts have already been stressed, but they are so crucial that they bear repeating. The final step is the essential radiographic follow-up, which is the only true indicator of whether the work has been carried out properly.

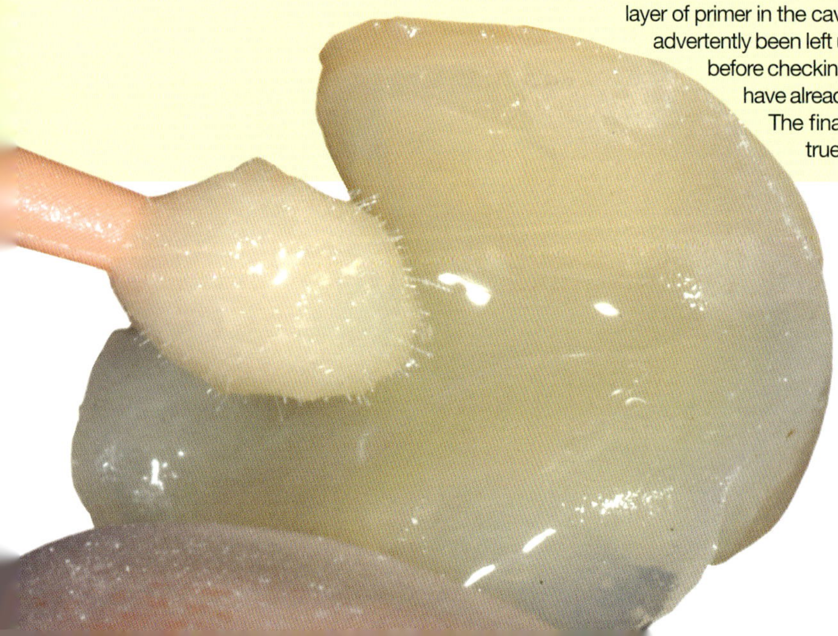

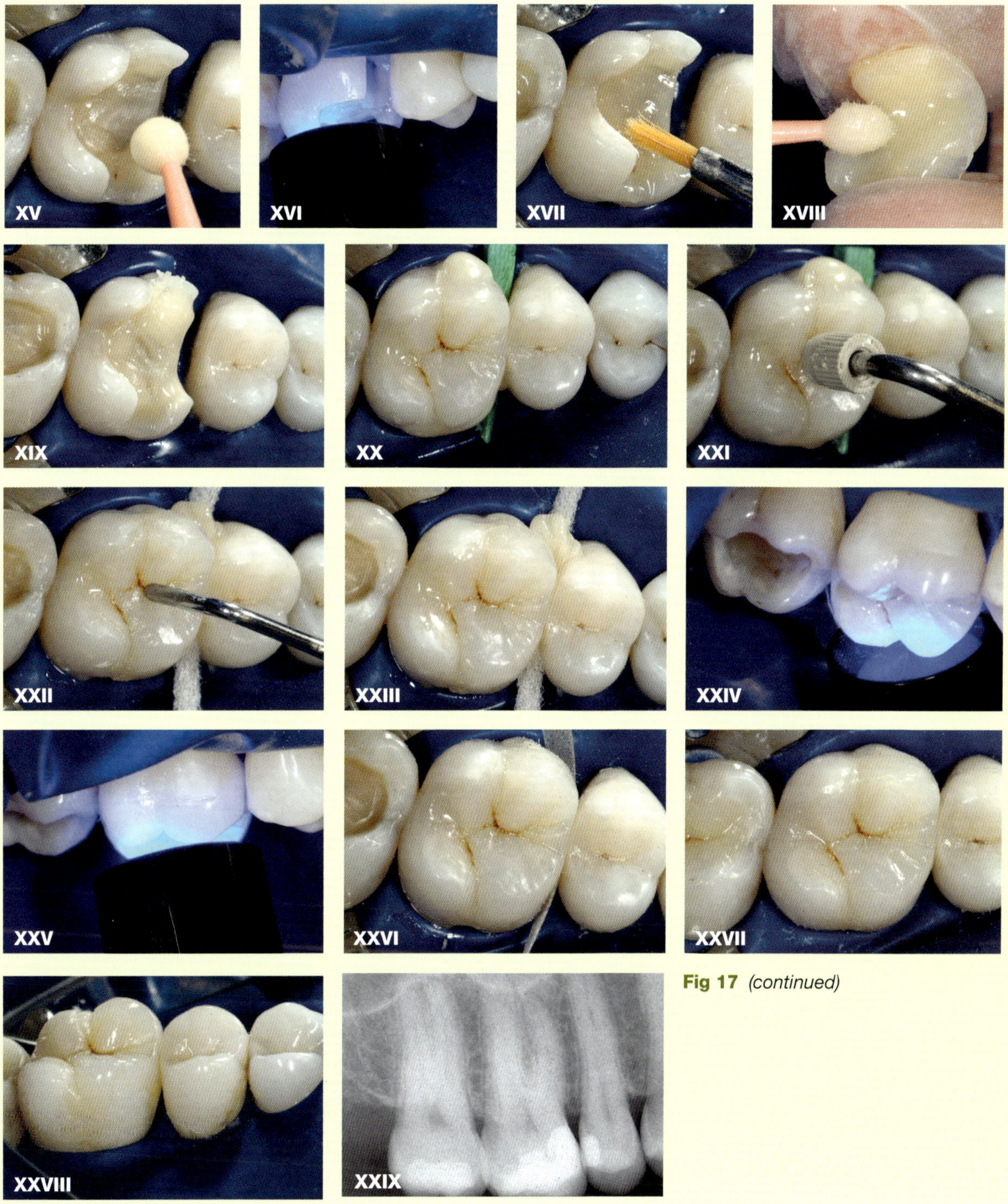

Fig 17 *(continued)*

Clinical case 4

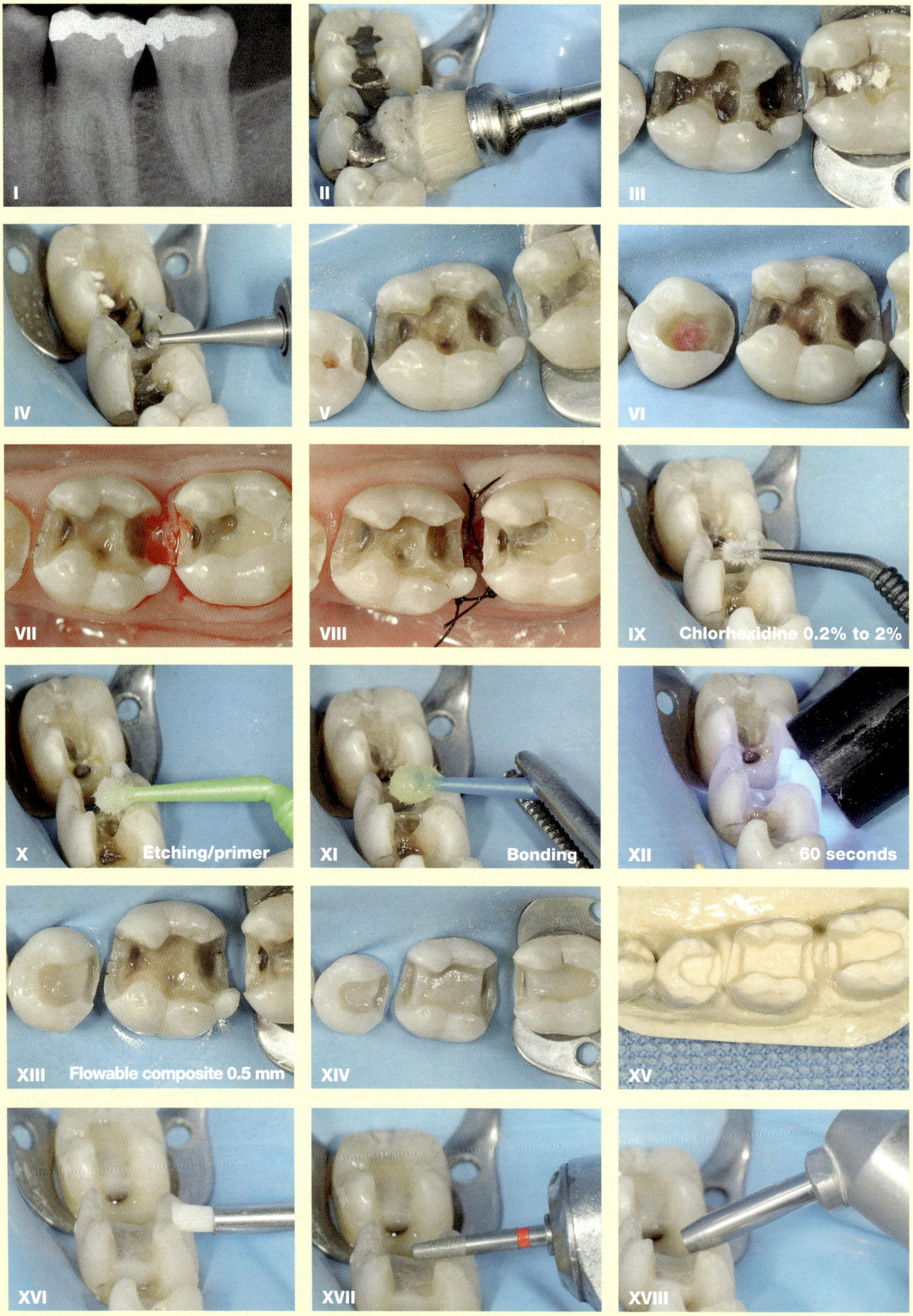

Fig 18 Another interdisciplinary step-by-step guide, with the use of a two-step self-etching adhesive system, showing all stages of reconstructing a quadrant with indirect restorations, followed by images of the results after periodontal surgery and at follow-up in 2012. Treatment was carried out in the left maxilla in 2003, in the right maxilla and mandible in 2008, and in the left mandible in 2009.

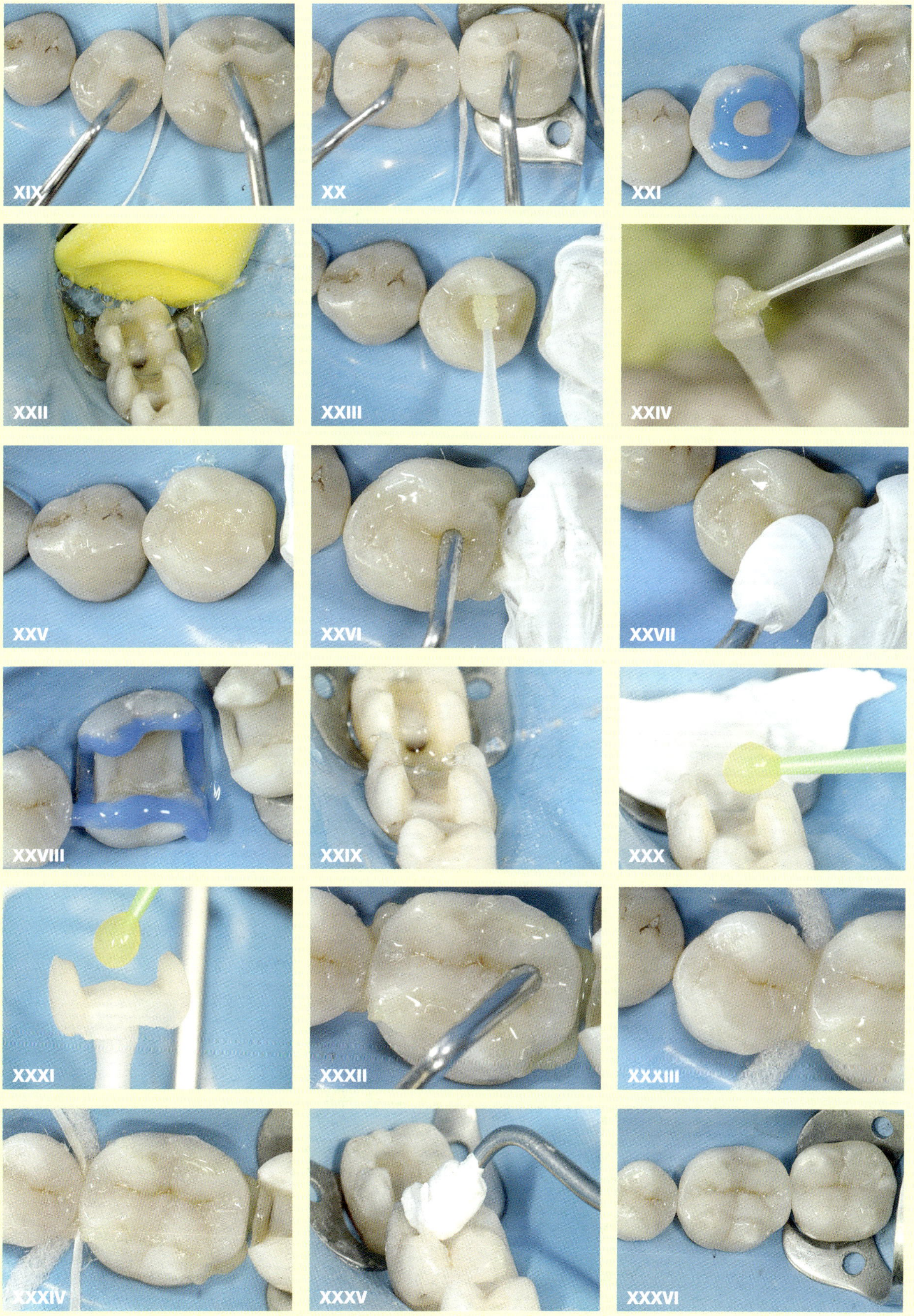

Fig 18 *(continued)*

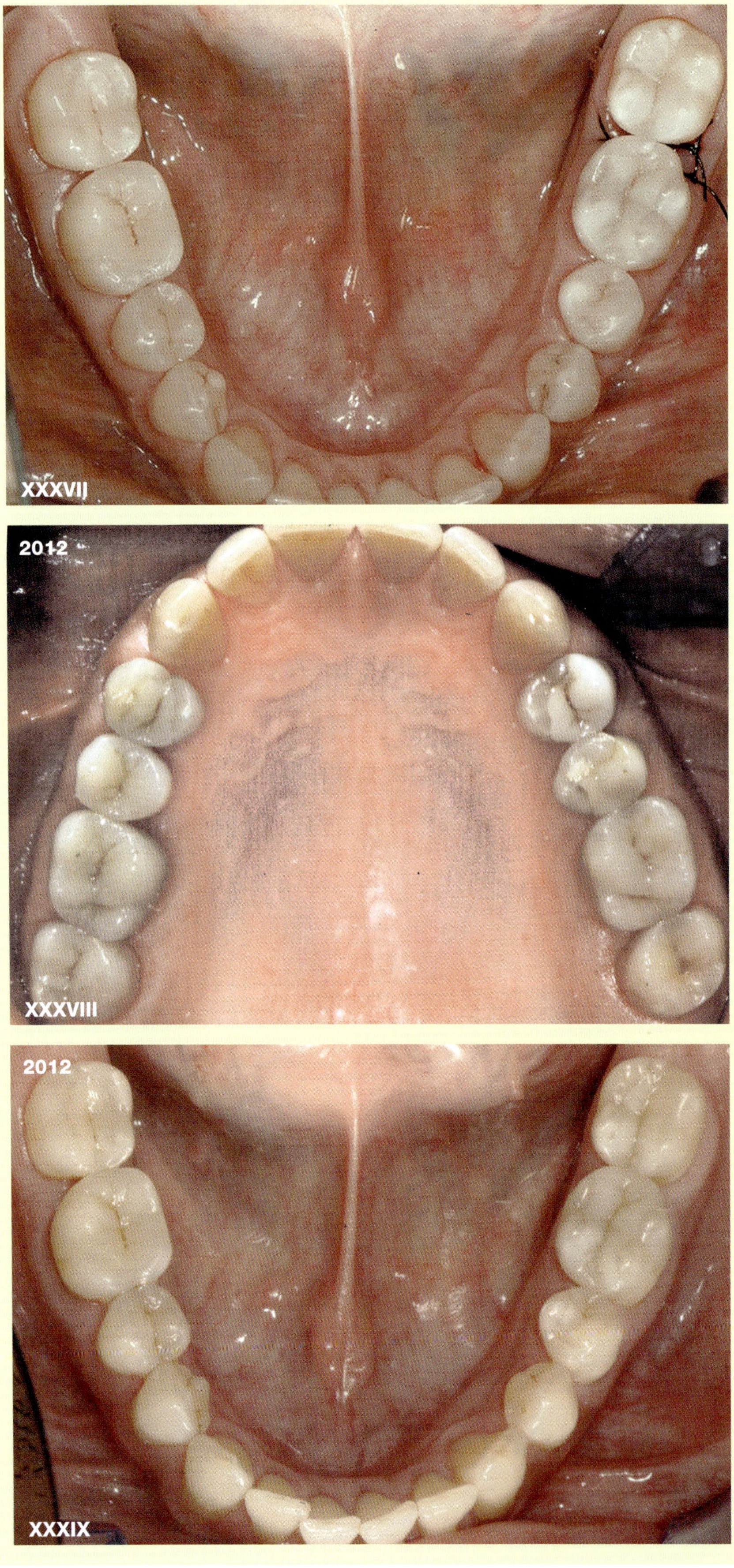

Fig 18 *(continued)*

Clinical case 5

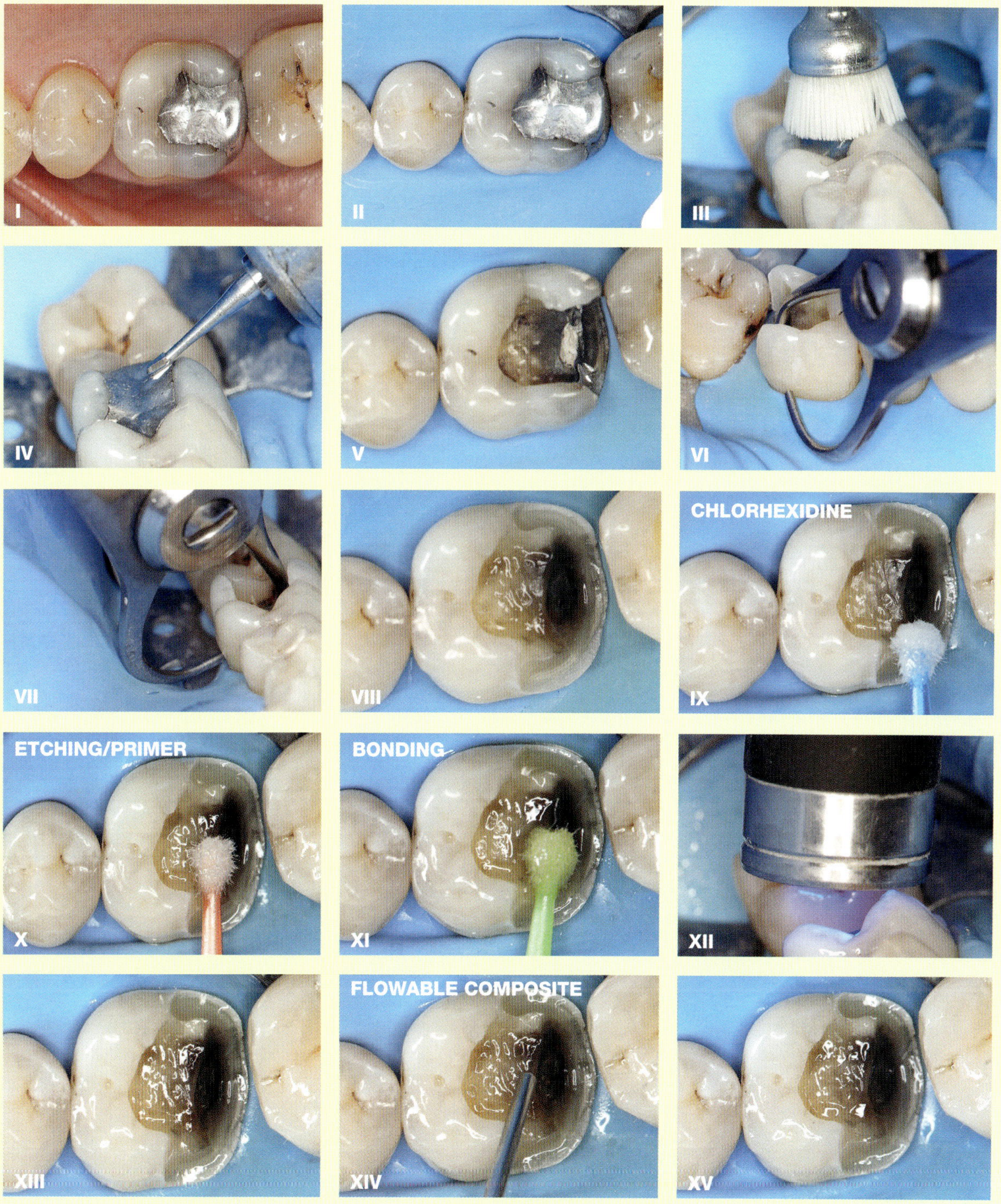

Fig 19 In this clinical case, the thicknesses at the base of the distobuccal and lingual cusps indicate that they should be removed and an onlay should be applied by means of cavity preparation. The adhesive system is again two-step self-etch. (Courtesy of Dr Lavinia Landi.)

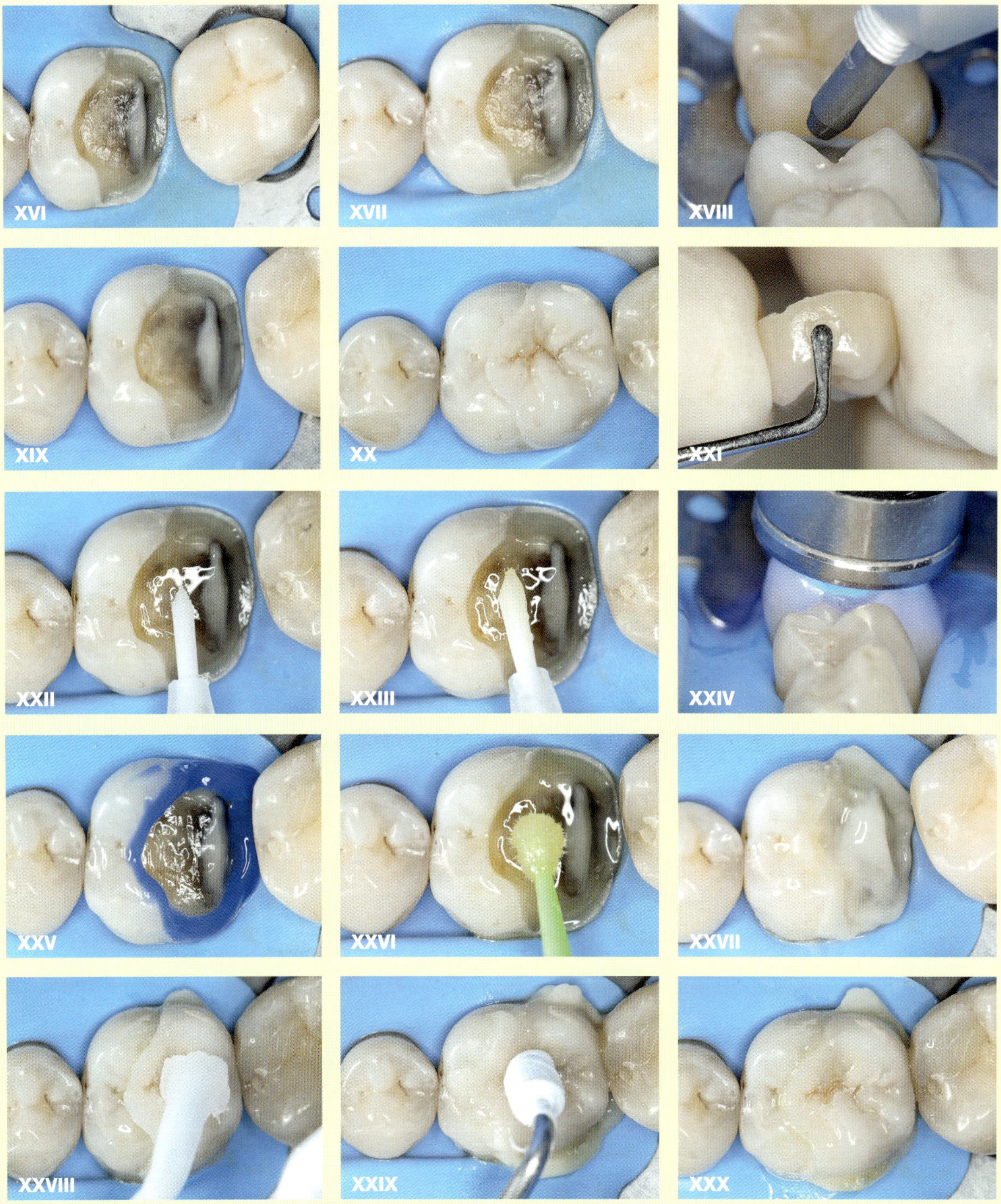

Fig 19 *(continued)*

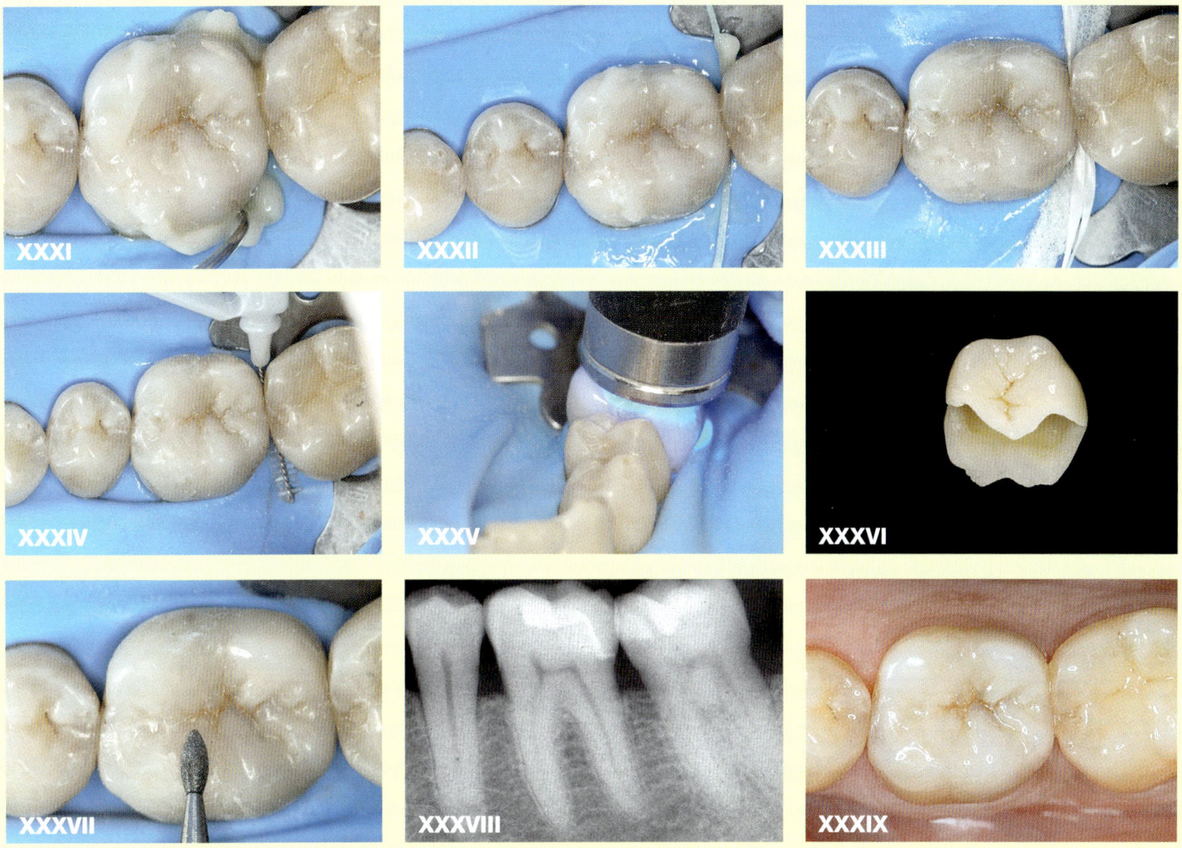

Fig 19 *(continued)*

References

1. Buonocore MG. A simple method of increasing the adhesion of acrylic filling materials to enamel surface. J Dent Res 1955;34:849–853.
2. Bowen RL. Properties of a silica-reinforced polymer for dental restorations. J Am Dent Assoc 1963;66:57–64.
3. Swift EJ, Perdigão J, Heymann HO. Bonding to enamel and dentin: A brief story and state of the art, 1995. Quintessence Int 1995;26:95–110.
4. Packham DE. Adhesion. In: Packham DE (ed). Handbook of Adhesion. Essex: Longman Scientific & Technical, 1992.
5. Sharma SJ, Roulet JF. Adhesion: The silent revolution. 2nd European Symposium on Adhesive Dentistry:7-9 May 1999. J Adhes Dent 1999;1:285–287.
6. Lutz F, Krejci I, Oddera M. Restauri Estetici nei settori posteriori. Manuale operative. Zurich: PPK, 1996.
7. Simmer JP, Hu JC. Dental enamel formation and its impact on clinical dentistry. J Dent Educ 2001;65:896–905.
8. Pashley DH. Dentin: A dynamic substrate—A review. Scanning Microsc 1989;3:161–176.
9. Mjör IA, Fejerskov O. Human Oral Embryology and Histology, ed 1. Copenhagen: Munksgaard, 1986.
10. Pashley DH, Carvalho RM. Dentine permeability and dentine adhesion. J Dent 1997;25:355–372.
11. Pashley DH, Tay FR, Yiu CK, et al. Collagen degradation by host-derived enzymes during aging. J Dent Res 2004;83:216–221.
12. Kinney JH, Oliveira J, Haupt DL, Marshall GW, Marshall SJ. The spatial arrangement of tubules in human dentin. J Mater Sci Mater Med 2001;12:743–751.
13. Bowen RL. Adhesive bonding of various materials to hard tooth tissues. XXII. The effects of a cleanser, mordant, and polySAC on adhesion between a composite resin and dentin. J Dent Res 1980;59:809–814.
14. Perdigão J. Dentin bonding—Variables related to the clinical situation and the substrate treatment. Dent Mater 2010;26:e24–e37.
15. Pashley DH. Smear layer: Physiological considerations. Oper Dent 1984;3:13–29.
16. Van Meerbeeck B, De Munck J, Yoshida Y, et al. Buonocore memorial lecture: Adhesion to enamel and dentin: Current status and future challenges. Oper Dent 2003;28:215–235.
17. Breschi L, Mazzoni A, Ruggeri A Jr, et al. Dental adhesion review: Aging and stability of the bonded interface. Dental Mater 2008;24:90–101.
18. Nakabayashi N, Kojima K, Mashuara E. The promotion of adhesion by the infiltration of monomers into tooth substrates. J Biomed Mater Res 1982;16:1240–1243.
19. Goracci G, Mori G, Casa De Martinis L, Bazzucchi M. Otturazioni in composito ed adesione alle strutture dentarie. 1994 Masson S.P.A- Milano.
20. Tay FR, Pashley DH. Have dentin adhesives become too hydrophilic? J Can Dent Assoc 2003;69:726–731.
21. Tay FR, Pashely DH, Suh BI, Carvahlo RM, Itthagarun A. Single step adhesives are permeable membranes. J Dent 2002;30:371–382.
22. Yiu CK, Pashley EL, Hiraishi N, et al. Solvent and water retention in dental adhesive blends after evaporation. Biomaterials 2005;26:6863–6872.
23. Mazzoni A, Pashley DH, Nishitami Y, et al. Reactivation of quenched endogenous proteolytic activities in phosphoric acid etched dentine by etch-and-rinse adhesives. Biomaterials 2006;27:4470–4476.
24. Carrilho MRO, Carvalho RM, de Goes MF, et al. Chlorhexidine preserves dentin bond in vitro. J Dent Res 2007;86:90–94.
25. Ito S, Tay FR, Hashimoto M, et al. Effects of multiple coatings of two all-in-one adhesives on dentin bonding. J Adhes Dent 2005;7:133–141.
26. Cadenaro M, Antoniolli F, Sauro S, et al. Degree of conversion and permeability of dental adhesives. Eur J Oral Sci 2005;113:525–530.
27. Breschi L, Cammelli F, Visintini E, et al. Influence of chlorhexidine concentration on the durability of etch-and-rinse dentin bonds: A 12 months in vitro study. J Adhes Dent 2009;11:191–198.
28. Breschi L, Suppa P, Mazzoni A, et al. Electric impulse-assisted application of a self-etch adhesives to dentin. J Dent Res 2006;12:1092–1096.
29. D'Arcangelo C, Vanini L. Effect of three surface treatments on the adhesive properties of indirect composite restorations. J Adhes Dent 2007;9:319–326.

Cavity preparation 3

It has already been stated that maximum preservation of healthy tissue is the goal that must be pursued when preparing a tooth for adhesive restoration (Fig 1), but it goes without saying that cavity design is dependent on the shape and volume of the restoration to be replaced and/or the extent of the caries lesions[1] (Figs 2 to 4).

Cavity preparation is of vital importance when producing indirect restorations. All subsequent treatment stages are dependent on the accuracy of this process: impression, preparation of study casts, prosthetic product, and cementation (Fig 5).

The choice of cavity preparation, ie, inlay, onlay, or overlay, must be based on a biomechanical analysis of the remaining healthy tooth tissue.

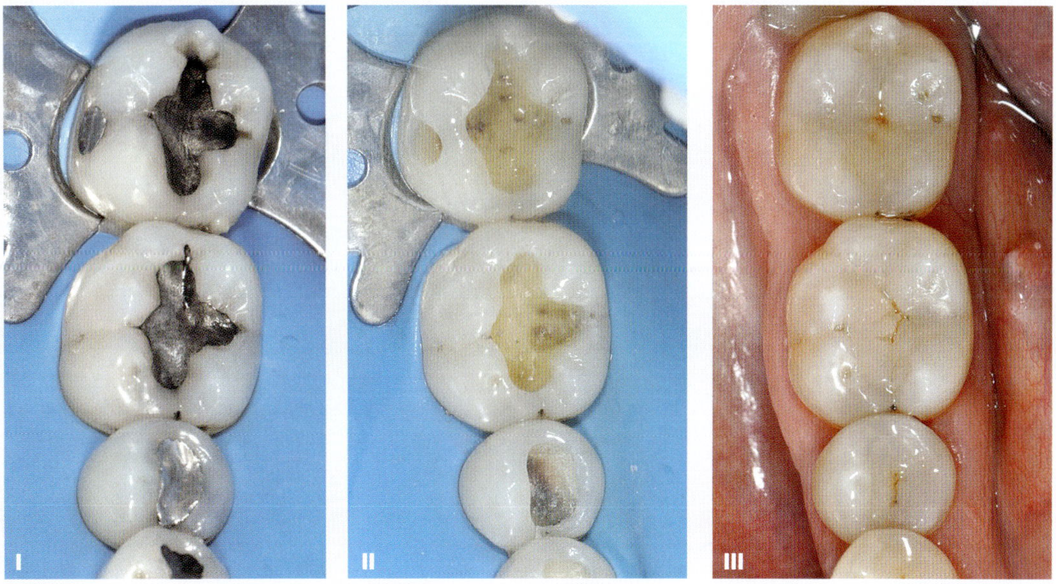

Fig 1 Direct restorations reflect maximum preservation of healthy tooth tissue.

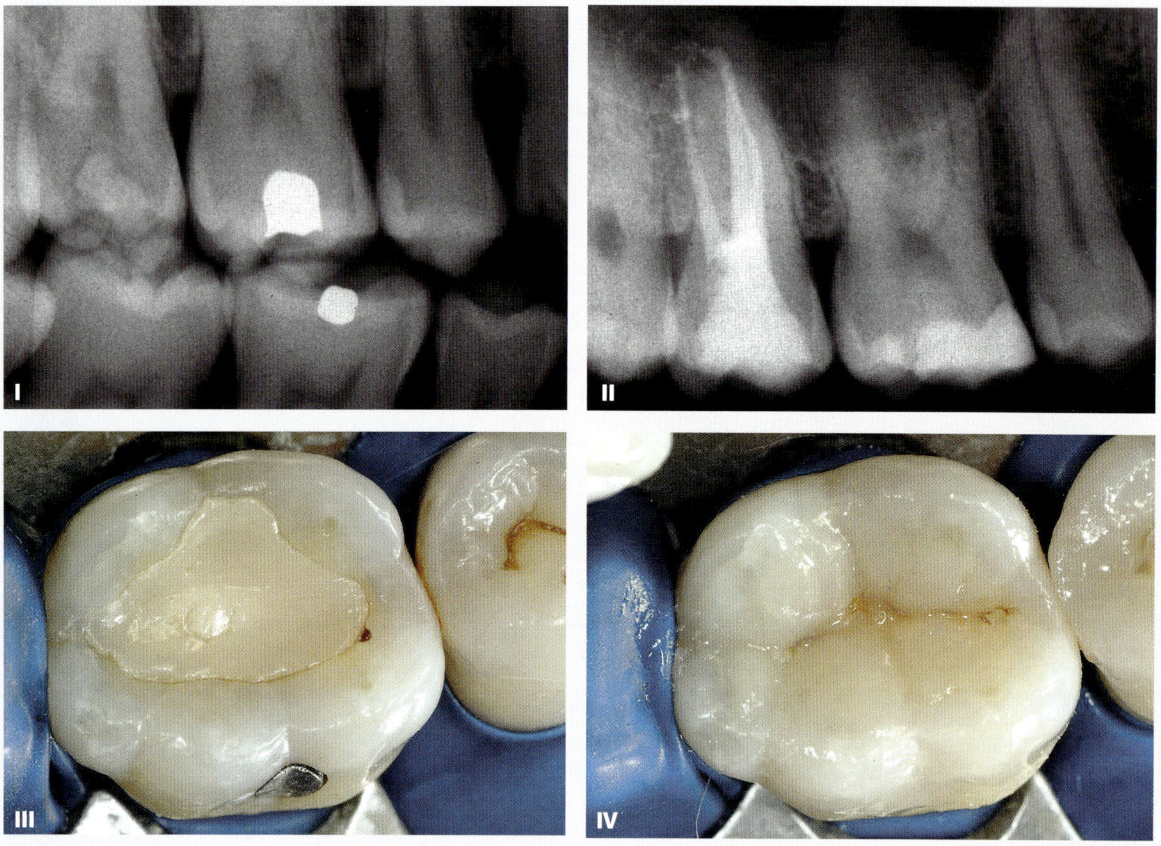

Fig 2 Endodontic treatment of the maxillary right second molar for pulpitis, showing preservation of four walls and the inlay of the adjacent first molar *(I, II)*. Reconstruction of a defective restoration using a direct technique *(III, IV)*.

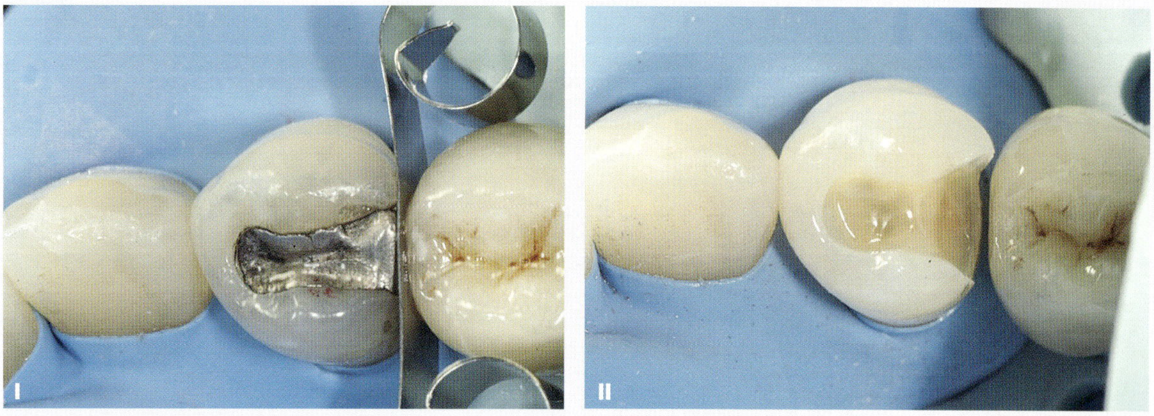

Fig 3 Protection of the adjacent tooth in a Class 2 cavity.

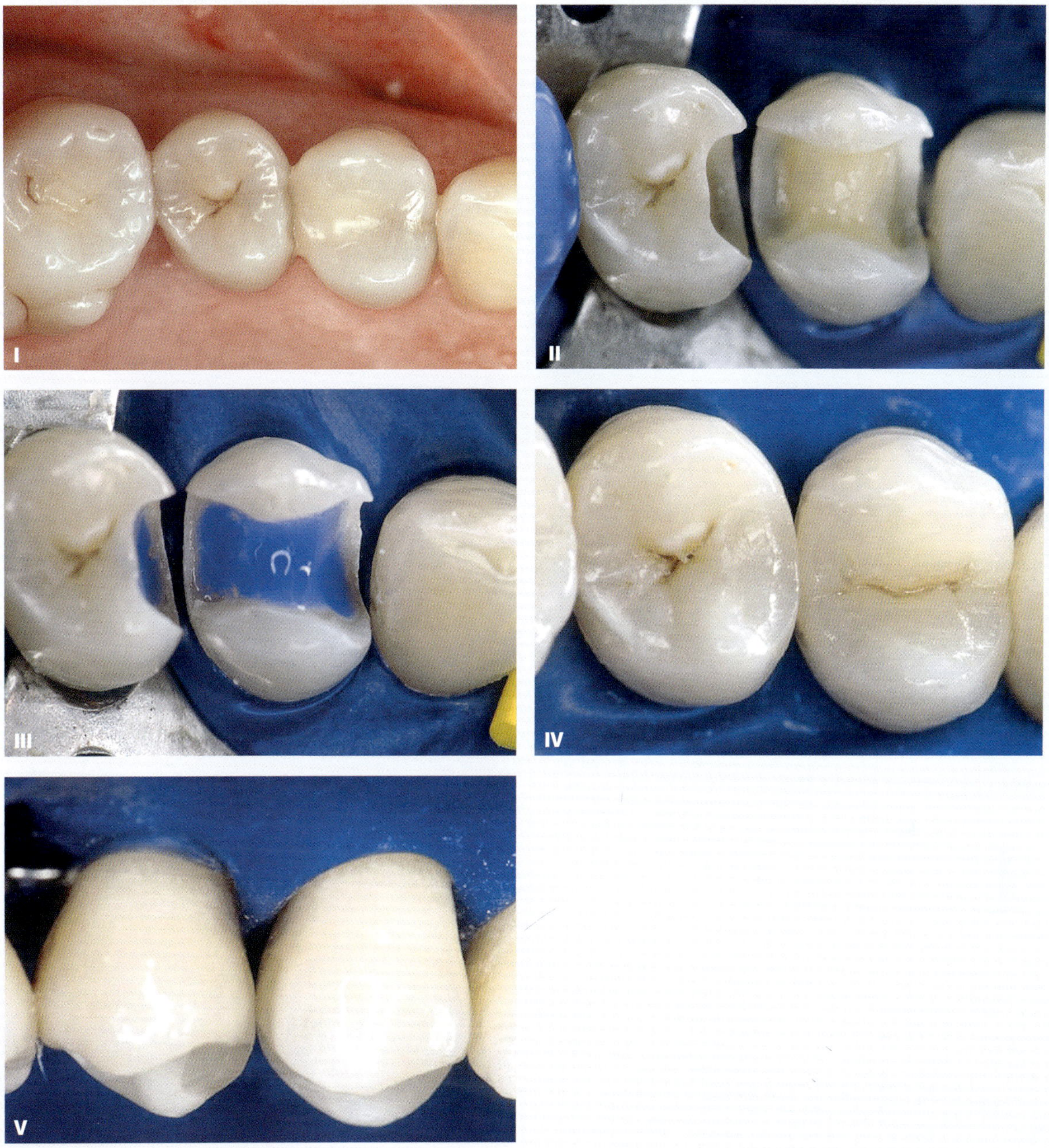

Fig 4 Preparation of mesio-occlusodistal and mesial cavities on two maxillary right premolars: direct restoration for the second premolar and an inlay for the first premolar.

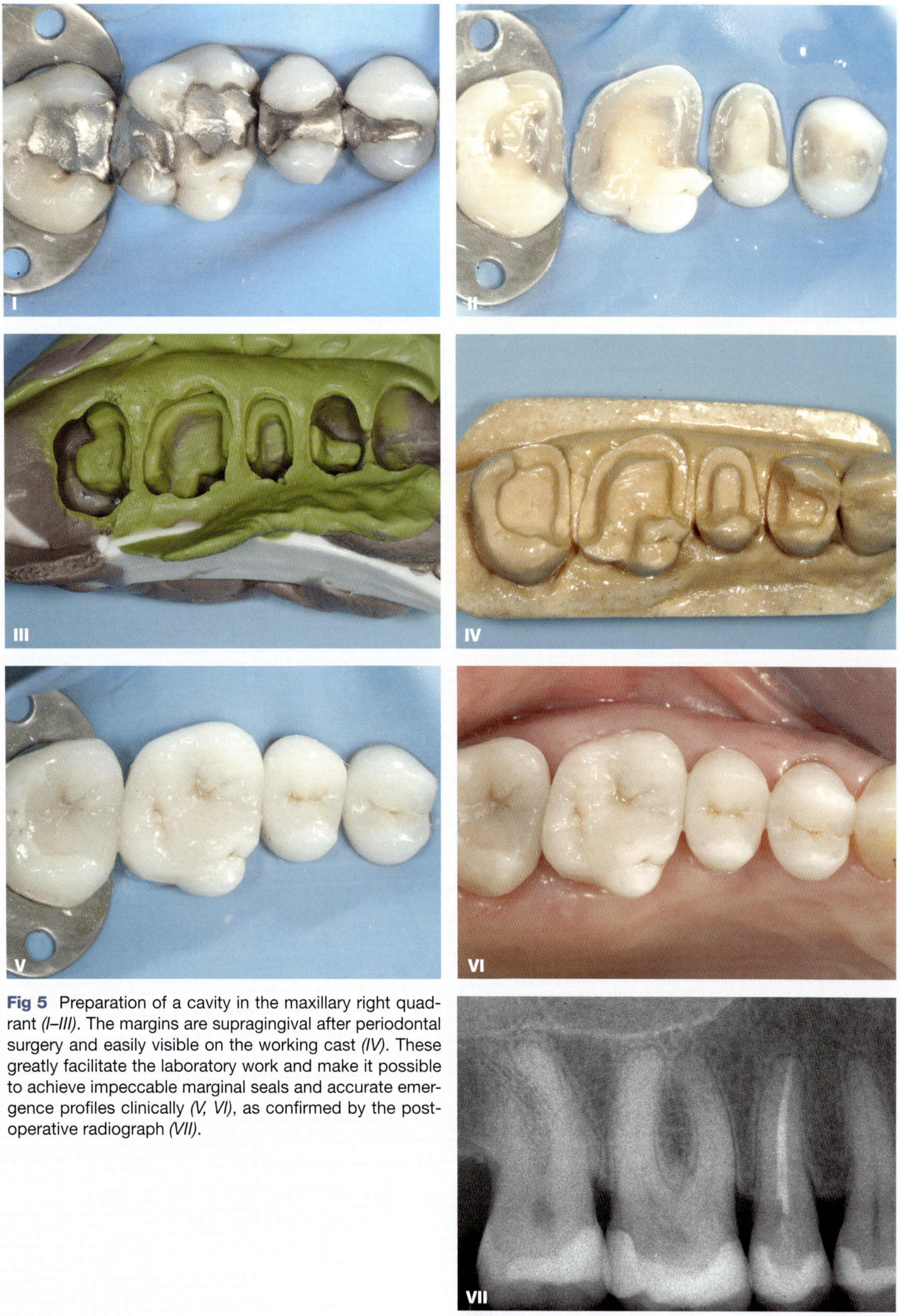

Fig 5 Preparation of a cavity in the maxillary right quadrant *(I–III)*. The margins are supragingival after periodontal surgery and easily visible on the working cast *(IV)*. These greatly facilitate the laboratory work and make it possible to achieve impeccable marginal seals and accurate emergence profiles clinically *(V, VI)*, as confirmed by the postoperative radiograph *(VII)*.

The treatment plan may be established only after removing all the decayed tissue and any defective restorations (Figs 6 and 7). Only at this time is it possible to examine the remaining healthy dental structure of the tooth. This analysis, and the subsequent preparation of a treatment plan, must include a multidisciplinary assessment (Figs 8 to 10).

When building a house, good sense suggests ensuring that the underlying land is sound before doing anything else. Only then is it logical to think about other matters, eg, shape and color (Fig 11).

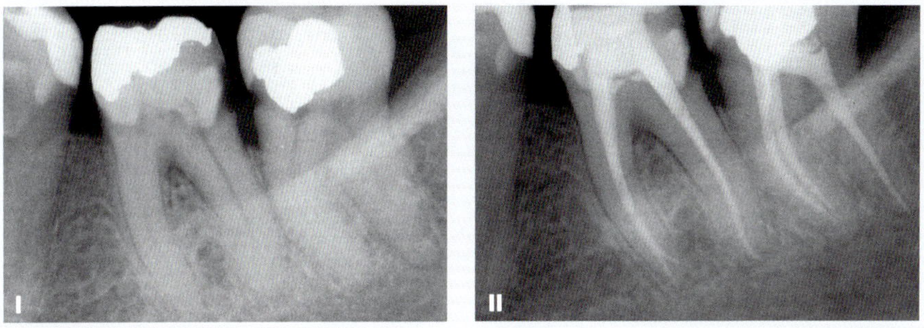

Fig 6 Endodontic treatment carried out impeccably, but without having previously assessed the remaining healthy dental tissue. The treatment plan for each individual tooth must be planned only after removing decay and defective restorations.

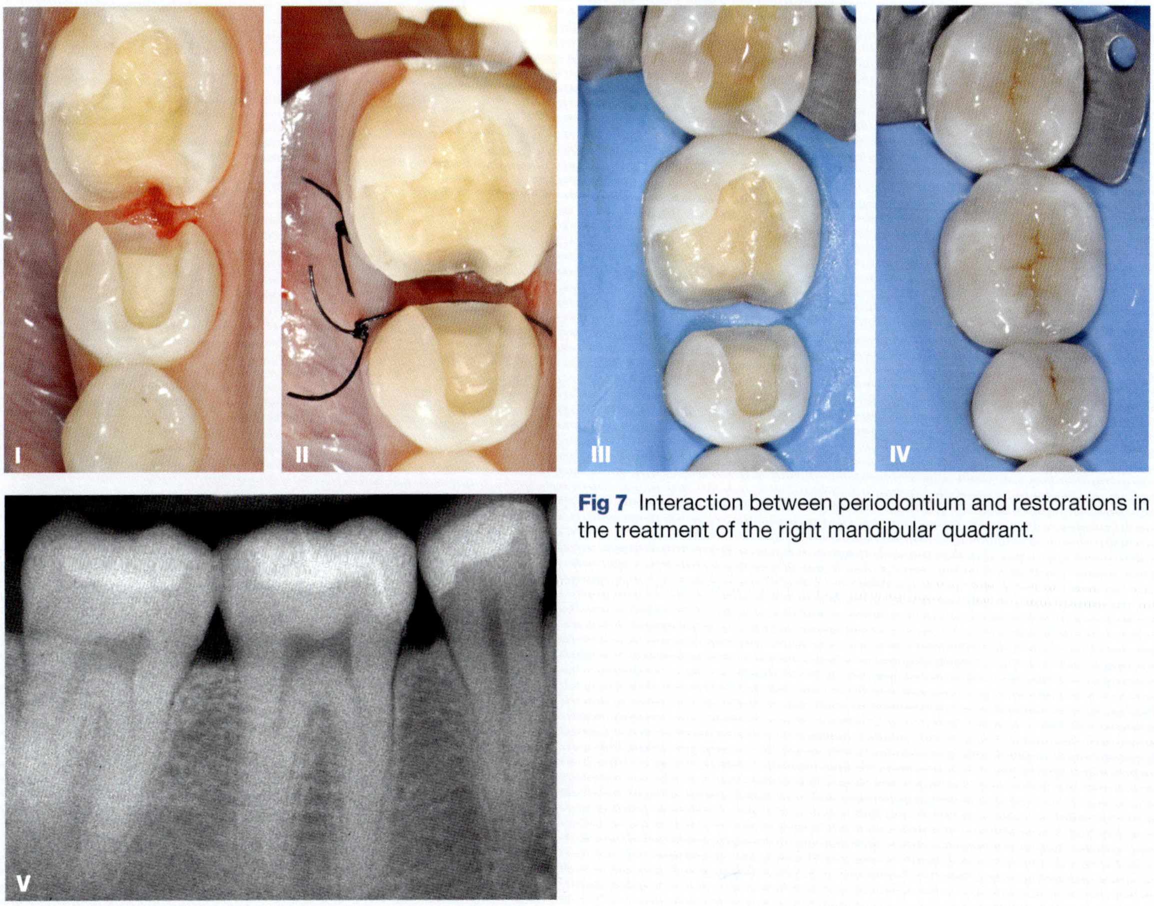

Fig 7 Interaction between periodontium and restorations in the treatment of the right mandibular quadrant.

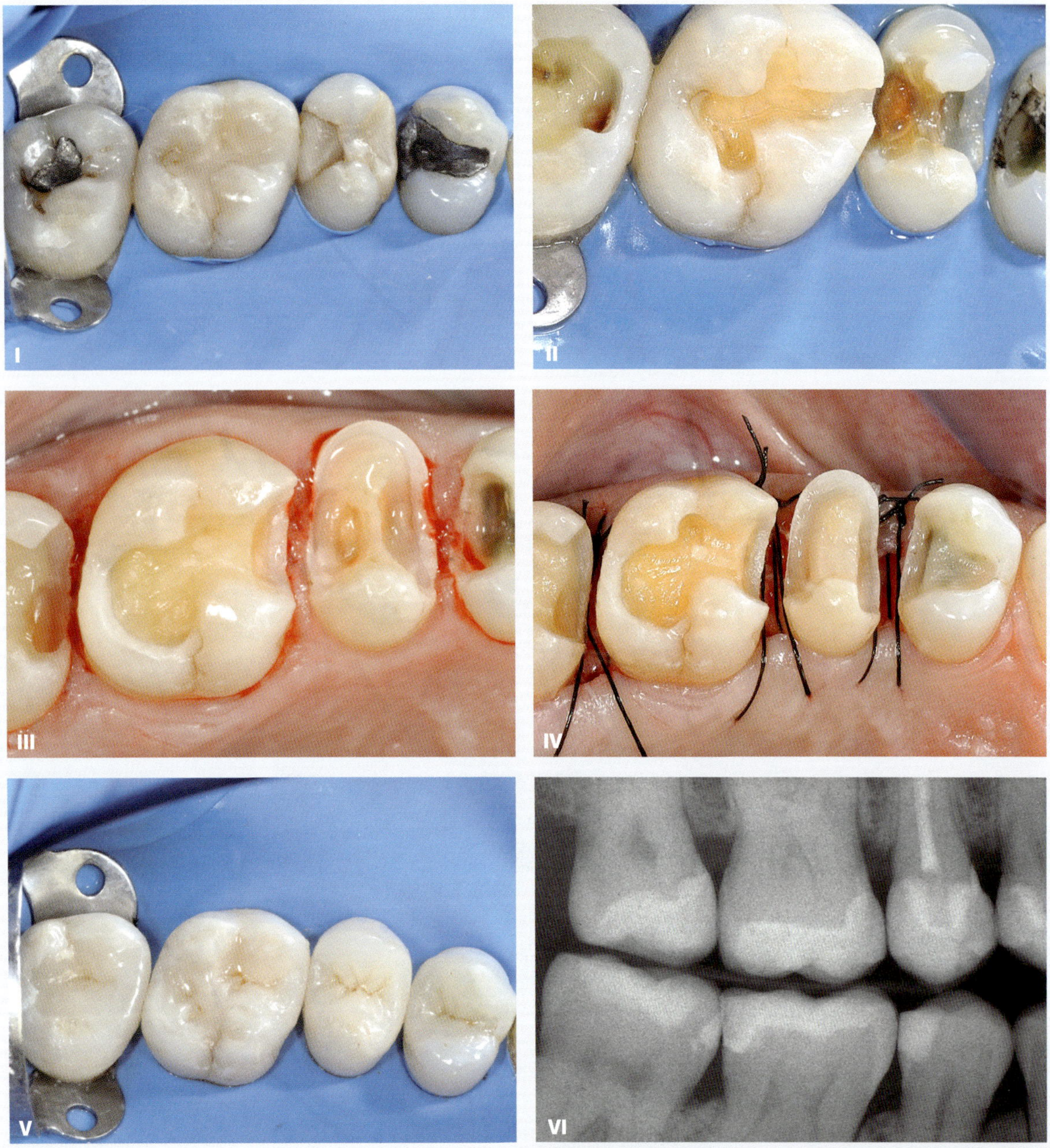

Fig 8 Interdisciplinary treatment plan for the maxillary right quadrant: synergy between endodontics, periodontology, and restoration *(I–V)*. Postoperative radiographs *(VI, VII)*.

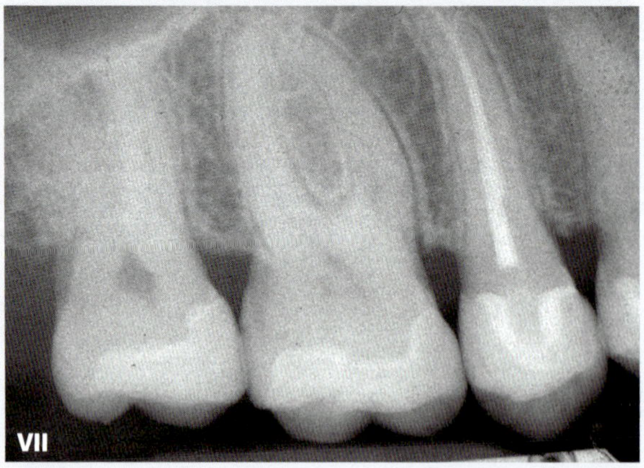

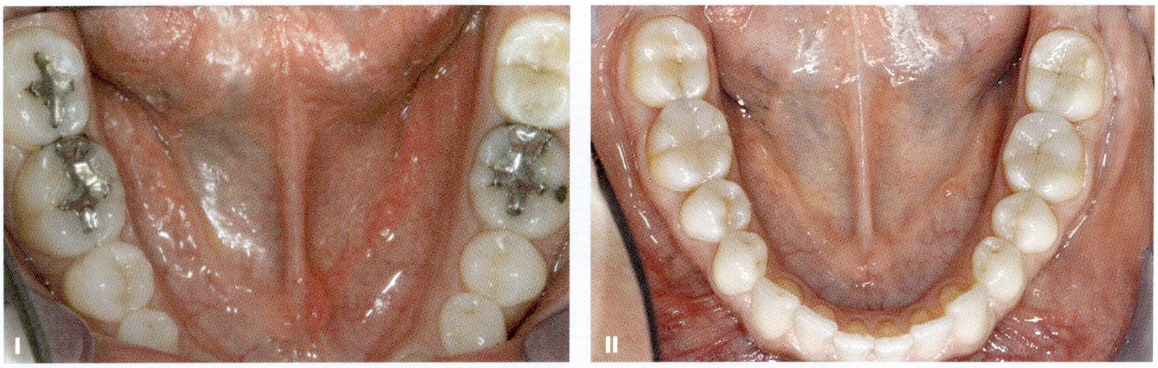

Fig 9 Before treatment *(I)* and clinical follow-up of two indirect restorations after 5 years *(II)*.

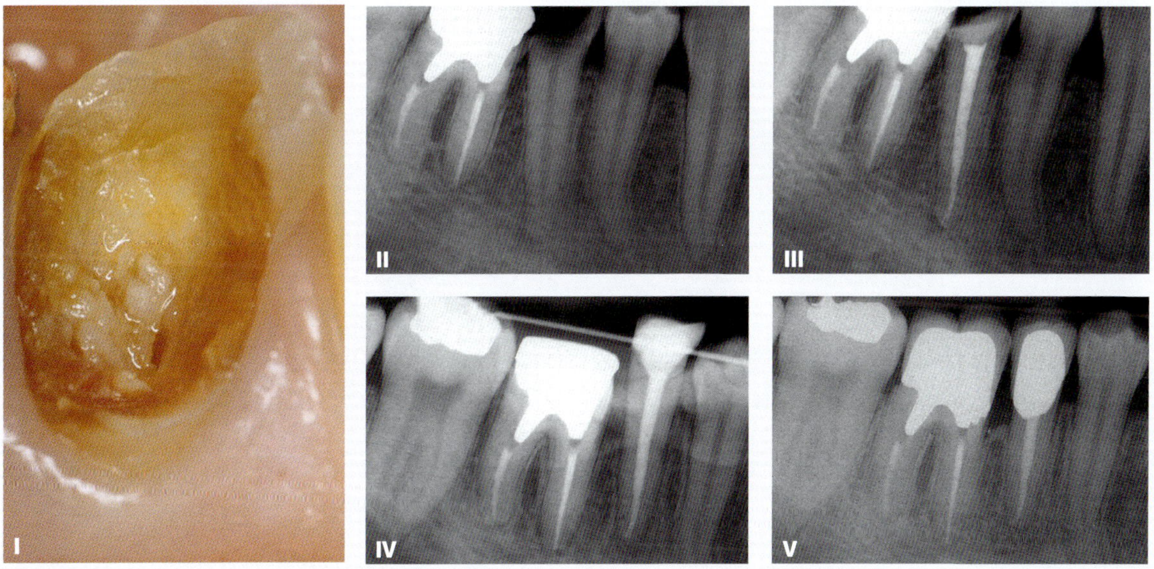

Fig 10 In this case, a restorative dentist, an endodontist, and an orthodontist (extrusion) contributed to the treatment of a mandibular premolar, which was completed with a metal-ceramic crown *(I–V)*. Radiographic follow-up after 14 years *(V)*.

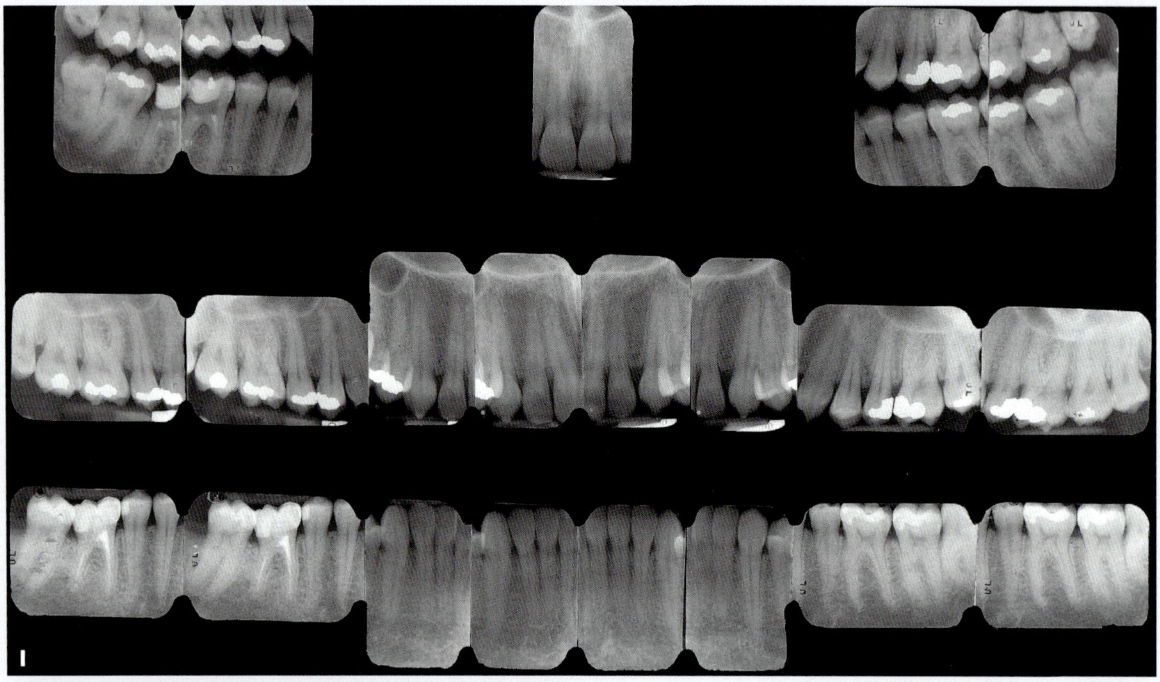

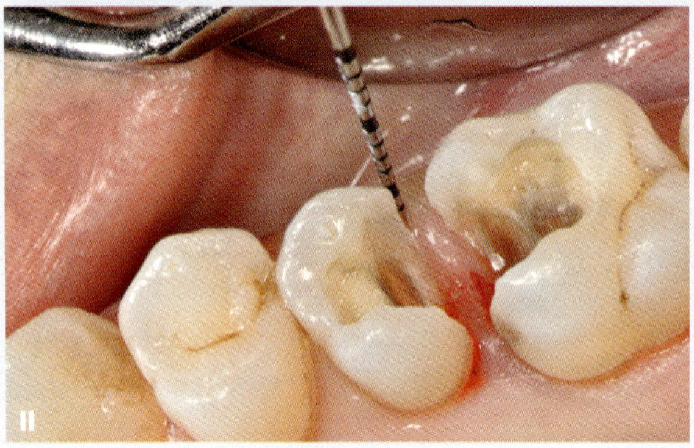

Fig 11 Radiographs and periodontal assessment: two essential tools for carrying out a proper treatment plan.

It is the author's firm conviction that one essential condition of a treatment plan must be a preliminary overview of the state of health of the periodontal support structure. Without this, even the most ideal restoration can only have an uncertain prognosis.

The treatment plan will therefore be drawn up by the team, who will work together to assess the structural, endodontic and functional aspects of the teeth to be treated from a clinical and radiographic viewpoint. An orthodontic evaluation of the arches also is important.

Indirect restorations in composite involve cavity preparations in which a part of the clinical crown remains intact, with the margins situated in a supragingival position.

When approaching a partial coronal preparation, attention must be paid to ensuring that the structural and biomechanical strength characteristics are such that, once the inlay is inserted, the tooth can perform its functions over time as effectively as possible (Fig 12).

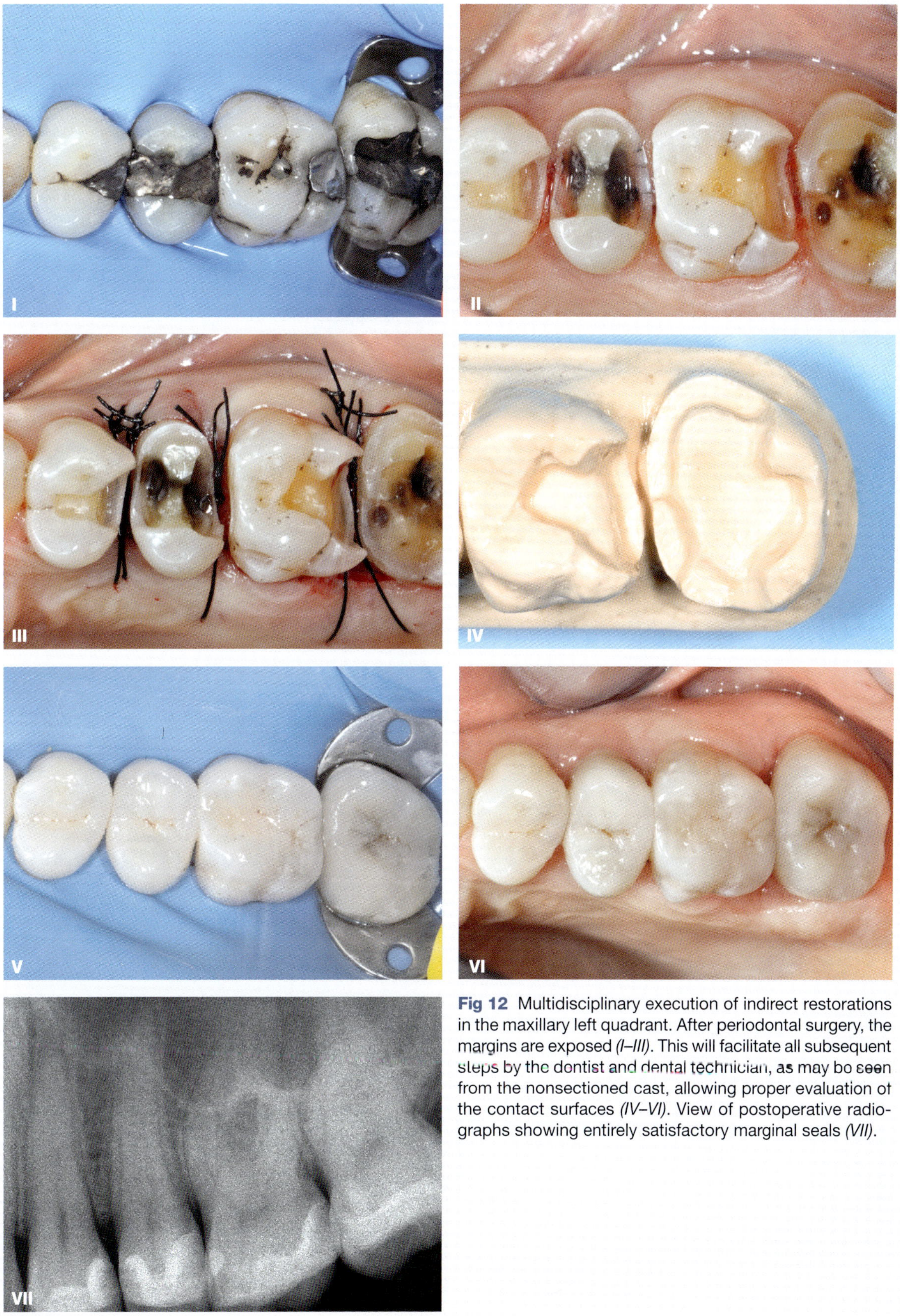

Fig 12 Multidisciplinary execution of indirect restorations in the maxillary left quadrant. After periodontal surgery, the margins are exposed *(I–III)*. This will facilitate all subsequent steps by the dentist and dental technician, as may be seen from the nonsectioned cast, allowing proper evaluation of the contact surfaces *(IV–VI)*. View of postoperative radiographs showing entirely satisfactory marginal seals *(VII)*.

The literature provides significant information on the biomechanical and structural analysis of the remaining healthy tooth tissue[2]: the presence or absence of marginal ridges, the dentinoenamel thickness at the base of the cusps, absence or presence of the pulp chamber roof, and thickness and depth of the interaxial dentin. Today it is also known that the mechanical failure of such restorations is attributable to incorrect cavity designs, eg, the restoration-cavity interface being located near the top of the cusp or insufficiently thick residual tooth walls (Fig 13).

When assessing the healthy remaining tooth structure clinically, attention must be focused on:

- The depth and width of the isthmus (interaxial dentin)
- Presence or absence of a proximal box (marginal ridge)
- Vitality or presence of endodontic treatment (pulp chamber roof)
- Thickness of the remaining cusp

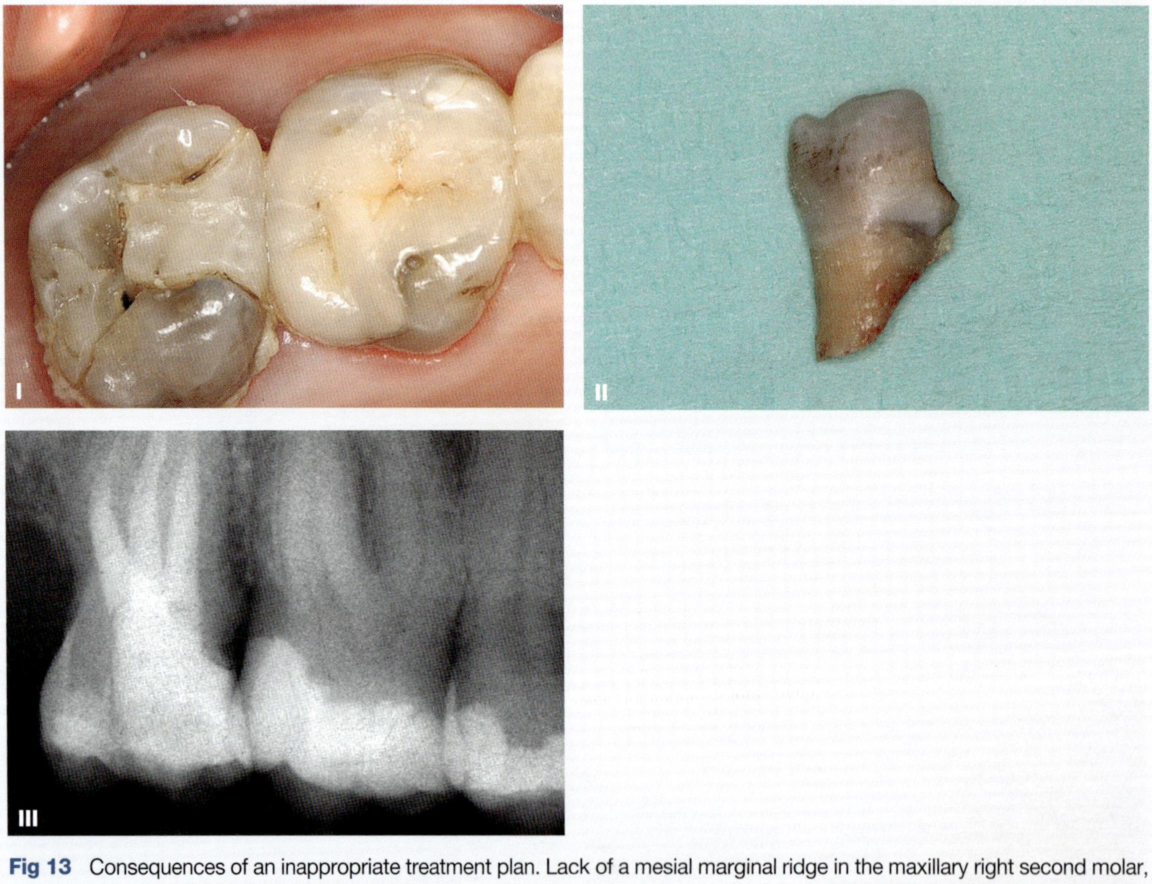

Fig 13 Consequences of an inappropriate treatment plan. Lack of a mesial marginal ridge in the maxillary right second molar, which is endodontically treated, should have suggested that the course of action was to remove the walls adjacent to the missing ridge and prepare an onlay. It was not possible to control the inflammation, which was probably a contributory factor to the mesial caries lesion.

Fichera et al[2] classified the structural factors of a tooth based on their topographic position as central or peripheral structural factors. The central factors are the interaxial dentin and the roof of the pulp chamber (Fig 14). The peripheral factors are the marginal ridge and the remaining cusp (Fig 15).

"The interaxial dentin is the occlusocervical continuation of the pulp chamber roof: dentin and roof may be treated as a single structure, but dividing them helps us in quantitative terms when assessing the remaining tooth tissue and appreciating the biomechanical and structural differences between a vital tooth and an endodontically treated tooth."

A vital tooth may lose more or less interaxial dentin, but it will always have a pulp chamber roof, while all the interaxial dentin and the pulp chamber roof will be irremediably lost in an endodontically treated tooth.

When evaluating the remaining interaxial dentin, the depth factor determines structural weakening to a significantly greater degree than does the width factor[3,4] (Fig 16).

Interaxial dentin joins the buccal wall to the lingual wall. This is the most important structural factor because if this is sound, structural problems in the other factors will not reduce the fracture resistance of the remaining healthy tooth tissue.[3,5]

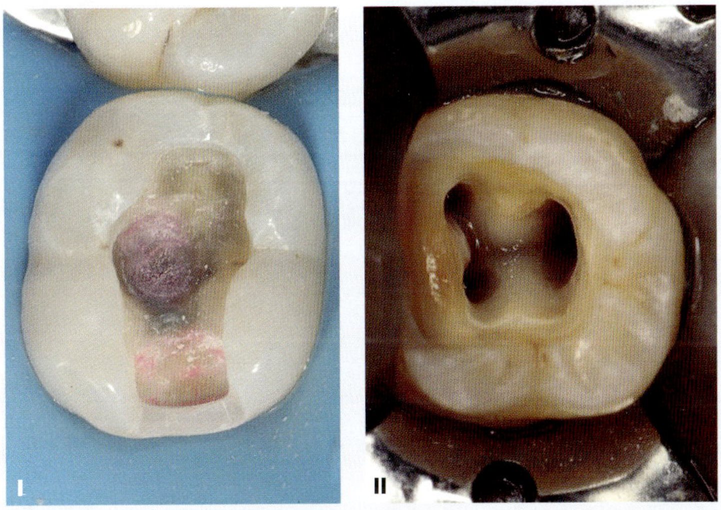

Fig 14 Interaxial dentin present in a vital tooth and absent in an endodontically treated tooth.

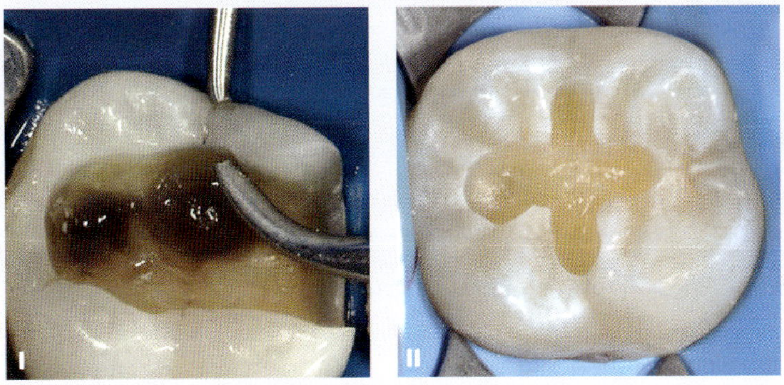

Fig 15 Residual cusp *(I)* and marginal ridge *(II)*, which exercise a crucial role in determining the strength of a tooth. This strength is expressed in the quantity and quality of the healthy residual tooth structure.

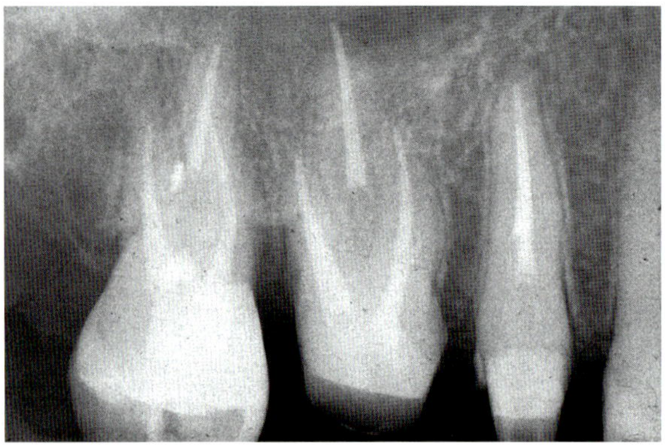

Fig 16 Radiographic view of a restoration on an endodontically treated tooth, therefore lacking interaxial dentin and a pulp chamber roof.

Mondelli et al[5] and Larson et al[6] demonstrated that the absence of a marginal ridge does not cause structural weakness if the occlusal isthmus is intact. Conversely, a defect in the interaxial dentin alone leads to a significant loss of structural strength.

Loss of the marginal ridge associated with loss of interaxial dentin leads to structural weakening.

That being said, the following clinical example shows two restored arches in which pulp vitality has been maintained and conservative preparations have been achieved (Fig 17).

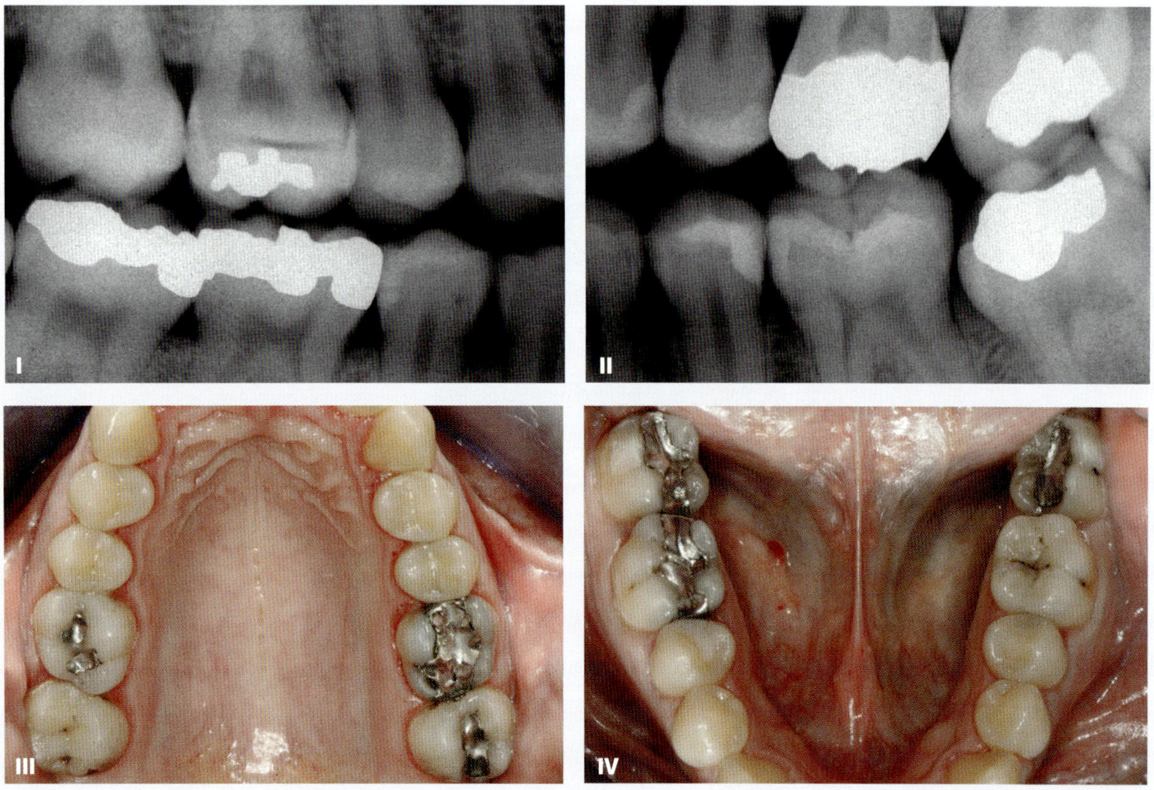

Fig 17 Preoperative radiographs and clinical views *(I–IV)*. Execution of a mesio-occlusodistal (MOD) inlay in the maxillary right quadrant *(V, VI)*. Execution of two MOD inlays in the mandibular right quadrant after checking thicknesses at the base of each cusp and direct restoration of the second premolar *(VII–IX)*. Preparation of a cavity in the mandibular left quadrant *(X–XIII)*. Partial restorations (inlay, overlay) in the maxillary left quadrant, with the situation after periodontal surgery and after taking an impression *(XIV–XVI)*. Radiographic and clinical situation at the end of treatment; it should be stressed that no teeth were endodontically treated *(XVII–XX)*. Radiographic and clinical follow-up after 3 years *(XXI–XXIII)*.

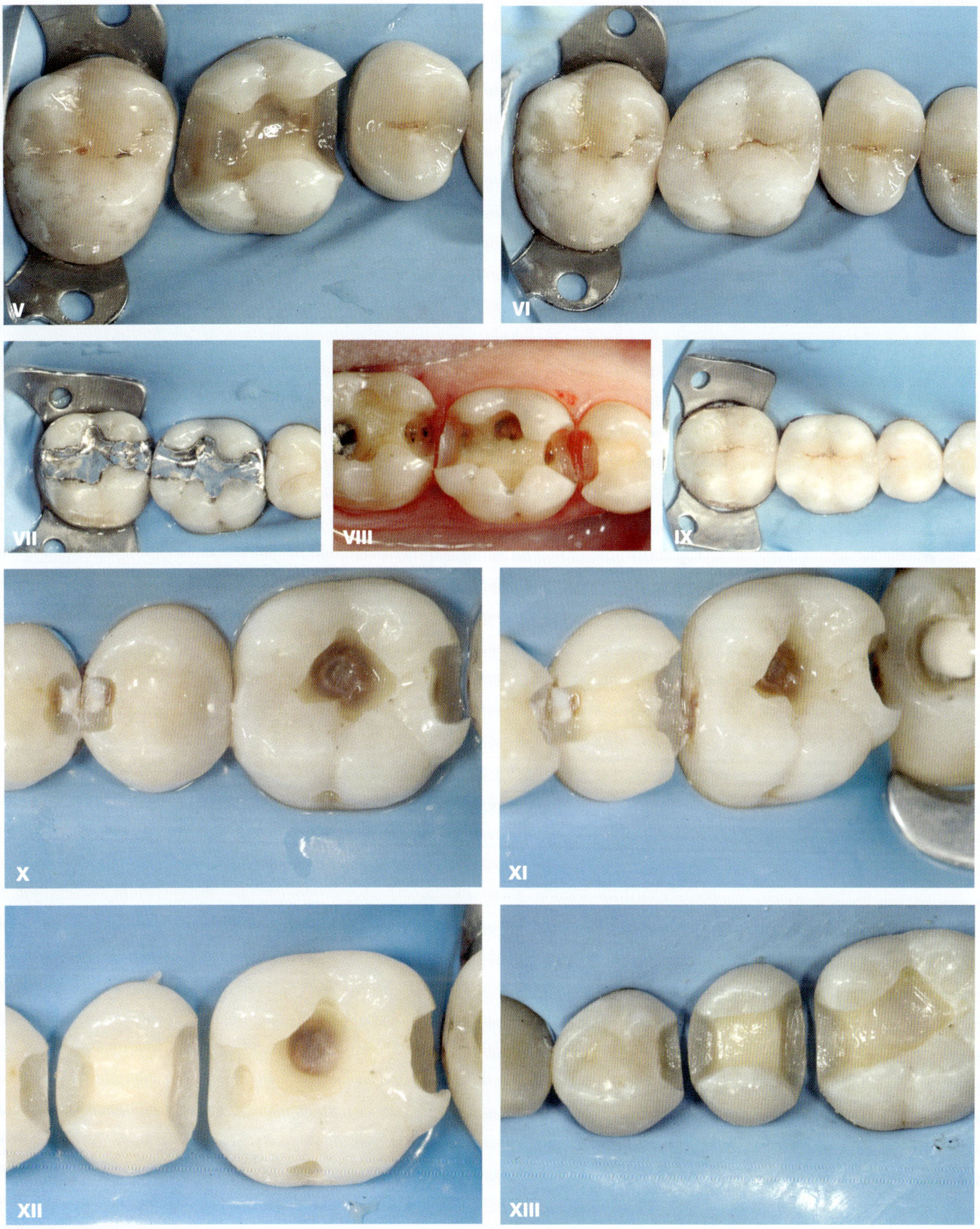

Fig 17 *(continued)*

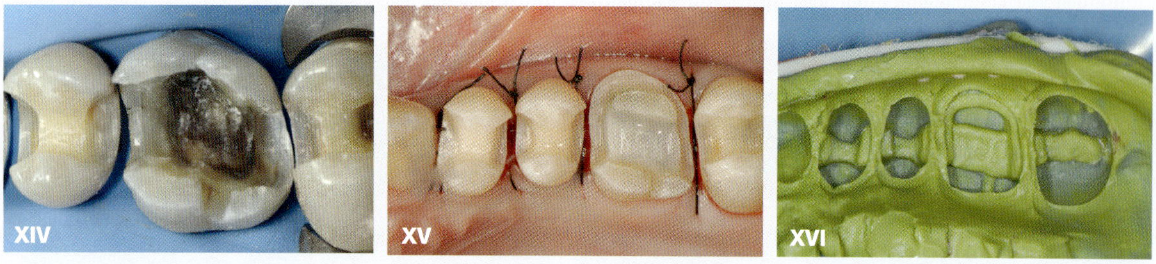

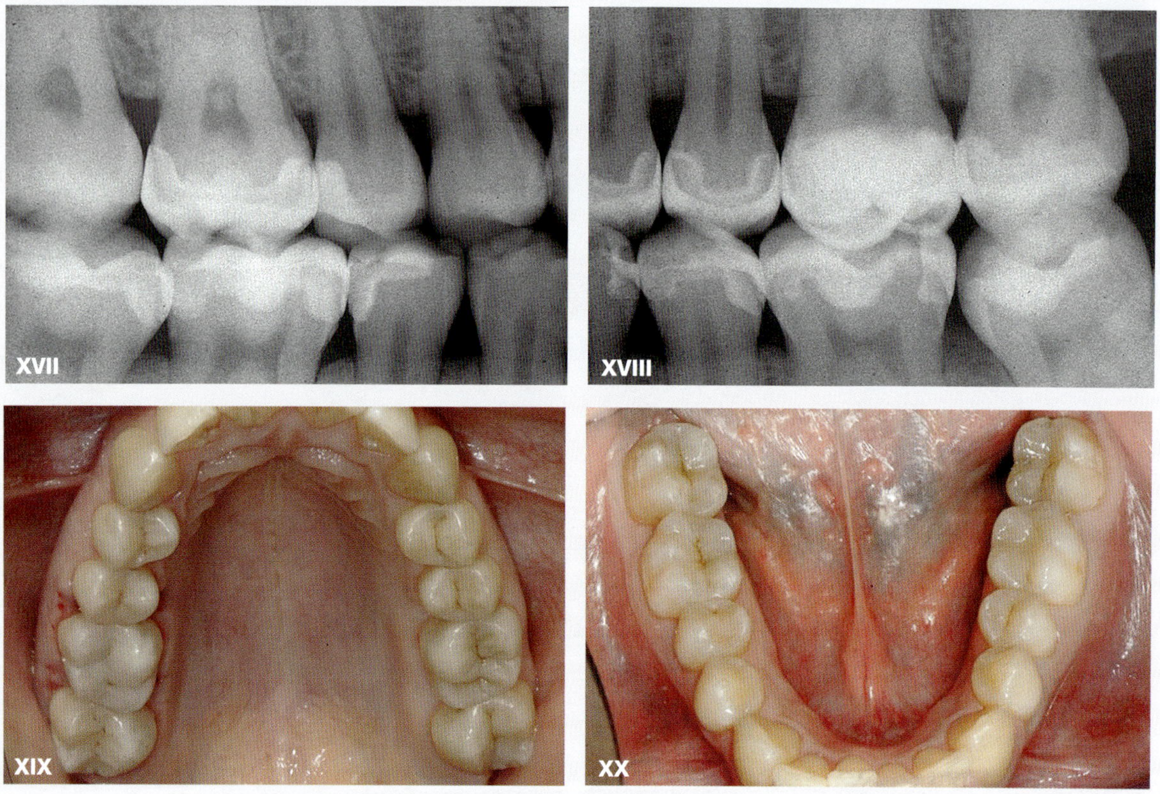

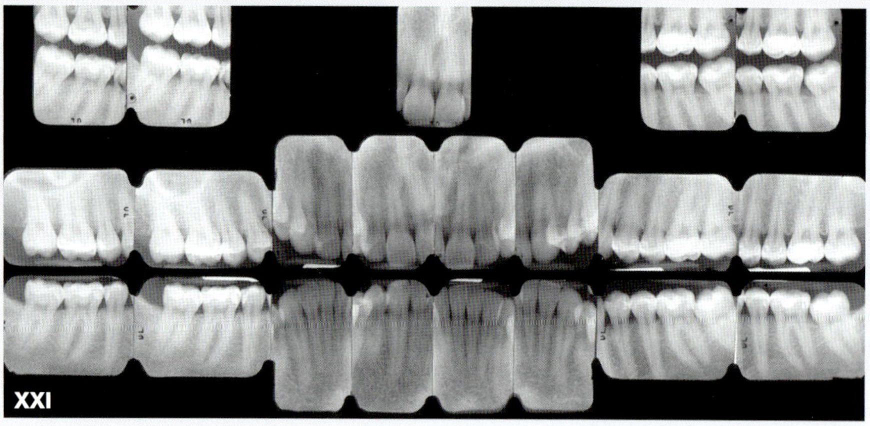

Fig 17 *(continued)*

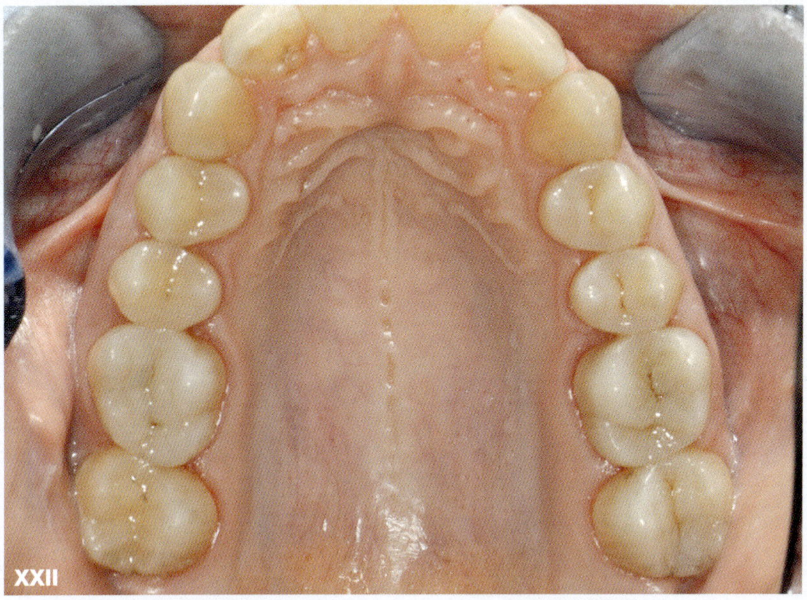

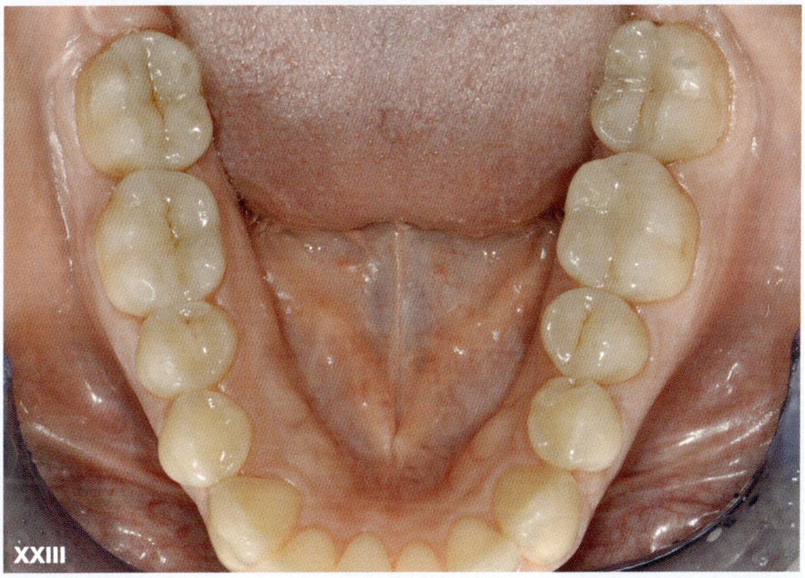

Fig 17 *(continued)*

The roof of the pulp chamber deserves a section to itself. An endodontically treated tooth that has maintained both of its marginal ridges is structurally stronger than a vital tooth with mesio-occlusal (MO), occlusodistal (OD), or mesio-occlusodistal (MOD) cavities, as demonstrated by Reeh et al in 1989.[7]
The above study by Reeh et al[7] is very important because it demonstrated a 5% loss of strength in a tooth that has been endodontically treated but has maintained both marginal ridges intact, while the loss of strength would be 35% in the same tooth without endodontic treatment and lacking one marginal ridge but 55% if both marginal ridges were lost. In other words, a vital tooth with an MO, OD, or MOD restoration is much weaker than the same devitalized tooth with a single access cavity in which both marginal ridges are maintained intact (Fig 18).

A hierarchical order of structural factors may be deduced from this:

- Interaxial dentin (isthmus depth and width)
- Marginal ridge (presence or absence, depth and width of the proximal box)
- Pulp chamber roof (presence or absence)
- Remaining cusp (evaluation of thicknesses)

Moving on from the central factors (interaxial dentin and pulp chamber roof) to peripheral factors (marginal ridge and residual cusp), it may be observed that loss of a marginal ridge leads to the presence of a box. This should be assessed in terms of occlusocervical depth, mesiodistal depth, and buccolingual width.
It has already been demonstrated that the depth of a proximal box has a greater weakening effect than box width. In the same way, its mesiodistal depth gives rise to a reduction in interaxial dentin width, a primary factor in determining tooth strength[4,8] (Figs 19 to 21).
It is also already known from the literature that the residual cusp thickness of the dentinoenamel structure has a clinical impact on the decision to maintain or remove a cusp. This observation demonstrates that the remaining cusp is biomechanically independent of the adjacent and opposing cusps, while it is dependent on the adjacent marginal ridge.[9–11]

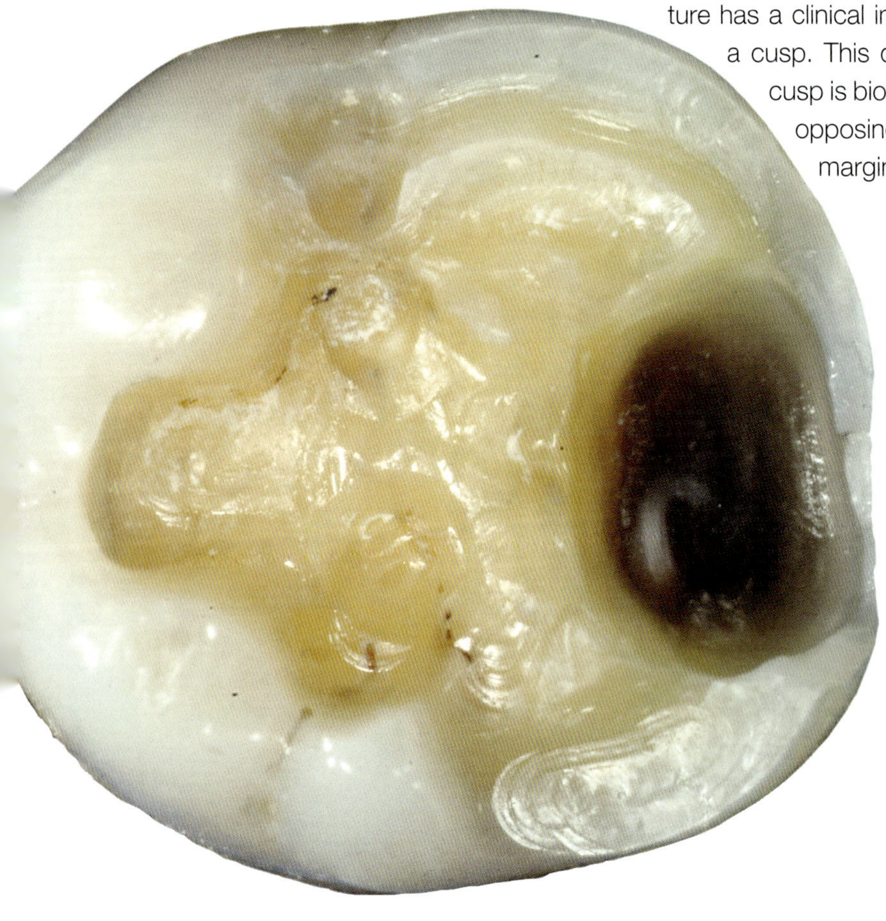

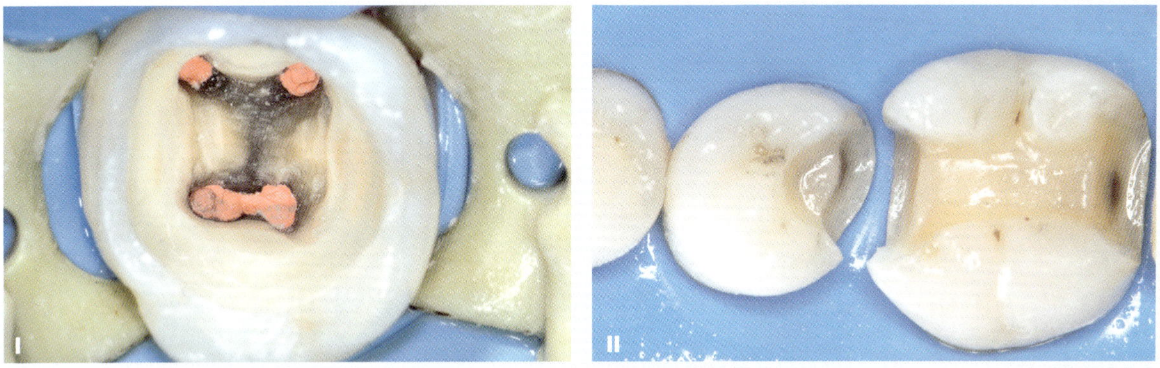

Fig 18 Loss of strength in different clinical situations.

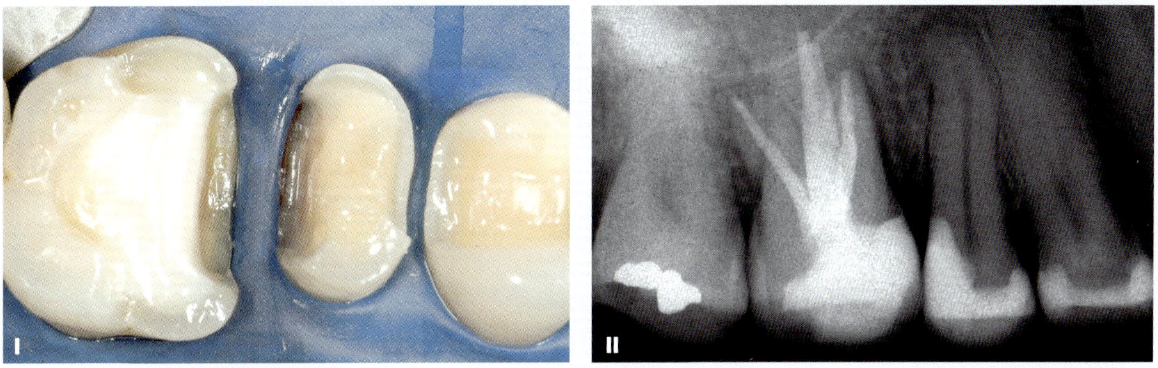

Fig 19 Clinical and radiographic views of proximal boxes with depth at the limit at which use of dam is possible.

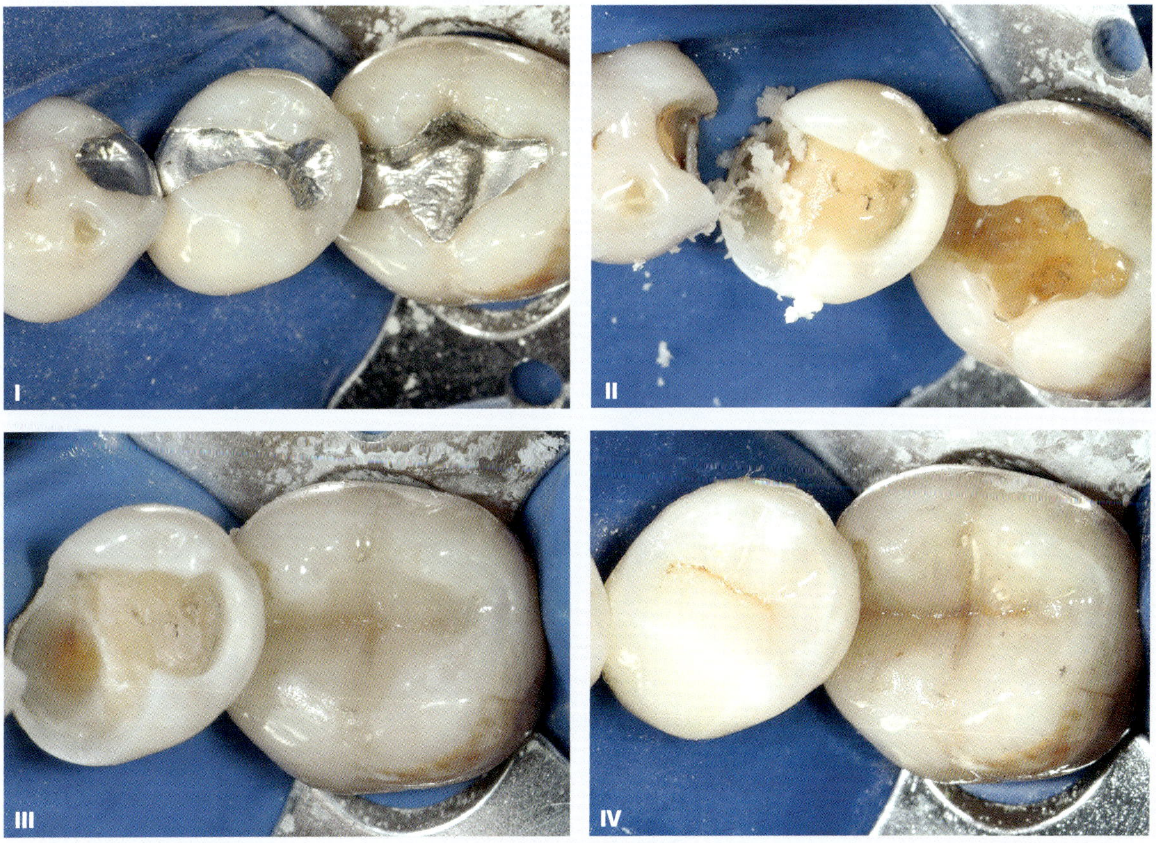

Fig 20 Preparation of a box in the mandibular left second molar with an unusual shape dictated by the anomalous tooth position. The patient had refused very necessary orthodontic treatment.

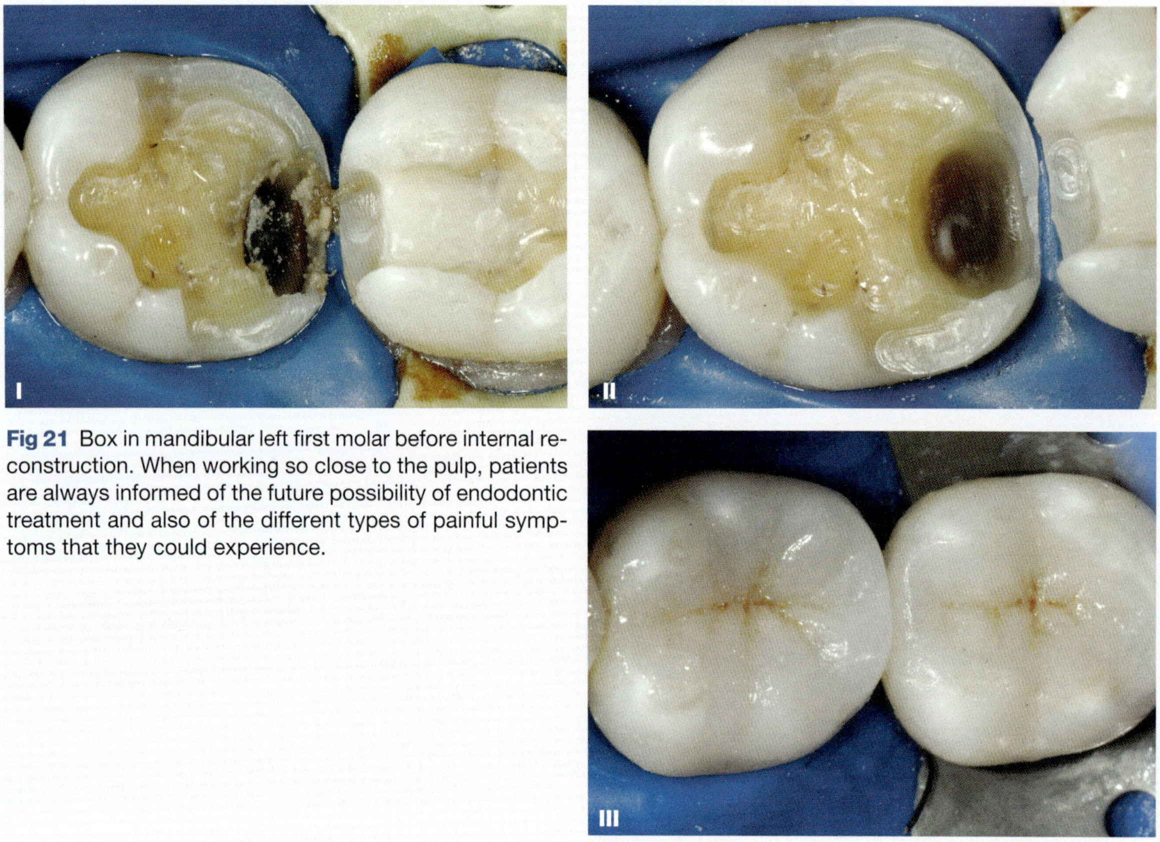

Fig 21 Box in mandibular left first molar before internal reconstruction. When working so close to the pulp, patients are always informed of the future possibility of endodontic treatment and also of the different types of painful symptoms that they could experience.

A study by Hood[12] teaches us that the greater the increase in the depth of the remaining cusp base, the more its thickness must increase proportionately for the cusp deformation value to stay the same. In numeric terms, this means that saving the cusp requires a thickness of 2 mm in a vital tooth and 3 mm in an endodontically treated tooth (Figs 22 to 24).

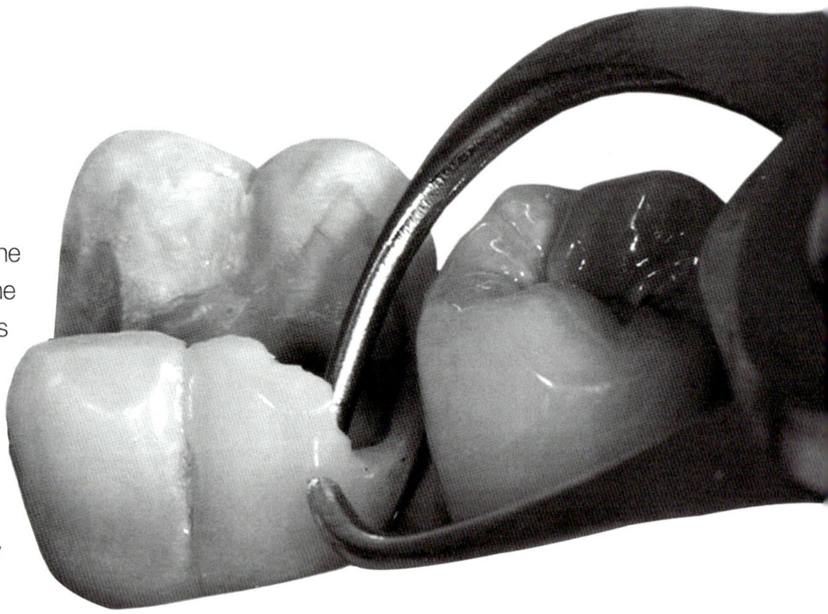

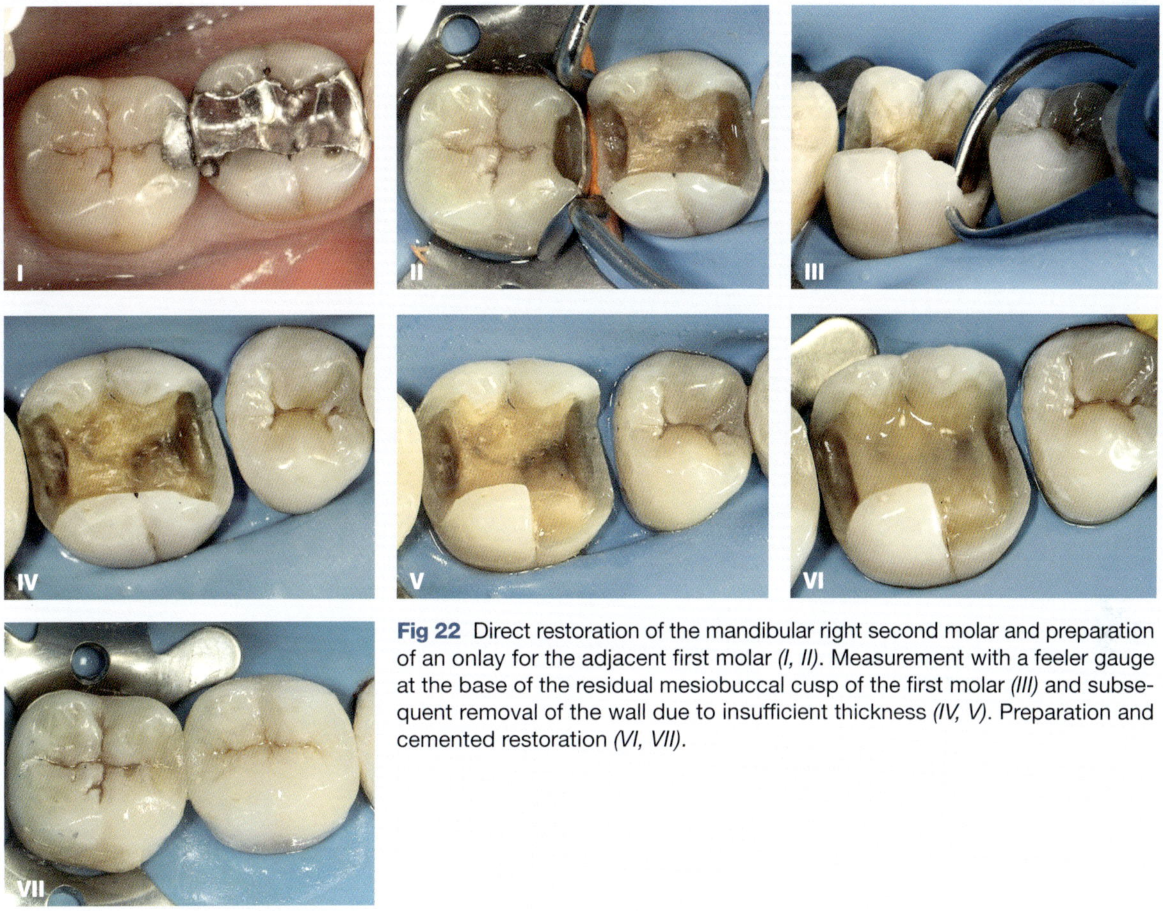

Fig 22 Direct restoration of the mandibular right second molar and preparation of an onlay for the adjacent first molar *(I, II)*. Measurement with a feeler gauge at the base of the residual mesiobuccal cusp of the first molar *(III)* and subsequent removal of the wall due to insufficient thickness *(IV, V)*. Preparation and cemented restoration *(VI, VII)*.

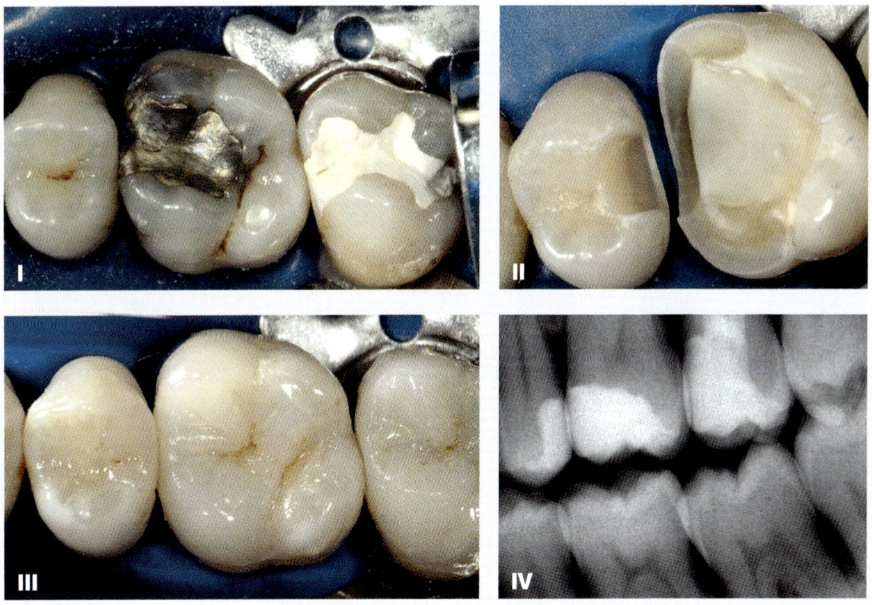

Fig 23 Another case with insufficient thickness, this time of the mesiobuccal and mesiopalatal walls of the maxillary left first molar, leading to preparation of an onlay and coverage of the mesial cusps.

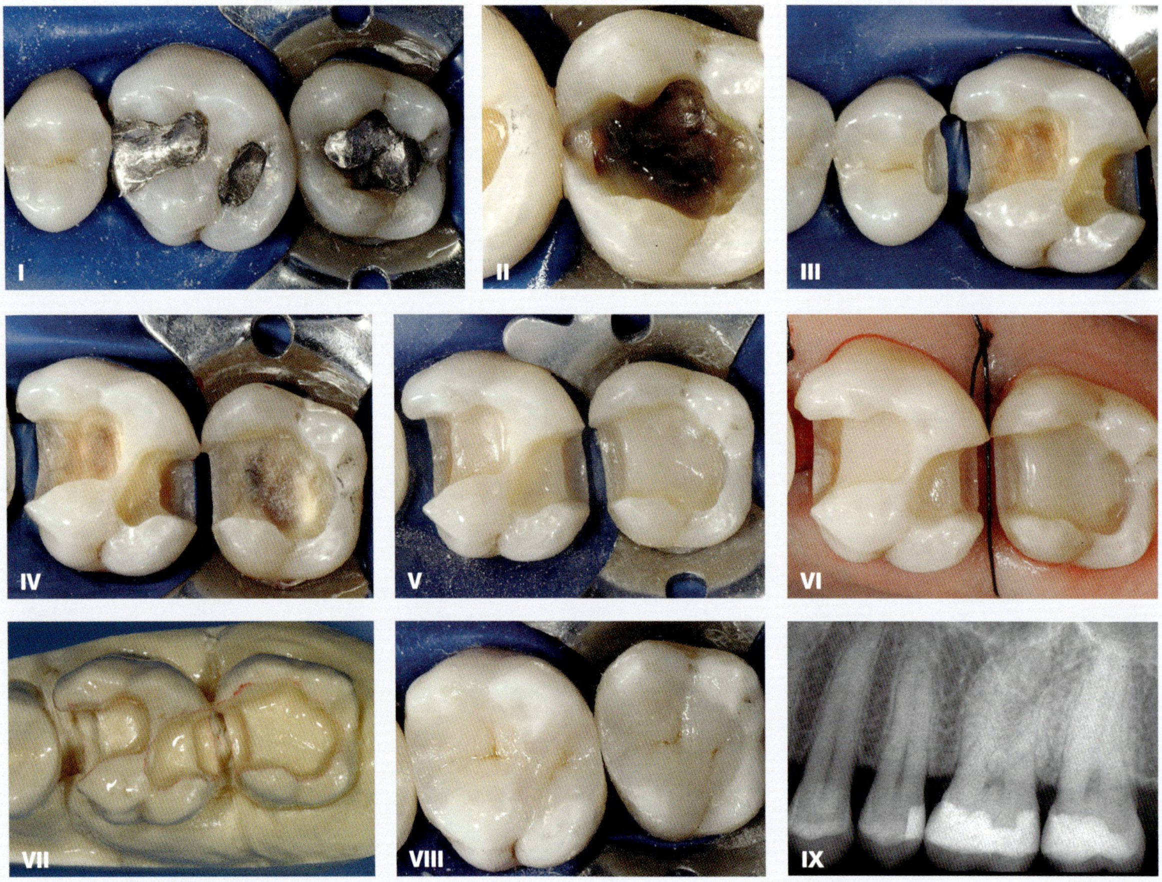

Fig 24 Sufficient thicknesses, on the other hand, allow maintenance of all walls and execution of simple inlays.

These measurements should be carried out using a feeler gauge at the base of the remaining cusp and after removal of any restorations, eg, previous Class 5 restorations (Fig 25).

For the case of an endodontically treated tooth, the literature suggests that the physical, chemical, and histologic consequences are not clinically significant after pulp removal.[13,14]

Conversely, the structural changes due to endodontic treatment, eg, proximal decay with obvious loss of the marginal ridge and interaxial dentin, removal of the pulp chamber roof, and instrumental modification of the root dentin, are extremely significant changes due to weakening of the endodontically treated tooth.

An MOD cavity is the type with the greatest negative impact on the structure of a tooth with regard to masticatory load, significantly impairing fracture resistance. It goes without saying that the risk will increase in the case of an endodontically treated tooth[15] (Figs 26 to 29).

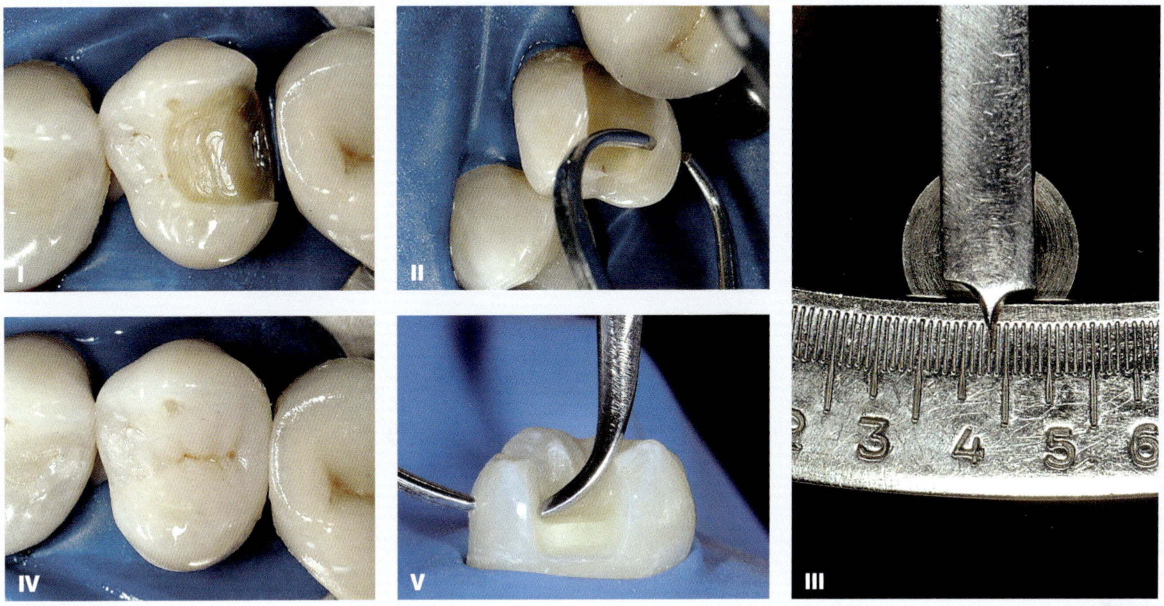

Fig 25 Measurement of thicknesses using a feeler gauge.

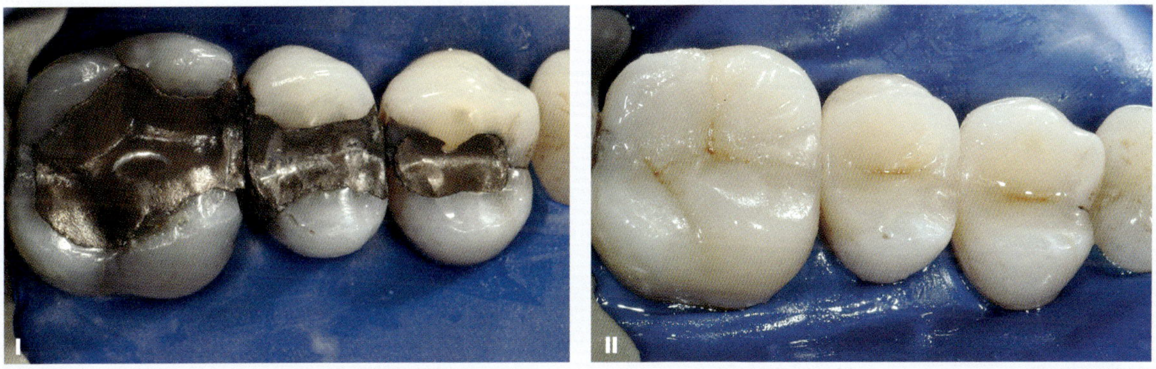

Fig 26 Reinforcement of weak walls with execution of composite partial restorations. This approach rules out or minimizes the possibility of fracture, which is a typical event when the enamel is not supported by healthy dentin.

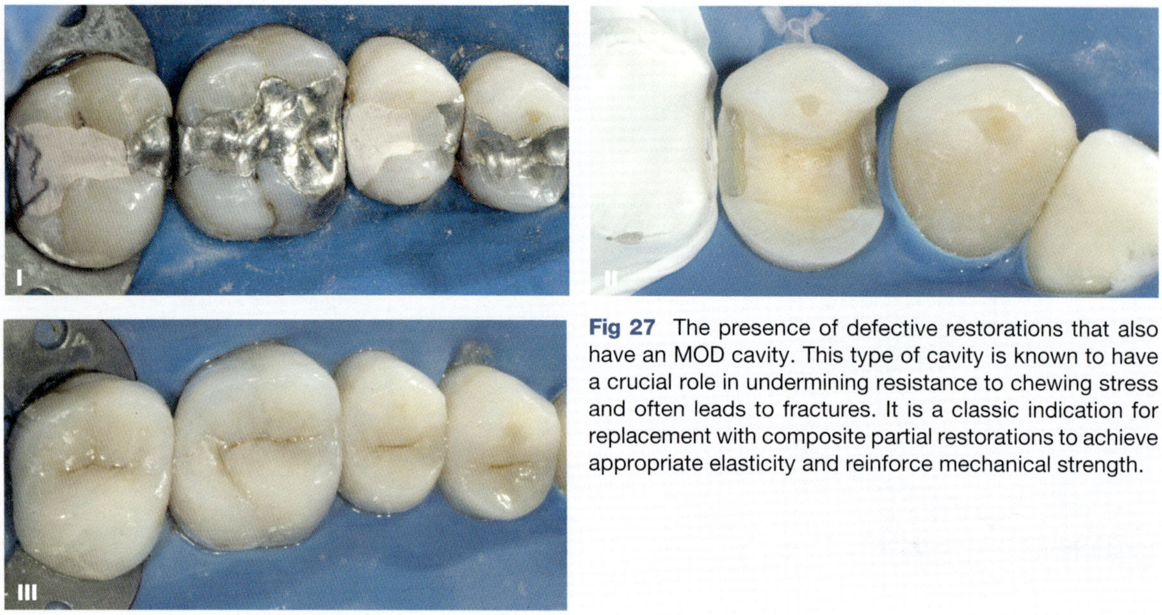

Fig 27 The presence of defective restorations that also have an MOD cavity. This type of cavity is known to have a crucial role in undermining resistance to chewing stress and often leads to fractures. It is a classic indication for replacement with composite partial restorations to achieve appropriate elasticity and reinforce mechanical strength.

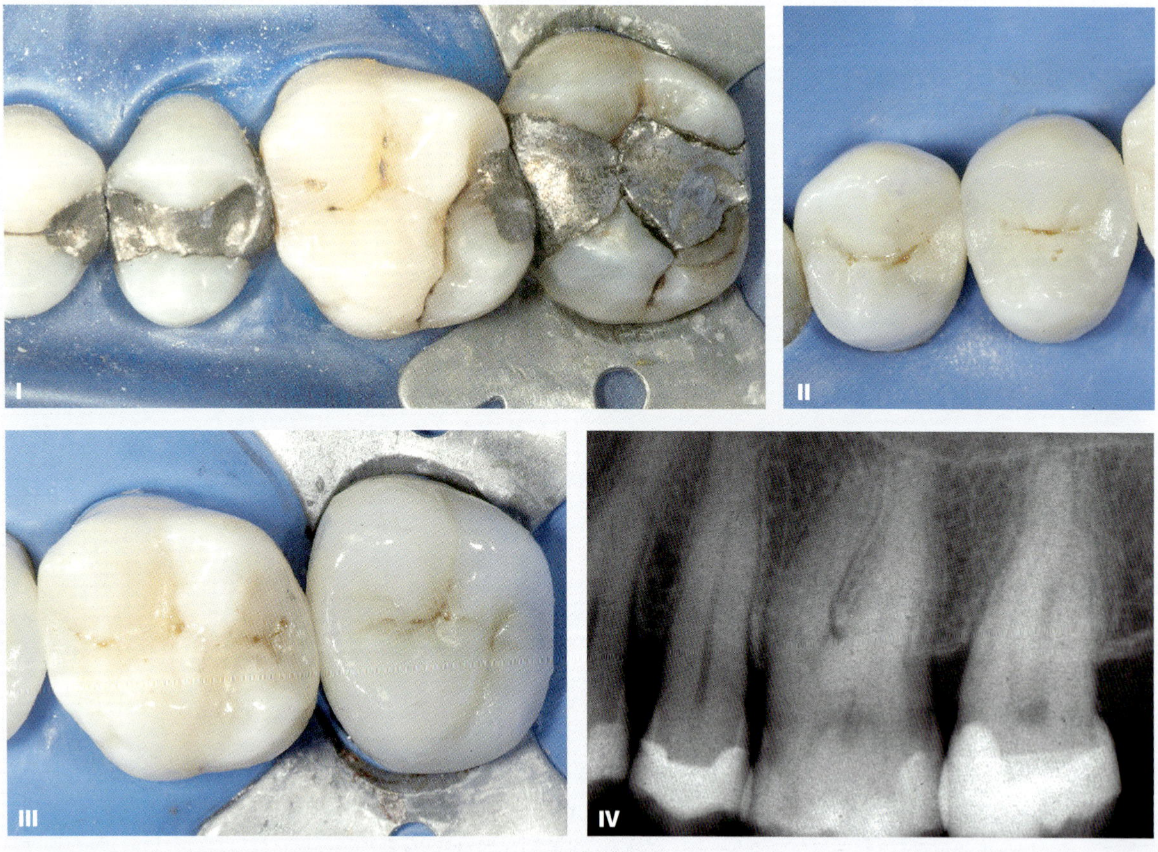

Fig 28 Another case presenting defective restorations with very weak walls. The state of the maxillary left second molar was an indication for replacing the old amalgam reconstructions with composite partial restorations to achieve mechanical reinforcement with consequent reduction of the fracture risk.

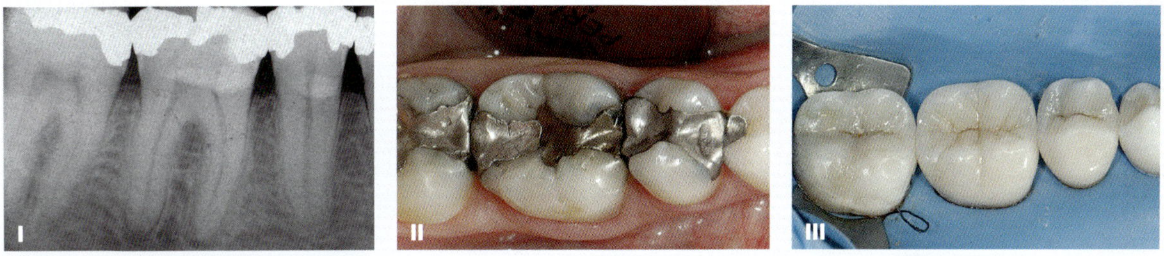

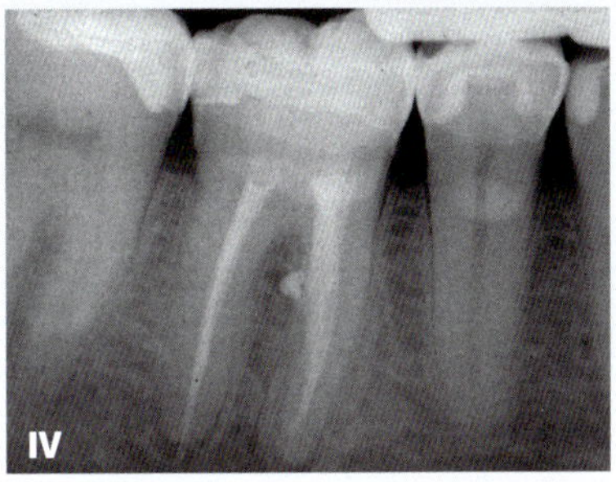

Fig 29 Absolute indication for execution of an overlay in order to reconstruct an endodontically treated tooth with a previous MOD cavity.

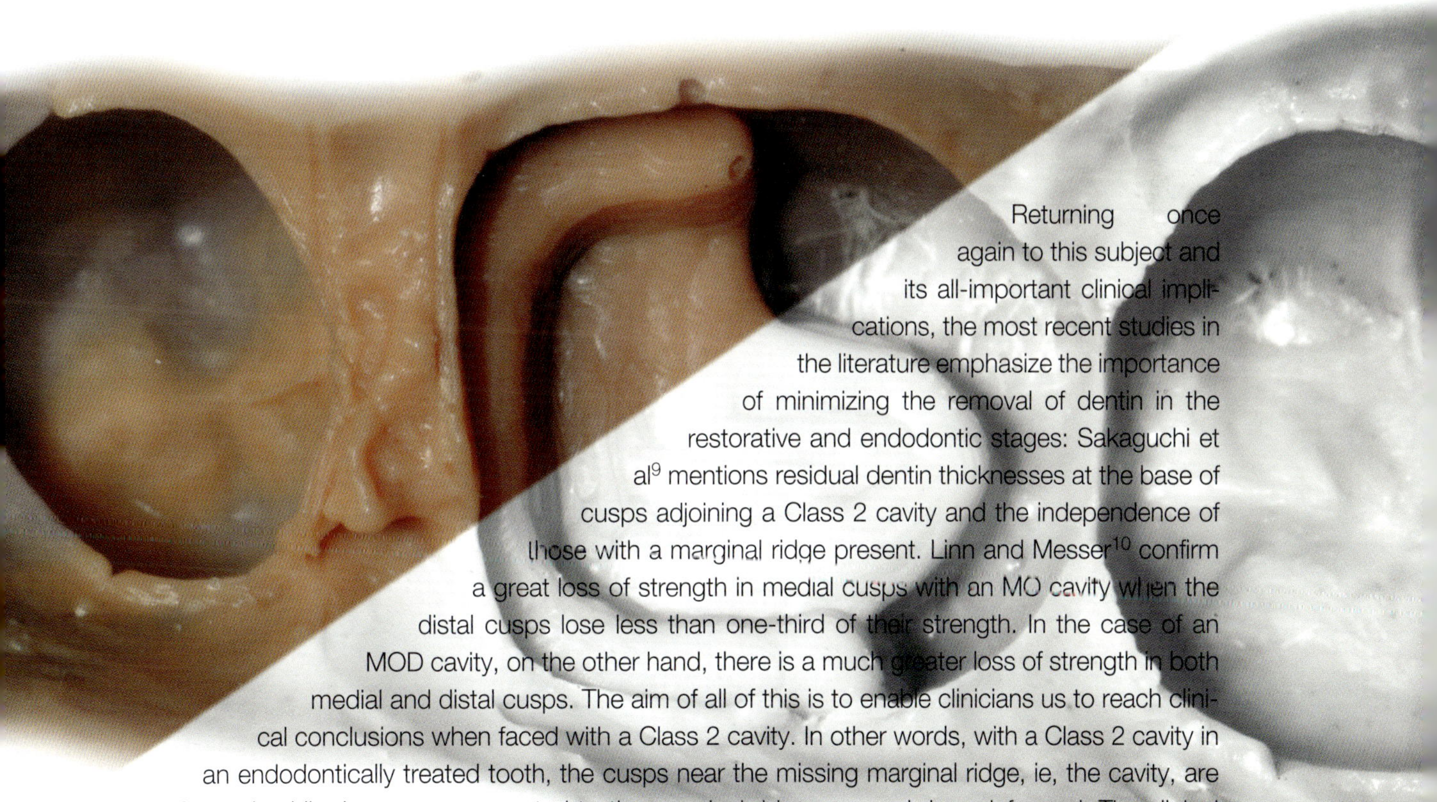

Returning once again to this subject and its all-important clinical implications, the most recent studies in the literature emphasize the importance of minimizing the removal of dentin in the restorative and endodontic stages: Sakaguchi et al[9] mentions residual dentin thicknesses at the base of cusps adjoining a Class 2 cavity and the independence of those with a marginal ridge present. Linn and Messer[10] confirm a great loss of strength in medial cusps with an MO cavity when the distal cusps lose less than one-third of their strength. In the case of an MOD cavity, on the other hand, there is a much greater loss of strength in both medial and distal cusps. The aim of all of this is to enable clinicians us to reach clinical conclusions when faced with a Class 2 cavity. In other words, with a Class 2 cavity in an endodontically treated tooth, the cusps near the missing marginal ridge, ie, the cavity, are deformed, while the cusps connected to the marginal ridge are much less deformed. The clinical implications of this are that in an endodontically treated tooth with an MO cavity, eg, only the mesial cusps need to be prepared, leaving the distal cusps intact, thus giving rise to a restoration with partial cusp coverage. Add to all this the consistent presence of preparation margins in a supragingival position and one has achieved nirvana—at least in terms of conservative dentistry (Figs 30 and 31).

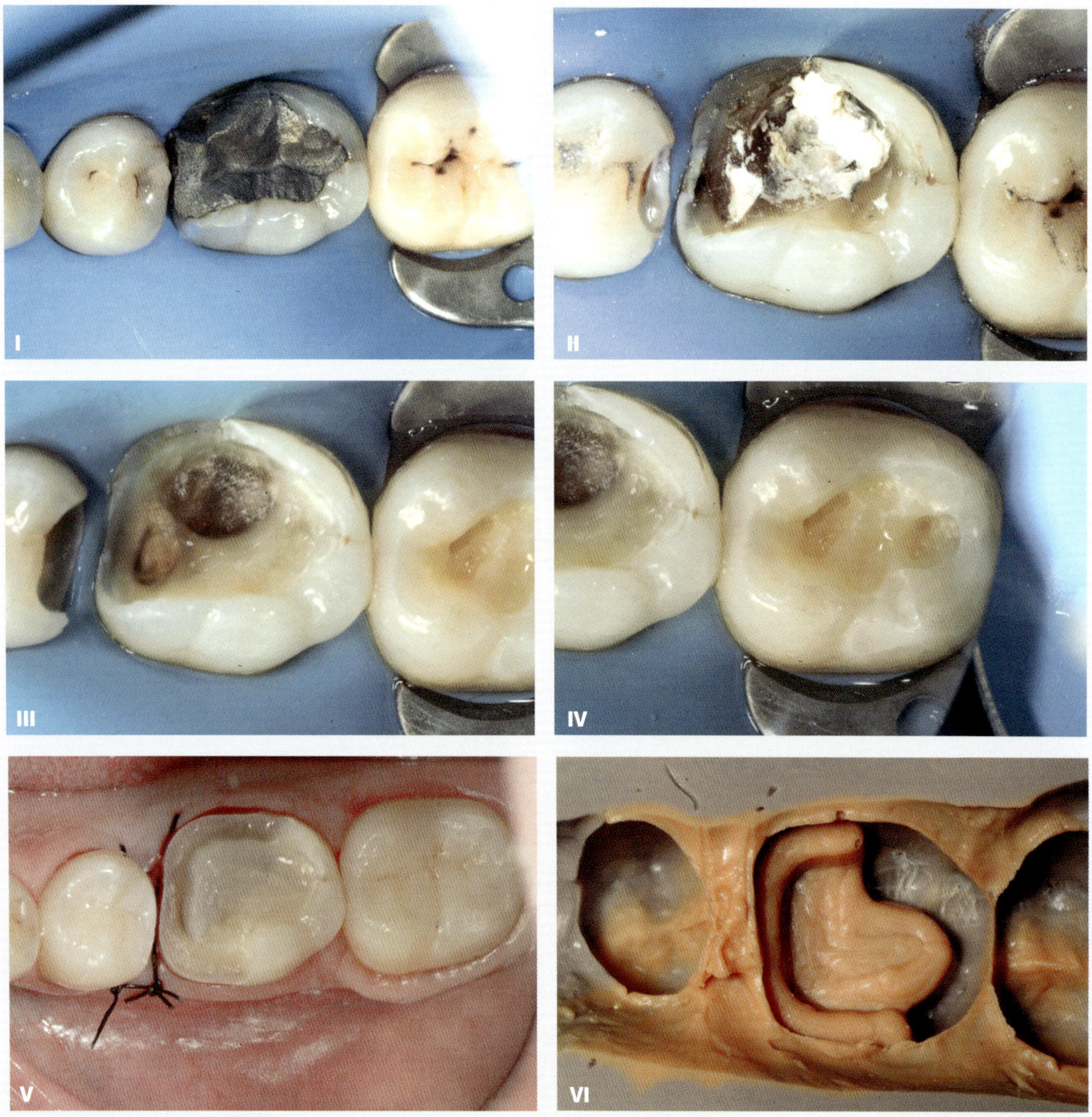

Fig 30 Taking an accurate impression after exposing the margins by means of an extremely conservative clinical crown lengthening procedure.

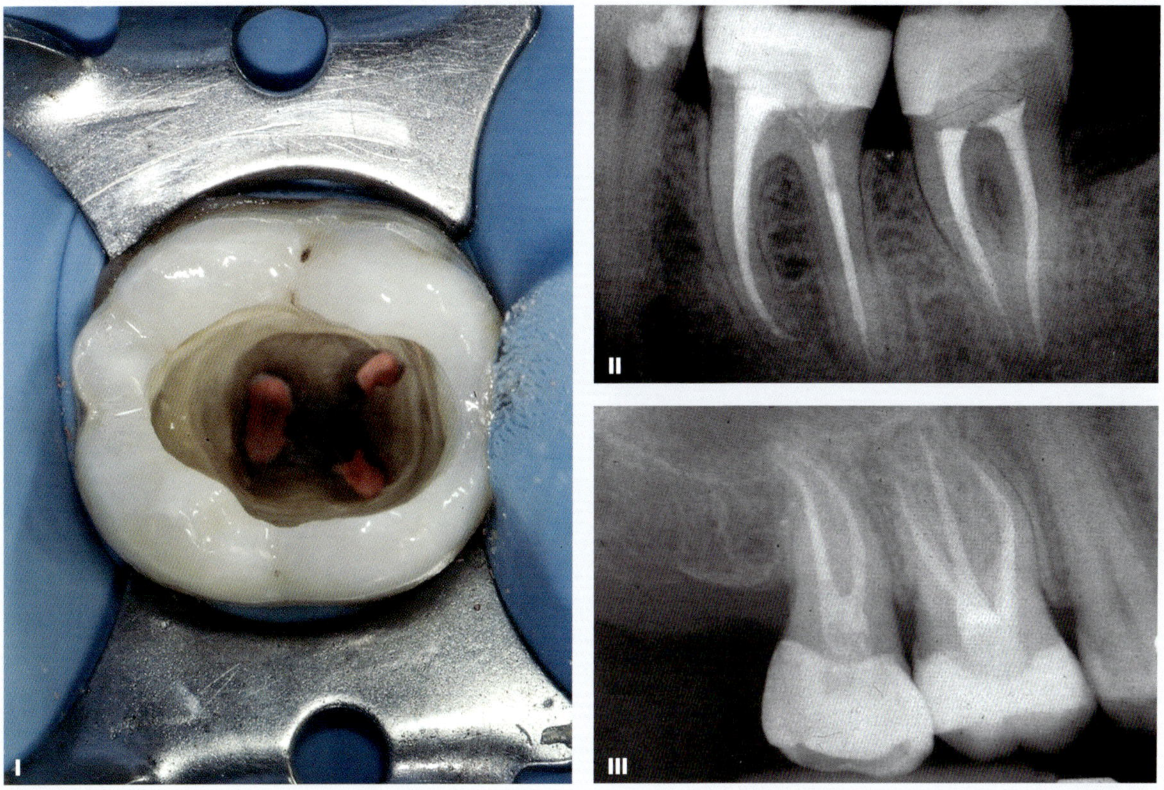

Fig 31 Indications for a direct restoration in an endodontically treated tooth with four walls present *(I)*. A restoration with partial coverage of cusps in an MO cavity of an endodontically treated mandibular left second molar *(II)* and a full-coverage restoration in an MOD cavity *(III)*.

These studies illustrate that present-day cavity design is moving in a more conservative direction, and after having completed approximately 3,000 indirect restorations, the author has absolutely no reservations in confirming the extreme ease of preparing a cavity for indirect composite restorations; however, cementing them is quite another matter.

Internal reconstruction (buildup)

Internal reconstruction of the cavity after the complete—with an emphasis on complete—removal of decayed tissue is performed with the aim of:

- Protecting the pulp-dentin complex by sealing the dentinal tubules[16]
- Creating consistent thicknesses[17–19]
- Removing undercuts, making it easier to take impressions and allowing more conservative cavity design (Figs 32 to 39).

For the buildup, cavity size is assessed on a case-by-case basis:

- ***In small cavities:*** one adhesive system only
- ***In medium-sized cavities:*** one adhesive system + flowable composite
- ***In large cavities:*** adhesive system + flowable composite + composite

Materials used:

- Adhesive system (three-step or two-step self-etch)
- Fine layer (0.5 mm) of flowable composite to coat the base of the cavity and the walls
- Microhybrid or nanohybrid composite (Fig 40)

Very elastic, flowable composite makes for a more effective gradient of elasticity, leading to a reduction of 20% to 50% in contraction stress due to polymerization.[20]
Traditional microhybrid composite is used in the geometric finishing of the cavity with the aim of achieving consistent, uniform thicknesses that will allow the curing light to reach the cement, ie, the composite, during curing at the inlay cementation stage. Studies in the literature suggest that proper curing cannot take place when inlay thickness is greater than 3 mm.[19]
One fundamental requirement for building a structure that is highly resistant to loads is homogeneity, and this requirement is met because the material used for the buildup is a microhybrid composite, the material used in the process of manufacturing the inlay is also microhybrid composite, and the material used for cementation is the very same microhybrid composite.
To summarize this concept, the thickness of all preparations must simultaneously satisfy requirements of mechanical strength and curing.

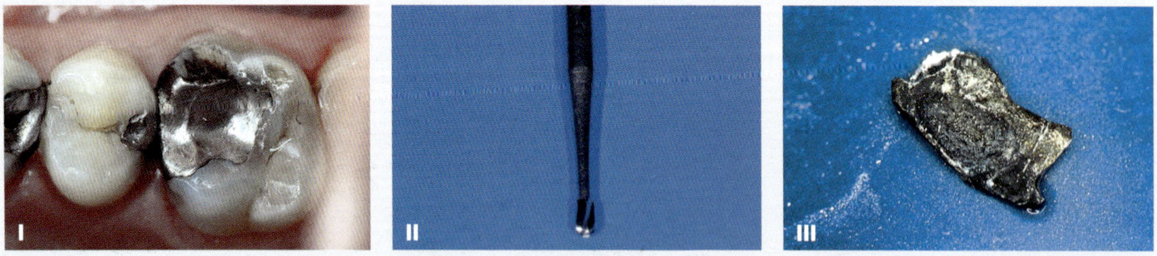

Fig 32 Removal of the amalgam restoration with a new bur and abundant water jet, seeking to remove the metal in blocks to avoid prolonged grinding.

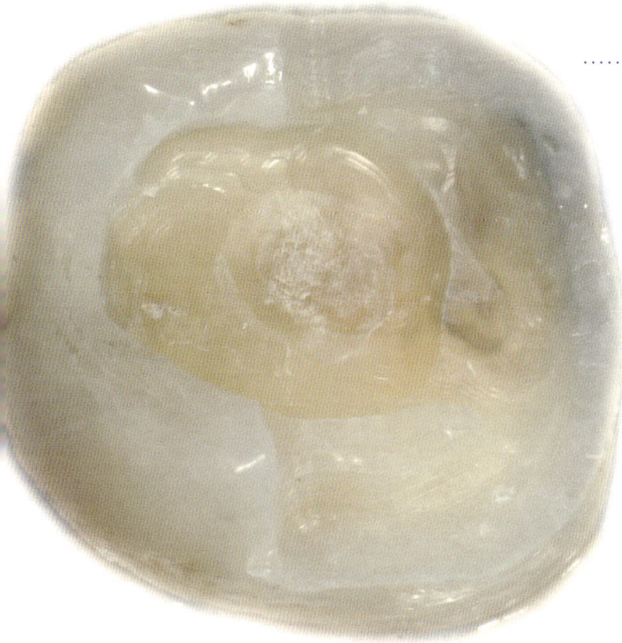

Fig 33 Cavity after complete removal of decayed tissue.

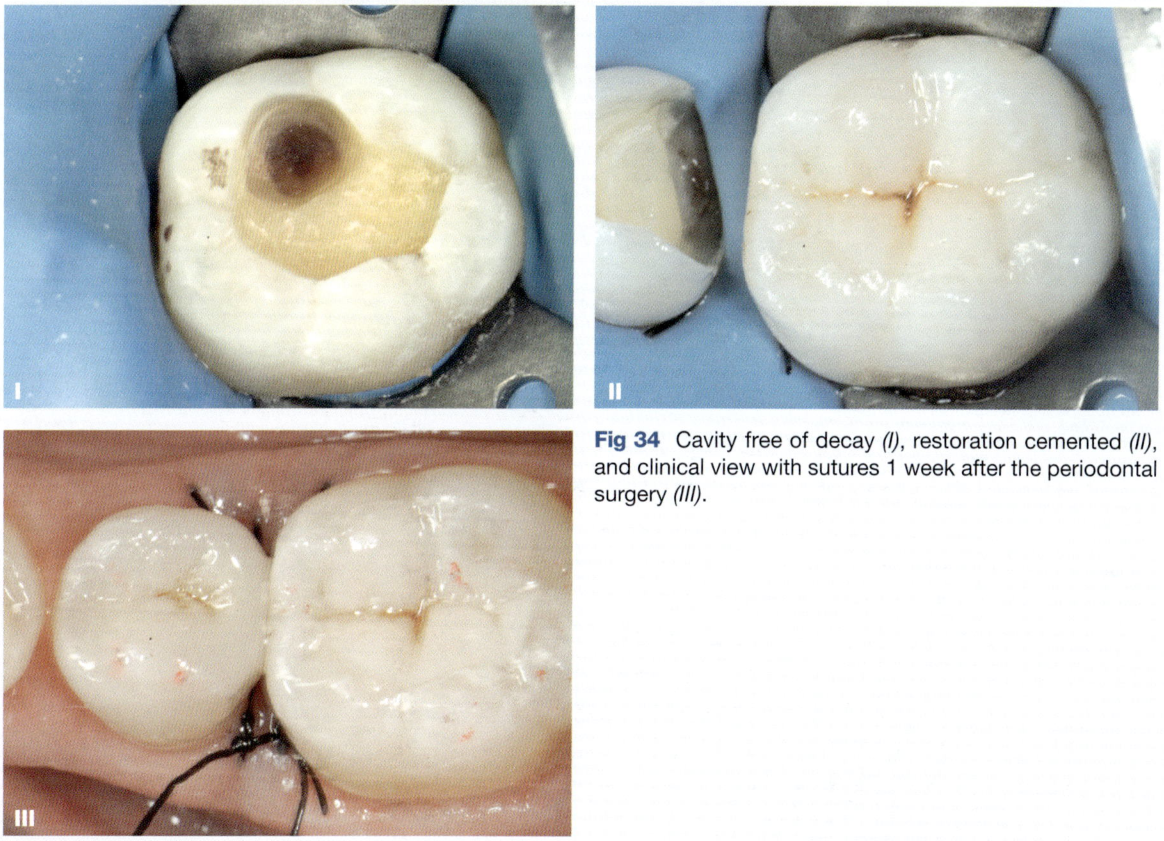

Fig 34 Cavity free of decay *(I)*, restoration cemented *(II)*, and clinical view with sutures 1 week after the periodontal surgery *(III)*.

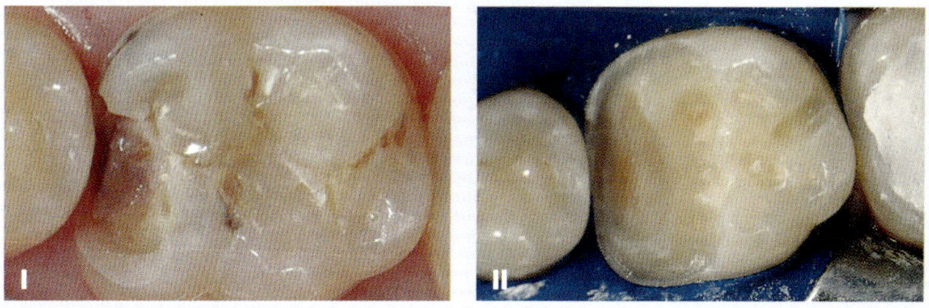

Fig 35 Removal of the decay and application of rubber dam to the tooth made possible by periodontal surgery. This allows the buildup to be carried out with a fully isolated operative field.

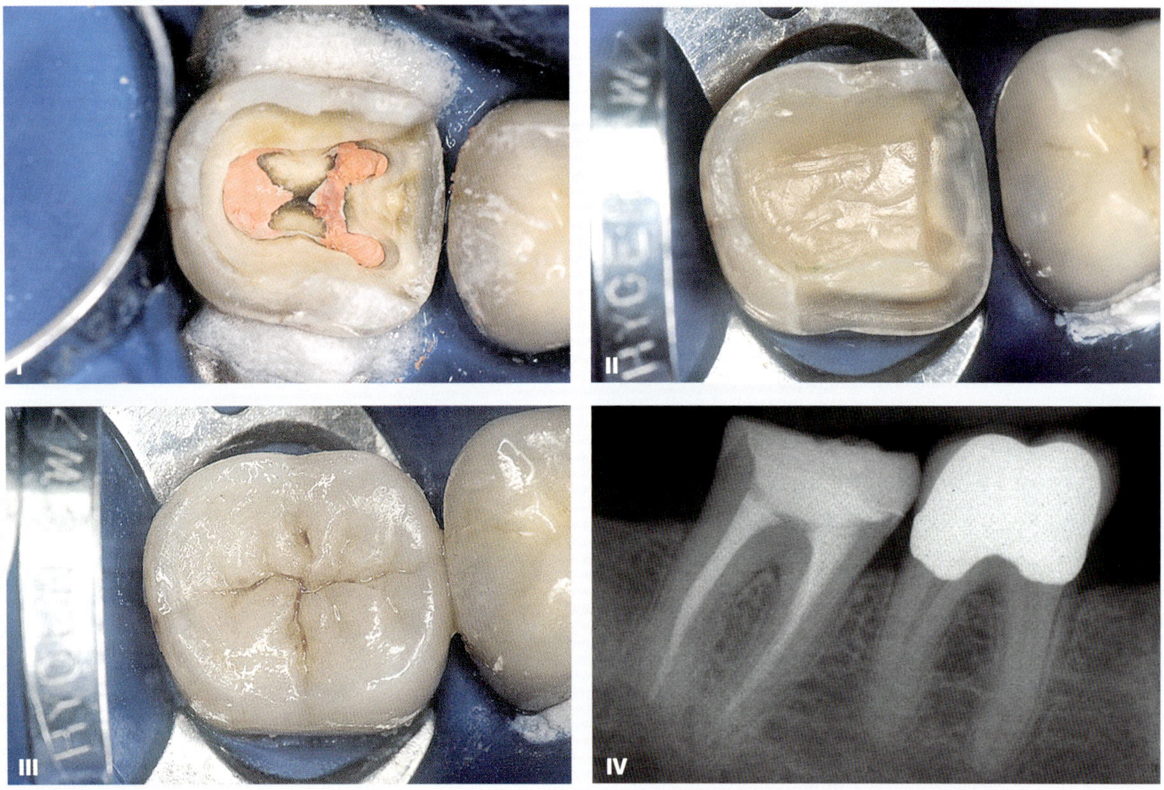

Fig 36 Intraoperative stages in execution of buildup and cemented inlay.

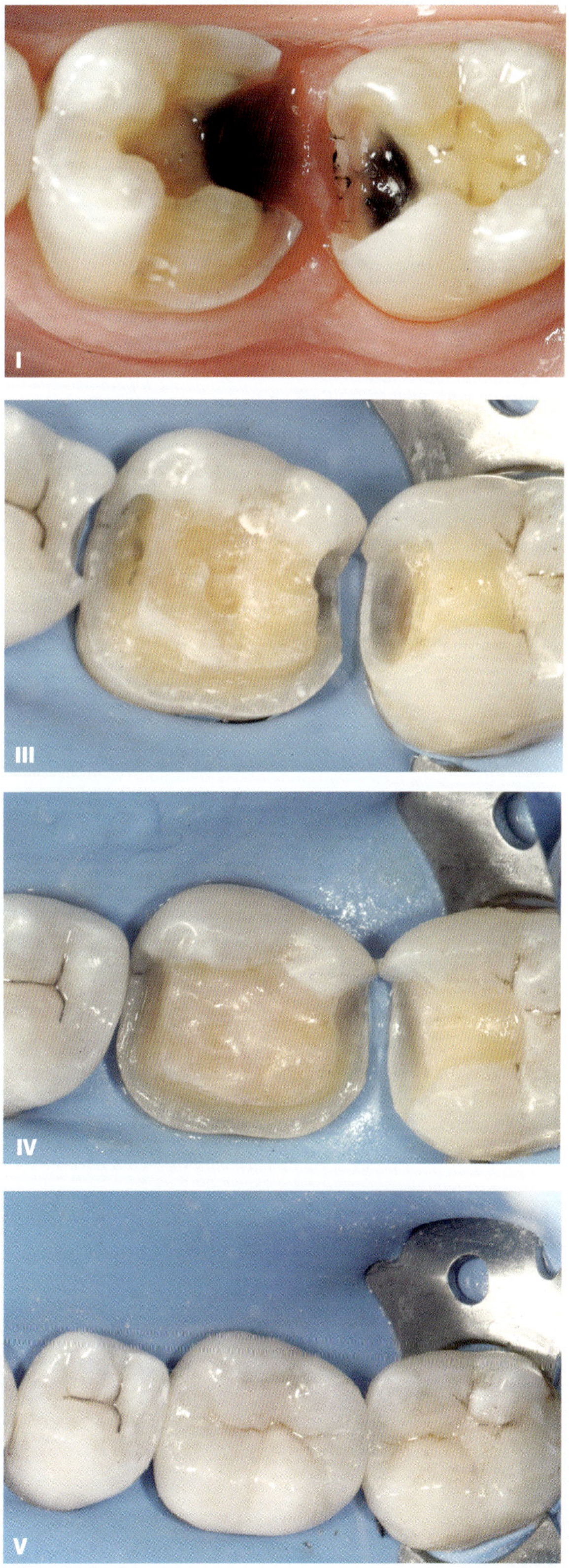
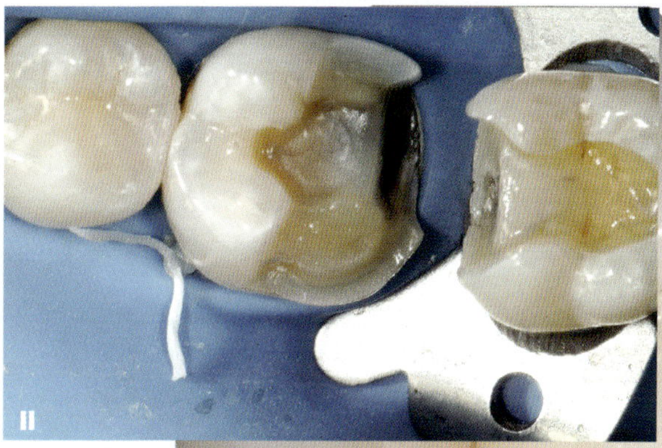

Fig 37 Intraoperative view of internal reconstructions. The importance of periodontal intervention for proper exposure of the margins is indisputable.

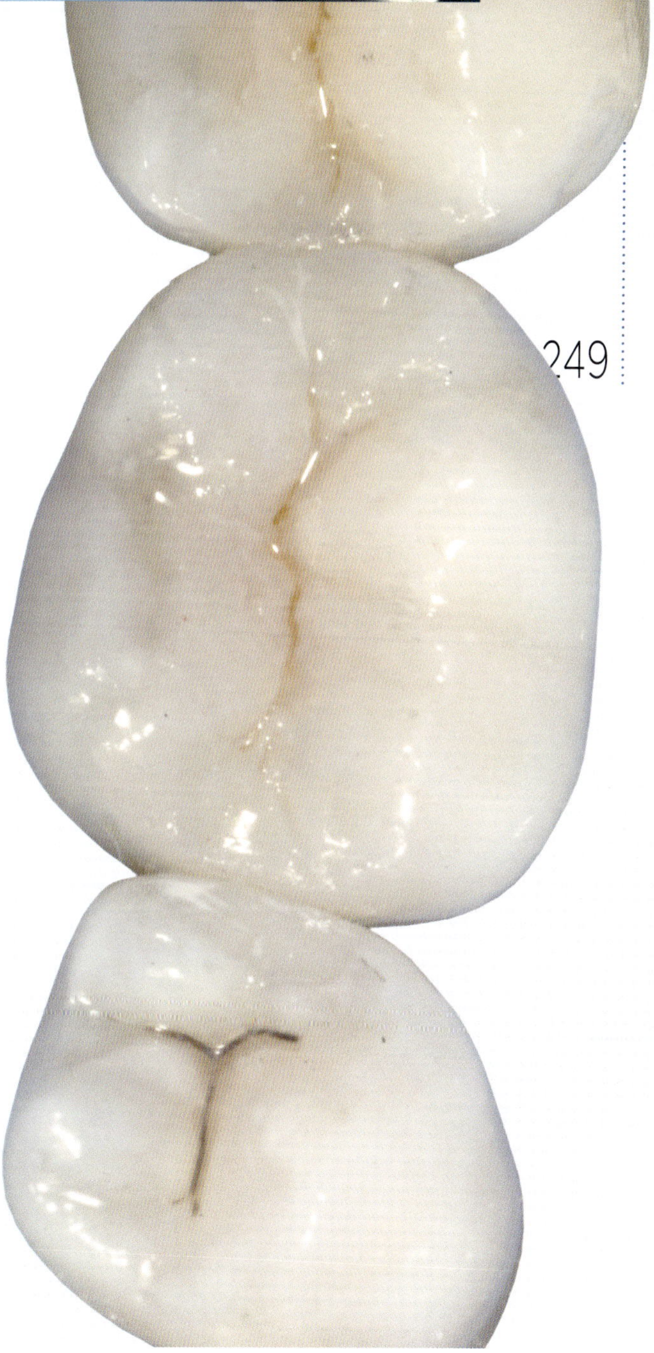

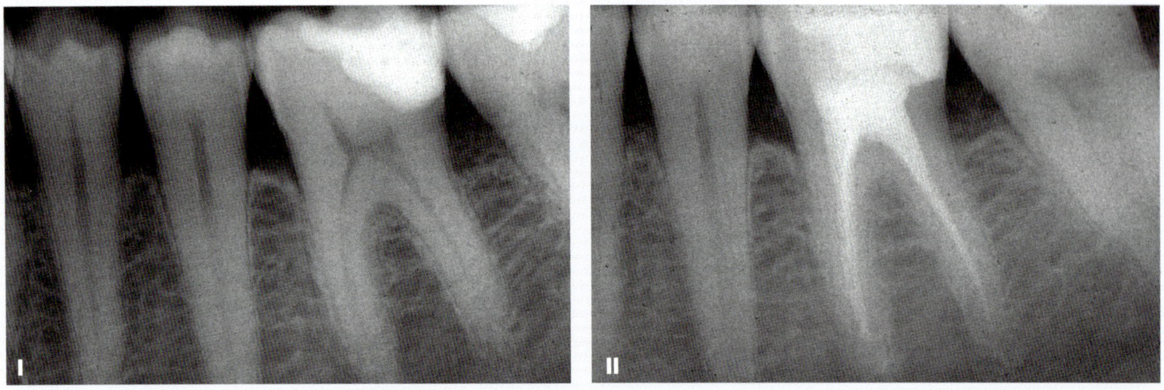

Fig 38 An incorrect internal filling and imperfect margin are evident in the preoperative radiograph *(I)*, while a postoperative follow-up after preparation of an indirect restoration reveals a successful buildup and marginal seal *(II)*. The tooth was treated endodontically for pulpitis.

Fig 39 Buildup and preparation for an onlay on an endodontically treated tooth, highlighting the concept of preserving as much healthy residual structure as possible with full respect for the tooth's biomechanical properties.

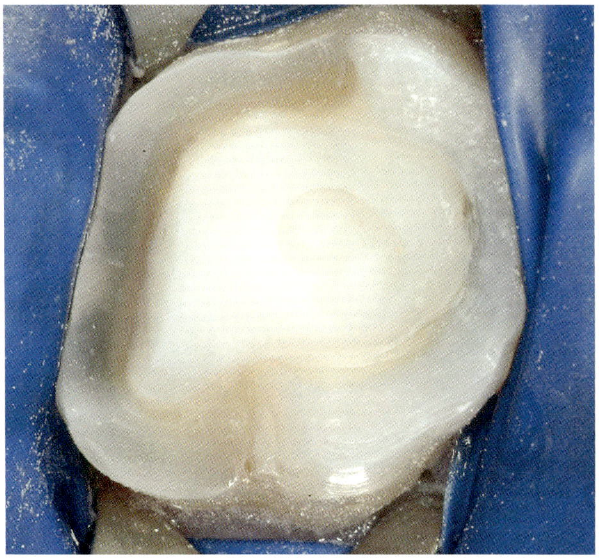

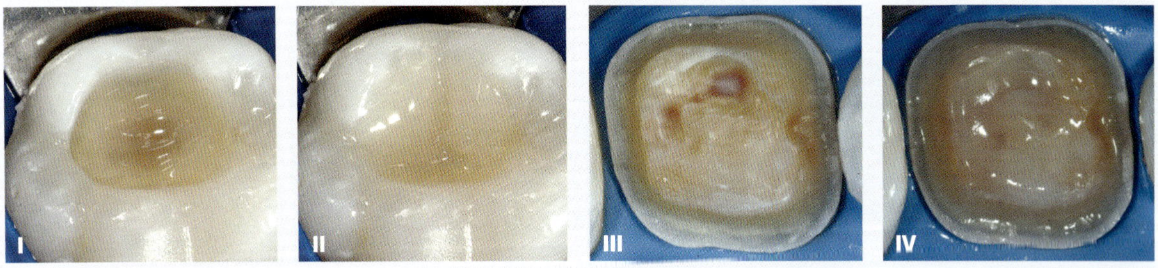

Fig 40 Clinical view showing addition of flowable composite and traditional composite in a direct restoration *(I, II)* and preparation of an overlay with 0.5 mm of flowable composite as a base layer prior to placement of the traditional composite *(III, IV)*.

Cavity geometry

Cavity preparation affects the subsequent treatment stage: the impression. The accuracy of this process determines the success of the working cast and hence construction of the inlay and cementation, with the latter being favorably affected by supragingival positioning of the margins.
Before preparation, it is worth remembering yet again to assess the tooth from a periodontal, structural, and endodontic viewpoint.
Complete removal of decayed tissue, as already stated, is such a fundamental requirement that it needs no further mention. There are so many different clinical situations that it is not always possible to come up with a specific protocol for determining cavity geometry. Clinical experience is naturally the best benchmark.

In 1978, Shillingburg et al[21] focused attention on principles of preserving the structure, durability, and strength of the teeth and the durability and structural integrity of the margins. Still today, these principles must be respected when forming a cavity, also taking into account developments in techniques and materials.

Certain preliminary evaluations must be taken into consideration:

- Condition of the pulp
- Presence or absence of marginal ridges
- Residual thickness at the base of the cusps, in the knowledge that the cusps that support 85% of masticatory actions are the distolingual cusps of the mandibular molars and the mesiobuccal cusps of the maxillary molars[22,23]
- Presence or absence of dentinal fracture lines
- Presence or absence of painful symptoms
- Position of occlusal contacts, taking the greatest care to ensure that the restoration margins do not coincide with the occlusal contacts
- Presence of any premature contacts and interferences
- Extension of the preparation into esthetically critical areas

Only when it is certain that the best design for the cavity has been selected can the clinical stage be initiated, with the intention of constructing a cavity that (Figs 41 and 42):

- Has the simplest possible geometry
- Is nonretentive, with walls diverging by 10 to 15 degrees
- Features an isthmus at least 3 mm wide
- Contains rounded internal angles
- Has a minimum depth of 2 mm
- Presents a box that is 2.5 mm wide and 3 mm high
- Features a prepared cervical margin of 90 degrees
- Has occlusal cusp reduction of at least 2 mm according to the various indications
- Presents a knife-edge or shoulder preparation

A separate chapter will be devoted to the clinical preparation of subgingival margins.

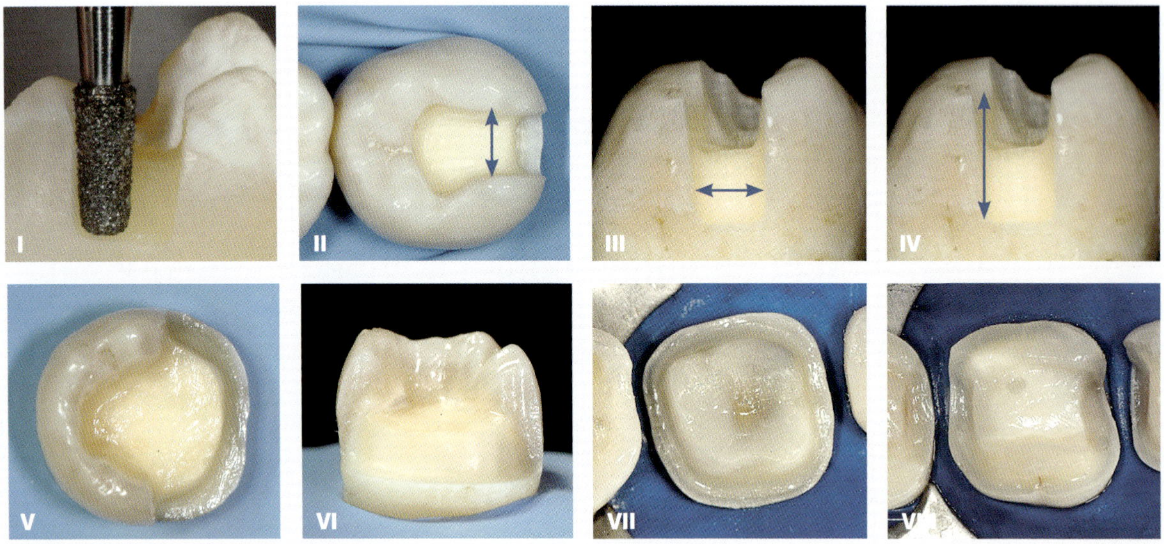

Fig 41 Walls diverging 10 to 12 degrees *(I)*. A 3-mm isthmus and rounded internal angles *(II)*. A 2.5-mm-wide box *(III)*. A 3-mm box height *(IV)*. Cervical margins at 90 degrees and view of shoulder preparation *(V–VII)*. Shoulder and lingual knife-edge preparation *(VIII)*.

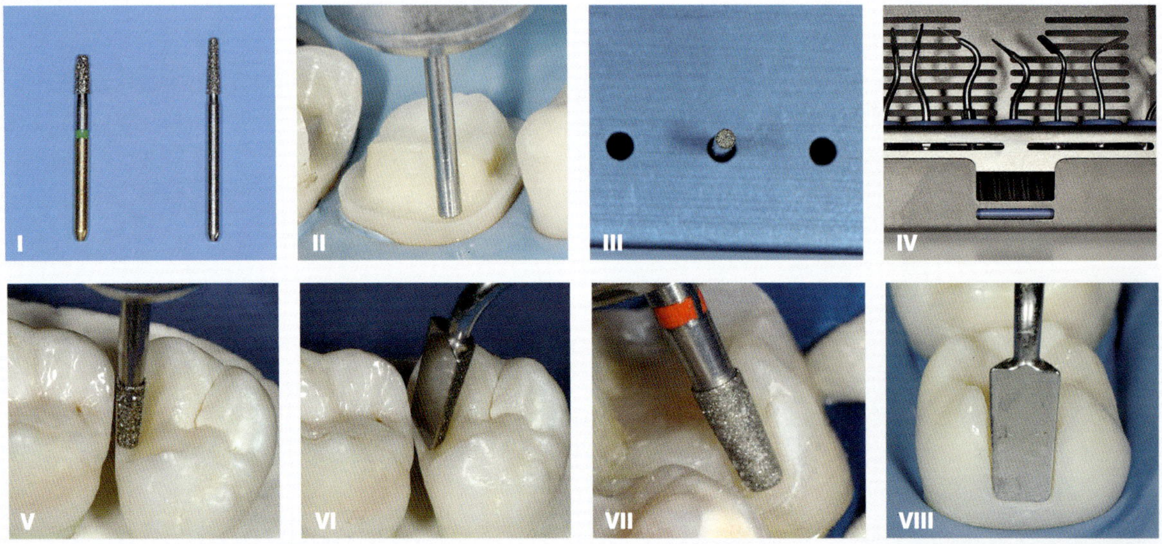

Fig 42 Preparation and finishing with rotary and subsonic burs.

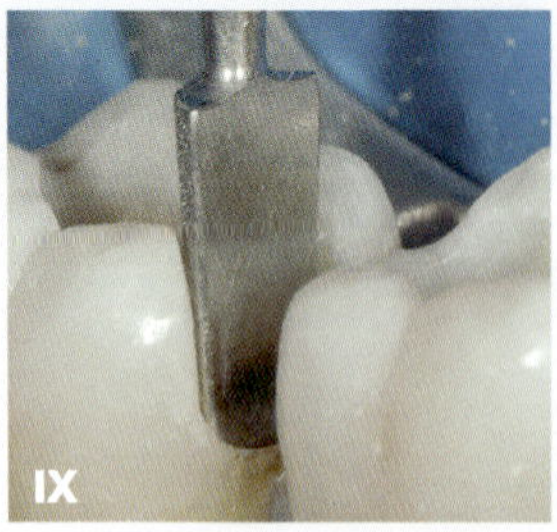

Vital tooth

OCCLUSAL CAVITIES

Large cavities in the same quadrant: DIRECT RESTORATION, but sometimes also INDIRECT, above all if associated with large fracture lines.

MO, OD CAVITIES

Well-supported cusps near a missing marginal ridge (2.5 to 3 mm): MO INLAY, OD INLAY (Figs 43 to 57).
Cusps near a missing marginal ridge with residual base thickness of under 2 mm: MO ONLAY, OD ONLAY (Figs 58 to 74).

MOD CAVITY

INLAY: In very rare cases, when all the thicknesses are highly reassuring (from 4 to 6 mm) (Figs 75 to 83).
ONLAY: When one or two cusps on the same side (mesial or distal) display insufficient remaining cusp material, eg, for an MO cavity with one or both of the mesial cusps displaying base thicknesses of under 2 mm, the indication is naturally for an ONLAY with coverage of one or both of the mesial cusps (Figs 84 to 94).
OVERLAY: When the thicknesses in two or more of the remaining cusps are insufficient; above all when the tooth in question is at great risk of endodontic treatment in the future (Figs 95 to 113).

MO, OD cavity: Inlay

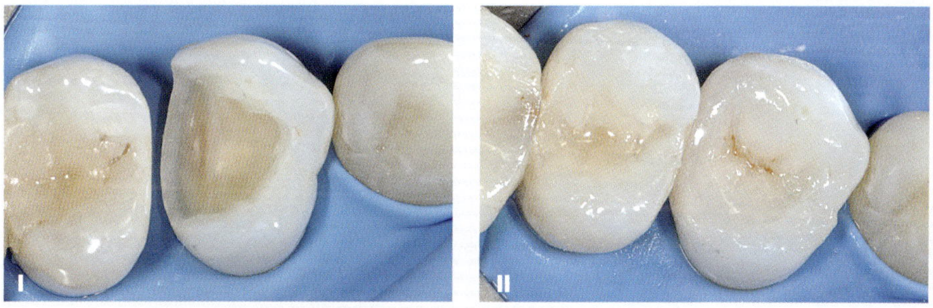

Fig 43 The indication dictated by the cavity after measuring thicknesses at the cusp bases is an inlay *(I)*. View of cemented restoration *(II)*.

MO, OD cavity: Inlay

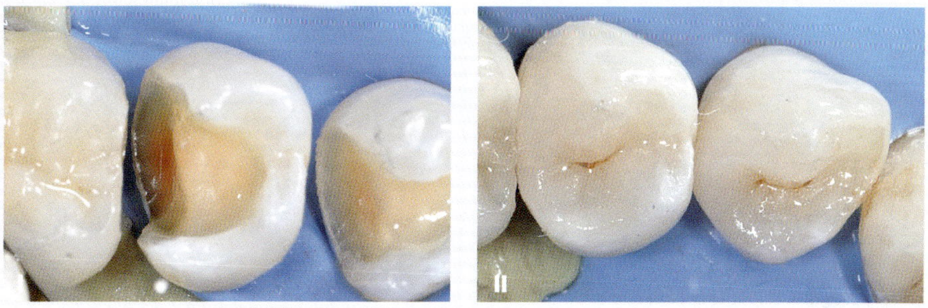

Fig 44 In these two premolars with OD cavities *(I)*, the application of two inlays is again the correct solution *(II)*.

MO, OD cavity: Inlay

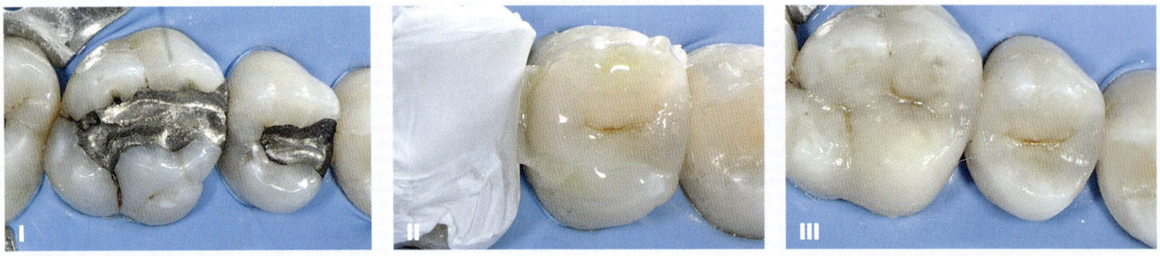

Fig 45 Intraoperative view showing cementation of an inlay before and after removal of excess composite used as cement.

MO, OD cavity: Inlay

Fig 46 Reconstruction of defective restorations with OD inlay for maxillary left first and second premolars.

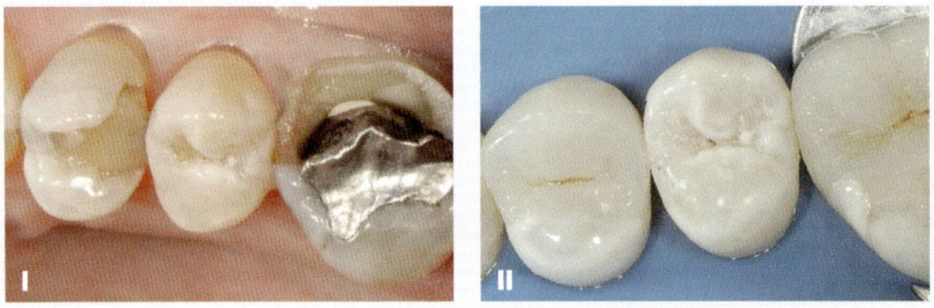

MO, OD cavity: Inlay

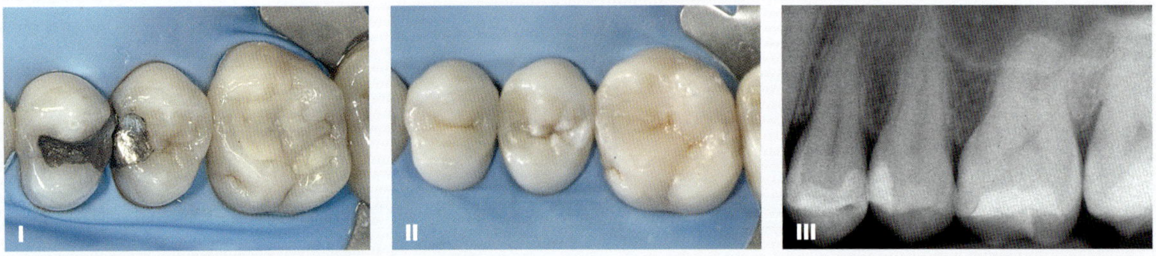

Fig 47 Replacement of two amalgam restorations requested by the patient for cosmetic reasons with an inlay on the maxillary left first premolar and direct technique for the adjacent second premolar *(I, II)*. Follow-up radiograph *(III)*.

MO, OD cavity: Inlay

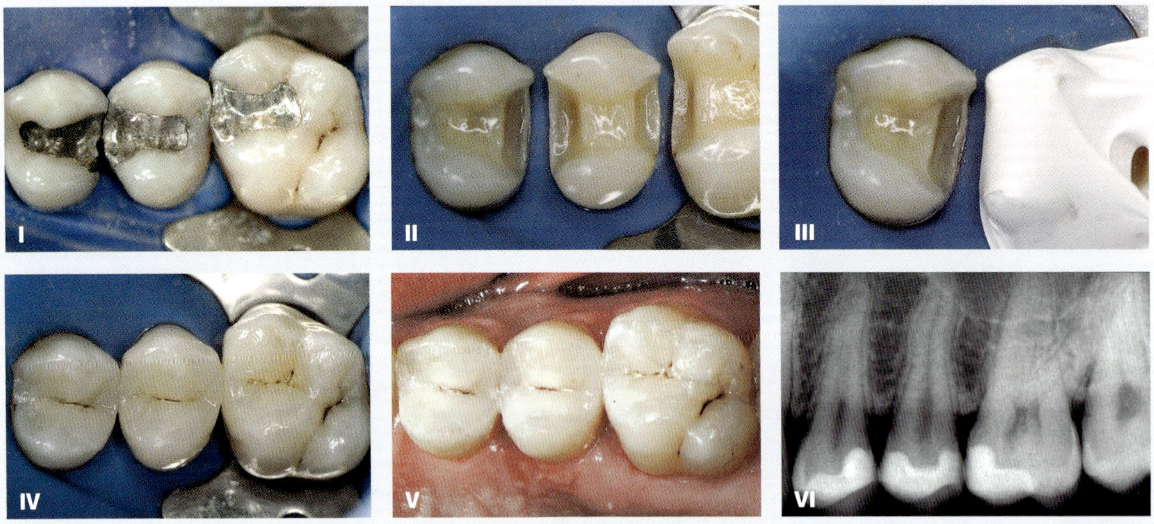

Fig 48 Cavity preparations of a quadrant with inlay in composite, again requested by the patient for cosmetic reasons *(I–V)*. Follow-up radiograph *(VI)*.

MO, OD cavity: Inlay

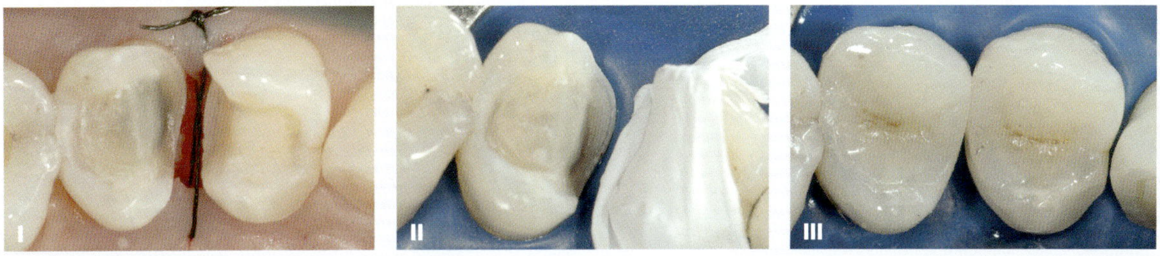

Fig 49 Exposure of margins after periodontal surgery *(I)* allows correct positioning of rubber dam. During cementation, the cavity in the proximal tooth is protected by simply using polytetrafluoroethylene *(II)*. Definitive restorations *(III)*.

MO, OD cavity: Inlay

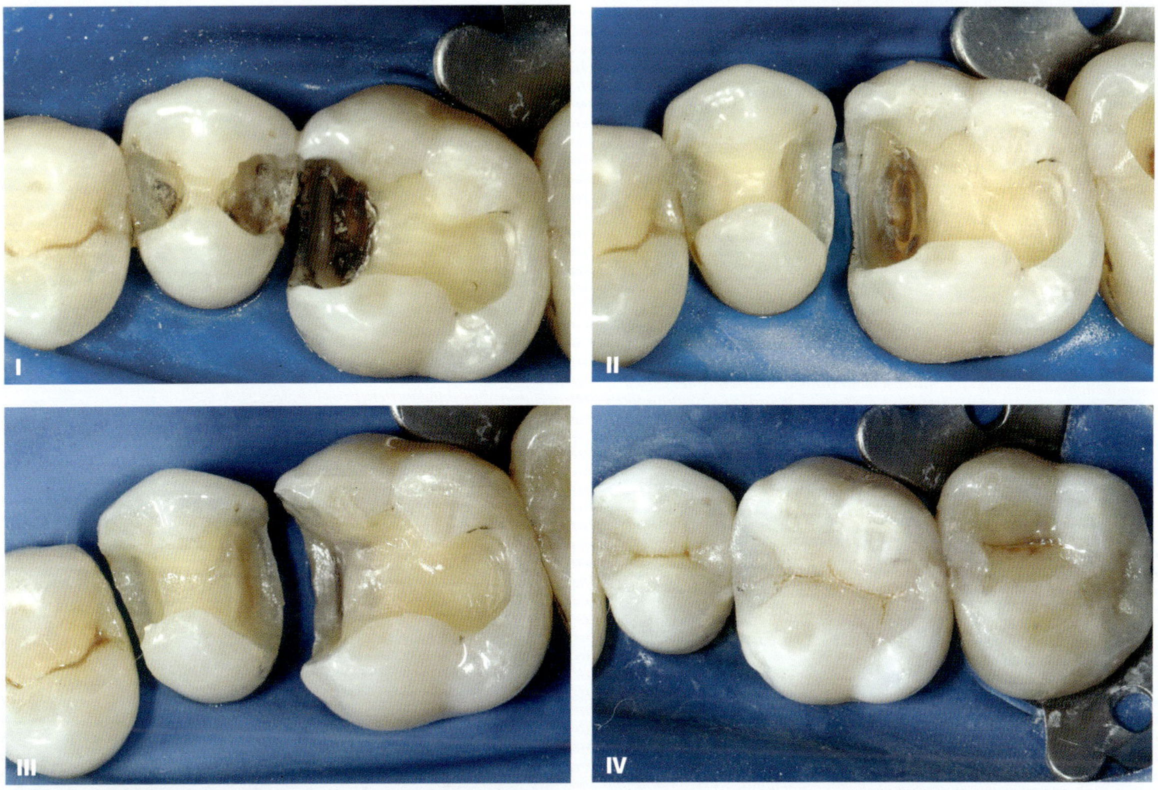

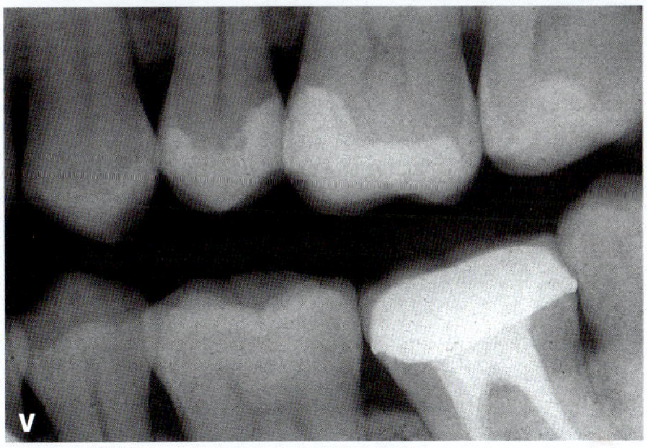

Fig 50 View of two deep caries lesions in the molar near the pulp complex *(I, II)*. After ablating the decayed tissue, buildup was performed with flowable composite and traditional composite *(III)*, and both inlays were cemented *(IV)*. Follow-up radiograph *(V)*.

MO, OD cavity: Inlay

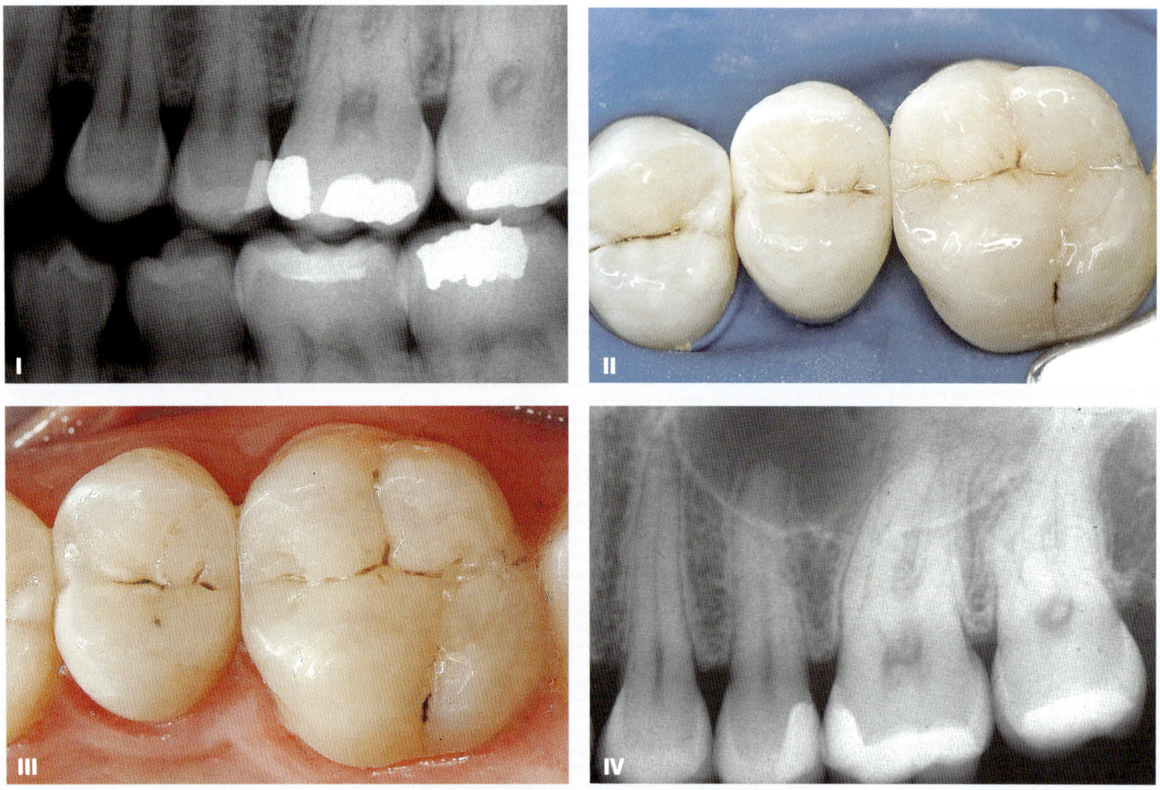

Fig 51 The patient complained of difficulties in passing dental floss between the maxillary left second premolar and first molar *(I)*. A leak is evident in the second premolar at the marginal level. Two inlays restored appropriate contact surfaces *(II, III)*. Follow-up radiograph at the end of treatment *(IV)*.

MO, OD cavity: Inlay

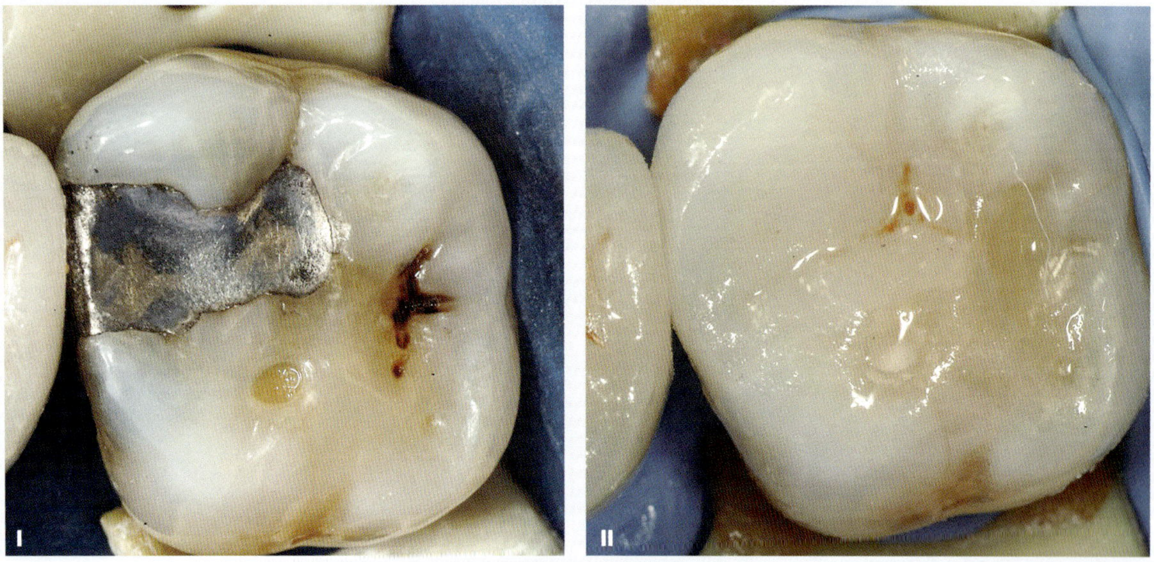

Fig 52 A simple inlay was performed in order to treat the maxillary left first molar, which was affected by pain on pressure and an occlusal caries lesion. The new contact surfaces appear consistent.

MO, OD cavity: Inlay

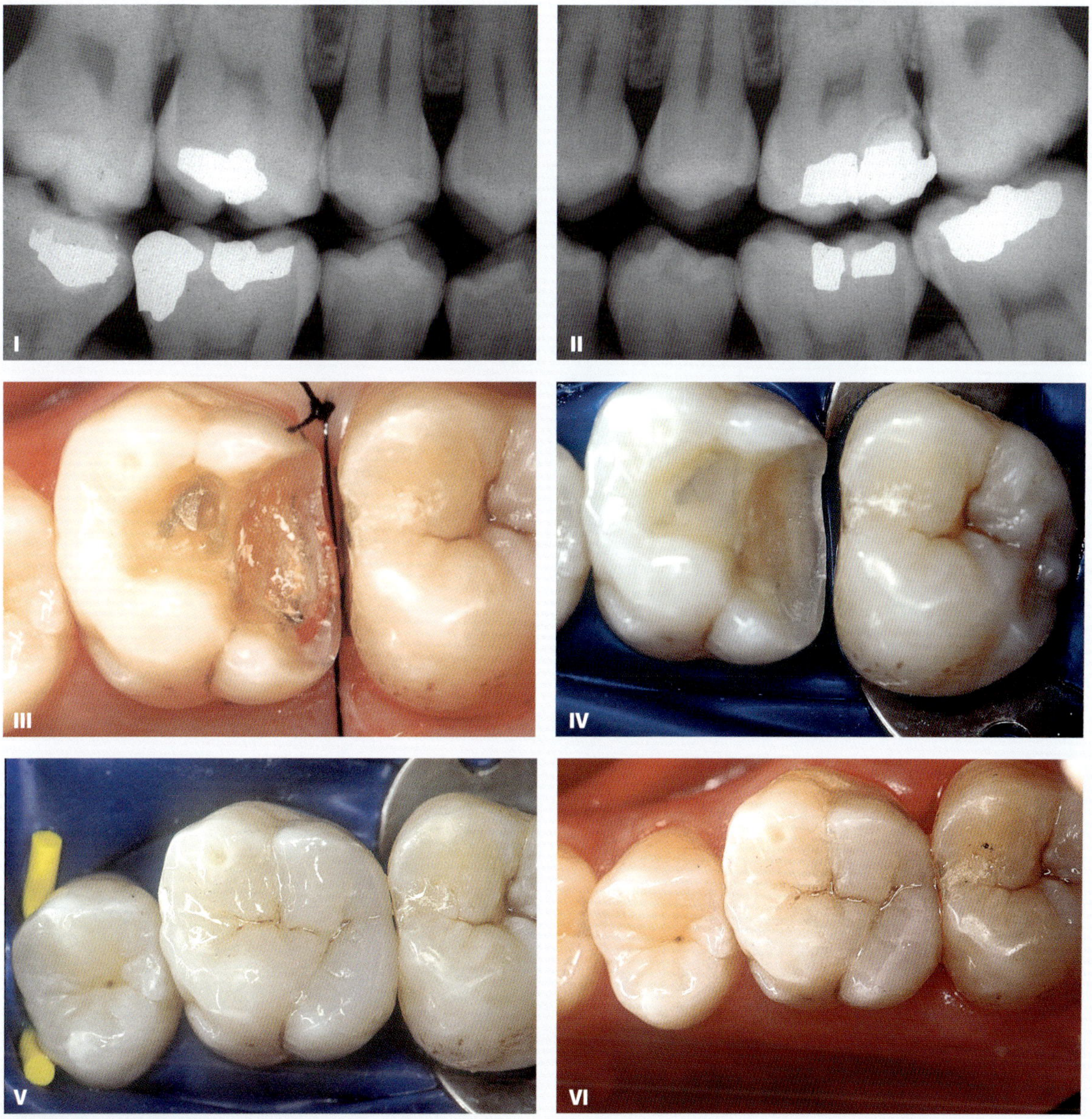

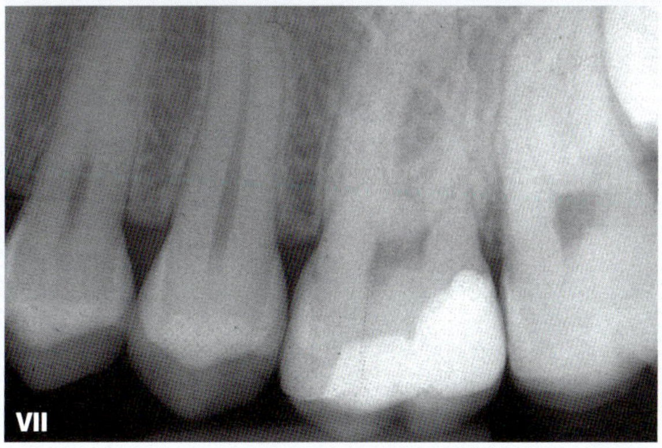

Fig 53 Preoperative bitewing radiographs *(I, II)* showing caries lesions and old metal restorations. Painful symptoms affecting the maxillary left first molar were characterized by spontaneous twinges and pain on pressure. After a positive pulp vitality test on the first molar and removal of very deep decay, clinical crown lengthening by means of periodontal surgery *(III)* allowed correct exposure of the distal margin and positioning of rubber dam *(IV)* in order to carry out internal reconstruction in accordance with protocol. View of the first molar *(V, VI)* and radiograph *(VII)* after cementing the inlay. View of both arches after treatment *(VIII, IX)* and radiographic follow-up *(X, XI)*.

Fig 53 *(continued)*

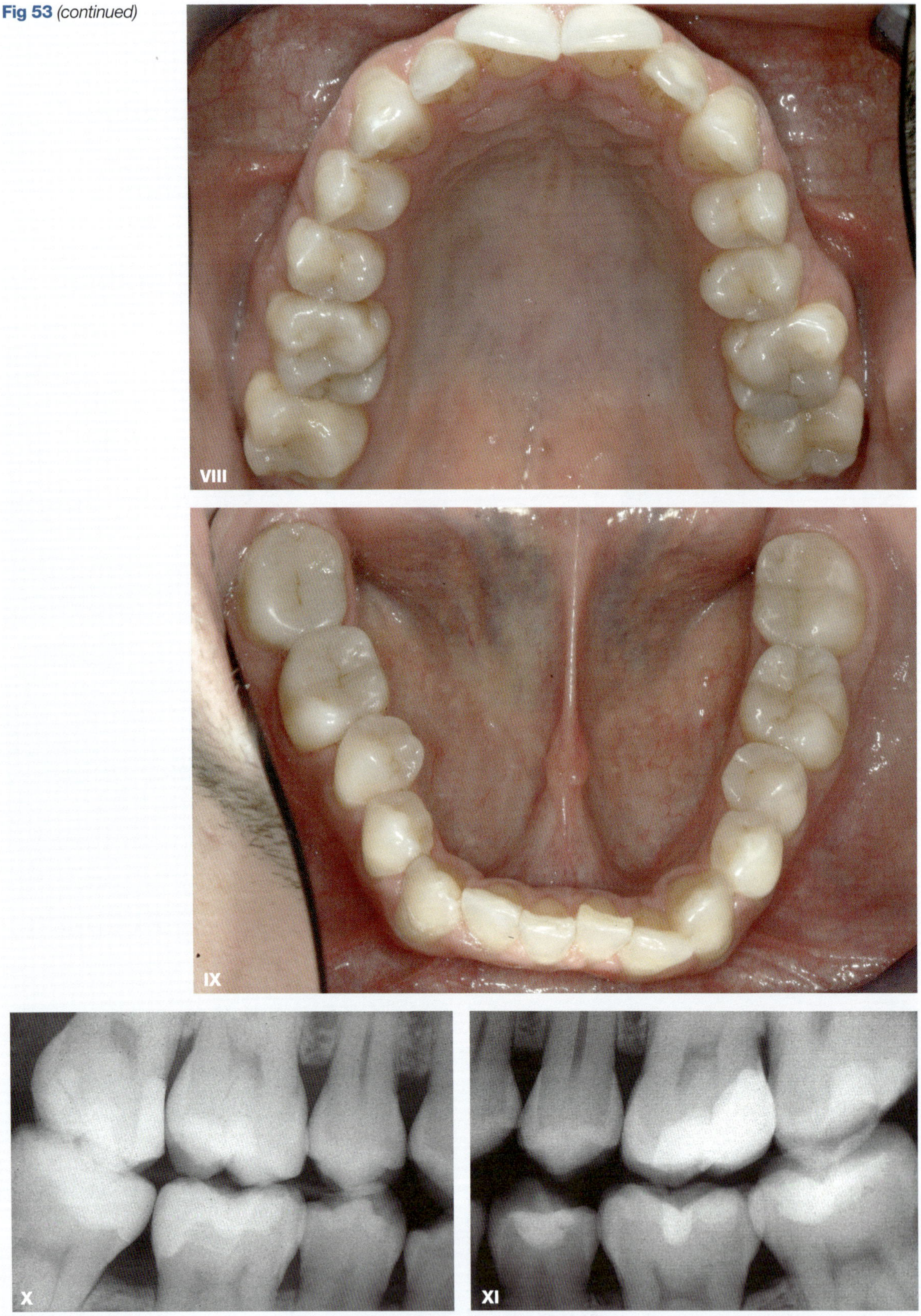

MO, OD cavity: Inlay

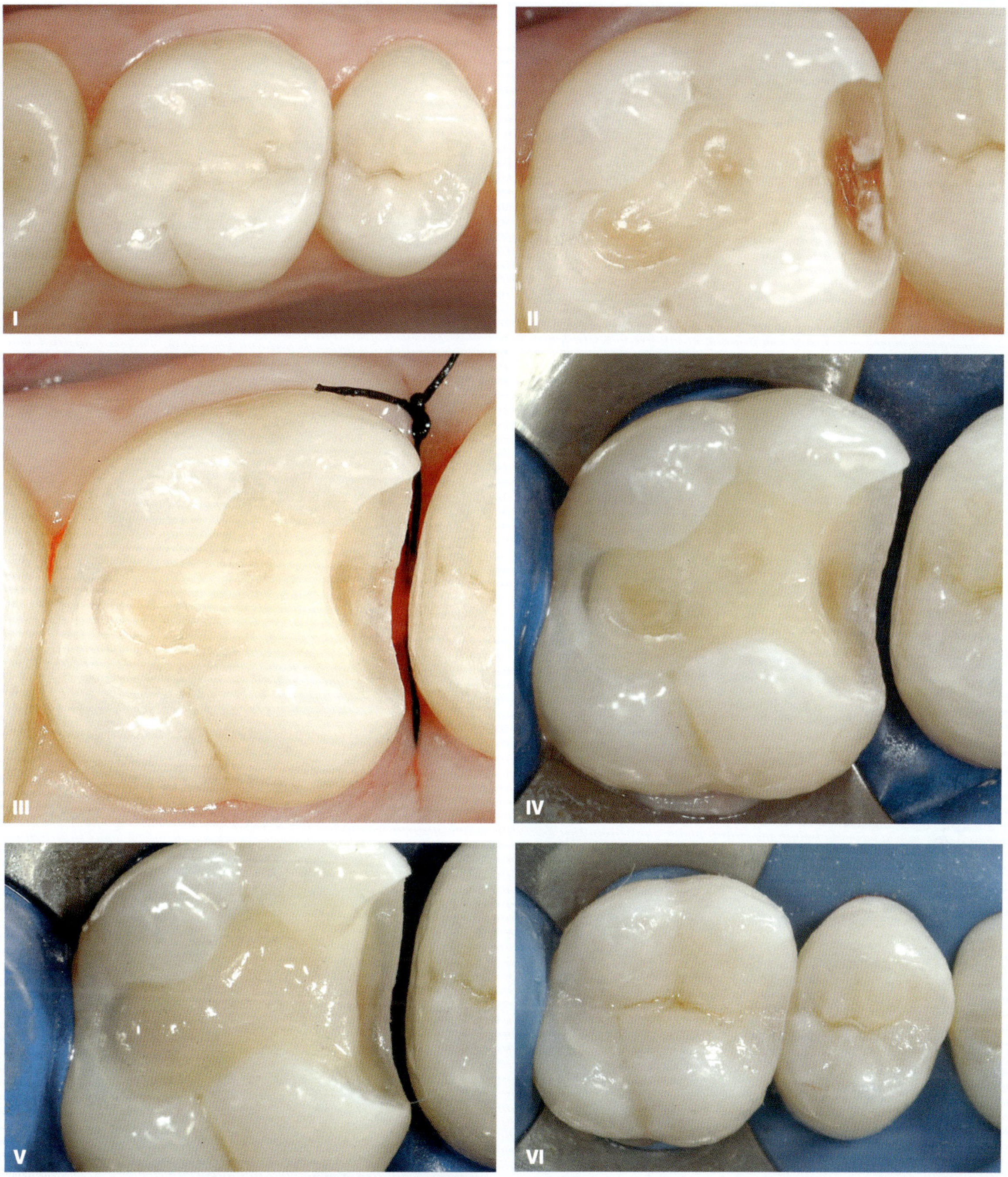

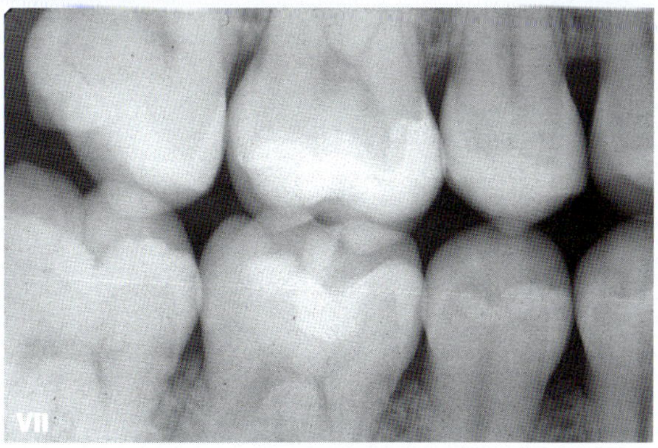

Fig 54 This clinical case is yet another example of the importance of periodontal-restorative action *(I–VI)*. The follow-up radiograph again clearly reveals the accuracy of the marginal seal and the emergence profile *(VII)*.

MO, OD cavity: Inlay

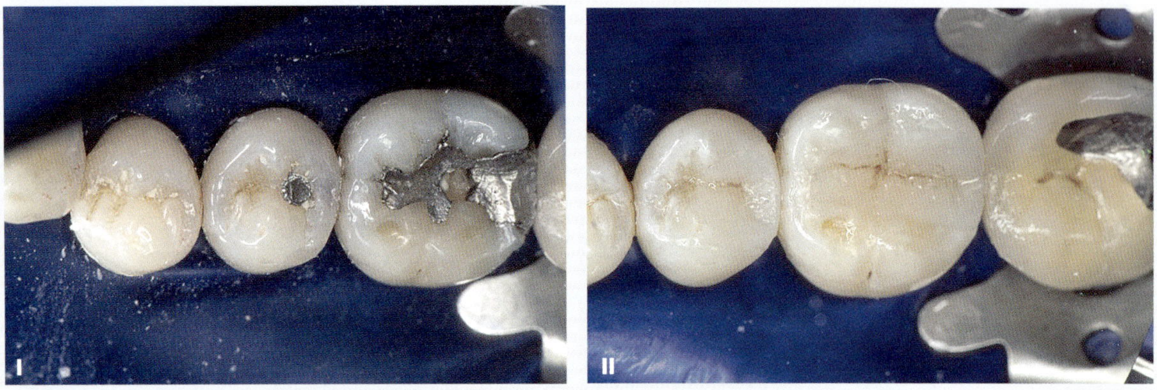

Fig 55 Dentin exposure caused by fracture of the amalgam in the mandibular left first molar had led to dentinal hypersensitivity and pain on pressure *(I)*. Replacement of the metal restoration with an inlay in composite caused the painful symptoms to stop *(II)*.

MO, OD cavity: Inlay

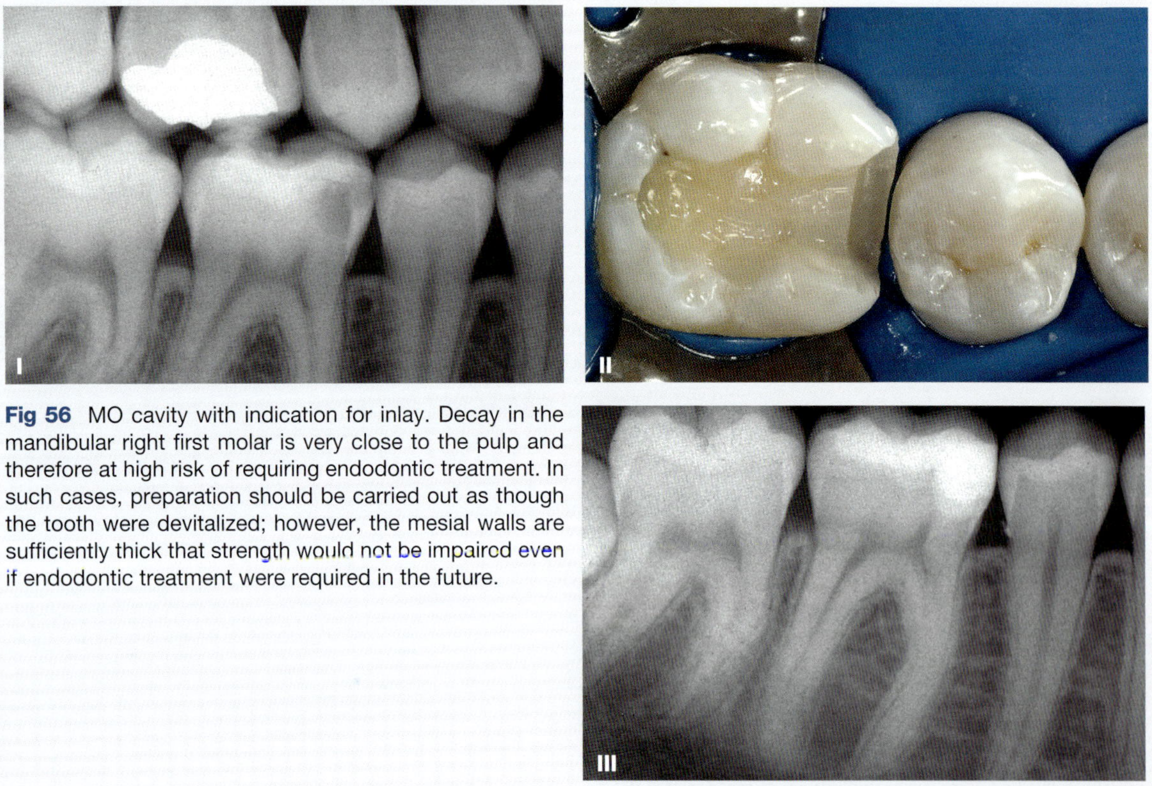

Fig 56 MO cavity with indication for inlay. Decay in the mandibular right first molar is very close to the pulp and therefore at high risk of requiring endodontic treatment. In such cases, preparation should be carried out as though the tooth were devitalized; however, the mesial walls are sufficiently thick that strength would not be impaired even if endodontic treatment were required in the future.

MO, OD cavity: Inlay

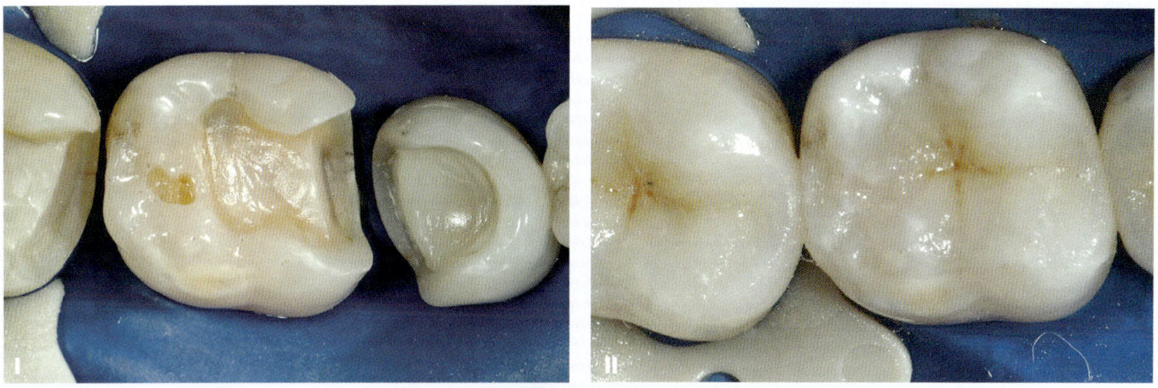

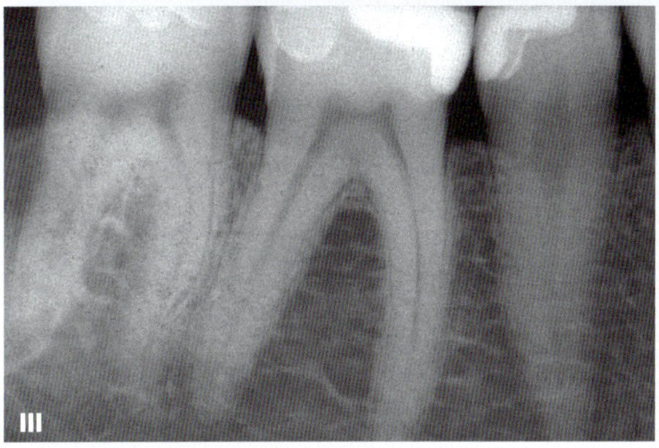

Fig 57 Cavity preparations for three inlays in the mandibular right quadrant *(I)*. Cemented inlay *(II)* and follow-up radiograph *(III)*.

MO, OD cavity: Onlay

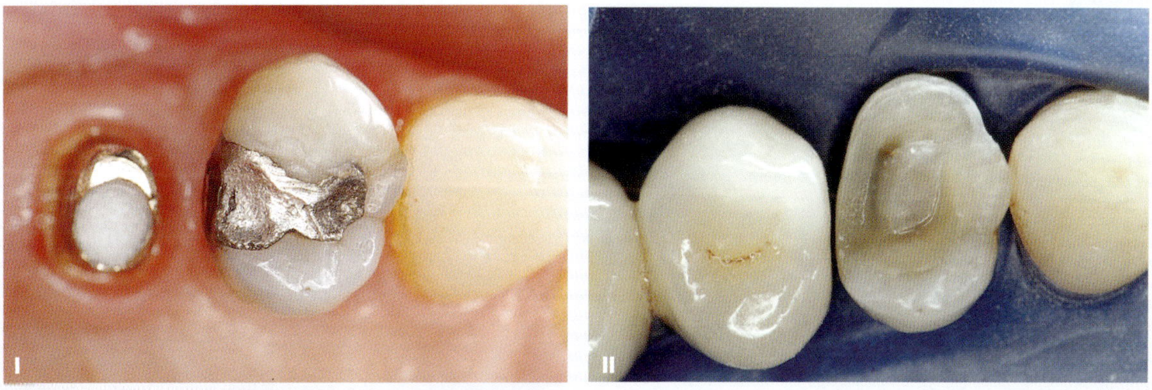

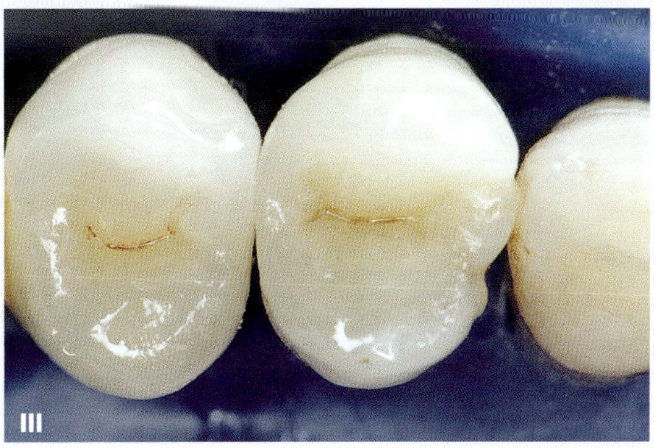

Fig 58 Fracture of the buccal wall with a temporary filling is a specific indication for an onlay.

MO, OD cavity: Onlay

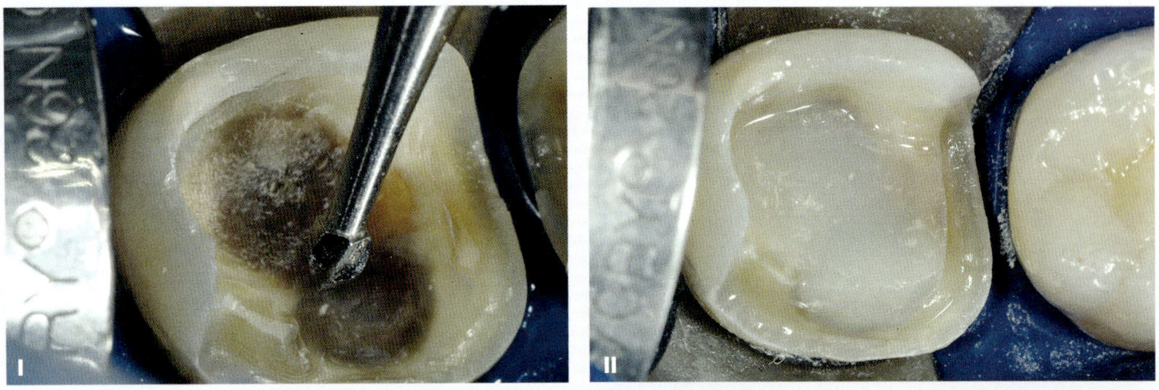

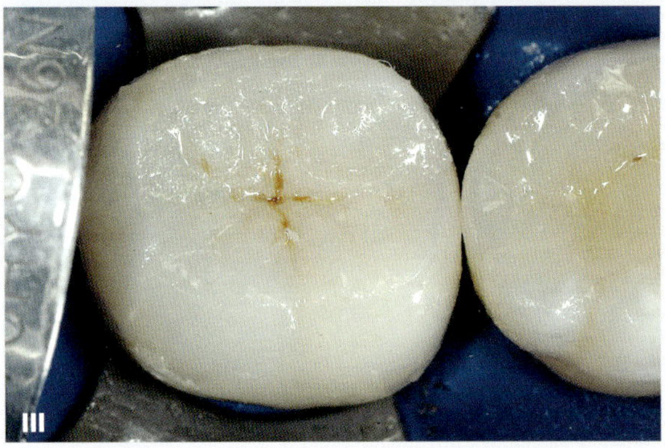

Fig 59 Removal of decayed tissue with a very low speed bur *(I)*, execution of buildup and preparation of an onlay *(II)*, and view of restoration after cementation *(III)*.

MO, OD cavity: Onlay

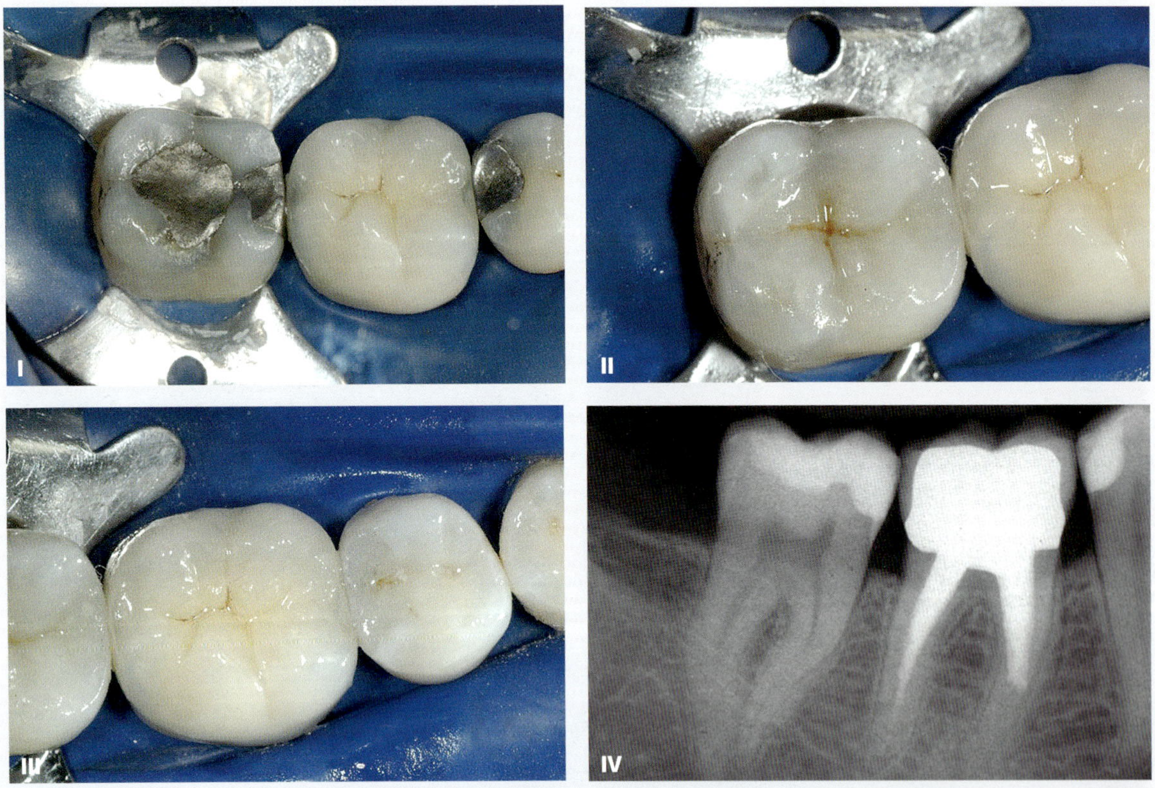

Fig 60 Indirect restorations (mandibular right second molar) and direct restorations (mandibular right second premolar) for replacement of defective amalgam fillings *(I–III)*. A post-cementation radiograph clearly shows correct marginal seals and ideal emergence profiles *(IV)*.

MO, OD cavity: Onlay

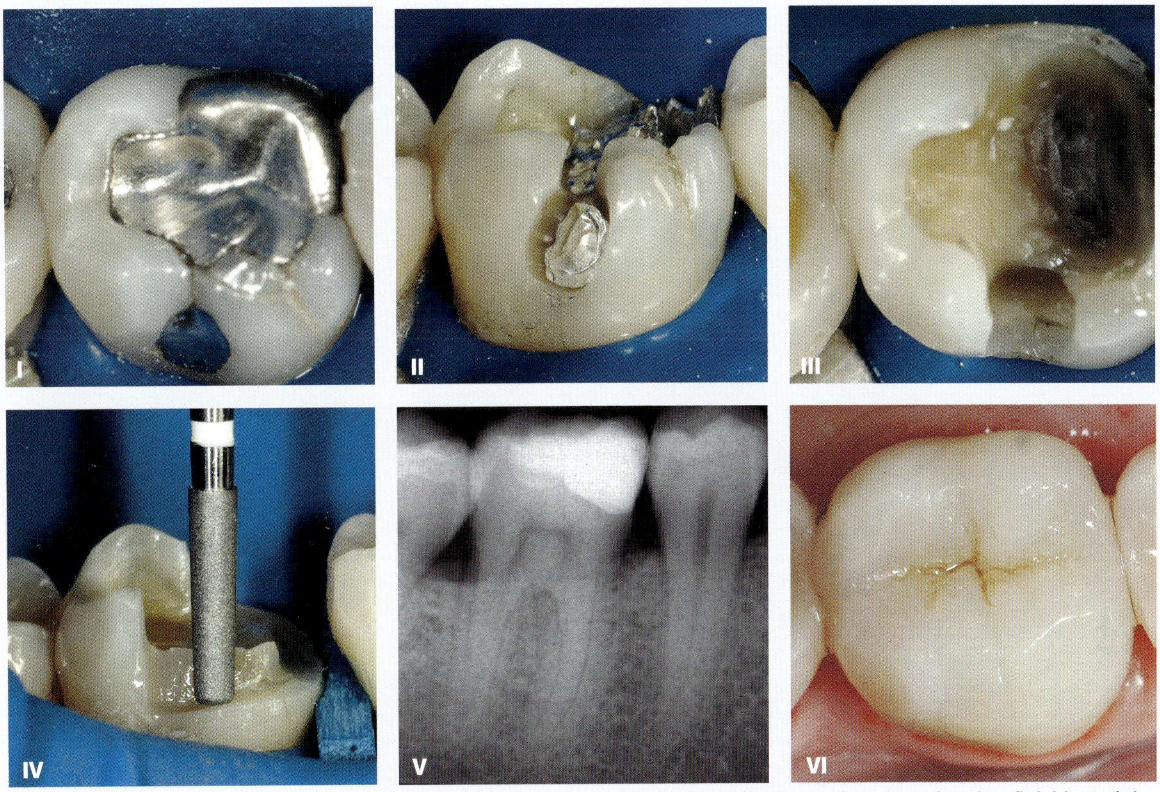

Fig 61 A leaking amalgam onlay *(I–III)* is replaced by a composite onlay. Intraoperative view showing finishing of the cavity with a bur *(IV)*, postoperative radiograph *(V)*, and cemented restoration *(VI)*.

MO, OD cavity: Onlay

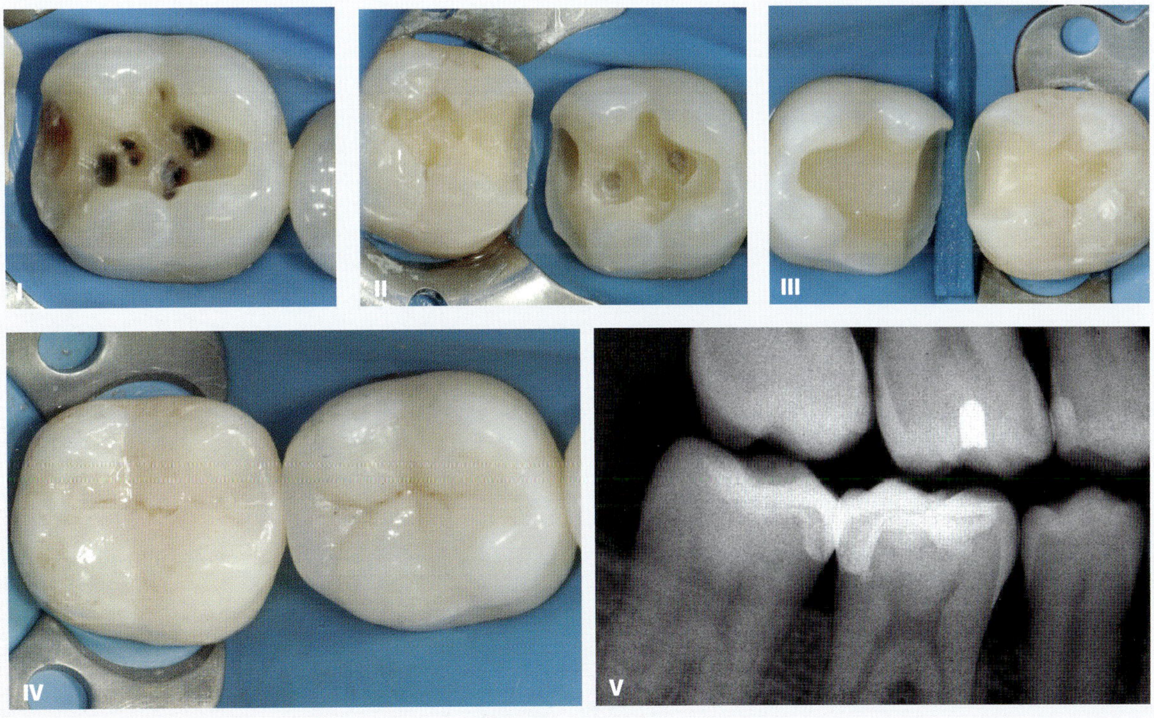

Fig 62 Removal of decay in the mandibular left second molar *(I, II)*, preparation of cavities after buildup with insertion of a wooden wedge to facilitate cementation of the restorations *(III)*, cemented inlay and onlay *(IV)*, and follow-up radiograph *(V)* showing cemented restorations and caries lesions in the maxillary teeth, which clearly require monitoring.

MO, OD cavity: Onlay

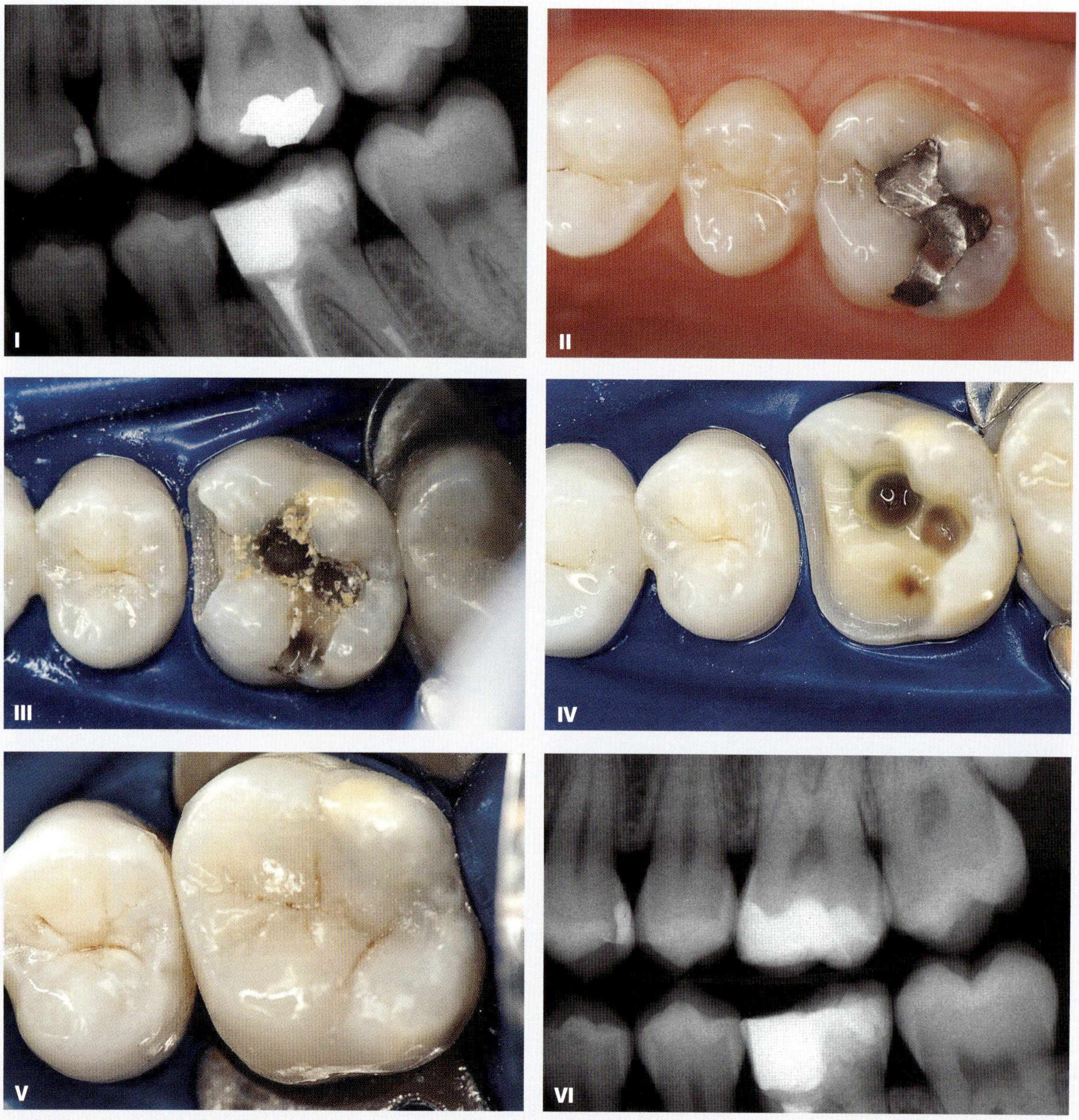

Fig 63 The maxillary left first molar shows a mesial caries lesion and infiltration of the old occlusopalatal restoration *(I, II)*. After the cavity was cleaned, an onlay was prepared with removal of the mesiopalatal wall because the thicknesses were insufficient *(III)*. Preparation of a 90-degree shoulder margin *(IV)*. Clinical and radiographic views following cementation *(V, VI)*.

MO, OD cavity: Onlay

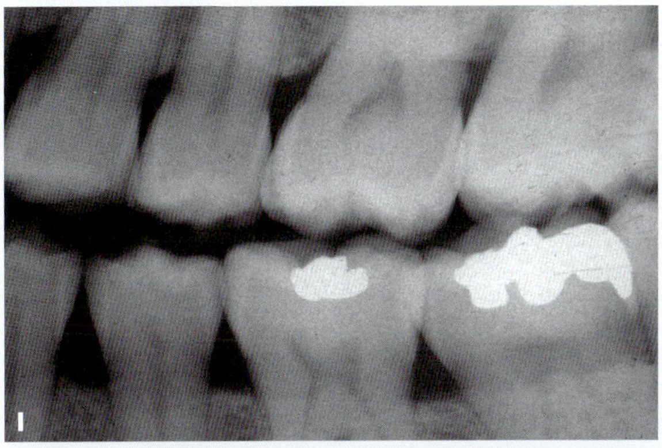

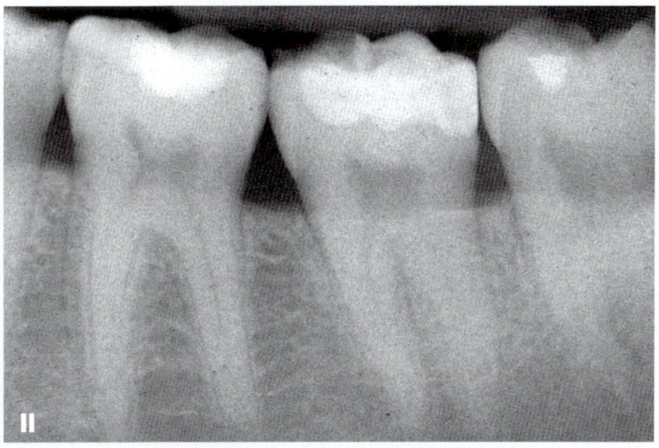

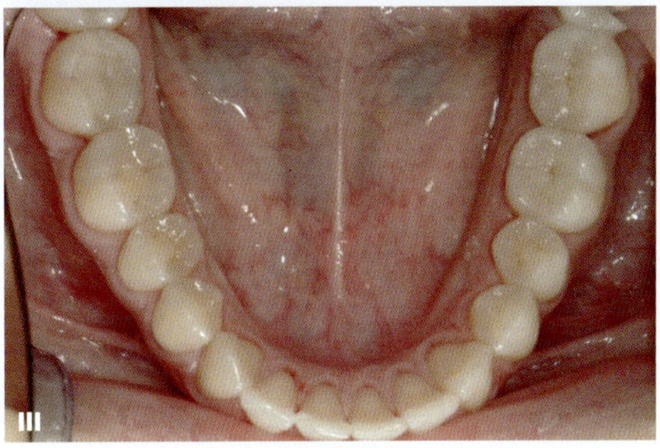

Fig 64 Mandibular arch 5 years after carrying out direct and indirect restorations in both quadrants.

MO, OD cavity: Onlay

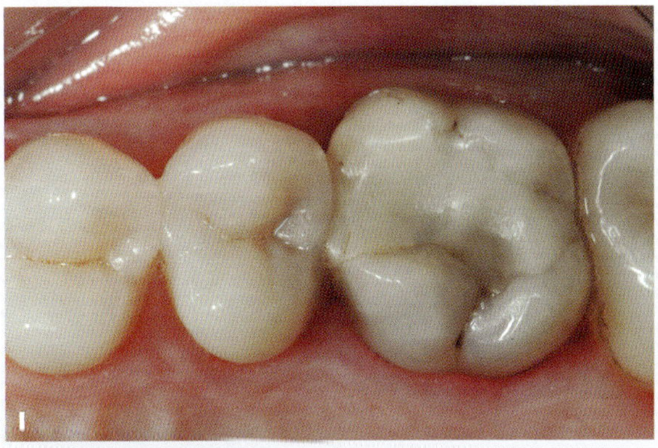

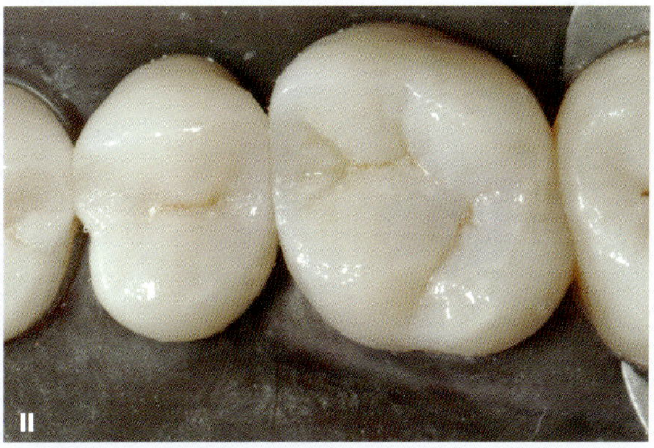

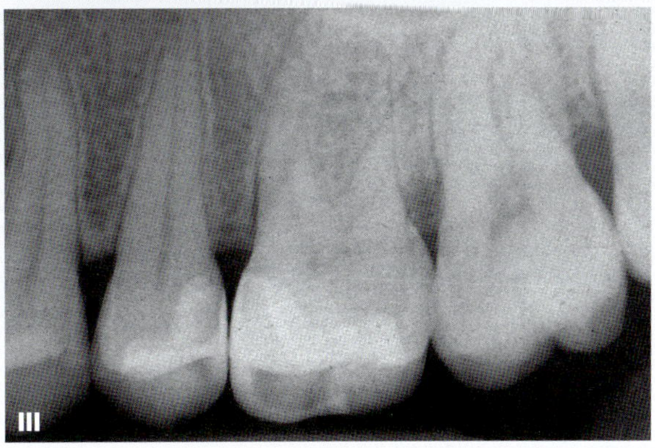

Fig 65 The composite restorations of the maxillary left second premolar and first molar are absolutely defective *(I)*. The clinical view shows the new composite inlays *(II)* to be much more satisfactory, while the follow-up radiograph reveals impeccable emergence profiles and marginal seals *(III)*.

MO, OD cavity: Onlay

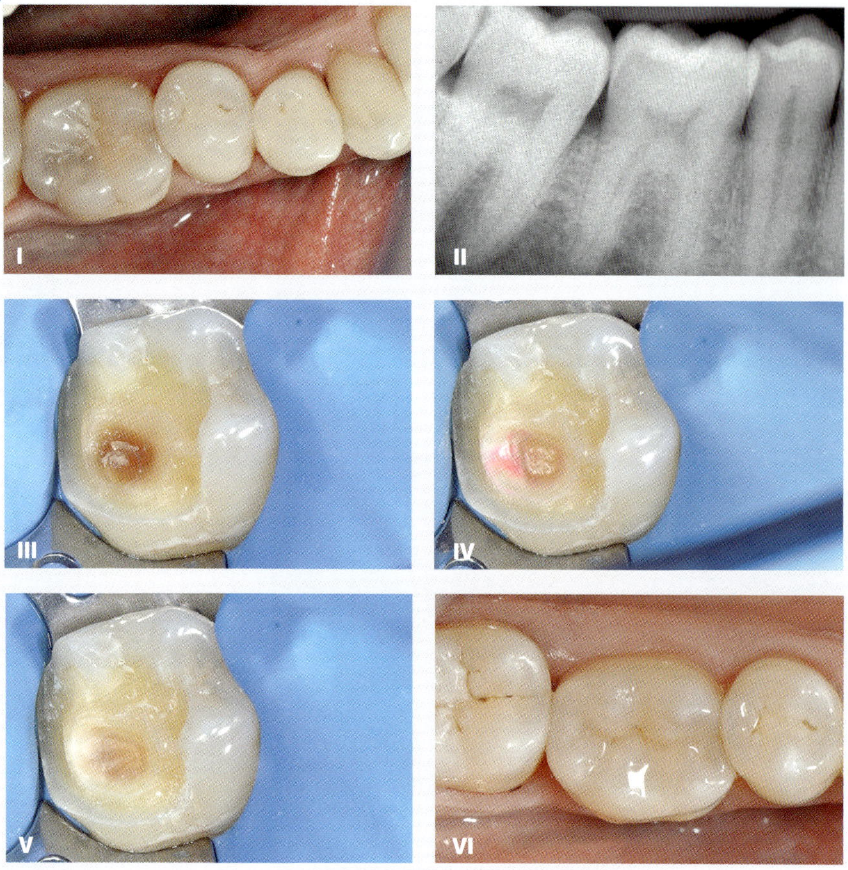

Fig 66 Very deep decay in the mandibular right first molar *(I–III)*. The aid of a caries detector is useful in providing an extra check that all the soft tissue has been removed *(IV)*. Final preparation *(V)* and clinical view of result *(VI)*.

MO, OD cavity: Onlay

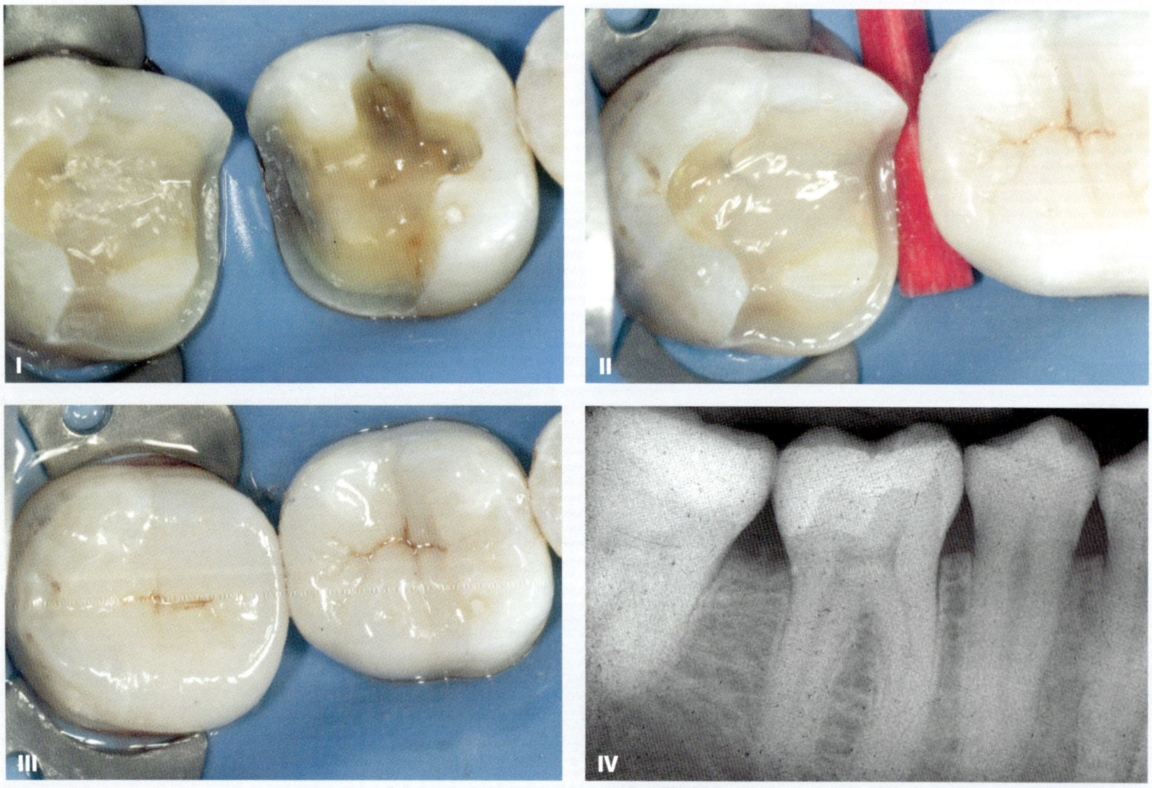

Fig 67 Classic preparation with shoulder margins for the onlays *(I, II)*. Restorations cemented and follow-up radiograph *(III, IV)*.

MO, OD cavity: Onlay

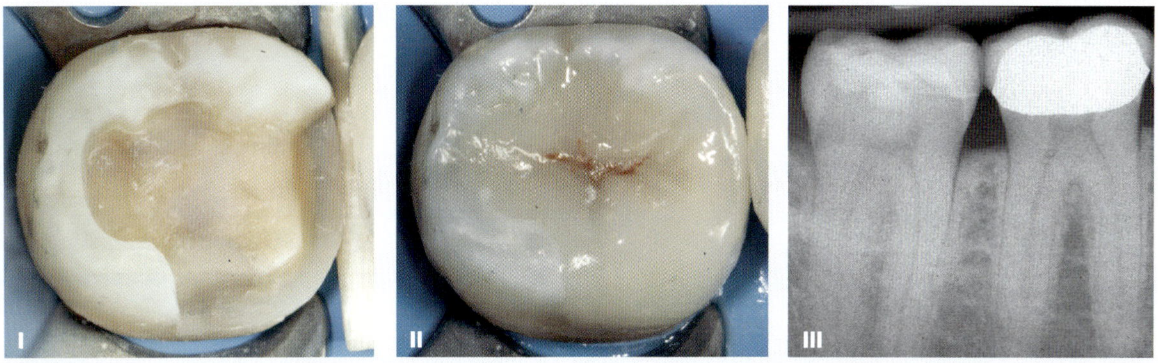

Fig 68 Yet another demonstration that the results are routinely very satisfactory when the protocol is followed.

MO, OD cavity: Onlay

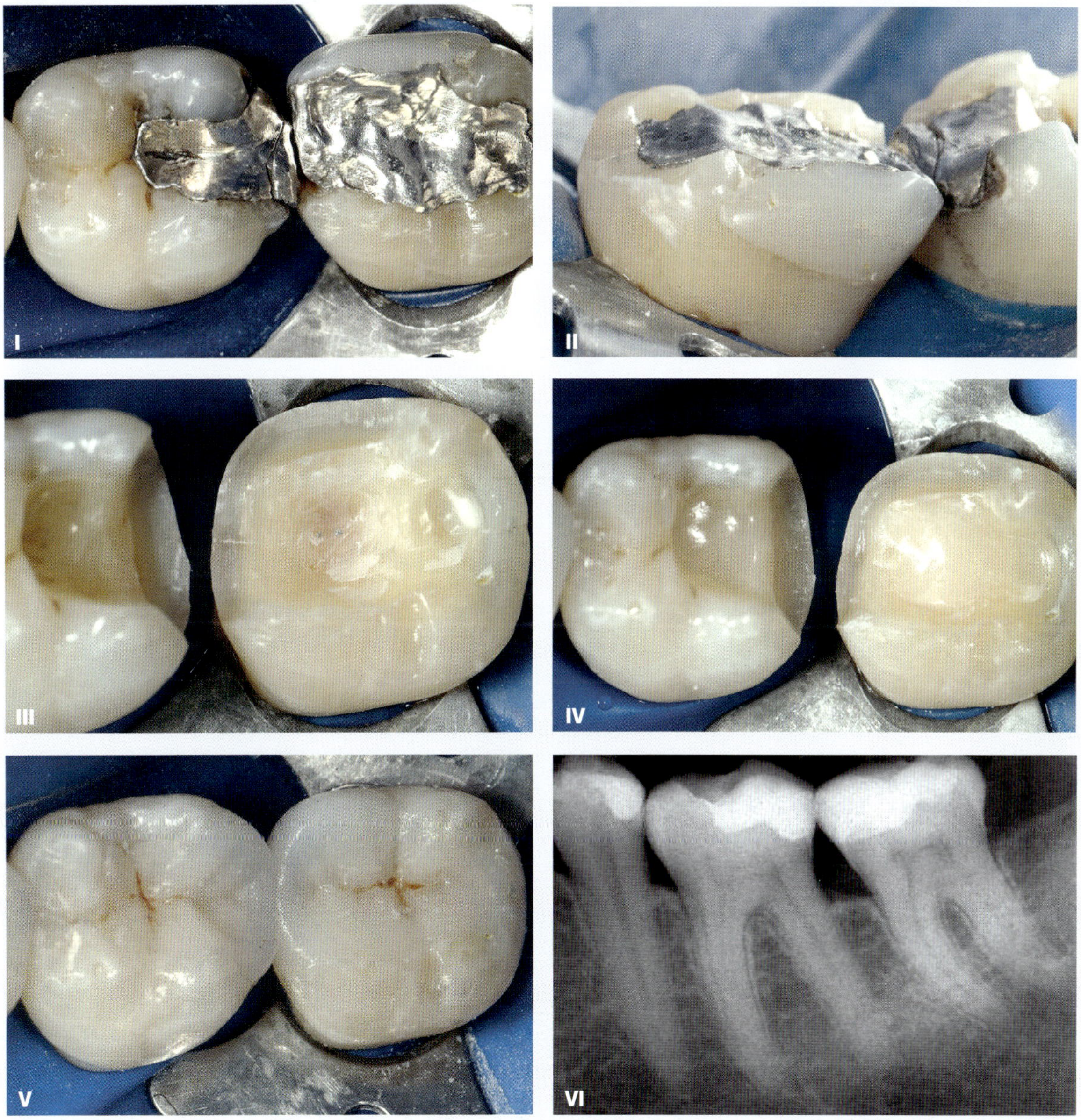

Fig 69 Two mandibular left molars with suboptimal amalgam restorations and a previous fracture of the lingual wall of the second molar. After preparation of the cavity and cementation of the partial restorations, the postoperative radiograph shows a very successful outcome.

MO, OD cavity: Onlay

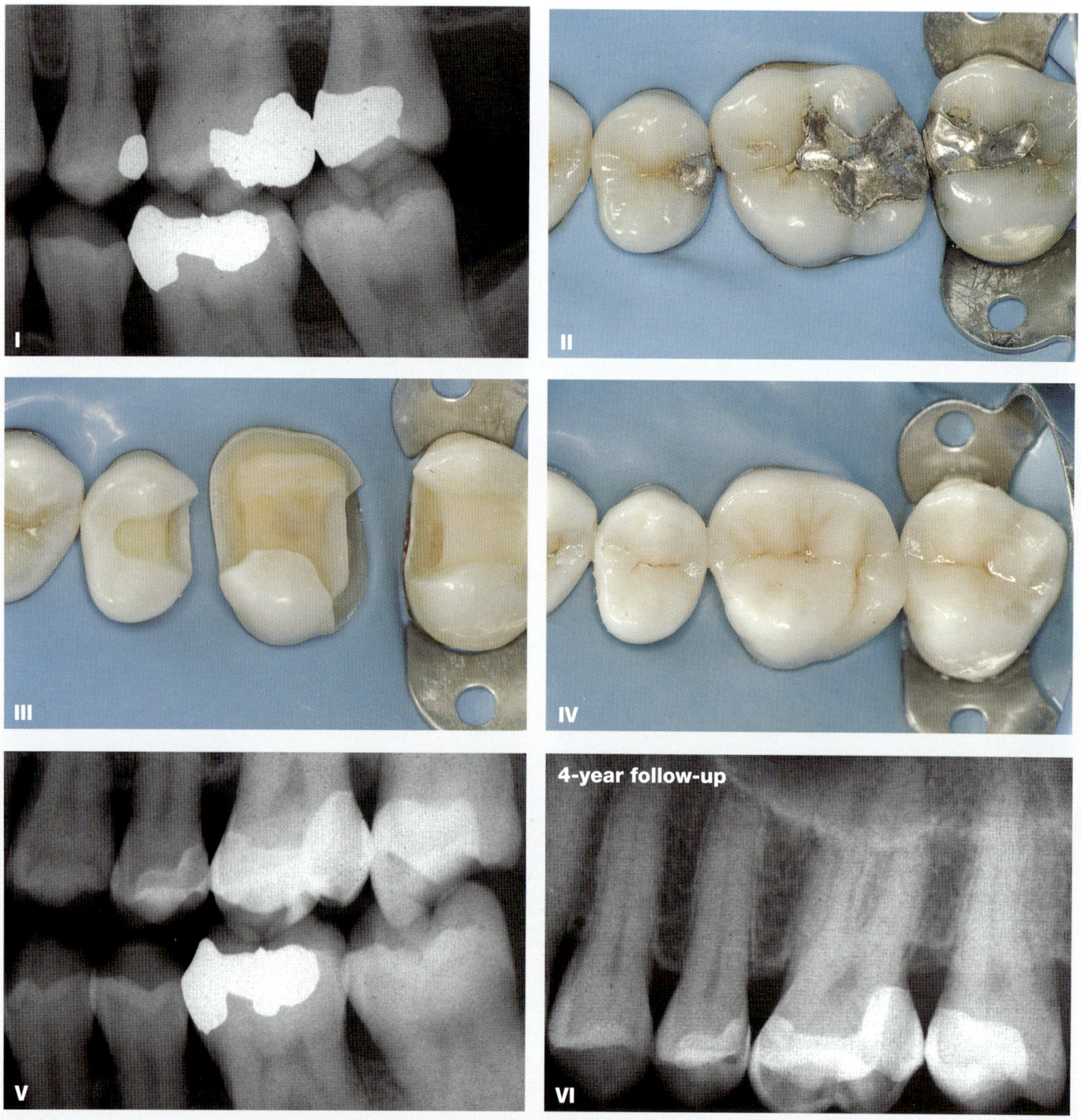

Fig 70 Replacement of three poor amalgam restorations *(I, II)* in the maxillary left quadrant (deep decay on the first molar), with two inlays for the second premolar and second molar and an onlay for the first molar. The depth of the margin of the first molar is evident, leading to consequent difficulties in isolation with rubber dam despite previous periodontal surgery *(III)*. Inlays cemented *(IV)* with satisfactory contact surfaces. The bitewing radiograph at the end of treatment *(V)* and periapical radiograph at 4-year follow-up *(VI)* reveal the absence of pulp lesions, an effective marginal seal, and accurate emergence profiles. (Courtesy of Dr Lavinia Landi.)

MO, OD cavity: Onlay

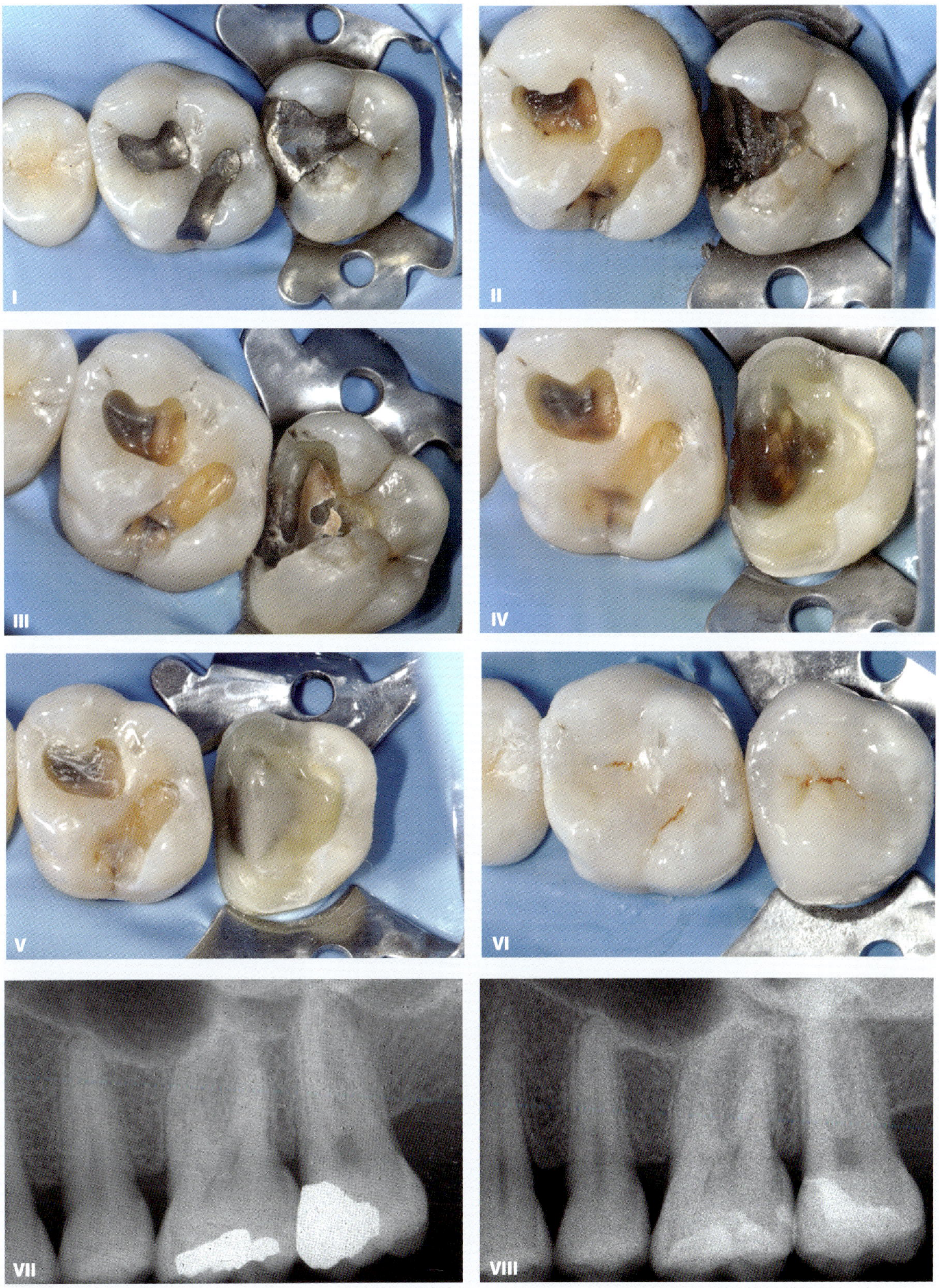

Fig 71 A positive vitality test for the second molar led to an attempt to execute an onlay after duly informing the patient of the possible risks of future endodontic treatment in view of the depth of the caries lesion *(I–VII)*. Follow-up radiograph after 3 years *(VIII)*.

MO, OD cavity: Onlay

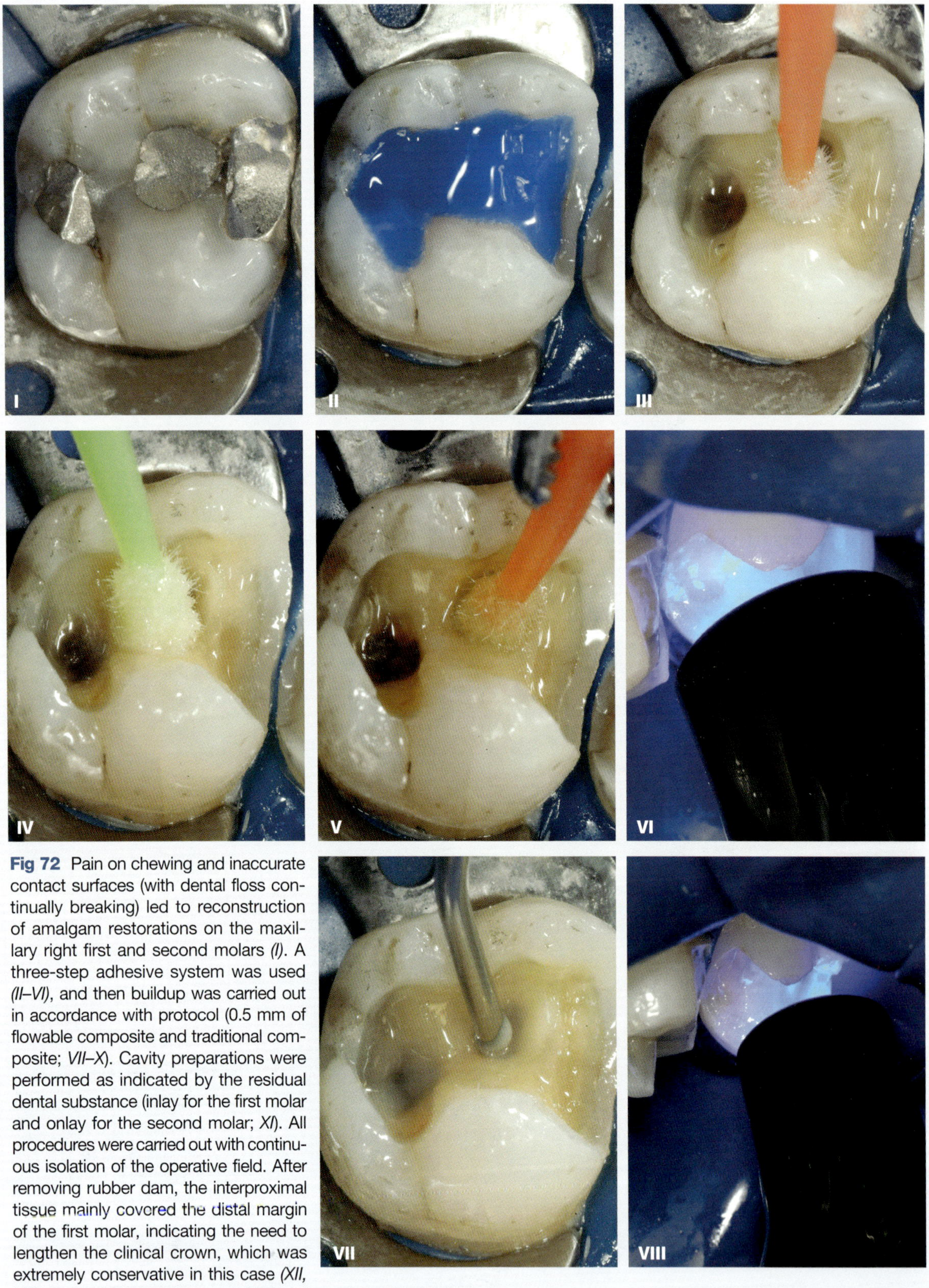

Fig 72 Pain on chewing and inaccurate contact surfaces (with dental floss continually breaking) led to reconstruction of amalgam restorations on the maxillary right first and second molars *(I)*. A three-step adhesive system was used *(II–VI)*, and then buildup was carried out in accordance with protocol (0.5 mm of flowable composite and traditional composite; *VII–X*). Cavity preparations were performed as indicated by the residual dental substance (inlay for the first molar and onlay for the second molar; *XI*). All procedures were carried out with continuous isolation of the operative field. After removing rubber dam, the interproximal tissue mainly covered the distal margin of the first molar, indicating the need to lengthen the clinical crown, which was extremely conservative in this case *(XII, XIII)*. A view of the working cast *(XIV)* and teeth isolated by dam before cementation *(XV)* shows the extent to which periodontal surgery complements restorative surgery. Intraoperative stage of cementation *(XVI, XVII)* and cemented inlays *(XVIII)*. Radiograph at the end of treatment *(XIX)*.

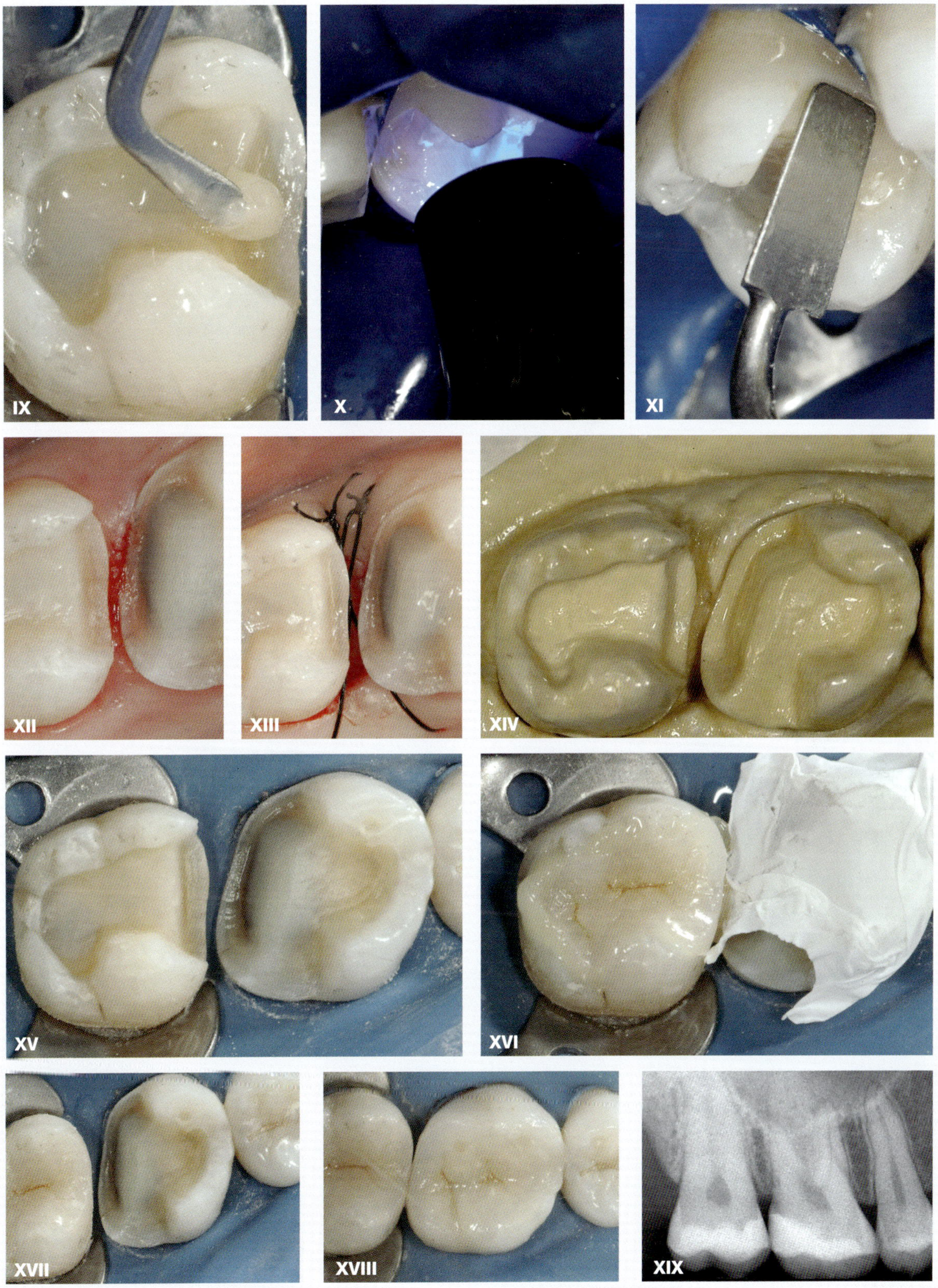

Fig 72 *(continued)*

MO, OD cavity: Onlay

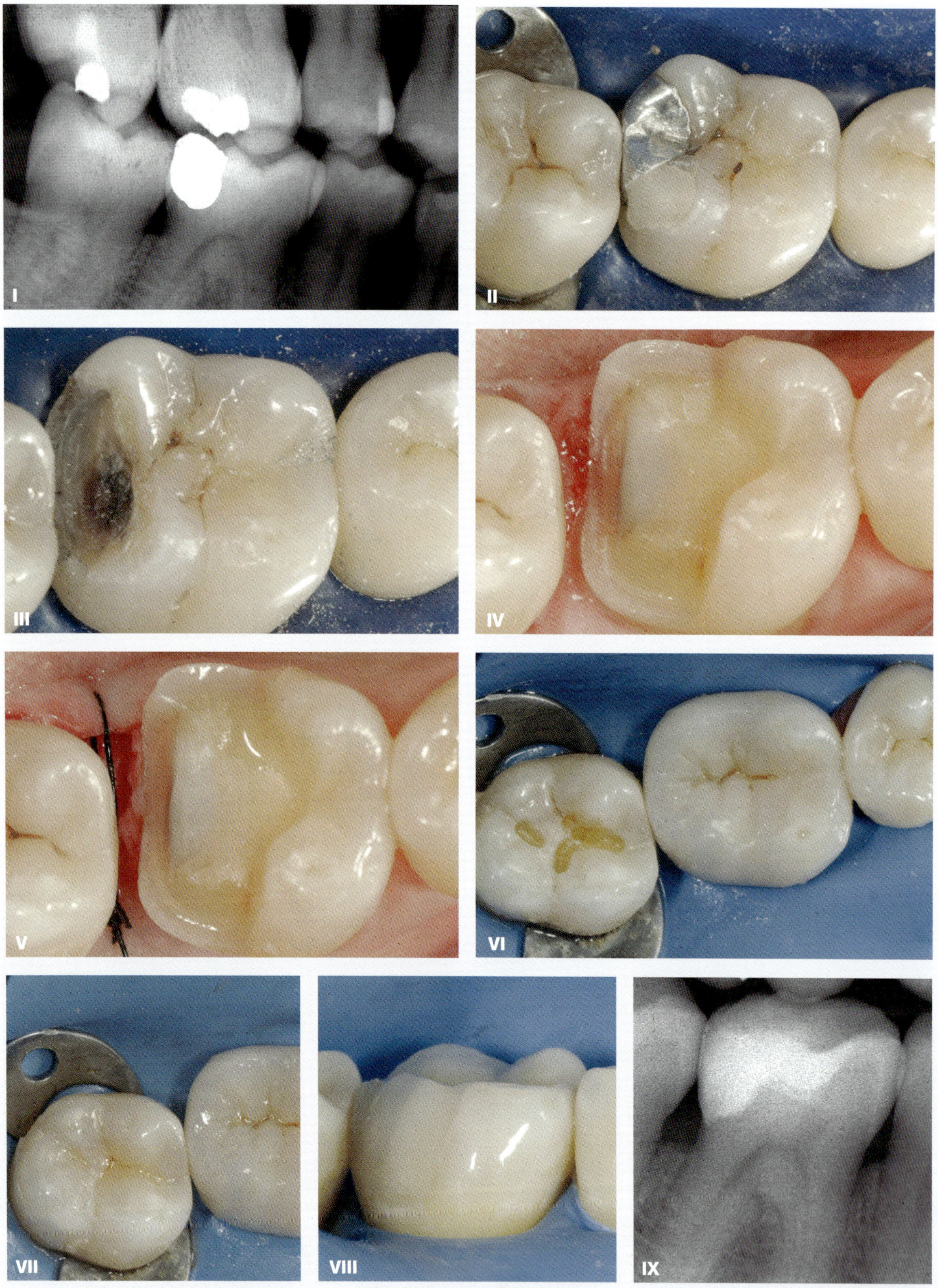

Fig 73 Fracture of the buccal cusp, temporarily repaired with resin *(I, II)*, led to preparation of a cavity with coverage of the distobuccal and distolingual cusps *(III)*. Lengthening of the clinical crown, advisable in order to expose the distal margin, was very conservative in this case as well *(IV, V)*. View of cemented restoration and follow-up radiograph *(VI–IX)*.

MO, OD cavity: Onlay

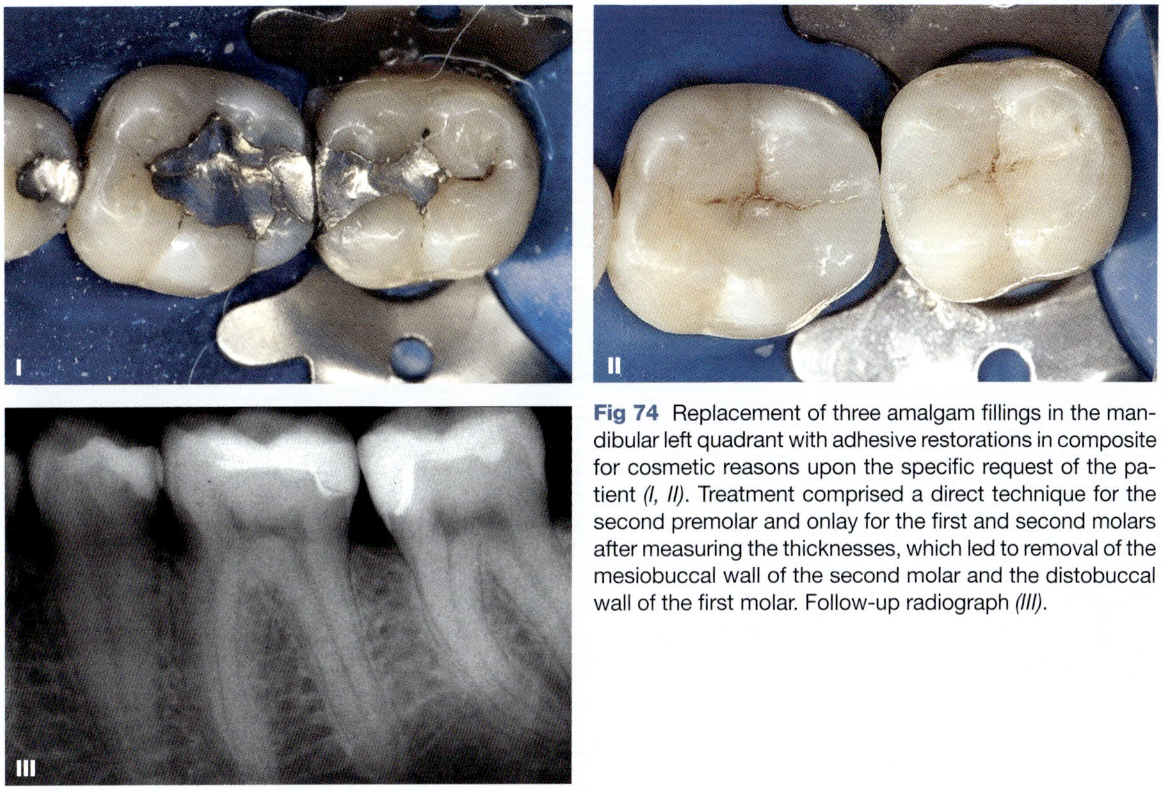

Fig 74 Replacement of three amalgam fillings in the mandibular left quadrant with adhesive restorations in composite for cosmetic reasons upon the specific request of the patient *(I, II)*. Treatment comprised a direct technique for the second premolar and onlay for the first and second molars after measuring the thicknesses, which led to removal of the mesiobuccal wall of the second molar and the distobuccal wall of the first molar. Follow-up radiograph *(III)*.

MOD cavity: Inlay

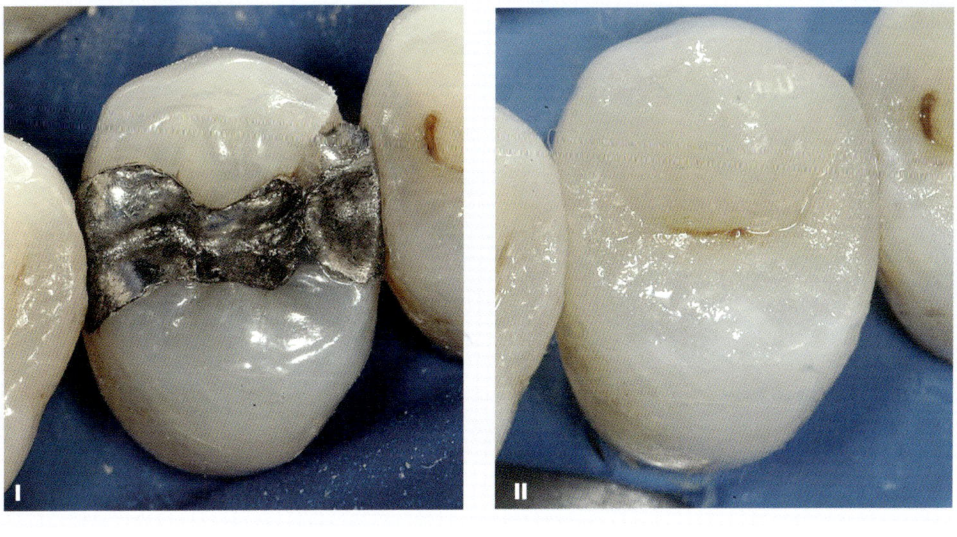

Fig 75 Fracture of the old amalgam restoration made it advisable to position a composite MOD inlay in view of the residual thicknesses.

MOD cavity: Inlay

Fig 76 A completely defective composite-amalgam restoration was removed and replaced by an MOD inlay in composite.

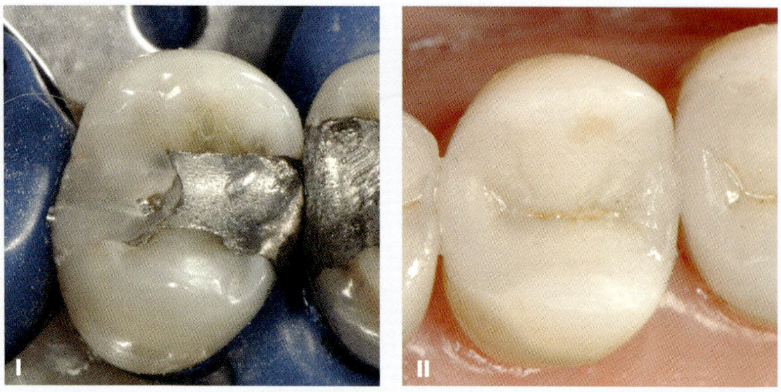

MOD cavity: Inlay

Fig 77 Typical cavity preparation for an MOD inlay. Use of interdental wedge to facilitate insertion of the inlay.

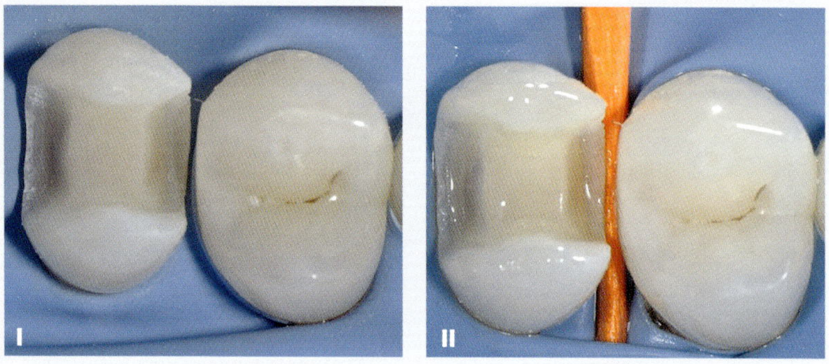

MOD cavity: Inlay

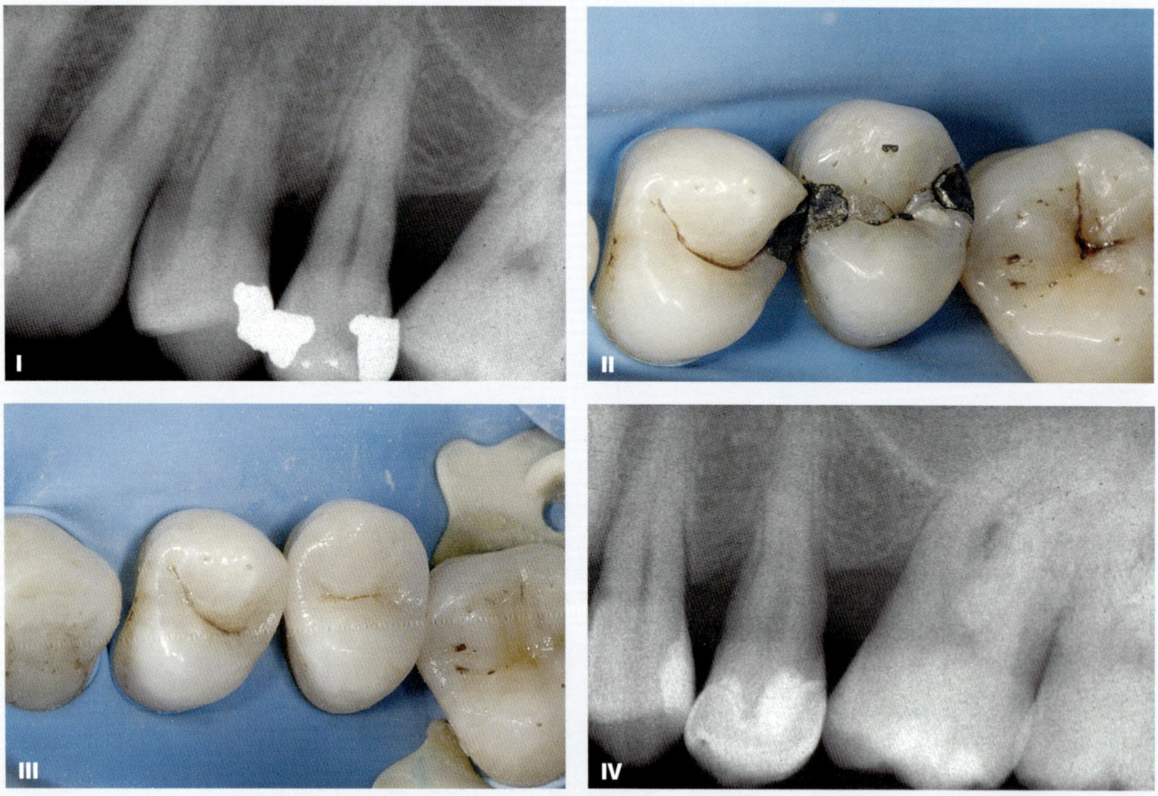

Fig 78 In a clear case of periodontal disease, the maxillary left second premolar shows deep decay and two amalgam restorations. An MOD inlay was constructed for the second premolar, and direct restoration was performed for the first molar. The follow-up radiograph 3 years later shows entirely satisfactory marginal seals and a stable periodontal situation due to regular dental hygienist visits.

MOD cavity: Inlay

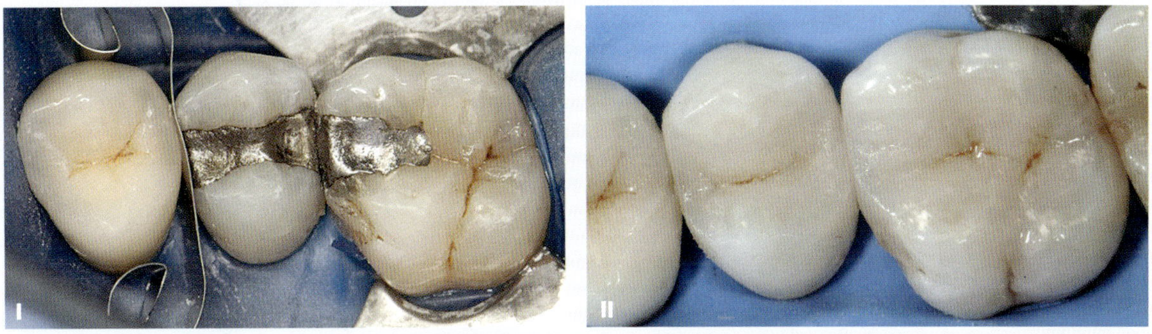

Fig 79 Another example of an inlay in an MOD cavity for a premolar and in an MO cavity for a molar. A separator was used to protect the adjacent teeth during preparation.

MOD cavity: Inlay

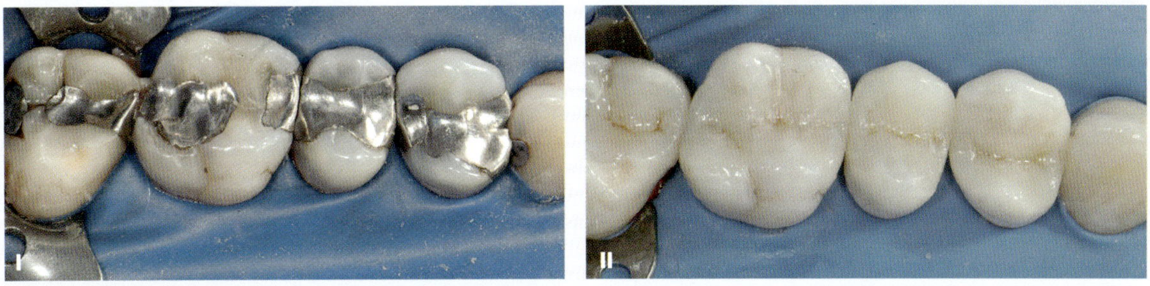

Fig 80 Defective MOD restorations in amalgam are replaced with an MOD inlay in composite. The inlays clearly display good morphology with appropriate contact surfaces.

MOD cavity: Inlay

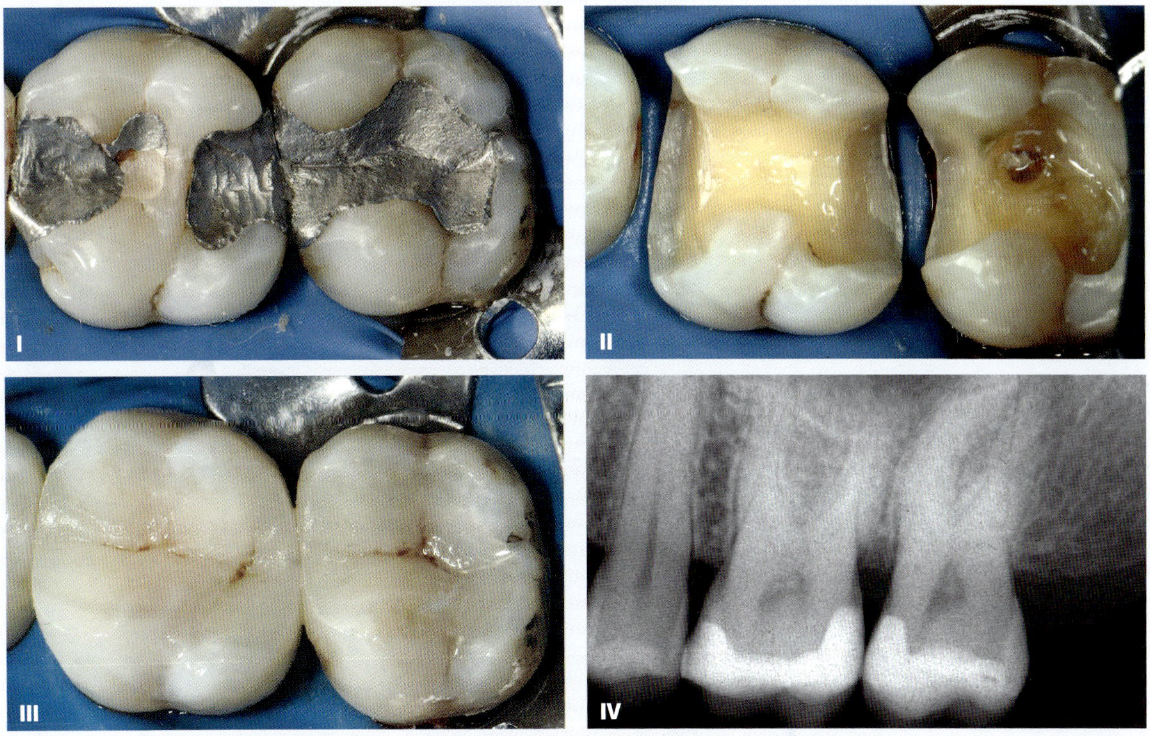

Fig 81 When replacing old amalgam restorations and after removing any decay, the next step is to measure the thicknesses at the cusp bases, which determine whether or not the walls should be removed. Clinical experience has led the author to be increasingly conservative as medium-term results emerge over the years, reflecting the performance of the materials used for the adhesive techniques.

MOD cavity: Inlay

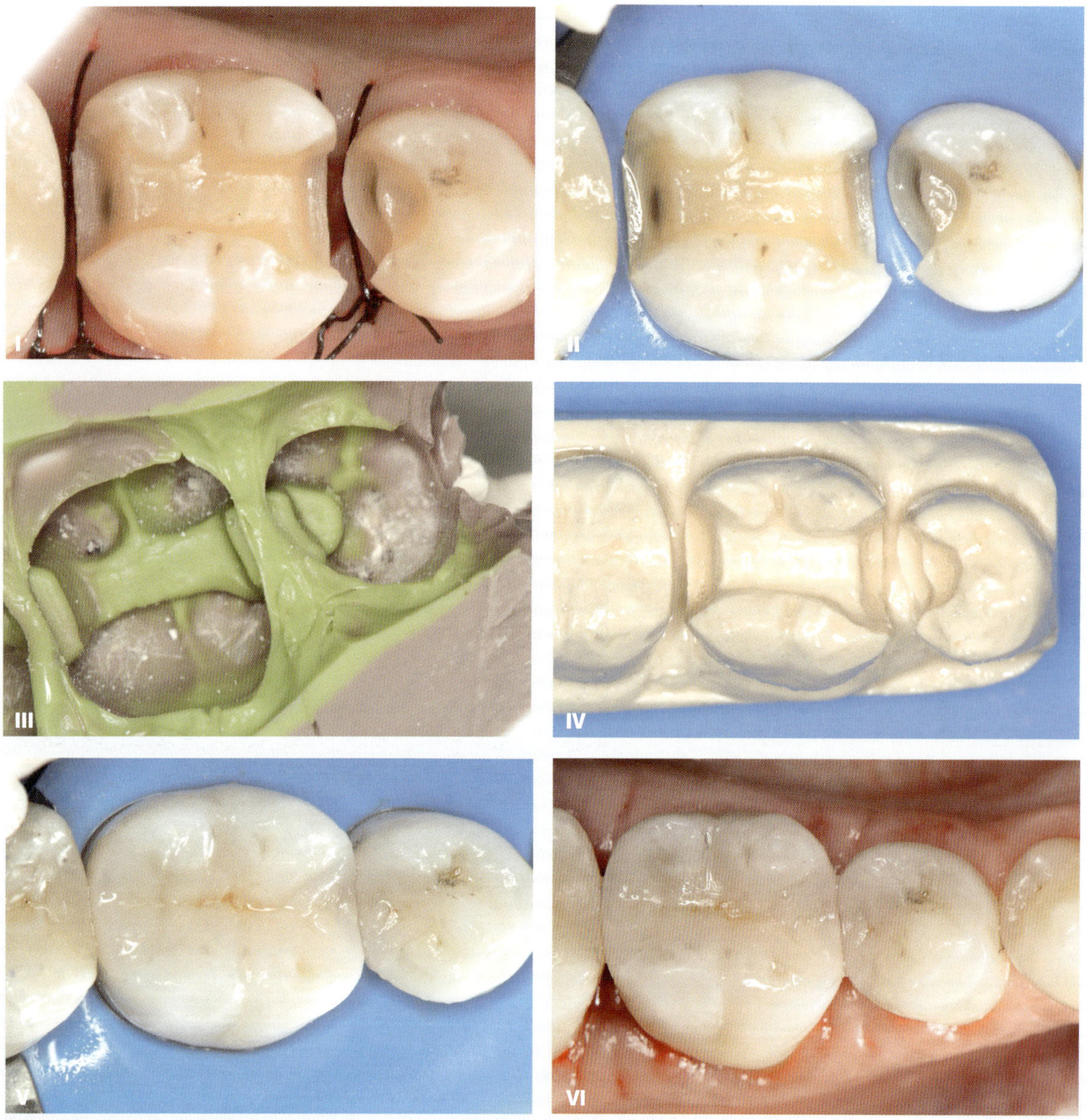

Fig 82 MOD cavity of a molar with thicknesses that indisputably suggest cavitational preparation for an inlay. The premolar clearly could have easily been treated with a direct technique, but because the patient no longer had the patience to undergo periodontal surgery or the preparation, the author opted to speed up the process, treating the small inlay with a simple Class 2 filling for purely financial reasons.

MOD cavity: Inlay

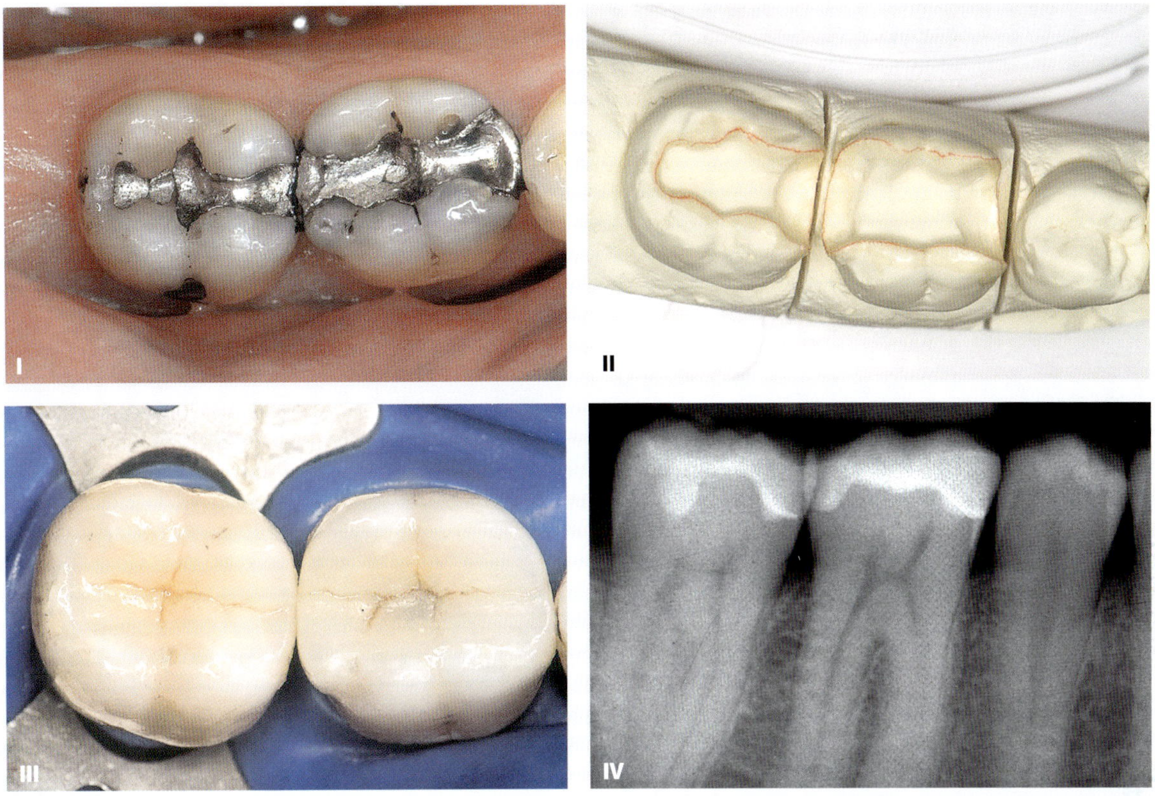

Fig 83 MOD and MO preparations were also used in this case. The follow-up radiograph shows successful marginal seals.

MOD cavity: Onlay

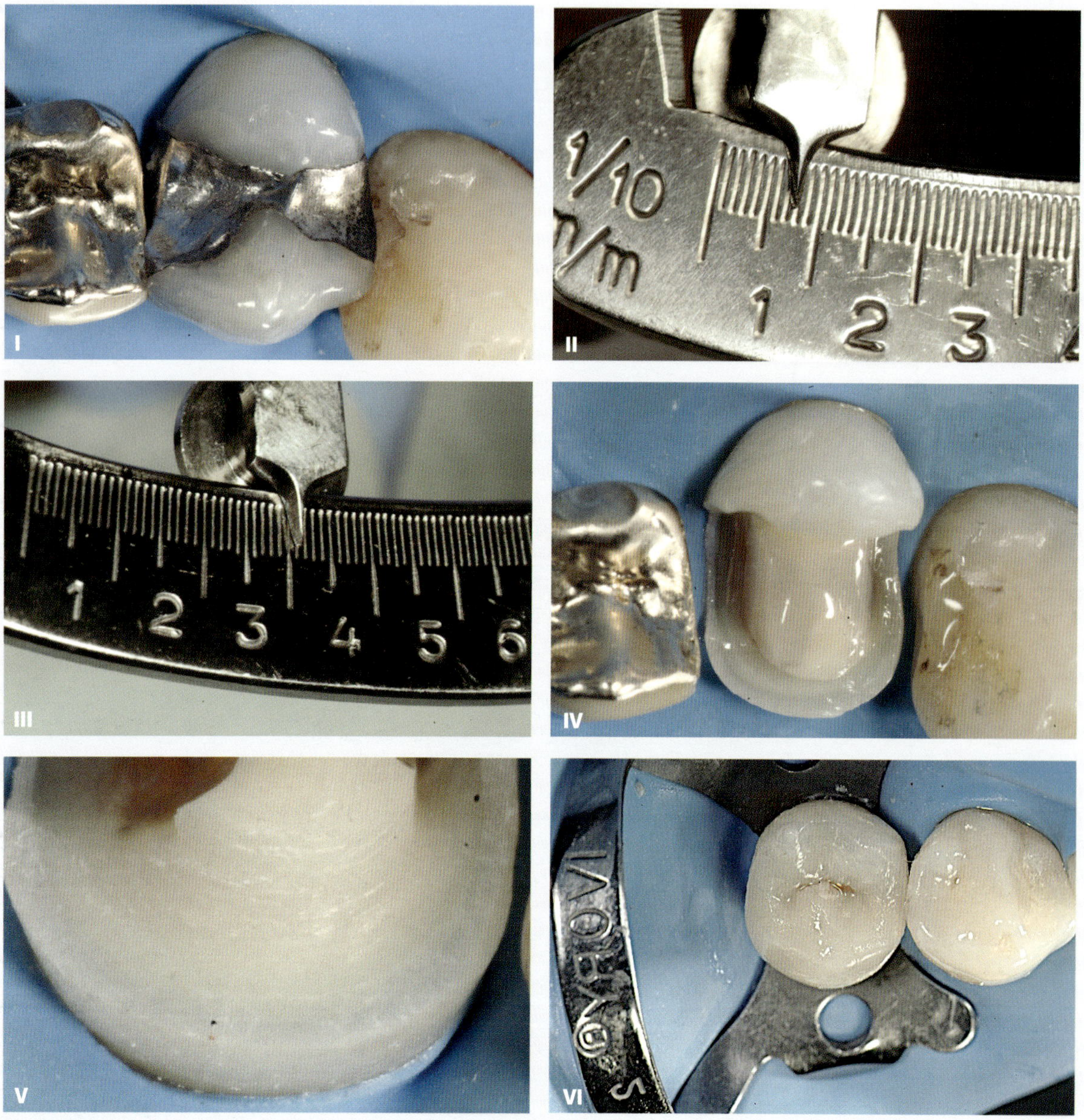

Fig 84 Typical example of how thickness measurement affects cavity preparation. In this premolar *(I)*, the values are entirely insufficient as far as the buccal aspect is concerned *(II)*. The palatal wall, on the other hand, meets all the requirements *(III)* to be left in place. Detail of the 90-degree preparation *(V)* and view of the completed restoration *(VI)*.

MOD cavity: Onlay

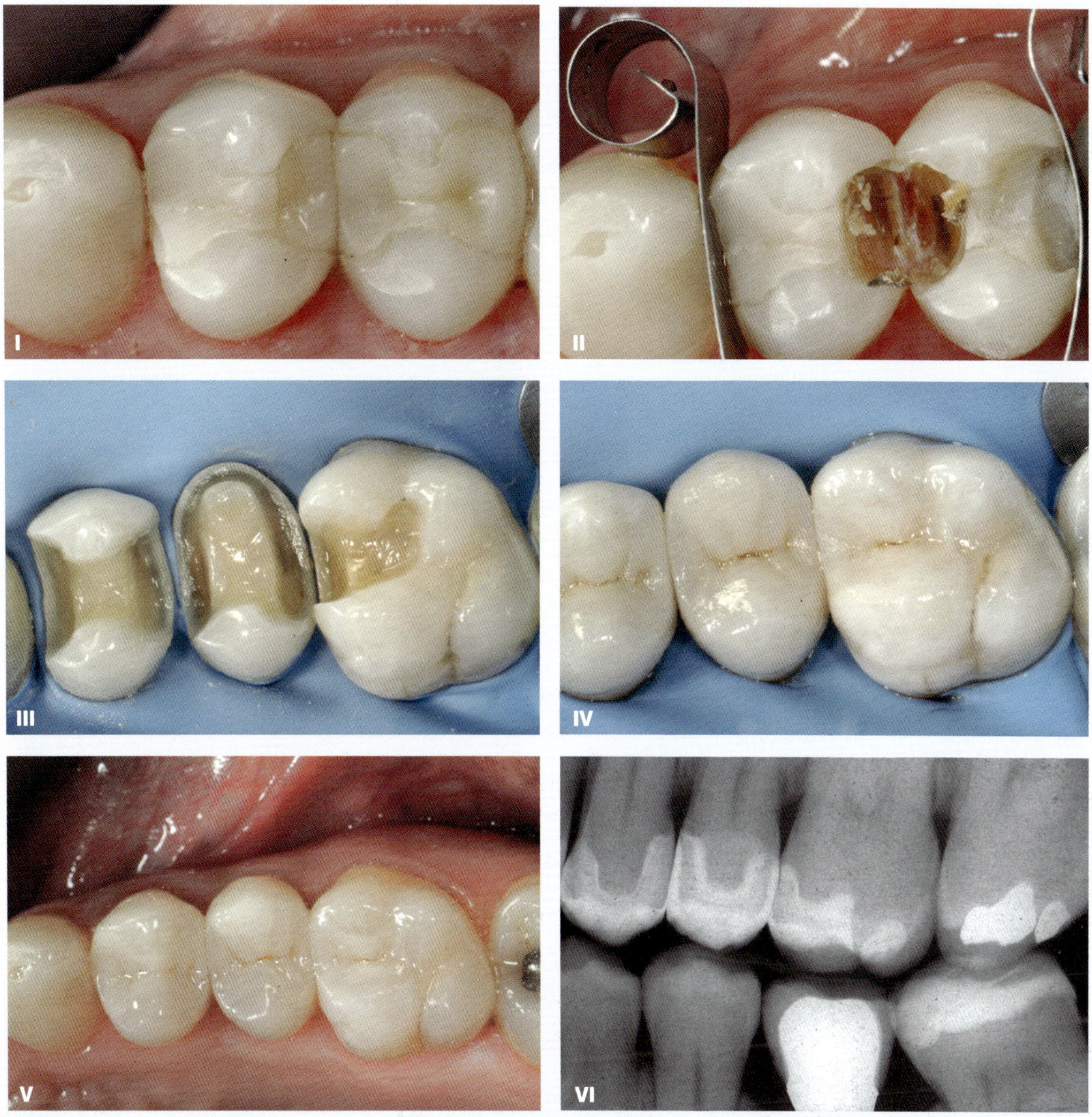

Fig 85 Restorations very recently performed by a colleague unfortunately led to sensitivity to heat and discomfort on chewing. It was inevitably necessary to repeat the restorations, which showed significant remains of caries lesions, among other things. An inlay was applied to the maxillary left first premolar and first molar, and an onlay was applied to the second premolar. A radiograph taken at the end of treatment is shown.

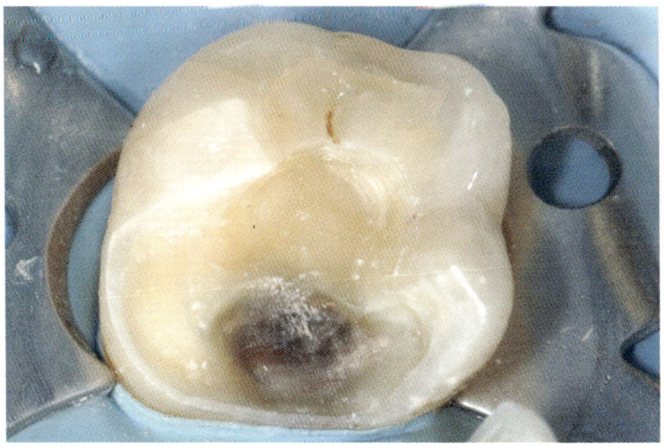

Fig 86 Example of how a cavity with deep decay should be cleaned.

MOD cavity: Onlay

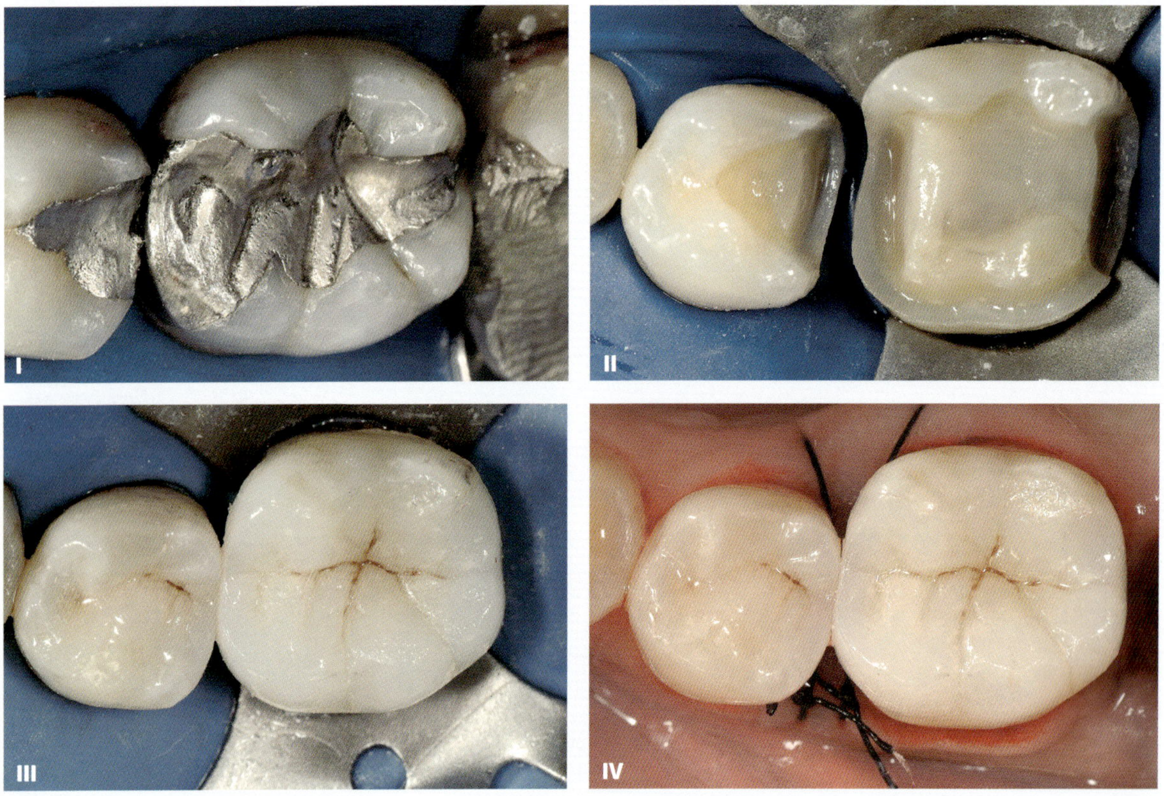

Fig 87 Preparations of cavities for an onlay and an inlay dictated by the design of previous restorations. Points to note include the effective isolation of the operative field a few minutes after the end of the periodontal surgery and the successful contact surfaces.

MOD cavity: Onlay

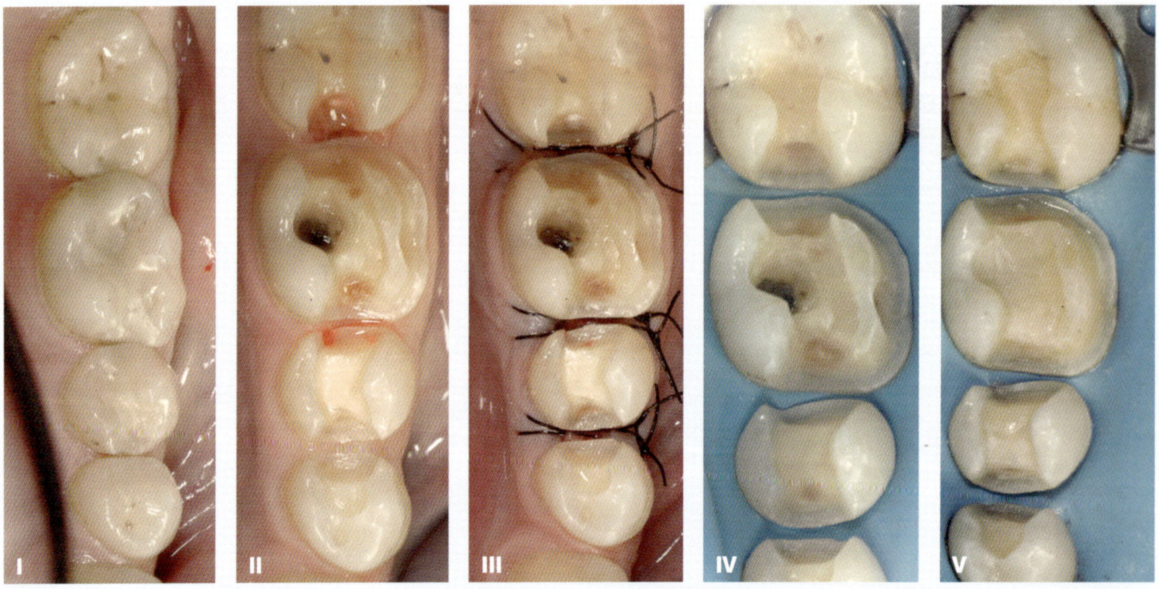

Fig 88 Importance of the interaction between periodontal and restorative surgery. Once again extremely conservative surgery allows effective isolation of the operative field, which is an essential condition for the use of adhesive techniques.

MOD cavity: Onlay

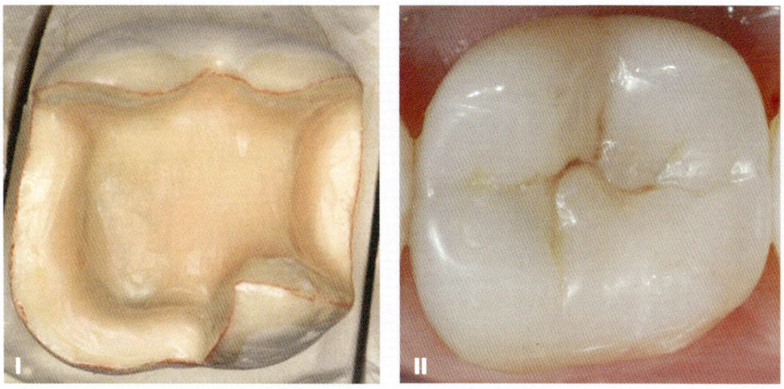

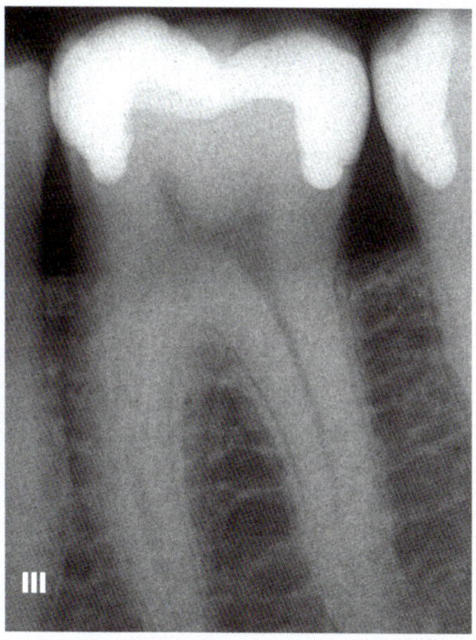

Fig 89 Working cast, onlay after cementation, and 7-year follow-up radiograph.

MOD cavity: Onlay

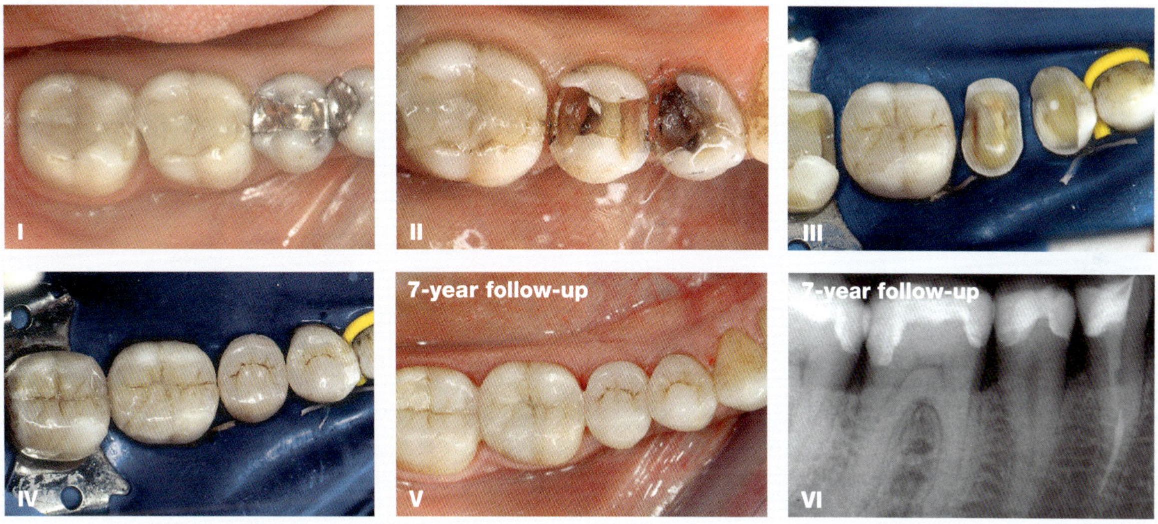

Fig 90 Restoration of a quadrant with leaking, decayed amalgam and composite *(I, II)*. Restorative treatment *(III, IV)* and 7-year clinical and radiographic follow-up *(V, VI)*.

MOD cavity: Onlay

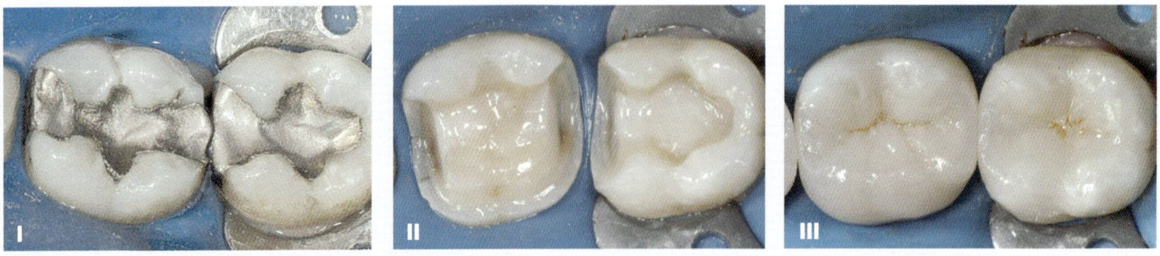

Fig 91 After routine measurement of thicknesses, leaking amalgam restorations are replaced with an onlay for the mandibular left first molar and an inlay for the second molar.

MOD cavity: Onlay

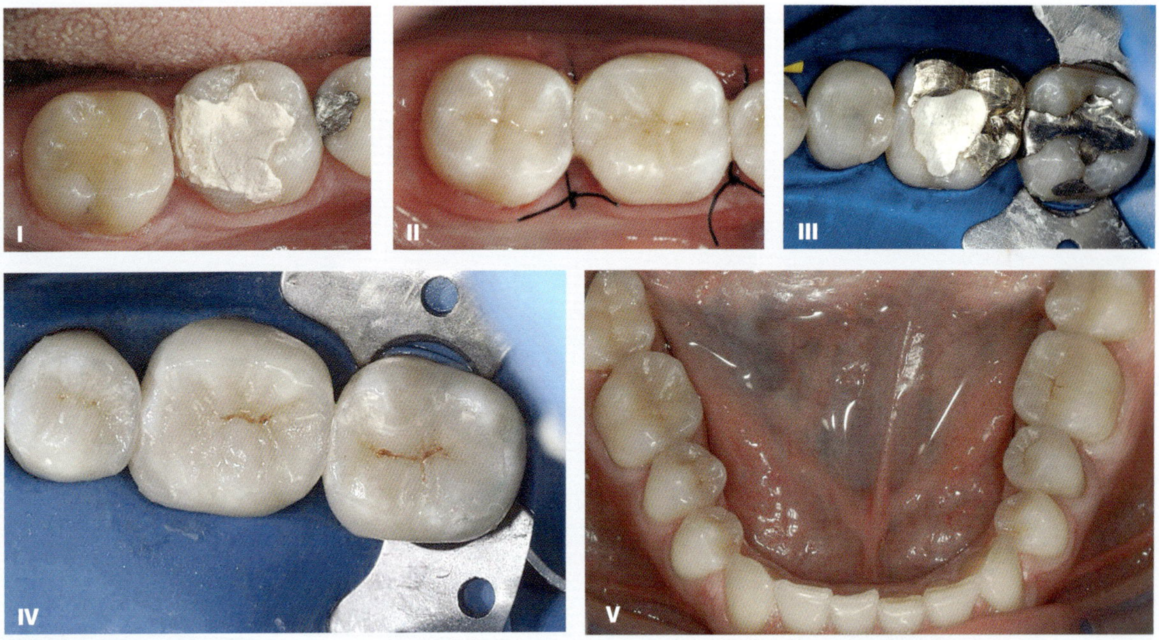

Fig 92 In this somewhat compromised mandible, interdisciplinary therapy allowed restoration of the patient's masticatory function through adhesive restorations, which were both direct (on the right second premolar) and indirect (MOD onlay for molars), and eliminated all painful symptoms.

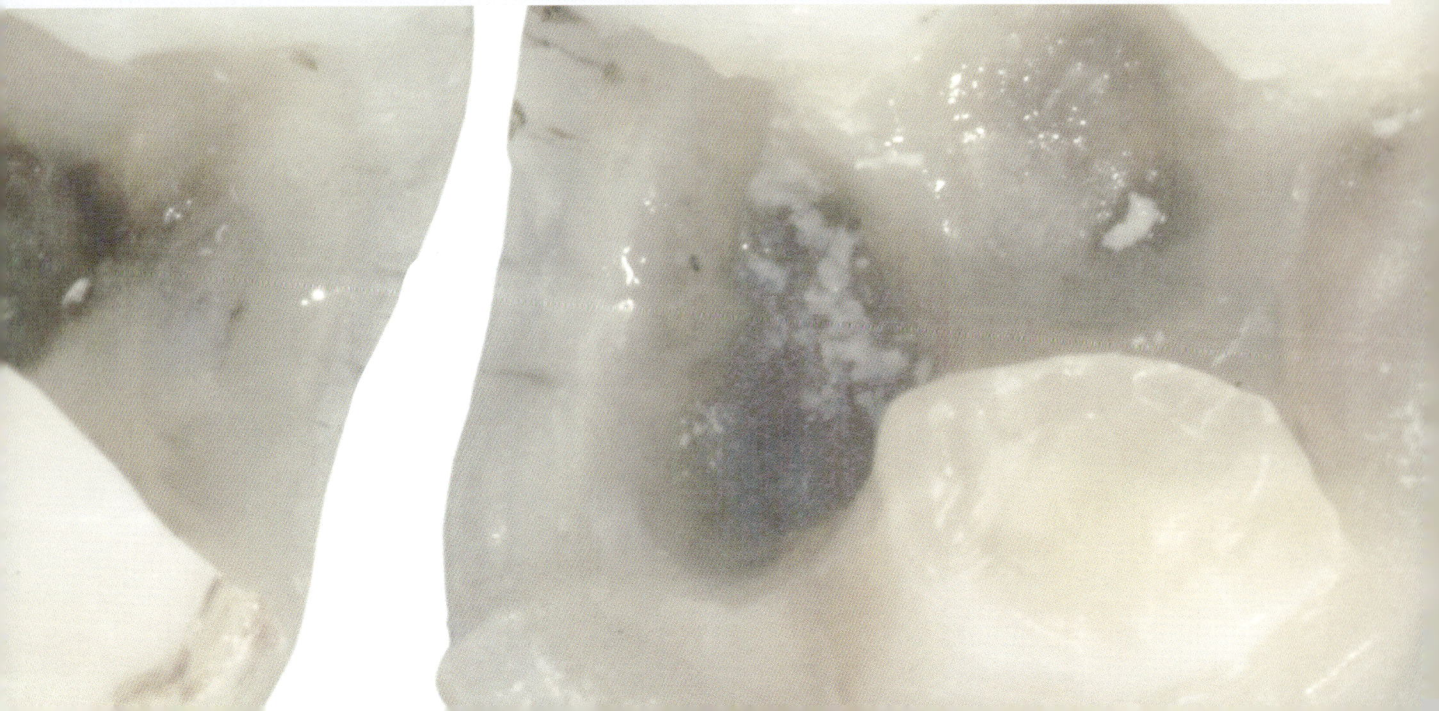

MOD cavity: Onlay

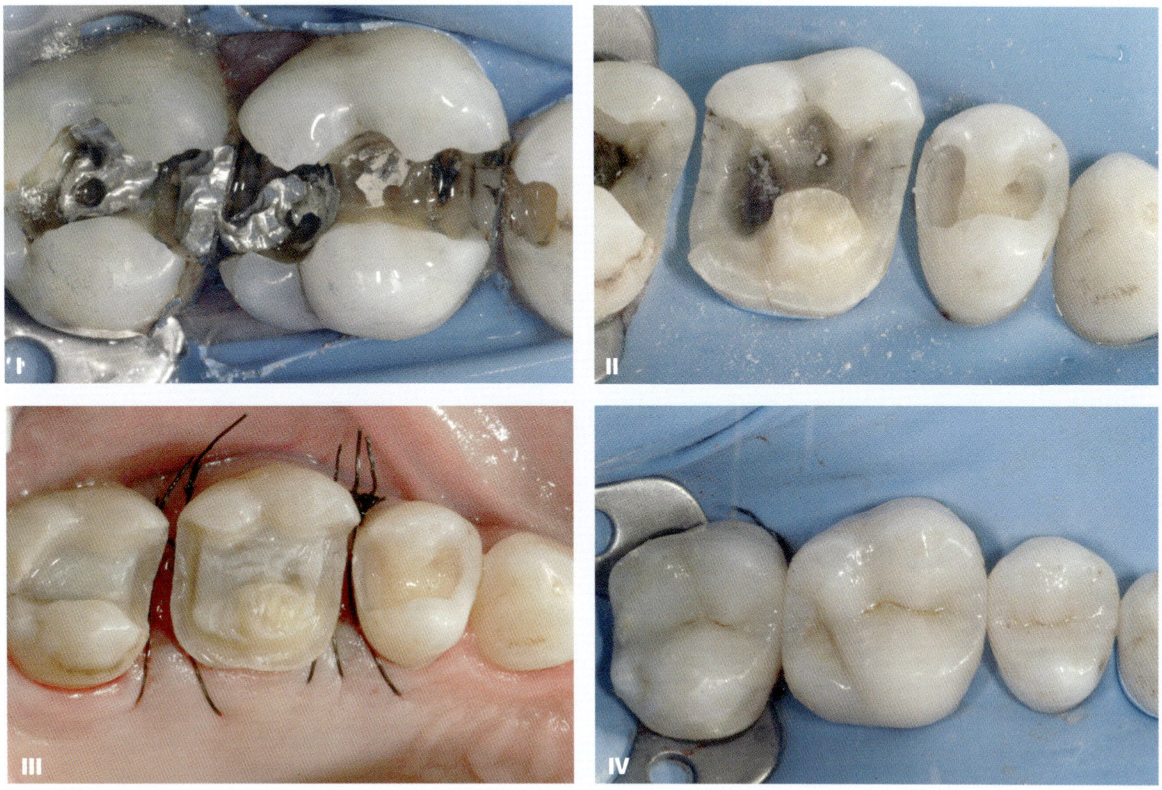

Fig 93 Removal of the buccal wall of the maxillary right first molar due to insufficient thickness followed by elimination of decayed tissues, periodontal surgery (very conservative), buildup, and cementation of the restorations.

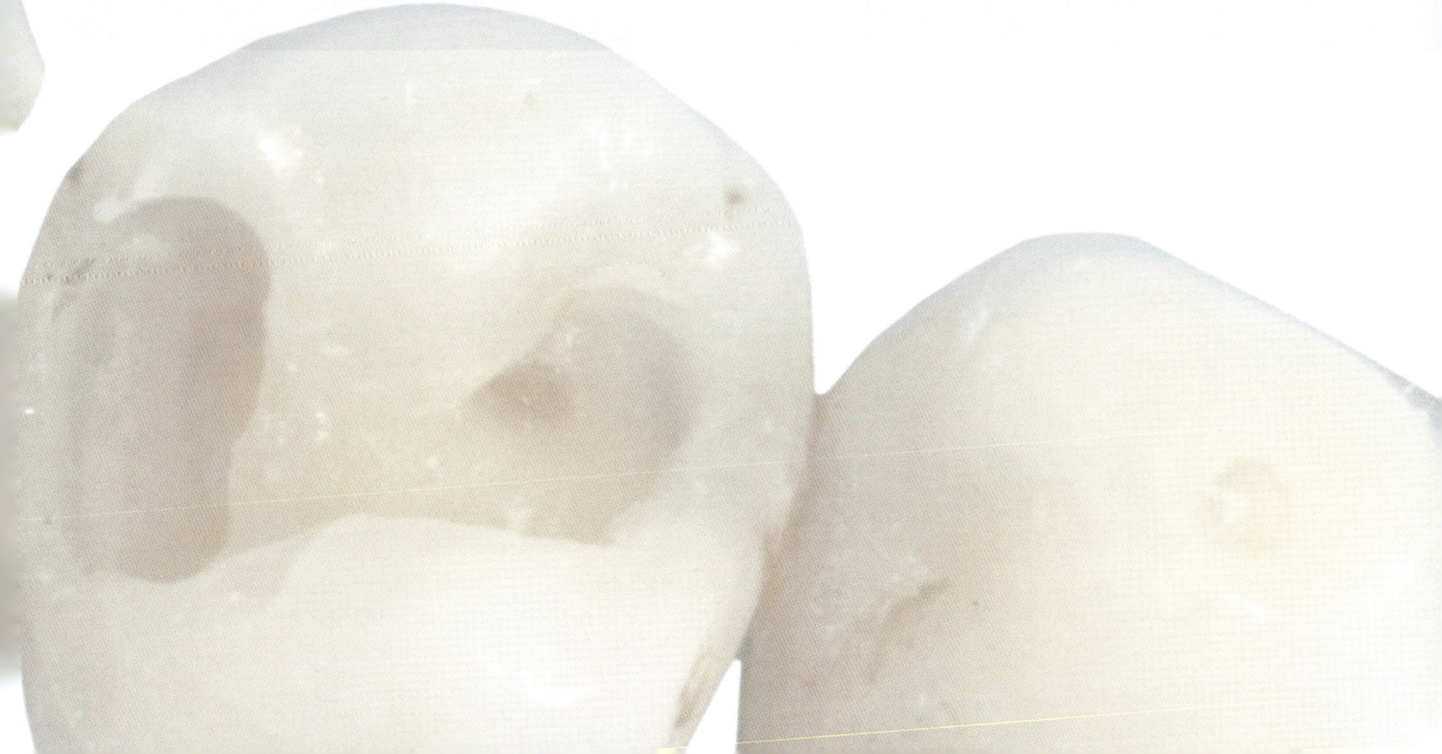

MOD cavity: Onlay

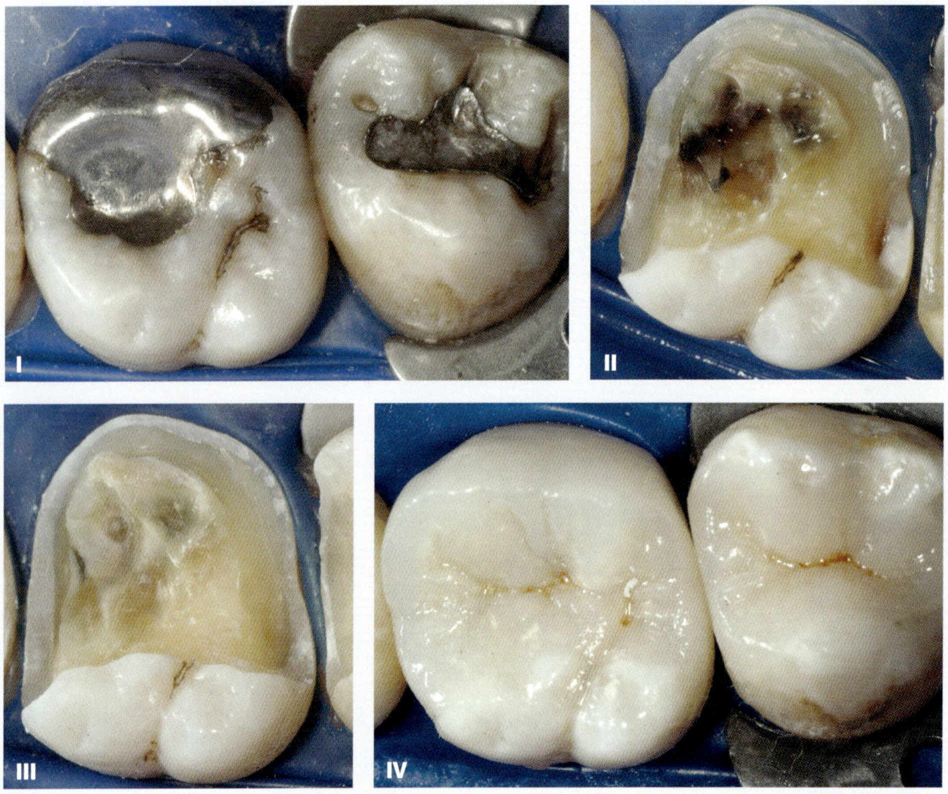

Fig 94 Very deep decay under an old amalgam filling. Removal of softened tissue and execution of an MOD onlay with maintenance of the palatal wall.

MOD cavity: Overlay

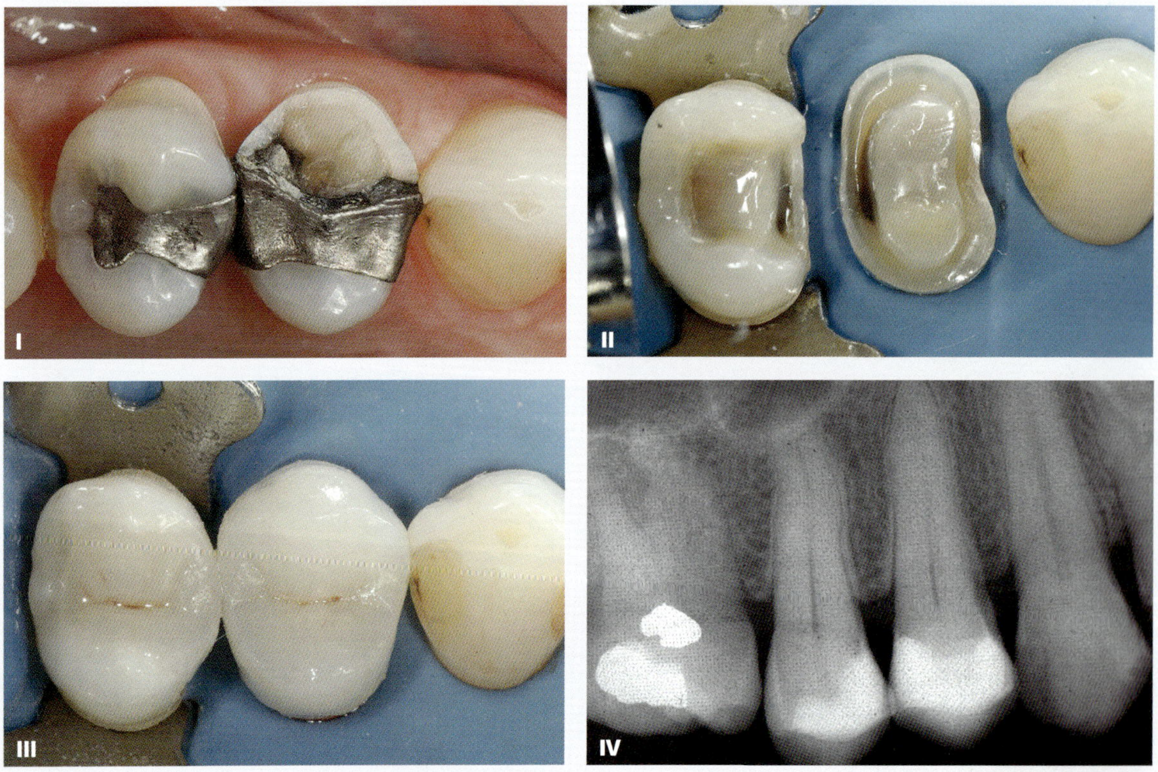

Fig 95 The fracture in the buccal wall of the maxillary premolar and the inadequate thicknesses of the palatal walls indicated preparation of an overlay *(I, II)*. View of cemented inlays *(III)* and follow-up radiographs after 8 years *(IV)*.

MOD cavity: Overlay

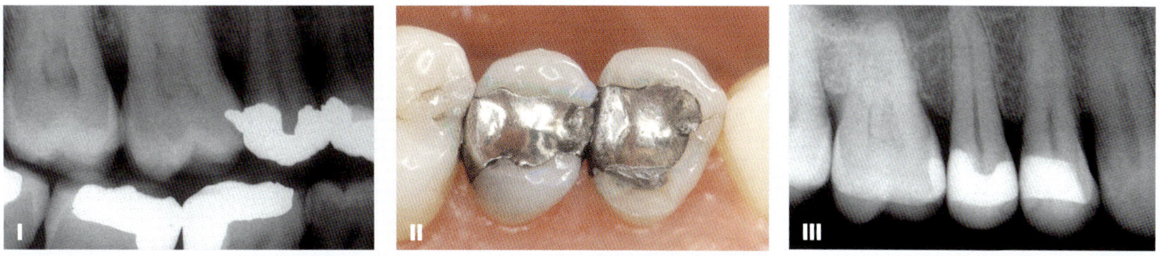

Fig 96 Two maxillary premolars with MOD and OD amalgam *(I, II)*. An MOD cavity has the greatest detrimental effect on tooth integrity with regard to masticatory load. It goes without saying that an overlay is indicated when the residual thicknesses are insufficient as in this MOD cavity. Radiograph at the end of treatment *(III)*.

MOD cavity: Overlay

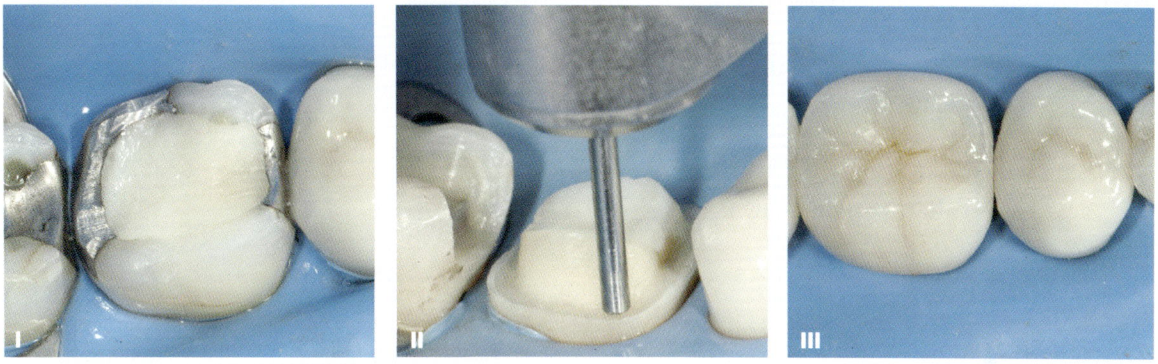

Fig 97 Intraoperative view of a preparation for overlay on an MOD cavity *(I, II)*. Cemented restoration *(III)*.

MOD cavity: Overlay

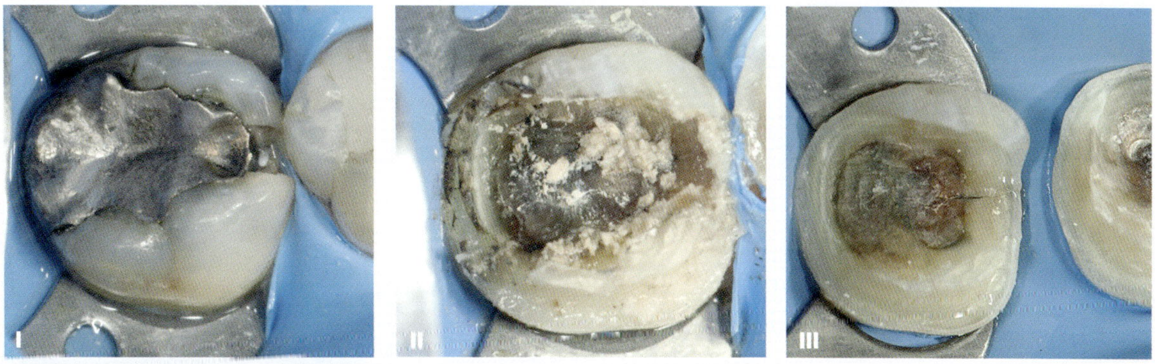

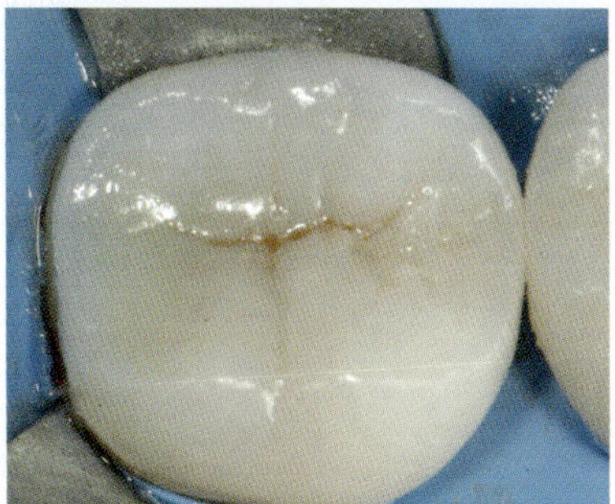

Fig 98 Presence of deep decay under an MOD amalgam restoration. Removal of the decayed tissue and application of an overlay.

MOD cavity: Overlay

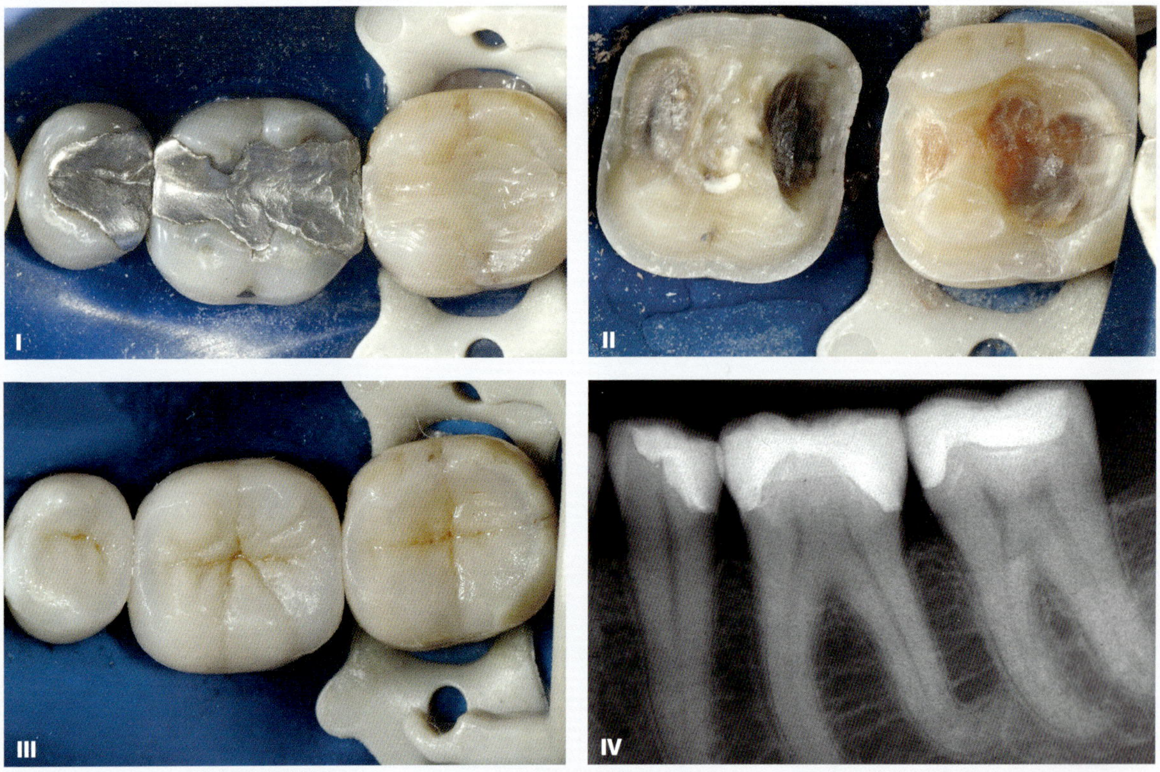

Fig 99 Unsatisfactory amalgam and composite fillings in the mandibular left quadrant *(I)*: after cleaning the cavities, an inlay, an overlay, and an onlay were applied to the second premolar and first and second molars, respectively *(II, III)*. A follow-up radiograph after 6 years *(IV)* and pulp vitality tests showed maintenance of vitality despite the depth of the caries lesions.

MOD cavity: Overlay

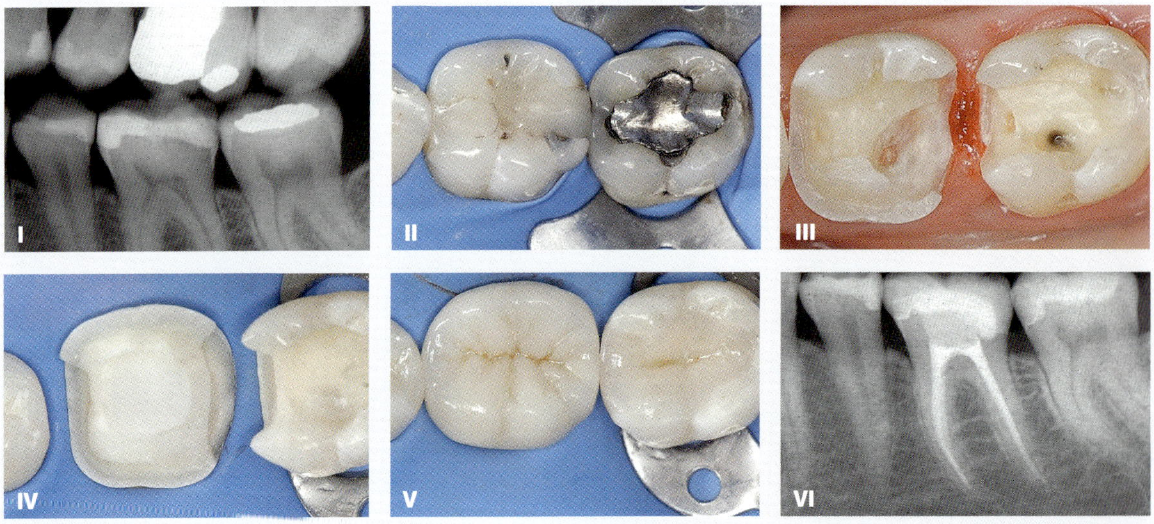

Fig 100 Endodontic treatment for penetrating decay in a mandibular left first molar *(I–III)* that was reconstructed by preparing an overlay *(IV)*. Treatment also included an inlay for the second molar and direct restoration of the second premolar *(V)*. Radiograph at the end of treatment *(VI)*. (Courtesy of Dr Lavinia Landi.)

MOD cavity: Overlay

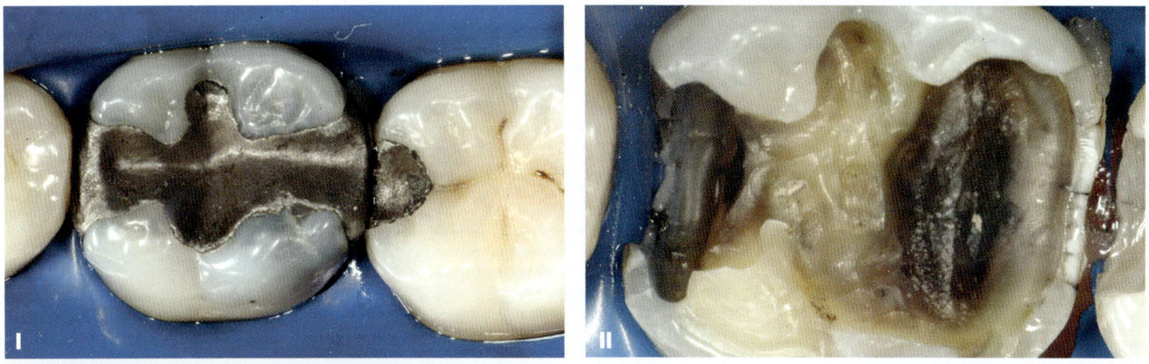

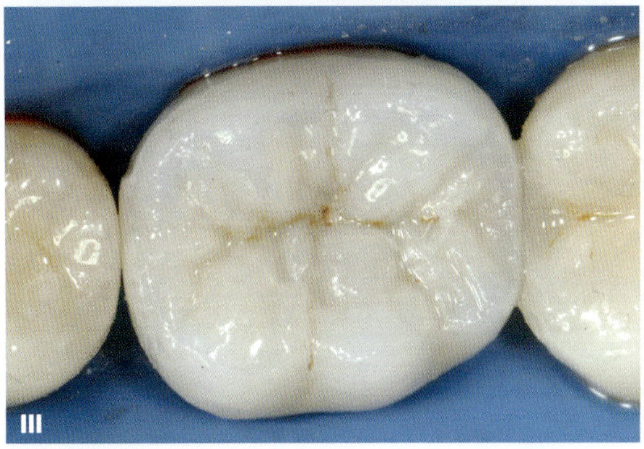

Fig 101 The patient complained of pain on chewing in the mandibular left first molar. A composite overlay quickly removed the painful symptoms.

MOD cavity: Overlay

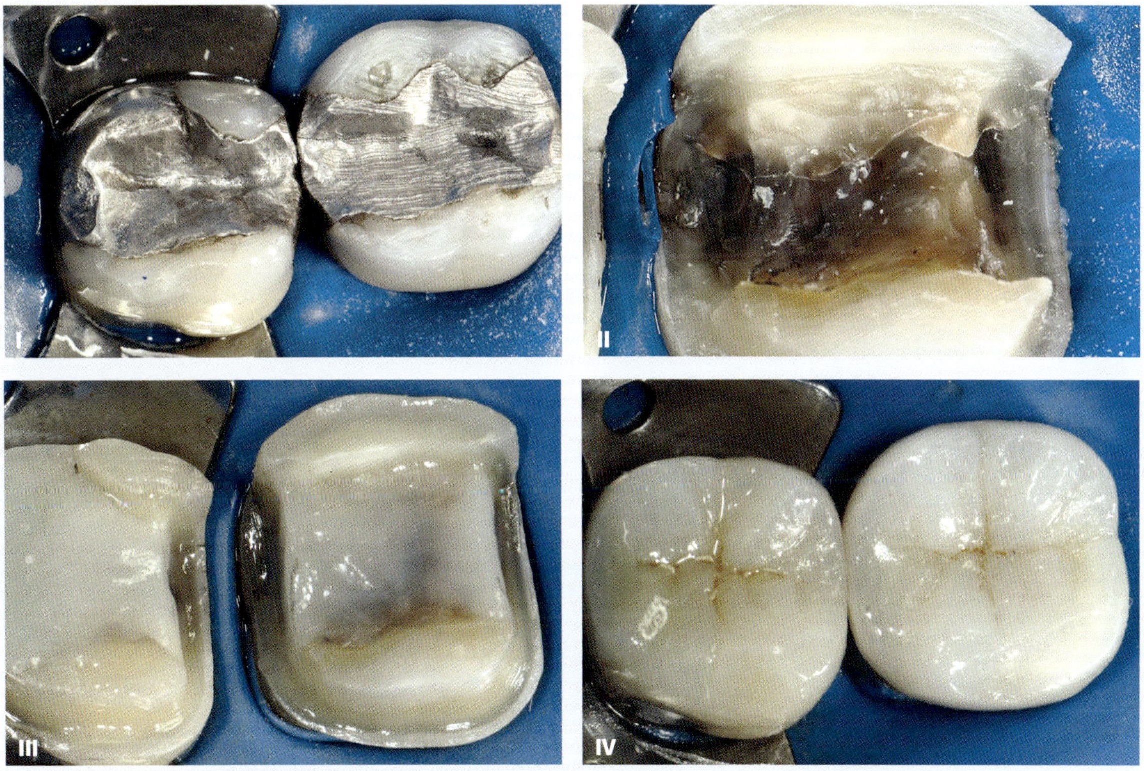

Fig 102 Very painful twinges on chewing in the mandibular right quadrant led the patient to consult the author's practice *(I)*. After removing the old restorations, clear MOD fracture lines could be seen in the first molar *(II)*. The decayed tissue was removed, the fracture lines were treated conservatively, an overlay was prepared with a 90-degree shoulder for the interproximal and buccal margins and a knife-edge margin for the lingual wall *(III)*, and the procedure was finished with cementation of the inlays *(IV)*. The twinges disappeared within a few weeks. A pulp vitality test was positive 4 years later. Chapter 6 is devoted to management of fracture lines.

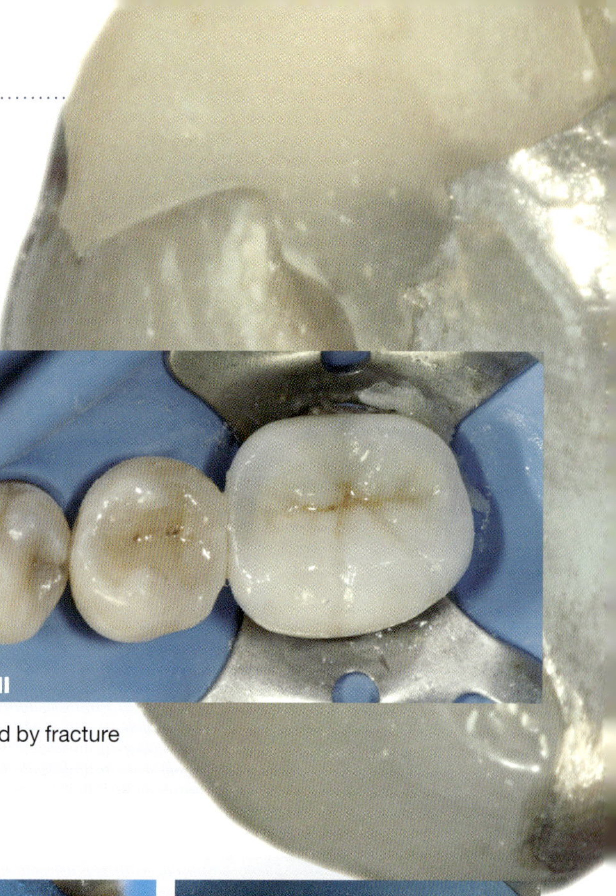

MOD cavity: Overlay

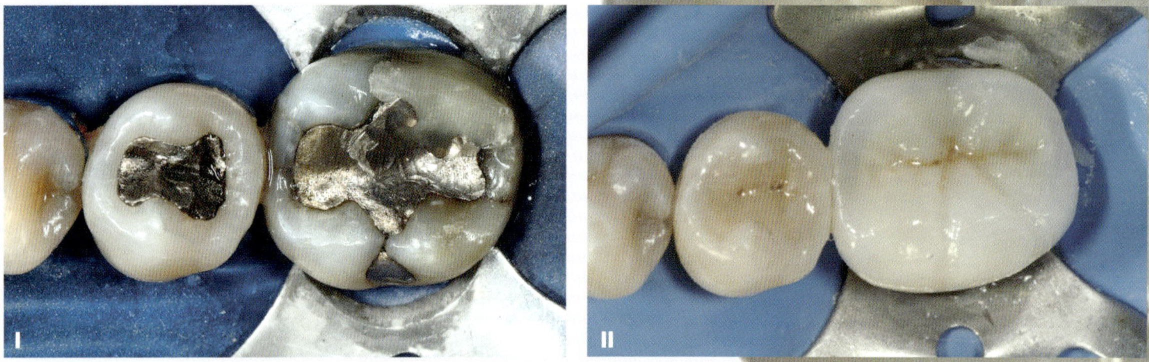

Fig 103 Yet another case of a defective restoration aggravated by fracture of the lingual wall, managed by preparation of an overlay.

MOD cavity: Overlay

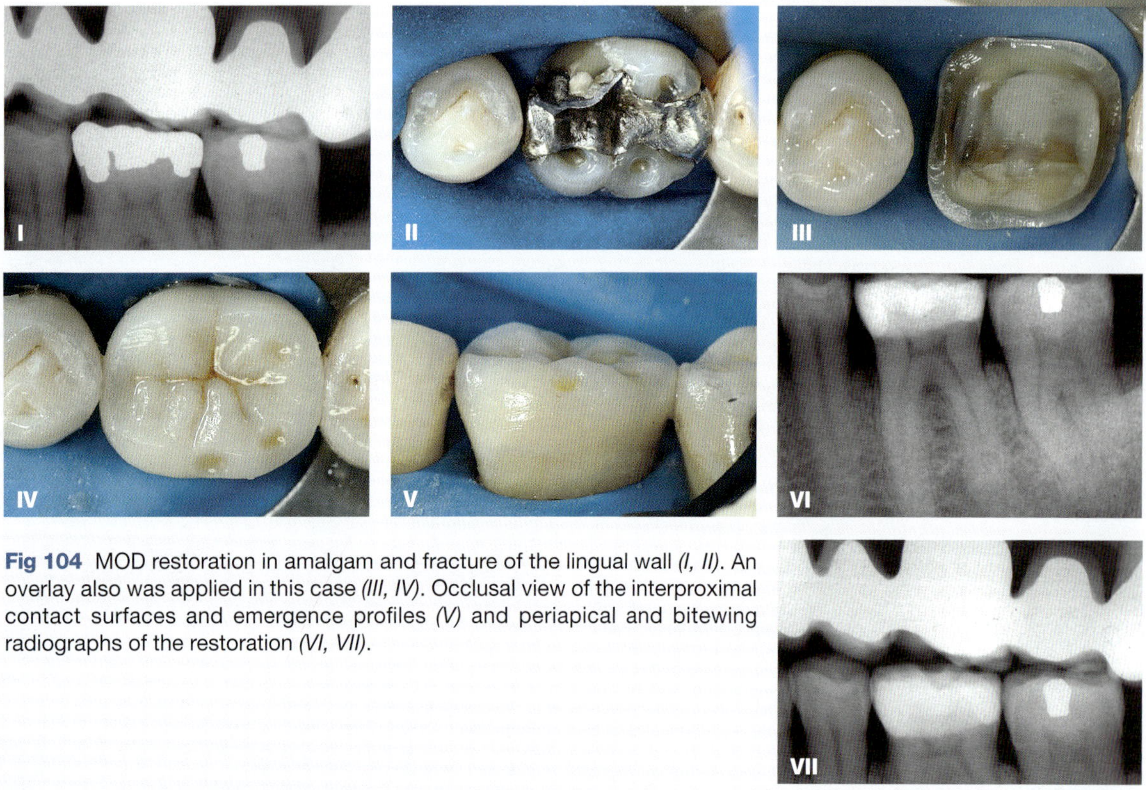

Fig 104 MOD restoration in amalgam and fracture of the lingual wall *(I, II)*. An overlay also was applied in this case *(III, IV)*. Occlusal view of the interproximal contact surfaces and emergence profiles *(V)* and periapical and bitewing radiographs of the restoration *(VI, VII)*.

MOD cavity: Overlay

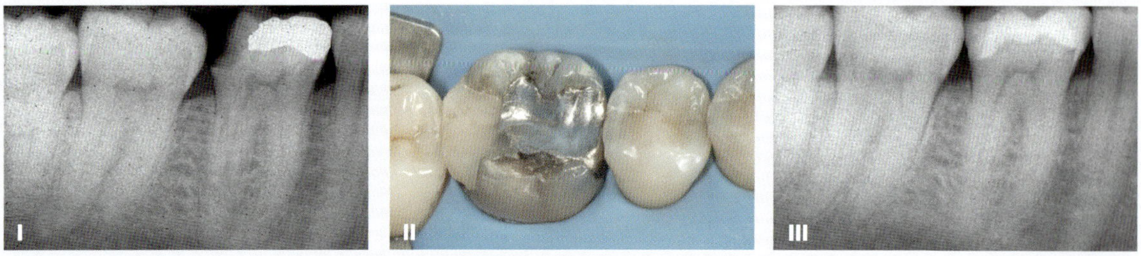

Fig 105 Another similar case with a radiograph at the end of treatment. Some might justifiably criticize this repetition of cases, but the author feels it is necessary in order to convey the fundamental principle underlying this book, ie, that the same satisfactory result can routinely be obtained by applying proper protocol. (Courtesy of Dr Lavinia Landi.)

MOD cavity: Overlay

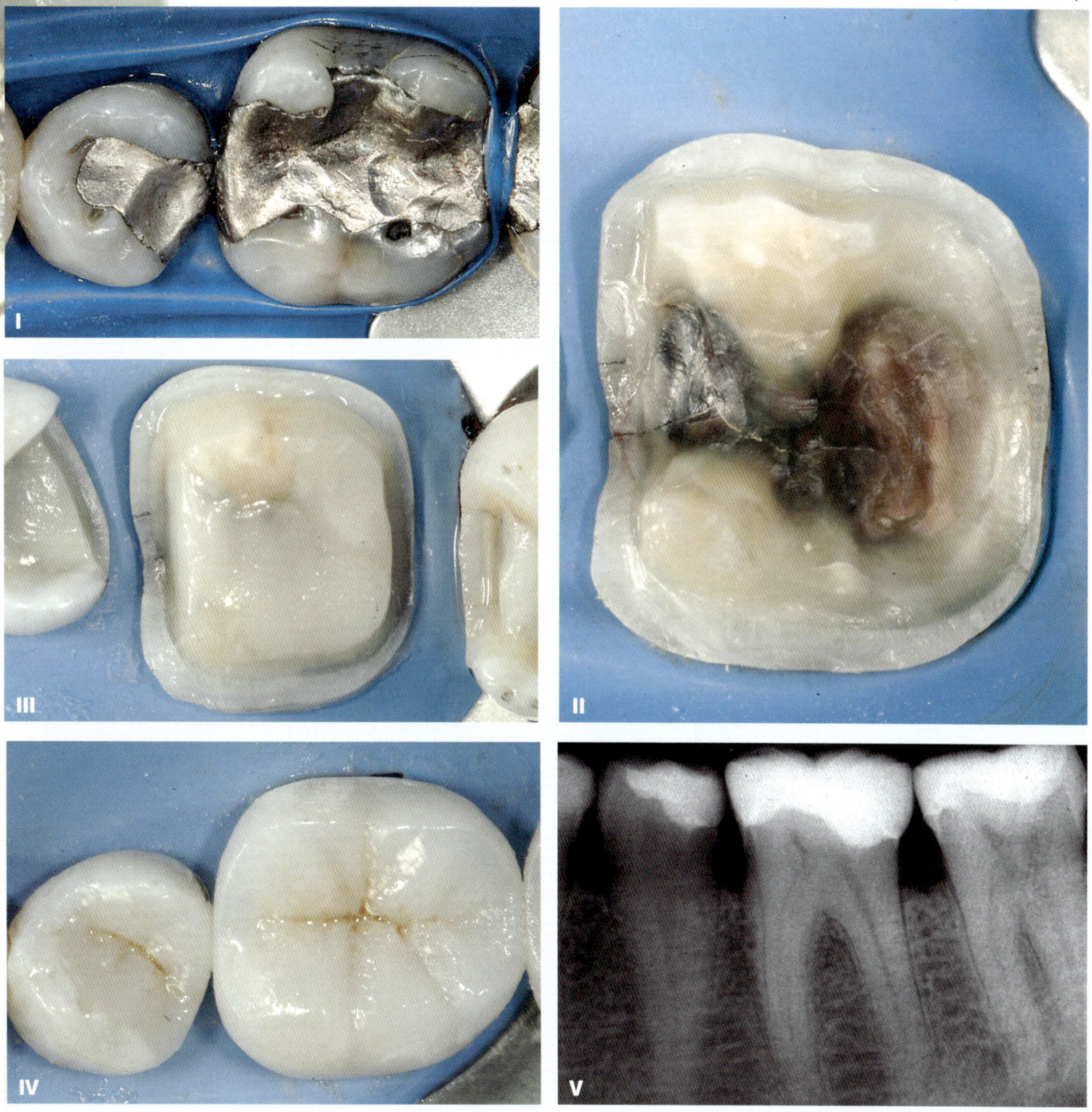

Fig 106 In this case, removal of leaking amalgam restorations on the mandibular left first molar *(I, II)* reveals fracture lines. There is distal communication with the pulp but no signs and symptoms of irreversible pulp disease, which is the only indication for endodontic treatment. The pulp test was also positive. Everything was built up *(III)*, and lastly the overlays were cemented *(IV)*. At the 6-year follow-up (the most recent; in such cases the tooth is monitored two to three times a year when the patient visits the hygienist), the vitality test was positive, the radiograph *(V)* did not show any radiolucency, and the patient did not complain of any discomfort—what more could be asked?

MOD cavity: Overlay

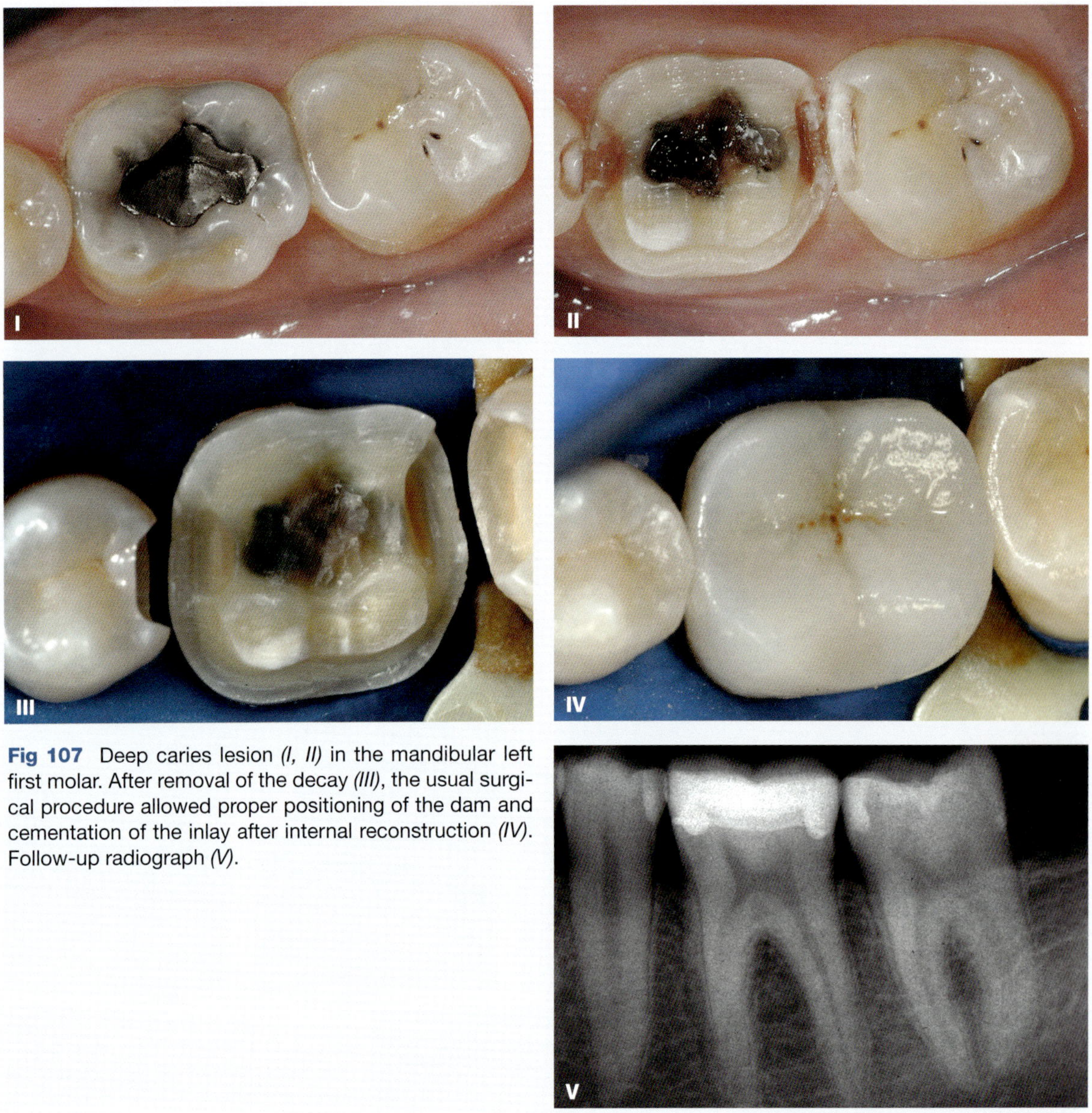

Fig 107 Deep caries lesion *(I, II)* in the mandibular left first molar. After removal of the decay *(III)*, the usual surgical procedure allowed proper positioning of the dam and cementation of the inlay after internal reconstruction *(IV)*. Follow-up radiograph *(V)*.

MOD cavity: Overlay

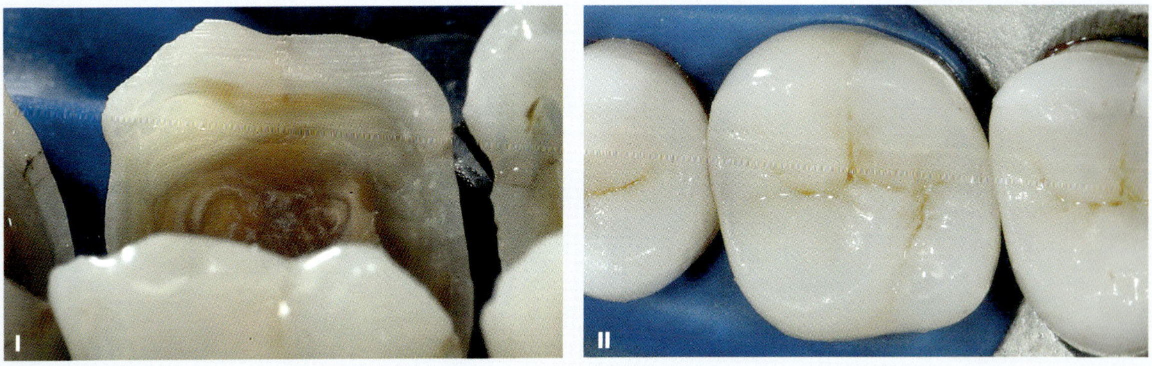

Fig 108 Enamel not supported by dentin: Indication for removal of walls and execution of an overlay.

MOD cavity: Overlay

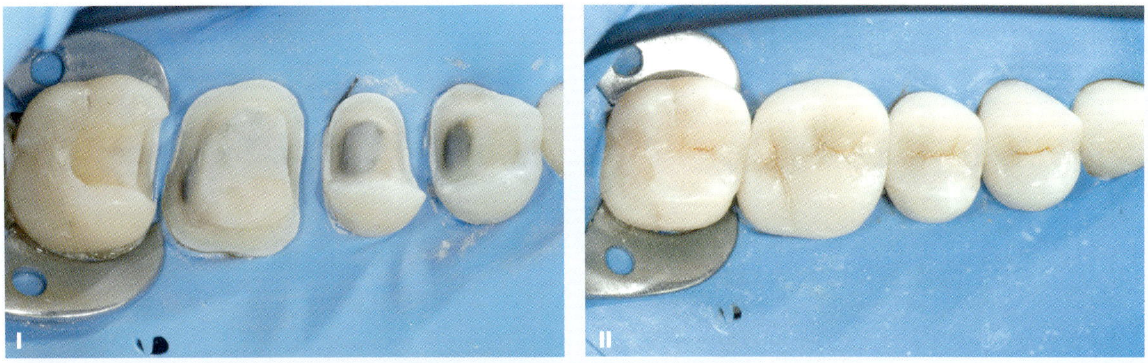

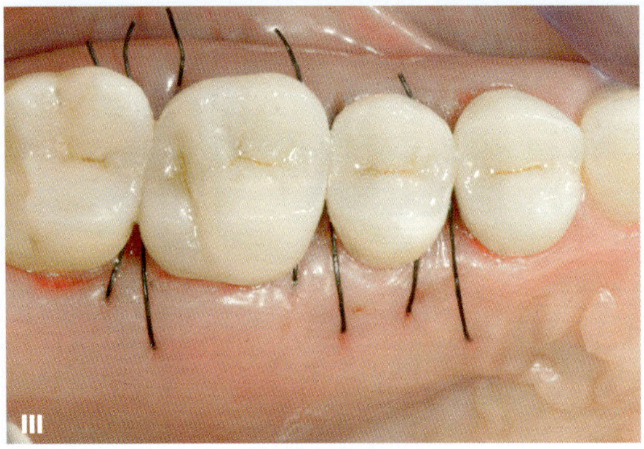

Fig 109 View of the maxillary right quadrant with inlay, onlay, and overlay. The sutures would be removed in 1 week or less.

MOD cavity: Overlay

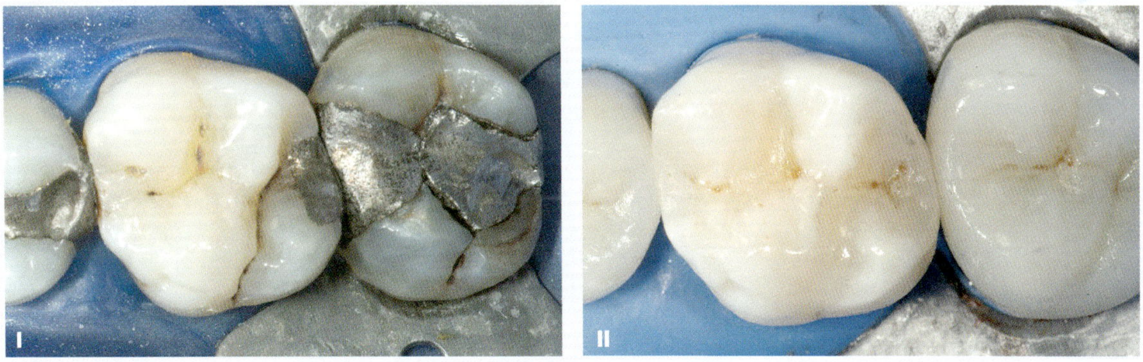

Fig 110 Another overlay for the morphofunctional restoration of the maxillary left second molar.

MOD cavity: Overlay

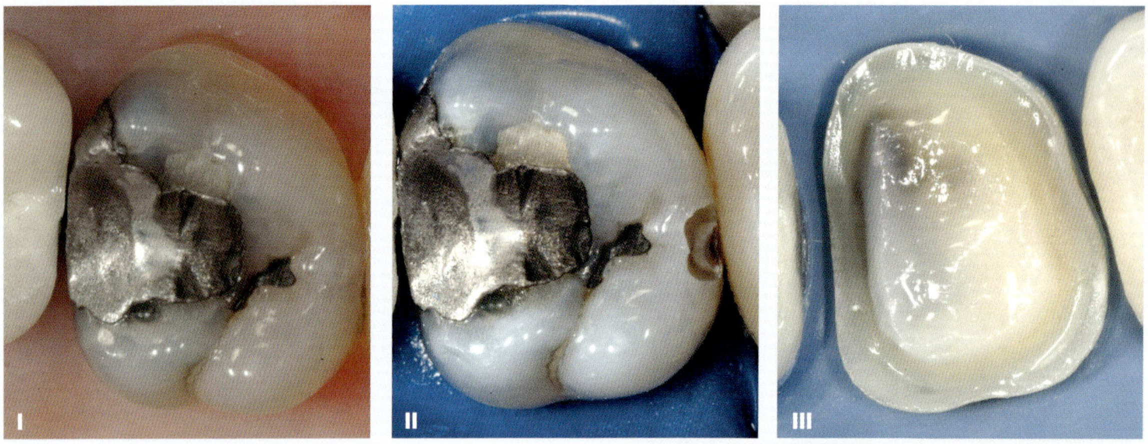

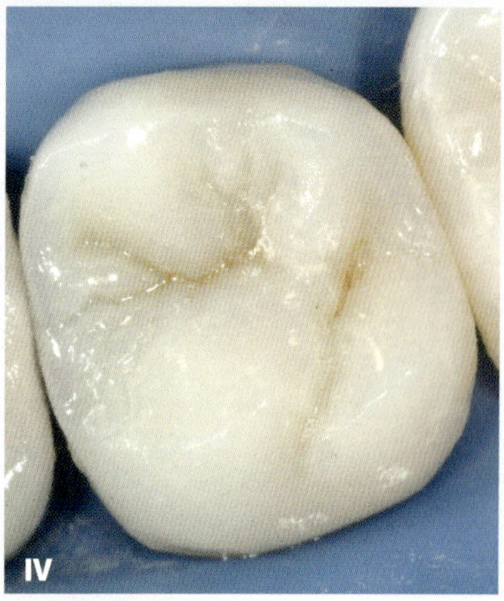

Fig 111 Preparation of an overlay after buildup and cemented restoration.

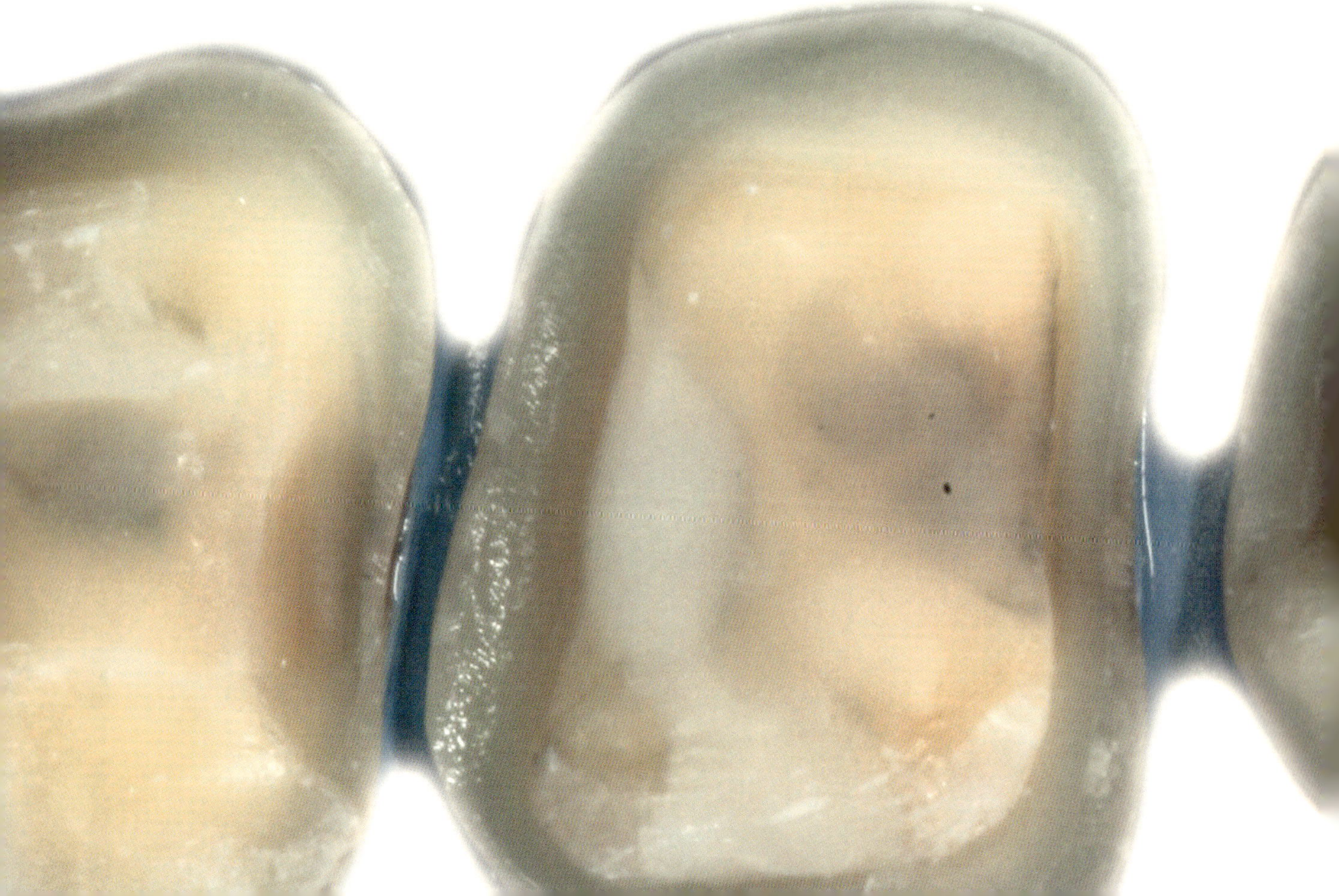

MOD cavity: Overlay

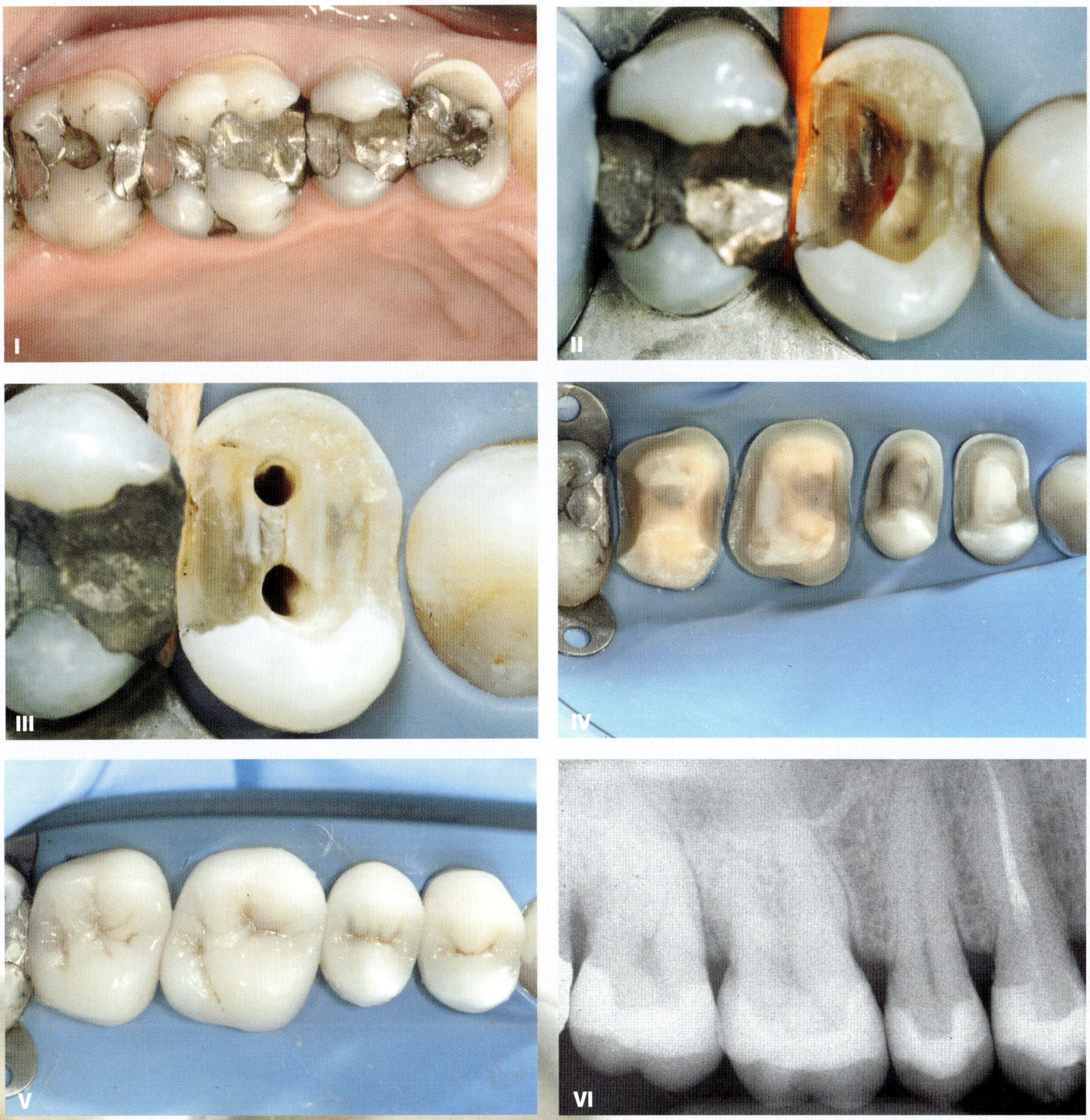

Fig 112 Multiple fractures of defective old restorations *(I)*. Endodontic treatment had to be carried out on the maxillary right first premolar because of penetrating decay *(II, III)*. This was completed, and the first and second premolars were prepared for two onlays, and, after evaluating the residual thicknesses, the two molars were prepared for overlays *(IV)*. View of the quadrant after cementation of the indirect restorations *(V)*. The radiograph illustrates the marginal seals *(VI)*. The treatment plan subsequently included removal of the maxillary right third molar.

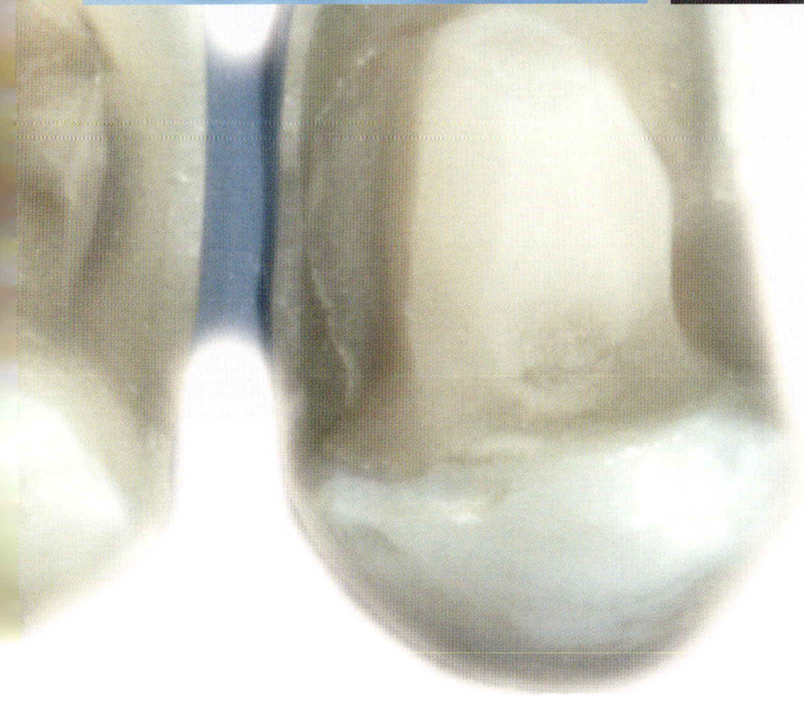

MOD cavity: Overlay

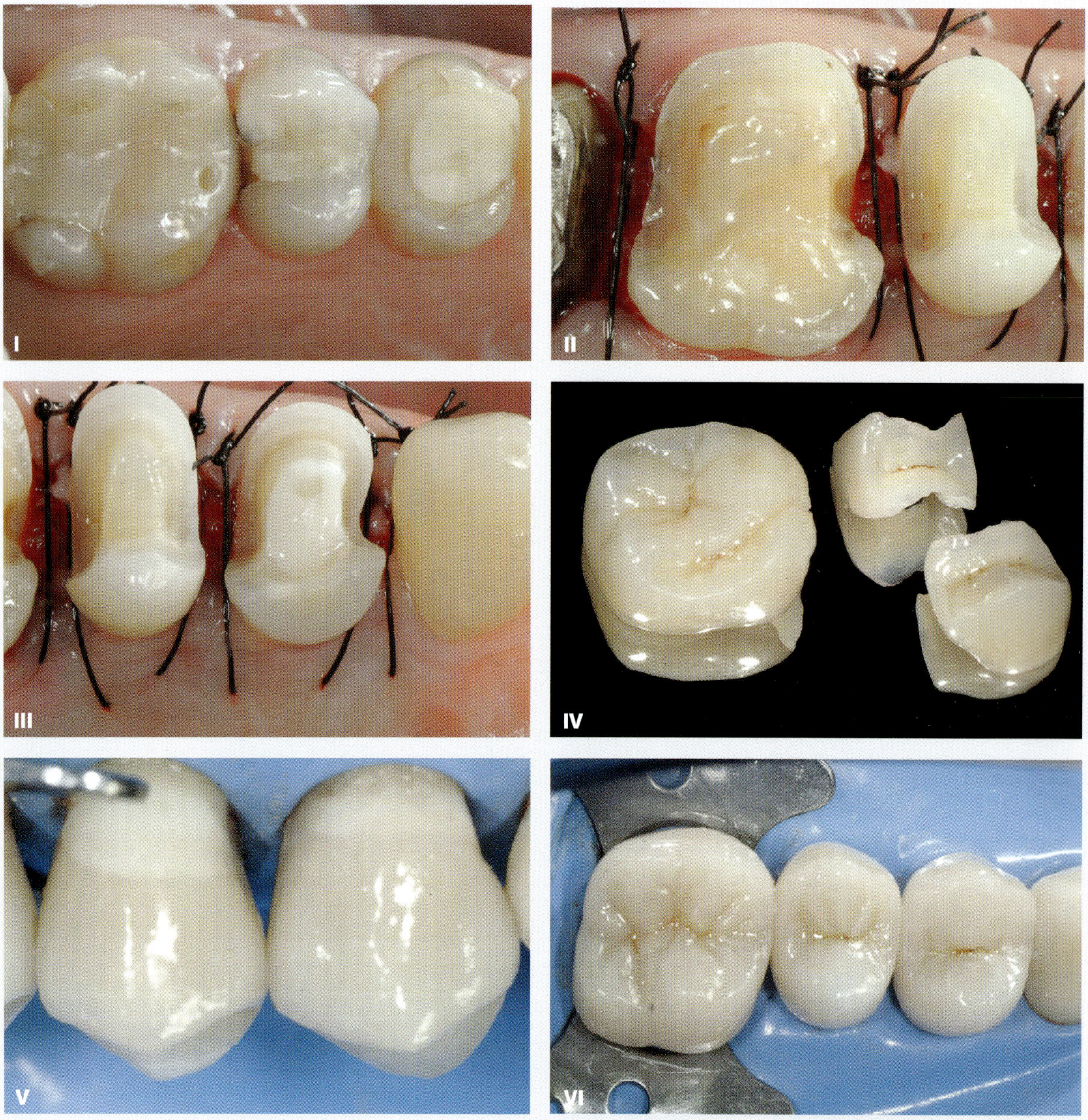

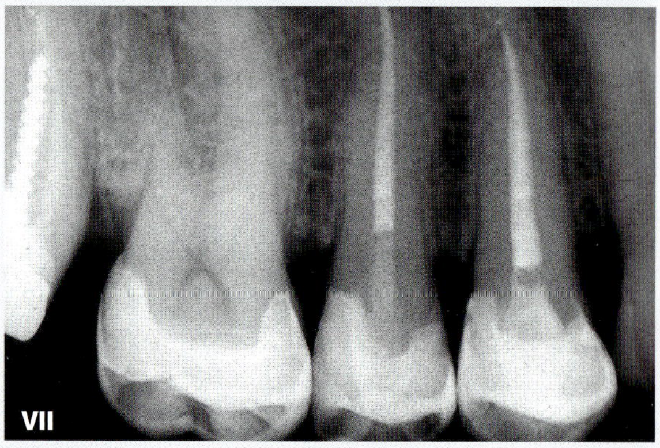

Fig 113 Leaking composite restorations of highly debatable quality in the maxillary right quadrant *(I)*. Multidisciplinary treatment *(II, III)* culminated in the positioning of two onlays on endodontically treated premolars and an overlay on the molar. Views of the restorations before cementation *(IV)*, of the interproximal contact surfaces and emergence profiles *(V)*, and of the occlusal aspect of the quadrant *(VI)*. Follow-up radiograph *(VII)*.

Endodontically treated teeth

Decades ago, a study by Sorensen and Martinoff[24] concluded that endodontically treated posterior teeth should be covered with a prosthesis, but recent biomechanical studies have led to a structural change toward more conservative methods. Partial adhesive restorations perform the function of restoring an endodontically treated tooth superlatively well in the great majority of cases, while prosthetic solutions are increasingly less common.

Reconstruction of an endodontically treated tooth must avoid sacrificing additional healthy structure but at the same time protect against fracture risks. Today, adhesive techniques offer the opportunity to achieve conservative restoration of these teeth without increasing the risk of fracture.

Cusp flexion increases in direct proportion to cavity size and the C-factor; the use of an incremental technique and indirect restorations reduces cusp flexion.[25]

In 2007, González-López et al[26] stressed that cusp flexion, which occurs as the result of contraction due to curing of the composite and occlusal load, is significantly greater in MOD composite restorations than in MO or OD composite restorations.

This demonstrates the fundamental importance of biomechanical knowledge when determining the most appropriate design for a cavity. All too often one sees far from conservative preparations involving structural parts that could easily be preserved. The most classic example of this in an endodontically treated tooth is involvement of healthy marginal ridges in the preparation. Twenty years ago Sakaguchi et al[9] and Linn and Messer[10] demonstrated—and this is so important that it bears repetition—that the cusps of a posterior tooth under load deform differently according to whether the marginal ridge is present or absent: Those with a missing ridge deform much more than those where a ridge is present. This being stated, clinicians must be aware that if a single marginal ridge is lost, they must cover only the cusps adjacent to the missing marginal ridge and save the cusps near the existing ridge after assessing the thicknesses at the base of those cusps (Fig 114).

Only the simultaneous opening of two marginal ridges in an endodontically treated tooth is an indication for total cusp coverage (overlay) (Fig 115).

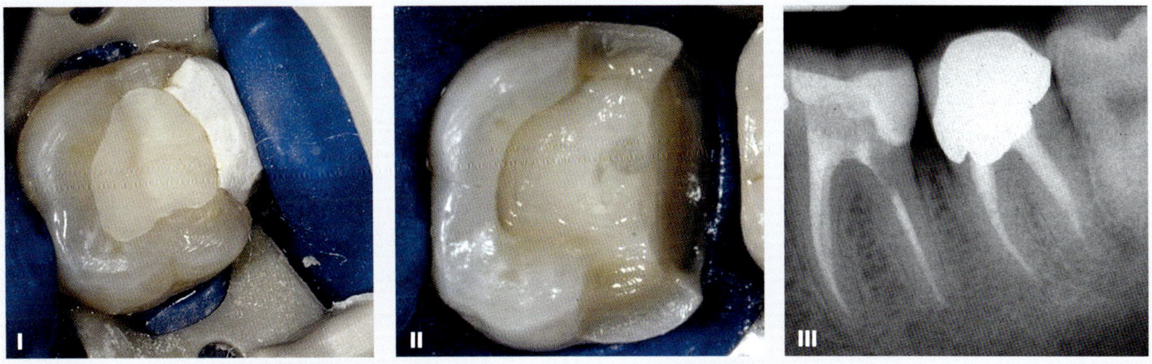

Fig 114

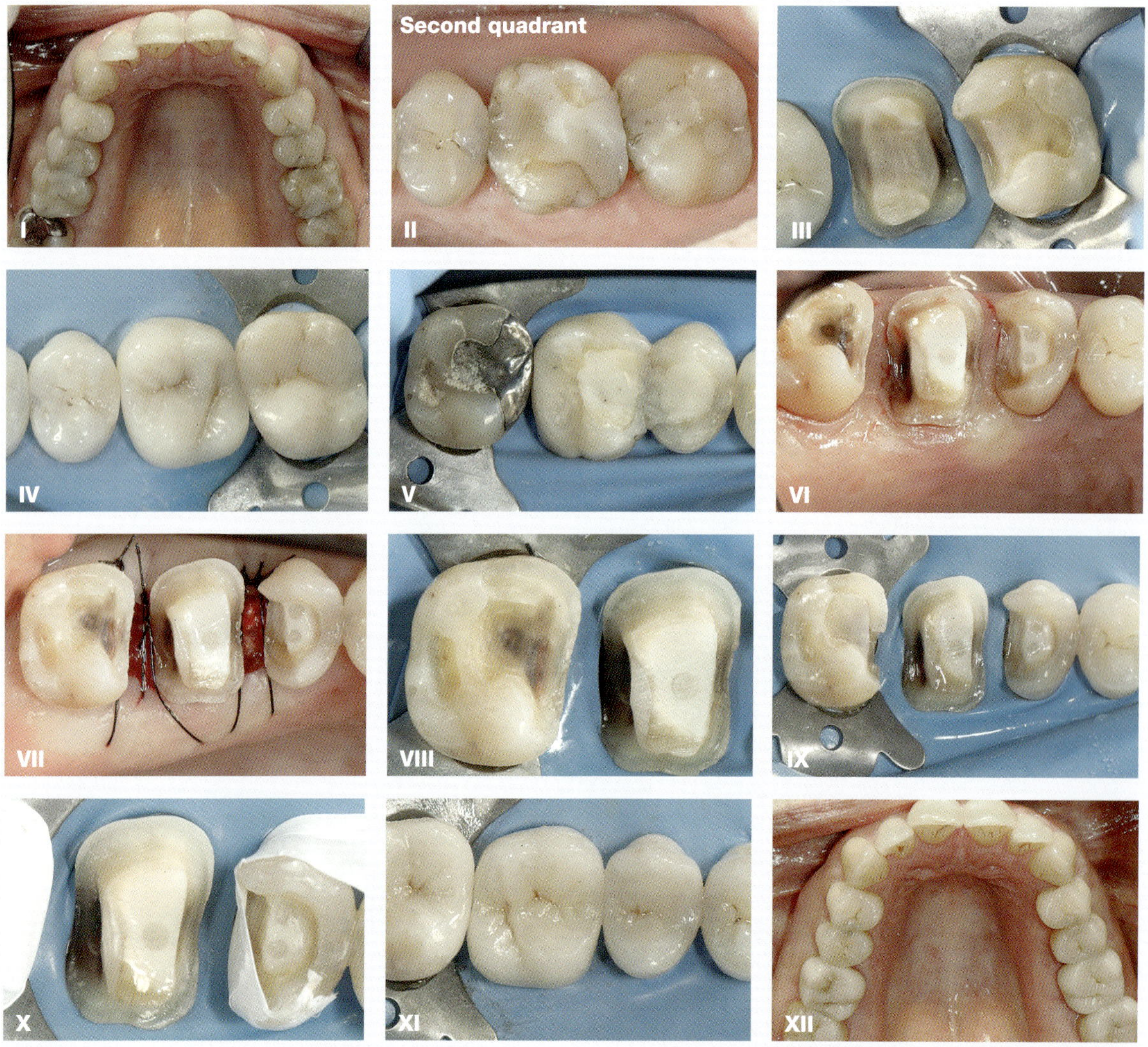

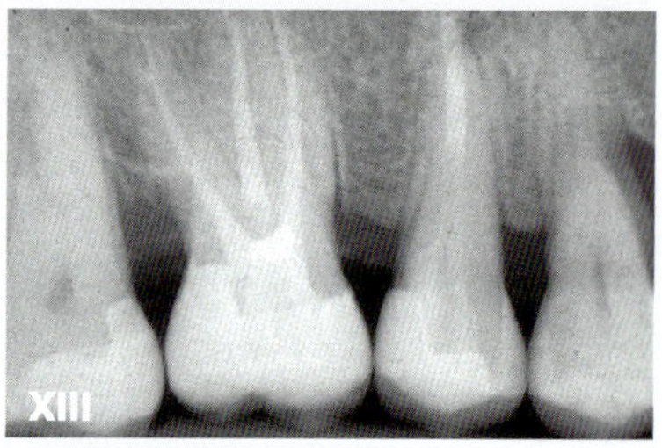

Fig 115 Absolutely unacceptable restorations required restoration of the posterior sectors of the maxillary arch *(I)*. In the maxillary left (second) quadrant, direct restoration of the second premolar, overlay on the first molar, and inlay on the second molar *(II–IV)*. A multidisciplinary approach was adopted in the treatment plan for the maxillary right quadrant *(V)*, with endodontic treatments for the second premolar and first molar and periodontal surgery for the correct exposure of the preparation margins *(VI, VII)*, which made it possible to proceed with the tricky procedure of isolating the operative field and cementing the prostheses *(VIII–XII)*. Postoperative radiograph of the maxillary right quadrant *(XIII)*.

In this case too, for the sake of accuracy, it should be emphasized that adhesive techniques should be used alongside—not replace—prosthetic solutions. Positioning of an endodontically treated tooth in an arch is another important factor when it comes to deciding the approach to take when faced with the choice of a direct or indirect restoration. The more mesially the tooth is located, the more it will be protected against wear and functional stresses.

When restoring endodontically treated anterior teeth, direct restorations will naturally be the approach of choice; however, care should be taken with the canine teeth when they are subject to strong tangential stresses in canine-guided lateral occlusion.

The maxillary premolars have a high risk of fracture due to their very pronounced interproximal concavities, particularly at the cervical level. These risks are reduced when restoring mandibular premolars.
Particular attention should be paid to the restoration of endodontically treated mandibular molars because the lingual angle of the nonsupporting cusps makes these teeth particularly vulnerable.
The quality of endodontic treatment, the use of intraradicular anchorages when strictly indicated, respect for root dentin during endodontic operations, and the timeliness and quality of the restoration, all within the context of a healthy, maintainable periodontium, naturally play a fundamental role in the quality of endodontic treatment.
During the 1980s, Trope et al[27] and Robbins[28] demonstrated that excessive removal of root dentin considerably compromises the root. Sorensen and Martinoff[24] demonstrated that tooth strength is directly connected to the quantity of residual dentin and, along with Guzy and Nicholls[29] and Reeh et al,[7] concluded that teeth without posts are stronger than those with posts.
All works in the literature agree that an endodontically treated tooth is more fragile and therefore at a greater risk of fracture than a vital tooth.
Even though it is not universally accepted, there is a growing belief that this fragility is a consequence of loss of tooth structure, ie, architectural changes associated with pulpectomy (interaxial dentin and pulp chamber roof) are the true culprits responsible for reducing the strength of an endodontically treated tooth[30,31] and not changes in water content,[32] changes in collagen ultrastructure,[33] or loss of proprioceptors.[34]
Furthermore, due consideration should be given to the fact that an endodontically treated tooth is more subject to fracture because it undergoes greater deformation and returns more slowly to normal stress resistance than a vital tooth. Such stresses give rise to small deformations that place the tooth in a situation of fatigue that leads to fracture if allowed to continue (Figs 116 and 117), hence the clinical advice to protect an endodontically treated tooth with appropriate restorations as quickly as possible.

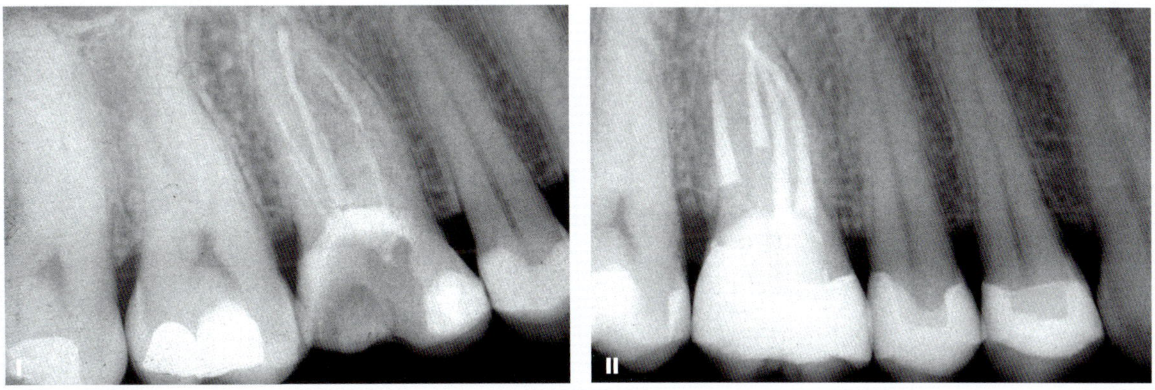

Fig 116

Given the independence of cusp deformation,[2,9,10] the fact that endodontic procedures are now much more conservative because of the advent of nickel-titanium rotary instruments, and the author's clinical results, a new protocol for cavity preparations in an endodontically treated tooth can now be devised.

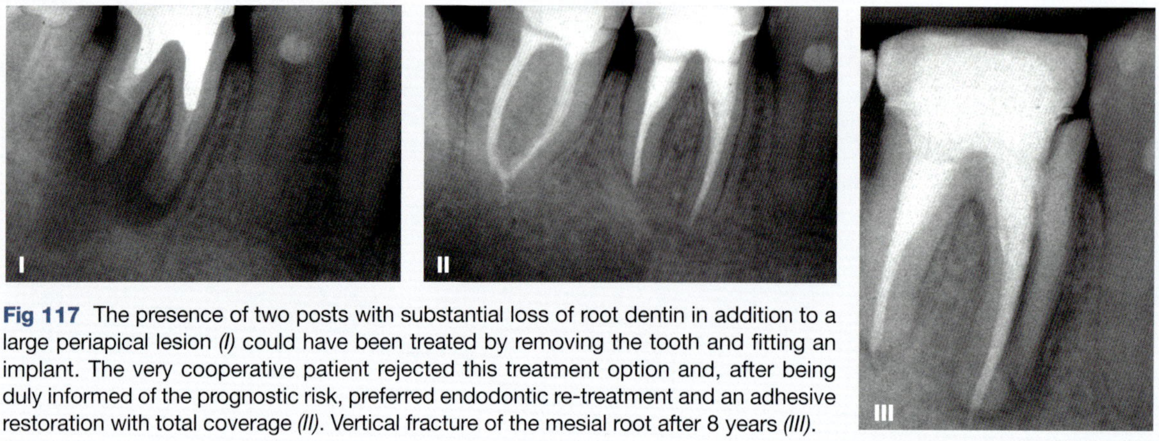

Fig 117 The presence of two posts with substantial loss of root dentin in addition to a large periapical lesion *(I)* could have been treated by removing the tooth and fitting an implant. The very cooperative patient rejected this treatment option and, after being duly informed of the prognostic risk, preferred endodontic re-treatment and an adhesive restoration with total coverage *(II)*. Vertical fracture of the mesial root after 8 years *(III)*.

OCCLUSAL CAVITY
Direct restoration (Fig 118)

OCCLUSAL CAVITY
Indirect restoration (when the remaining cusp is less than 2 mm) (Fig 119)

MO OR OD CAVITY
INLAY (Figs 120 and 121)
MO and OD ONLAY (Figs 122 to 126)

MOD CAVITY
OVERLAY in all cases (Figs 127 to 138)

Teeth restored using adhesive techniques have long shown reduced cusp deformation. In 1988 Hansen[35] showed that for endodontically treated and restored premolars in amalgam and composite, the incidence of fracture after 3 years was one-third for amalgam and none for composite. However, these figures have been simplified for educational purposes; the truth is that each case should be evaluated individually, as is evident from the clinical photographs, naturally giving close consideration to guidelines in the literature. There are so many different clinical situations that it is not possible to come up with a specific protocol for determining cavity geometry: clinical experience is clearly the best guide. It is important to stress that during preparations for adhesive techniques, each restoration to be replaced should be fully removed after isolating the operative field using rubber dam. The final cavity should be free of decay and, after applying an adhesive system determined in accordance with protocol, the internal buildup should be performed using incremental layers of composite applied 1 mm or at most 2 mm at a time, always within an isolated operative field.

Occlusal cavity: Direct restoration

Fig 118 Indication for a direct restoration with both marginal ridges present and upper walls thicker than 2 mm.

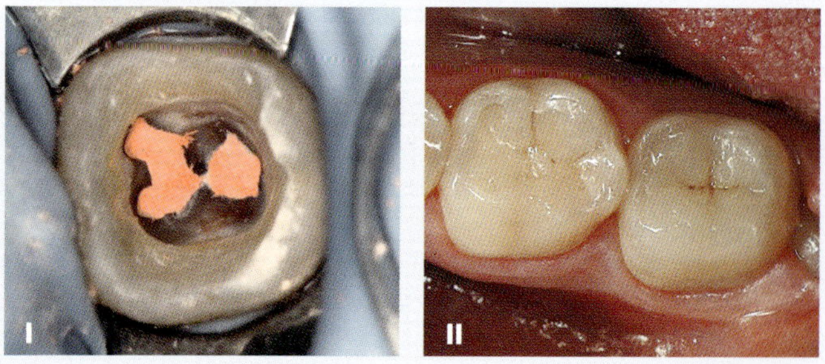

Occlusal cavity: Indirect restoration

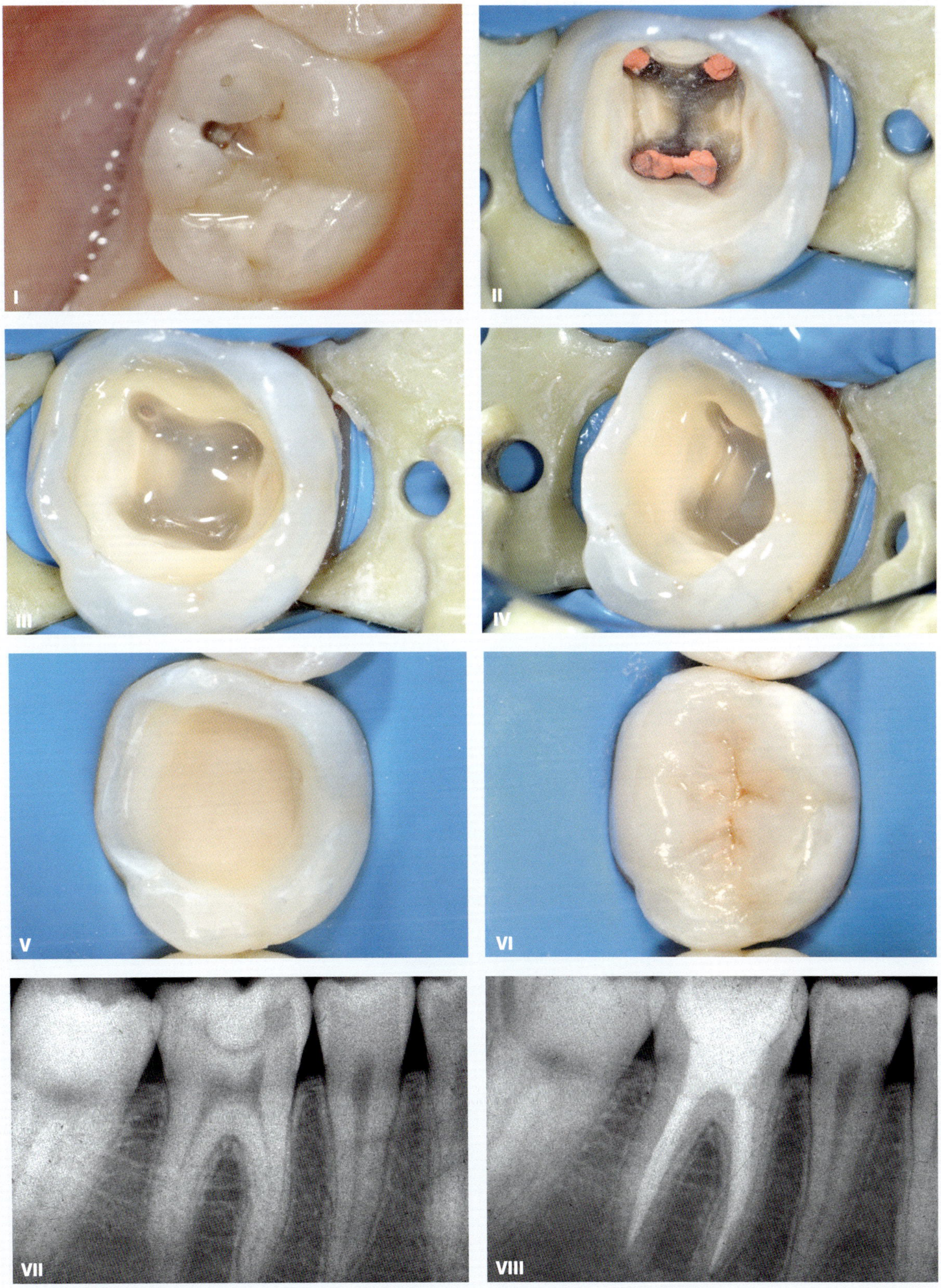

Fig 119 Indication for occlusal indirect restoration due to wall thicknesses of less than 2 mm. This somewhat debatable choice was dictated by the fact that the patient was very young, and it was therefore desirable to avoid the intraradicular anchorage necessary to retain the buildup required for an overlay and to avoid the high stress due to polymerization shrinkage arising as a result of a direct restoration. This procedure, incidentally the most conservative, does not rule out the possibility of a full-coverage restoration in the future, if necessary.

MO/OD cavity: Inlay

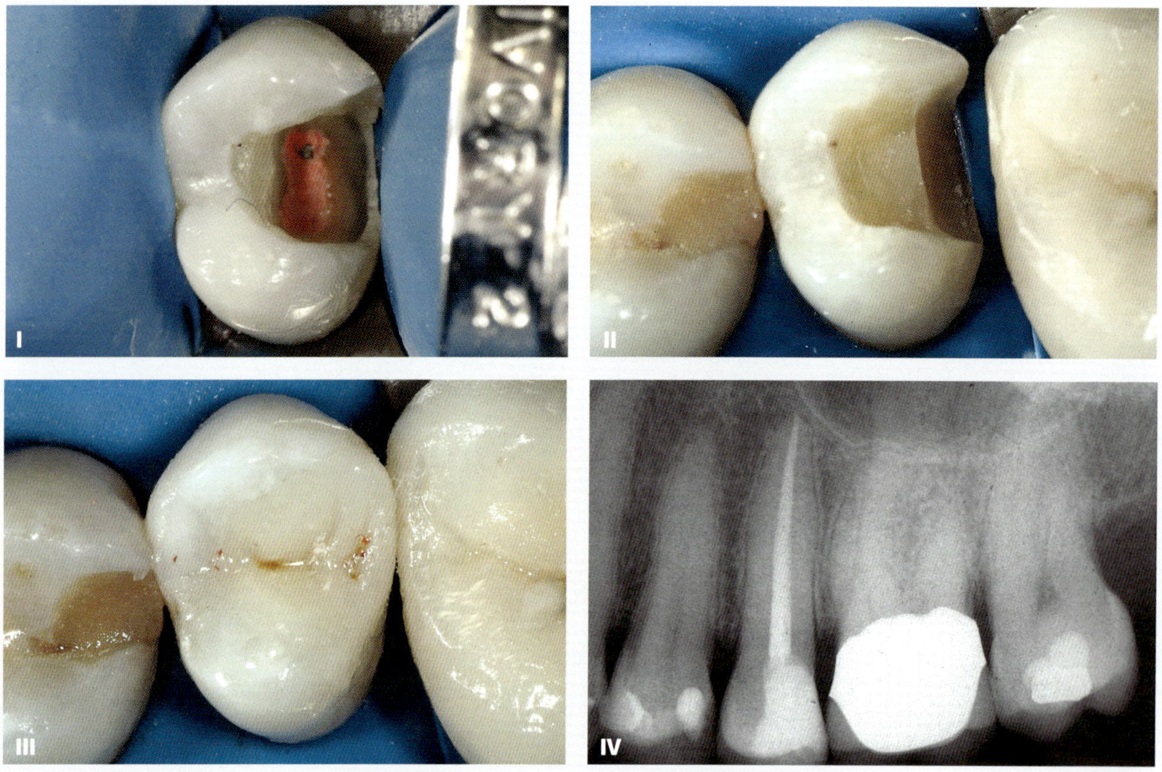

Fig 120 Endodontically treated maxillary premolar. The thicknesses at the cusp bases exceed 3 mm. In this case a simple inlay is the correct indication for reconstruction *(I–III)*. Follow-up radiograph *(IV)*.

MO/OD cavity: Inlay

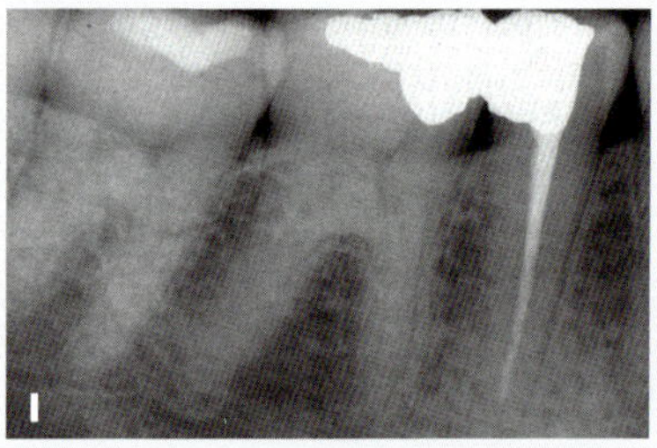

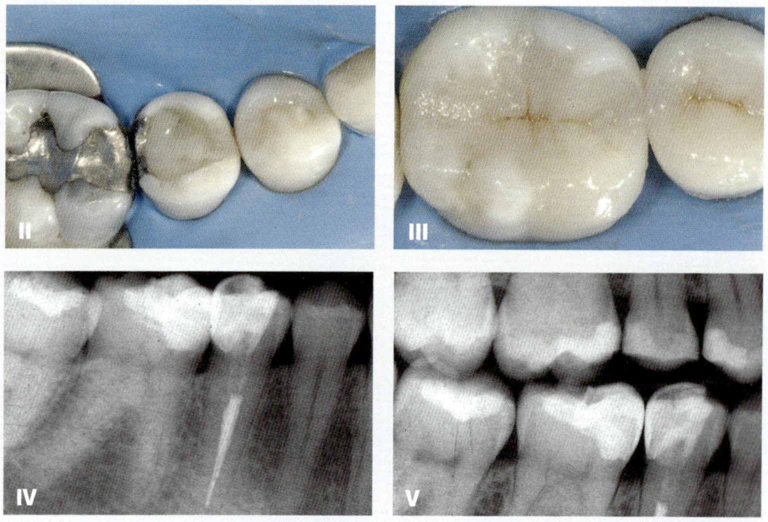

Fig 121 Nonvital mandibular premolar with thicknesses of 2.5 mm. Reconstruction with an inlay after positioning of an intraradicular post.

MO/OD cavity: Onlay

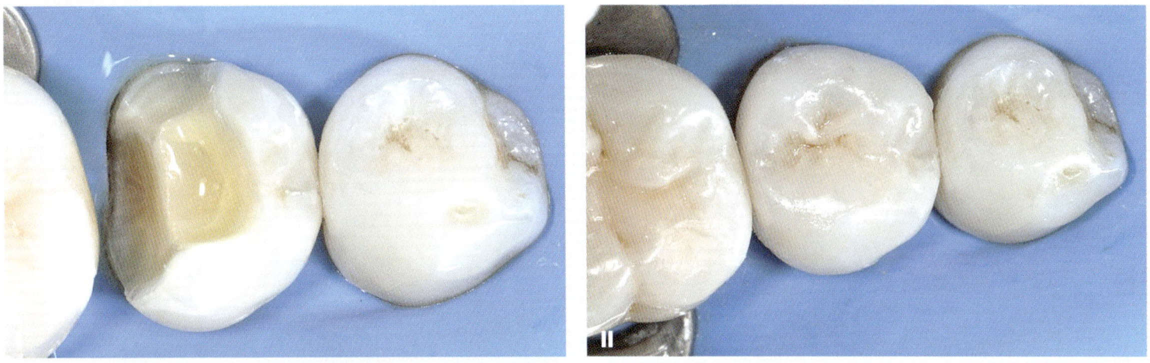

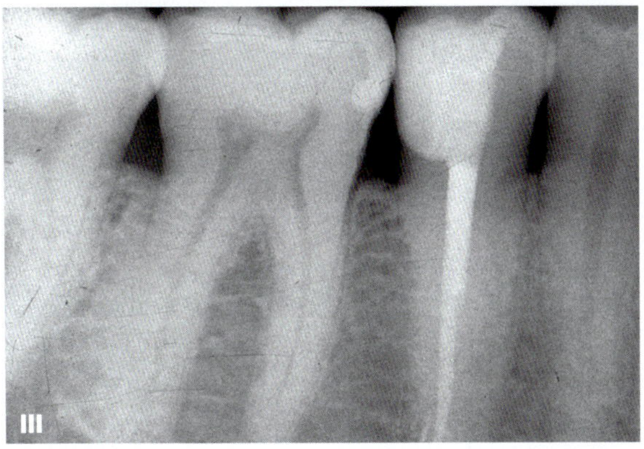

Fig 122 Loss of a wall is a clear indication for protecting the tooth with an onlay *(I, II)*. Postoperative radiograph *(III)*.

MO/OD cavity: Onlay

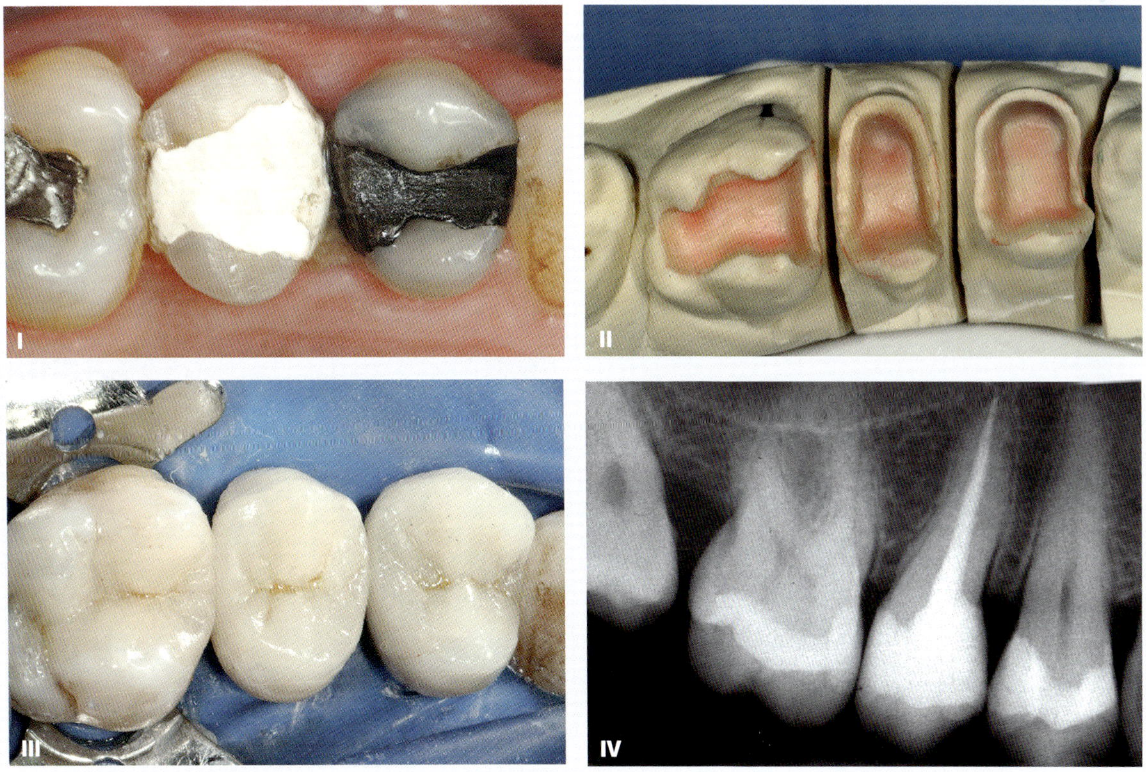

Fig 123 Preparation of two onlays for MOD cavities in two premolars, leading to endodontic treatment in one case *(I–III)*. The accuracy of the marginal seals is visible on the follow-up radiograph *(IV)*.

MO/OD cavity: Onlay

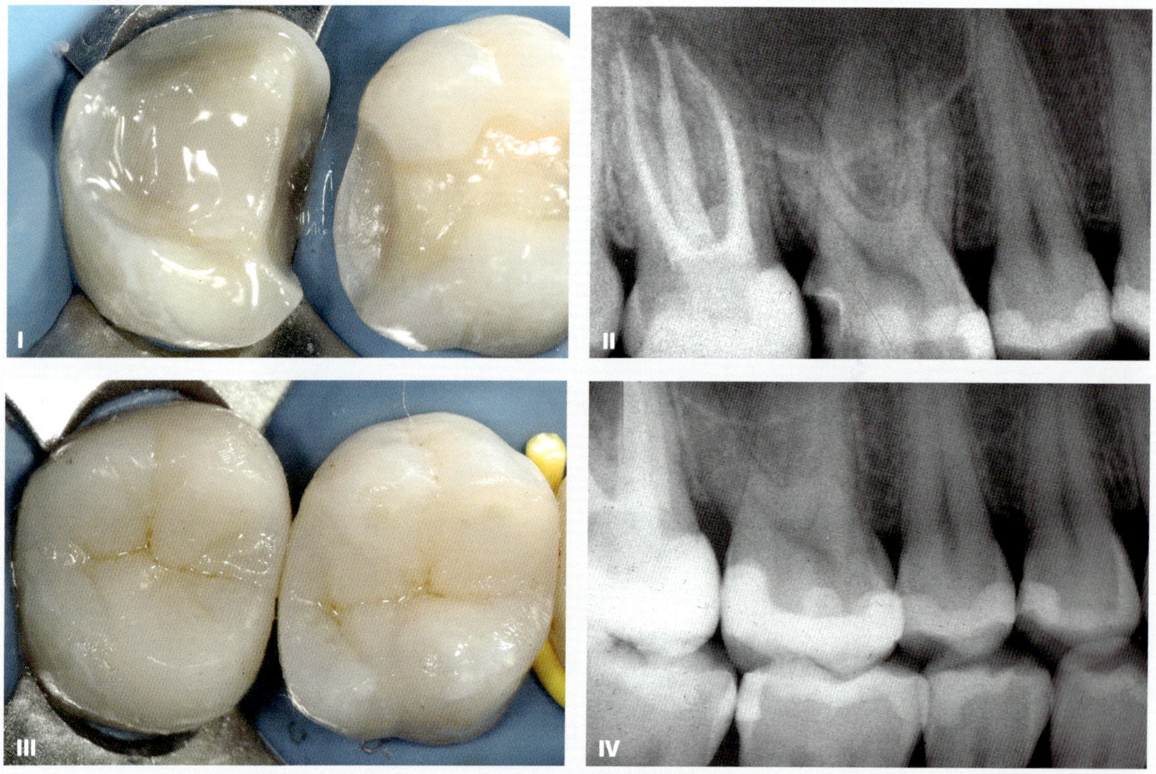

Fig 124 Onlay for a maxillary right second molar following endodontic treatment. Despite the depth of the box and the consequent difficulty in isolating the operative field *(I–III)*, the post-cementation radiograph shows adequate marginal closure *(IV)*. To achieve this, after cementation at the second molar, rubber dam was removed to facilitate procedures to finish the margin before cementation of the restoration for the first molar, which was performed after repositioning the dam.

MO/OD cavity: Onlay

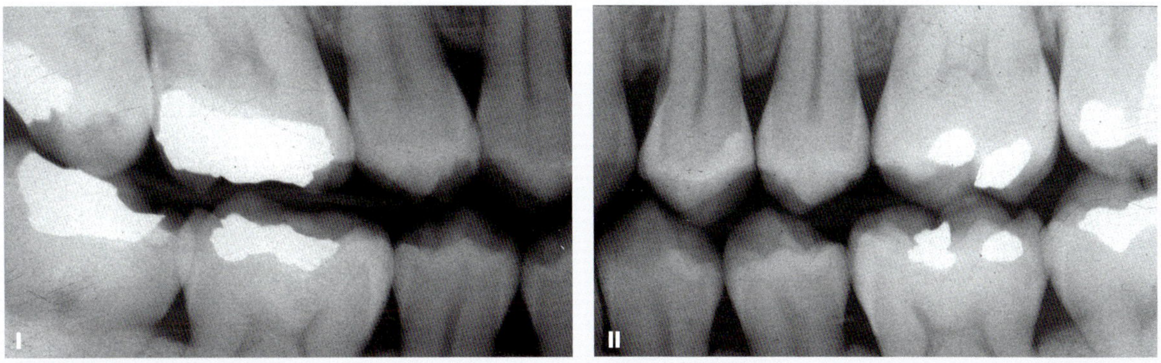

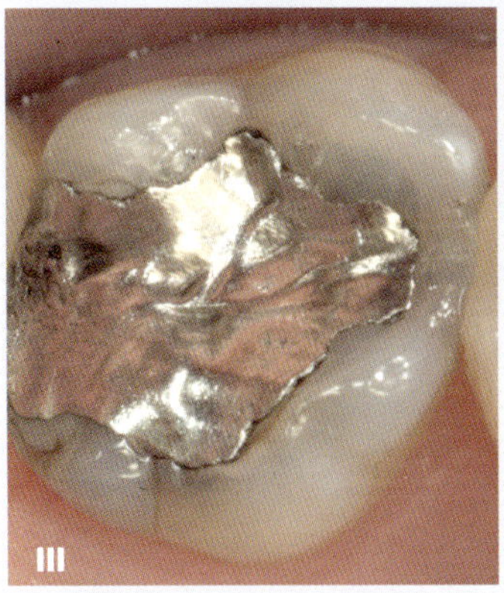

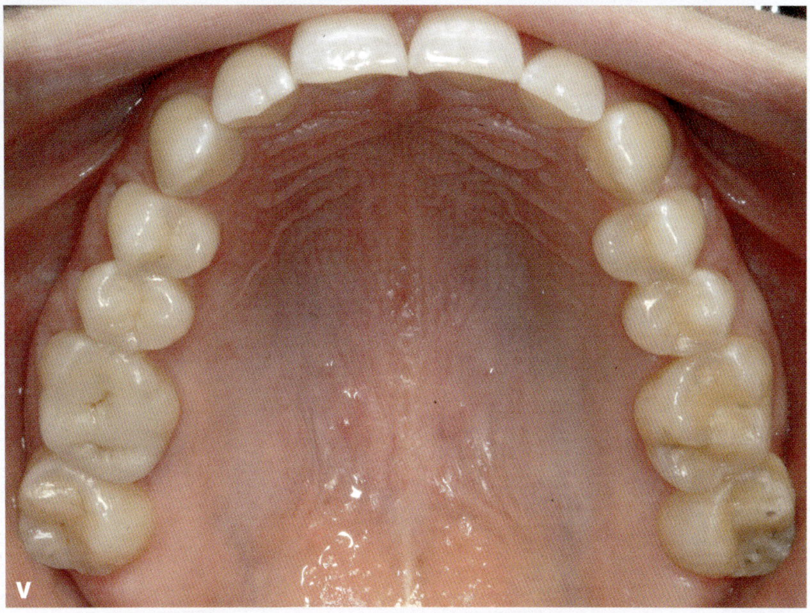

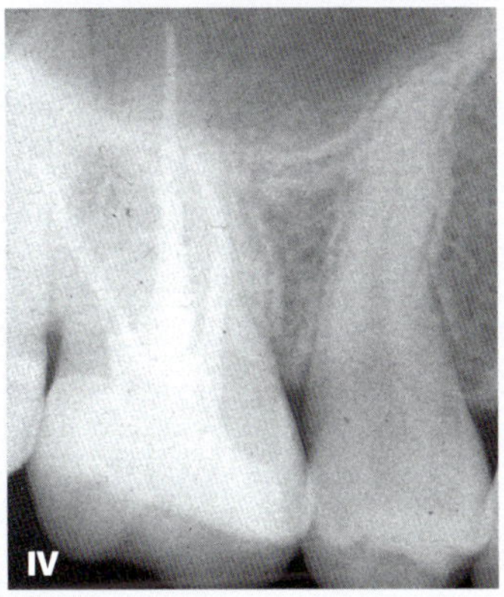

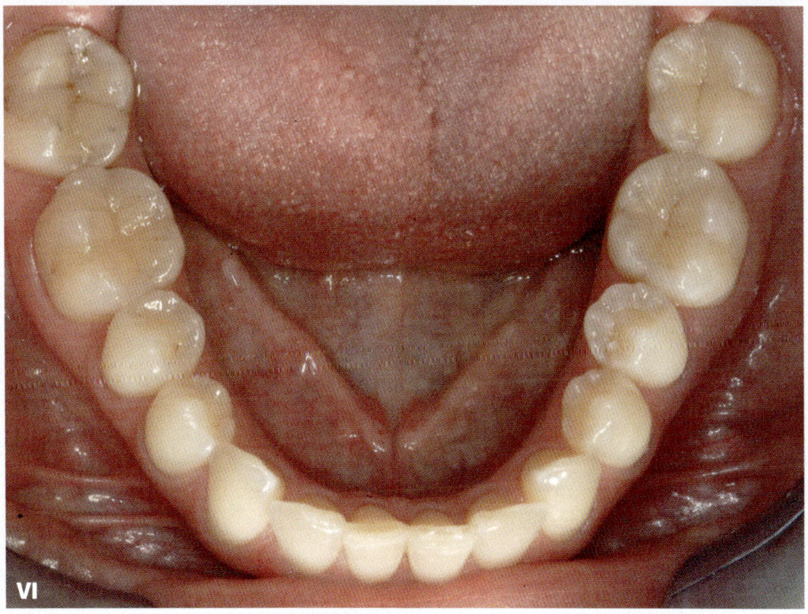

Fig 125 View of two arches restored using direct techniques, with the exception of the maxillary right first molar, which was endodontically treated for pulpitis and reconstructed with an onlay.

MO/OD cavity: Onlay

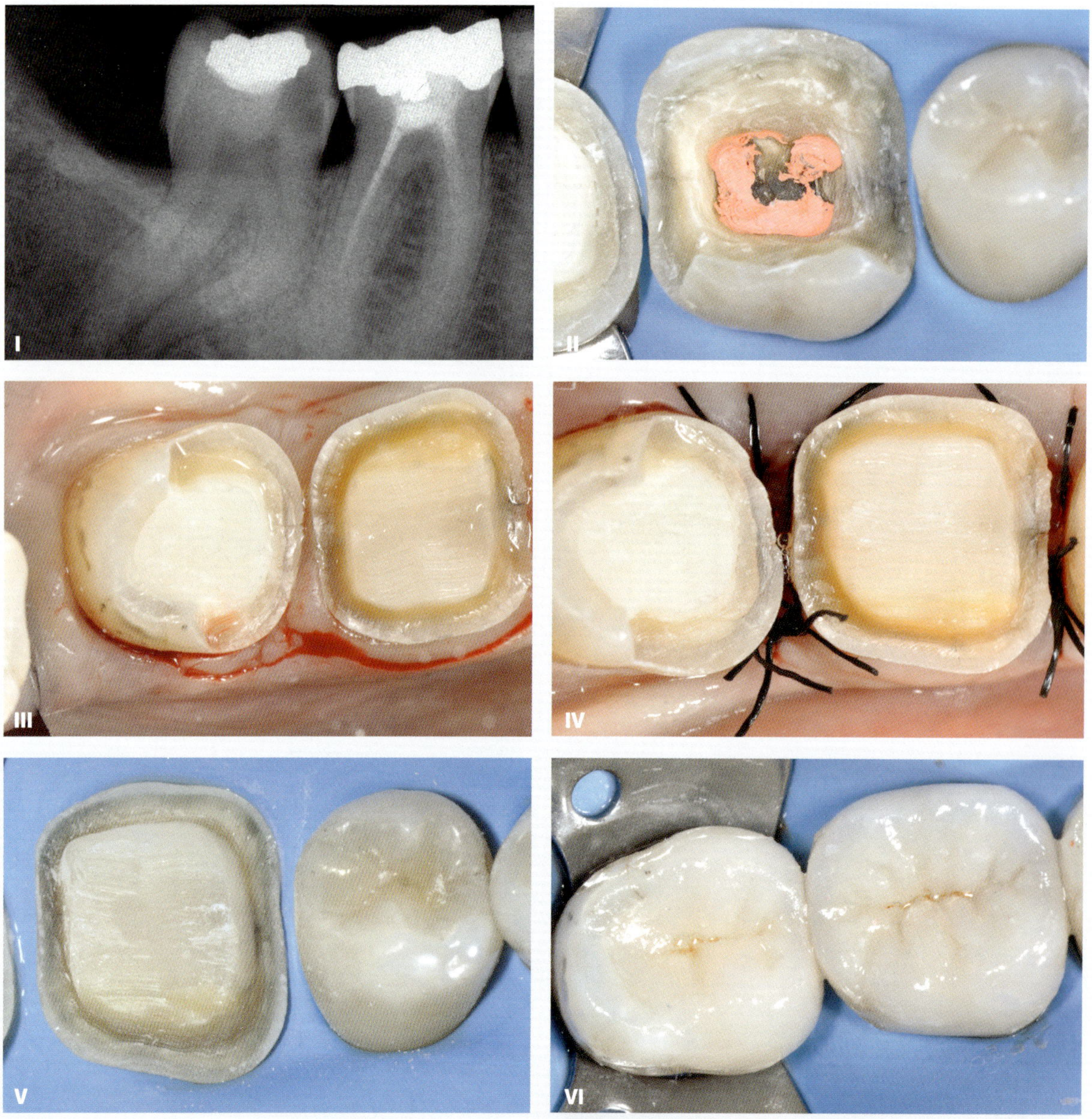

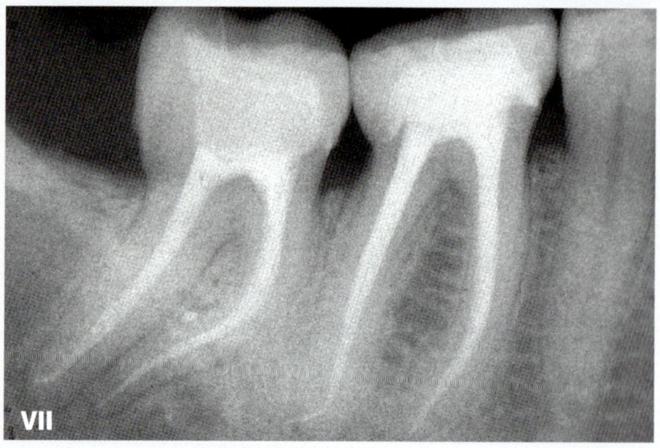

Fig 126 Penetrating decay and defective endodontic treatment for mandibular right second and first molars, respectively *(I, II)*. After the endodontic stage and periodontal surgery *(III, IV)*, the teeth were reconstructed with an onlay for the second molar and an overlay for the first molar *(V, VI)*. Follow-up radiograph showing the marginal seals and endodontic treatments performed by Dr Marco Forestali *(VII)*.

MOD cavity: Overlay

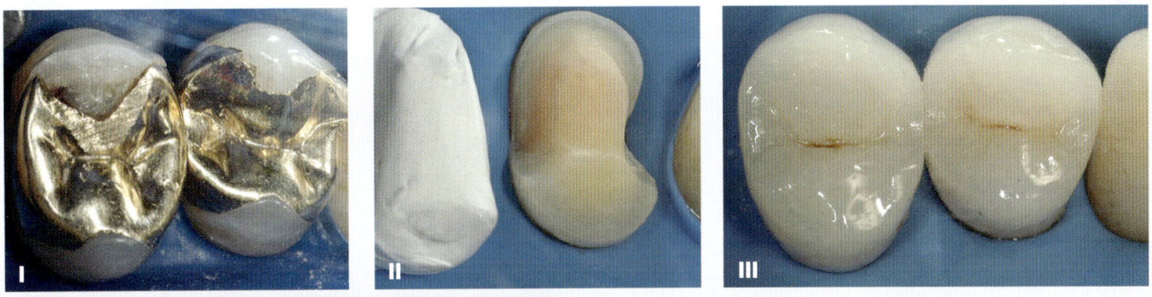

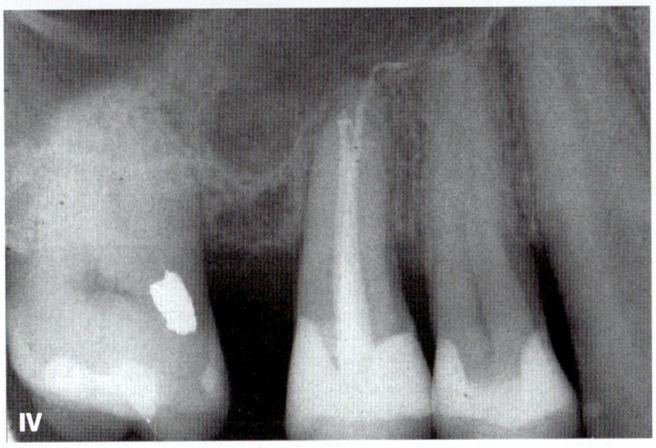

Fig 127 Morphofunctional restoration of two leaking maxillary premolar restorations after 20 years of service *(I)*. Endodontic treatment for penetrating decay of the second premolar and maintenance of pulp vitality in the first premolar. View showing preparation of the overlay *(II)* and cemented inlays *(III)*. Postoperative radiograph *(IV)*.

MOD cavity: Overlay

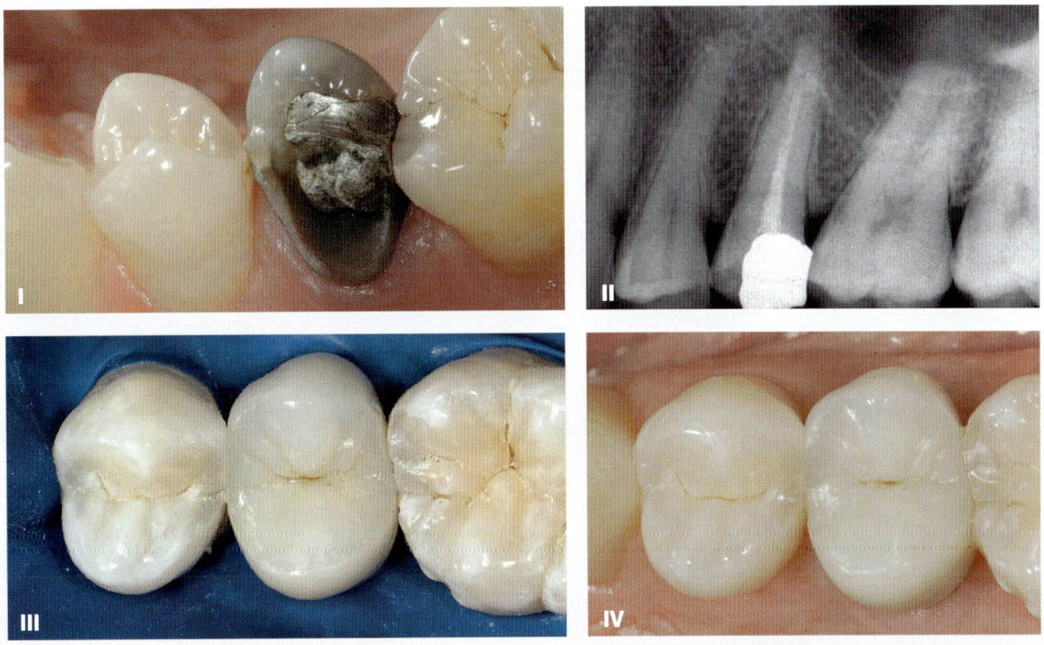

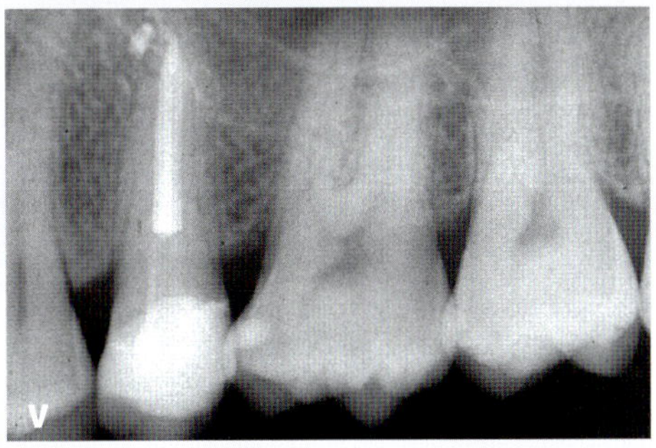

Fig 128 Fracture of the lingual wall of the maxillary left second premolar, which had received suboptimal endodontic treatment *(I, II)*. After the necessary endodontic re-treatment and positioning of a post for reconstruction, the restoration was finalized with an overlay *(III, IV)*. The patient wished to postpone treatment of the caries lesions in the distal aspect of the first premolar and the mesial aspect of the first molar. Postoperative follow-up radiograph *(V)*.

MOD cavity: Overlay

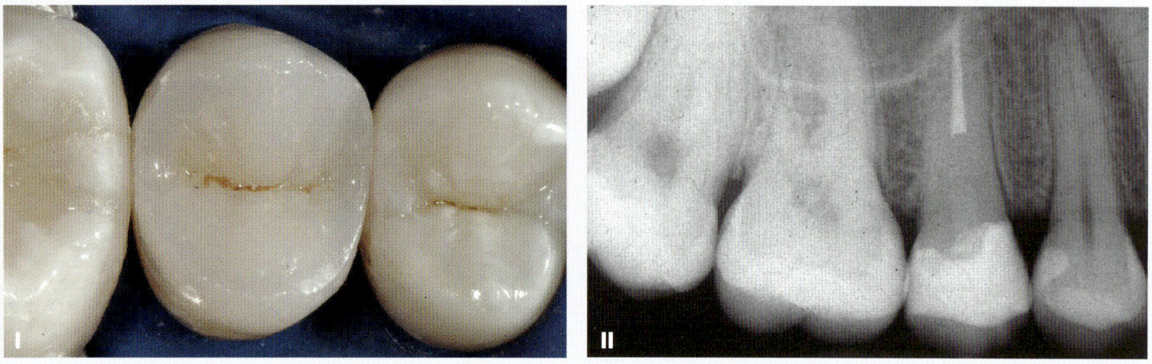

Fig 129 Clinical and radiographic views of an overlay on an endodontically treated premolar. The appearance of the marginal seals is good.

MOD cavity: Overlay

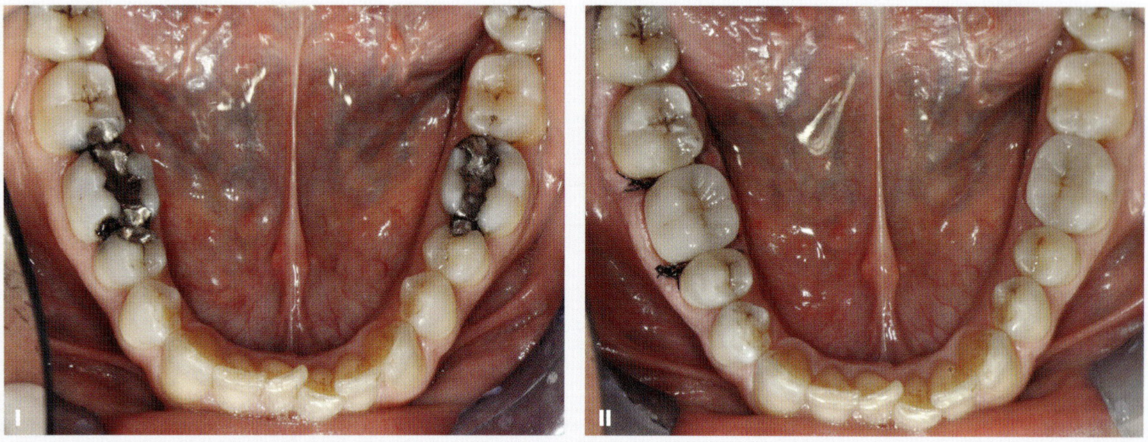

Fig 130 Pre- and postoperative clinical view of an arch with an overlay in the mandibular right first molar and direct and indirect restorations.

MOD cavity: Overlay

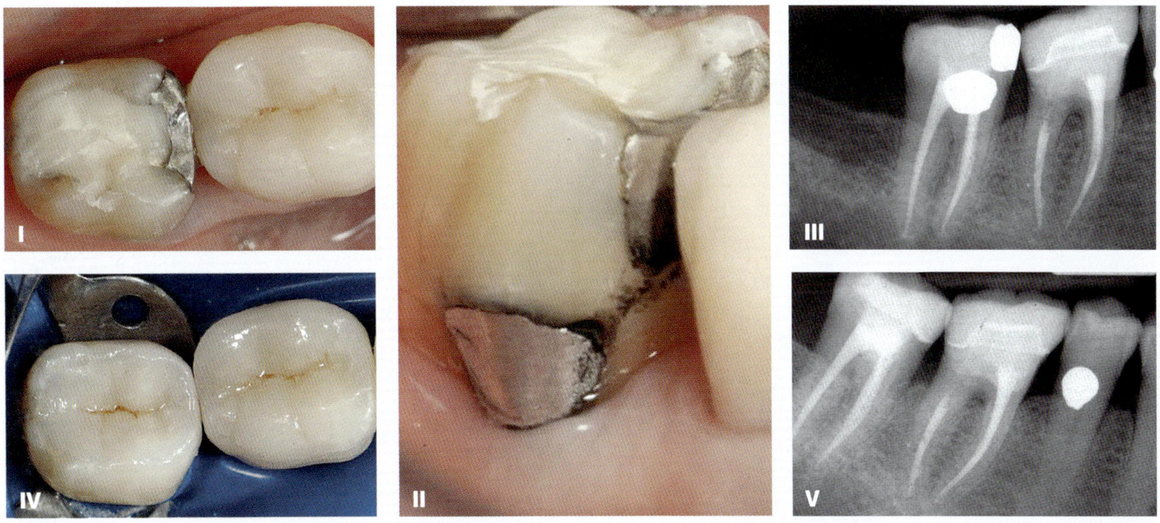

Fig 131 Overlay on the MOD cavity of the mandibular right second molar after endodontic treatment. The adjacent first molar had previously been treated in the same way.

MOD cavity: Overlay

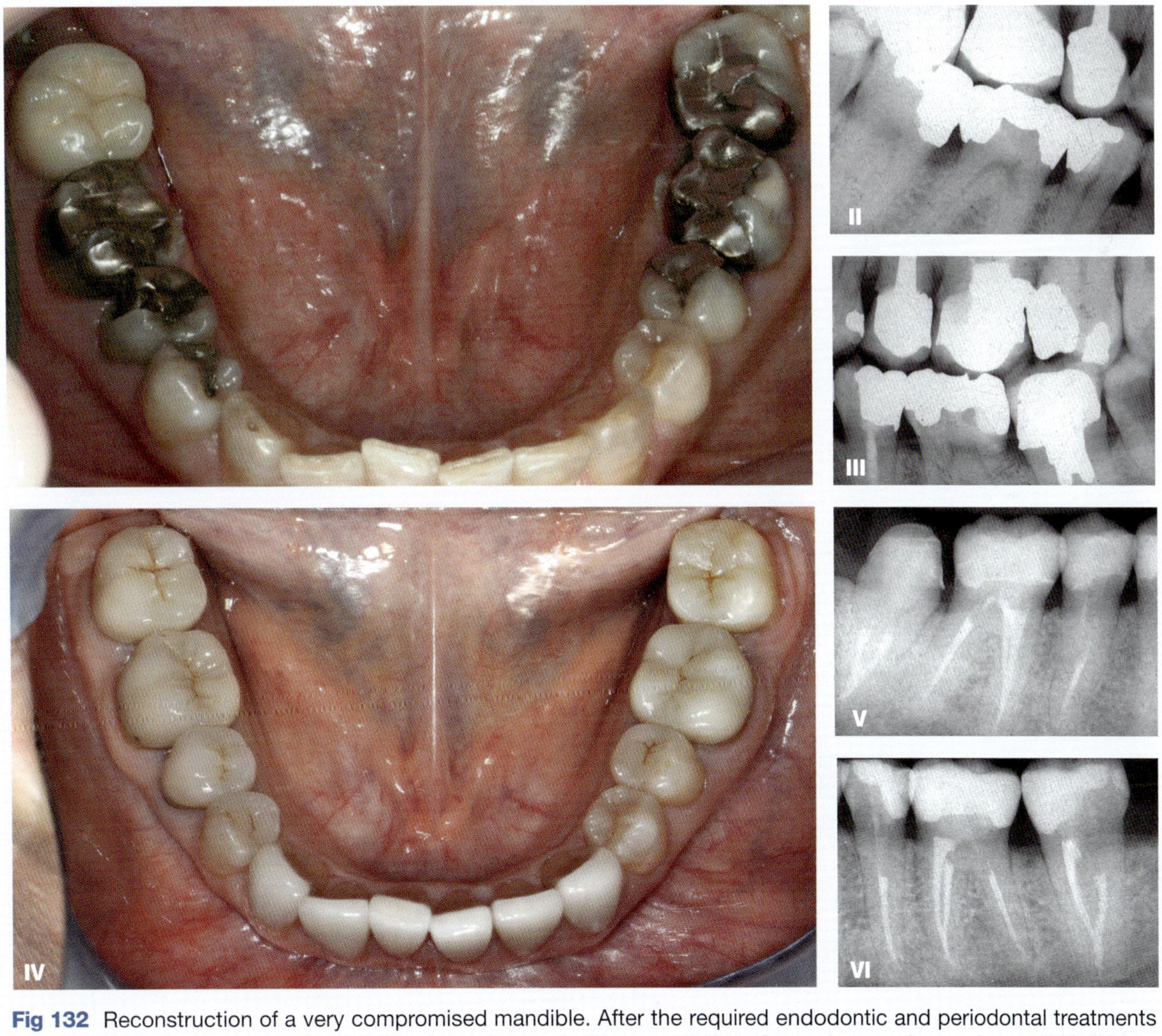

Fig 132 Reconstruction of a very compromised mandible. After the required endodontic and periodontal treatments in both quadrants, the restorative treatment was finalized with cementation of an onlay, overlay, and monolithic lithium disilicate crown.

MOD cavity: Overlay

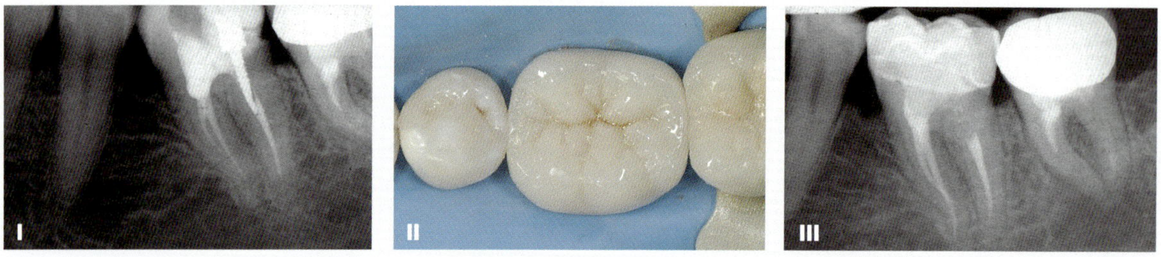

Fig 133 Overlay on a somewhat compromised left mandibular molar. The patient wished to put off treatment of the last molar.

MOD cavity: Overlay

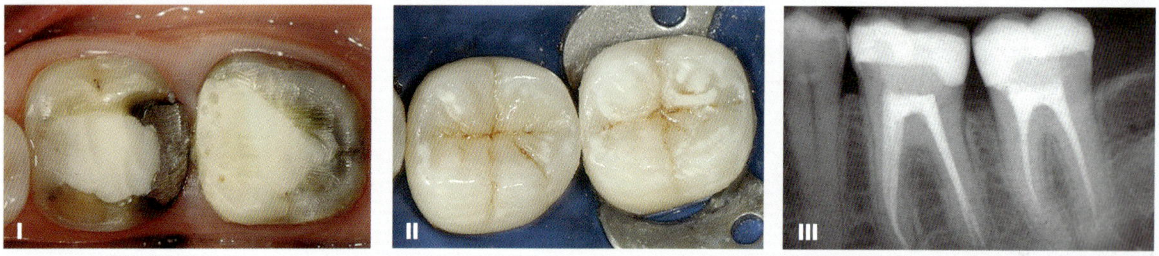

Fig 134 Entirely insufficient thicknesses required protection of these endodontically treated mandibular molars by means of two overlays.

MOD cavity: Overlay

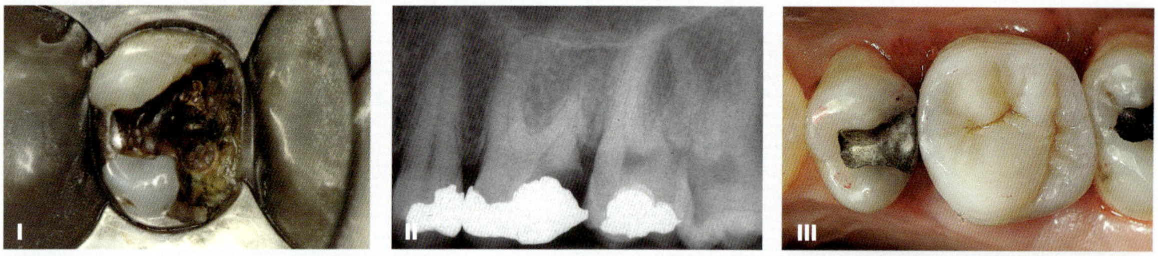

Fig 135 The maxillary left first molar showed extremely deep penetrating decay. Endodontic and periodontal treatments were essential before performing an overlay. The follow-up radiograph showed entirely satisfactory marginal seal of the inlay.

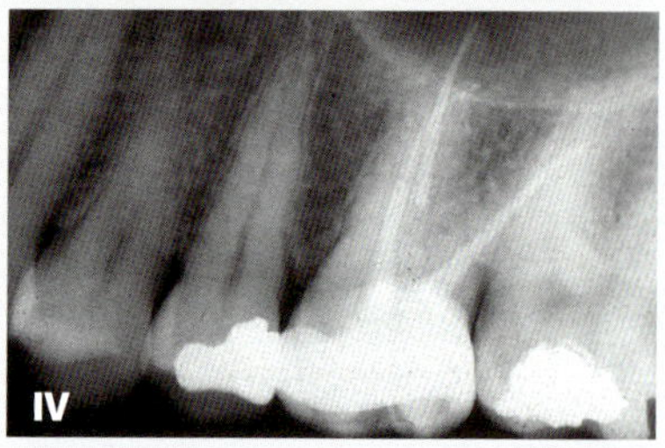

MOD cavity: Overlay

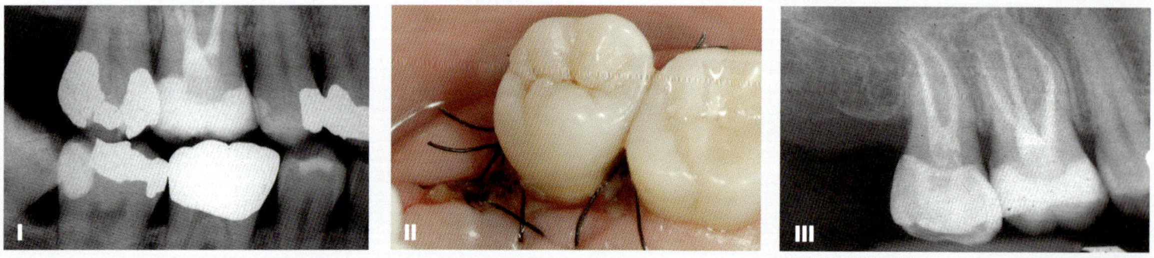

Fig 136 Diagnosis of pulpitis and consequent endodontic treatment for the maxillary right second molar *(I)*. Again, lengthening of the clinical crown *(II)* makes it possible to appreciate the impeccable margins of the overlay on the follow-up radiograph *(III)*.

MOD cavity: Overlay

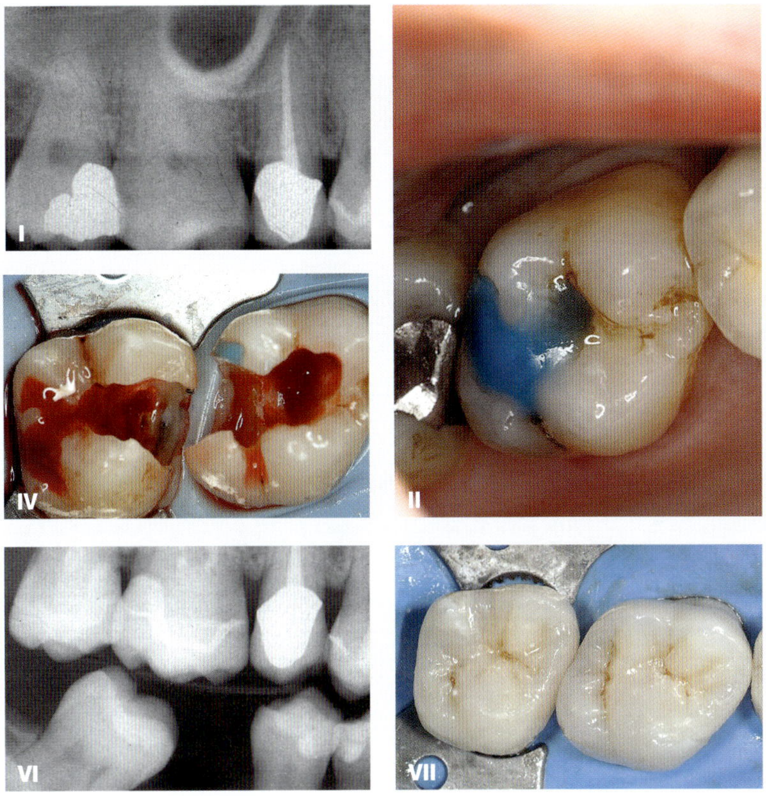

Fig 137 The overlay for the maxillary right first molar and onlay for the adjacent second molar represent the solution for the reconstruction of these severely compromised teeth, following endodontic and periodontal treatment *(I–V)*. View of the marginal seals *(VI)* and the cemented restorations *(VII)*.

MOD cavity: Overlay

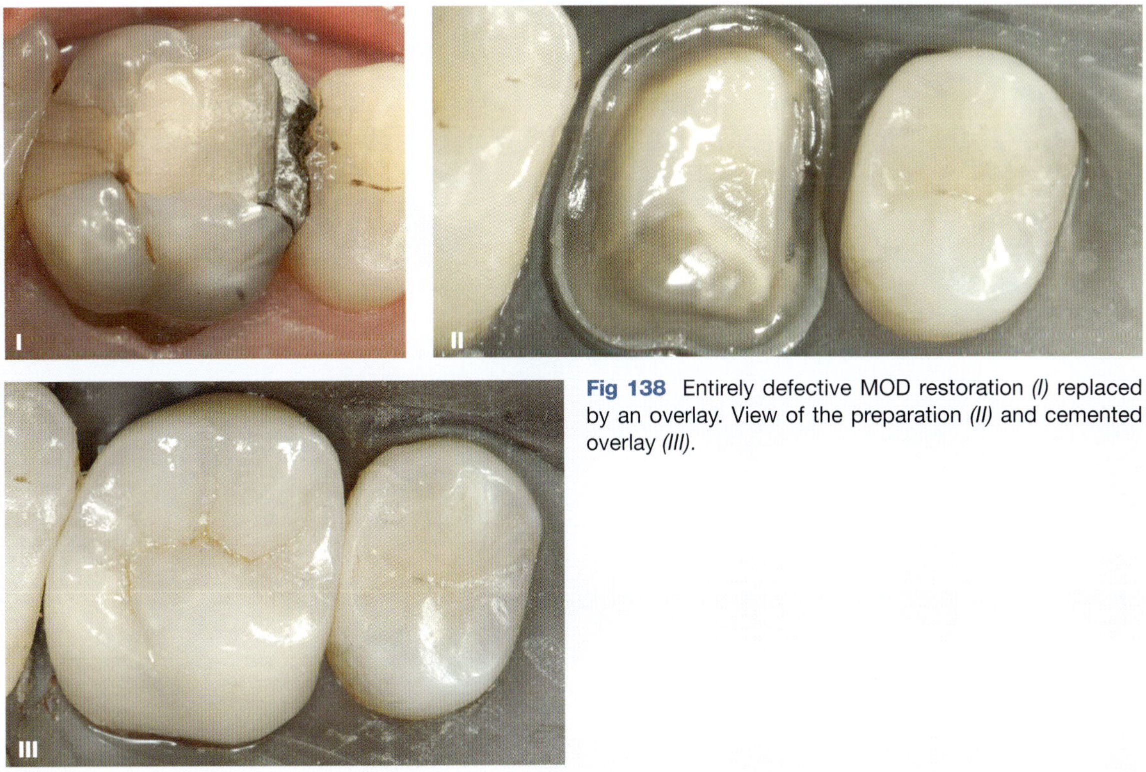

Fig 138 Entirely defective MOD restoration *(I)* replaced by an overlay. View of the preparation *(II)* and cemented overlay *(III)*.

Covering the cusps

It is known that the minimum thicknesses for cusp maintenance corresponds to 2 mm for a vital tooth and 3 mm for an endodontically treated tooth. At this point, the decision regarding whether or not to opt for a cavity is very simple; it only remains to decide whether the indication should be to cover a cusp by encircling it (ie, with a 90-degree shoulder preparation) or adopt a knife-edge preparation (Fig 139).

Research conducted by Fichera et al[2] suggests that a shoulder margin is indicated:

- With major loss of tooth substance from the cusp, with the involvement of the middle and/or cervical third
- In mandibular buccal cusps, irrespective of the extent of lost tooth tissue (Figs 140 to 147)

The characteristics of this procedural choice may be summarized as:

- Occlusoaxial reduction of the cusp with the cervical margin located at the supragingival level
- Less conservative preparation
- Technically more difficult preparation (even though it is still extremely simple in the author's opinion)
- Preparation with superior biomechanical characteristics in terms of retention, stability, and stress redistribution

Here the author would like to make one entirely personal comment on the breadth of the shoulder, since the clinical photographs show that the shoulders are all decidedly broad. This could give the impression of an aggressive, not very conservative preparation; in actual fact, the disadvantage of losing more tooth tissue during the preparation is more than outweighed by the gains made in terms of long-term maintenance; healthy, distinct margins without microfractures or microleaks; and no trace of caries lesions. The author believes that this is simply another way of being extremely conservative.

Fichera et al[2] furthermore suggests that coverage with a knife-edge margin is indicated:

- By the need to prevent the tooth-restoration margin coinciding with the occlusal contact
- By a structural deficiency in the occlusal third of the cusp
- By a structural weakening of the cusp that cannot be compensated for by the reinforcing action of the buildup (Figs 148 to 150)

The characteristics of a knife-edge preparation are:

- Exclusively occlusal reduction of the cusp
- A conservative preparation that is very simple to perform
- Lower biomechanical efficacy in terms of retention, stability, and stress redistribution

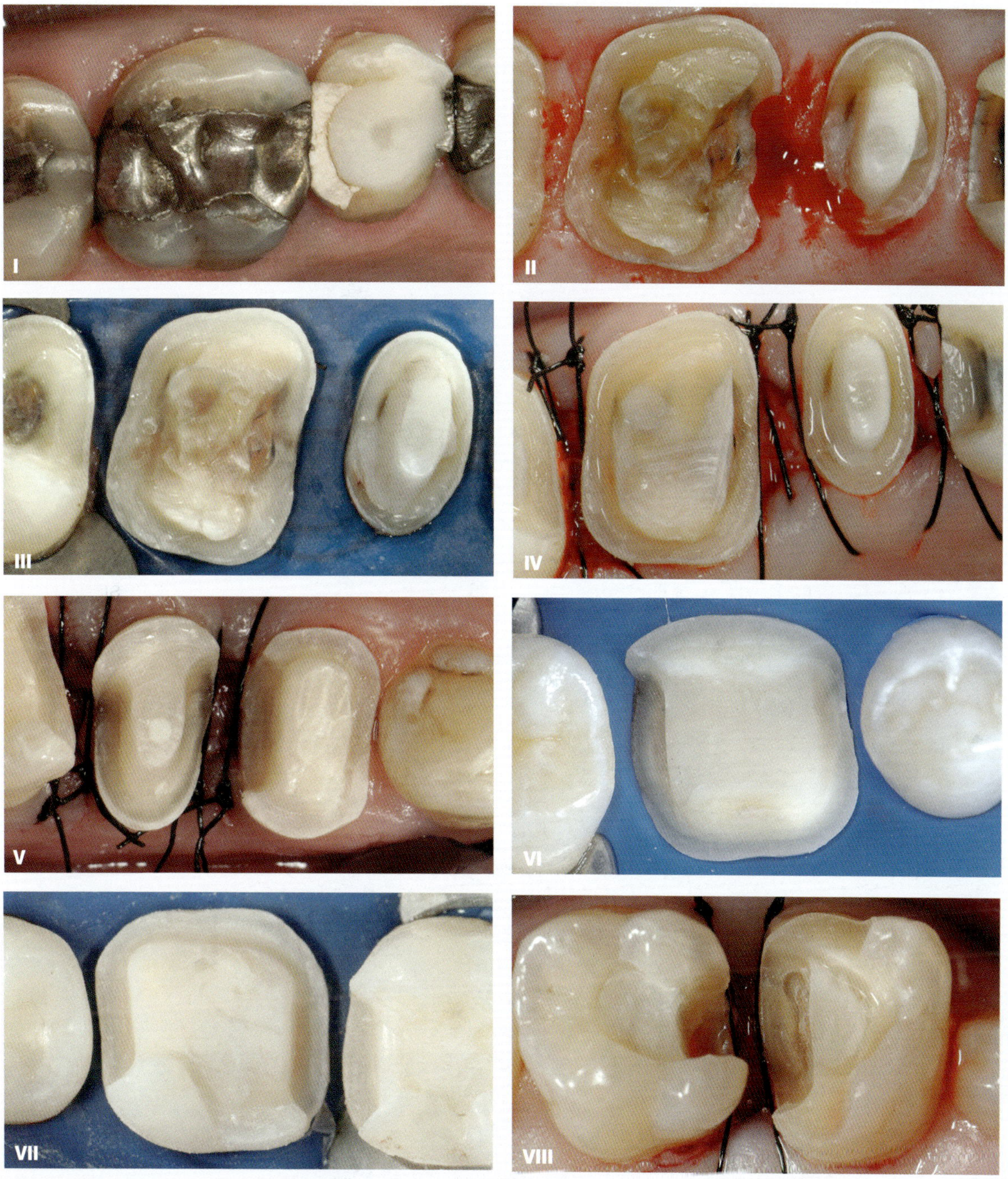

Fig 139 View of some preparations with shoulder and knife-edge margins.

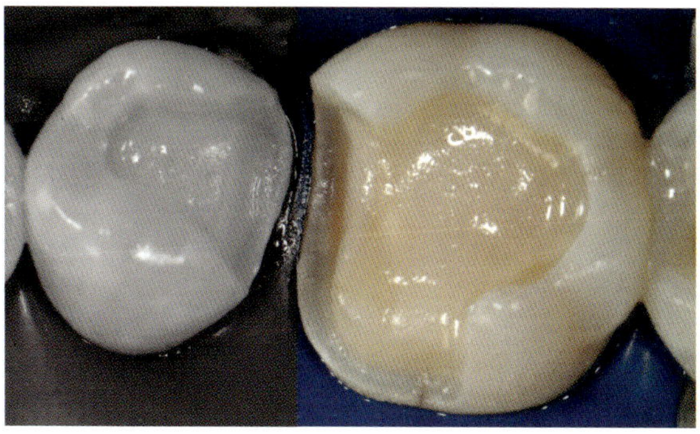

Fig 140 Typical shoulder preparation of a tooth with vital pulp: the thicknesses always determine whether or not the cusps should be maintained.

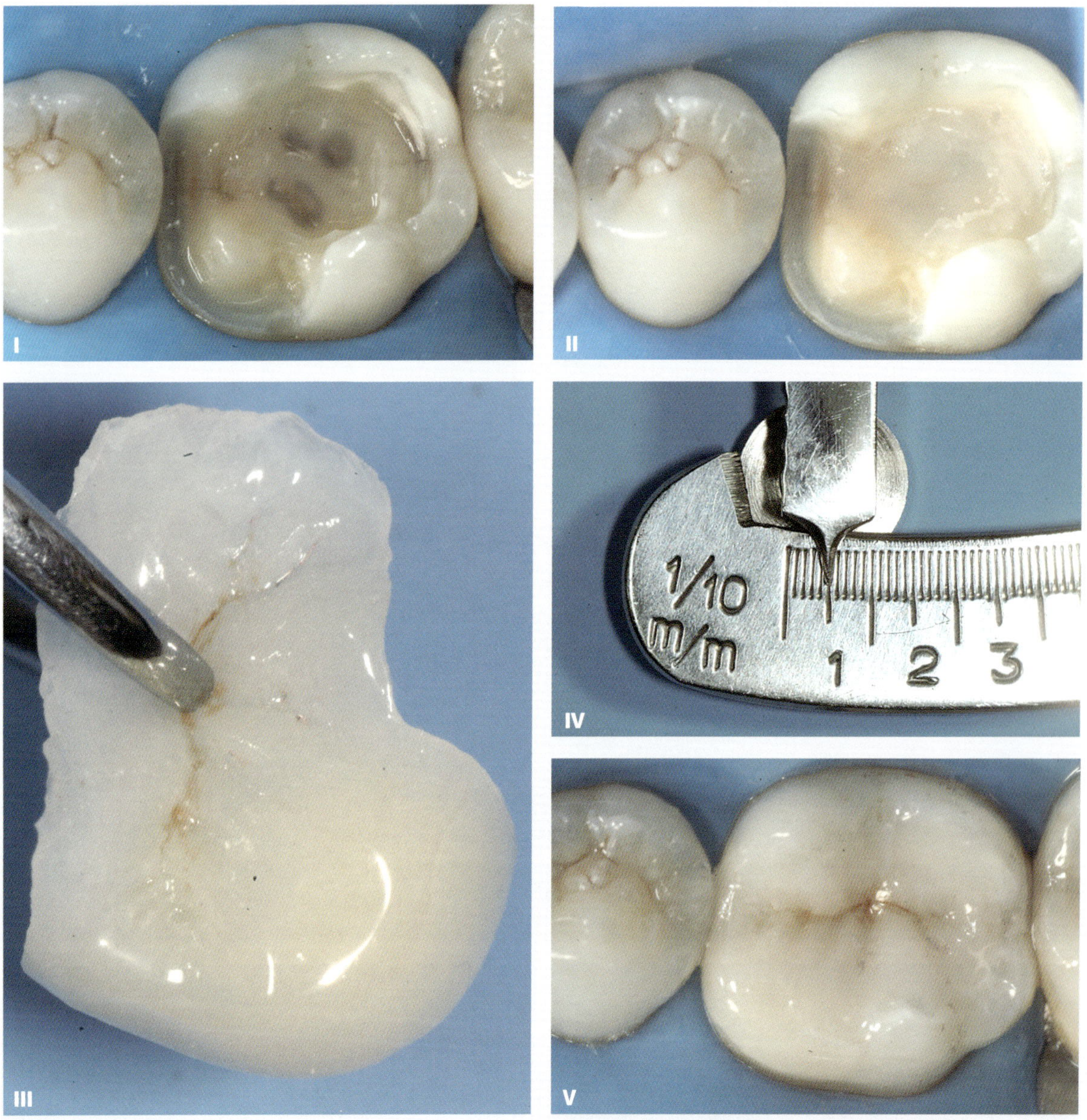

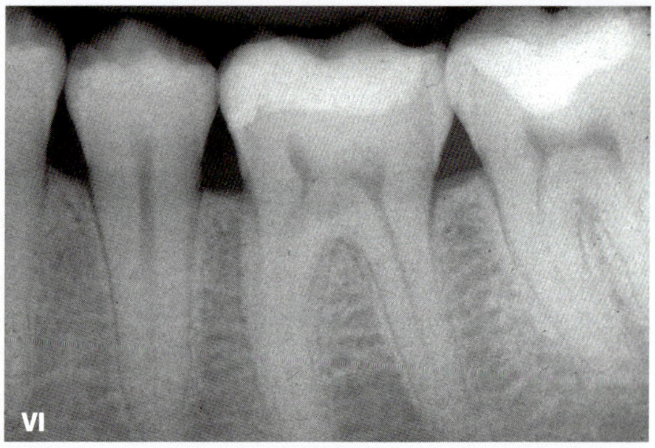

Fig 141 Onlay with mesiobuccal cusp coverage and shoulder preparation *(I, II)*. Note the minimum thickness of the inlay in its deepest groove *(III, IV)*; the inlay blends into the tooth perfectly in terms of its biomechanical resistance because the buildup, cement, and onlay are made out of the same material, ie, composite, which has elastic properties similar to those of dentin *(V, VI)*. It bears repeating that this wonderful material was chosen because it can be corrected during cementation and repaired over time.

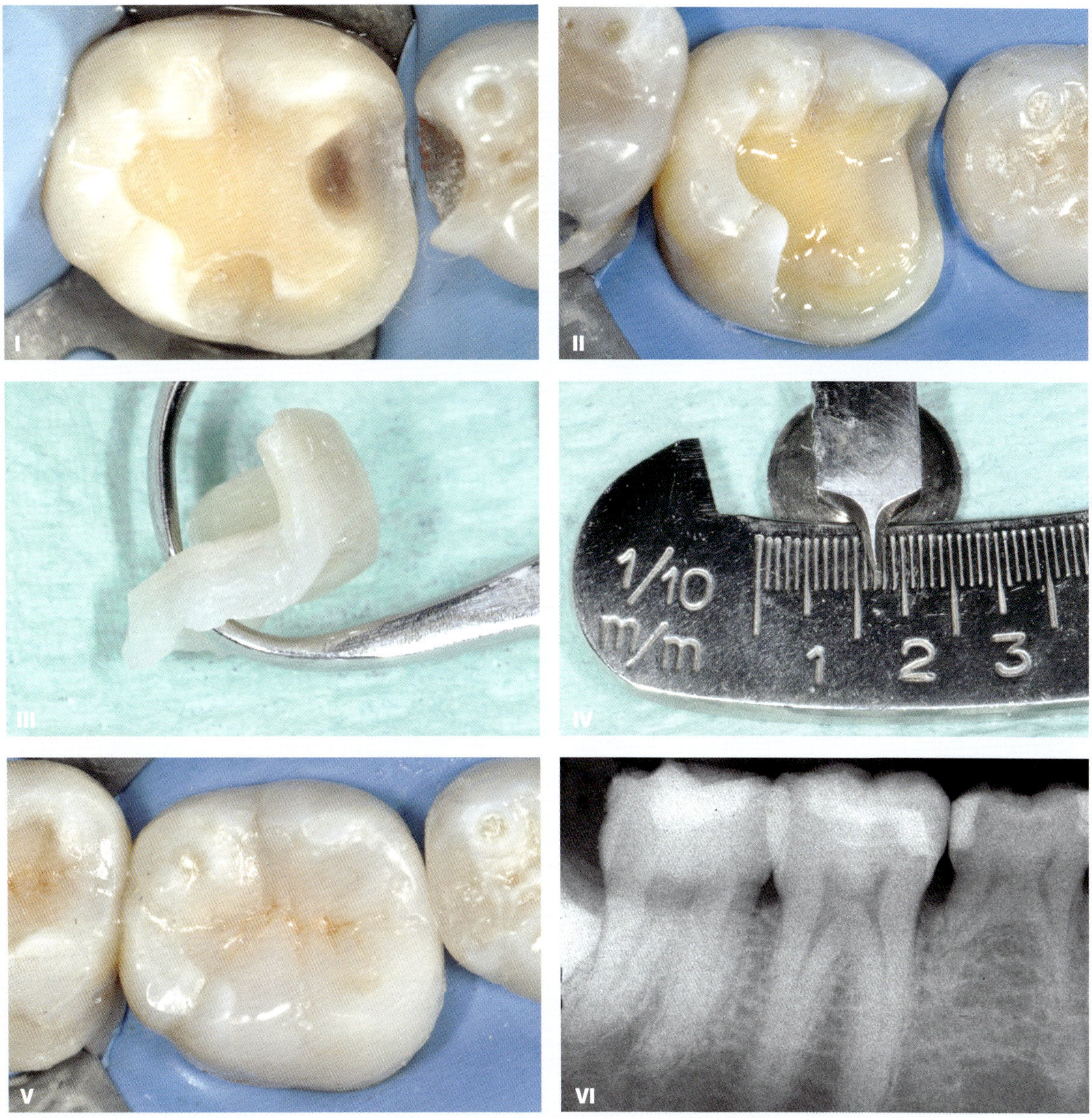

Fig 142 Classic shoulder preparation with intraoperative photographs during removal of decayed tissue *(I)* and execution of buildup *(II)*, demonstration of thickness of the inlay *(III, IV)*, cemented inlay *(V)*, and follow-up radiograph *(VI)*.

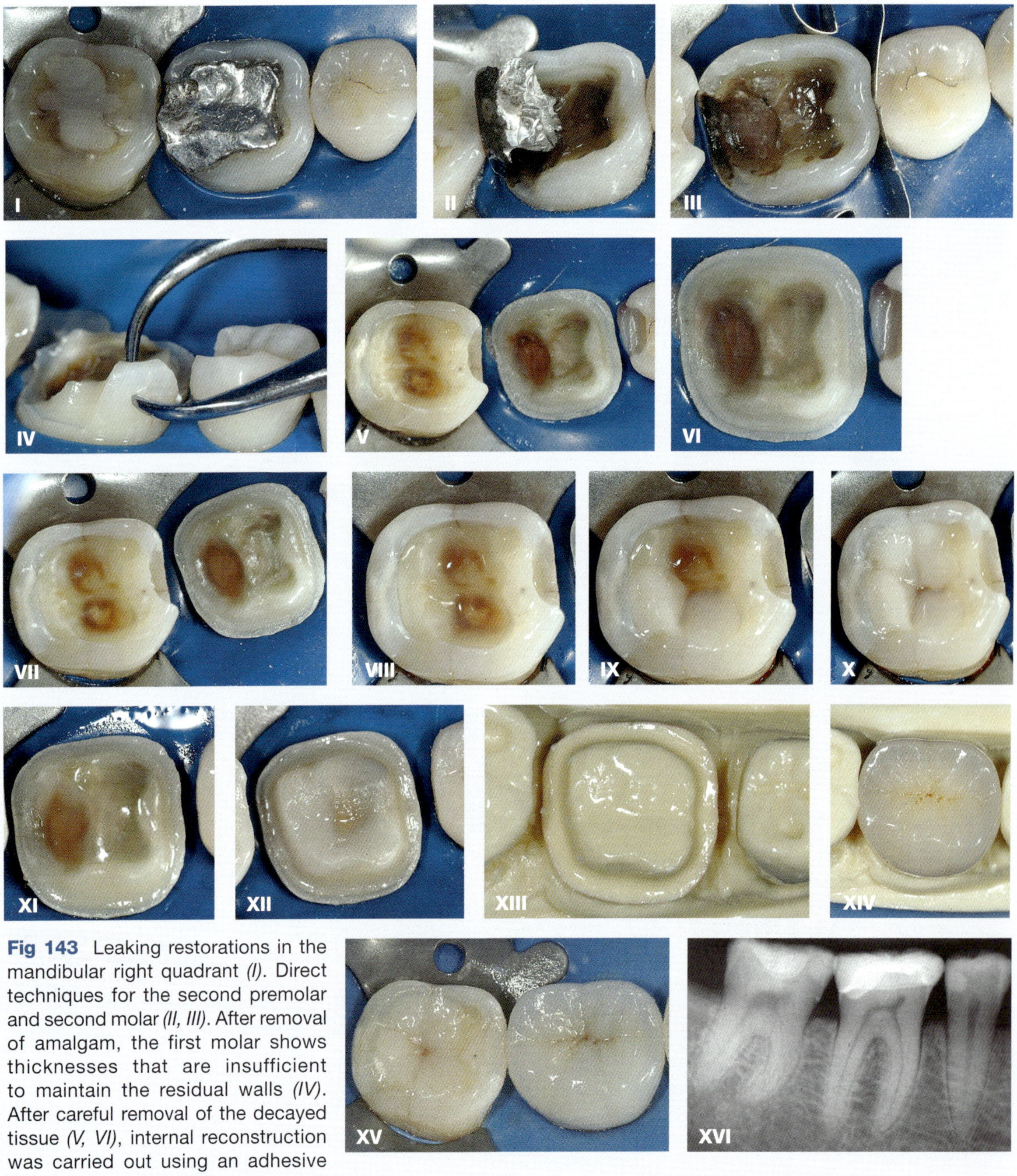

Fig 143 Leaking restorations in the mandibular right quadrant *(I)*. Direct techniques for the second premolar and second molar *(II, III)*. After removal of amalgam, the first molar shows thicknesses that are insufficient to maintain the residual walls *(IV)*. After careful removal of the decayed tissue *(V, VI)*, internal reconstruction was carried out using an adhesive system, flowable composite, and traditional composite *(VII–X)*, and an overlay was prepared with the usual 90-degree shoulder *(XI–XIV)*. View of the cemented inlay and follow-up radiograph *(XV, XVI)*.

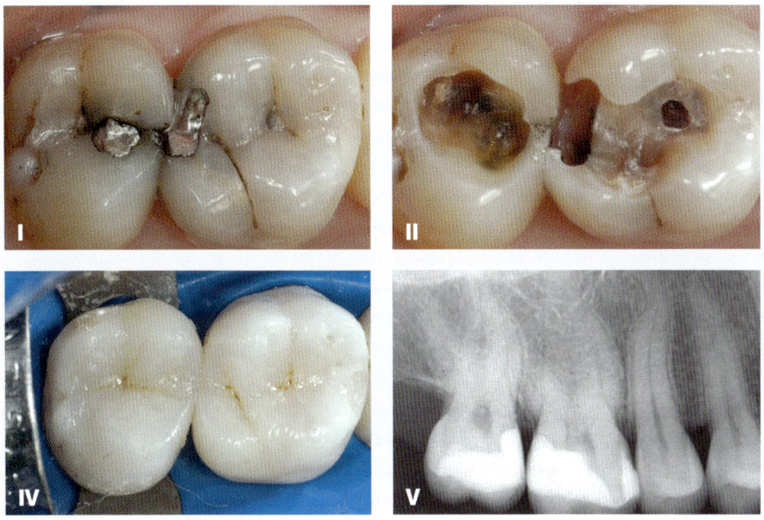

Fig 144 Preparation of two onlays with removal of walls after measuring the residual thicknesses *(I–III)*. Cemented inlays and follow-up radiograph *(IV, V)*.

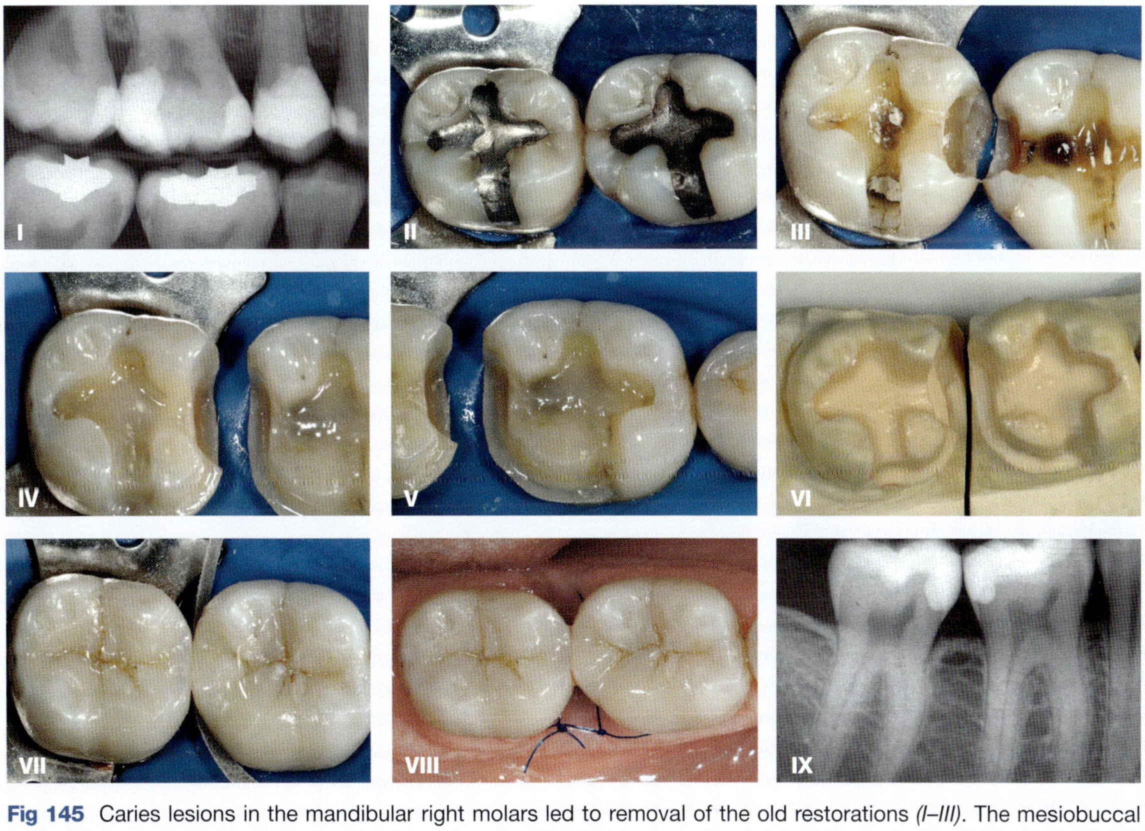

Fig 145 Caries lesions in the mandibular right molars led to removal of the old restorations *(I–III)*. The mesiobuccal wall of the second molar and the distobuccal wall of the first molar were removed because the usual thicknesses were insufficient. Views of the teeth after buildup and preparation *(IV, V)*, working casts *(VI)*, and cemented adhesive restorations *(VII, VIII)*. Follow-up radiograph *(IX)*.

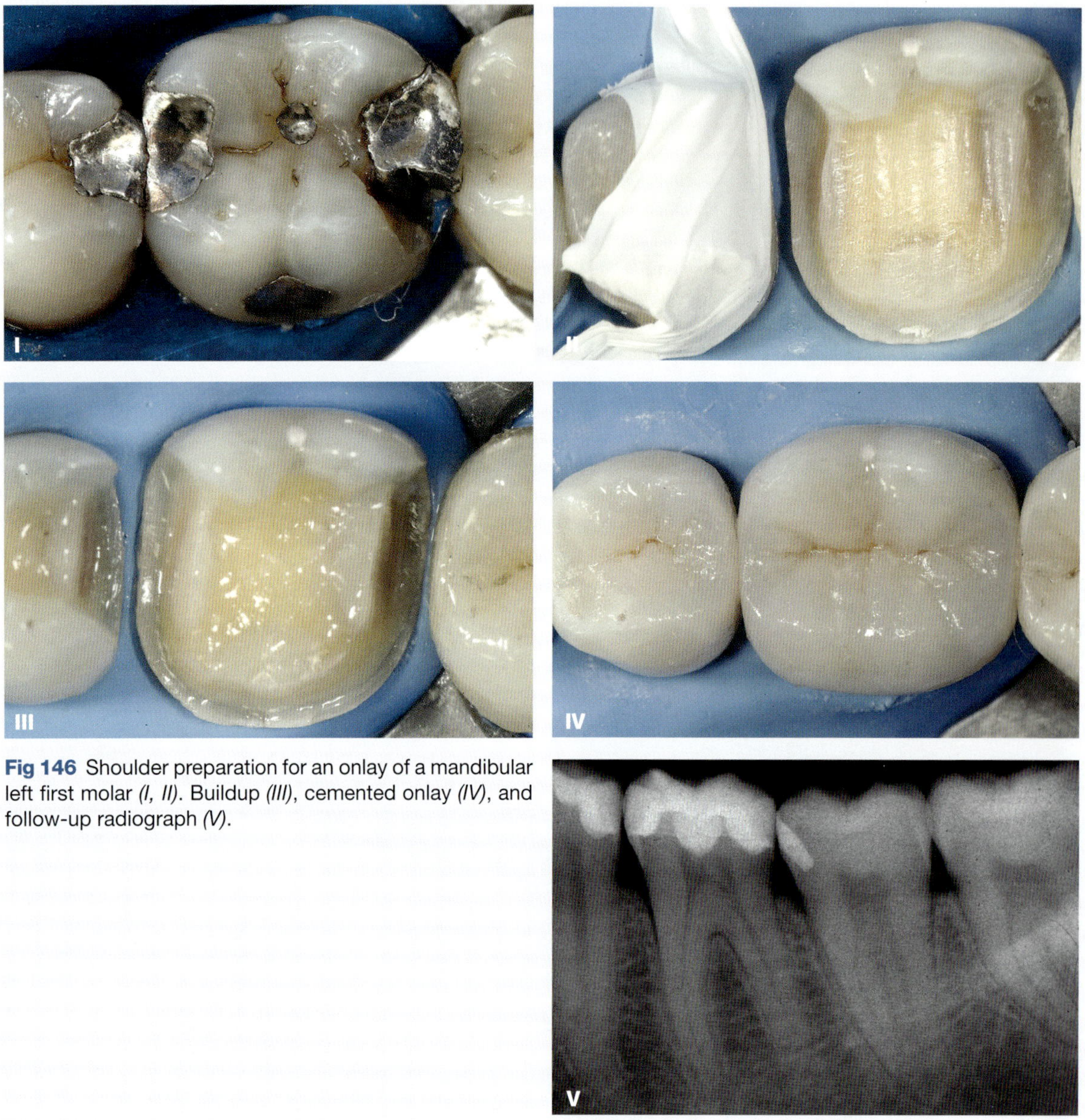

Fig 146 Shoulder preparation for an onlay of a mandibular left first molar *(I, II)*. Buildup *(III)*, cemented onlay *(IV)*, and follow-up radiograph *(V)*.

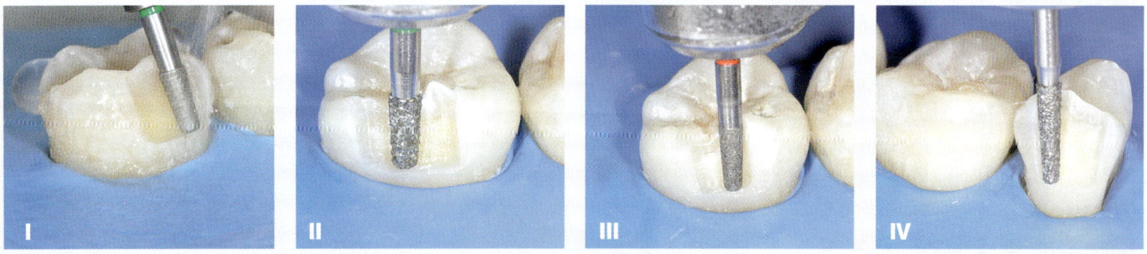

Fig 147 The author prefers a shoulder that corresponds to the entire diameter of the bur; being a few microns less conservative to obtain a broad shoulder has reaped rewards in terms of the negligible number of problems observed (eg, minor fractures, material scaling) over long-term follow-ups. Another consideration in terms of restoration-periodontium relationships is that the number of infiltrated margins has also been practically zero in the long term. This has been possible because the margins were always supragingival at the time of cementation, which was naturally carried out under rubber dam. This routinely allows their finishing to be optimized in accordance with protocol.

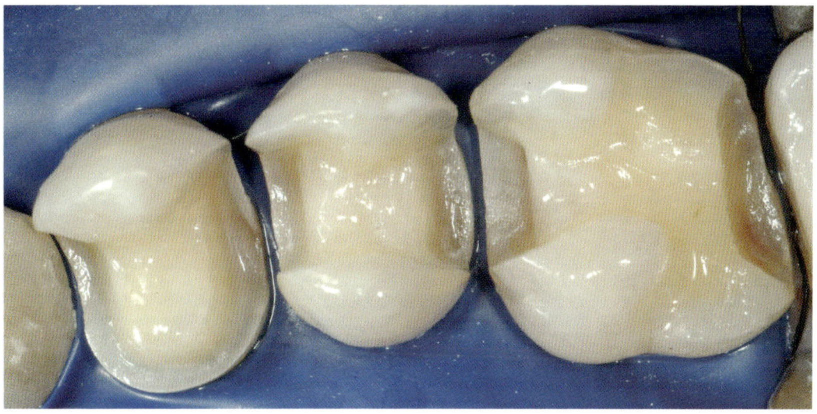

Fig 148 Preparation of an onlay for a maxillary left first molar with removal of the distal wall with a knife-edge preparation.

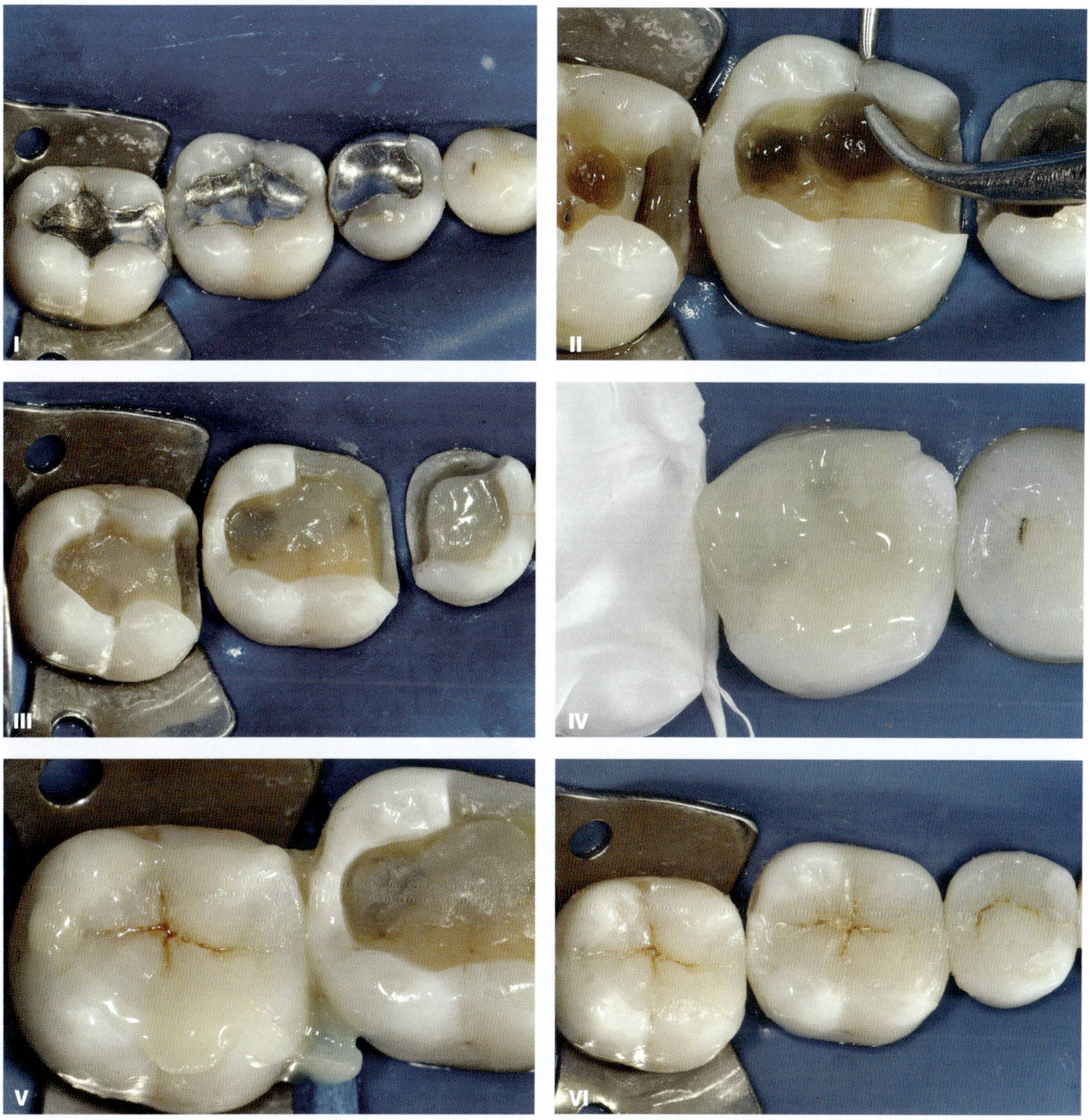

Fig 149 Preparation of indirect restorations in the fourth quadrant. An inlay is indicated for the mandibular right second molar, while the fact that the thickness is less than 2 mm suggests that the mesiobuccal wall of the adjacent first molar should be removed with a knife-edge preparation, and an onlay was performed for the second premolar *(I–III)*. Intraoperative view of cementation of the second premolar with protection of the first and second molars by a polytetrafluoroethylene strip *(IV)*. Build up of molars *(V)*. Cemented restorations *(VI)*.

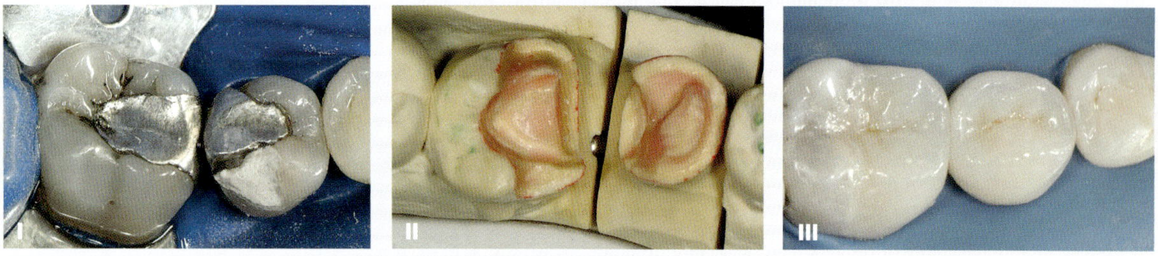

Fig 150 Knife-edge preparations and restorations after cementation.

Taking impressions

As already mentioned, taking an impression for partial restorations is made much easier by the supragingival positioning of preparation margins. If necessary, this can be achieved by lengthening the clinical crown, but obviously it is even more advantageous when the preparation margins are already located in a supragingival position without the need for intervention.

The material used to take the impression is polyvinyl siloxane positioned in an interocclusal record impression tray when one or two teeth are involved or in a full-arch impression tray when an entire quadrant is involved (Figs 151 and 152).

These topics are discussed in chapter 5.

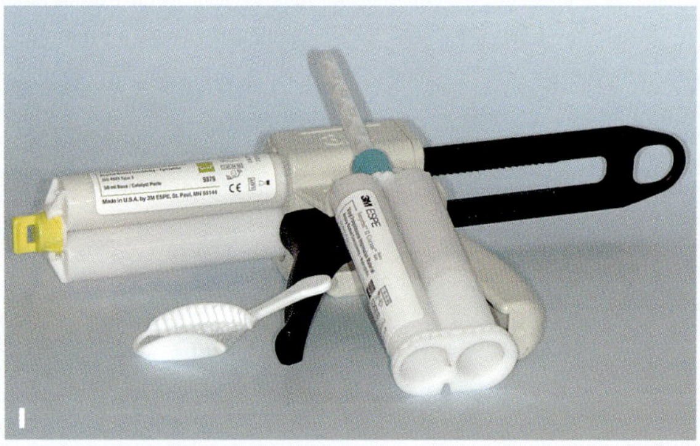

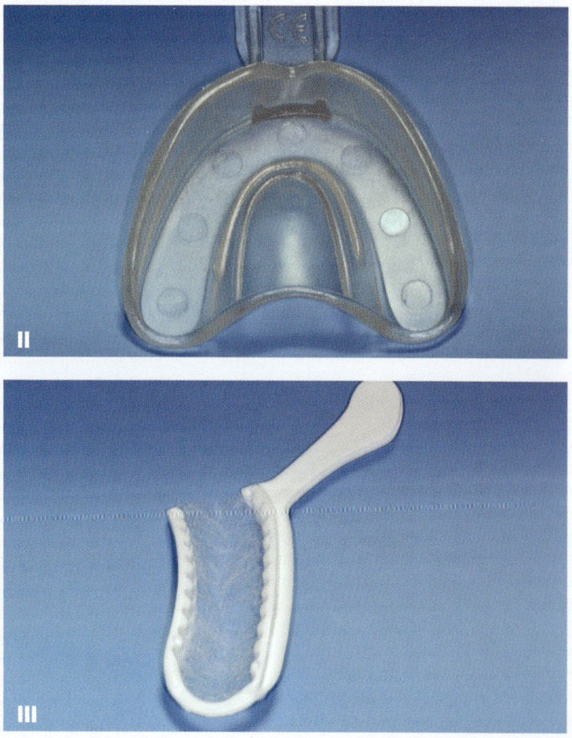

Fig 151 Material and impression tray.

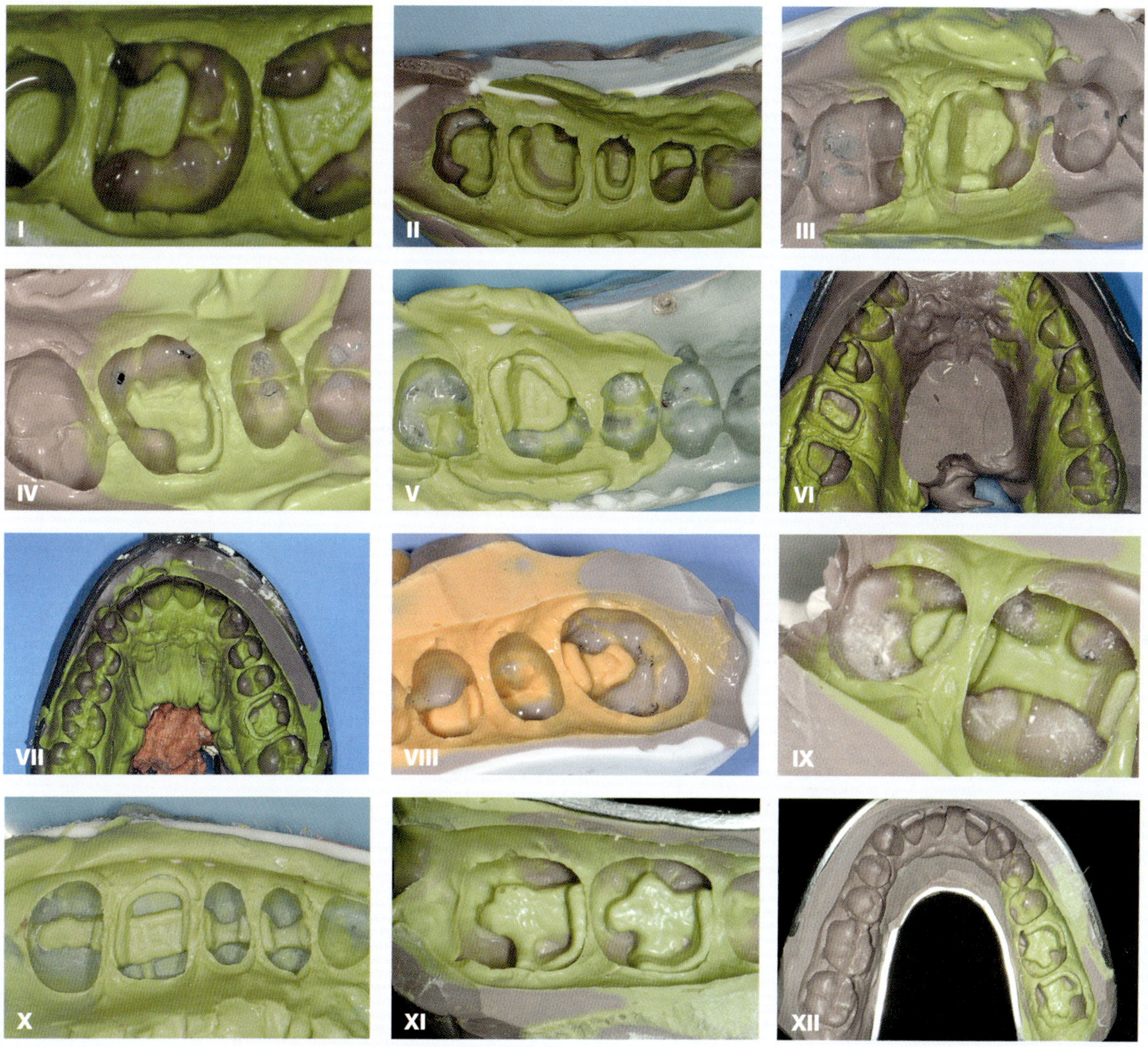

Fig 152 Examples of polyvinyl siloxane impressions.

Provisional restoration

The aim of a provisional restoration is to offer further protection to the pulp-dentin complex, which is already protected by the buildup. It must be designed in relation to the antagonist and proximal teeth and to allow proper function.

The material commonly used is Fermit N (Ivoclar Vivadent), applied in such a way as to allow the usual oral hygiene procedures to prevent tissue inflammation.

If cementation is due to take place within a very short time (1 to 3 days), a periodontal pack may be used as a temporary dressing (Figs 153 to 155).

Fig 153

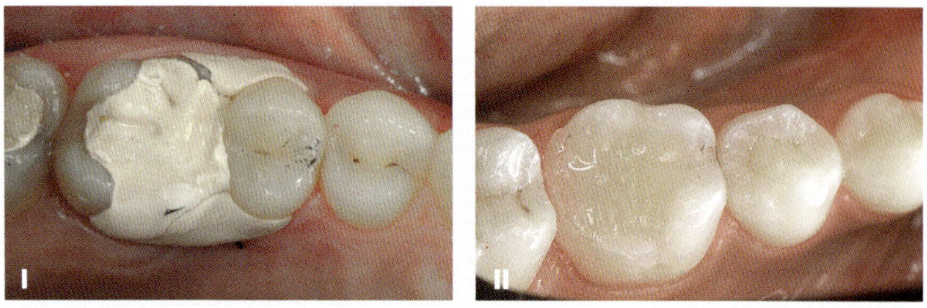

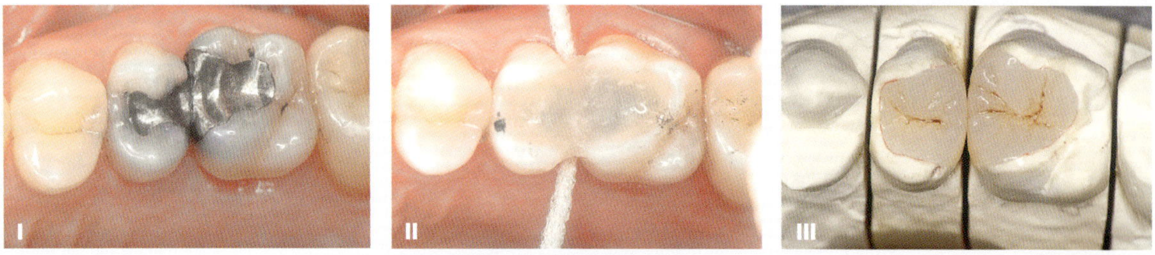

Fig 154

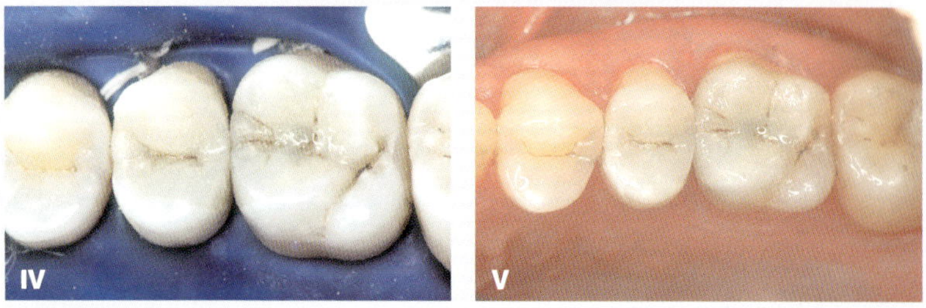

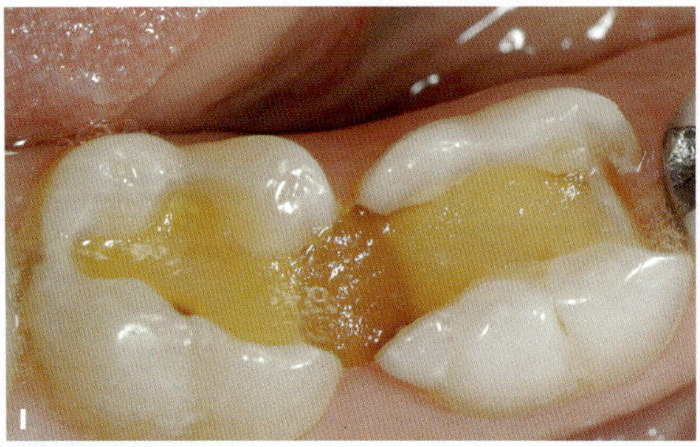

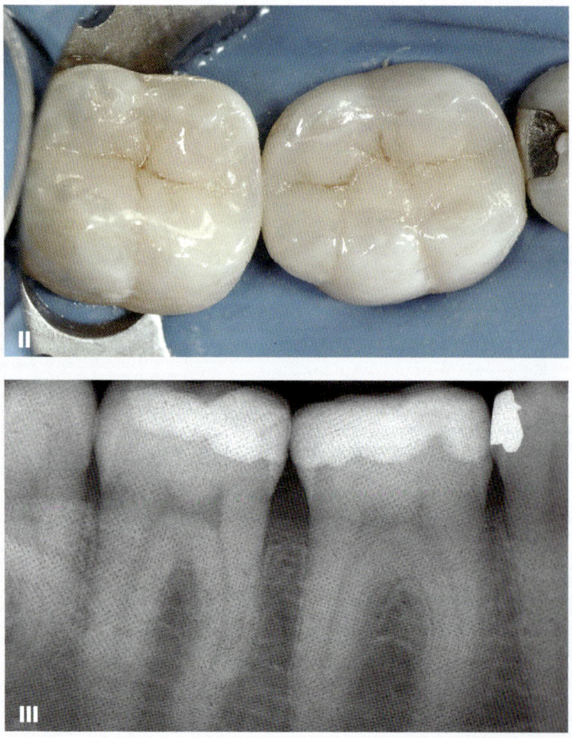

Fig 155 It should be noted that every so often patients fail to present for appointments, and sometimes cementation has to be carried out as long as 18 months after the preparation, as in this fine example. Fortunately, the preparation stood the test of time, and it was possible to carry out normal cementation in accordance with protocol.

Cementing adhesive restorations

This is certainly the most difficult stage of the entire process. As was discussed in chapter 2, the author's team uses the same material for cementation as for the buildup and for making the inlay in the laboratory. The composite cement is heated in a special warmer (Calset, AdDent) to make it more flowable; preheating light-cured composites to 54°C increases the monomer conversion level, which improves the properties of the cementing agent[36,37] (Figs 156 to 161).

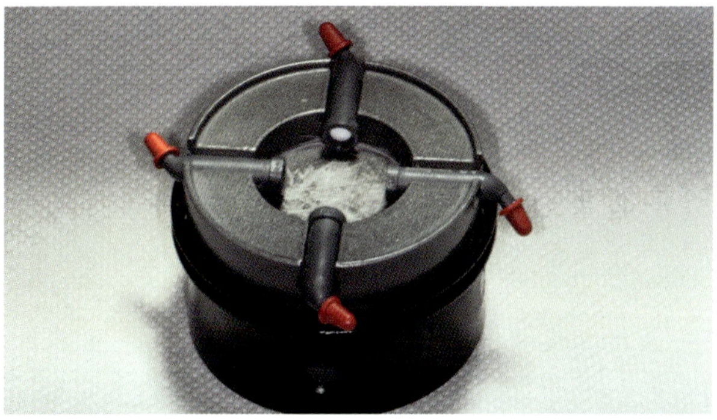

Fig 156 Warmer for heating the composite.

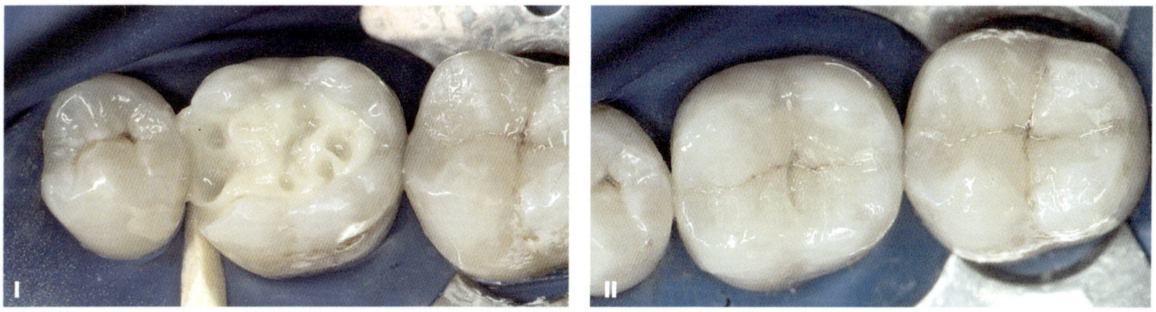

Fig 157 Filling the cavity with composite for cementation before applying the inlay.

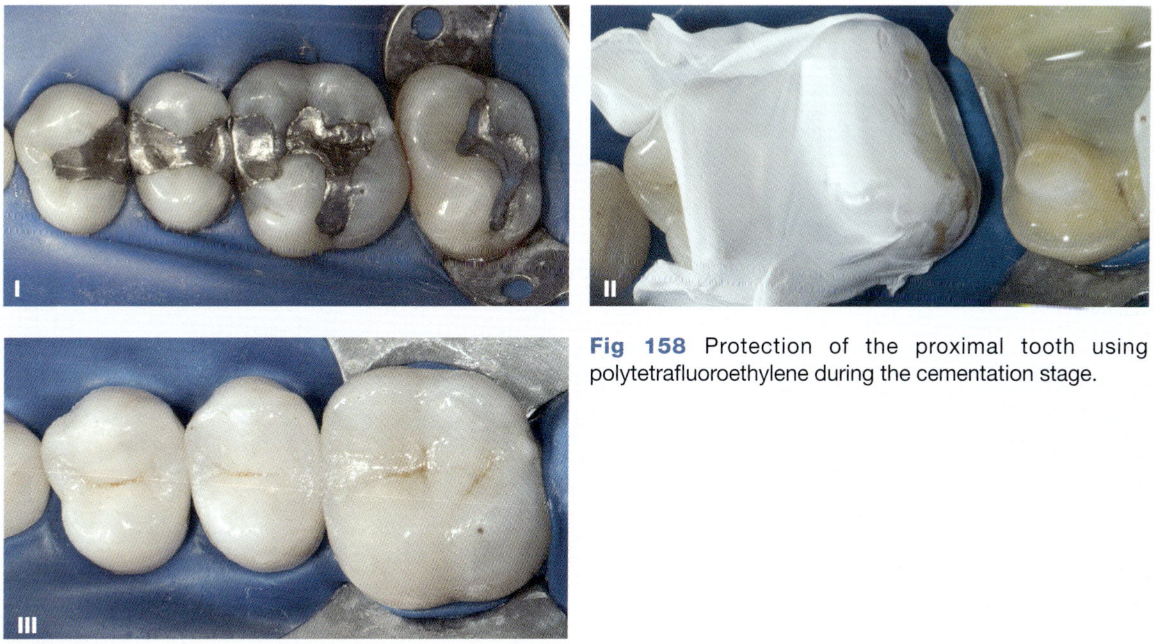

Fig 158 Protection of the proximal tooth using polytetrafluoroethylene during the cementation stage.

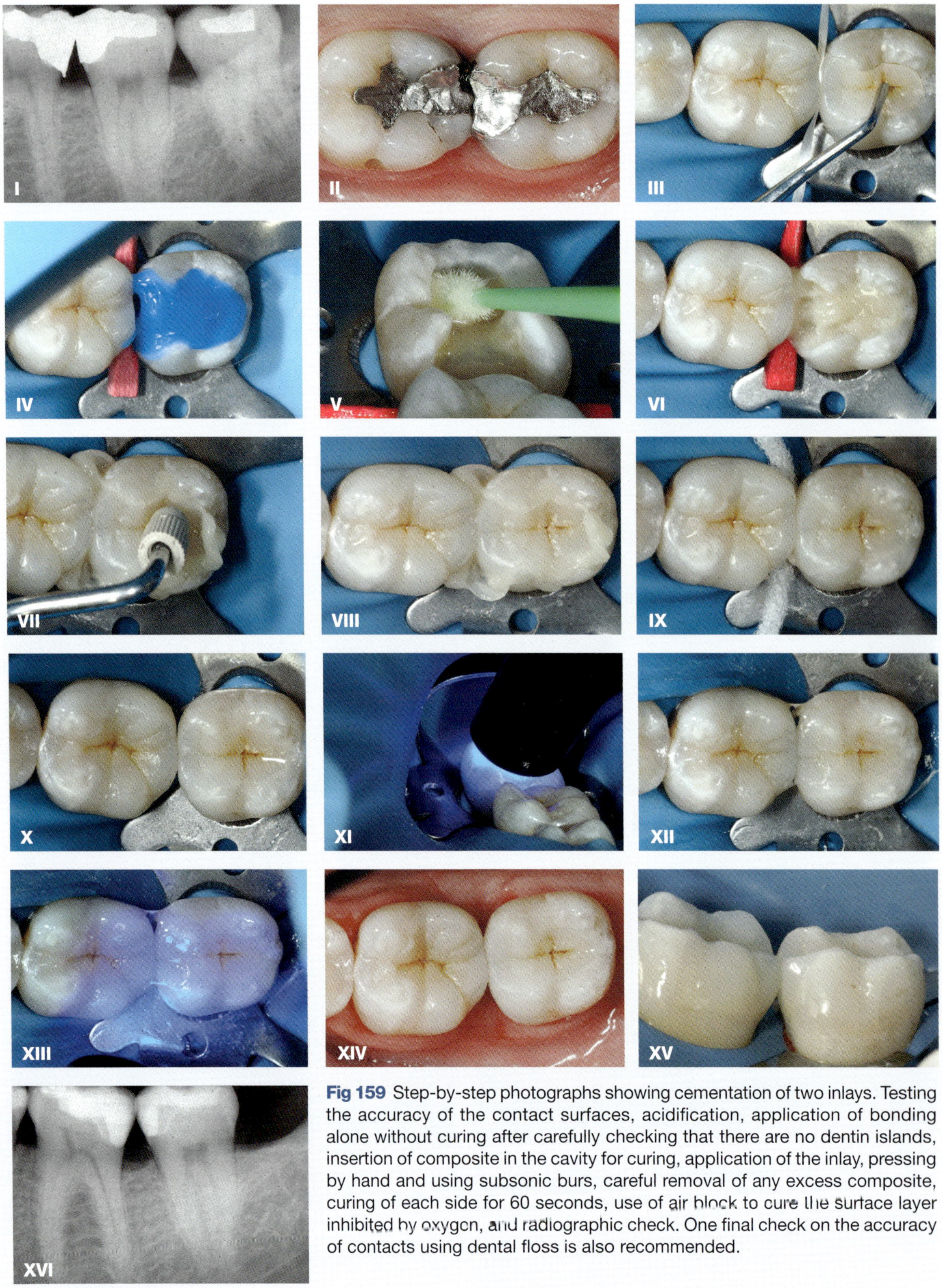

Fig 159 Step-by-step photographs showing cementation of two inlays. Testing the accuracy of the contact surfaces, acidification, application of bonding alone without curing after carefully checking that there are no dentin islands, insertion of composite in the cavity for curing, application of the inlay, pressing by hand and using subsonic burs, careful removal of any excess composite, curing of each side for 60 seconds, use of air block to cure the surface layer inhibited by oxygen, and radiographic check. One final check on the accuracy of contacts using dental floss is also recommended.

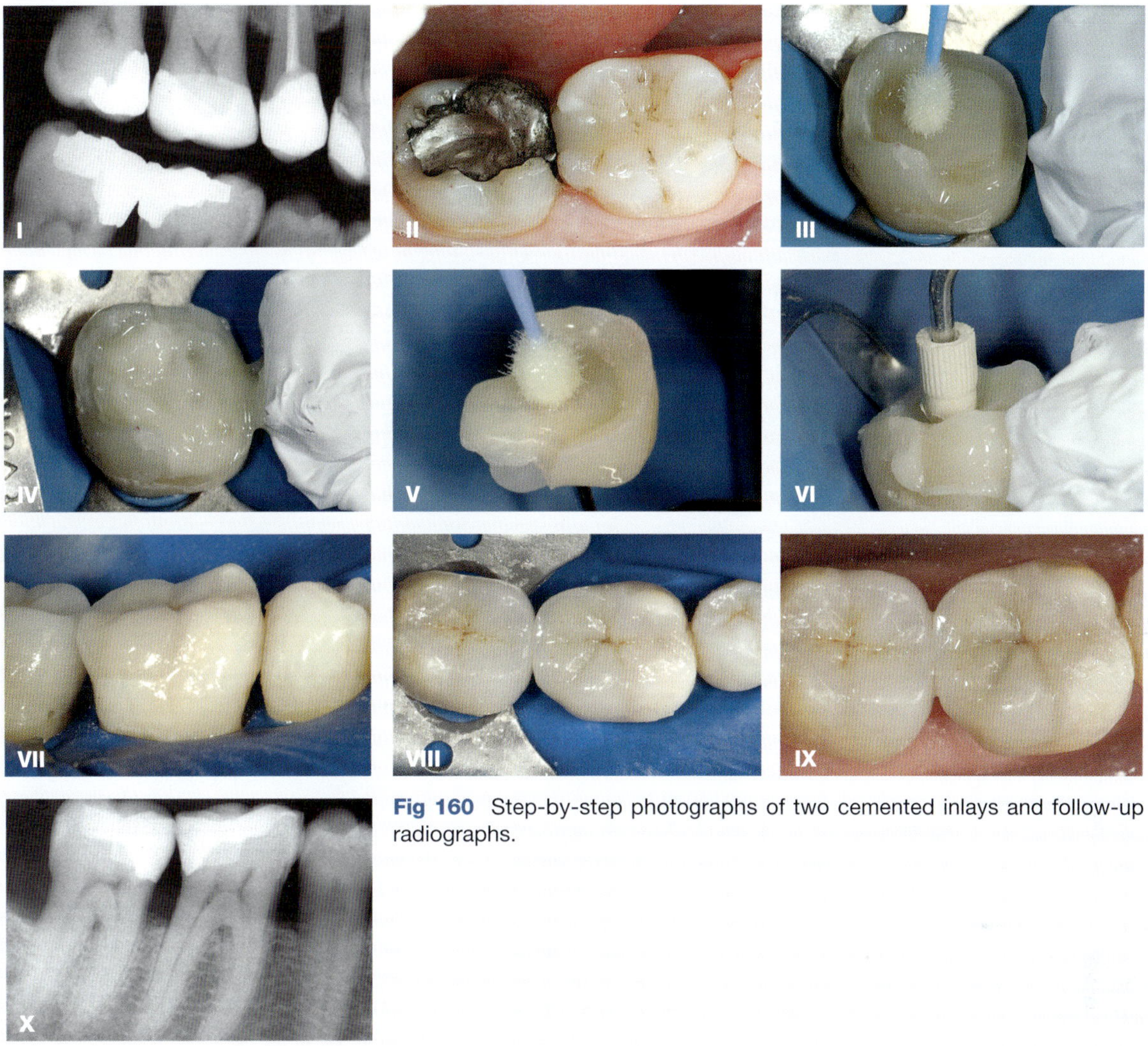

Fig 160 Step-by-step photographs of two cemented inlays and follow-up radiographs.

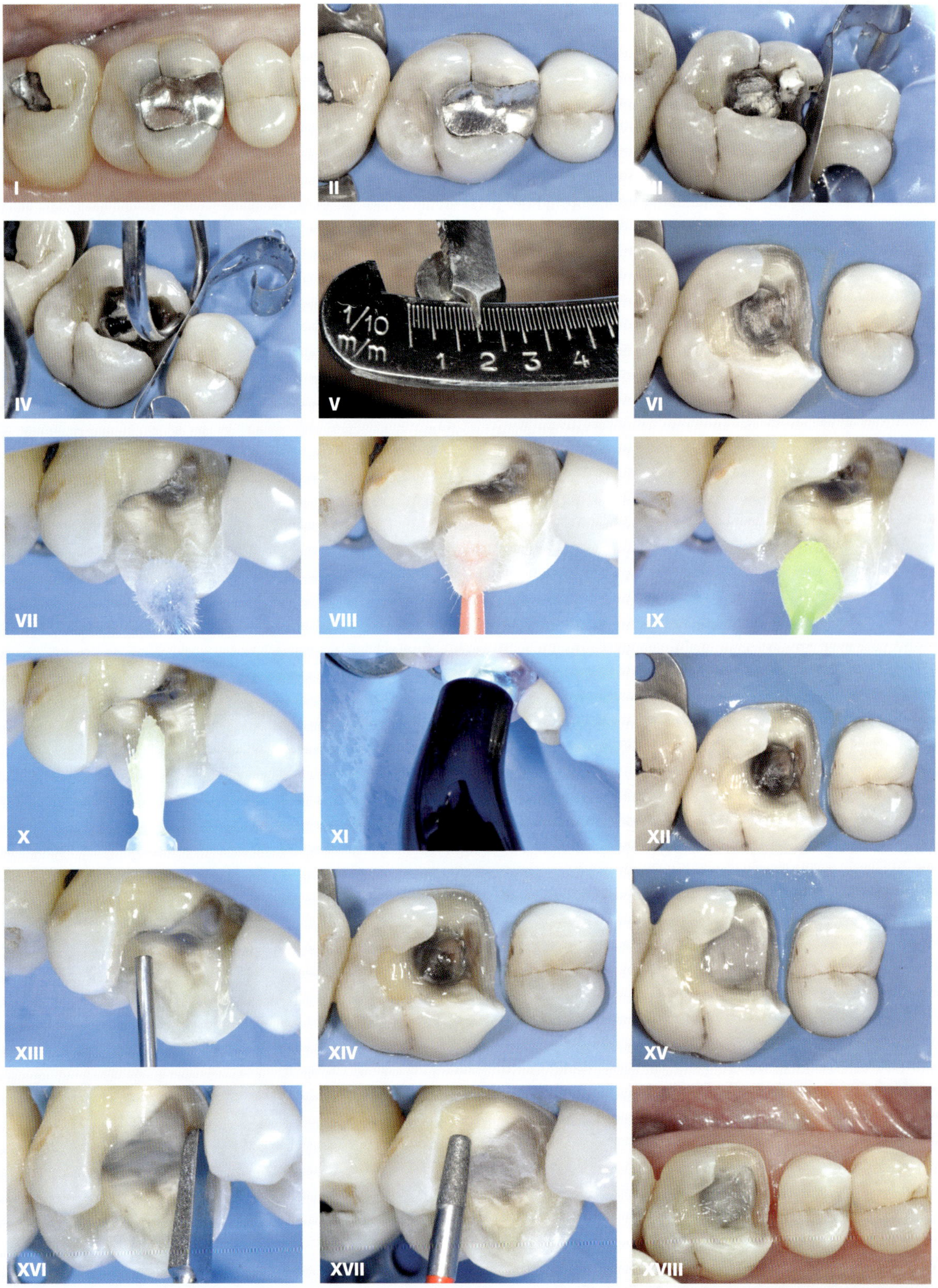

Fig 161 Step-by-step photographs of placement of an onlay. Removal of defective restoration, measurement of buccal wall thicknesses that were far too thin for wall maintenance to be considered even before removal of the decayed tissue, removal of the wall and shoulder preparation, thorough removal of decay, application of chlorhexidine, adhesion using two-step self-etch system, curing, application of flowable composite and traditional composite (buildup), cavity preparation and finishing, impression with polyvinyl siloxane with interocclusal record impression tray, working cast, and inlay prepared in the laboratory *(I–XXIII)*. The cementation stage started with cleaning the cavity after removal of the temporary dressing (Fermit),

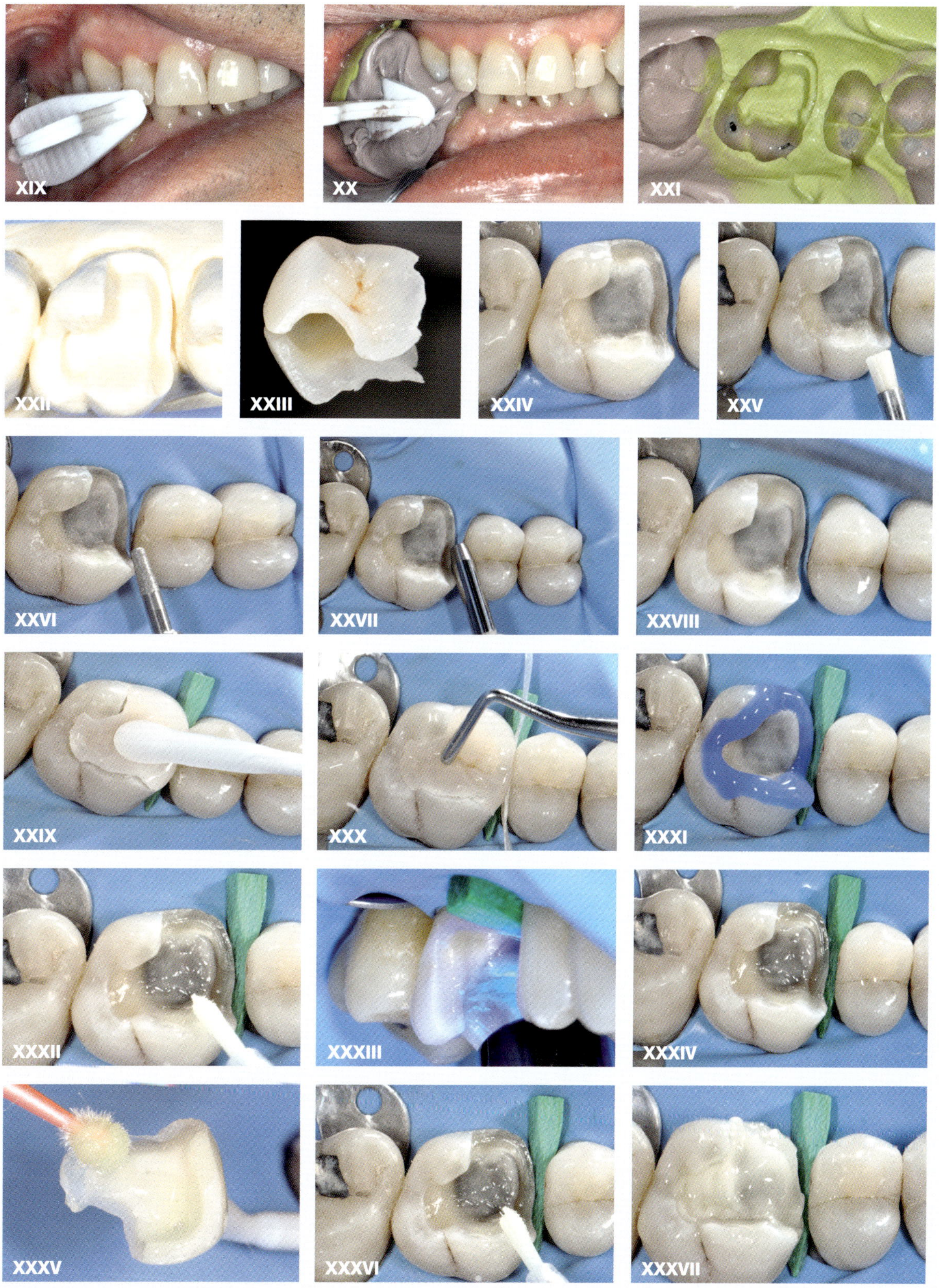

testing the inlay, selective acidification of the enamel and then re-application of fine layers of etching/primer and bonding for the hybridization of any dentin islands, curing, application of bonding to the internal part of the onlay and in the tooth cavity, filling of the cavity with composite, application of the inlay and very careful removal of all excess, curing of each surface of the tooth in accordance with protocol (60 seconds on each side), finishing of the strictly supragingival tooth-restoration margins with the aid of abrasive strips or dedicated burs, and lastly postoperative radiograph and occlusal check *(XXIV–XLV)*.

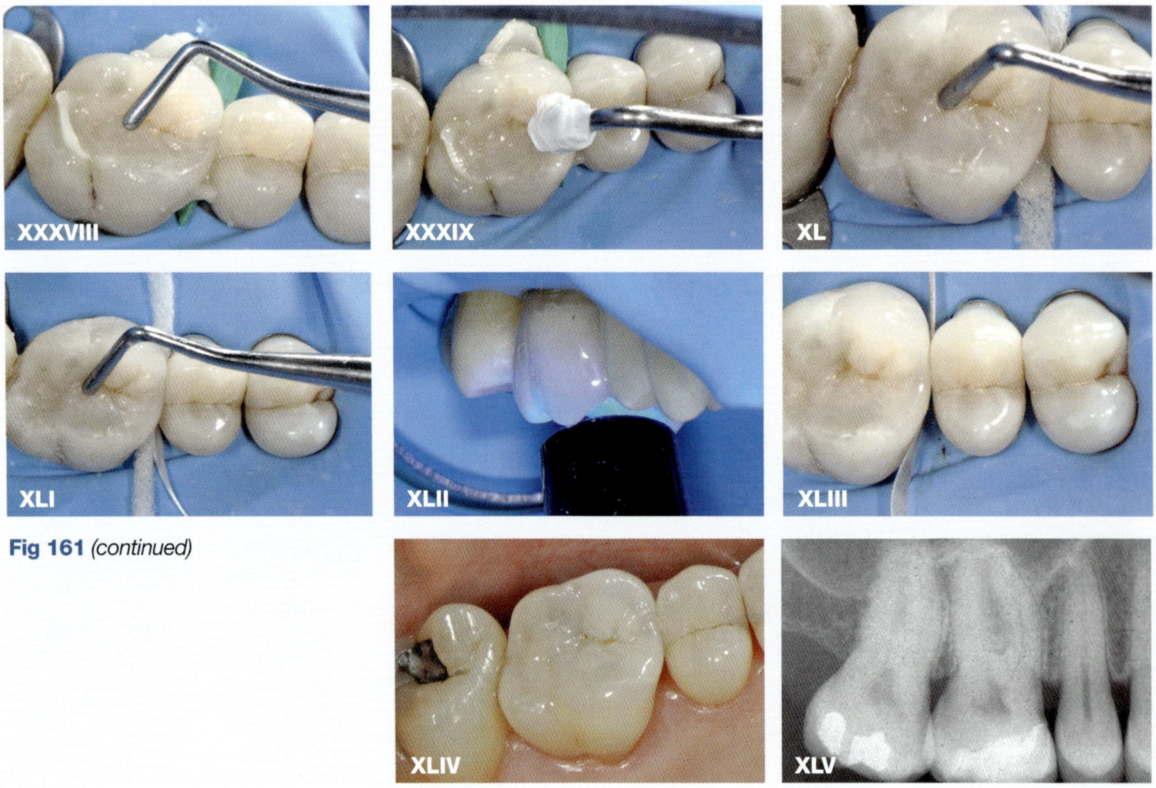

Fig 161 *(continued)*

Finishing

Finishing consists of removing any remaining excess composite using dedicated instruments and abrasive strips, followed by final polishing (Figs 162 to 164).
Clinical cases are shown in Figs 165 to 171.

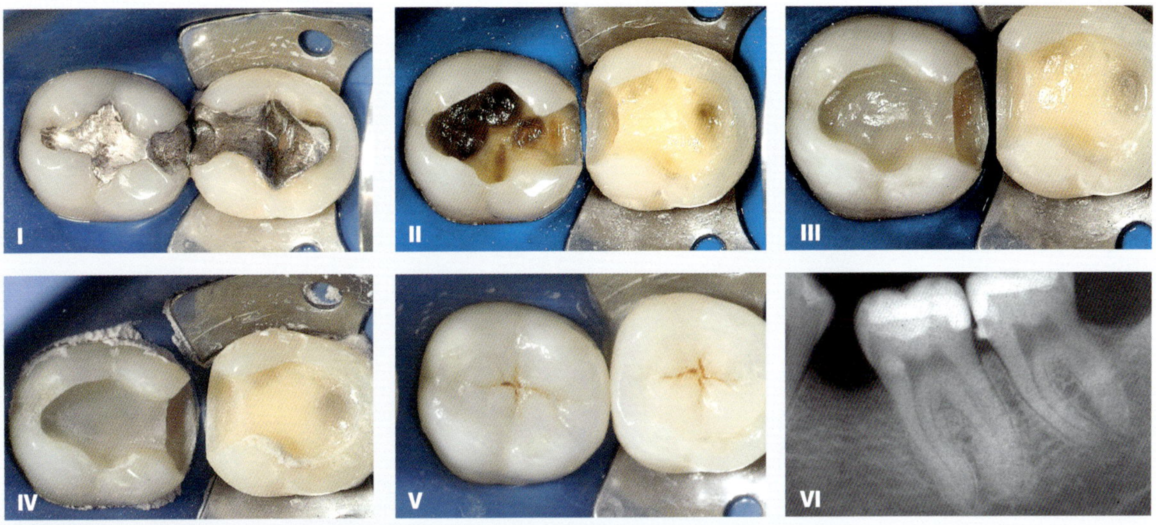

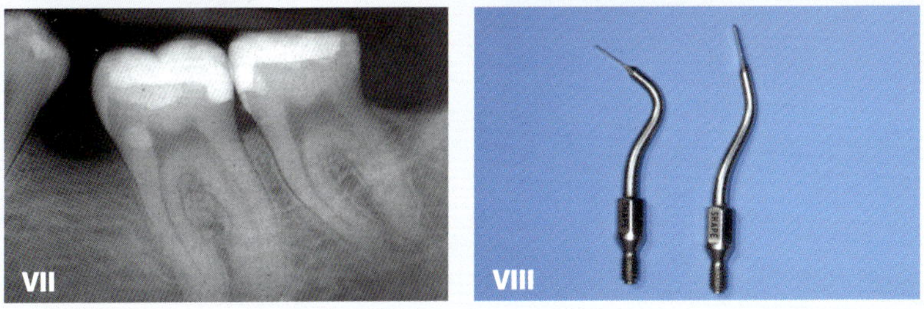

Fig 162 Clinical stages of cementation and removal of excess on the mandibular left second molar.

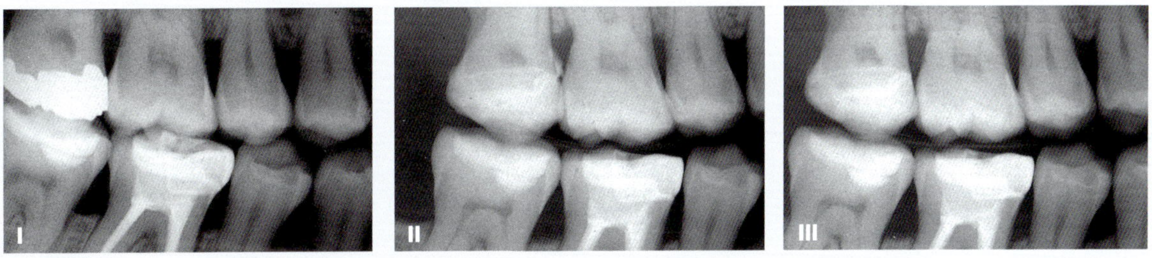

Fig 163 Removal of excess composite after cementation in the maxillary right second molar.

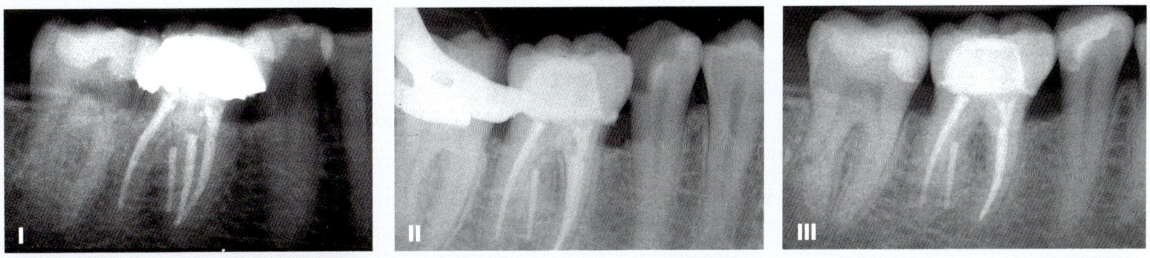

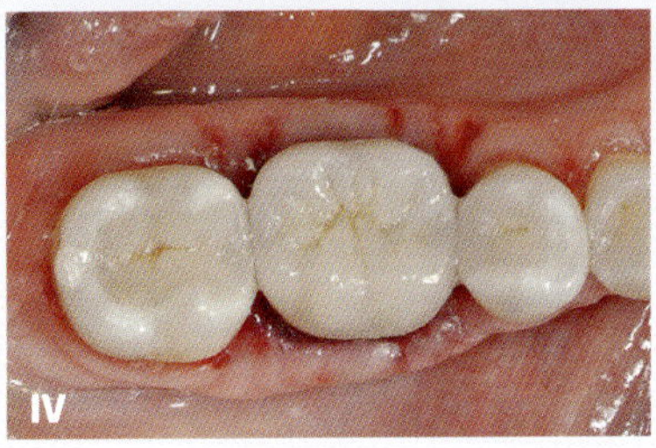

Fig 164 Replacement of the prosthetic crown of the mandibular right first molar with a fully adhesive composite restoration, reconstruction of defective restorations in the adjacent second premolar and second molar with partial composite restorations, and finishing of margins. Pre-, intra-, and postoperative radiographs and a postoperative clinical view are shown.

Clinical cases

Clinical case 1

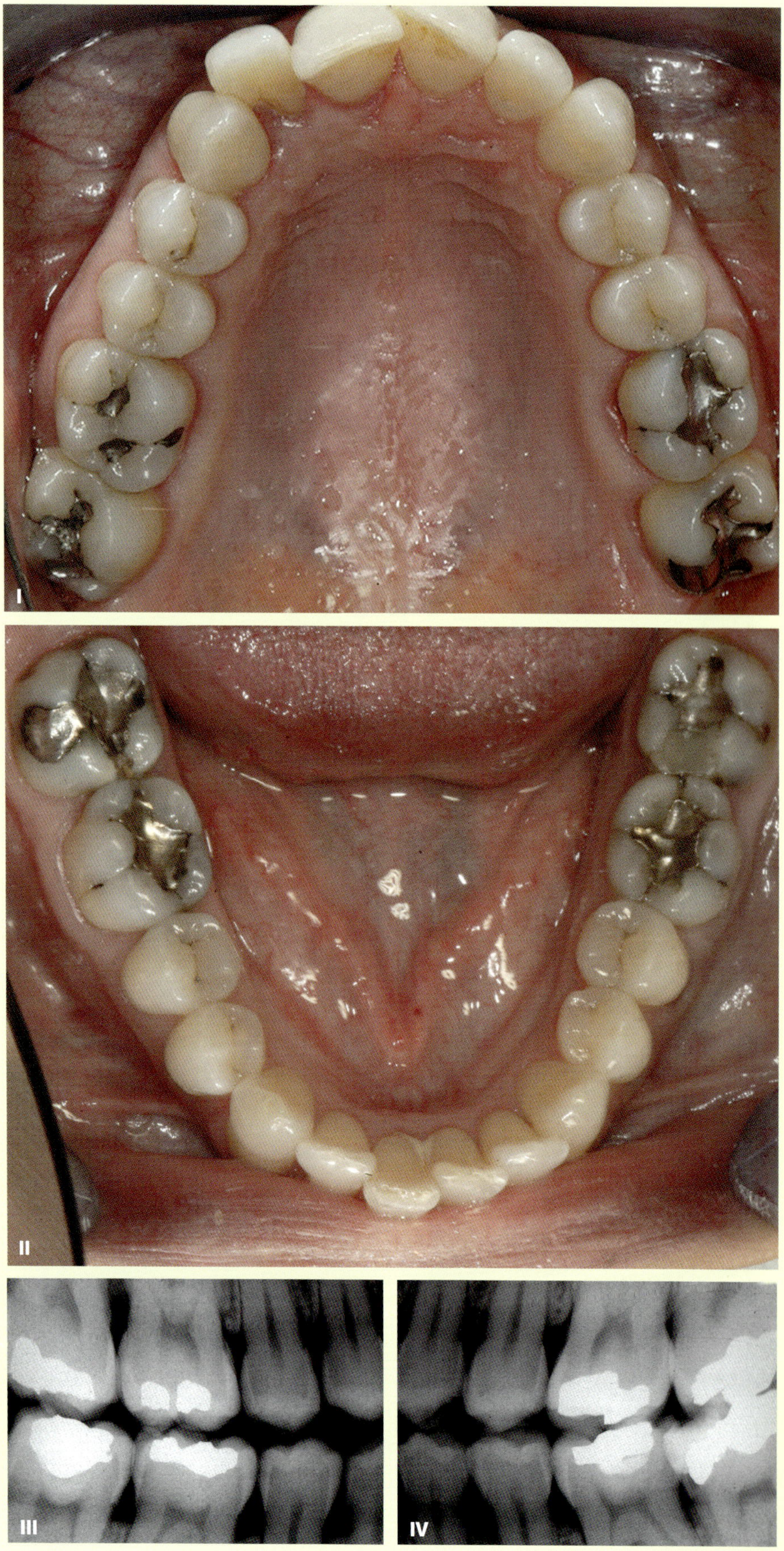

Fig 165 Preoperative clinical and radiographic view of both arches *(I–IV)*.

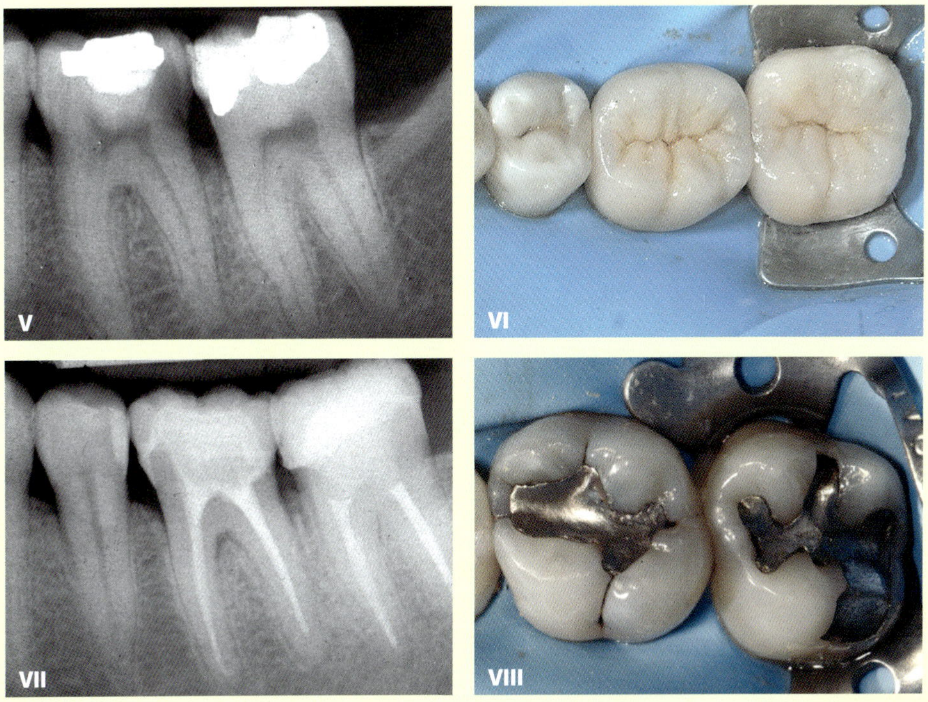

Fig 165 *(continued)* Endodontic treatment of the mandibular left first and second molars and adhesive composite restorations *(V–VII)*. Caries lesions of the maxillary left second premolar and first molar, fracture line of the first molar, and restoration of the second molar, which was defective from a biomechanical viewpoint *(VIII–XV)*: after removing the decay and cleaning the fracture line, surgical exposure of the margins and internal reconstruction (with flowable composite and traditional composite), cementation of partial adhesive restorations, and postoperative radiograph.

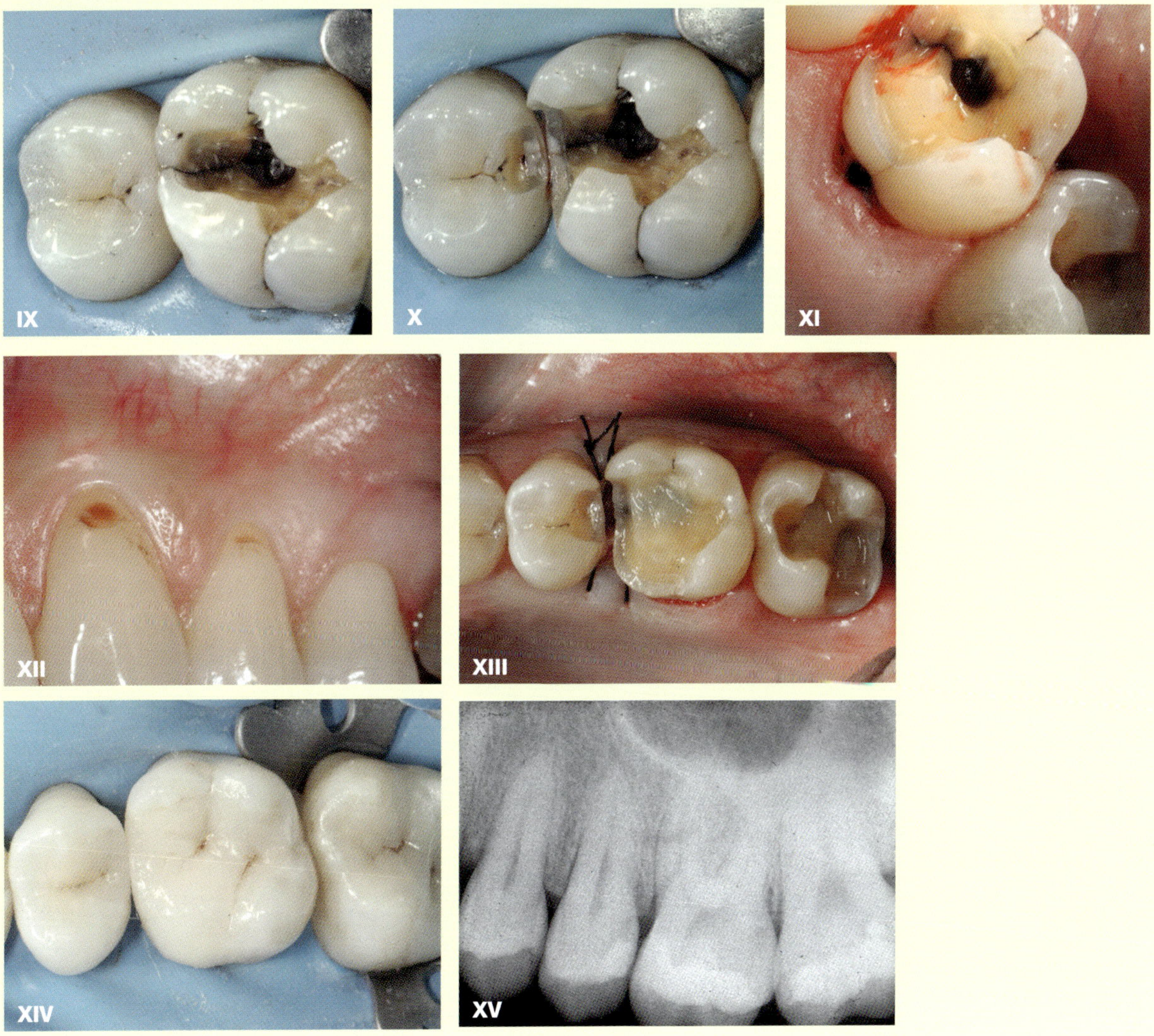

Fig 165 *(continued)* Also in this case the author's team opted for interdisciplinary management of the fourth quadrant. Preparations, impressions, cementation of the prostheses, and follow-up radiographs *(XVI–XXIV)*. Postoperative view of the arches following treatment *(XXV–XXVIII)*.

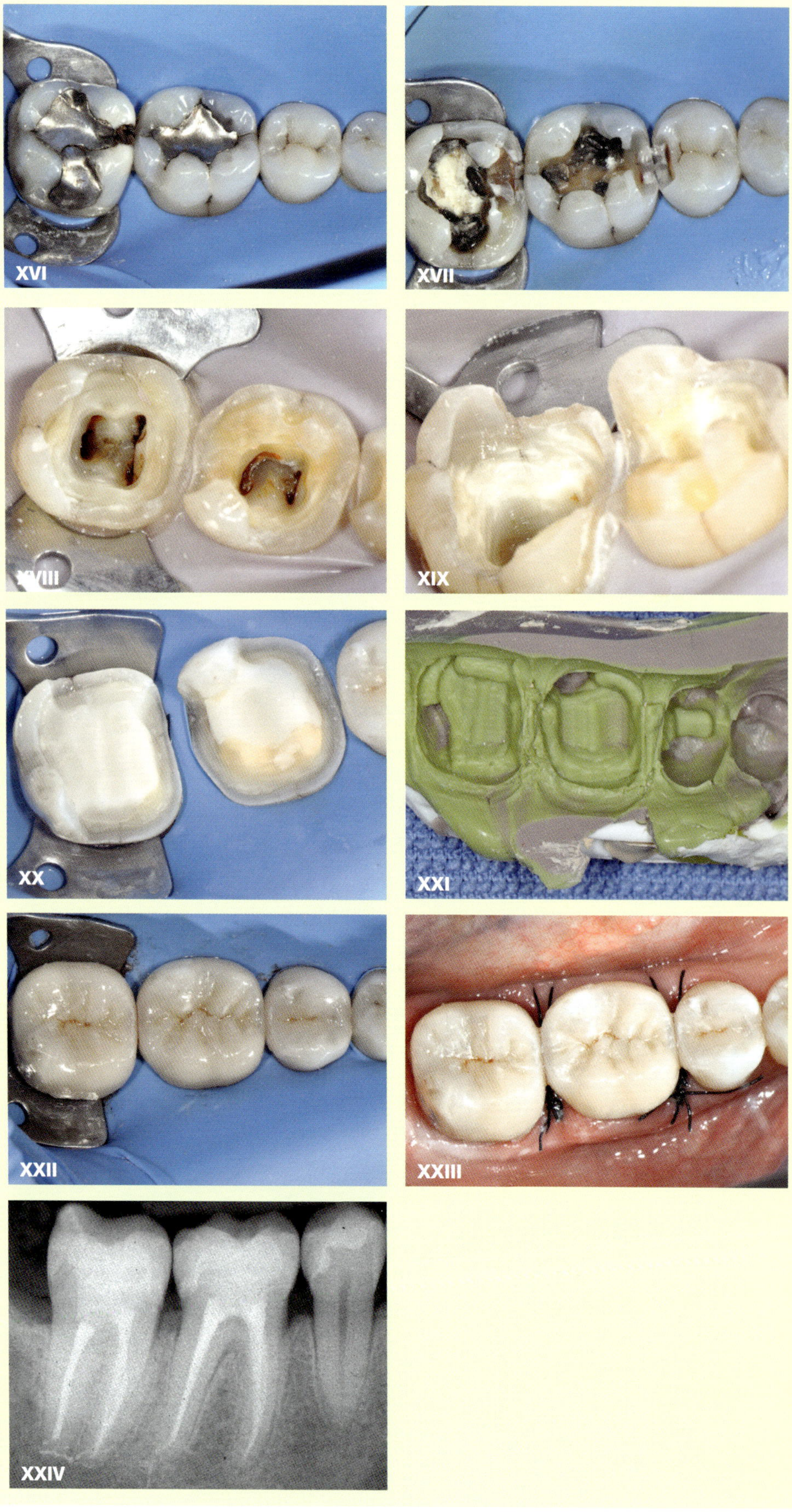

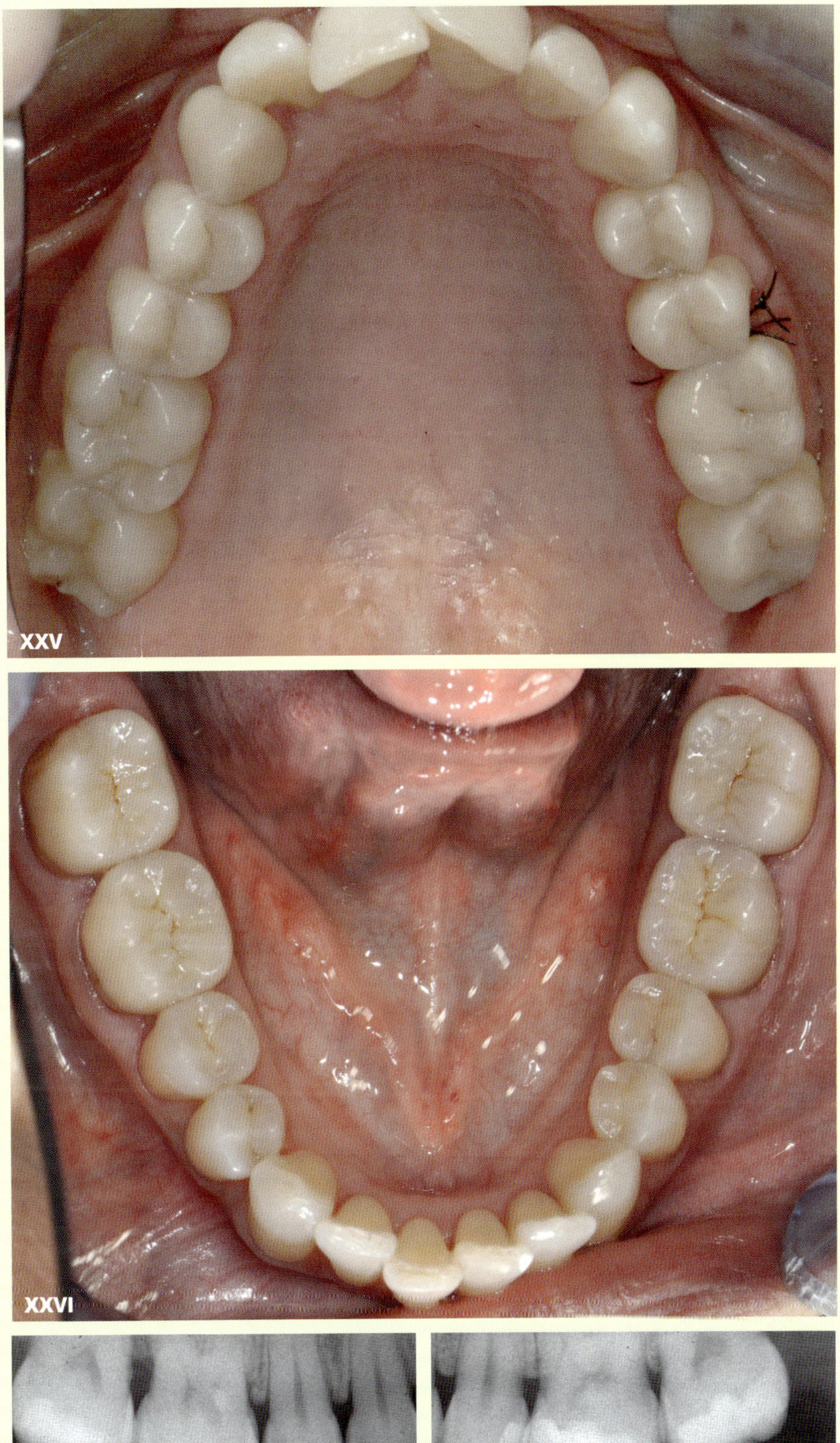

Fig 165 *(continued)*

Clinical case 2

Fig 166 Typical example of completely inappropriate tooth restorations. A clinical inspection and two bitewing radiographs revealed leaking restorations and multiple caries lesions *(I–IV)*. Multidisciplinary treatment of the maxillary right (first) quadrant by means of surgical exposure of the margins and direct and indirect adhesive restorations *(V–XXVIII)*.

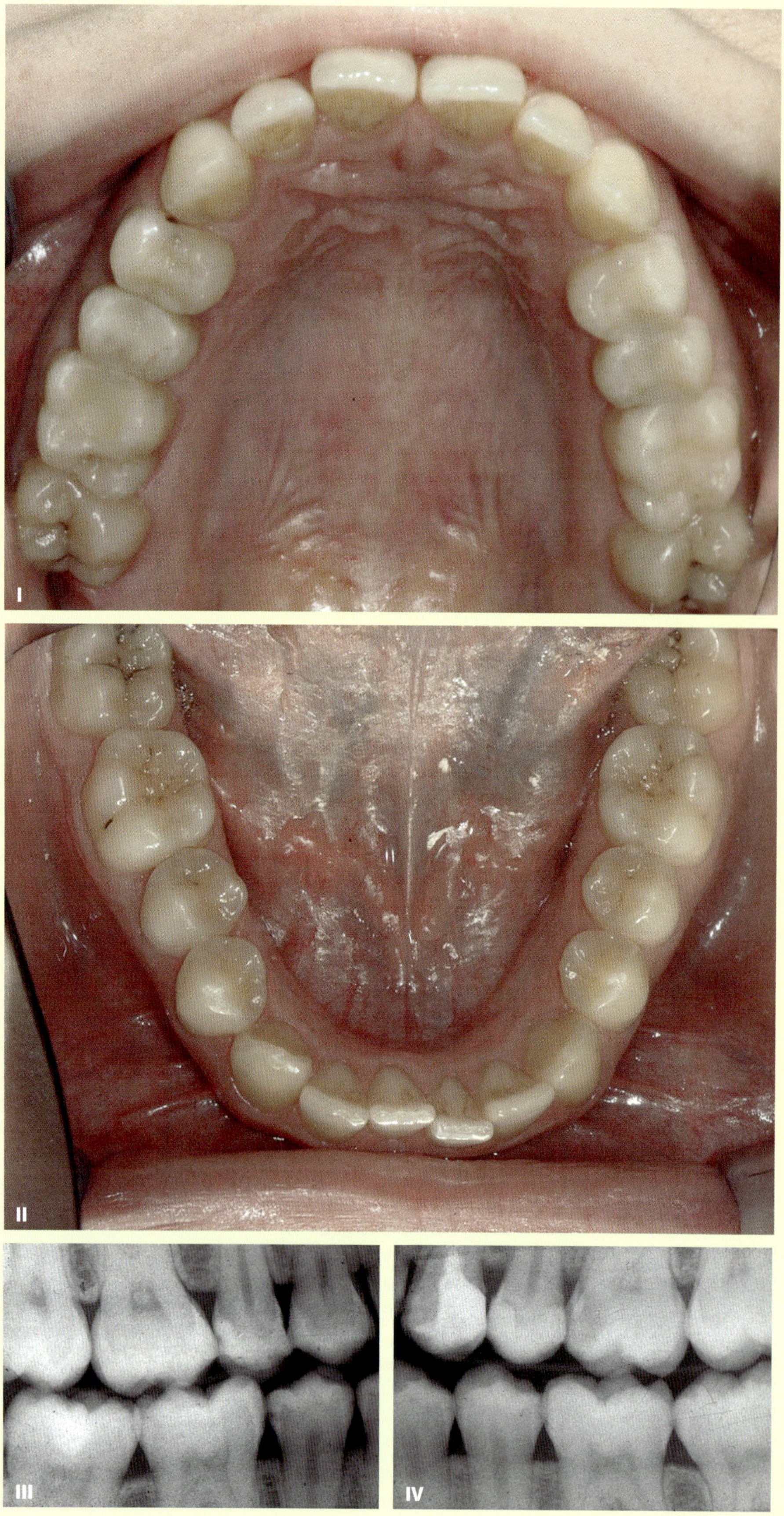

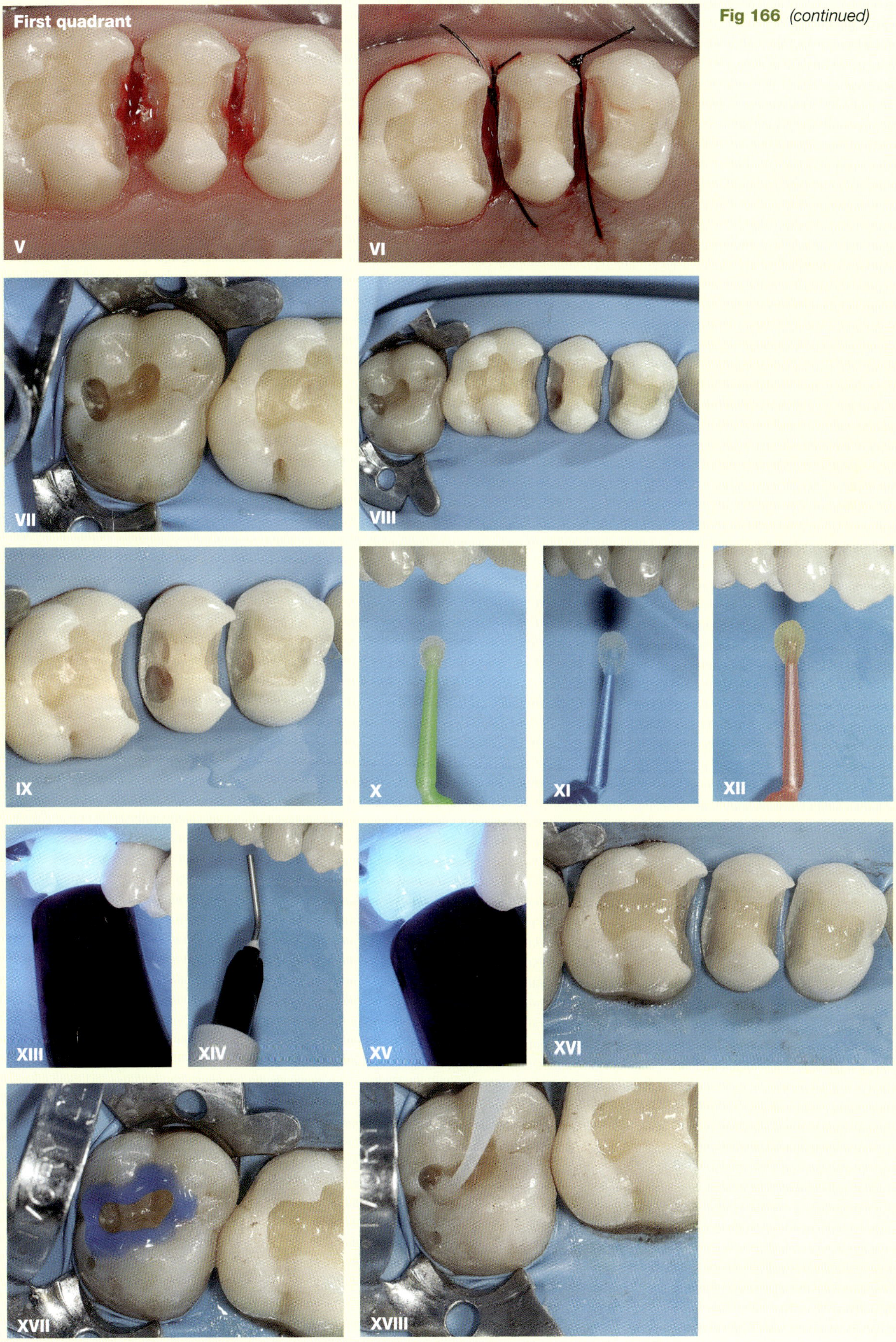

Fig 166 *(continued)*

Fig 166 *(continued)* In the maxillary left (second) quadrant, the presence of penetrating decay of the second premolar and first molar required endodontic treatment *(XXIX, XXX)* and reconstruction with an overlay for the premolars and an onlay for the molar *(XXXI, XXXII)*. Direct adhesive techniques were used for the small caries lesions of the mandibular left (third) quadrant *(XXXIII–XXXV)*. In the mandibular right (fourth) quadrant, direct restorations were placed on the molars, and the second premolar was prepared for an inlay *(XXXVI–XXXIX)*.

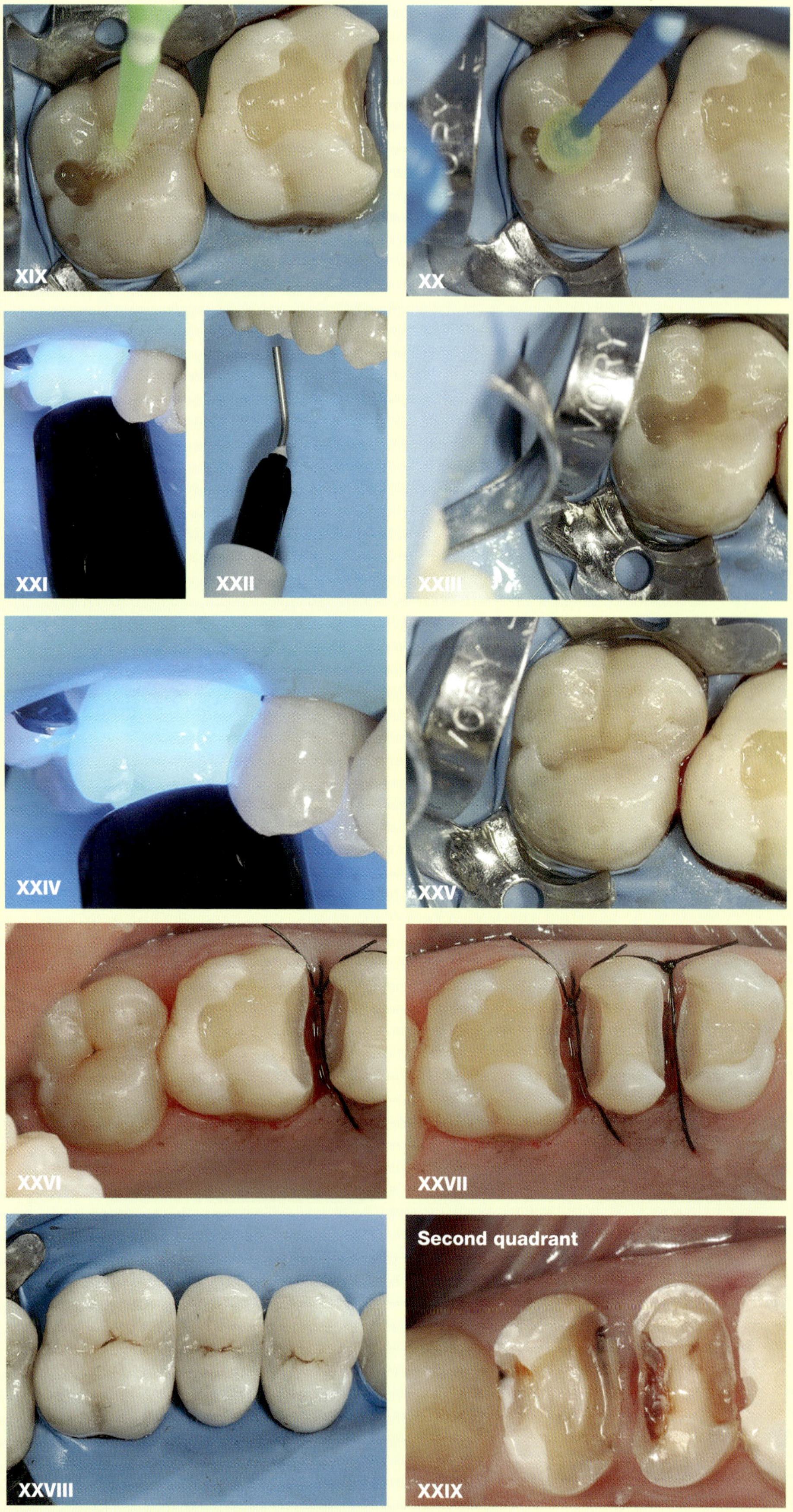

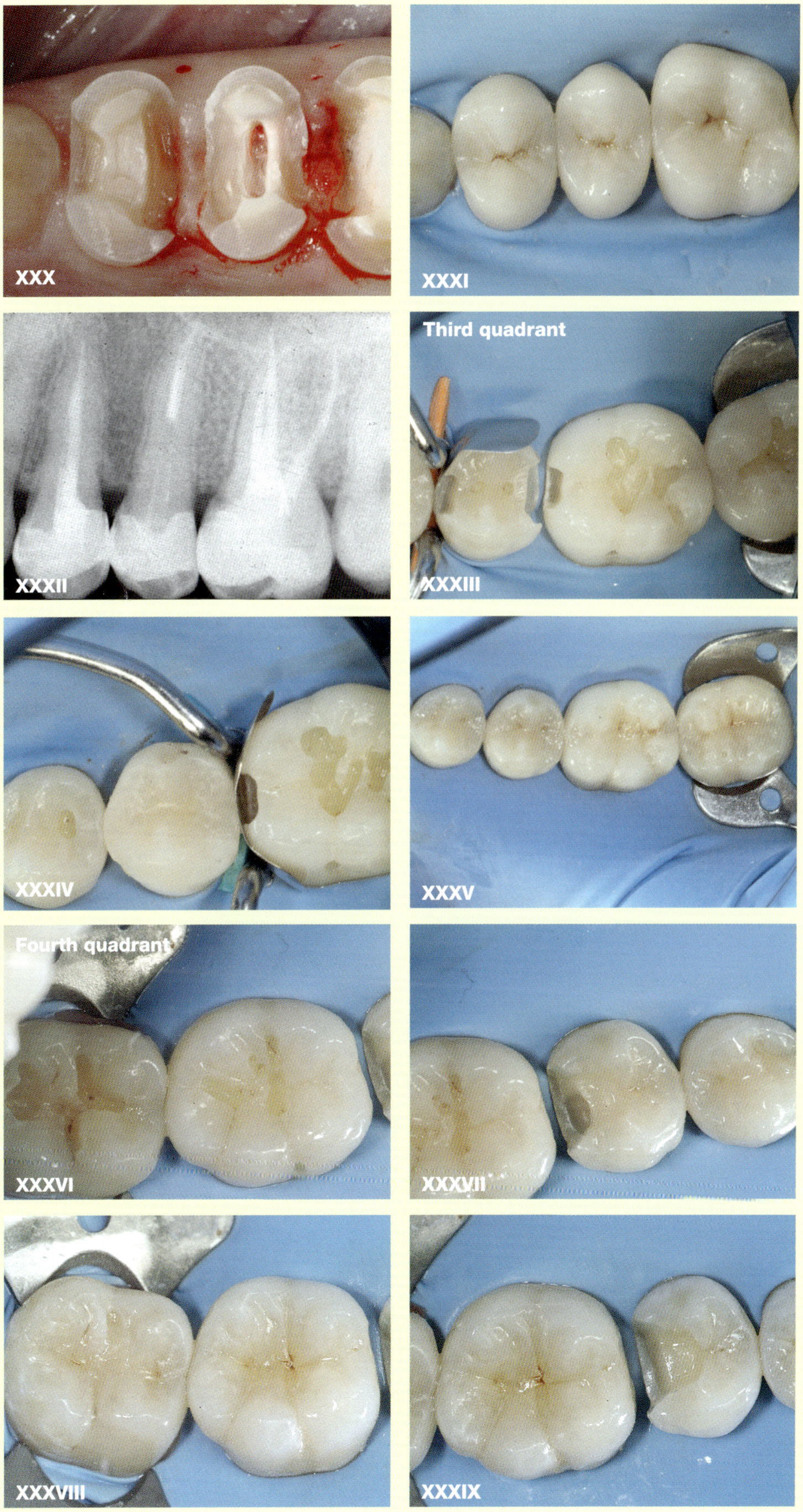

Fig 166 *(continued)*

Fig 166 *(continued)* View of the arches after treatment *(XL, XLI)*. View of arches after 3 years and follow-up radiographs *(XLII–XLVI)*.

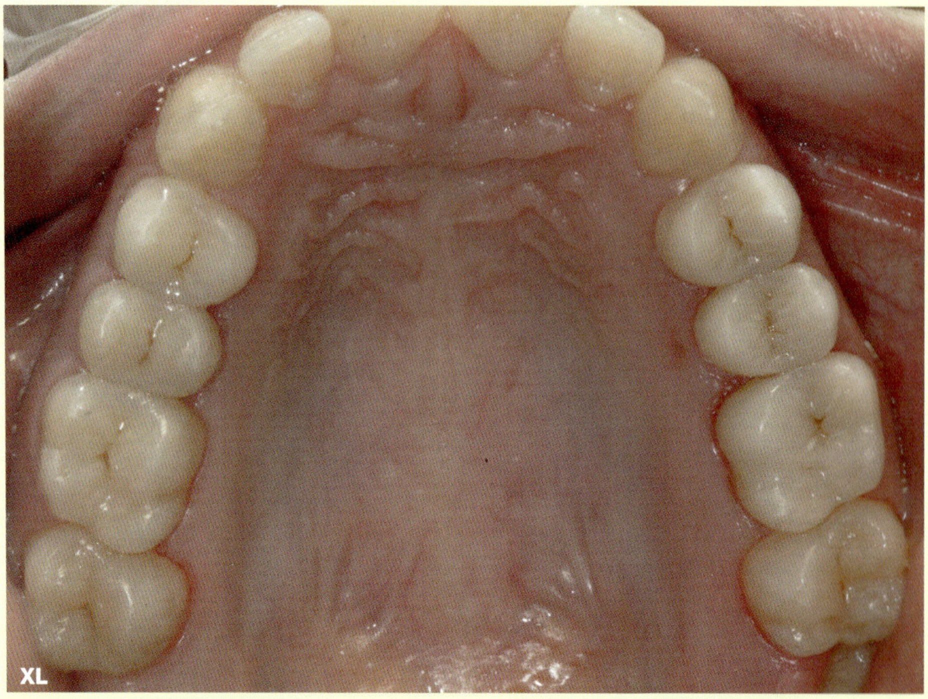

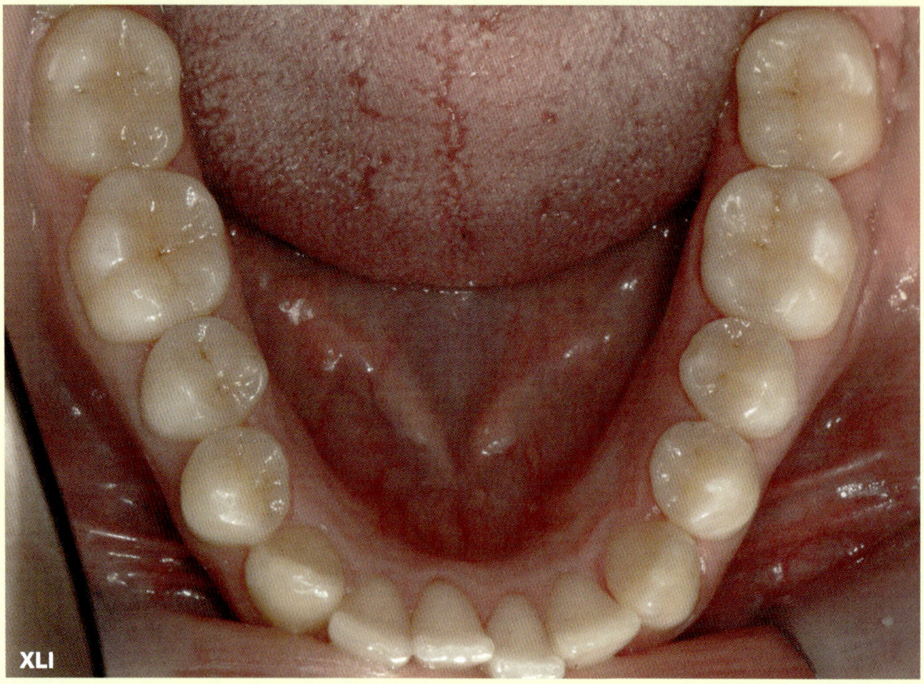

Fig 166 *(continued)*

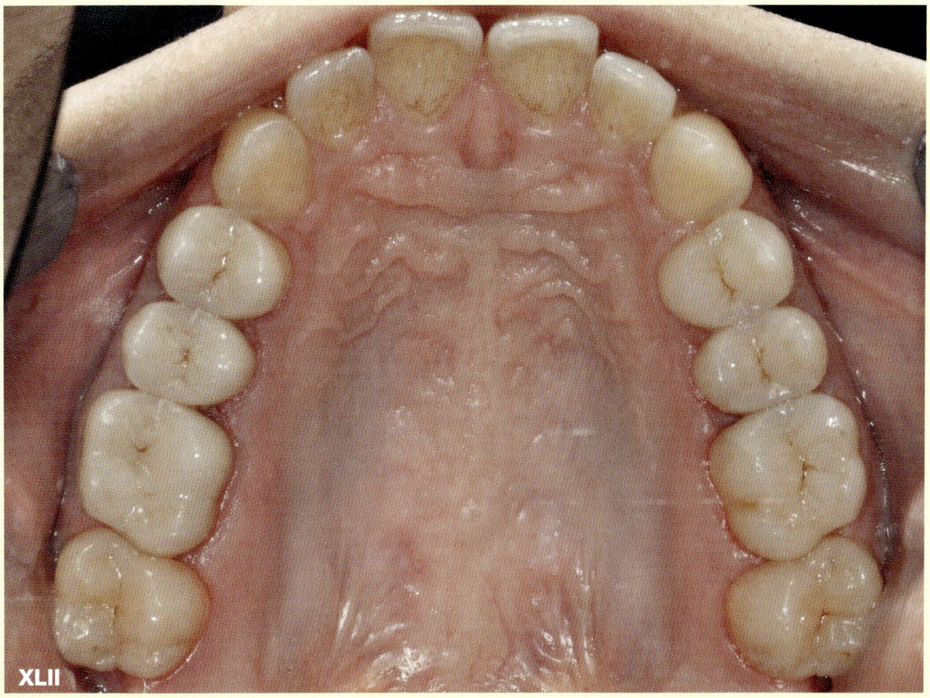

XLII

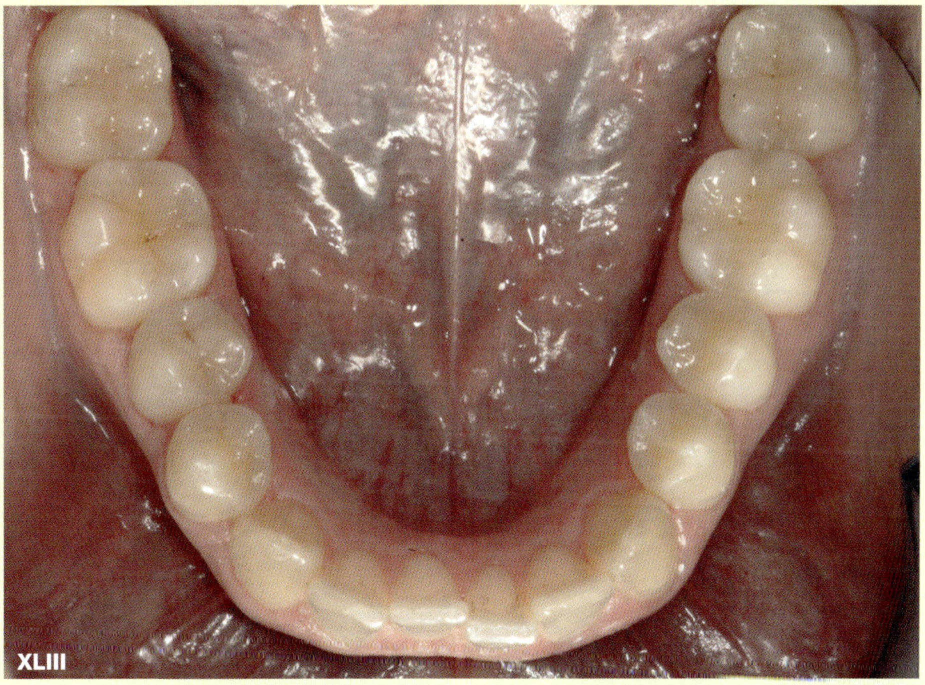

XLIII

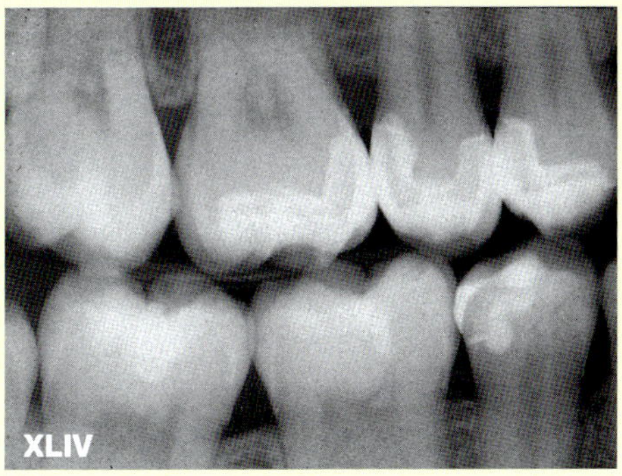

XLIV

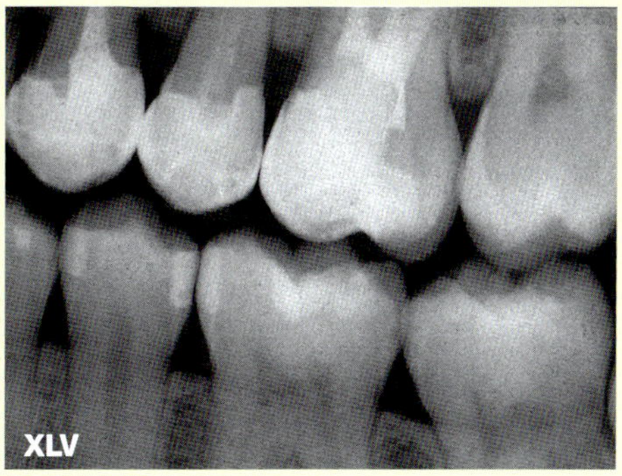

XLV

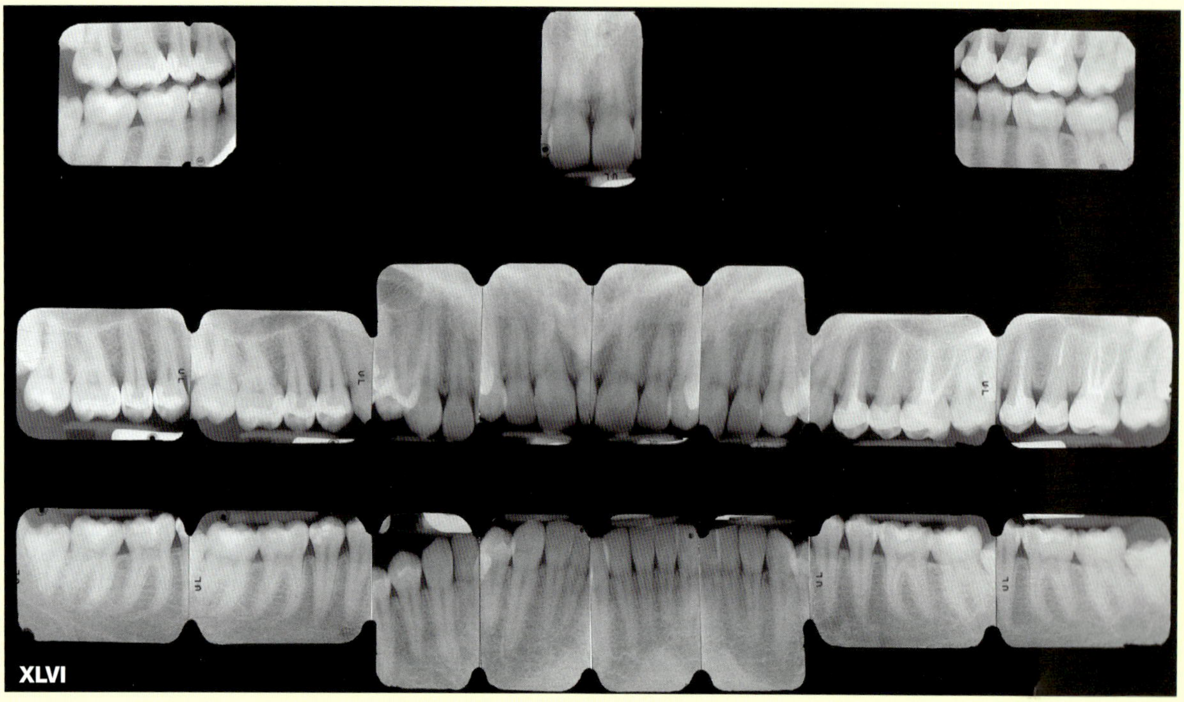

Fig 166 *(continued)*

Clinical case 3

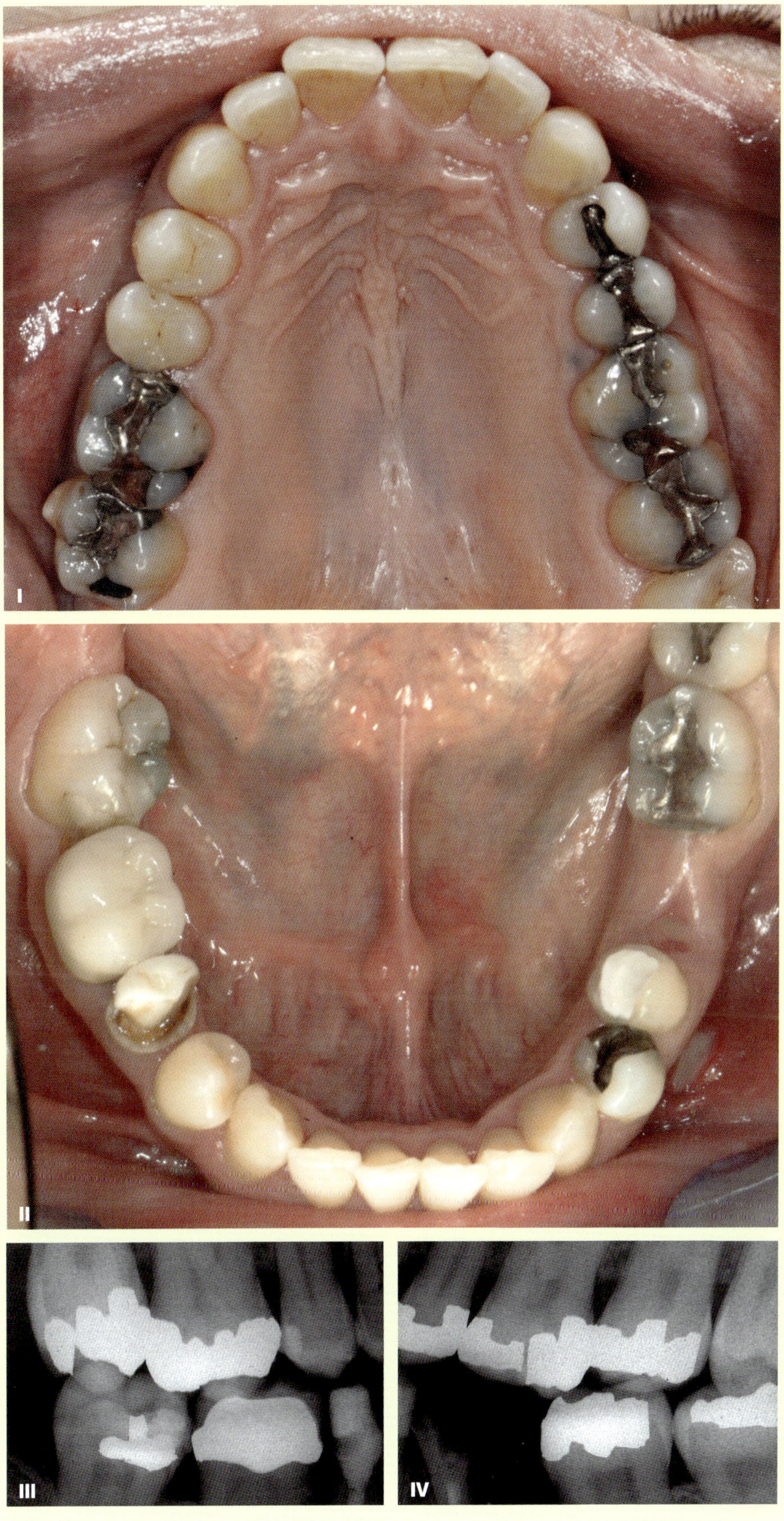

Fig 167 Restoration of both arches in a young patient with severe dental and functional problems *(I–XLVIII)*. As usual, multidisciplinary treatment was planned for each quadrant, including replacement of the defective prosthetic crown in the mandibular right second premolar position with an implant-supported adhesive restoration with supragingival margins *(XXI–XXXIII)*. The mandibular arch treatment would be completed with another implant for replacement of the left first molar.

Fig 167 *(continued)*

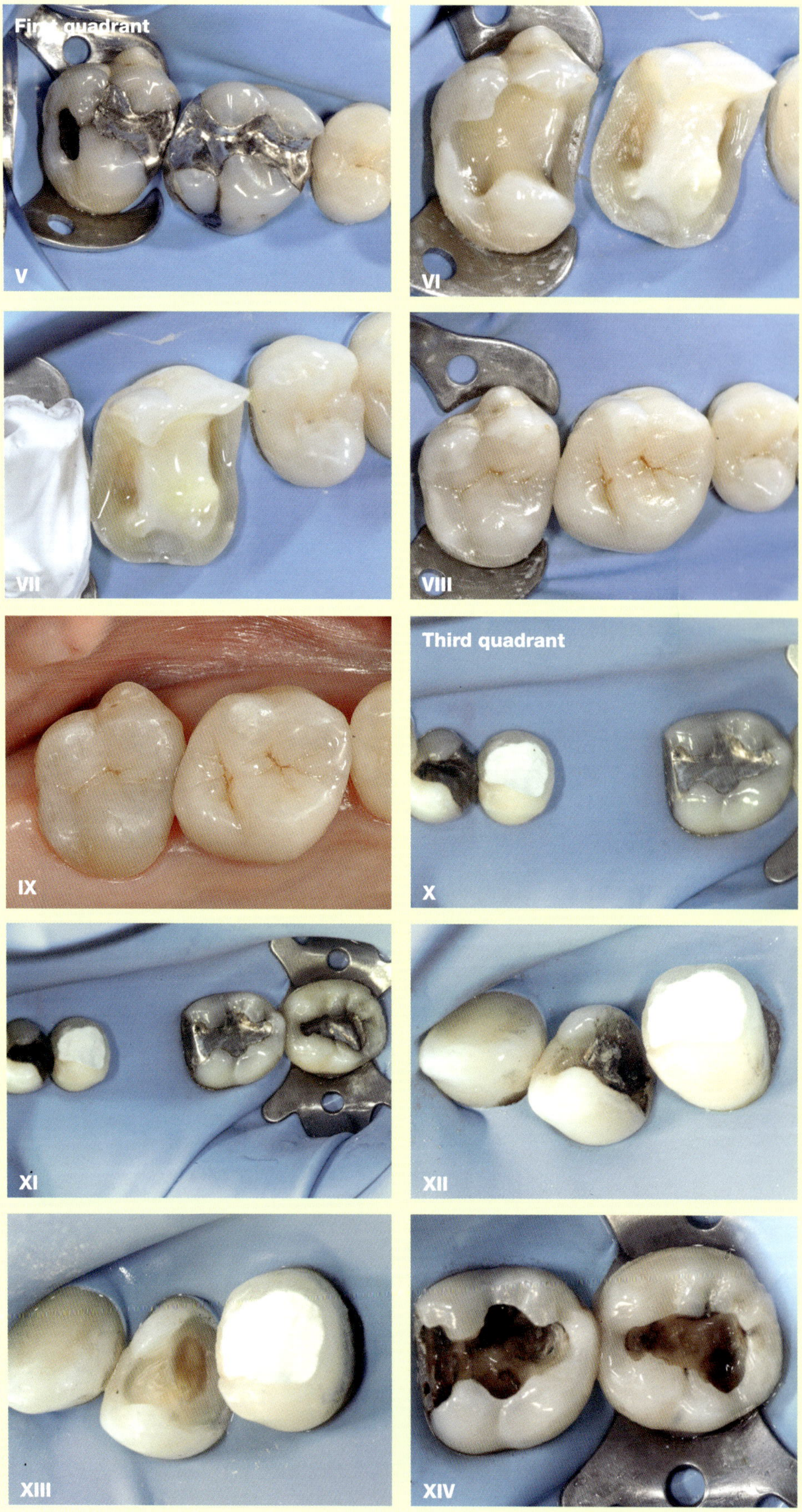

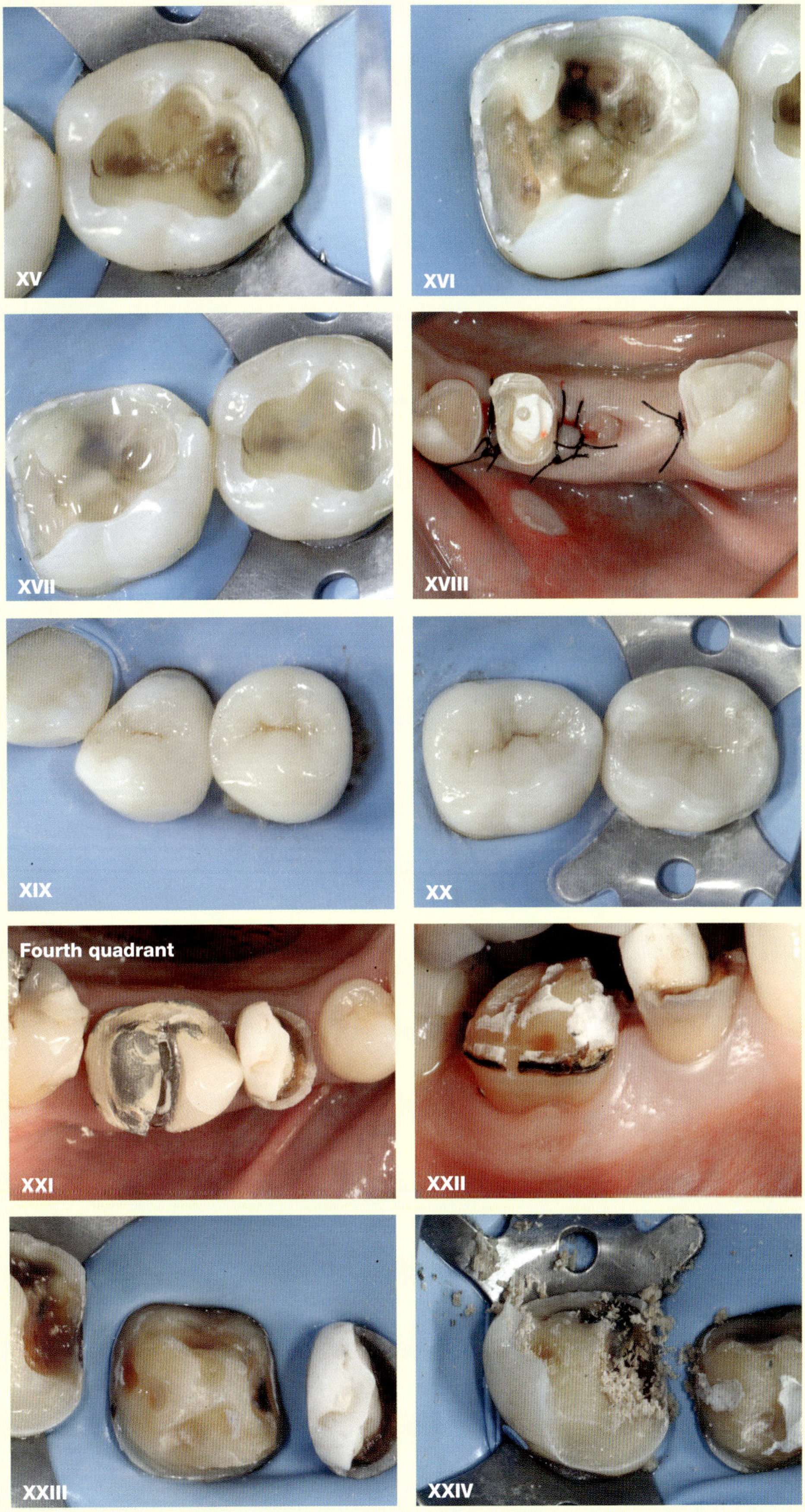

Fig 167 *(continued)*

Fig 167 *(continued)*

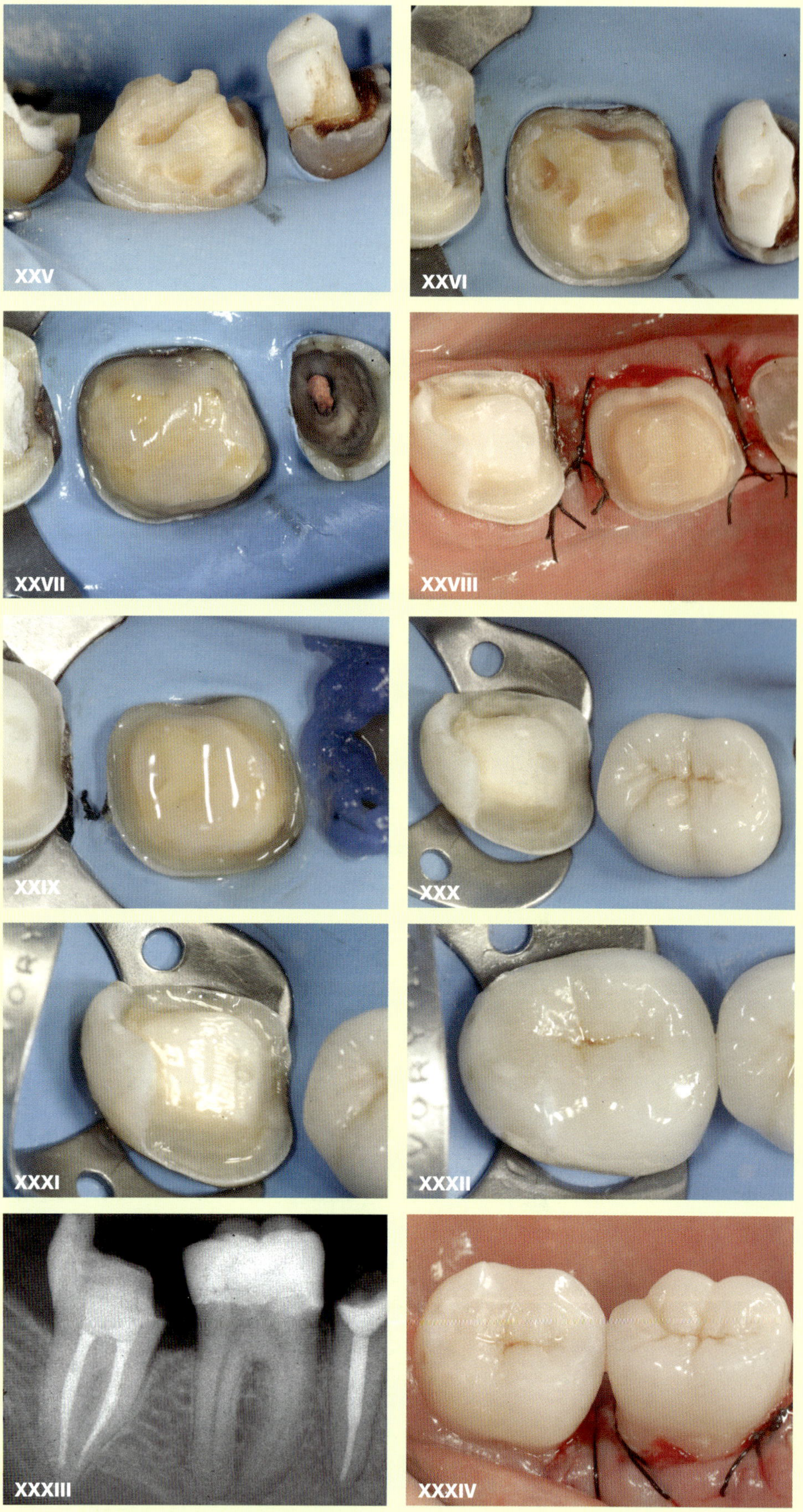

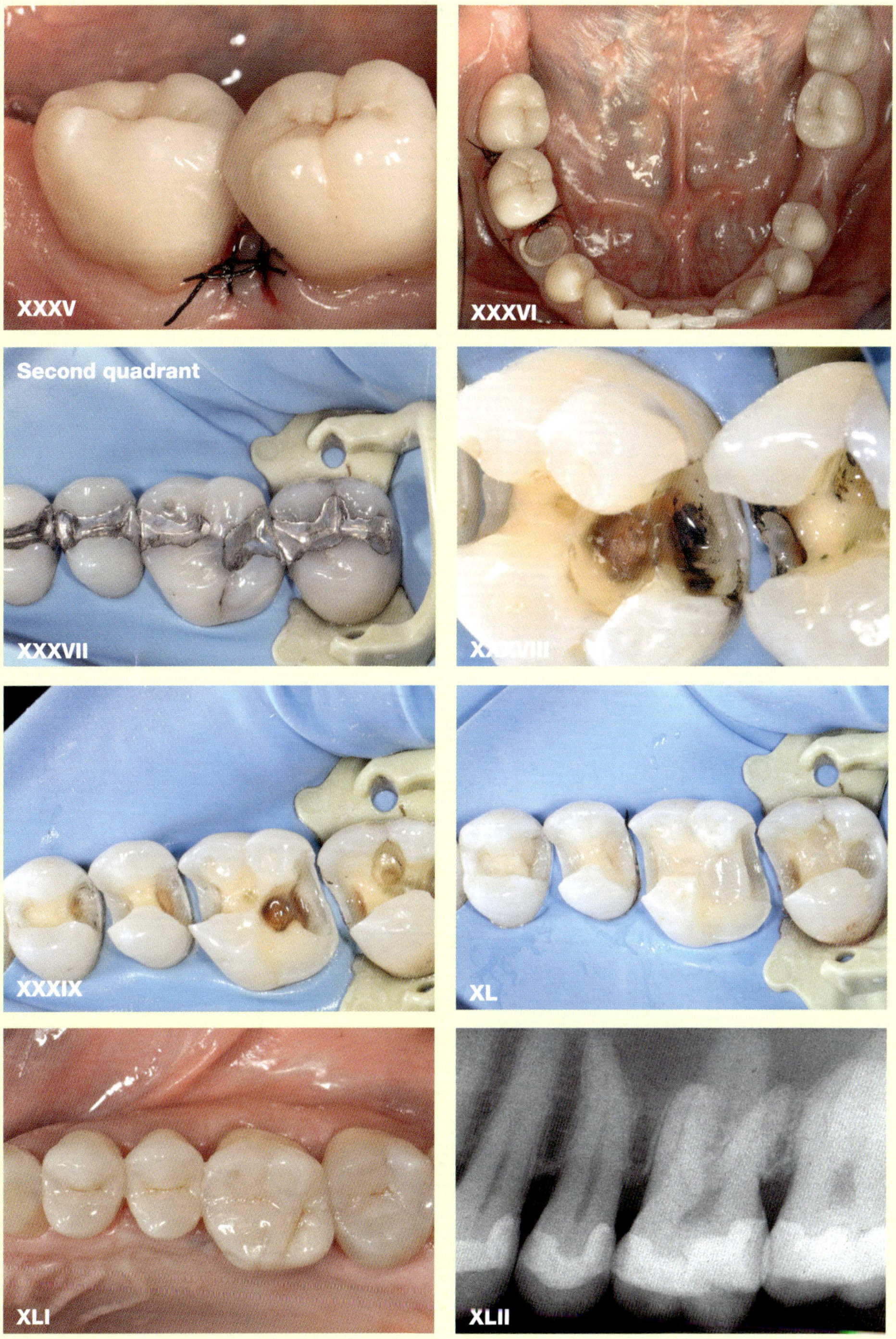

Fig 167 *(continued)*

Fig 167 *(continued)*

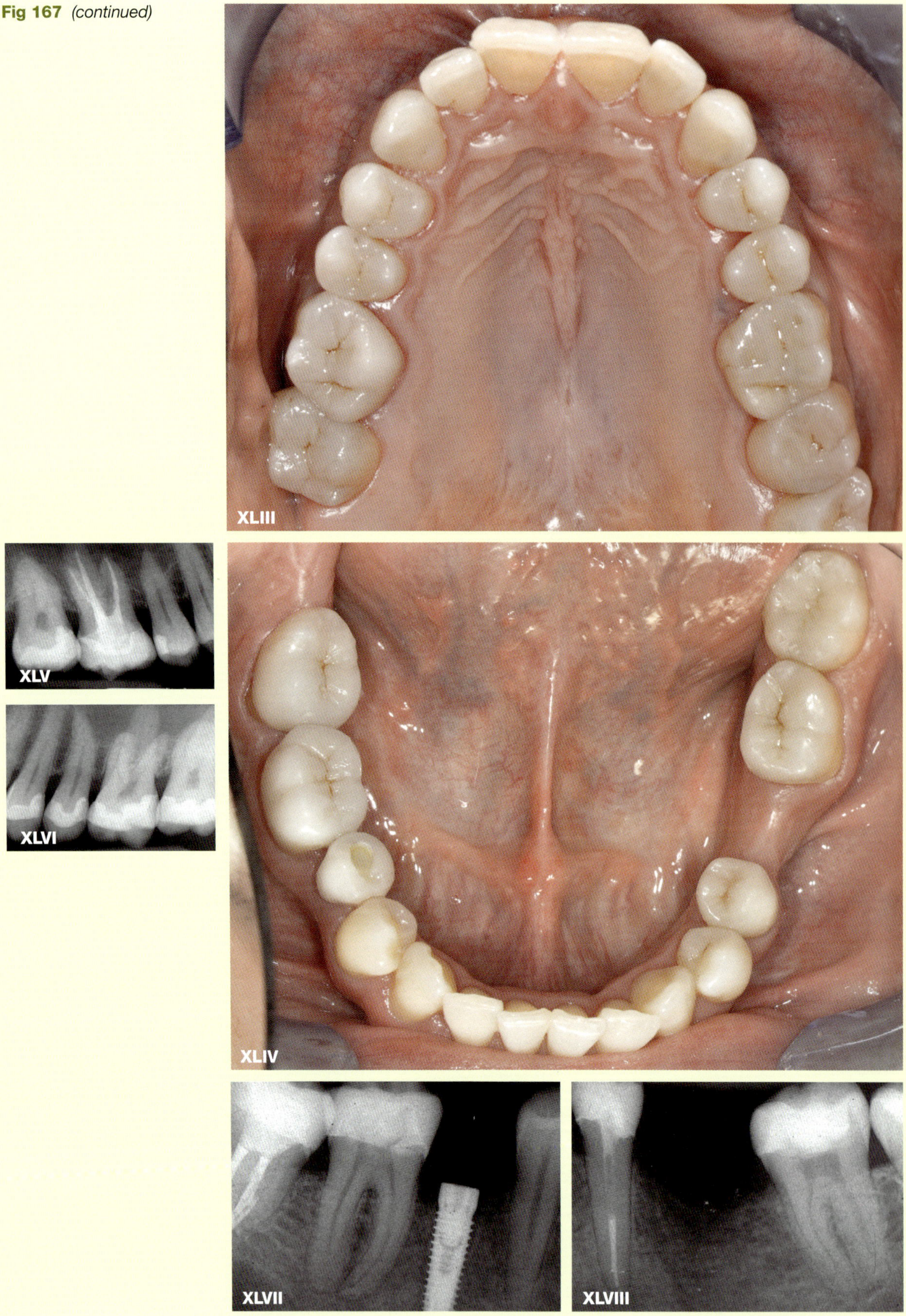

Clinical case 4

Fig 168 Restorations performed in all four quadrants using direct and indirect adhesive techniques *(I–XX)*. In the mandibular left (third) quadrant, adequate thicknesses at the base of the distobuccal cusp of the first molar, even after removing an old buccal restoration, indicated that the tooth should be saved and a simple inlay performed *(IX-XVII)*. Radiographic and clinical status after 3 years are shown *(XXI–XXV)*.

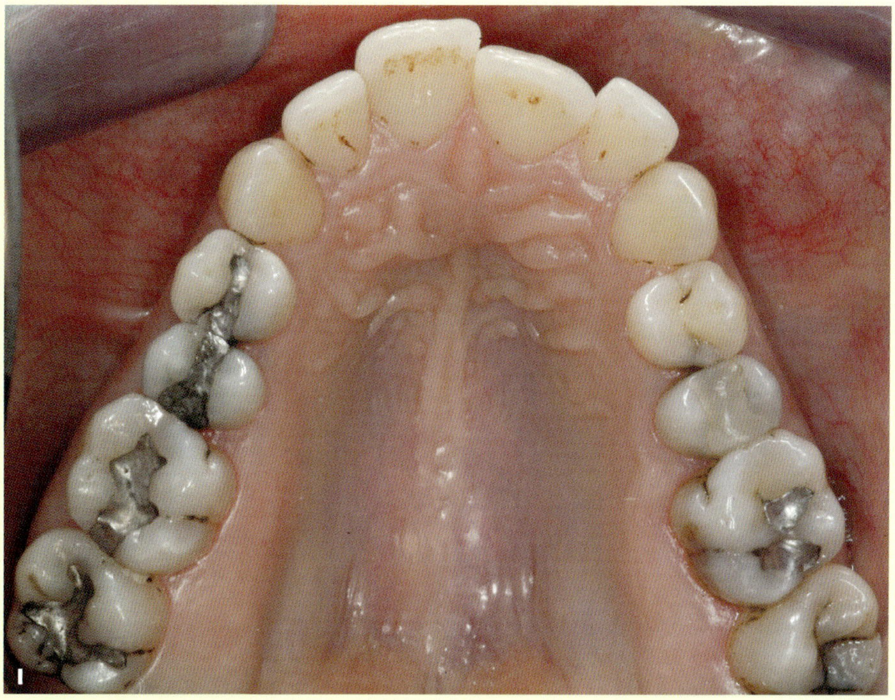
I

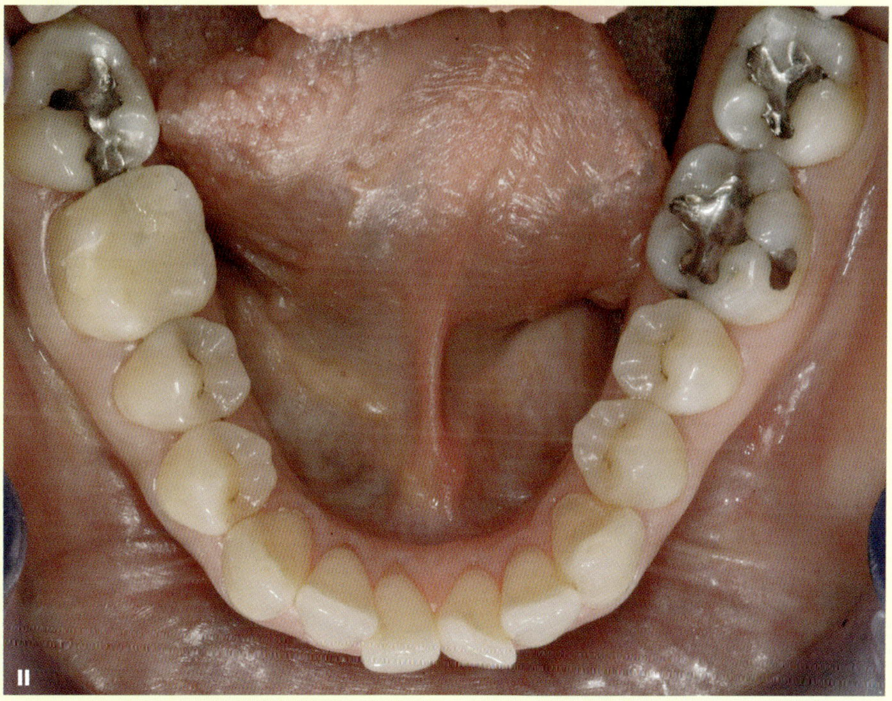
II

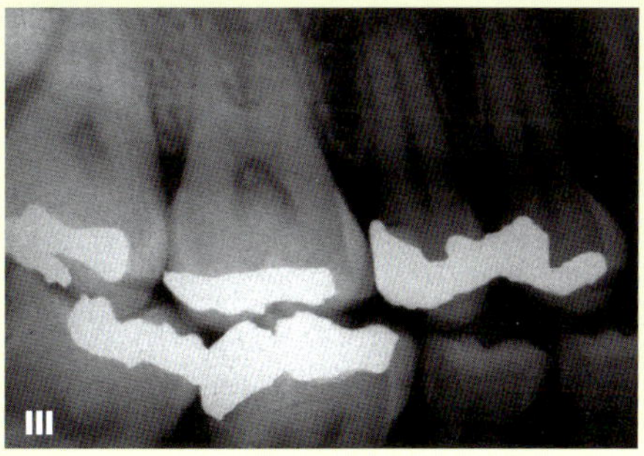
III

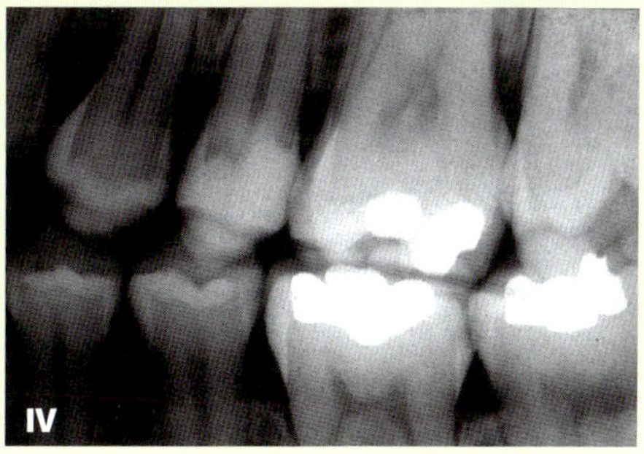
IV

Fig 168 *(continued)*

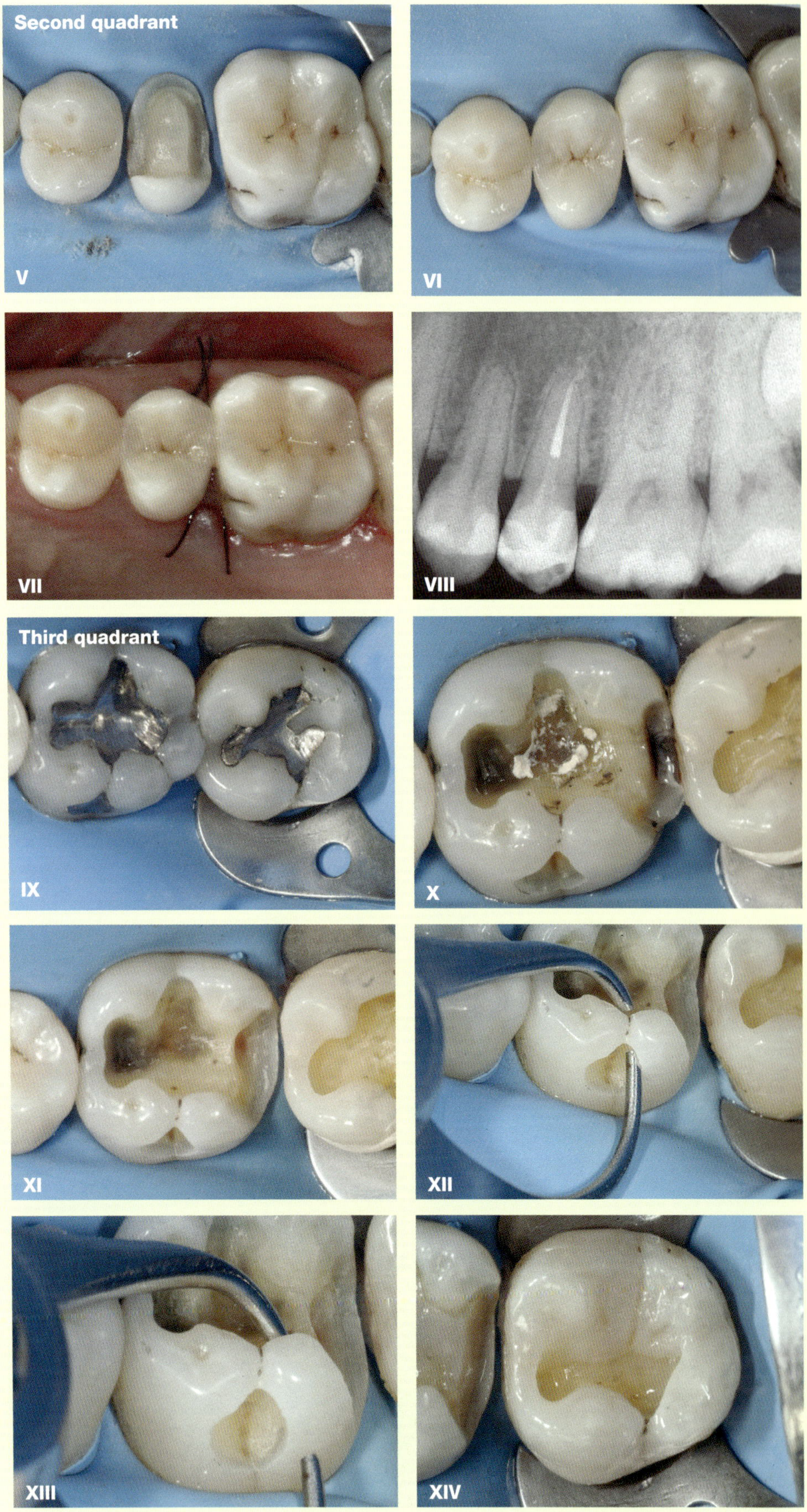

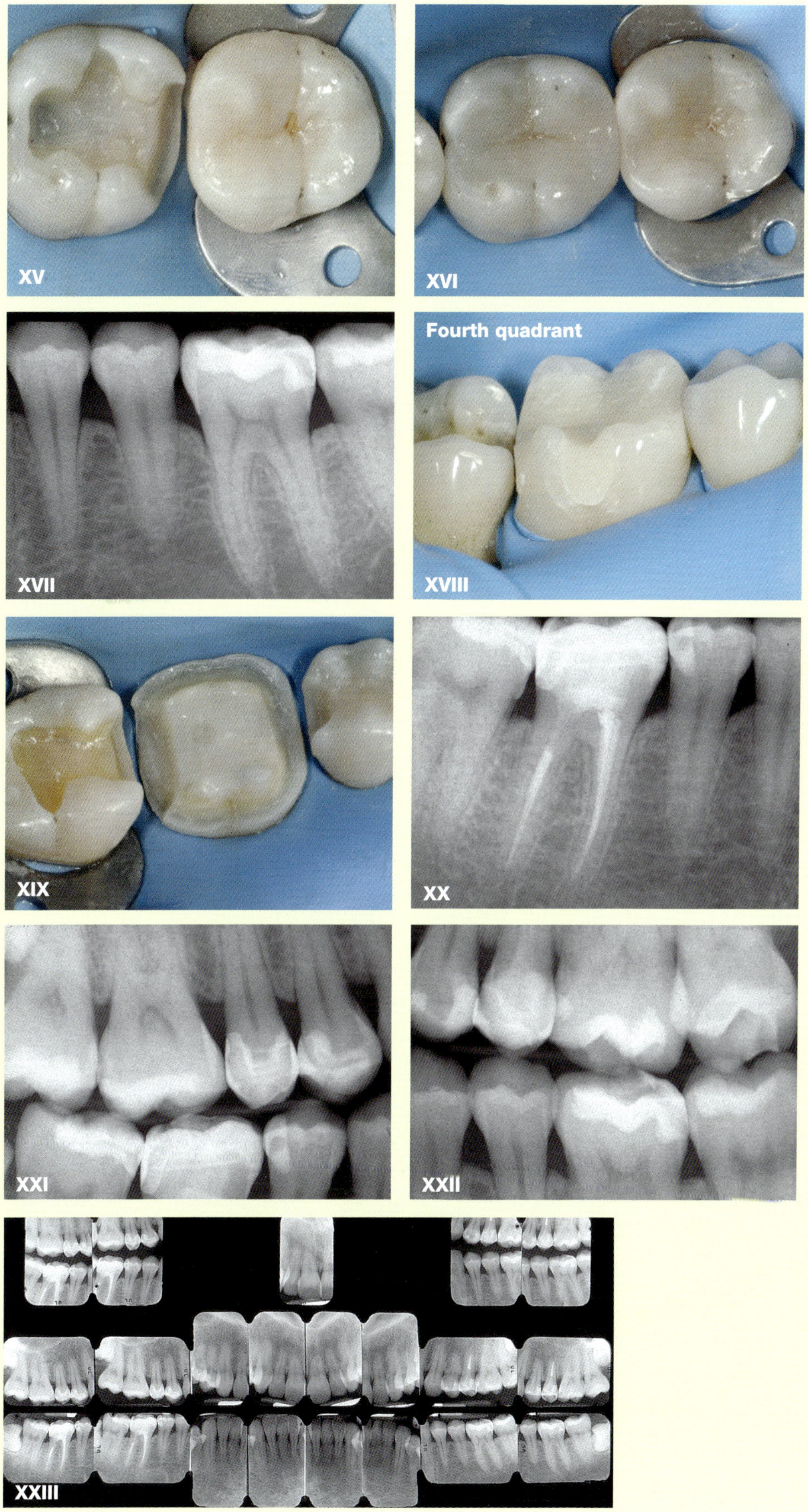

Fig 168 *(continued)*

Fig 168 *(continued)*

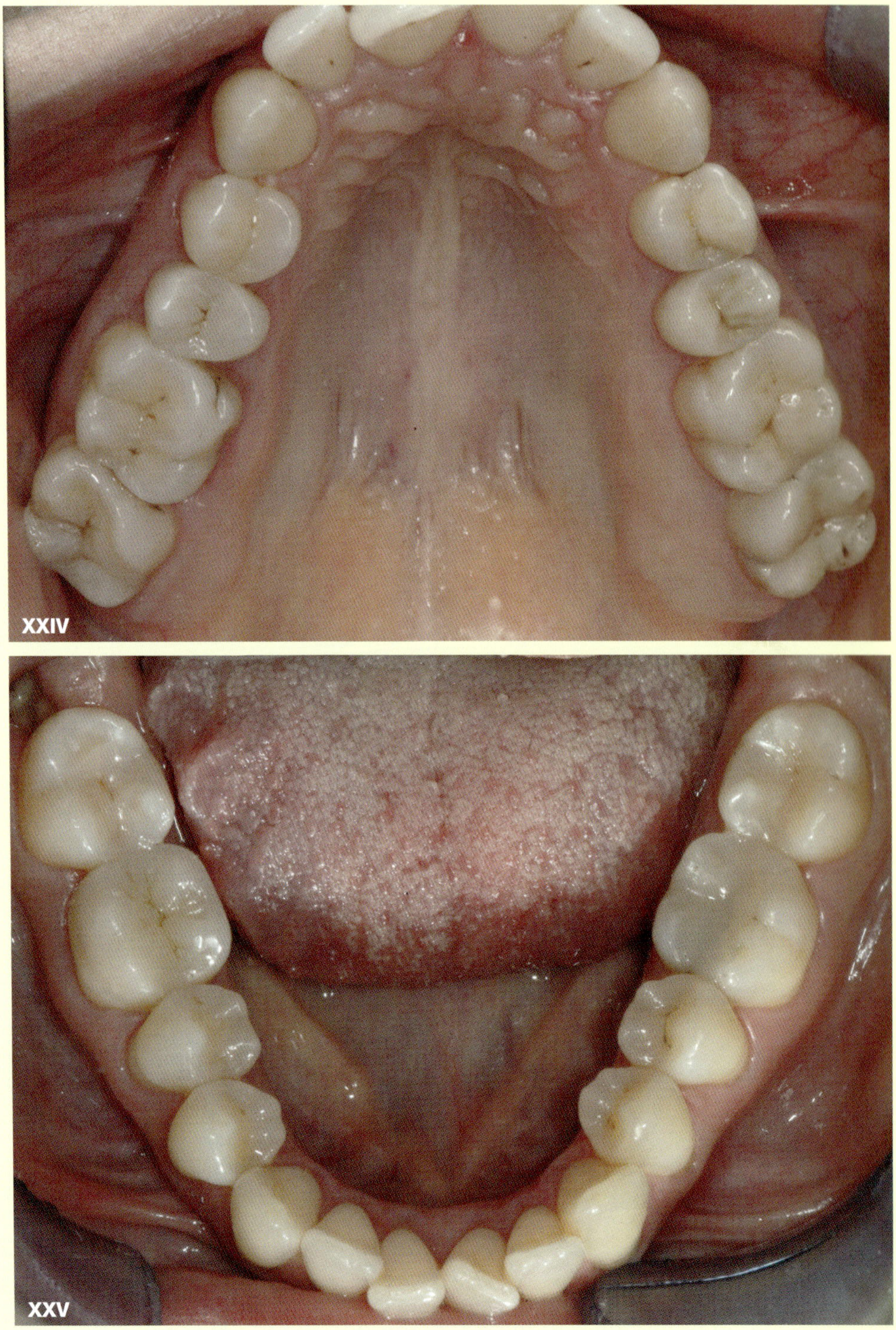

Clinical case 5

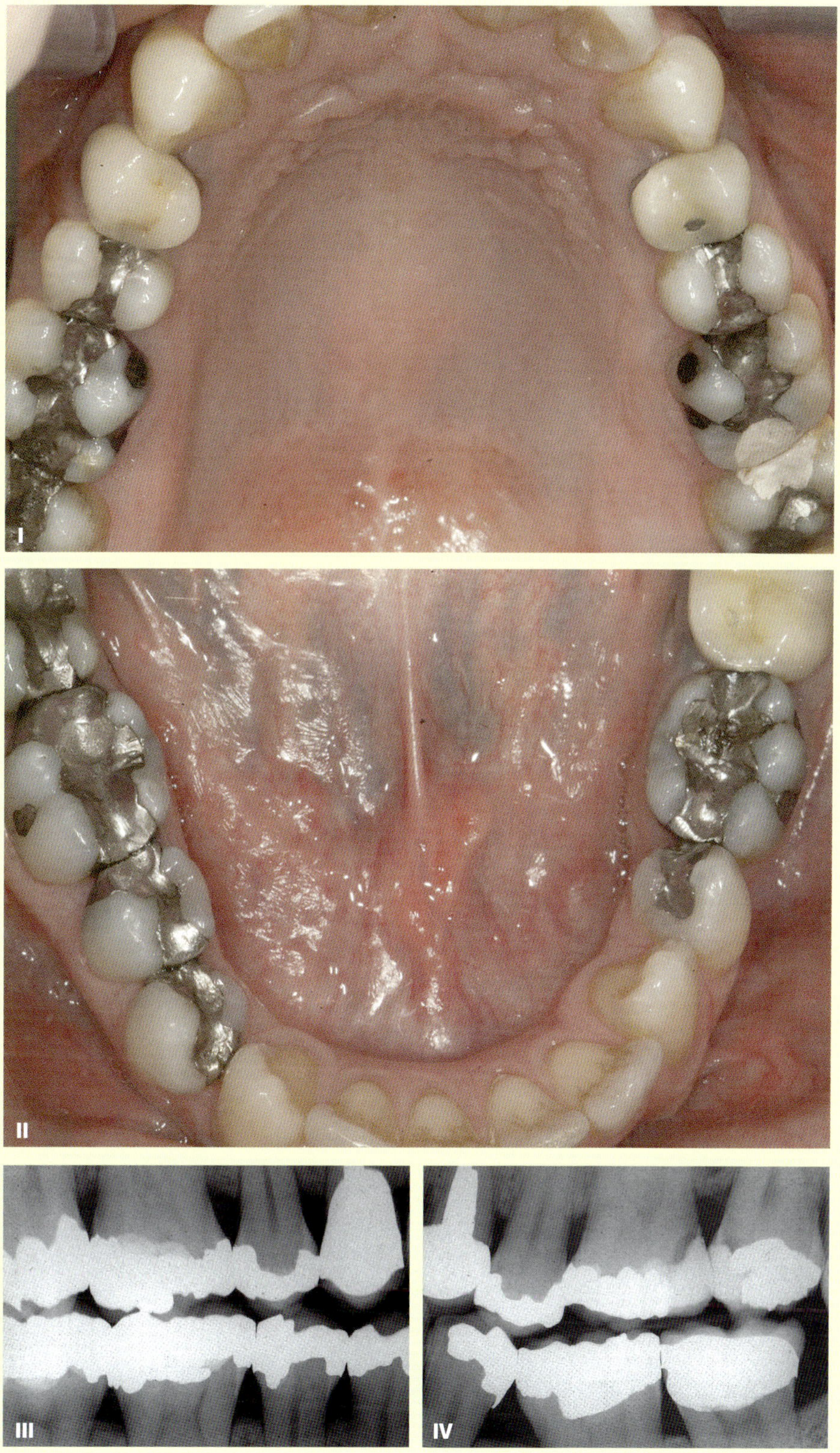

Fig 169 Another case of restoration of all four quadrants in a young patient *(I–IV)*. The routine difficulty in carrying out these very conservative techniques is effectively demonstrated by the intraoperative stages in the various quadrants *(V–XV)*. The final outcome *(XVI–XIX)* and follow-up radiographs after 5 years *(XX)* are shown.

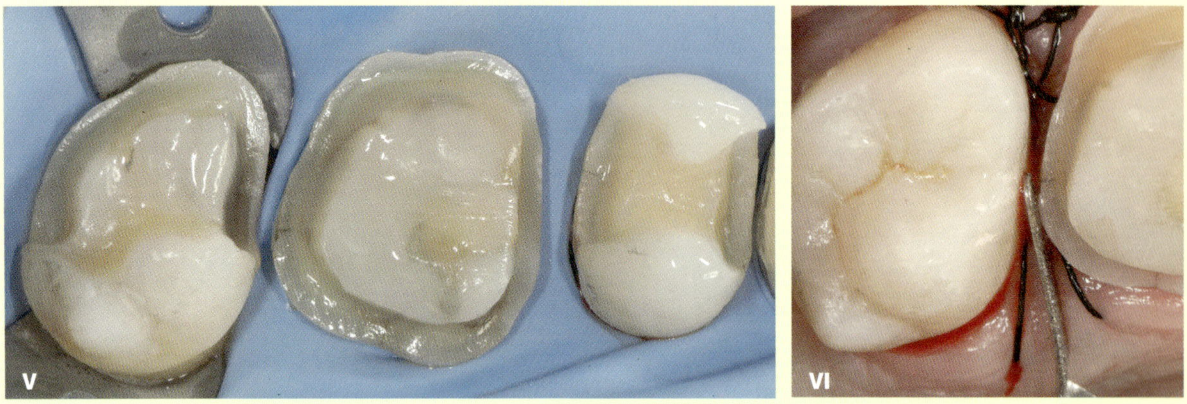

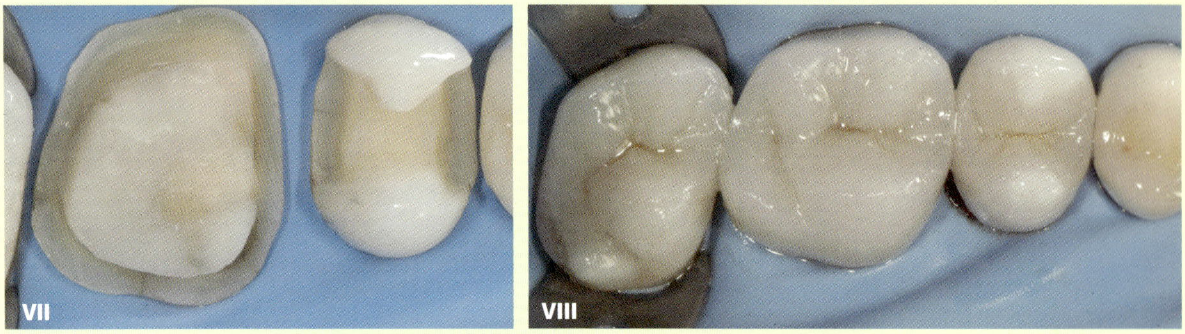

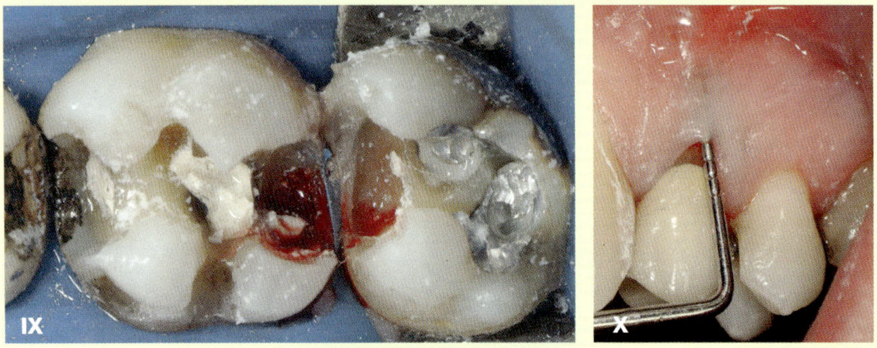

Fig 169 *(continued)*

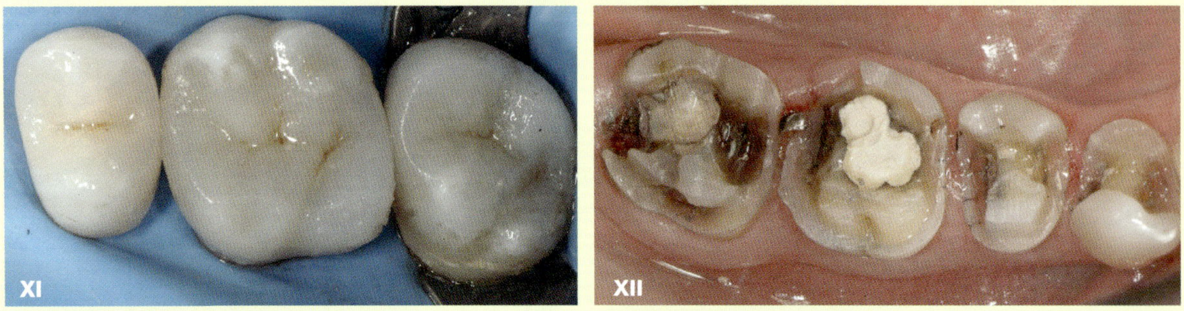

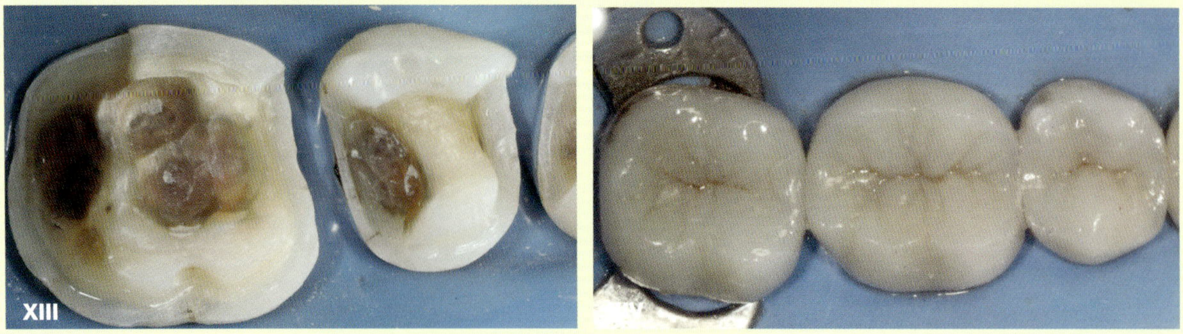

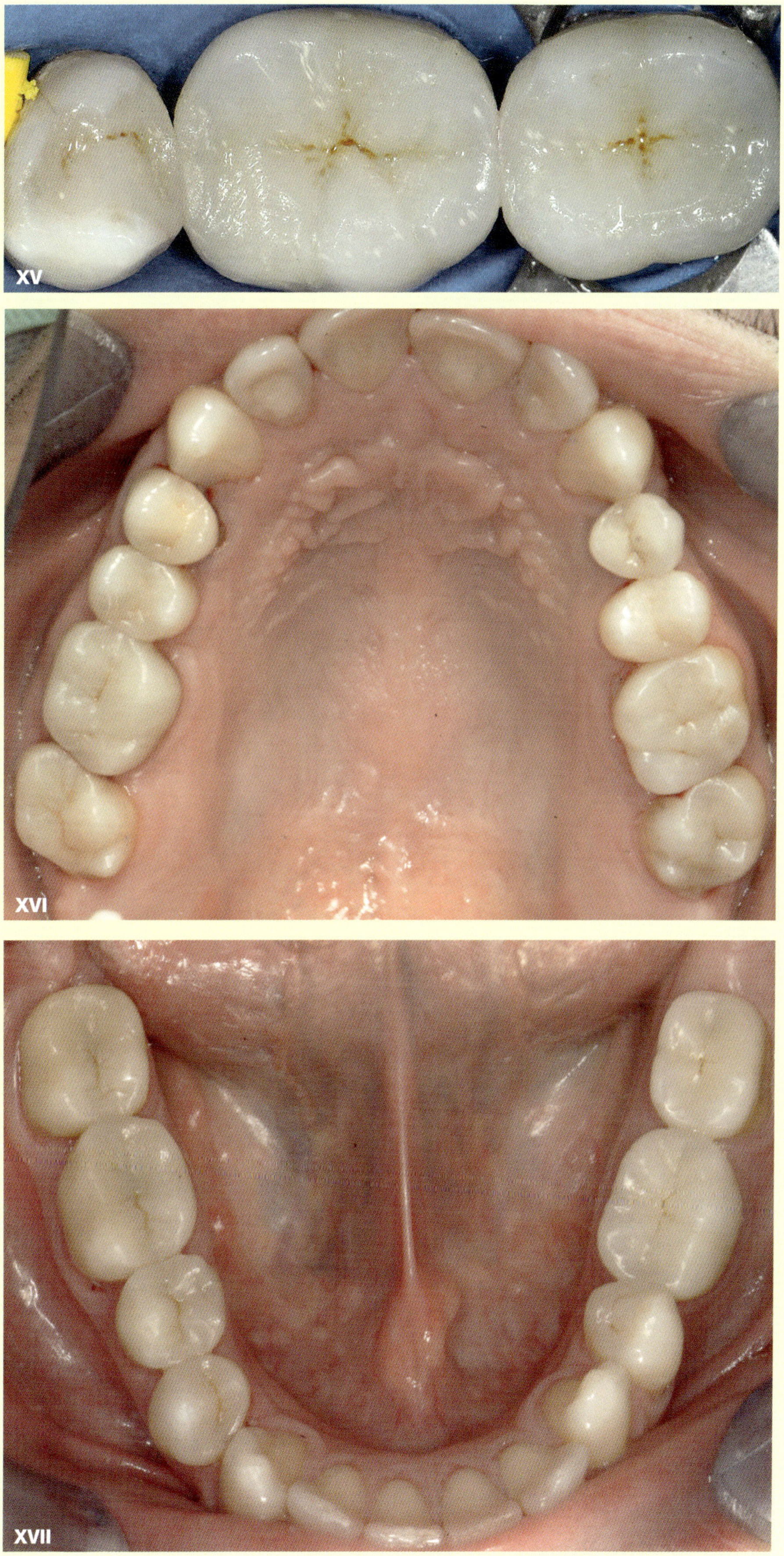

Fig 169 *(continued)*

Fig 169 *(continued)*

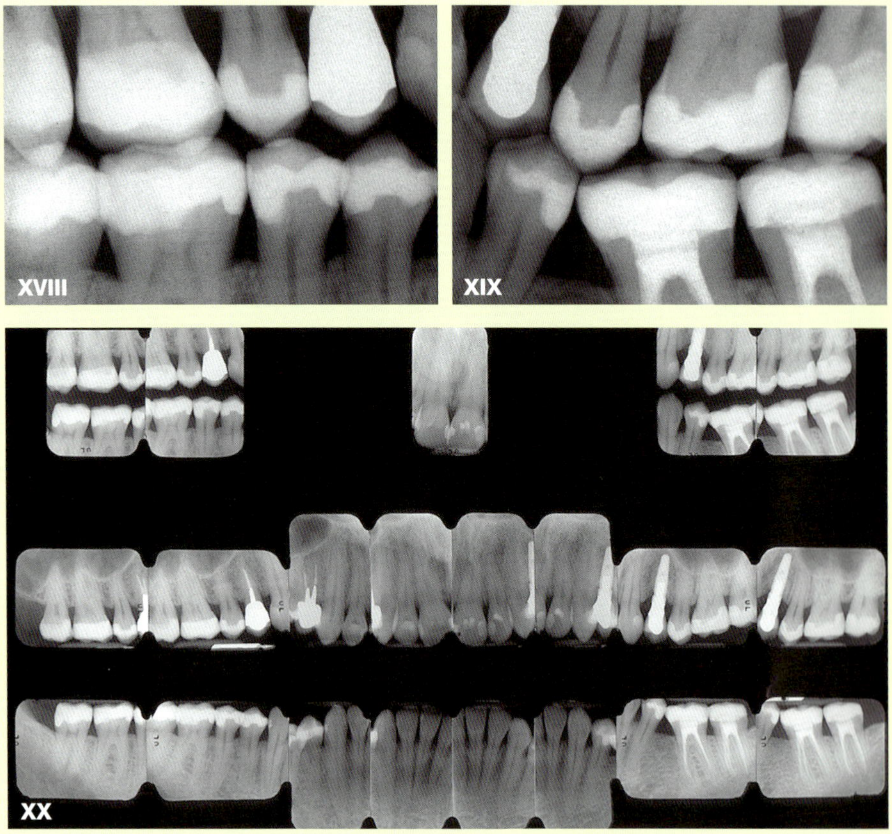

Clinical case 6

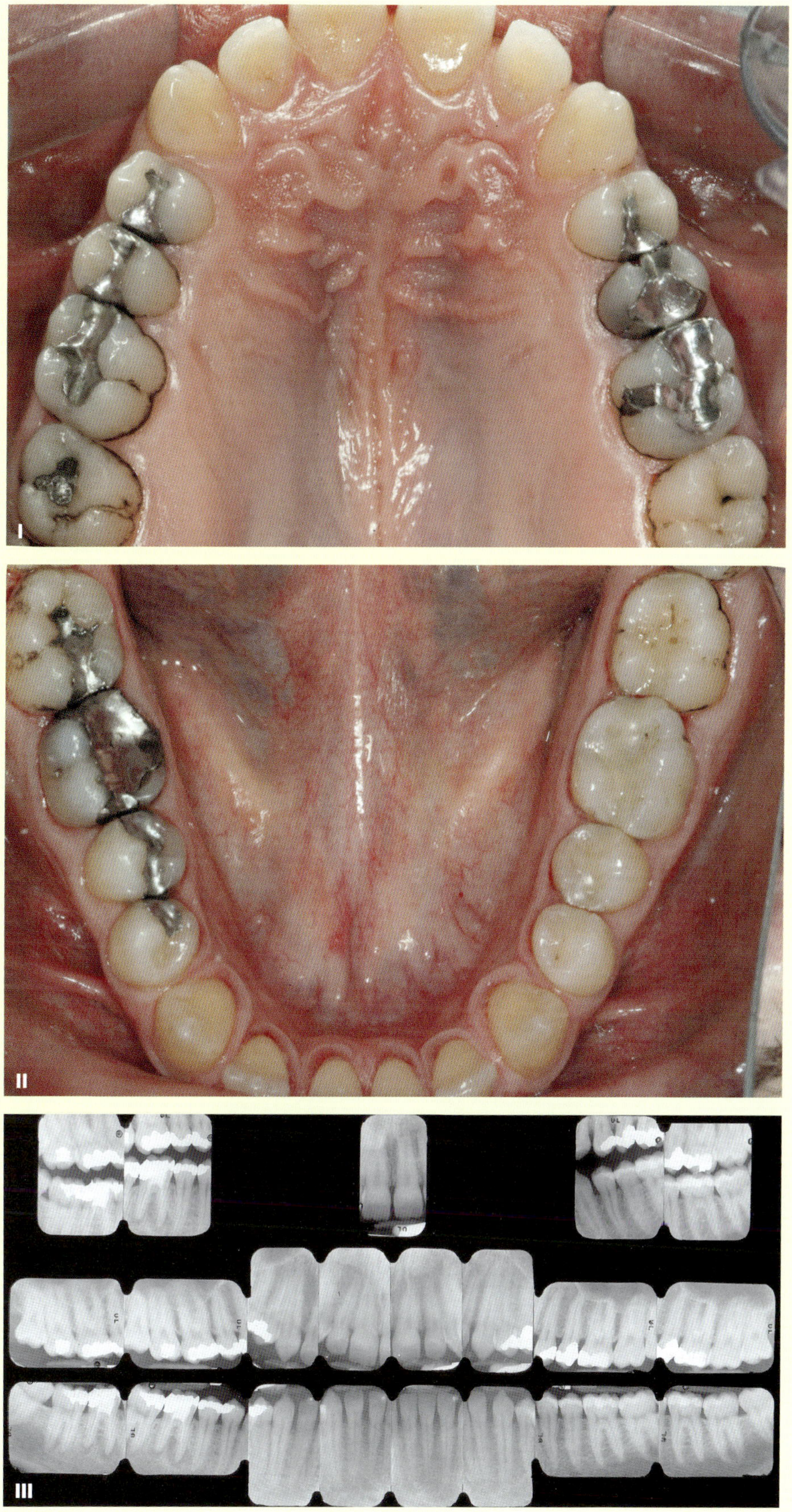

Fig 170 Preparation, buildup, and cementation of biologic and cosmetic restorations in both arches of a young patient *(I–XVII)*. Clinical follow-up of arches after 3 years *(XVIII, XIX)*. No follow-up radiographs showing the completed treatment are available because of patient refusal.

Fig 170 *(continued)*

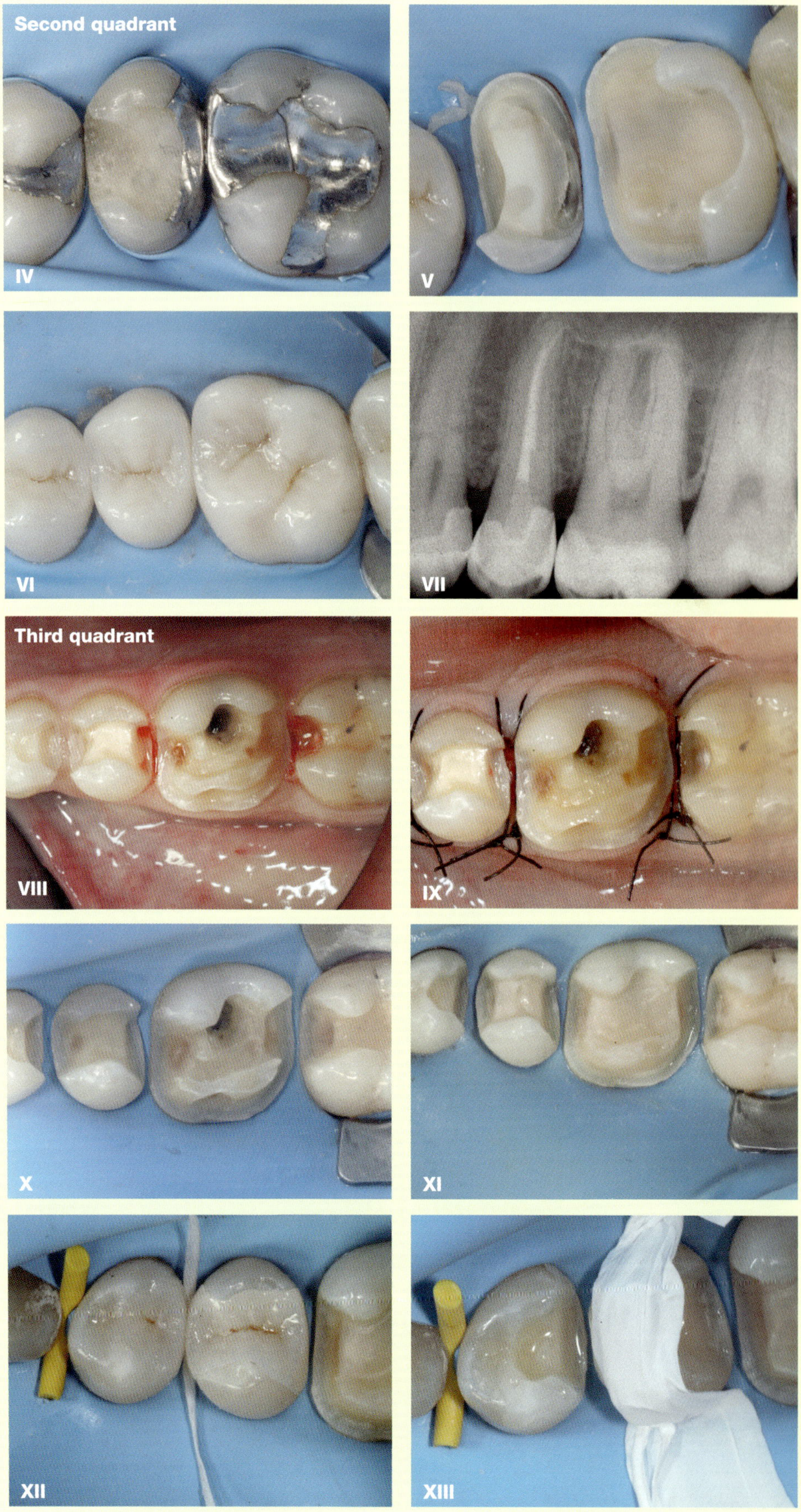

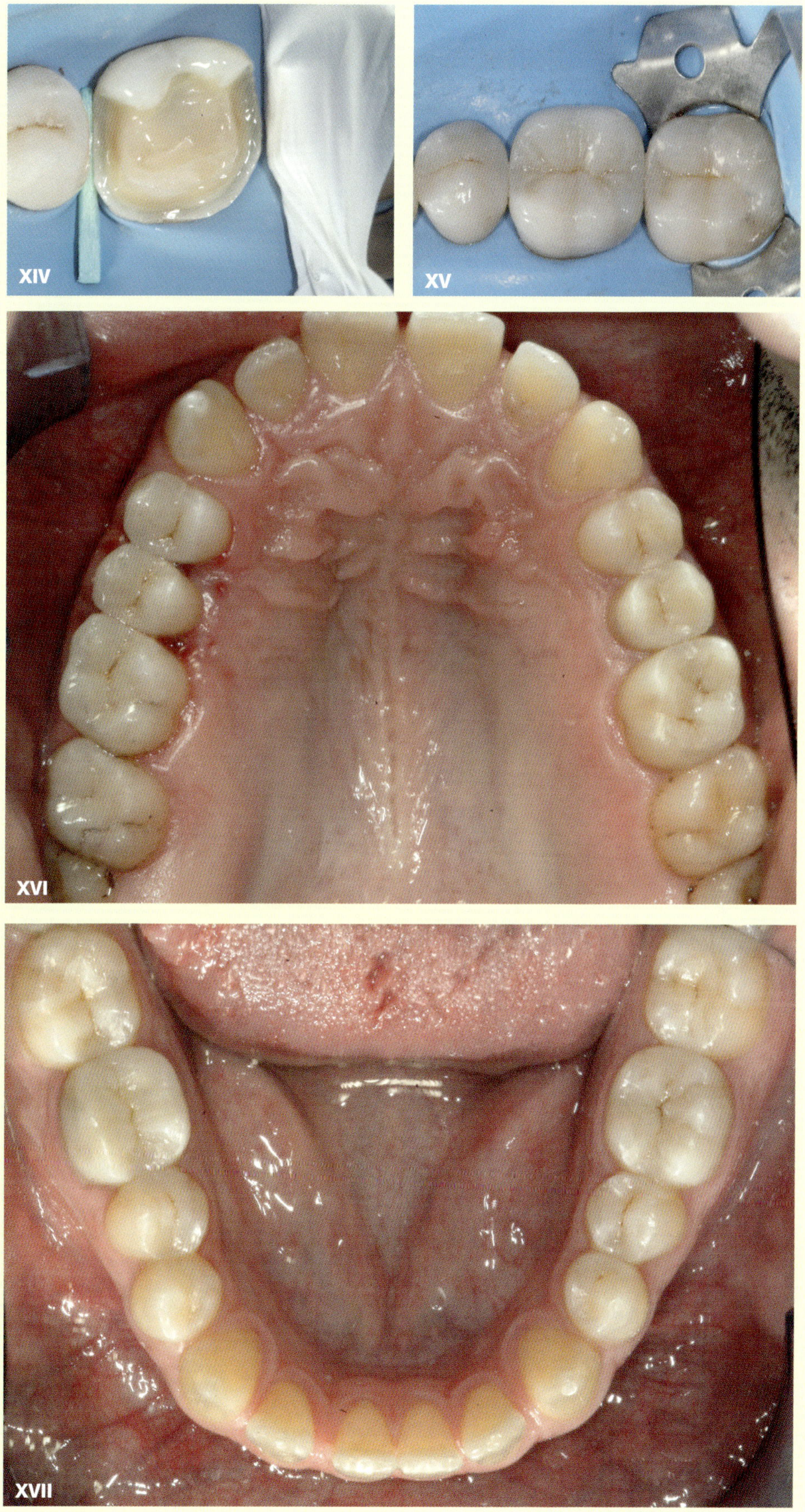

Fig 170 *(continued)*

Fig 170 *(continued)*

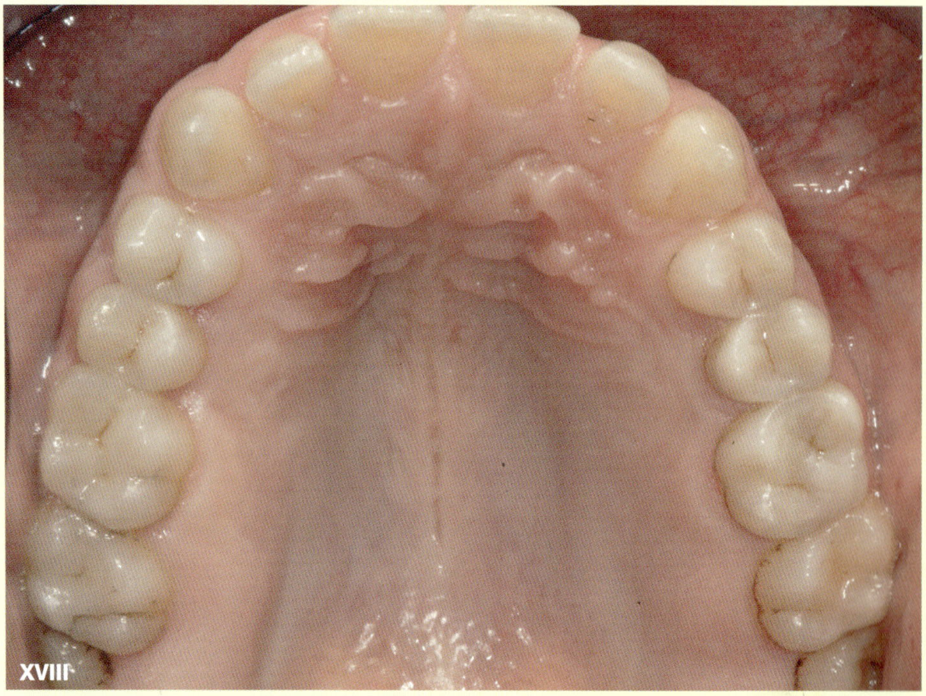

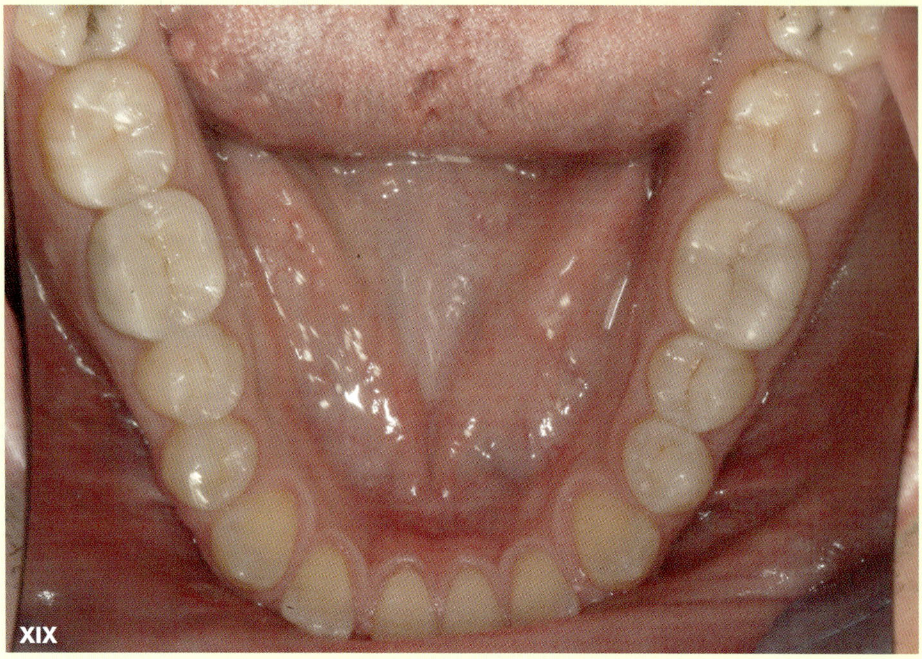

Clinical case 7

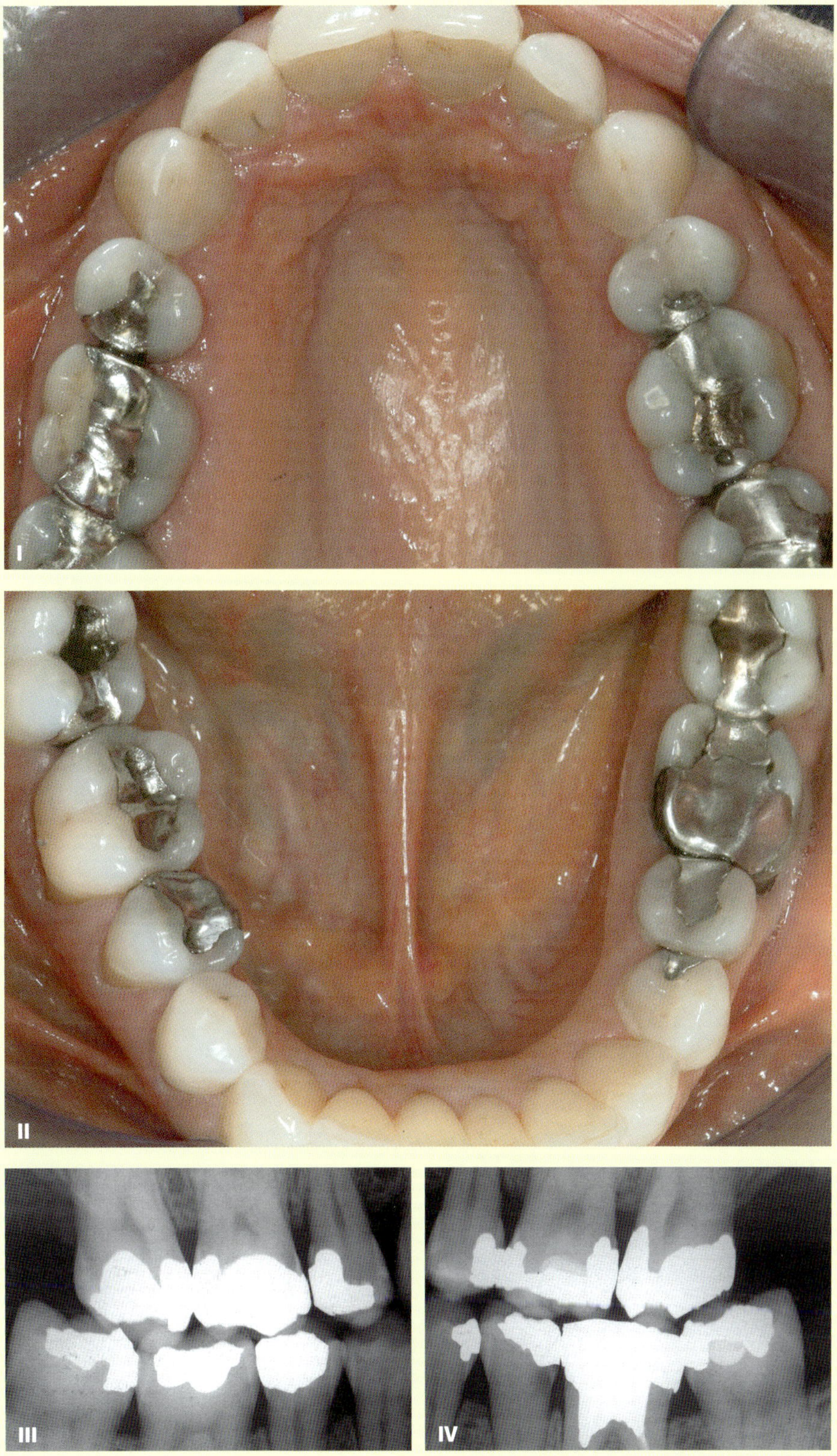

Fig 171 The reasons for restoring both arches were multiple caries lesions, infiltrated restorations, and fracture of the distobuccal wall of the mandibular left first molar *(I–VI)*. The periodontologist demonstrated considerable commitment and skill in making it possible to apply dam to this tooth *(VII, VIII)*. However, isolation of the operative field was still difficult *(IX–XII)*; nevertheless, the patient was willing to sacrifice a more cosmetic result in order to achieve supragingival margins. This topic deserves greater discussion, but this is not the ideal place for it. The margin may be unsightly, but it is nevertheless very biologically sound *(XIII)*. The other three quadrants were likewise restored *(XIV–XXXI)*. Follow-up radiographs performed after 3 years *(XXXII)* reveal that the pulp in the mandibular left second premolar was still vital and each individual tooth-restoration margin was still intact, although excessive wear has clearly been caused by parafunctions and inconsistent use of the duly recommended bite guard that was fabricated and given to the patient when the restorations were complete.

Fig 171 *(continued)*

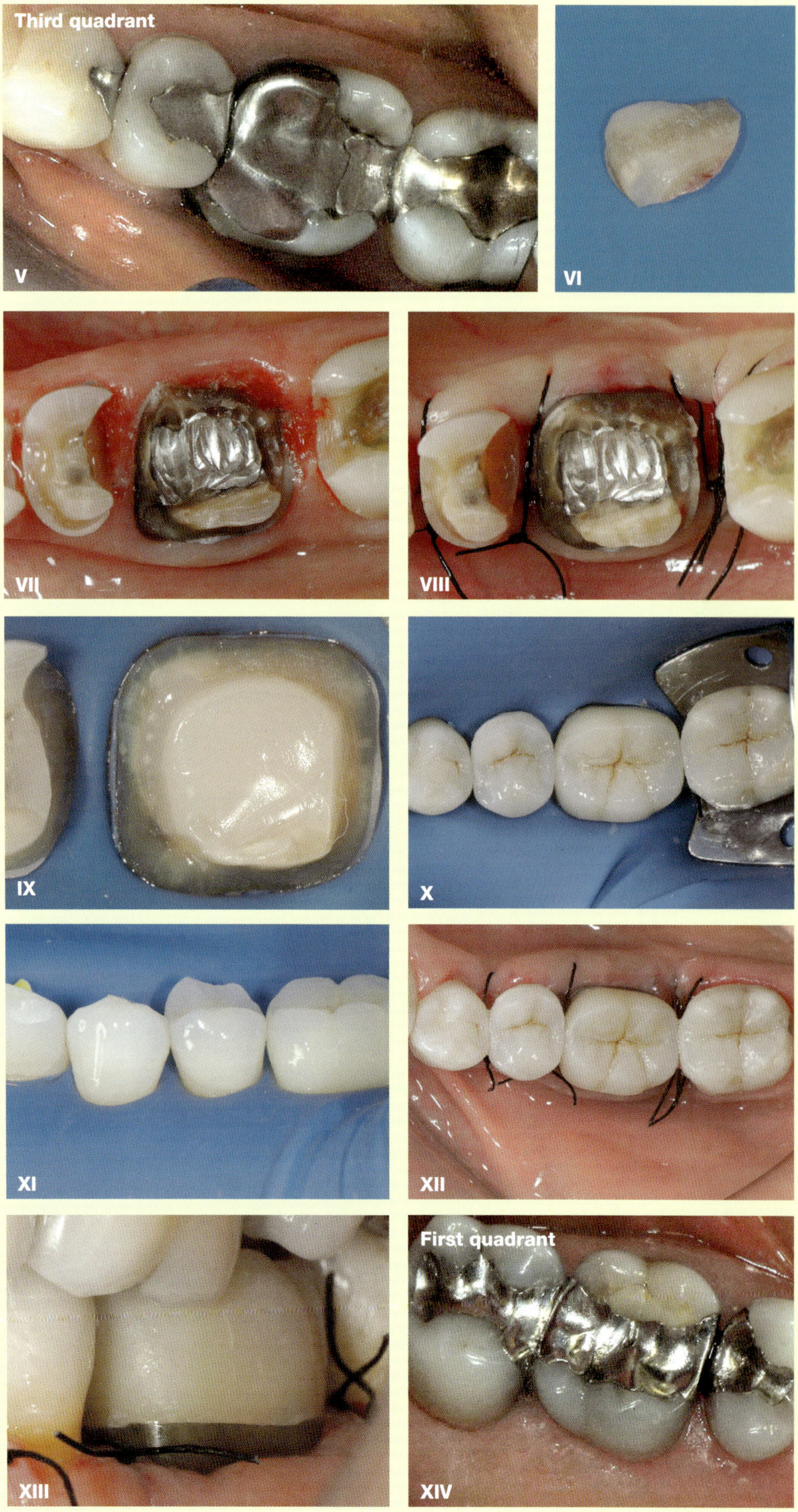

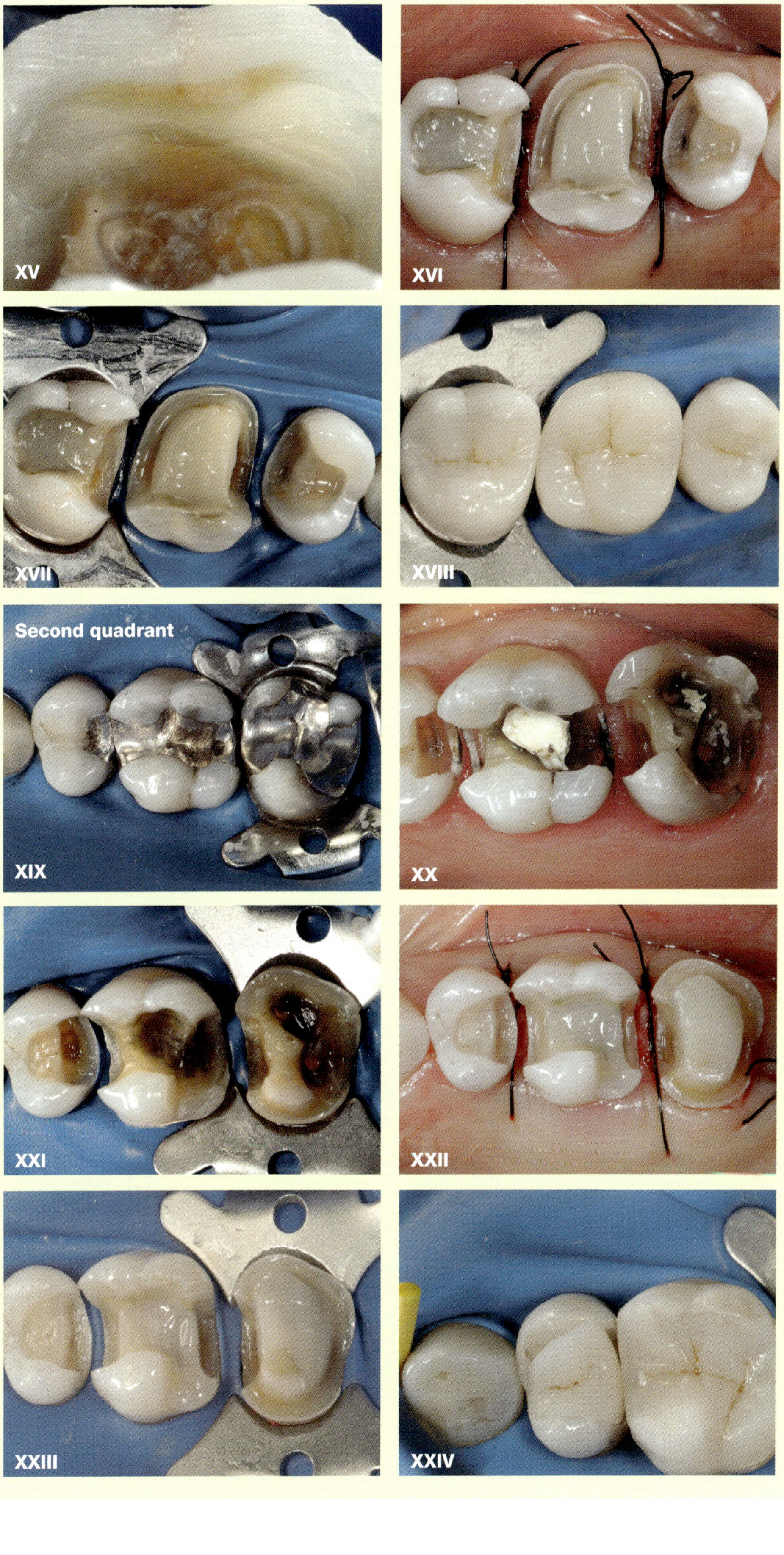

Fig 171 *(continued)*

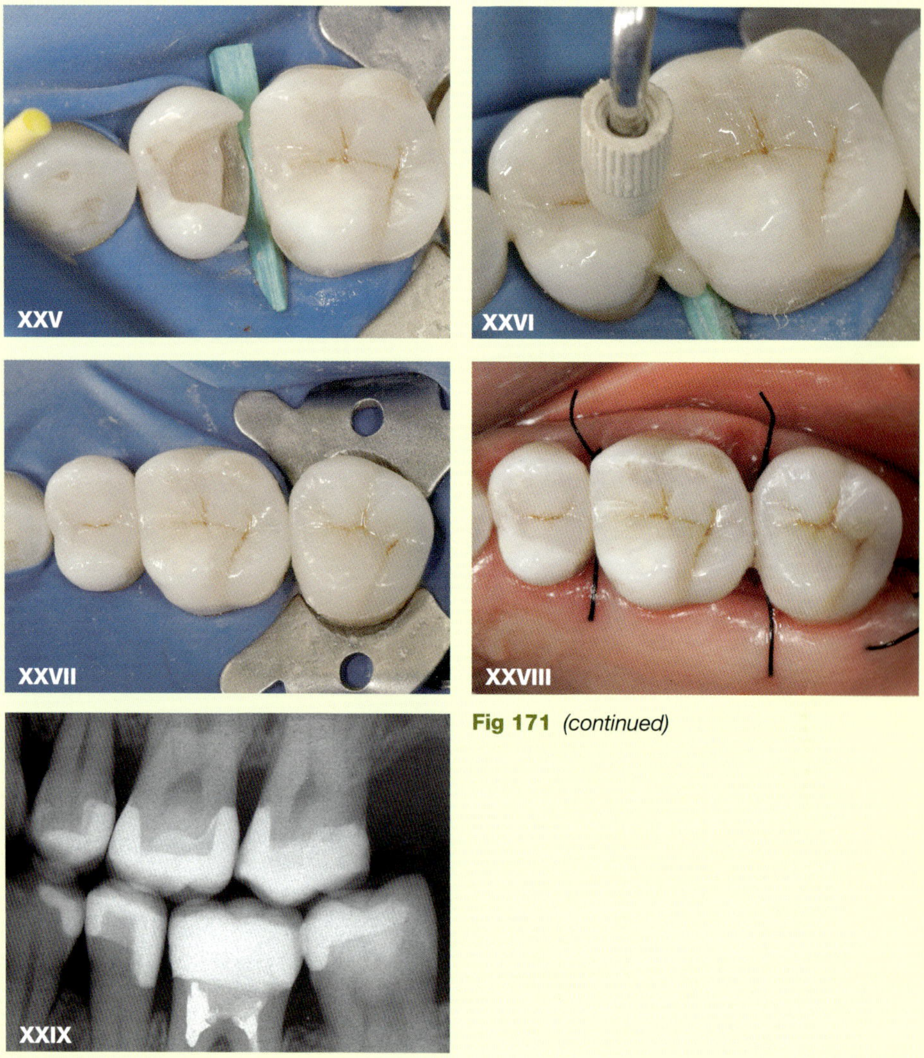

Fig 171 *(continued)*

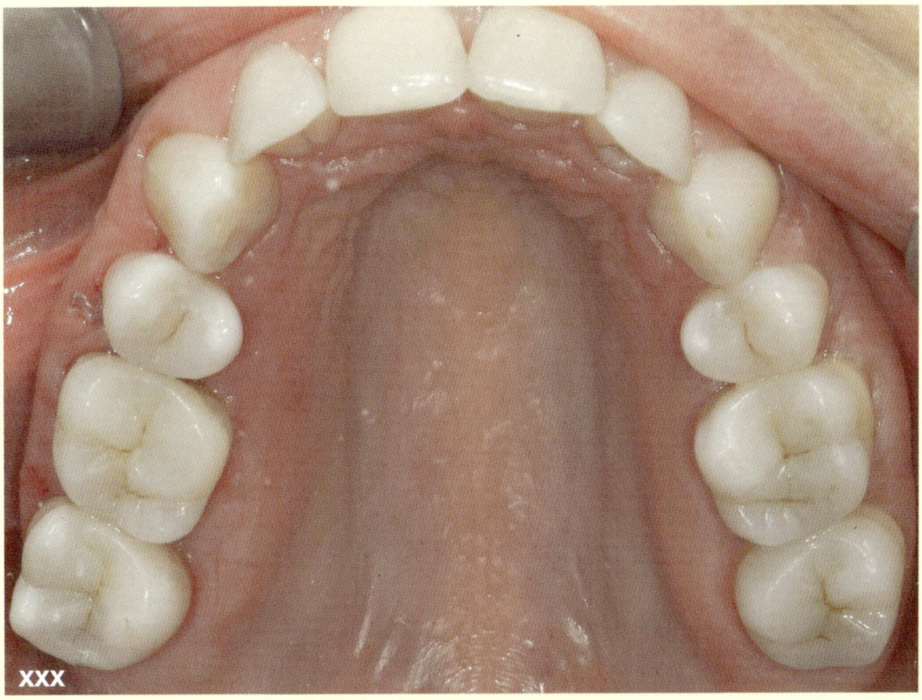

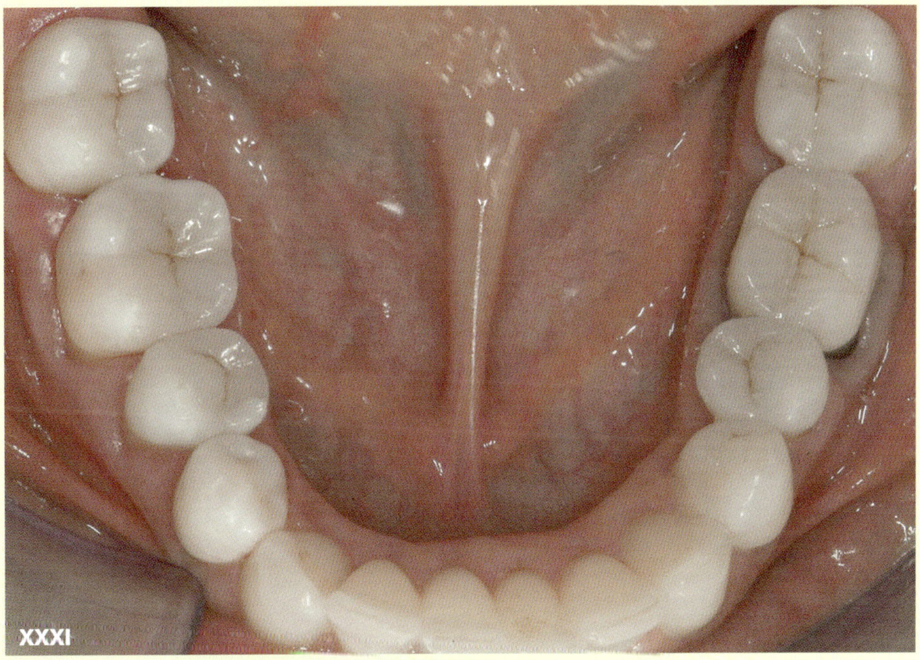

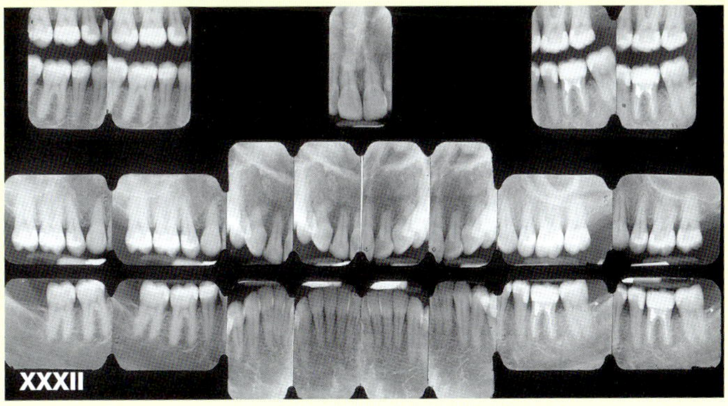

Fig 171 *(continued)*

References

1. Lasfargues JJ, Burkiet F, Tirlet G, Ducup F. Bonded partial restorations for endodontically treated teeth. In: Roulet JF, Wilson NHF, Fuzzi M (eds). Advances in Operative Dentistry. Vol 1: Contemporary Clinical Practice. Chicago: Quintessence, 2001:191–209.
2. Fichera G, Dinapoli C, Dino R. Restauri estetico-adesivi indiretti: modello per diagnosi di configurazione cavitaria. Il Dentista Moderno 2003;2:21–57.
3. Caron GA, Murchinson DF, Cohen RB, Broome JC. Resistance to fracture of teeth with various preparations for amalgam. J Dent 1996;6:407–410.
4. Khera SC, Goel VK, Chen RC, Gurusami SA. Paramater of MOD cavity preparation: A 3D FEM Study. Oper Dent 1991;16:42–54.
5. Mondelli J, Steagall L, Ishikiriama A, De Lima Navarro MF, Soares FB. Fracture strength of human teeth with cavity preparations. J Prosthet Dent 1980;43:419–422.
6. Larson TD, Douglas WH, Geistfeld RE. Effect of prepared cavities on strength of teeth. Oper Dent 1998;6:2–5
7. Reeh ES, Messer HH, Douglas WH. Reduction in tooth stiffness as a result of endodontic and restorative procedures. J Endod 1989;15:512–516.
8. Goel VK, Khera SC, Gurusami SA, Chen RC. Effect on cavity depth on stresses in a restored tooth. J Prosthet Dent 1992;2:174–183.
9. Sakaguchi RL, Brust EW, Cross M, Delong R, Douglas WH. Independent movement of cusps during occlusal loading. Dent Mater 1991;7:186–190.
10. Linn J, Messer HH. Effect of restorative procedures on the strength of endodontically treated molars. J Endod 1994;20:479–485.
11. Panitvisai P, Messer HH. Cuspal deflection in molar in relation to endodontic and restorative procedures. J Endod 1995;21:57–61.
12. Hood JAA. Methods to improve fracture resistance of teeth. In: Vanherle G, Smith DC (eds). Posterior Composite Resin Dental Restorative Materials. Utrecht, The Netherlands: Peter Szule Publishing, 1985:443–450.
13. Sedgley CM, Messer HH. Are endodontically treated teeth more brittle? J Endod 1992;7:332–335.
14. Assif D, Gorfil C. Biomechanical considerations in restoring endodontically treated teeth. J Prosthet Dent 1994;71:565–567.
15. Macpherson LC, Smith BG. Reinforcement of weakened cusps by adhesive restorative materials: An in-vitro study. Br Dent J 1995;178:341–344.
16. Magne P. Immediate dentin sealing: A fundamental procedure for indirect bonded restorations. J Esthet Restor Dent 2005;17:144–155.
17. Wassell RW, Walls AW, McCabe JF. Cavity convergence angles for direct composite inlays. J Dent 1992;20:294–297.
18. Burke FJ, Wilson NH, Watts DC. The effect of cavity wall taper on fracture resistance of teeth restored with resin composite inlays. Oper Dent 1993;18:230–236.
19. Aravamudhan K, Floyd CJ, Rakowski D, et al. Light-emitting diode curing light irradiance and polymerization of resin-based composite. J Am Dent Assoc 2006;137:213–223.
20. Kemp-Scholte CM, Davidson CL. Complete marginal seal of Class V resin composite restorations effected by increased flexibility. J Dent Res 1990;69:1240–1243.
21. Shillingburg HT, Hobo S, Whitsett LD. Fundamentals of Fixed Prosthodontics. Chicago: Quintessence, 1978.
22. Polz MH. Biomechanical basis of occlusal masticatory surface design [in German]. Zahntechnik (Zur) 1981;39:126–134.
23. Seubert G. Conoscenze basilari della tecnica di ceratura gnatologica naturale secondo D. Schulz. Villa Carcina, Brescia: Mea, 1996.
24. Sorensen JA, Martinoff JT. Intracoronal reinforcement and coronal coverage: A study of endodontically treated teeth. J Prosthet Dent 1984;51:580–584.
25. Lee MR, Cho BH, Son HH, Um CM, Lee IB. Influence of cavity dimension and restoration methods on the cusp deflection of premolars in composite restoration. Dent Mater 2007;23:288–295.
26. González-López S, Vilchez Díaz MA, de Haro-Gasquet F, Ceballos L, de Haro-Muñoz C. Cuspal flexure of teeth with composite restorations subjected to occlusal loading. J Adhes Dent 2007;9:11–15.
27. Trope M, Maltz DO, Tronstad L. Resistance to fracture of restored endodontically treated teeth. Endod Dent Traumatol 1985;1:108–111.
28. Robbins JW. Guidelines for the restoration of endodontically treated teeth. J Am Dent Assoc 1990;120:558,560,562.
29. Guzy GE, Nicholls JI. In vitro comparison of intact endodontically treated teeth with and without endo-post reinforcement. J Prosthet Dent.1979;42:39–44.
30. Hansen EK, Asmussen E, Christiansen NC. In vivo fractures of endodontically treated posterior teeth restored with amalgam. Endod Dent Traumatol 1990;6:49–55.
31. Fichera G, Dinapoli C, Ferrari P, Re D. Restaurativa postendodontica con perni in fibra. Indicazioni e tecnica operativa. Il Dentista Moderno 2005;9:23–51.
32. Helfer AR, Melnick S, Schilder H. Determination of the moisture content of vital and pulpless teeth. Oral Surg Oral Med Oral Pathol 1972;34:661–670.
33. Rivera E, Yamauchi G, Chasldler G. Dentin collagen cross-links of root-filled and normal teeth. J Endod 1988;14:195.
34. Randow K, Glantz PO. On cantilever loading of vital and non-vital teeth. An experimental clinical study. Acta Odontol Scand 1986;44:271–277.
35. Hansen EK. In vivo cusp fracture of endodontically treated premolars restored with MOD amalgam or MOD resin fillings. Dent Mater 1988;4:169–173.
36. Daronch M, Rueggeberg FA, Hall G, De Goes MF. Effect of composite temperature on in vitro intrapulpal temperature rise. Dent Mater 2007;23:1283–1288.
37. Stansbury JW. Curing dental resins and composites by photopolymerization. J Esthet Dent 2000;12:300–308.

Relationship between restorative dentistry and periodontology 4

A patient who has lost some or most of the structure of one or more teeth needs ideal morpho-functional and esthetic rehabilitation (Fig 1).
The loss may have occurred due to a caries lesion or trauma, and the treatment is based on a specific diagnosis (Fig 2).

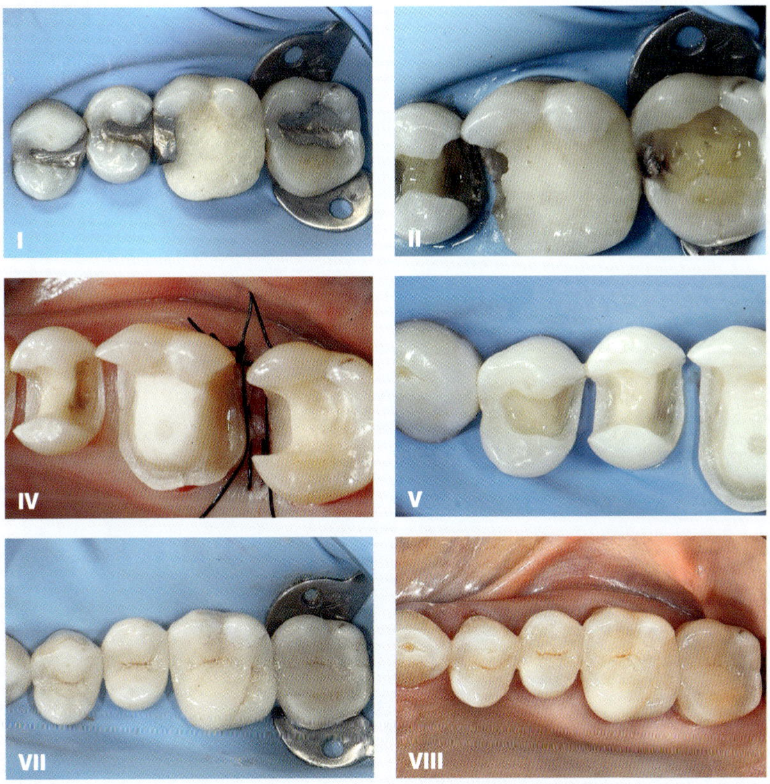

Fig 1 Periodontal and restorative treatment of a case *(I–VIII)*. Note the presence of abundant inflammatory tissue *(III)* and the correction of periodontal structures in a particularly critical area *(IV)*.

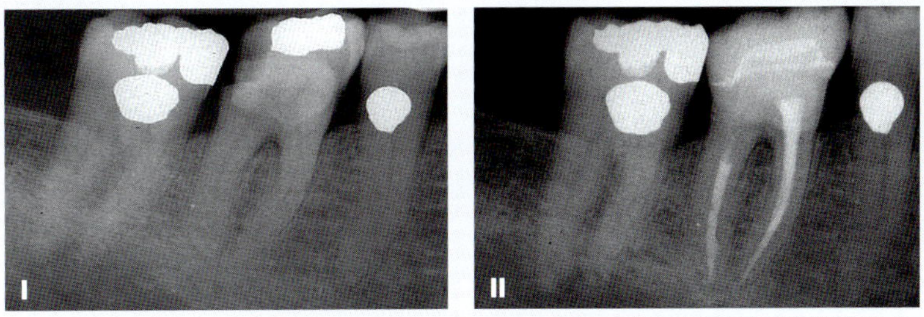

Fig 2 The treatment plan must be based on an evaluation of biologic parameters concerned with loss of tooth structure and maintainability of pulp vitality. Control of the periodontal support is of fundamental importance, and an evaluation of the furcations is essential. The restorability and maintainability of a tooth is based on these considerations.

The treatment must trace back all the stages of the abnormal event that gave rise to the damage and the deformities in each individual case.

The treatment plan must be multidisciplinary and clearly defined in full detail and in the correct sequence (Figs 3 to 6).

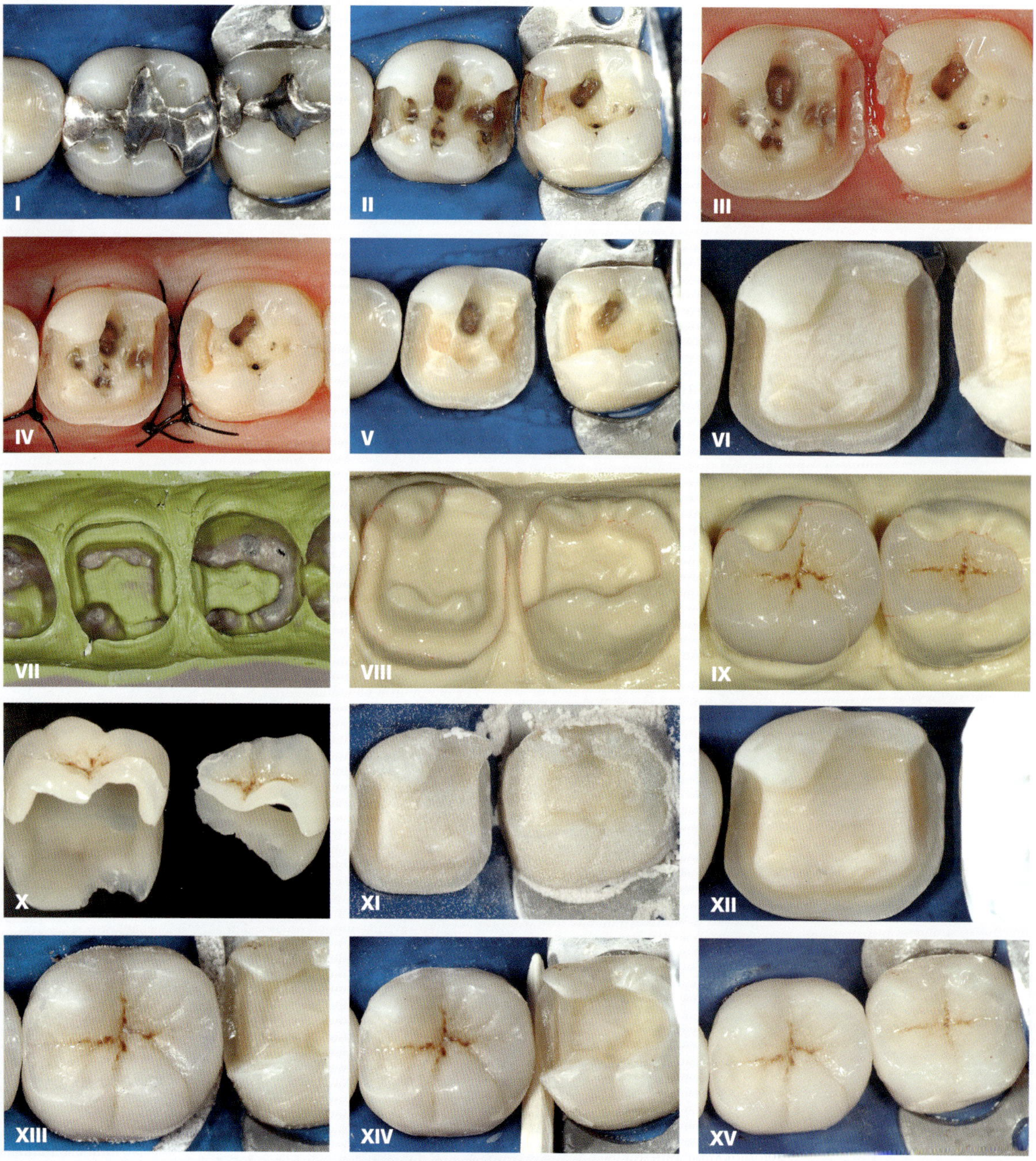

Fig 3 Inflammation and pits in the soft tissue obscure the margins of the lesions and dental preparations. Periodontal surgery removes the inflammatory tissue and exposes the lesion margins. In particular, it allows optimum control of all procedures necessary to achieve an accurate restoration.

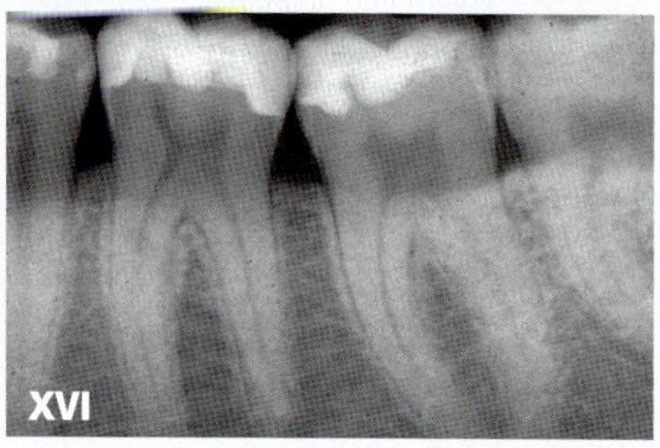

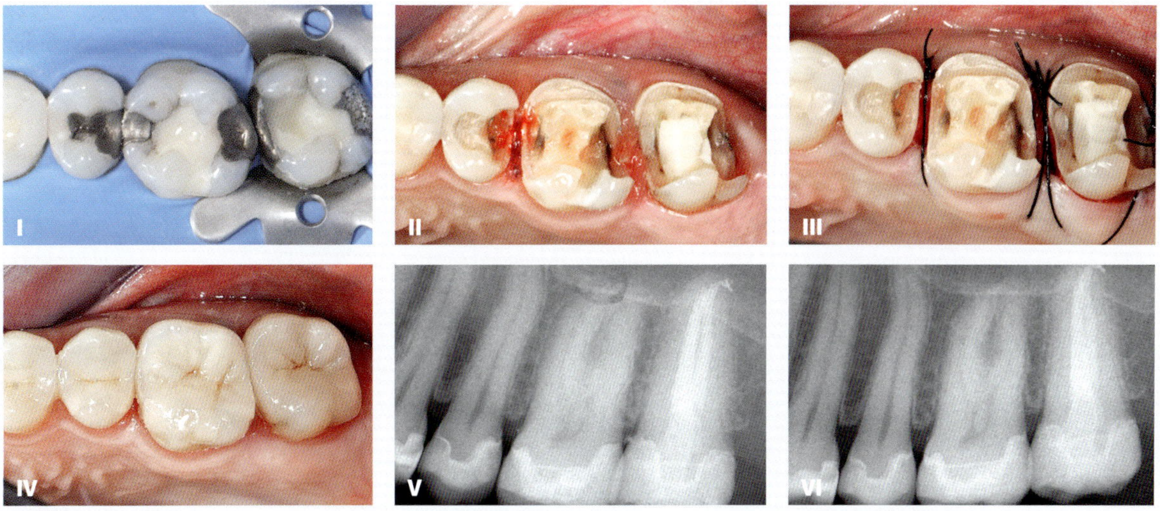

Fig 4 Inflammatory tissue corresponding to the interproximal spaces. The margins are not easily visible, and bleeding arises spontaneously or as a result of clinical procedures *(I, II)*. Surgical flap design is dependent on the relationship between dental lesions/preparations and periodontal structures. The purpose of periodontal surgery is to expose the preparation margins while complying with a positive periodontal architecture *(III, IV)*. Posttreatment radiographs, before and after removal of excess composite used as cement *(V, VI)*.

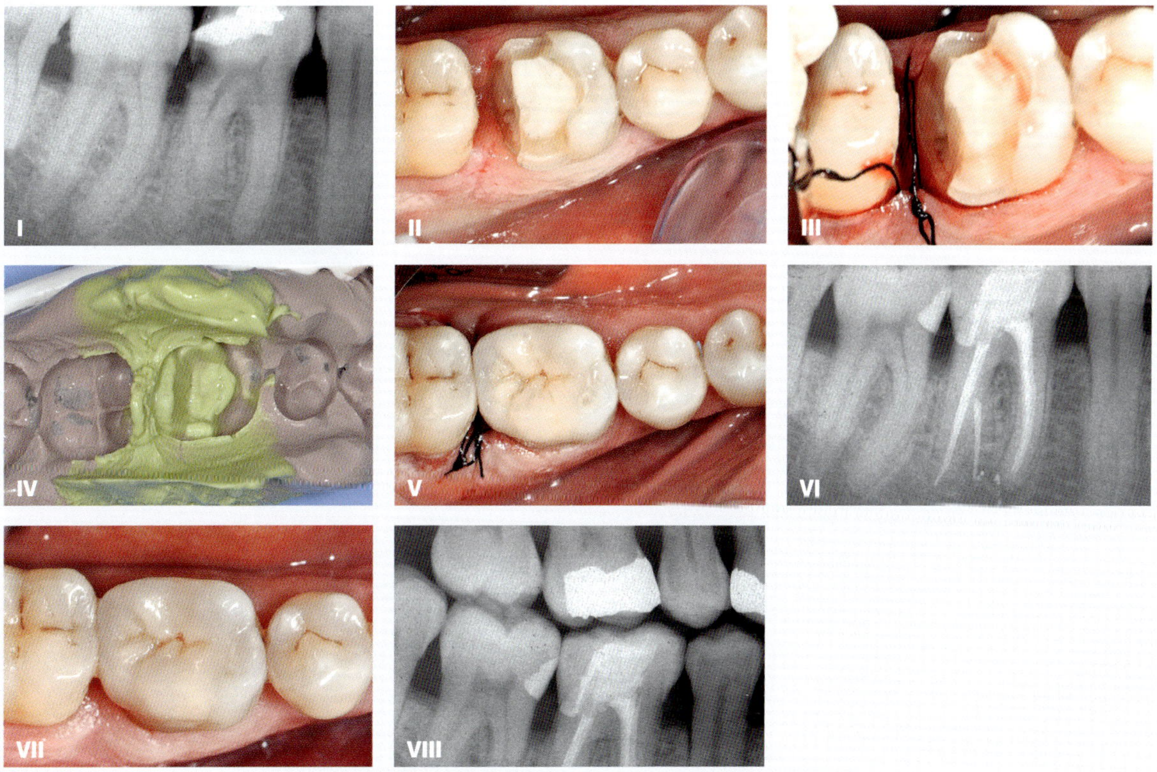

Fig 5 A deep caries lesion of the root of a multi-rooted tooth must be evaluated in relation to the root trunk and the furcations *(I, II)*. Exposure of preparation margins and protection of the furcations *(III–V)*. Appropriate control of restoration margins while ensuring periodontal biologic width *(VI)*. Clinical and follow-up radiographs after 4 months *(VII, VIII)*.

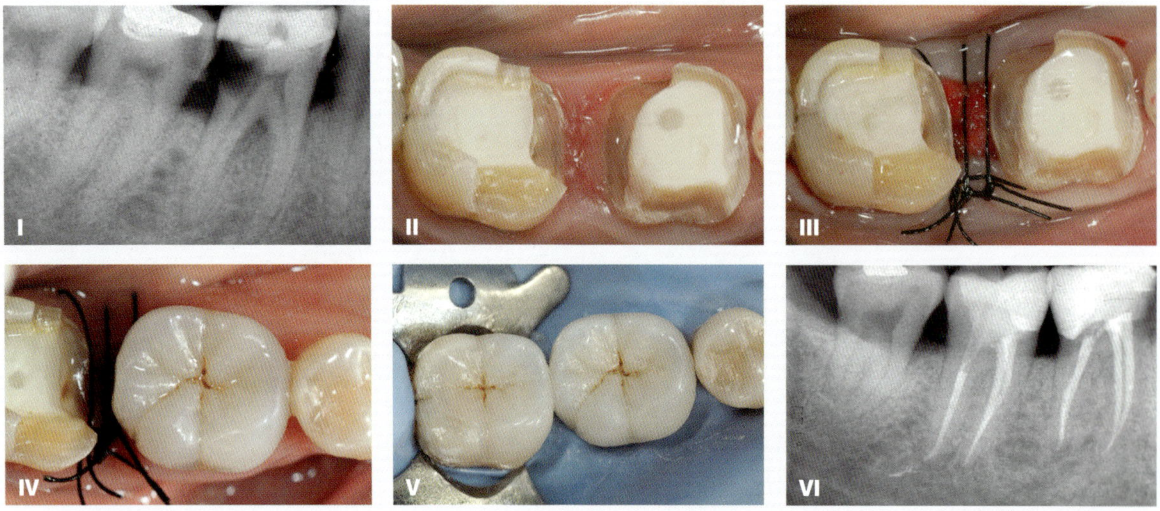

Fig 6 Concomitant caries lesion and periodontal damage affecting the mandibular right first and second molars *(I)*. Interference between inflammatory tissue and border of caries lesions *(II)*. Restoration of accurate tooth-periodontal ratios, an indispensable requirement in order for proper restorative maneuvers to be performed *(III–V)*. Follow-up radiograph after 6 years *(VI)*.

The operating protocols naturally must be strictly applied and take into account the individual characteristics of the case. This means that the protocols must be adapted to the case and appropriately tailored. According to Heraclitus, "Change is the only constant in life."

Multidisciplinary treatment must be based on and guided by a specific diagnosis.

The collection of all data in order to interpret the case in a specific manner must be very thorough and rigorous and will be confirmed and supported by the practitioner's fundamental knowledge of dental medicine. According to Kramer,[1] we can cure only what we see, and we see only what we know.

The results of instrumental tests must be combined with an objective examination of the case. Periapical and bitewing radiographic examination, periodontal probing, complete removal of decayed dental tissue, and, if necessary, a pulp vitality test, periodontal probing, and casts fitted on an articulator allow the clinician to accurately establish the dental and periodontal situation in each individual case (Fig 7).

Only after having established an accurate diagnosis is it possible to begin to formulate a correct treatment plan that, as already stated, must be multidisciplinary in nature (Fig 8).

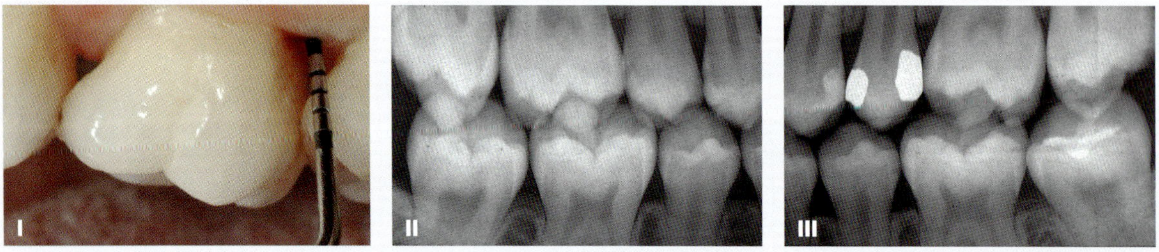

Fig 7 Periodontal probing and radiographic examination are the basic instrumental investigatory methods underlying diagnosis in periodontology. Their correlation is of utmost significance.

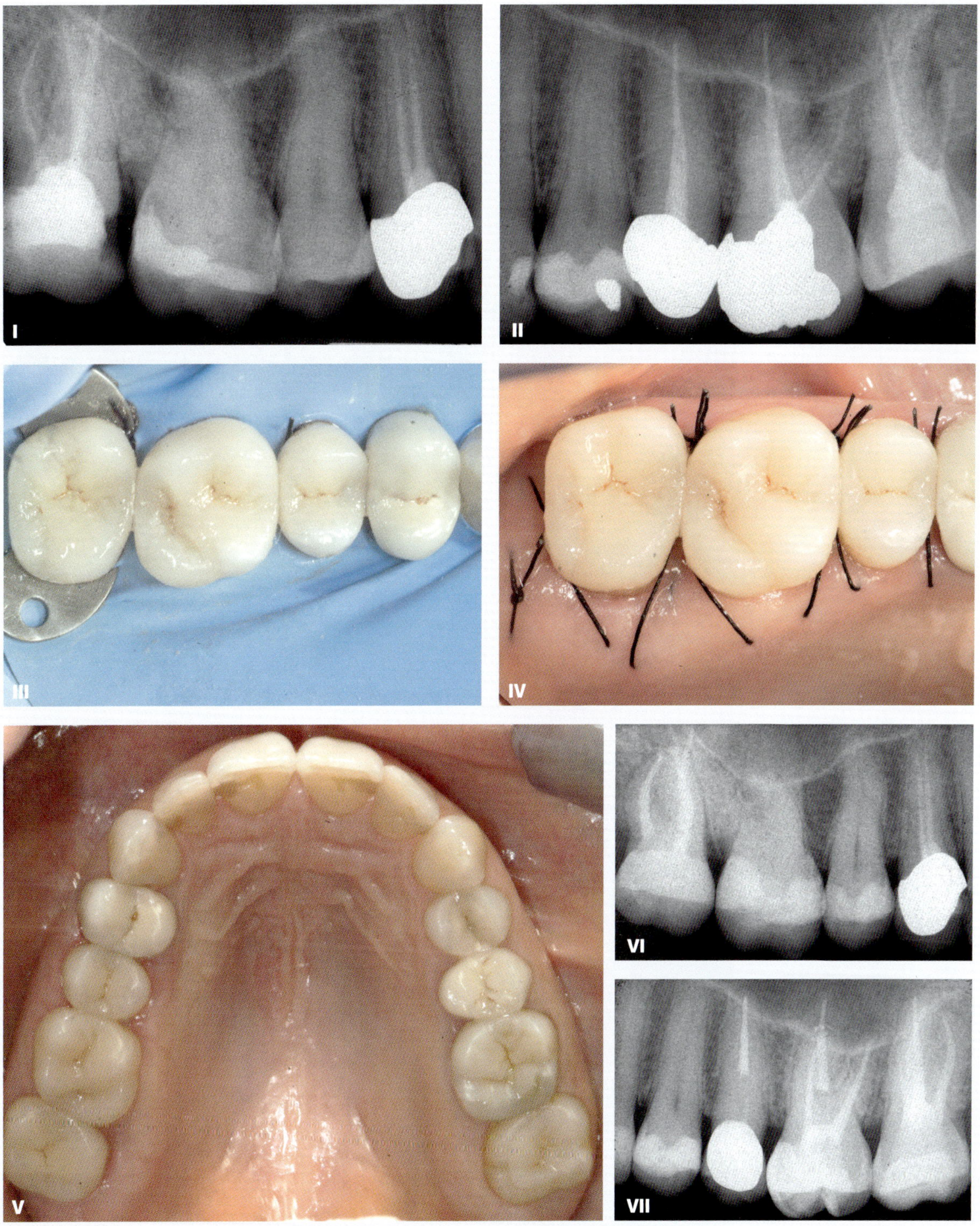

Fig 8 Clinical example of an arch restored in an interdisciplinary manner.

The focal point of treatment is the interface between the restoration and the periodontal structure, and biologic parameters must guide the accurate definition of the therapeutic procedure to be followed (Fig 9). In periodontology, Dr Harald Löe demonstrated the relationship between a buildup of plaque and the onset of a gingival inflammatory process.[2]

Fig 9 Restoration of two arches using adhesive techniques. Preoperative view of arches and radiographic status *(I–III)*.

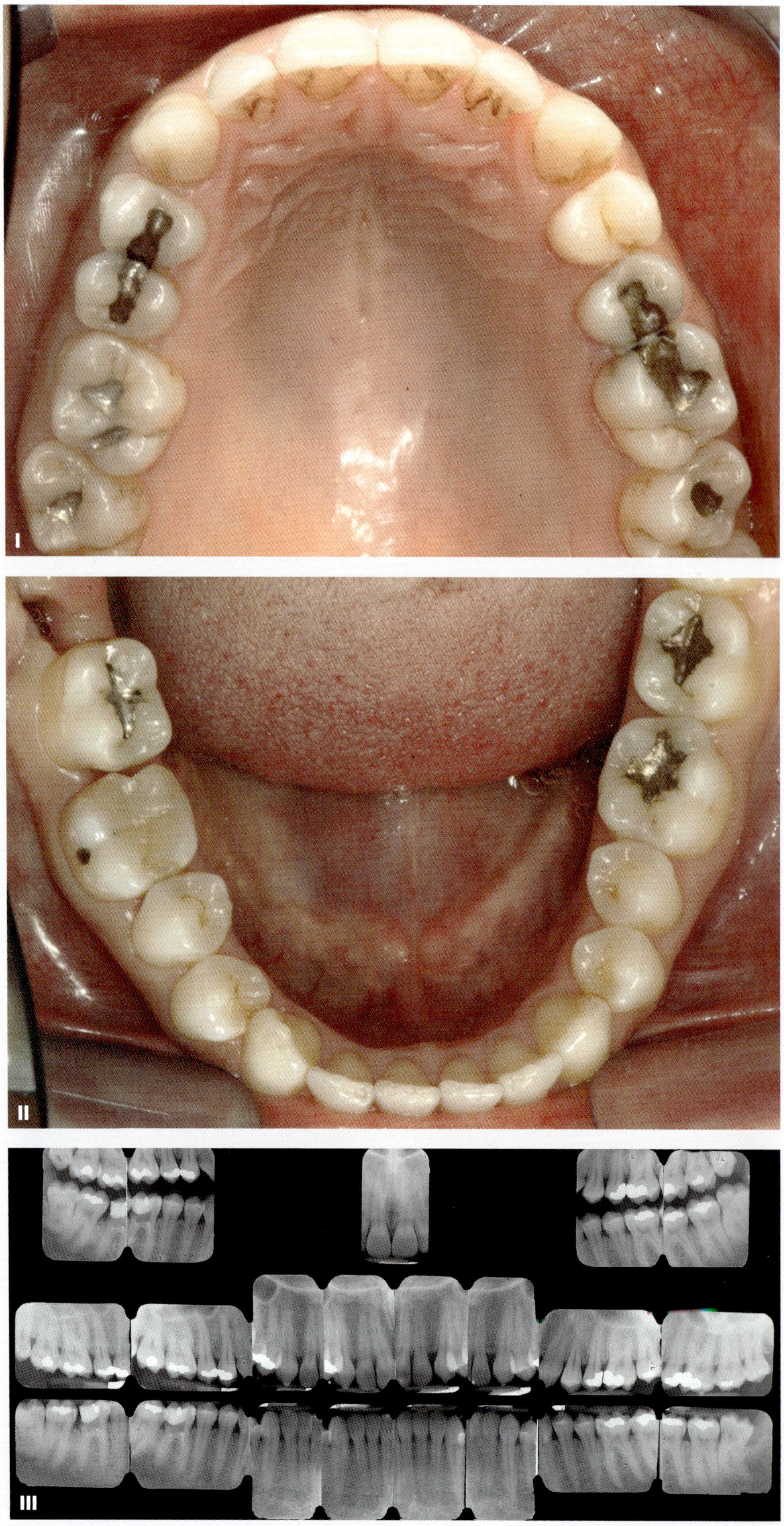

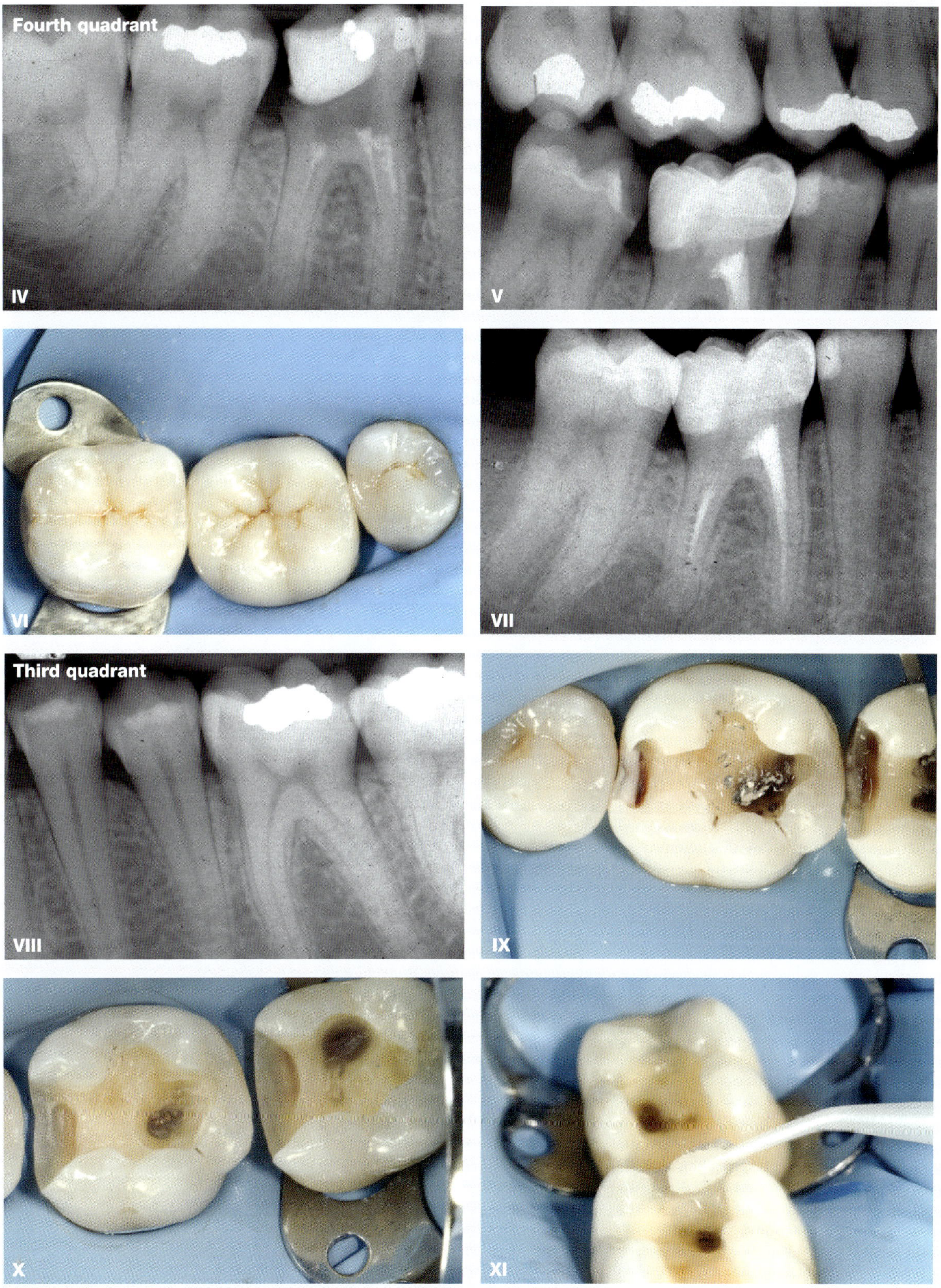

Fig 9 *(continued)* Intraoperative stages involving the mandibular right (fourth) quadrant *(IV–VII)* and left (third) quadrant *(VIII–XX)*.

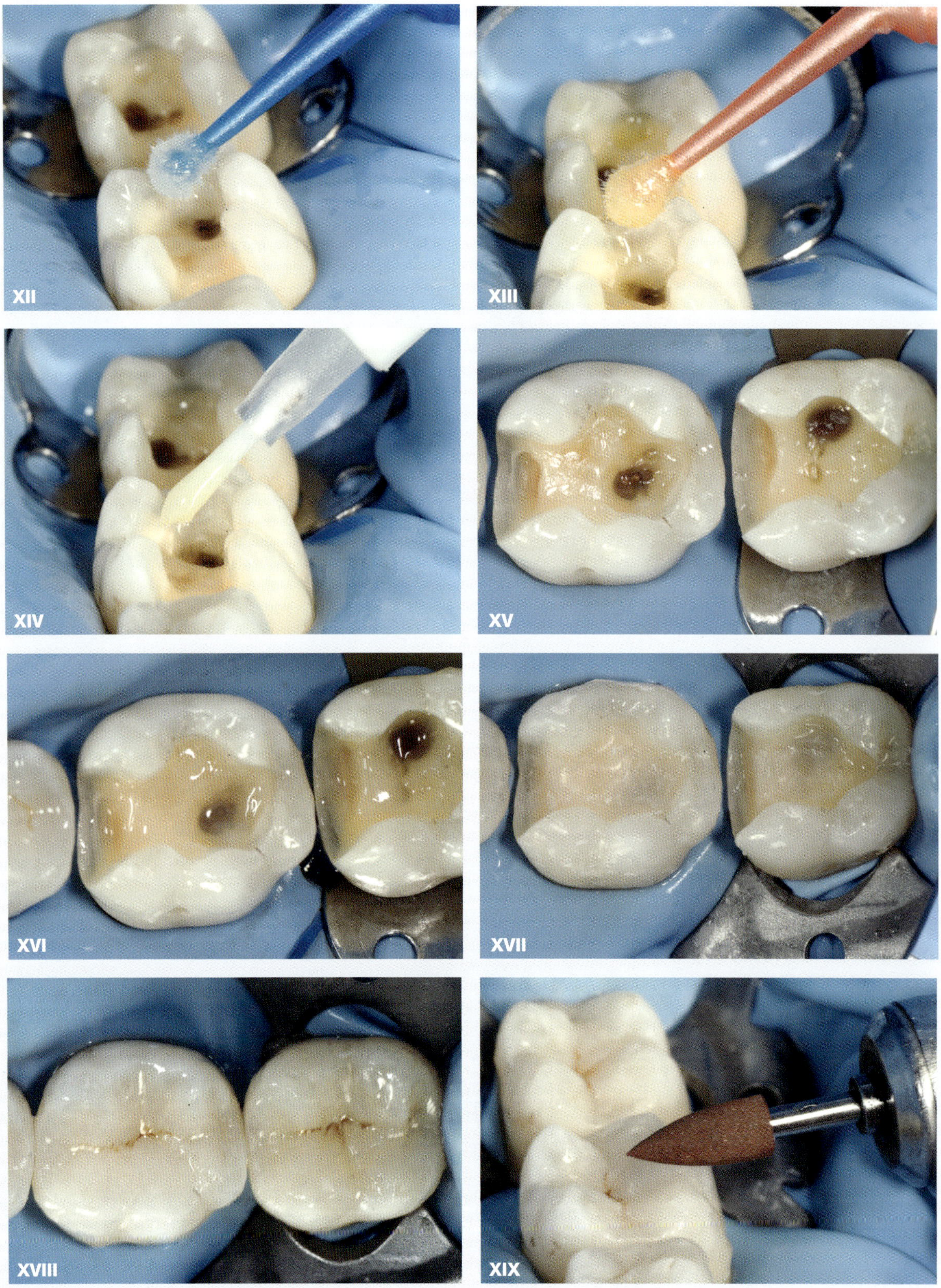

Fig 9 *(continued)*

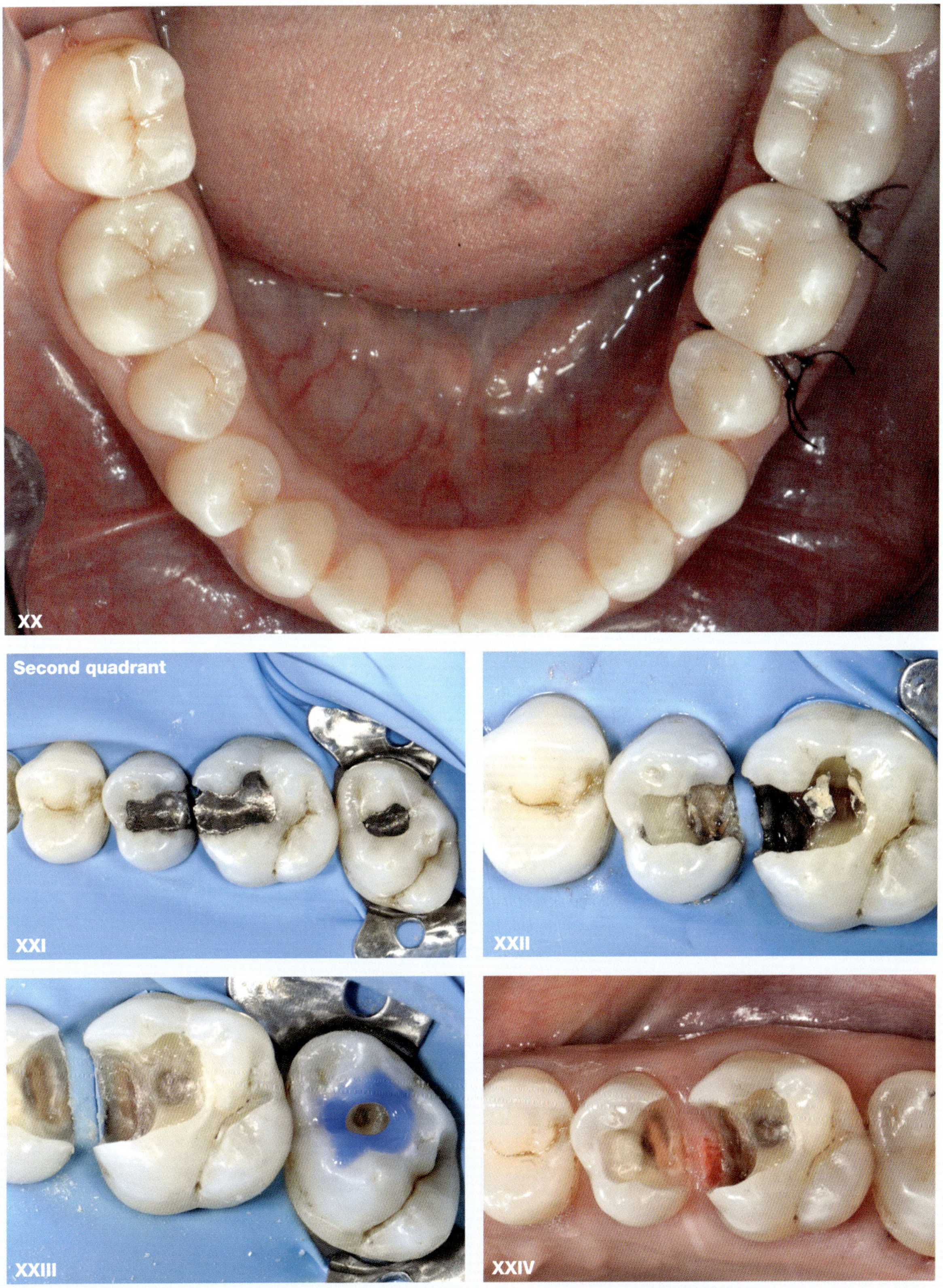

Fig 9 *(continued)* In the second quadrant, after removal of the old restorations and caries lesions, probing is carried out around the entire perimeter of each tooth to establish the relationship between the tooth and periodontium, and radiographs are taken of the region. These findings constitute the premise for a proper surgical treatment plan. When both instrumental examinations are correlated, it is possible to gain an impression of the relationships between the deep periodontium and the tooth *(XXI–XXIX)*.

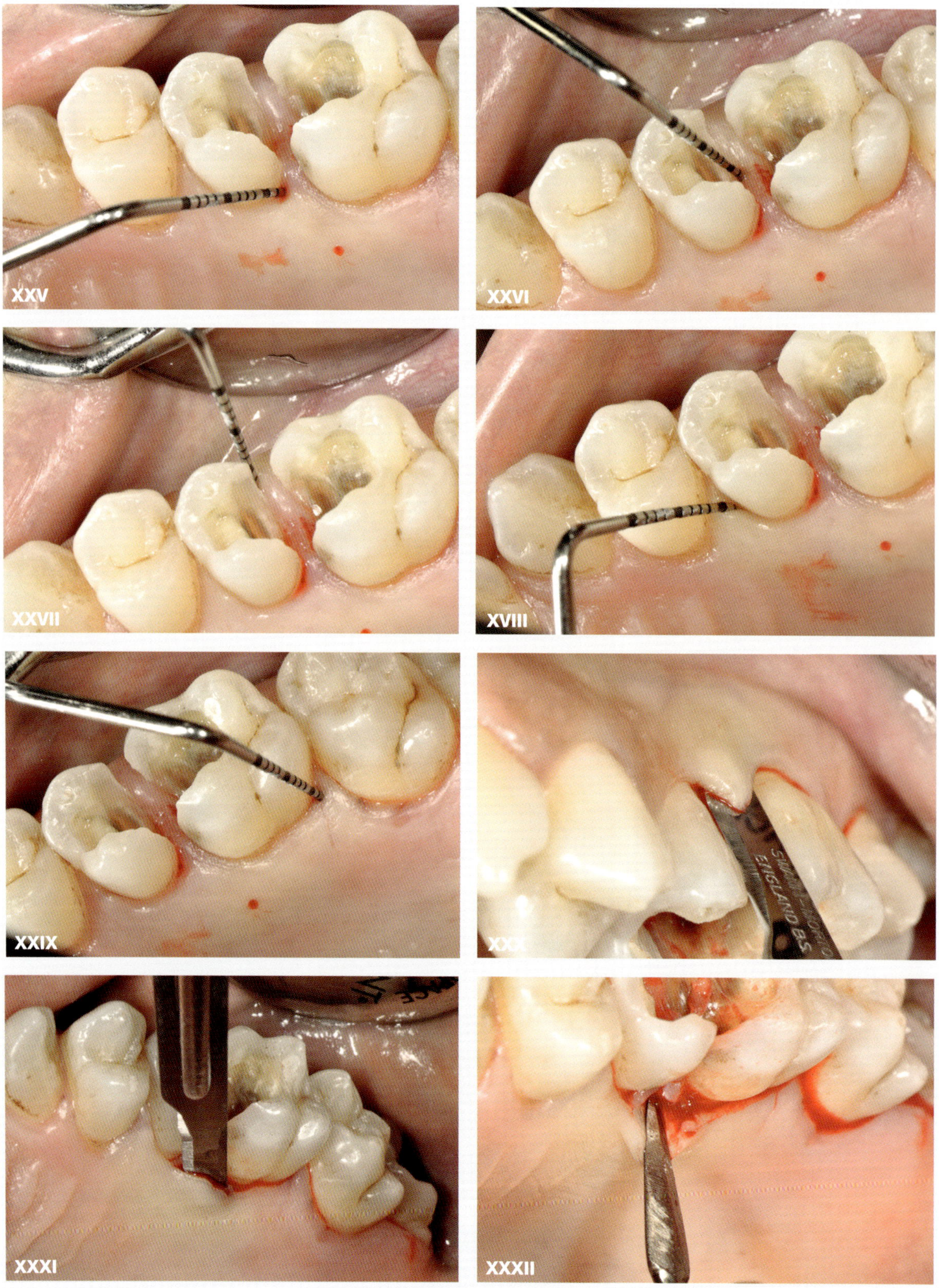

Fig 9 *(continued)* The thickness of the flap must be uniform, and its design must be appropriate *(XXX, XXXI)*. The incision of interproximal soft tissues takes into account the biologic width *(XXXII, XXXIII)*.

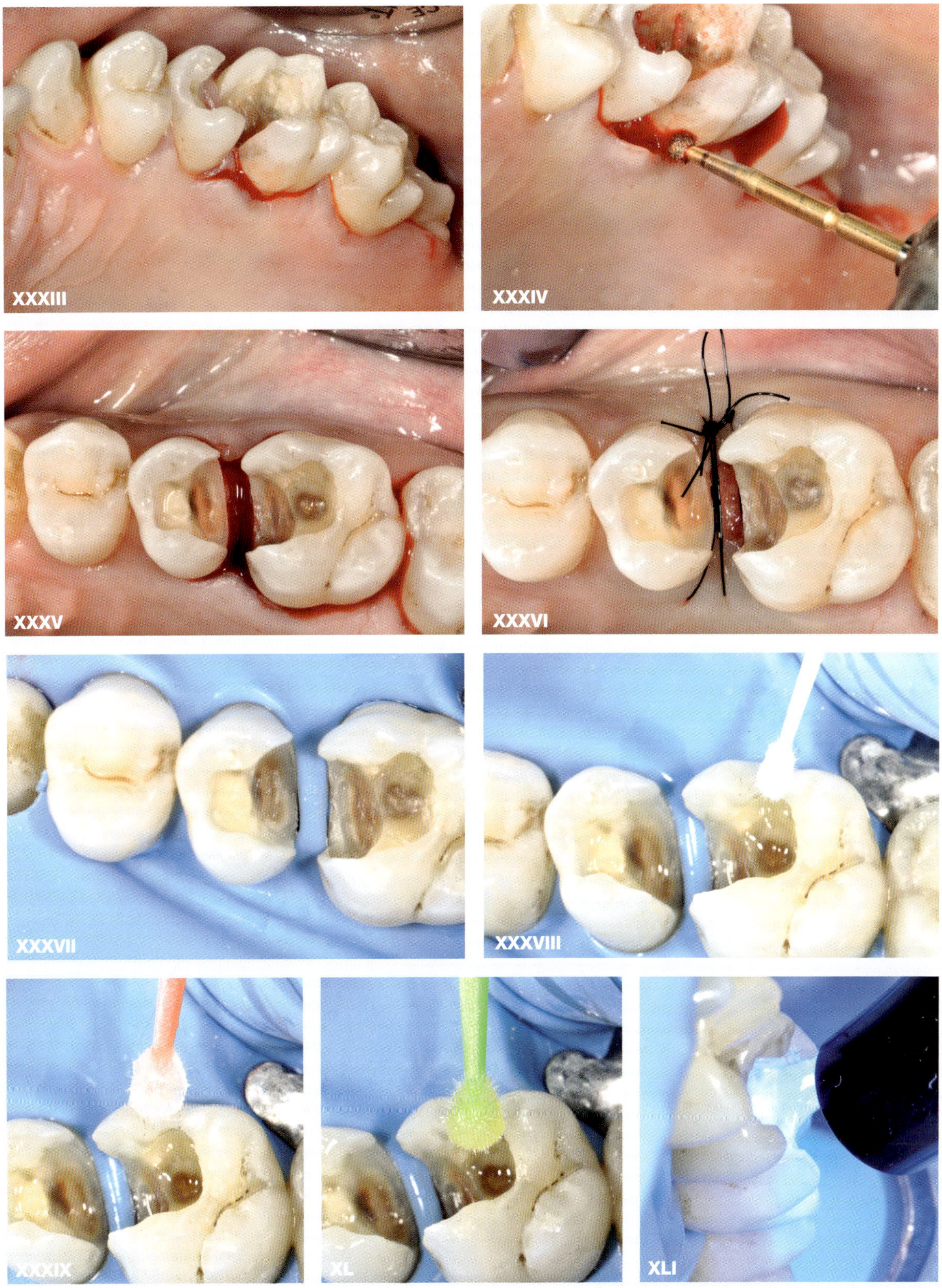

Fig 9 *(continued)* Osteoplasty procedures determine the morphology that the soft tissues will acquire when healed *(XXXIV–XXXVI)*. Stages of adhesion and cementation and view of arch *(XXXVII–XLVI)*.

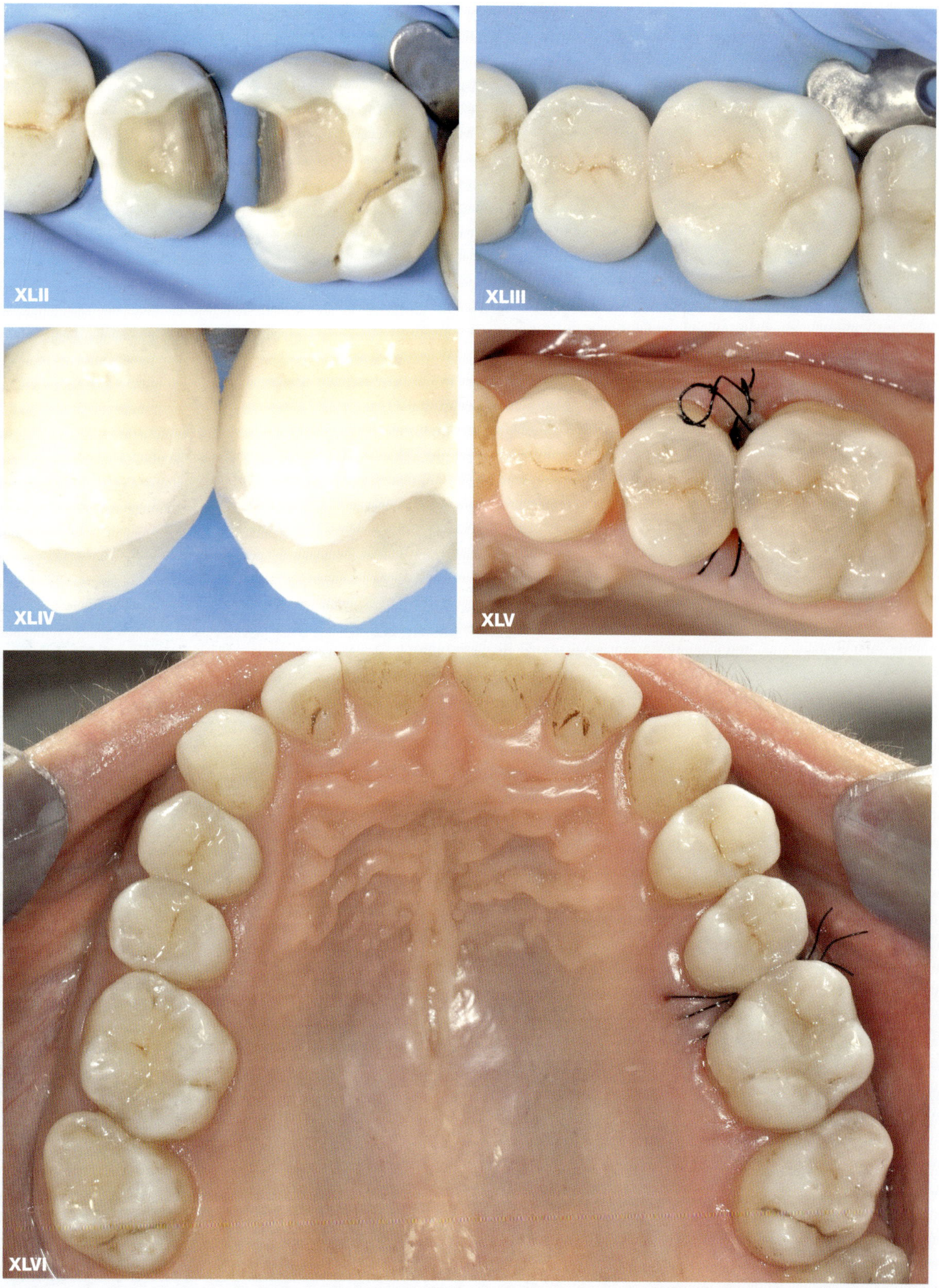

Fig 9 *(continued)*

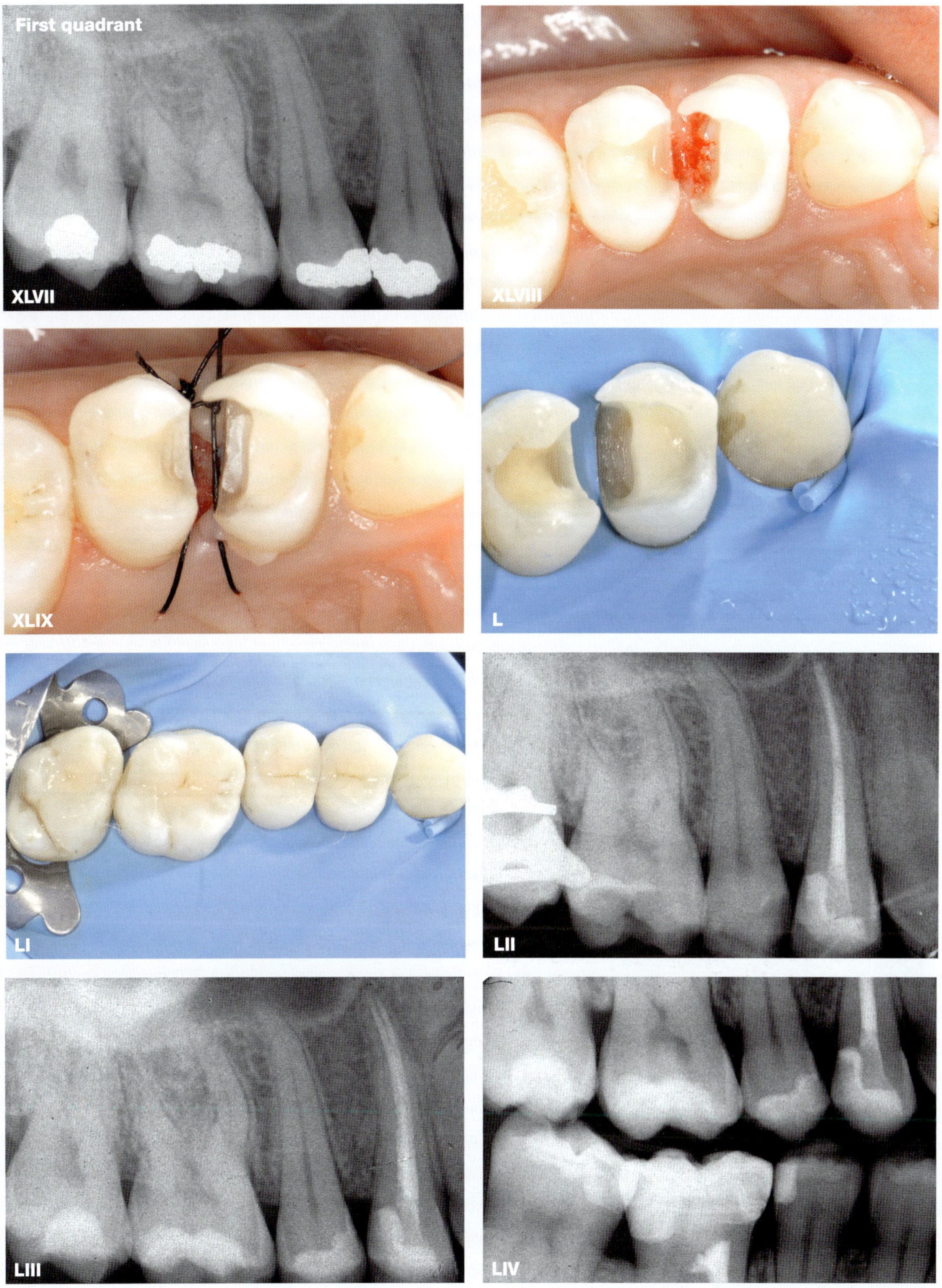

Fig 9 *(continued)* Intraoperative stages in the first quadrant *(XLVII–LI)*. Intraoperative radiographs to check the marginal seal *(LII–LIV)*.

Fig 9 *(continued)* Clinical and radiographic views of the arches at the end of treatment *(LV–LVIII)*.

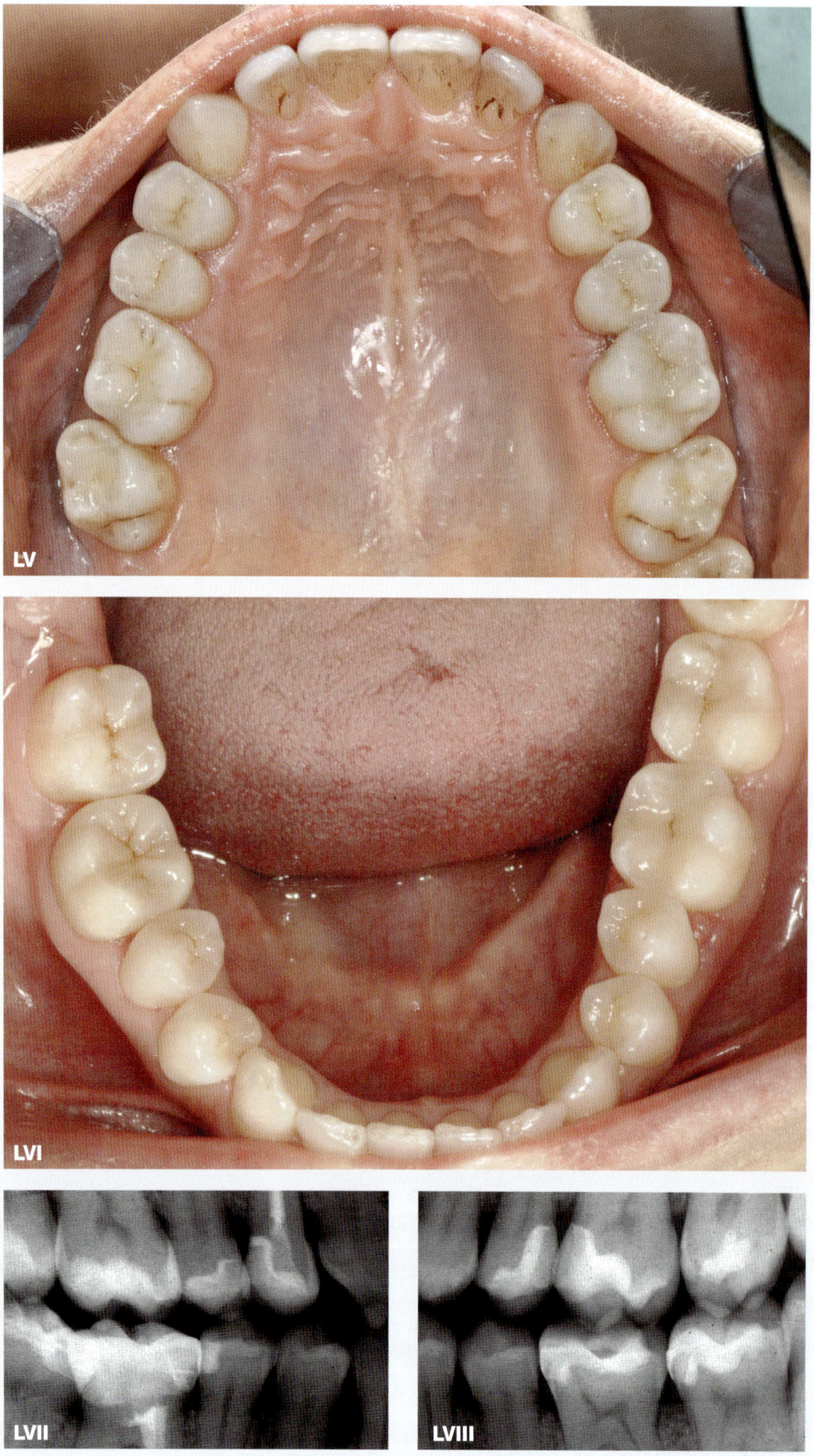

The susceptibility of the patient and the type of biofilm, as well as the amount of accumulated plaque and particularly the nature and virulence of its component microorganisms, lie at the basis of the gingival and periodontal inflammatory process.
Therefore the first biologic requirement is to achieve an ideal restoration that prevents plaque buildup and allows its removal (Figs 10 to 19).

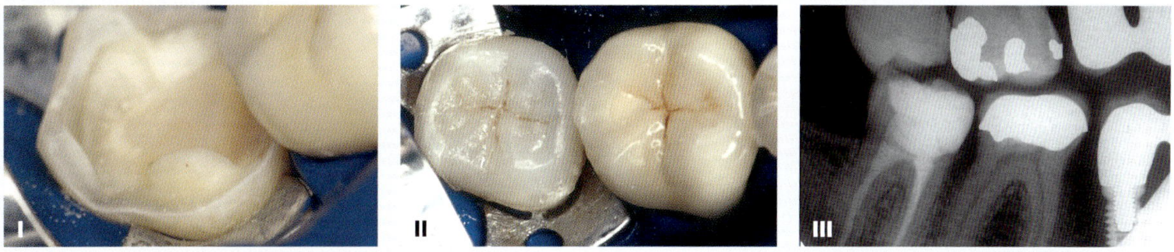

Fig 10 A supragingival margin allows ideal control of gingival tissue inflammation.

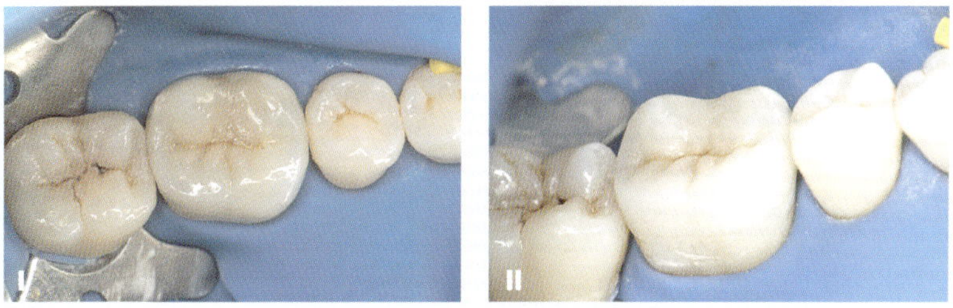

Fig 11 Accurate contact surfaces, ideal emergence profiles, and a supragingival margin are crucial to superficial and deep periodontal tissue health.

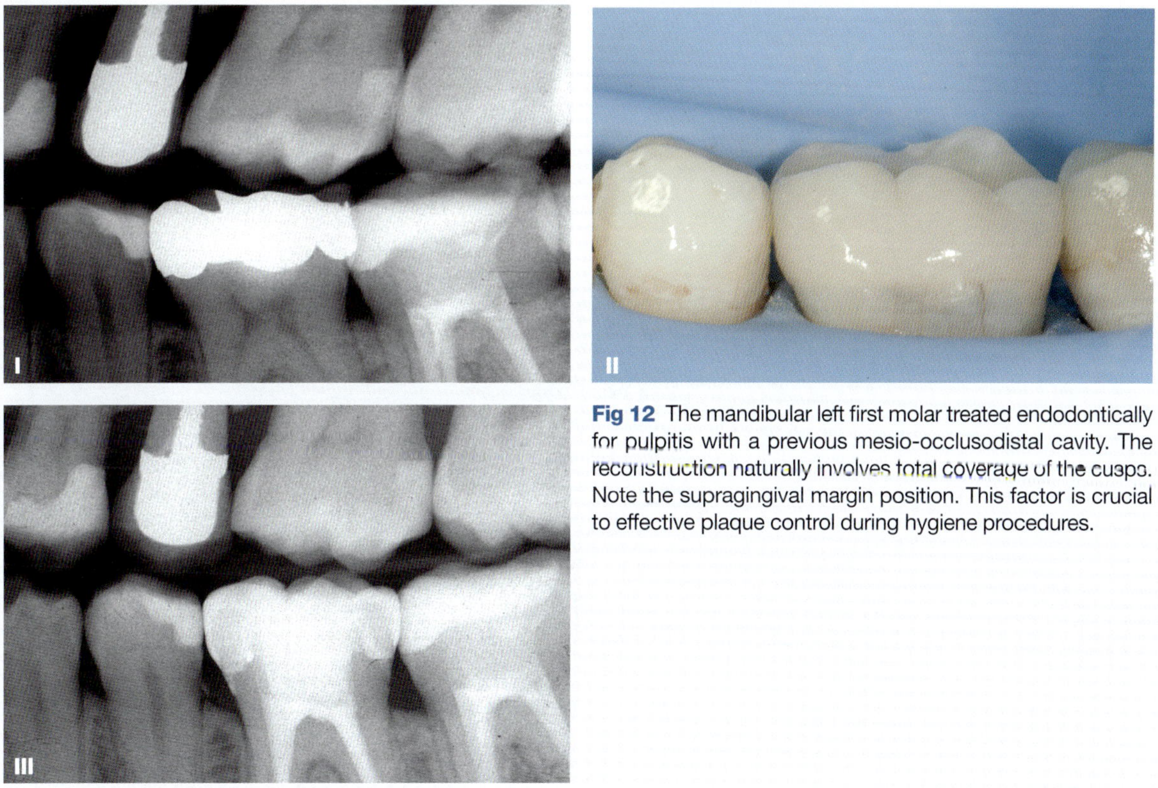

Fig 12 The mandibular left first molar treated endodontically for pulpitis with a previous mesio-occlusodistal cavity. The reconstruction naturally involves total coverage of the cusps. Note the supragingival margin position. This factor is crucial to effective plaque control during hygiene procedures.

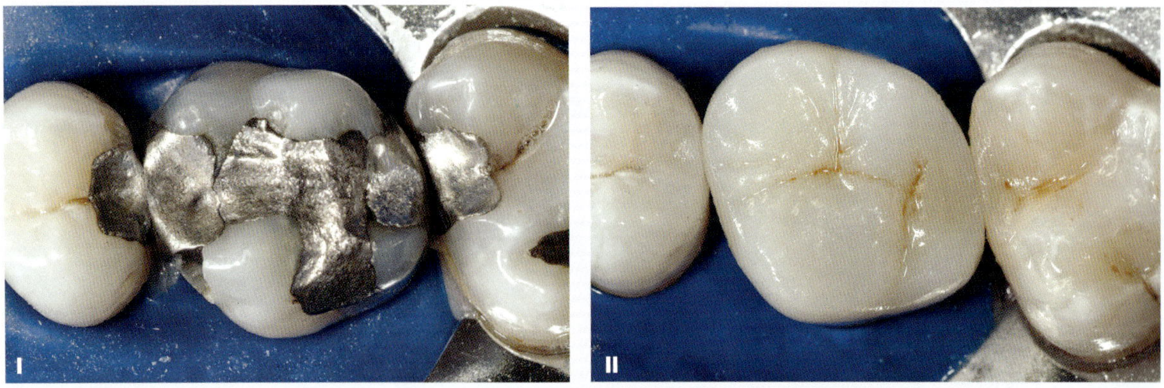

Fig 13 Maxillary left first molar with defective mesio-occlusodistal restoration and mesial wall fracture *(I)* restored with an overlay. Direct restorations in proximal teeth and view of interproximal contact surfaces *(II)*.

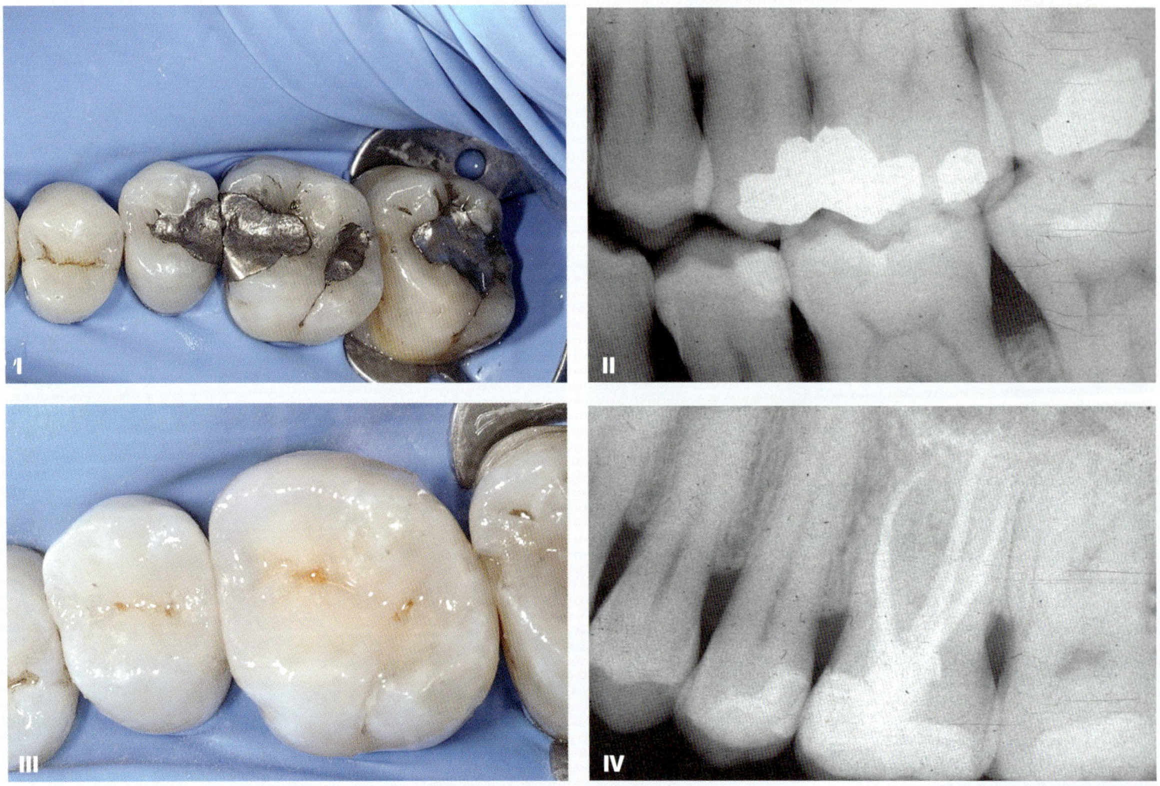

Fig 14 Maxillary left quadrant with leaking amalgam restorations *(I, II)*. After endodontic treatment of the first molar for penetrating decay, the teeth were reconstructed using direct (second molar) and indirect (second premolar and first molar) techniques *(III)*. The radiograph taken at the end of treatment reveals accurate emergence profiles and marginal seals *(IV)*.

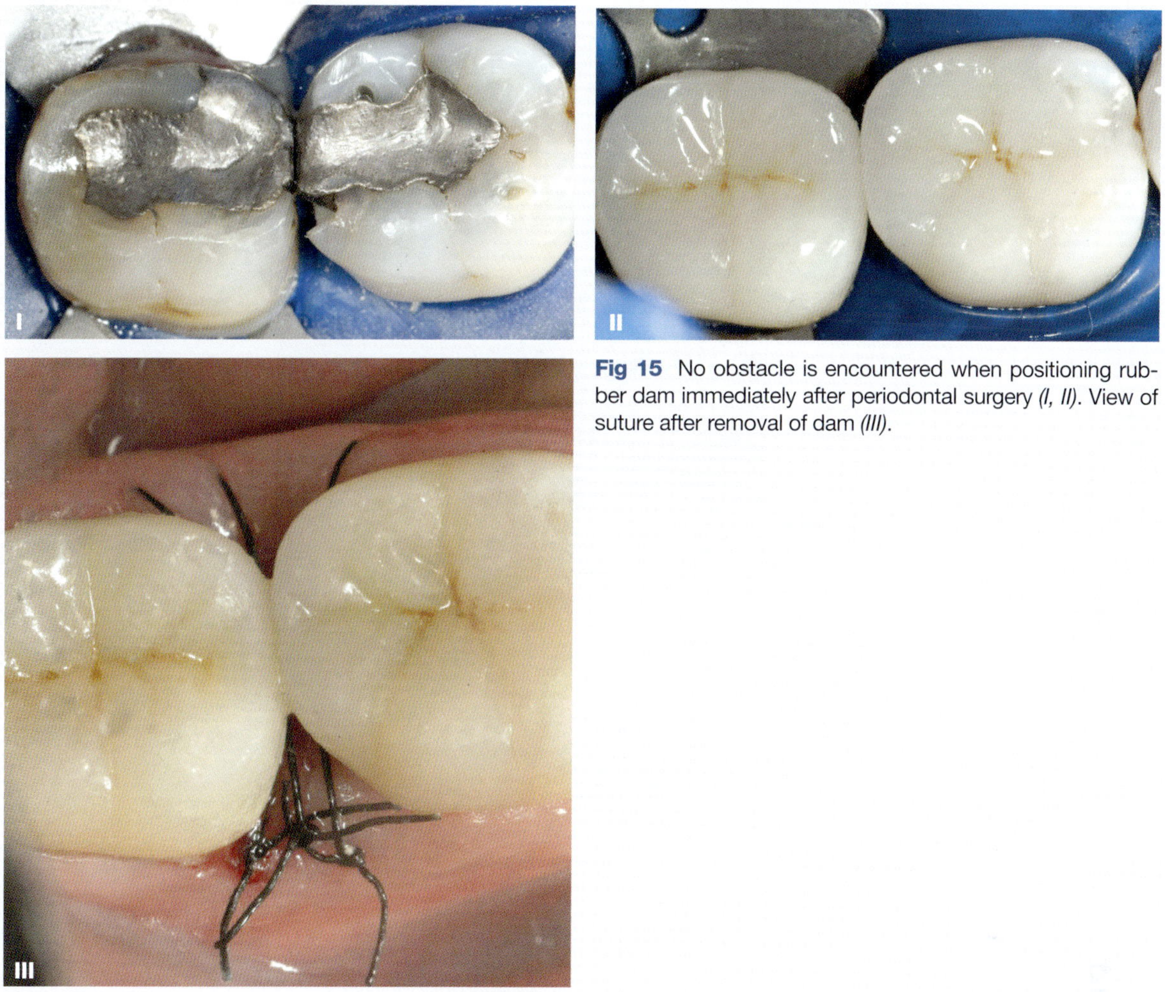

Fig 15 No obstacle is encountered when positioning rubber dam immediately after periodontal surgery *(I, II)*. View of suture after removal of dam *(III)*.

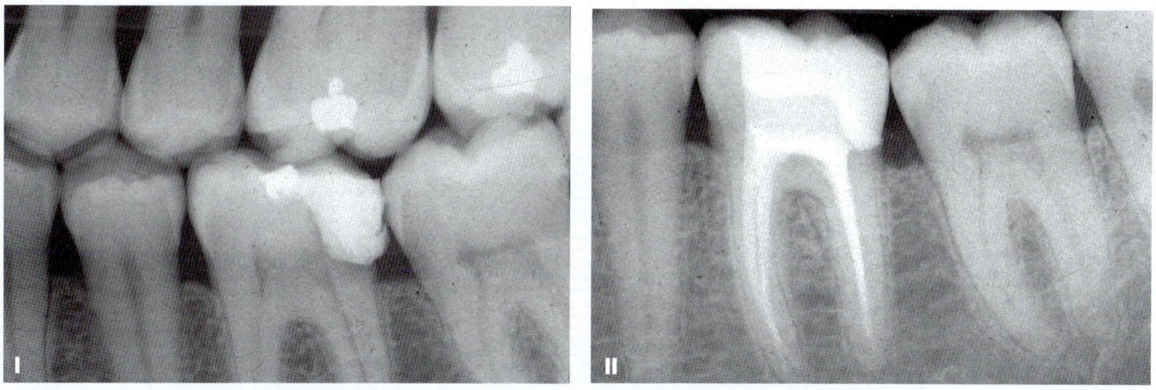

Fig 16 An entirely defective tooth-restoration seal causes bacterial infiltration into the pulp tissue with consequent pulpitis and endodontic treatment as well as invasion of the biologic space by the material *(I)*. Radiographic view of the cemented adhesive restoration with perfect marginal seal and restoration of an accurate emergence profile *(II)*.

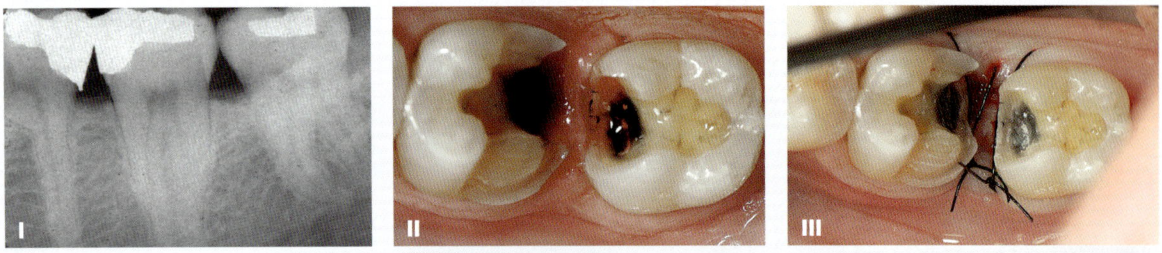

Fig 17 The lesions in the mandibular molars tend to be orientated in a lingual direction.

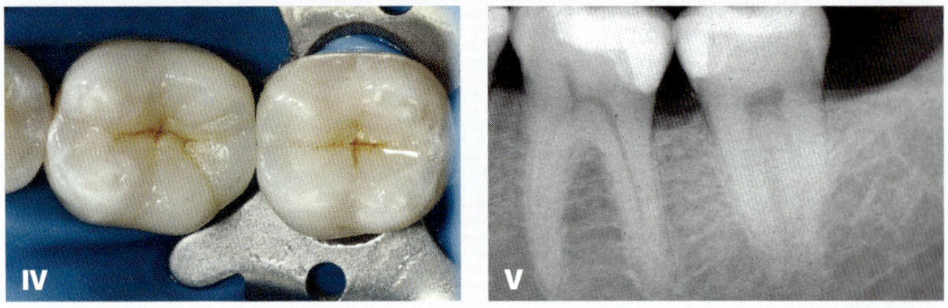

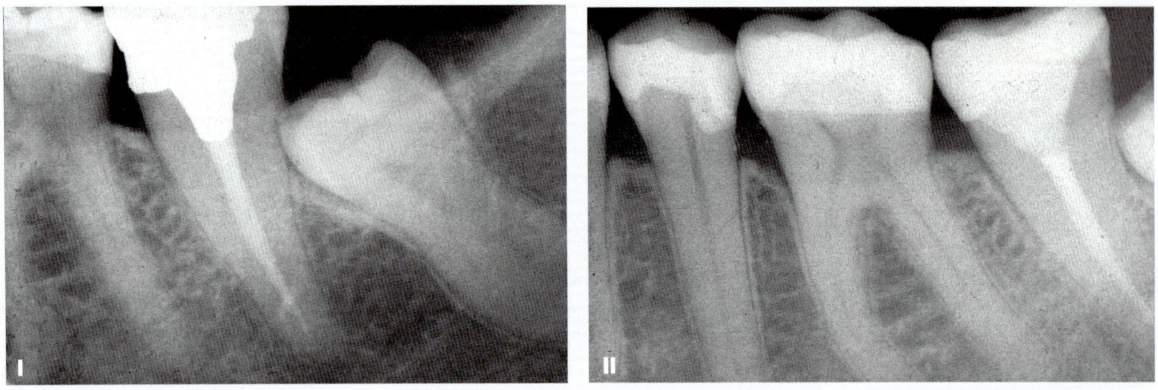

Fig 18 Restoration of an accurate emergence profile for the mandibular left second molar by replacing a defective amalgam restoration with a composite inlay.

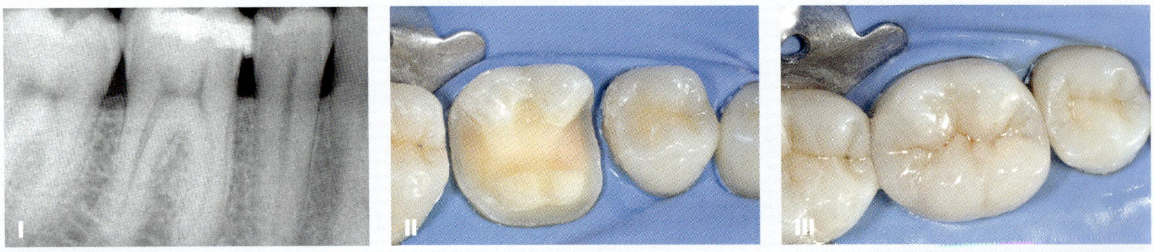

Fig 19 Preparation and before/after radiographs of a marginal seal where the previous periodontal conditions led to constant tissue inflammation.

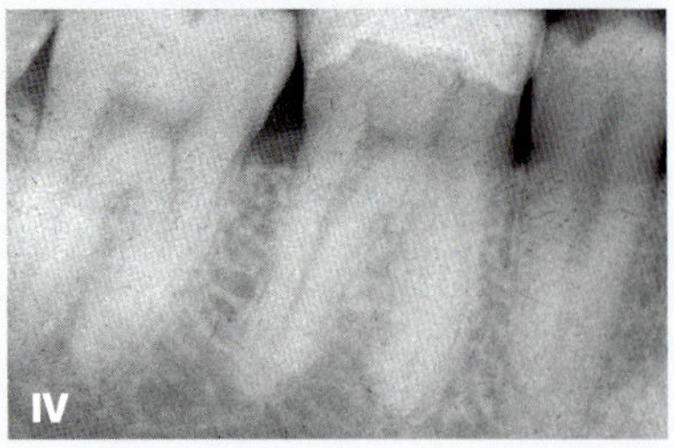

The various dental restoration materials have been extensively studied, and it is known that factors contributing to plaque formation and buildup include the nature of the material as well as its surface irregularity, porosity, and roughness.

The second biologic requirement to be met by a restoration is the accuracy and integrity of the margin (Figs 20 to 30).

Oral microorganisms measure between 1 and 5 μm, while the size of a restoration margin opening is between 50 and 100 μm; these figures indicate how easy it is for a microbial colony to develop, and this constitutes another risk factor in patients susceptible to severe loss of periodontal attachment.

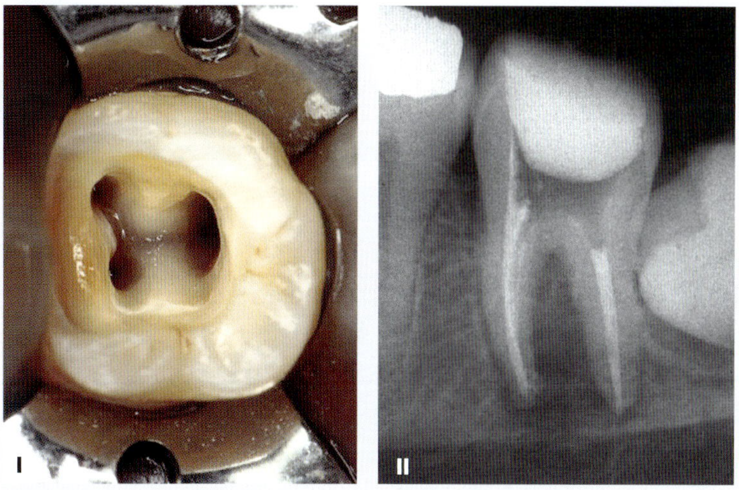

Fig 20 The importance of a proper view of the operative field naturally applies to all disciplines.

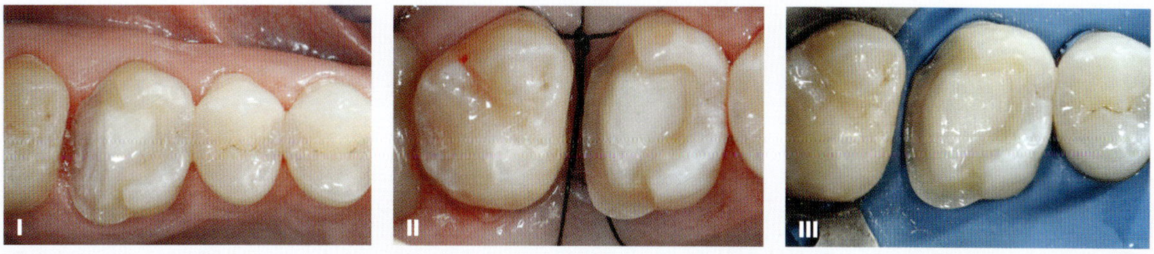

Fig 21 Illustration of the concept of periodontal surgery allowing placement of rubber dam. Extensive and deep caries lesion of the interdental space between two maxillary molars in a young patient *(I)*. The situation has high risk due to the presence of underlying furcations and the invasion of soft tissues into the caries lesion. After periodontal surgery, the preparation margins return to view and allow reconstruction procedures to be easily performed *(II, III)*.

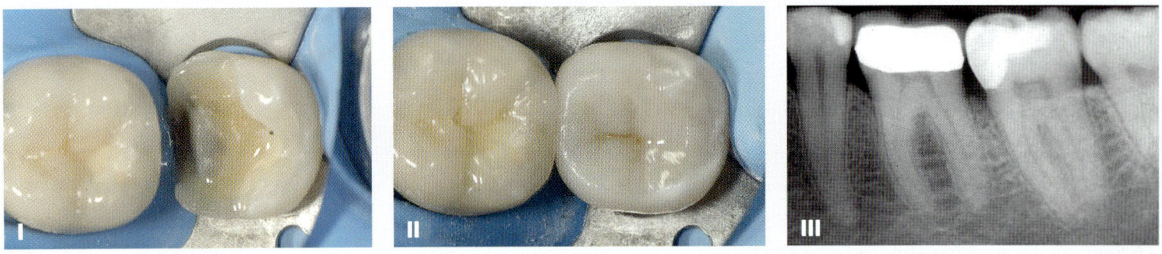

Fig 22 Operational difficulties in obtaining an effective seal of the tooth-restoration margin.

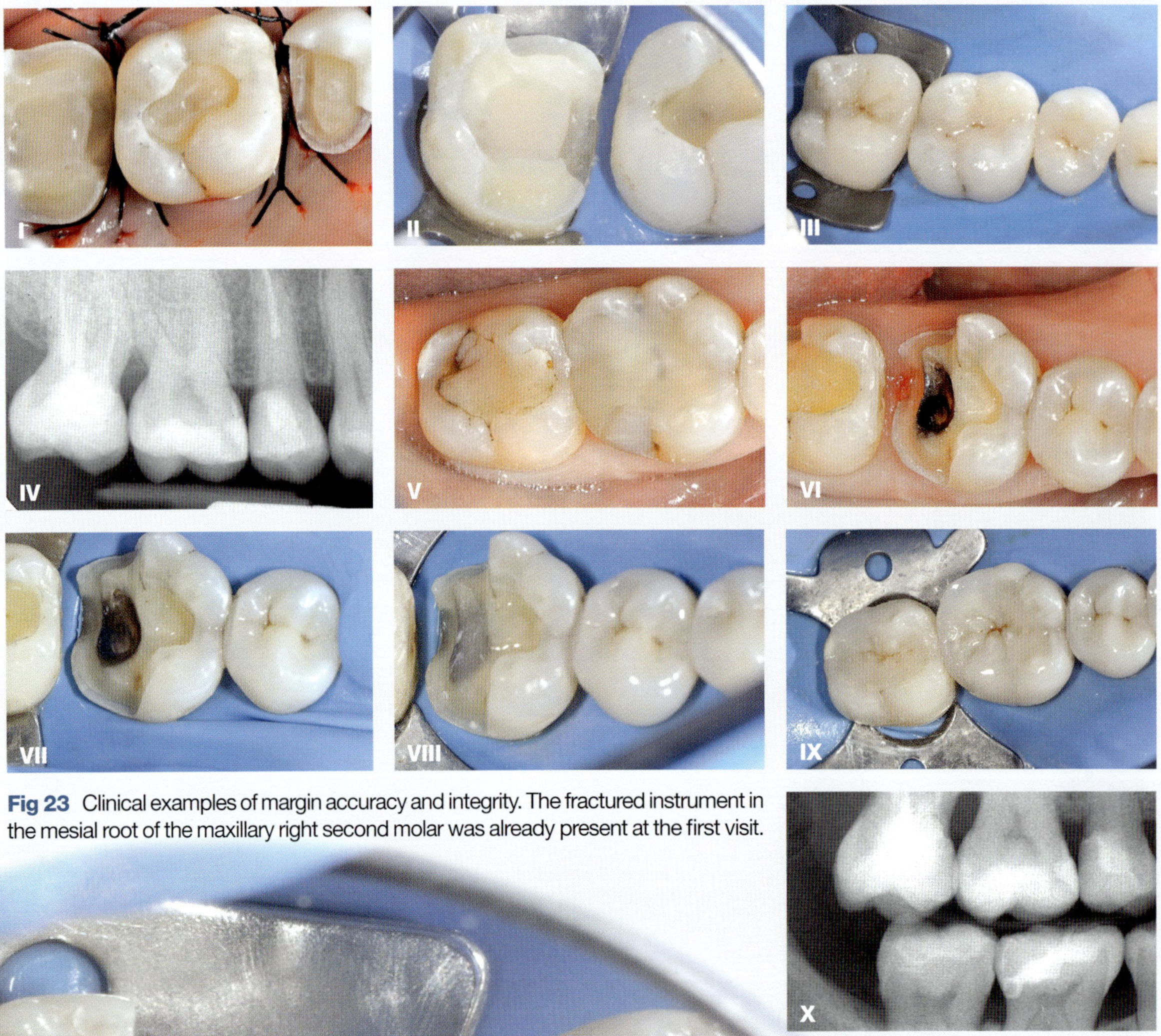

Fig 23 Clinical examples of margin accuracy and integrity. The fractured instrument in the mesial root of the maxillary right second molar was already present at the first visit.

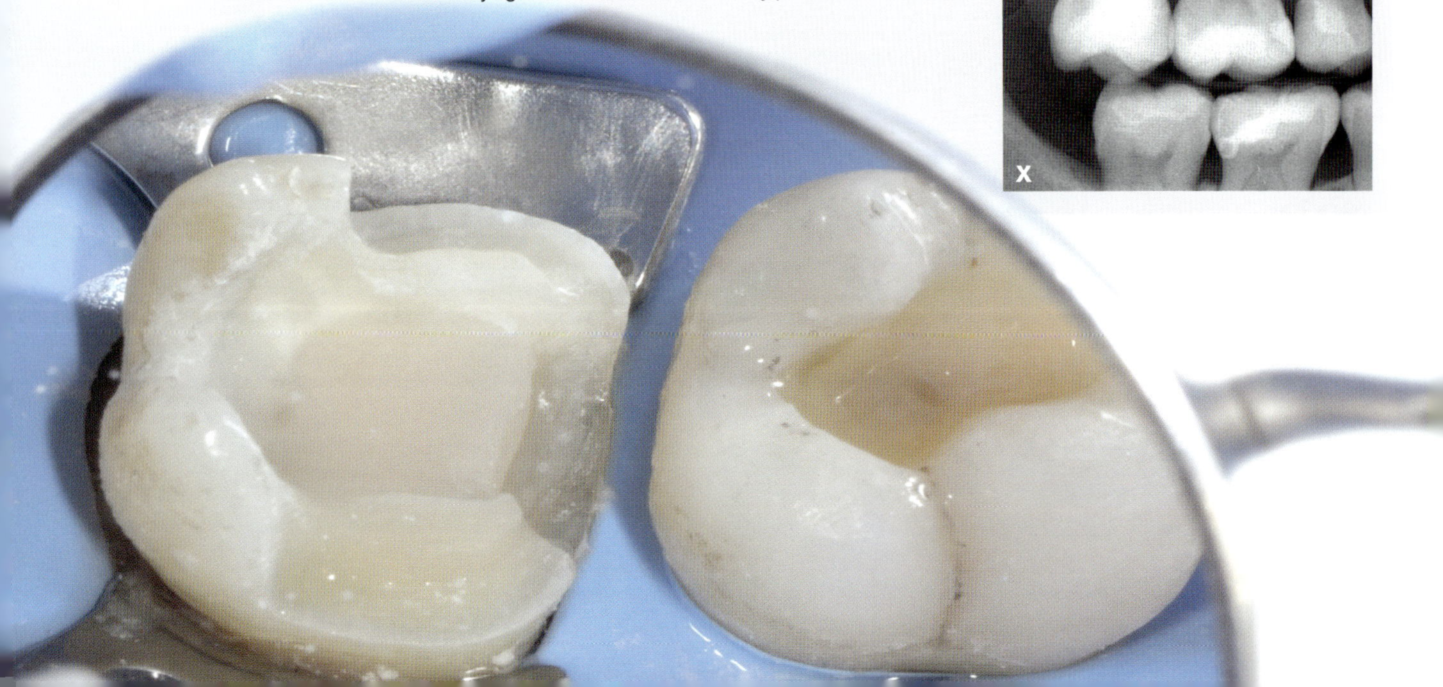

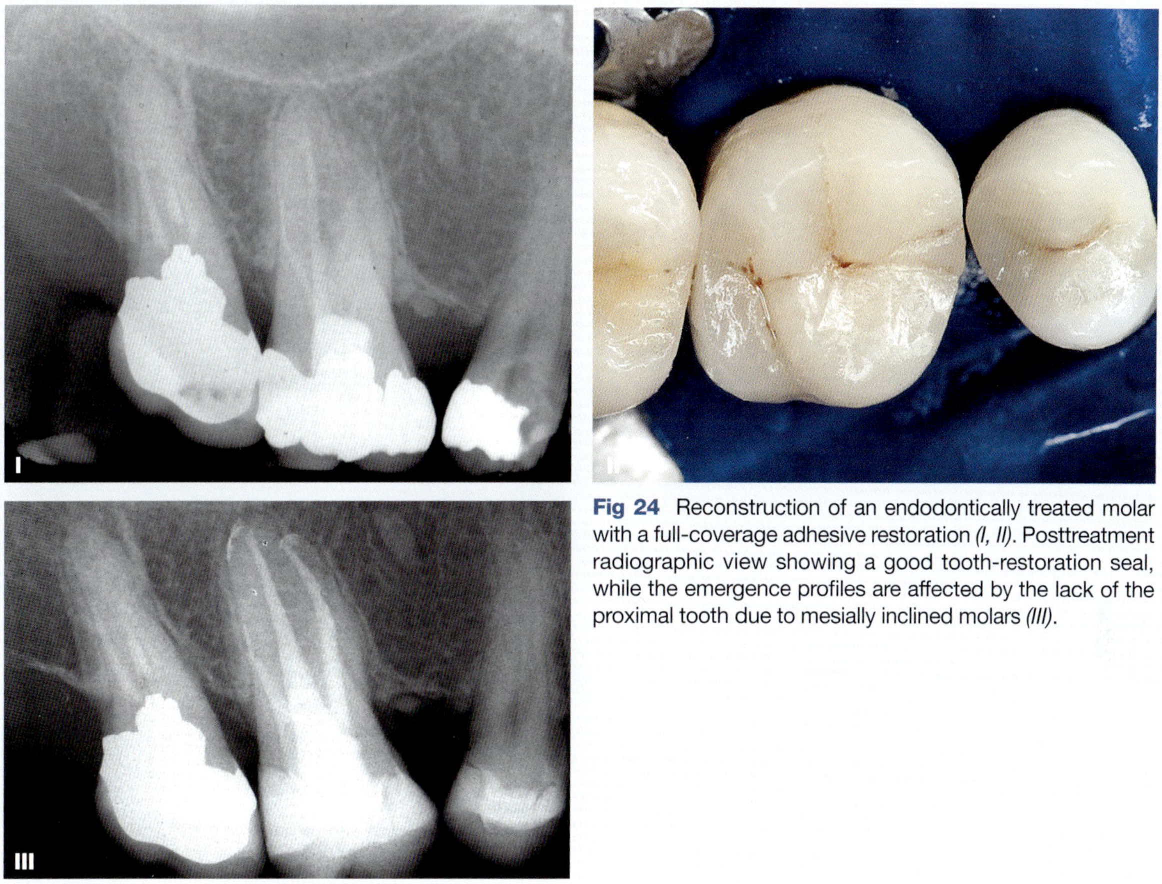

Fig 24 Reconstruction of an endodontically treated molar with a full-coverage adhesive restoration *(I, II)*. Posttreatment radiographic view showing a good tooth-restoration seal, while the emergence profiles are affected by the lack of the proximal tooth due to mesially inclined molars *(III)*.

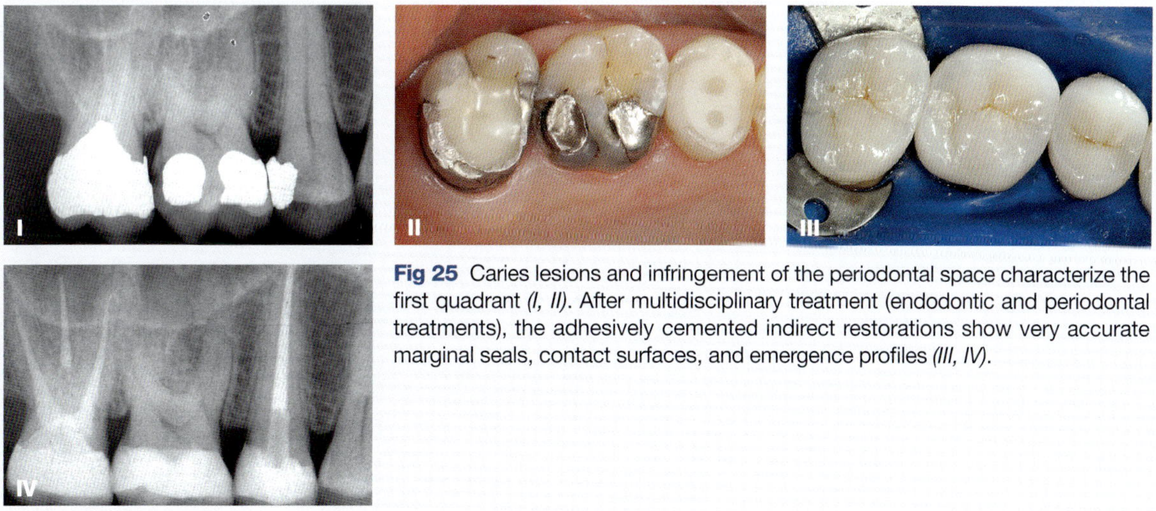

Fig 25 Caries lesions and infringement of the periodontal space characterize the first quadrant *(I, II)*. After multidisciplinary treatment (endodontic and periodontal treatments), the adhesively cemented indirect restorations show very accurate marginal seals, contact surfaces, and emergence profiles *(III, IV)*.

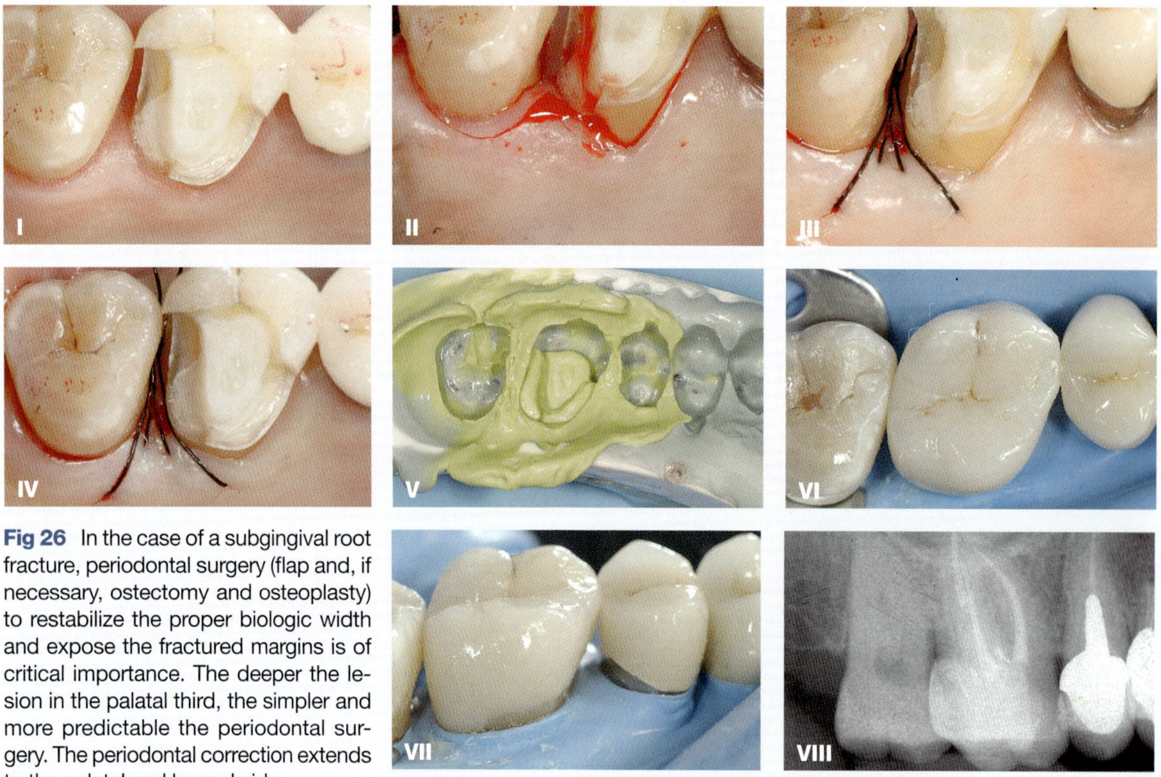

Fig 26 In the case of a subgingival root fracture, periodontal surgery (flap and, if necessary, ostectomy and osteoplasty) to restabilize the proper biologic width and expose the fractured margins is of critical importance. The deeper the lesion in the palatal third, the simpler and more predictable the periodontal surgery. The periodontal correction extends to the palatal and buccal side.

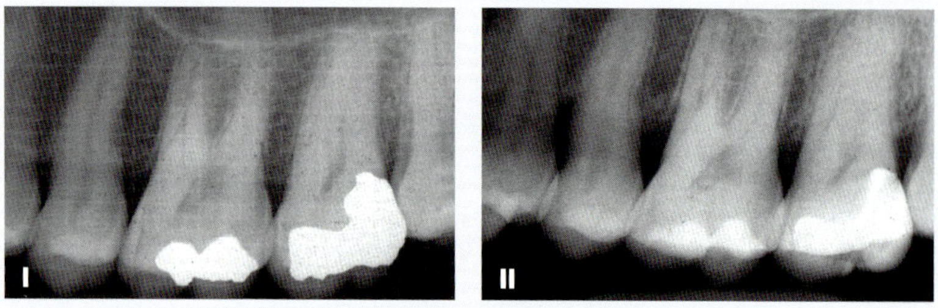

Fig 27 Twelve-year follow-up of an inlay on a maxillary left second molar with the adjacent third molar in situ.

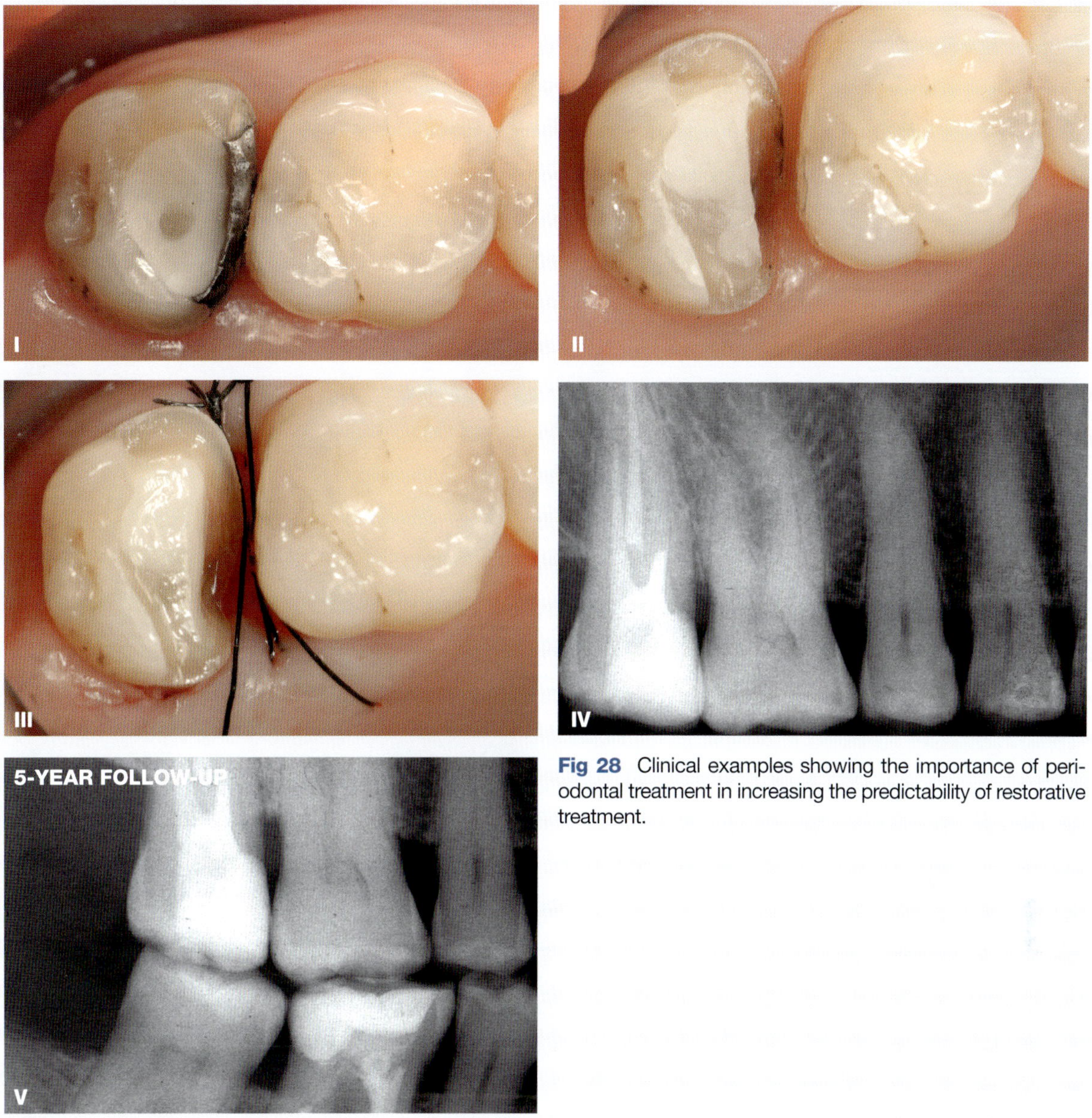

Fig 28 Clinical examples showing the importance of periodontal treatment in increasing the predictability of restorative treatment.

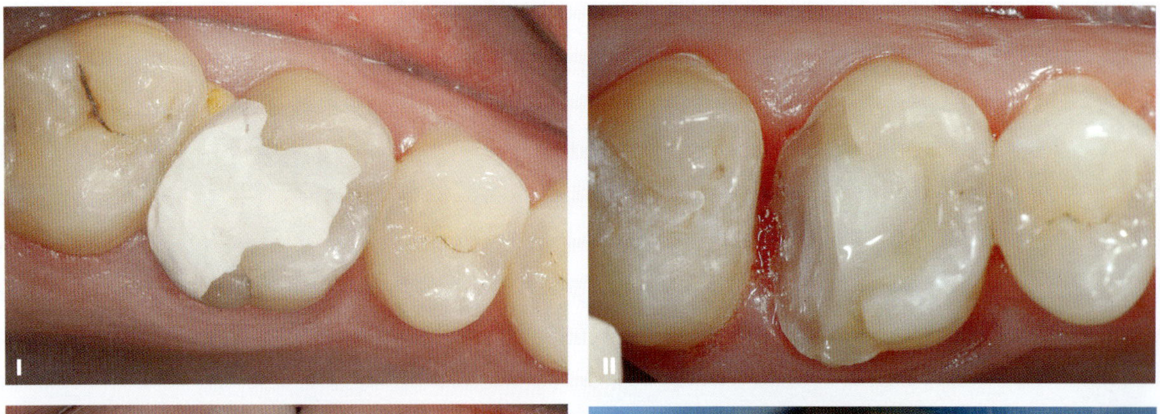

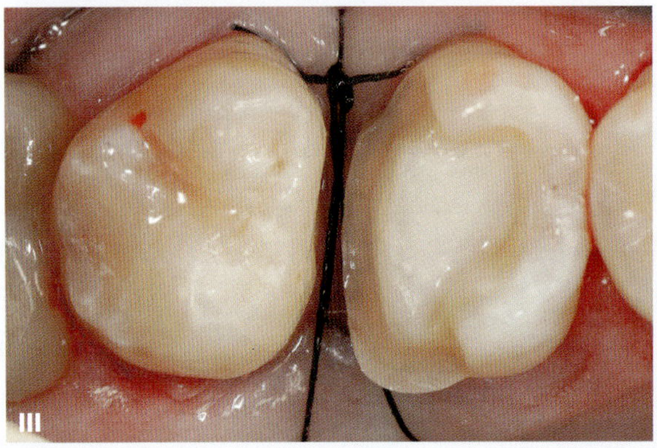

Fig 29 Very clear example of periodontal-restorative synergy. Immediately after clinical lengthening of the maxillary right first molar through highly conservative periodontal surgery *(I–III)*, it was possible to position rubber dam and finish preparing the cavity *(IV, V)*. Clinical view of the cemented restoration *(VI)* and follow-up radiograph *(VII)*.

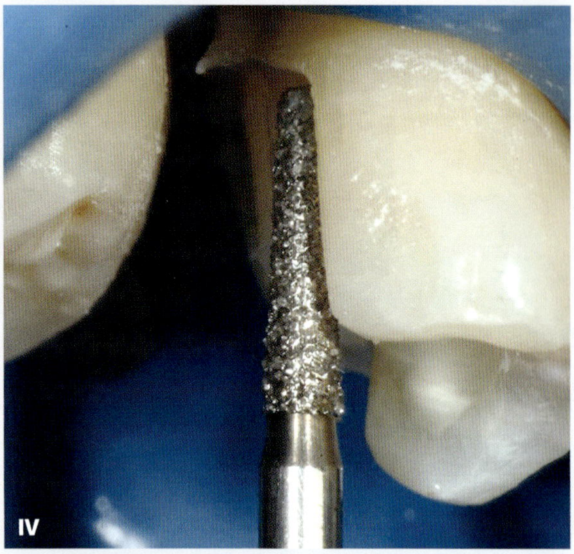

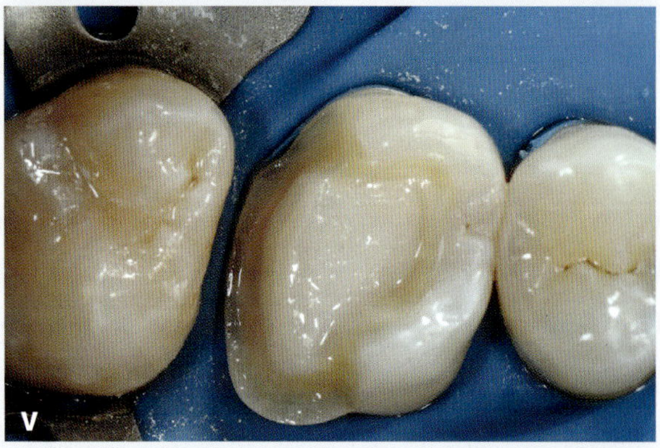

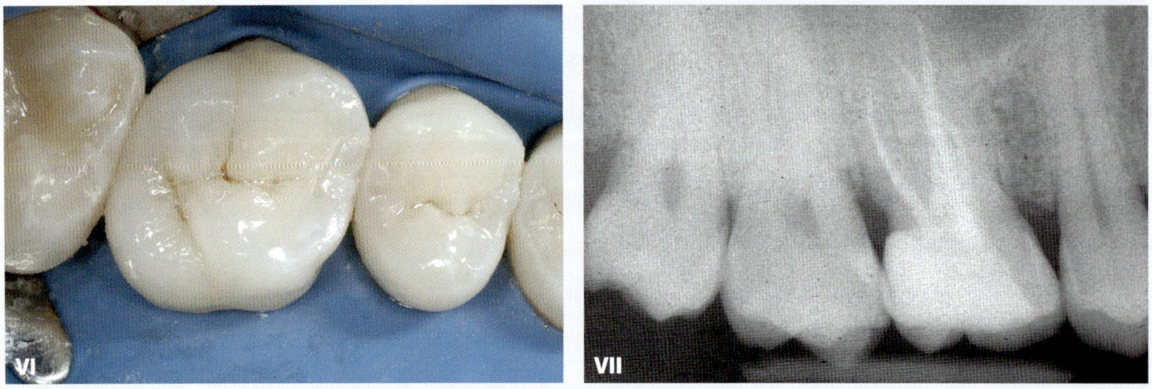

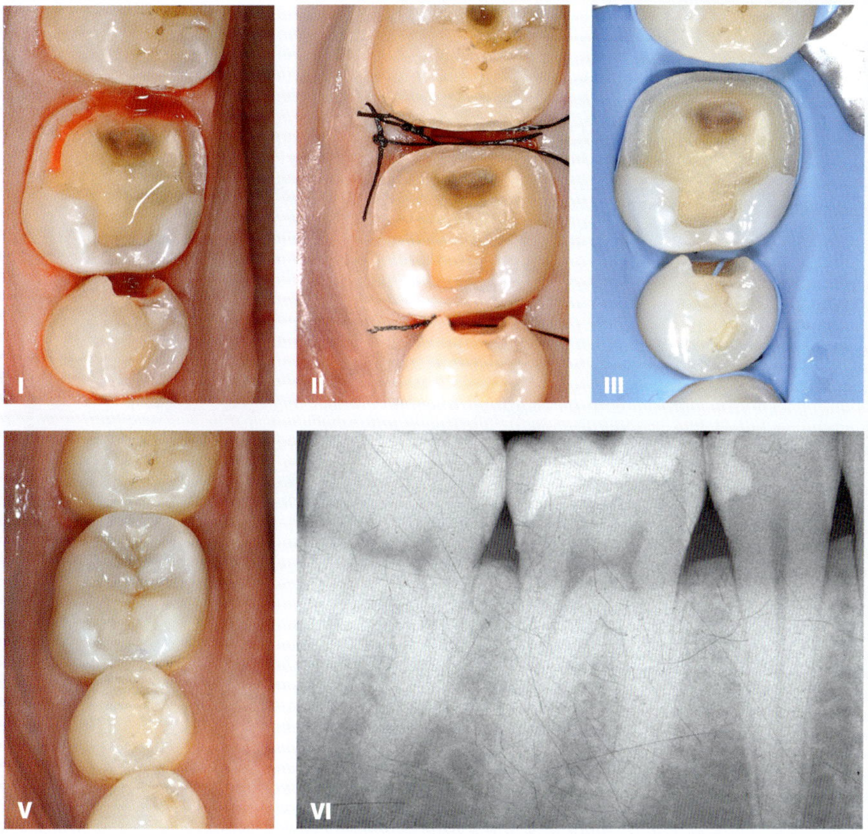

Fig 30 Another case showing surgical lengthening of the clinical crown of the molar *(I, II)*, buildup *(III, IV)*, and clinical view of the positioned inlay *(V)*. Naturally, before direct restoration of the mandibular right second premolar, torn dam was replaced. The post-cementation radiograph shows excellent tooth-restoration integration *(VI)*.

The third biologic requirement to be met by a restoration is its contour, the properties of which must be designed to ensure it is biologically accepted and integrated (Figs 31 to 45).

The ideal contour prevents plaque buildup and allows the patient easy access to carry out appropriate oral hygiene procedures while also allowing the normal development of the periodontal structures and potentially maintaining a state of health.

The relationship between restoration contour and gingival shape and health has been documented and analyzed by various authors and continues to be the subject of discussion and investigation.

In general, the location of the proximal surfaces of adjacent teeth constitutes a critical factor for the health of interdental gingival tissue.[3]

The closer the proximity of the roots, the greater their influence on gingival tissue. With minimal space between the roots, the smallest change in profile can have an impact on the integrity of the intervening soft tissue and the various components of periodontal structures[1] (Fig 46).

When the space between the roots increases, it is possible to achieve greater flexibility when changing the profile of the contour, maintaining the integrity of the soft tissue.

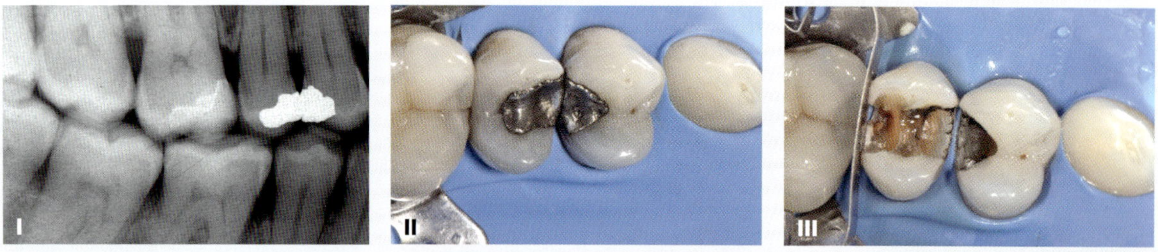

Fig 31 Decay and defective amalgam restorations on adjacent maxillary premolars *(I, II)*. Use of a separator to protect the proximal molar *(III)*. View of cemented restorations and follow-up radiograph *(IV, V)*.

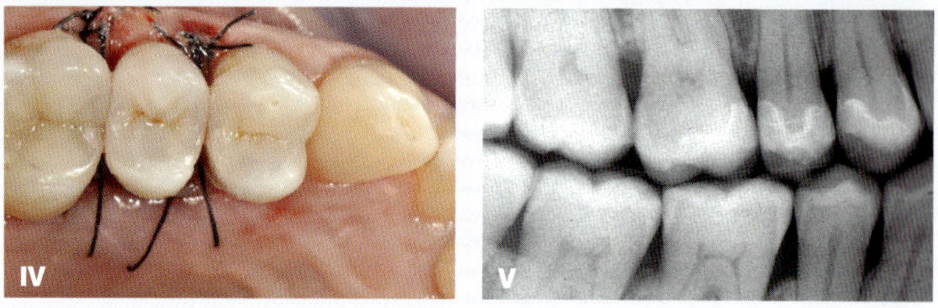

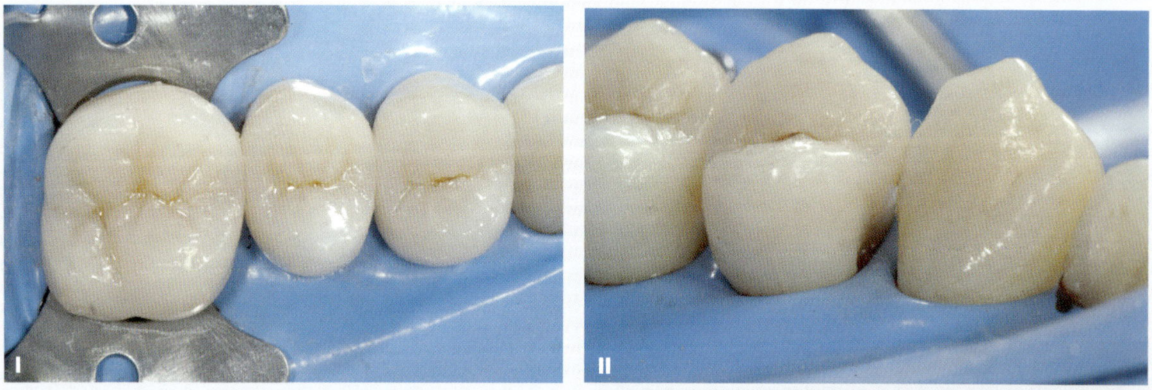

Fig 32 The emergence profiles, contact areas, and interdental alveolar ridge are the hard surfaces delimiting the interproximal space that is occupied by periodontal soft tissues. Incorrect emergence profiles alter the extent and morphology of the interproximal area and can cause inflammatory responses in the periodontal soft tissues that become altered in quantitative and qualitative terms. Oral hygiene maneuvers are made more difficult or impossible. It should be remembered that the interdental contact areas are located in the buccal two-thirds of the maxillary arch and in the lingual two-thirds of the mandibular arch.

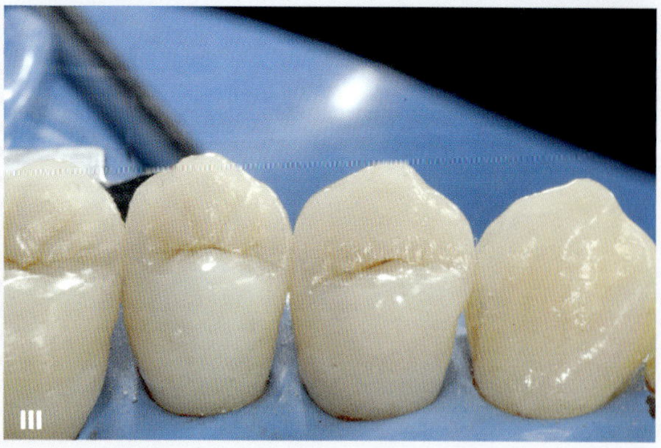

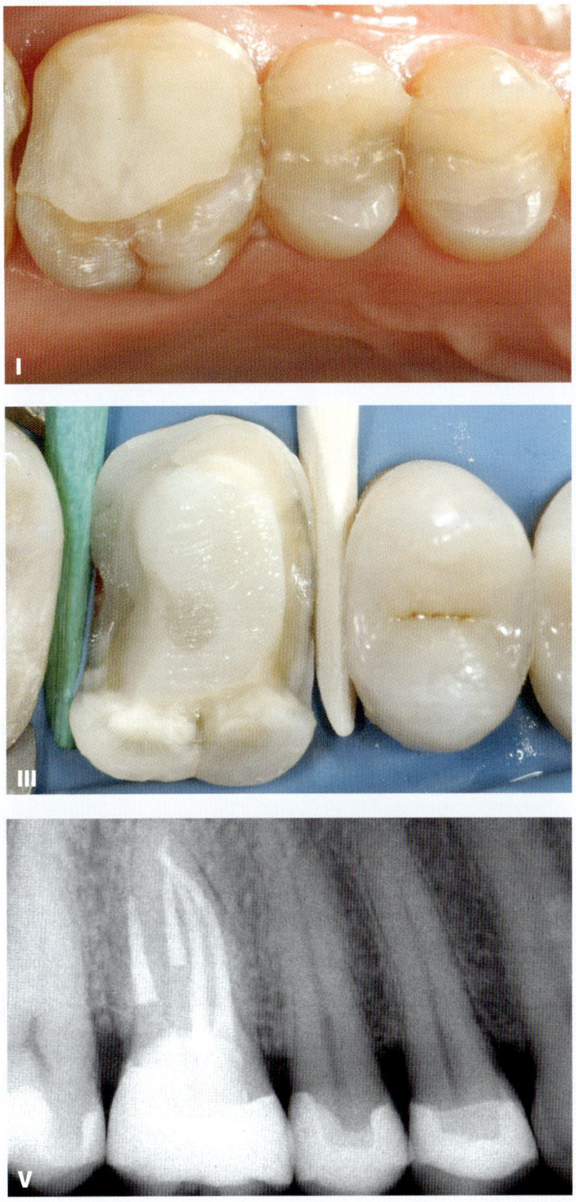

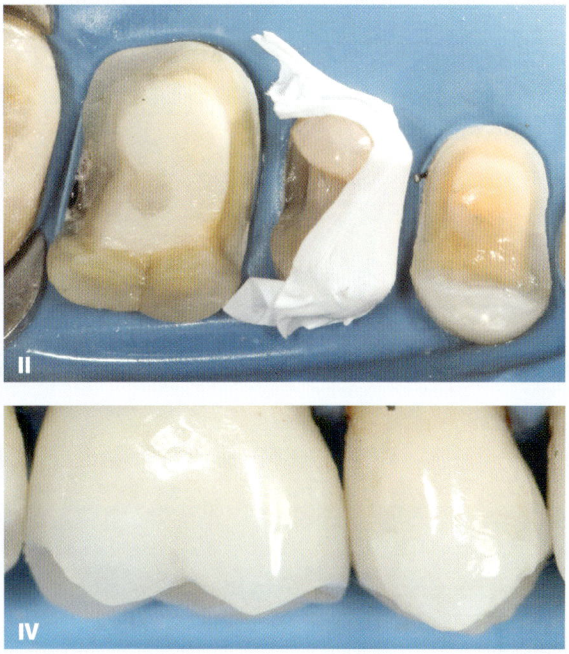

Fig 33 Contact surfaces and emergence profiles. Showing so many clinical examples may seem repetitive, and almost certainly is, although the author's aim is simply to emphasize that the results are routinely very satisfactory when a protocol is followed.

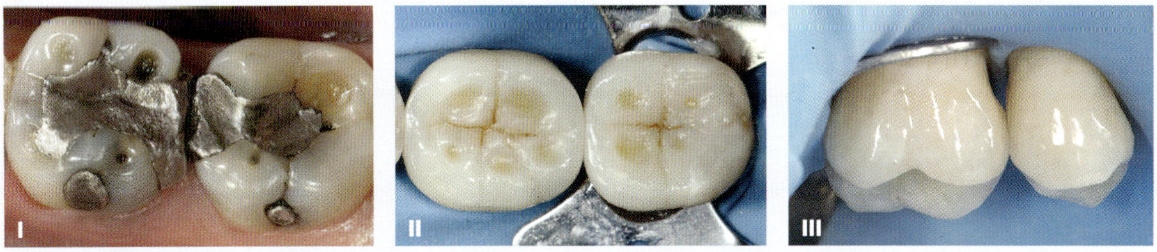

Fig 34 Occlusal view of the contact surfaces after cementation of two inlays on the mandibular left molars *(I, II)* and view of the interproximal contacts between the adhesive restorations on the maxillary right premolar and first molar *(III)*.

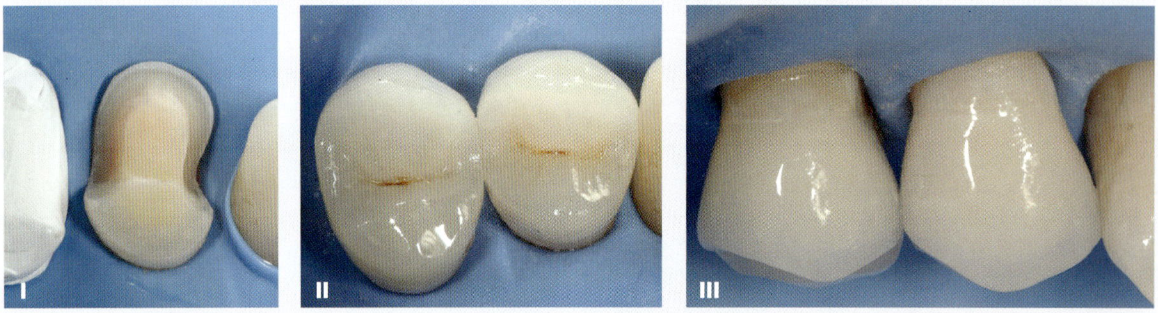

Fig 35 Completed preparation of a maxillary right first premolar *(I)*, occlusal and buccal views of cemented restorations on both premolars *(II, III)*.

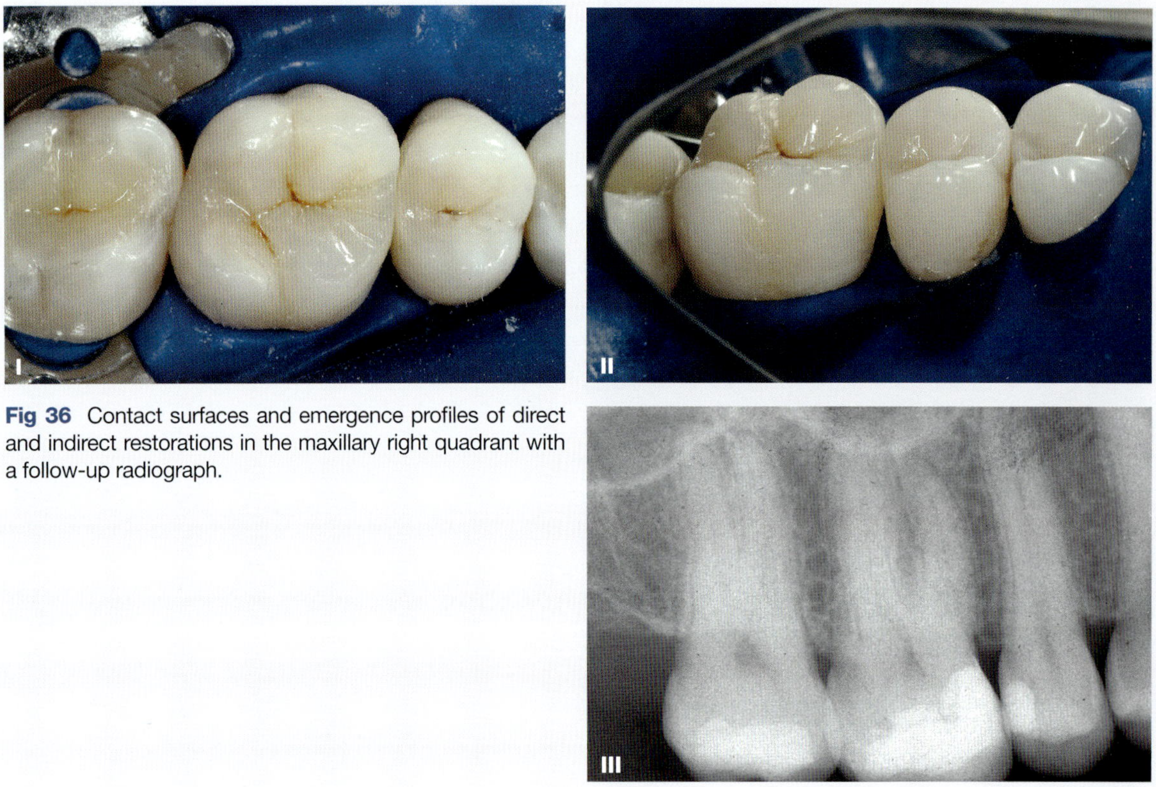

Fig 36 Contact surfaces and emergence profiles of direct and indirect restorations in the maxillary right quadrant with a follow-up radiograph.

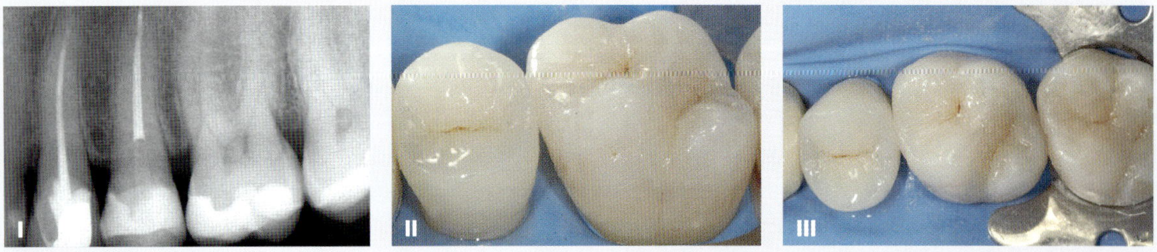

Fig 37 The marginal seals and profiles of the maxillary left second premolar and first molar are ideal from both a clinical and a radiographic viewpoint.

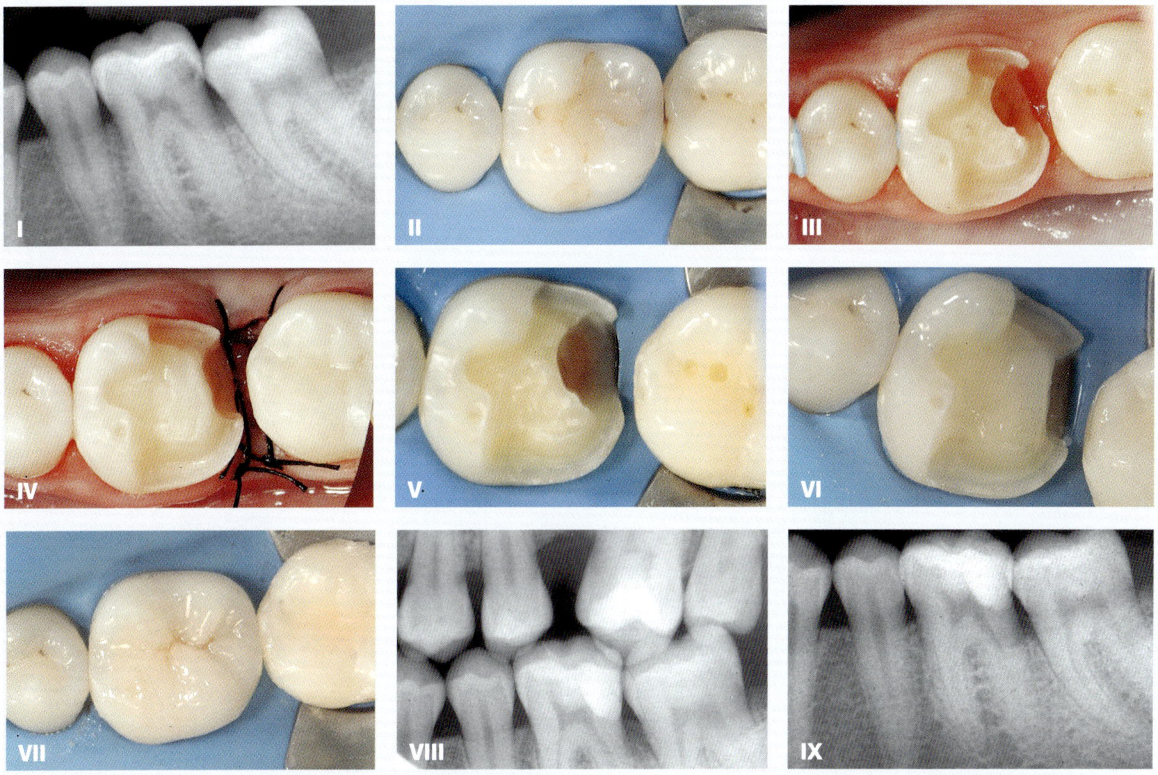

Fig 38 Very deep distal caries lesion on the mandibular left first molar *(I, II)*. After removal of the decayed tissue, the margin is in a subgingival position *(III)*, hence the need to lengthen the clinical crown *(IV)*, which makes it possible to position rubber dam, albeit with difficulty *(V)*. Execution of buildup *(VI)* and clinical and radiographic views of the cemented onlay *(VII–IX)*.

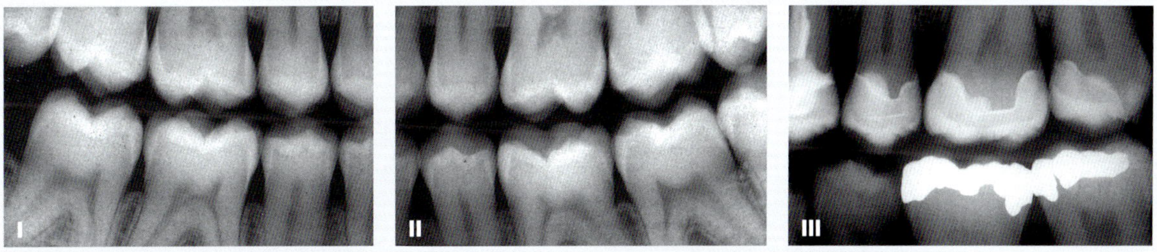

Fig 39 Emergence profiles of natural teeth *(I, II)* and teeth with adhesive composite restorations *(III)*.

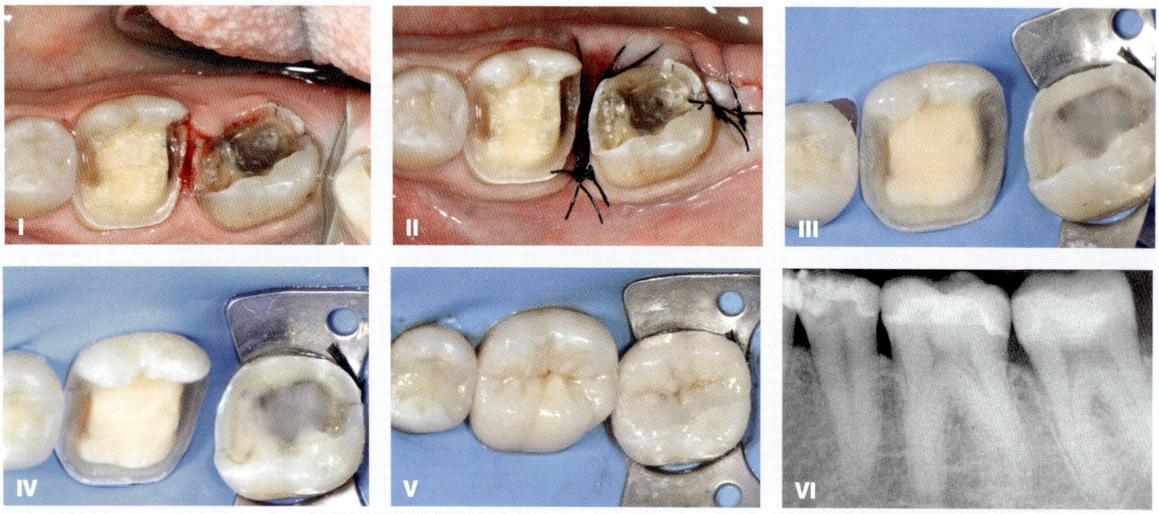

Fig 40 Somewhat difficult recovery of the lingual margin of the mandibular left second molar *(I, II)*. Isolation of the operative field, execution of buildup, cementation of inlays, and follow-up radiograph *(III–VI)*.

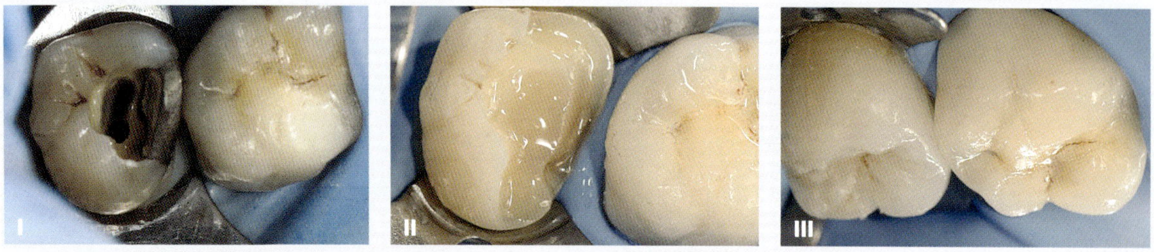

Fig 41 Isolation of the operative field is extremely difficult *(I, II)*. View of cemented restoration *(III)*.

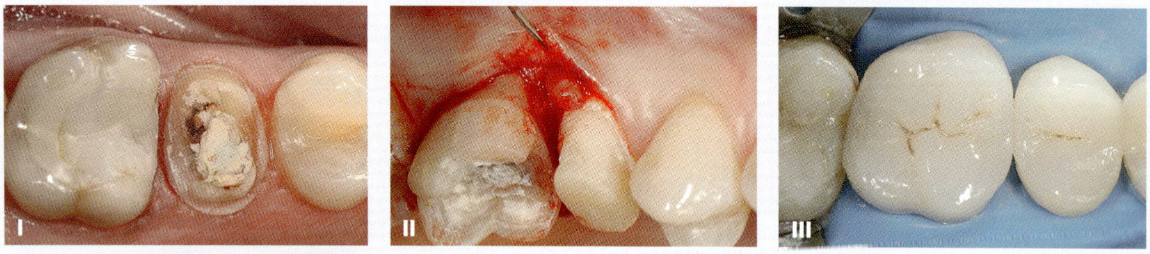

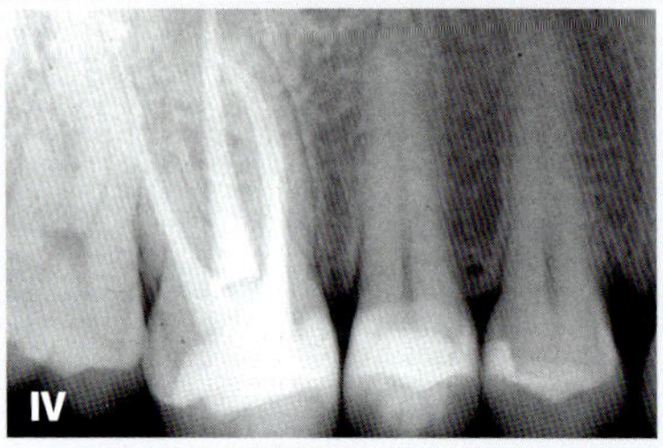

Fig 42 The remaining root of a primary tooth may change the interdental alveolar structure.

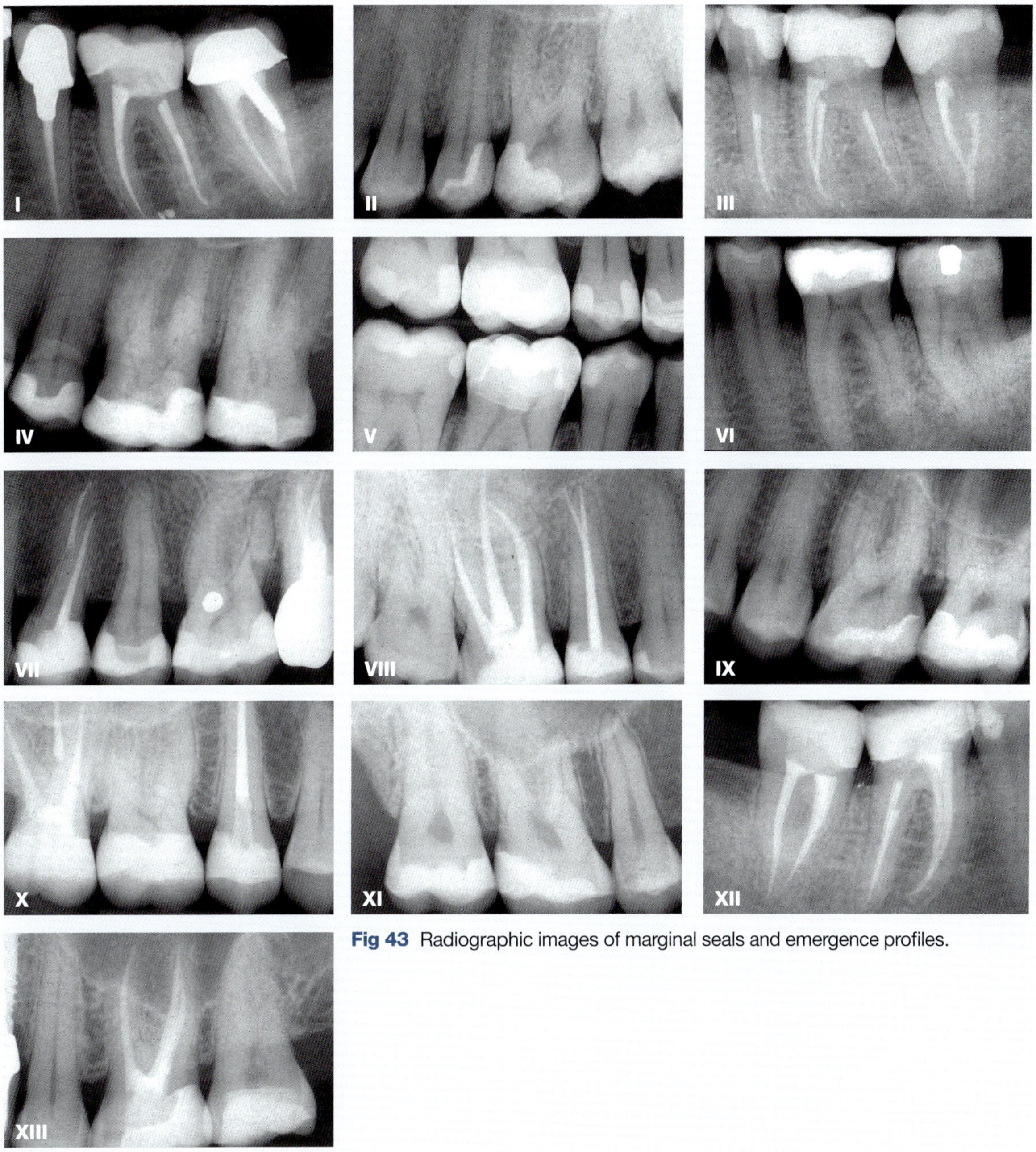

Fig 43 Radiographic images of marginal seals and emergence profiles.

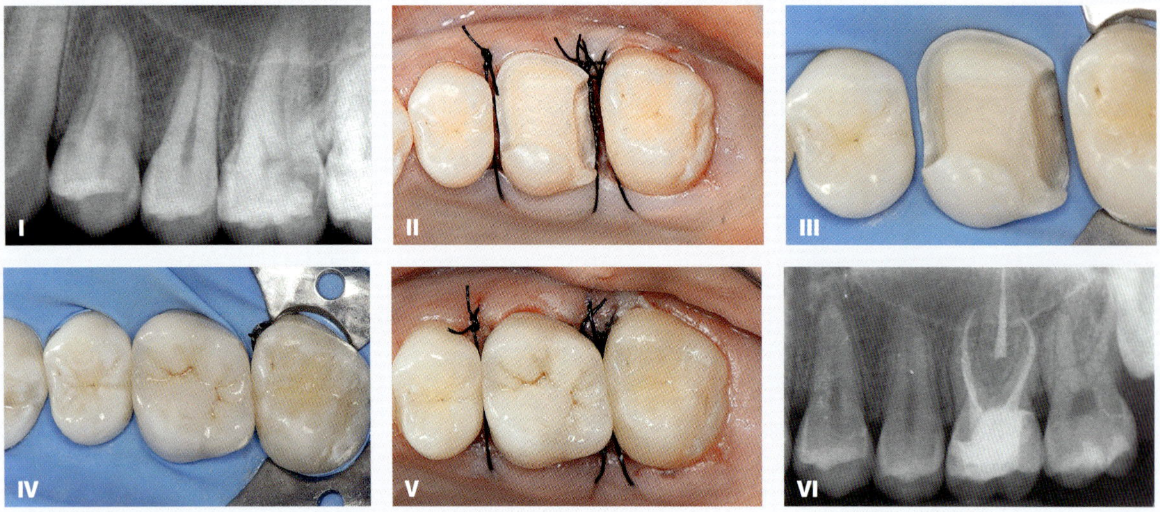

Fig 44 Periodontal surgical adaptation due to caries lesions at various levels. (Courtesy of Dr Lavinia Landi.)

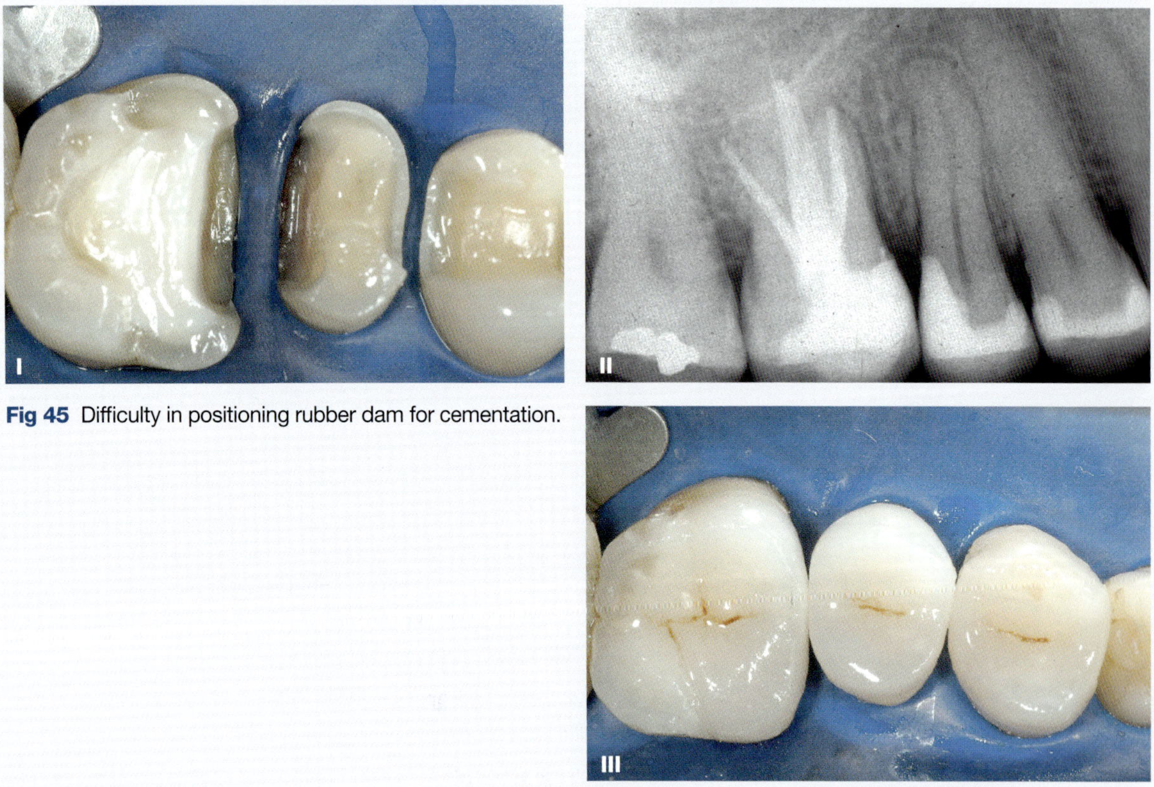

Fig 45 Difficulty in positioning rubber dam for cementation.

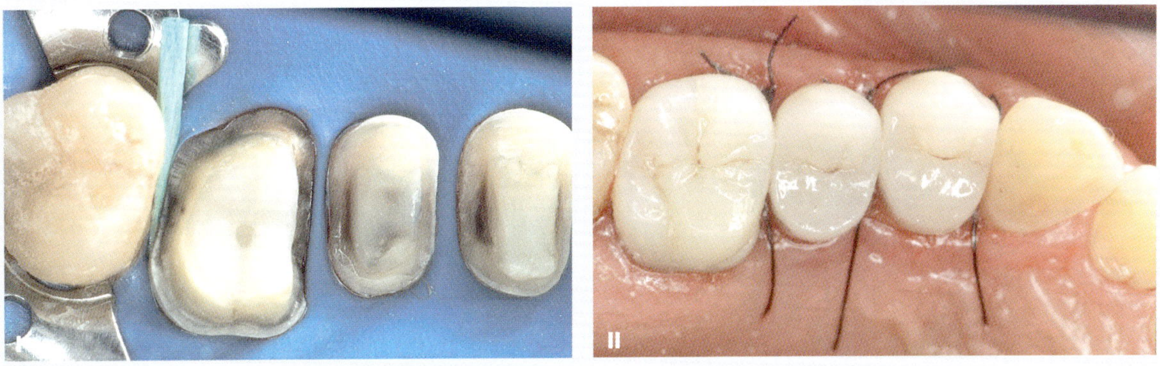

Fig 46 Another example of a somewhat complicated procedure required to isolate the operative field.

Interproximal spaces delimited by roots with concavities are particularly risky because restoration and plaque removal are much more difficult (Figs 47 to 51).

Periodontal surgery offers the option of increasing the interradicular space through dental preparation when flaps are opened, provided the roots are divergent. Another possibility is orthodontic movement.

The most complicated cases are those in which patients have experienced premature loss of the first molar. This causes the second and third molars to incline mesially, thus losing their normal contacts, altering the harmonious level of the marginal ridges and radically altering the interdental space with a consequent risk of root caries lesions and periodontal lesions (Fig 52).

Deep caries lesions extend to the root structure and in most cases are accompanied by gingival inflammation.

Interproximal gingival tissue develops classic soft crater lesions. Histologically, the epithelium appears ulcerated and hyperplastic, with fragmented connective fibers and showing massive infiltration of parvocellular inflammatory elements.

The inflammatory infiltrate tends to penetrate deep down, along the blood vessels, and involve the underlying bony tissue, which reacts with areas of resorption.

The positive periodontal architecture, which constitutes an indispensable premise for the health of supporting tissues, is altered, and the periodontal topography assumes negative architectural features.

Therefore what occurs is the onset of a typical chronic periodontal lesion that tends to be self-perpetuating, feeding on itself, and self-propagating.

The clinical periodontal attachment level begins to be lost, and an abnormal lesion described as a *periodontal pocket* becomes established.

Treatment involves removal of the pocket by means of regenerative or resective periodontal surgical techniques. A periodontal lesion may be buccal or lingual, in which case it is more easily recognizable by both the patient and the practitioner.

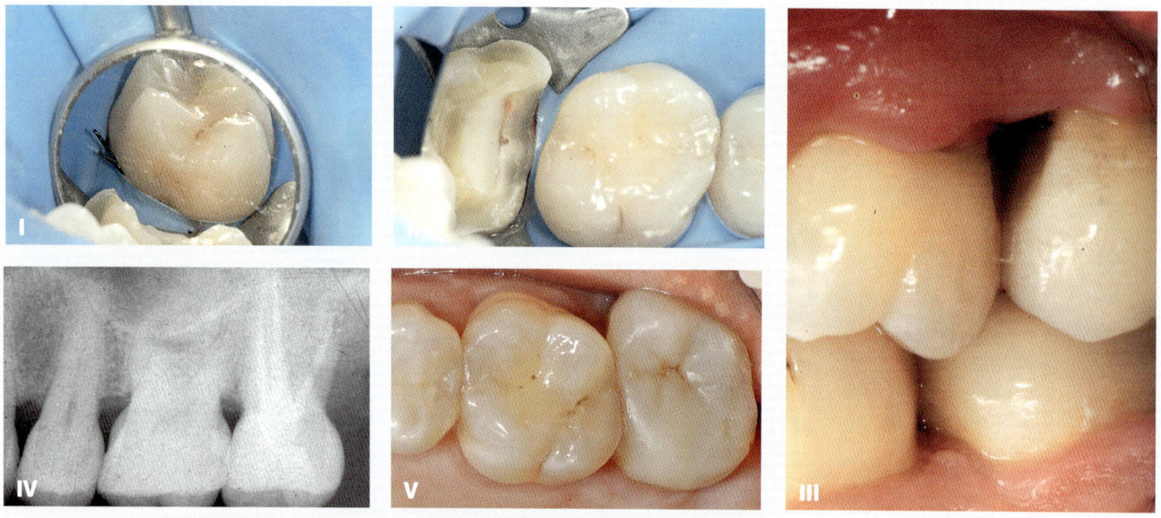
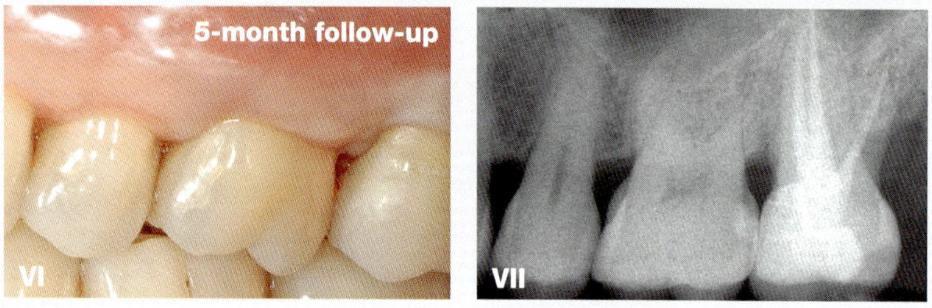

Fig 47 Unfavorable proximal anatomical changes make home hygiene procedures more complicated and delay soft tissue healing processes.

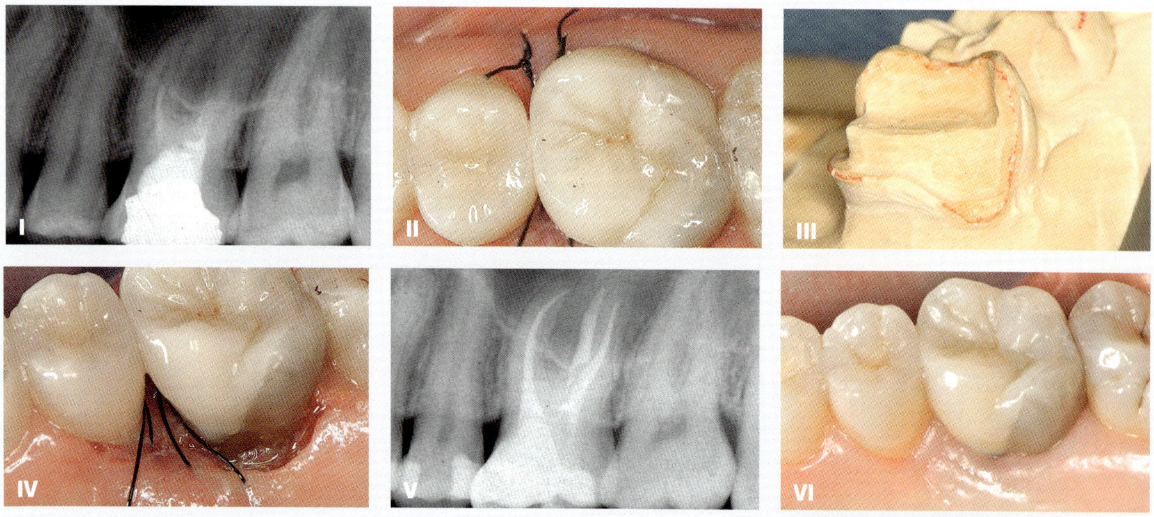

Fig 48 Periodontal surgery creates conditions for restorative recovery of root fractures *(I–V)*. Follow-up after 3 years *(VI, VII)*.

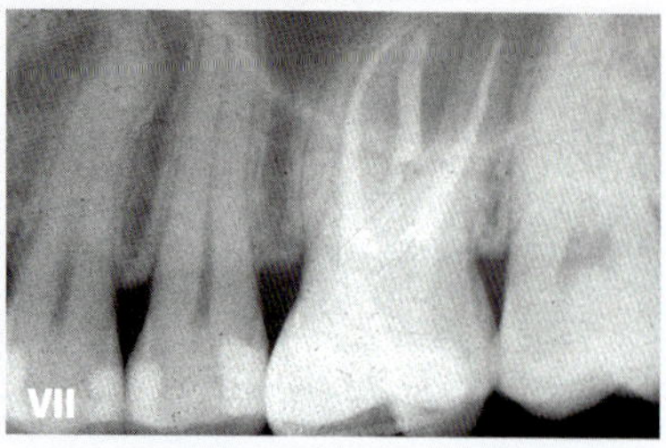

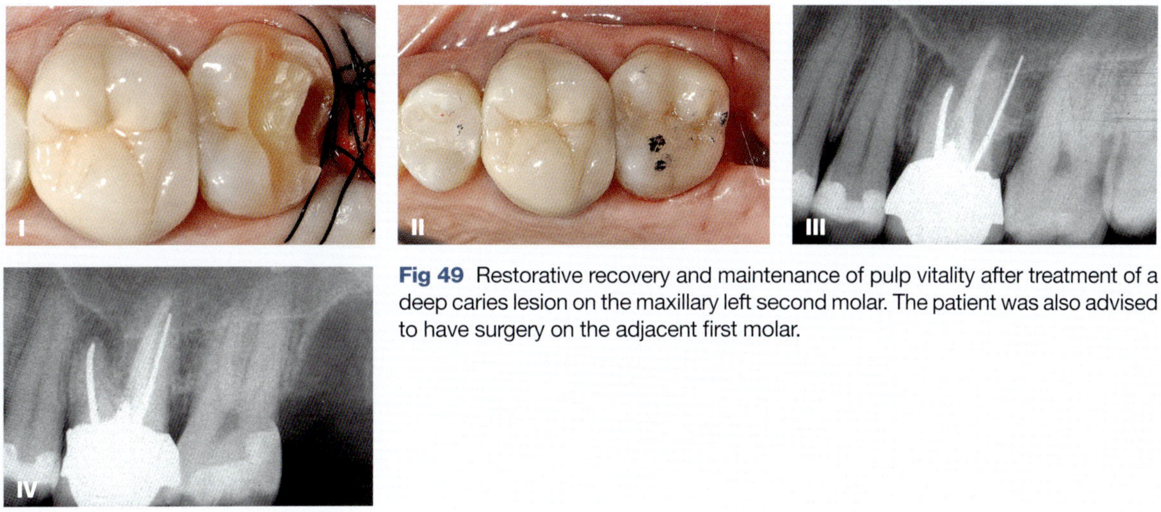

Fig 49 Restorative recovery and maintenance of pulp vitality after treatment of a deep caries lesion on the maxillary left second molar. The patient was also advised to have surgery on the adjacent first molar.

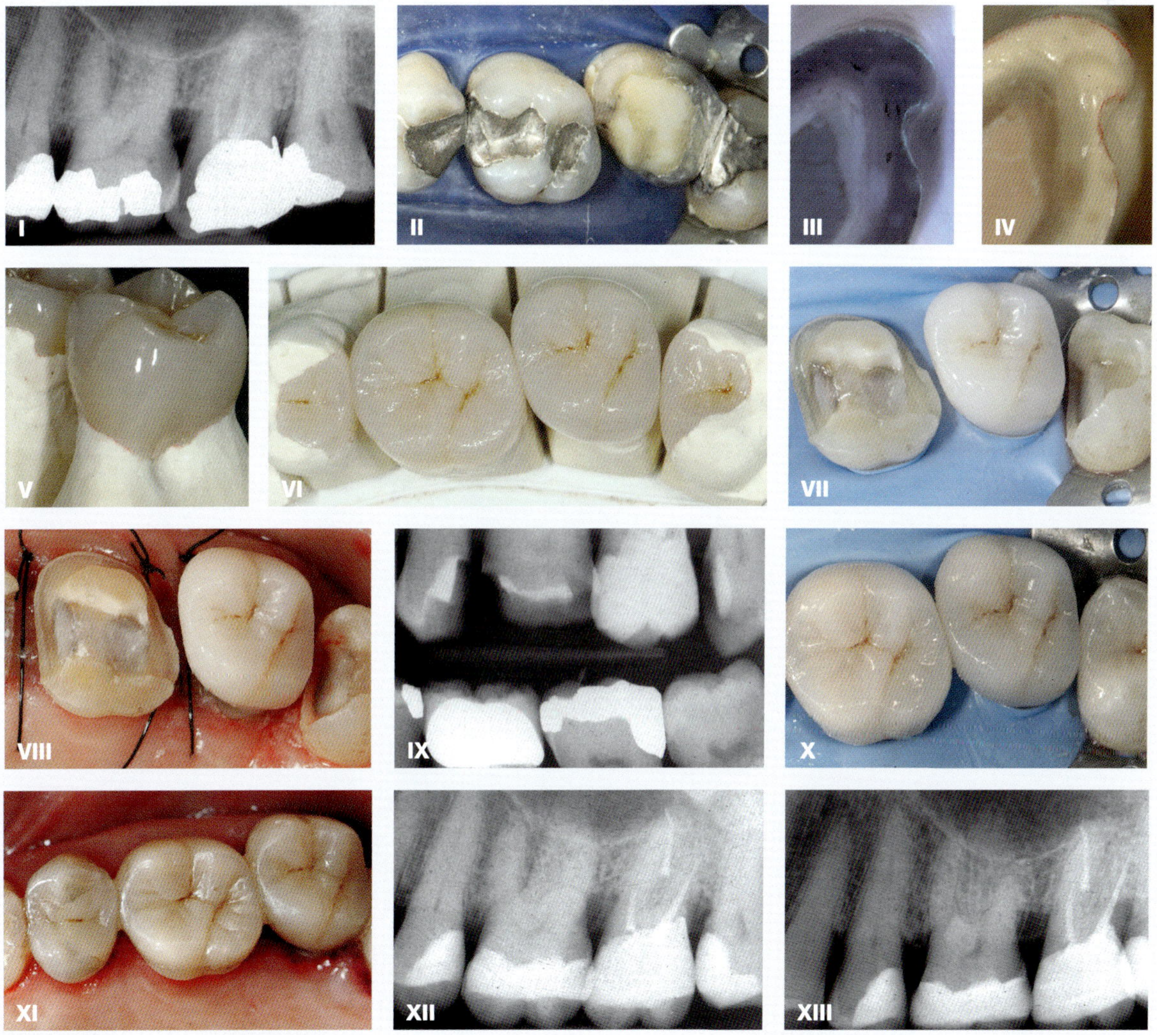

Fig 50 Restoration of a quadrant that was made extremely complicated by the patient's outright refusal to remove the third molar, which was considered necessary. The difficulty of making preparations in teeth with such pronounced concavities is evident.

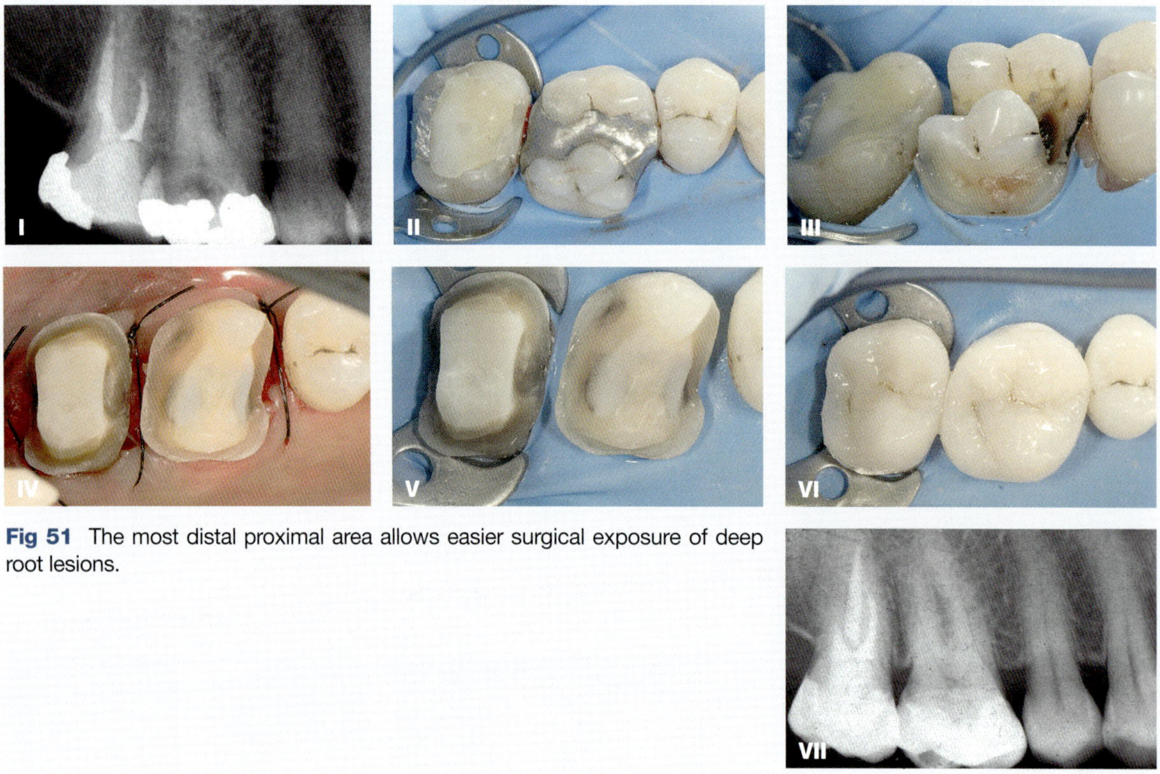

Fig 51 The most distal proximal area allows easier surgical exposure of deep root lesions.

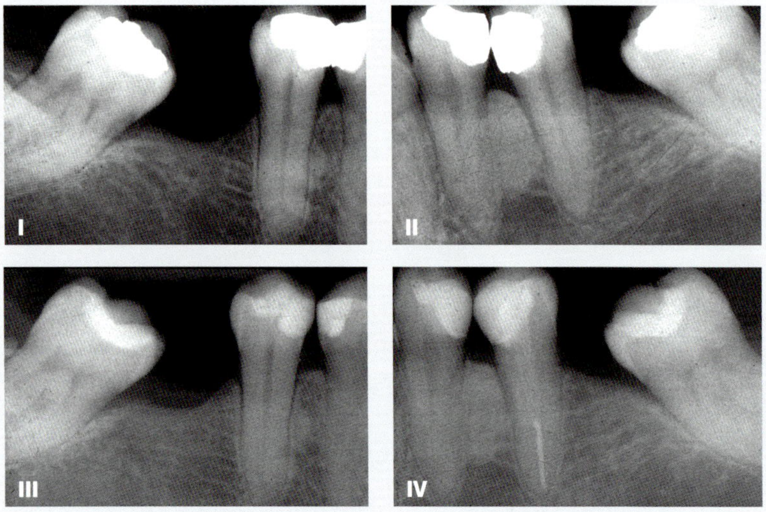

Fig 52 Inclination of second molars that, in the absence of the first molars, are subject to root decay and periodontal problems. The goal is achieved with the aid of orthodontic treatment and re-alignment of the arches.

If the lesion is interdental, it may be asymptomatic and thus insidious by nature. The most involved periodontal structures are generally located below the contact surfaces.
The fourth biologic requirement to be met by the restoration is connected to the position of the margin, which must allow normal development of periodontal biologic width in its relationship with the deep periodontium.[4]
The definition of biologic width appears to refer to a specific concept on a horizontal plane but actually relates to a measurement on a vertical plane and is clinically represented by approximately 1 mm of connectival attachment above the ridge, approximately 1 mm of epithelial junction, and lastly by a minimal sulcus depth. A classic restoration in metal or in metal and ceramic often requires approximately 2 mm of healthy dental tissue in order to achieve a ferrule effect.
When required, the surgical exposure must measure 3 to 5 mm from the lesion to the alveolar ridge.
The advent of adhesive dentistry has considerably reduced this distance to the minimum clinical level of 2.5 mm. Pre-restorative periodontal surgical techniques have therefore become less invasive and more conservative and are now the treatment of choice.
The tendency to replace these techniques with the cervical margin relocation method should be considered an unacceptable therapeutic compromise that does not resolve the restorative problem and completely ignores the periodontal problem (Figs 53 to 55).
When there is an indication to perform a dental restoration in a site beneath the gingival margin, an appropriate root area must be created that can be used to develop biologic width (Fig 56). This condition makes it possible to achieve a healthy support apparatus near a restoration.
Infringement of this fundamental biologic principle causes a highly destructive inflammatory lesion at the periodontal level[5,6] (Figs 57 to 61).
The crux of the matter is that if the margin can be fitted with dam, there is no reason for relocation. Conversely, when the cervical margin is borderline or subgingival, it is somewhat difficult to isolate the operative field perfectly, with all the attendant risks. Another outcome is having to carry out the adhesion in two sessions: one to position a little traditional composite or, worse still, flowable composite and then a second session for cementation of the prosthesis, thus making the whole process unnecessarily complicated.
The truth is that the margin either can or cannot be fitted with dam, and if it cannot, a periodontist can be called upon to resolve the problem. It is as simple as that.

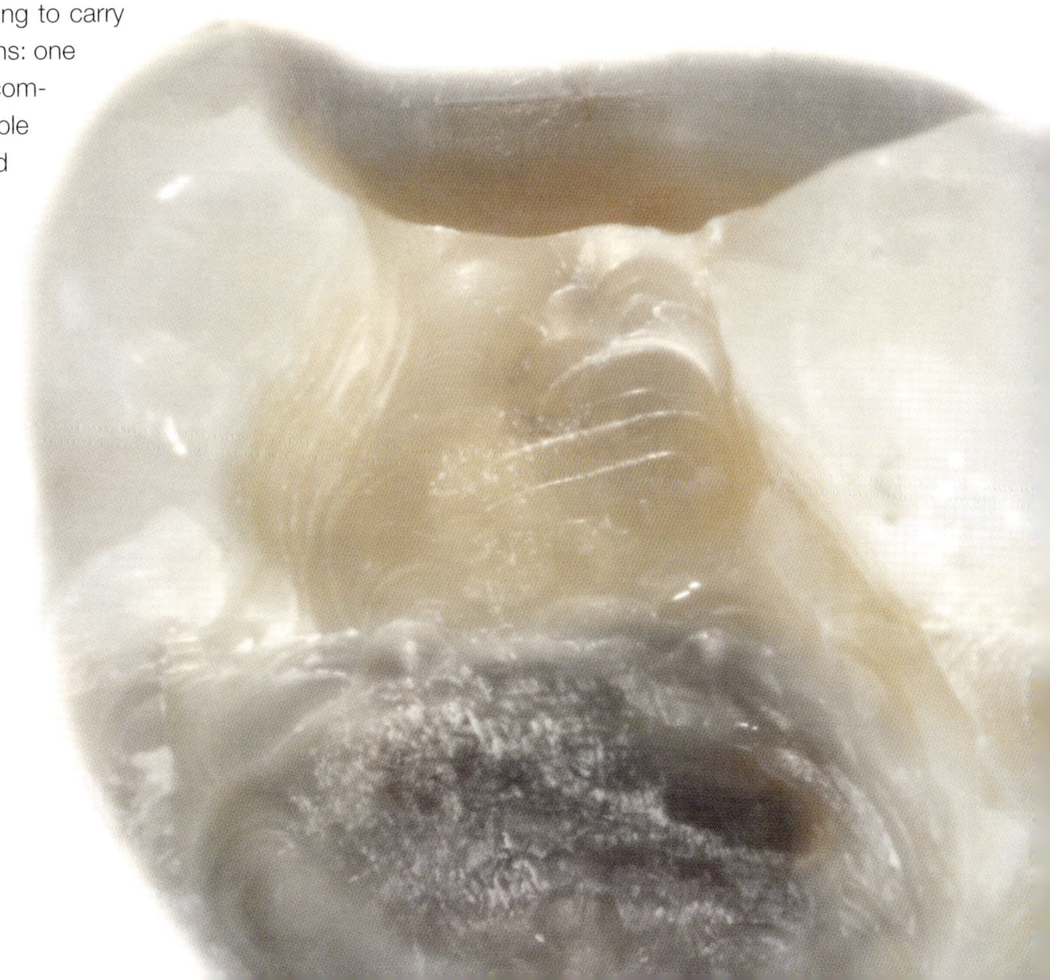

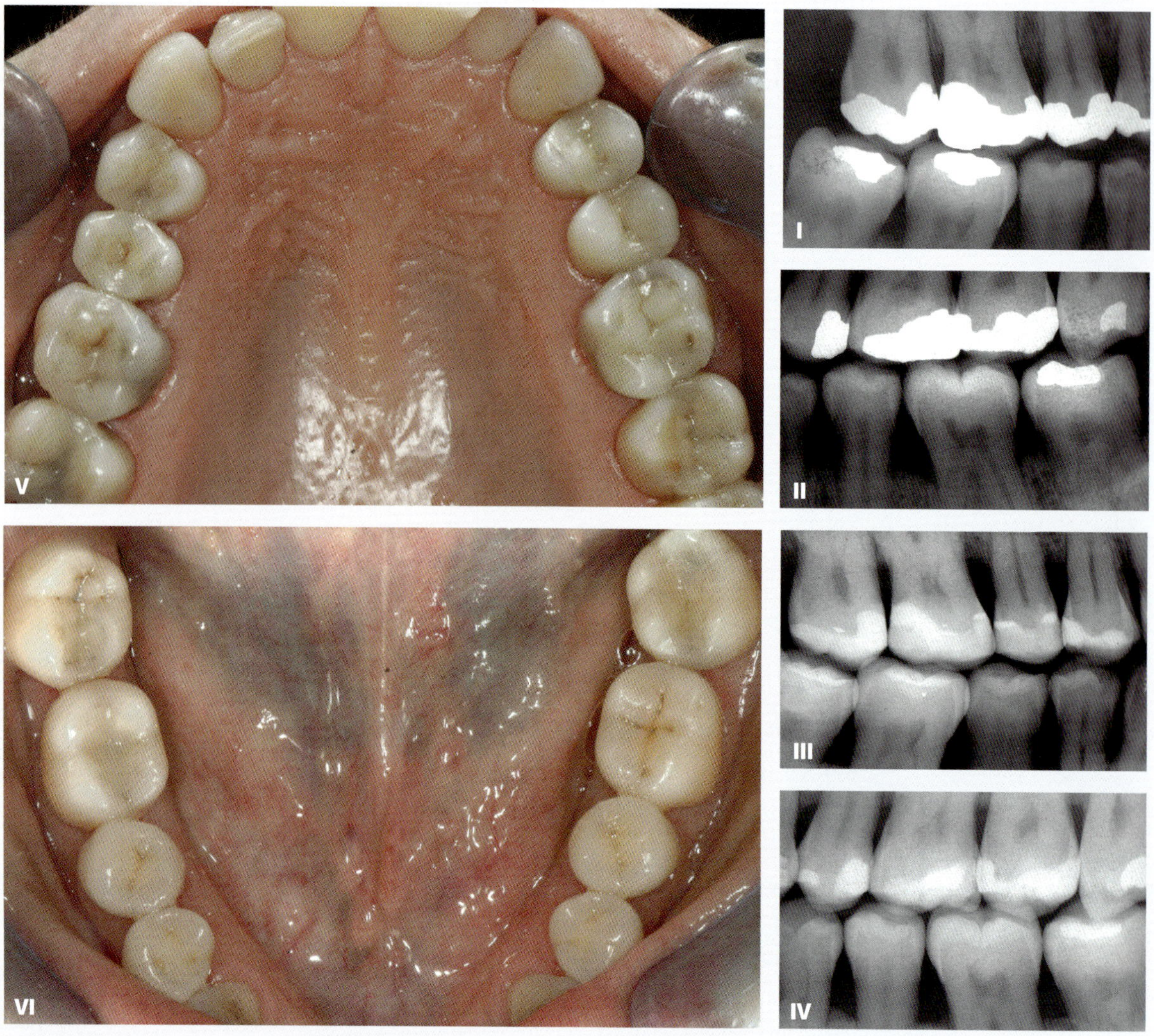

Fig 53 Clinical example of cervical margin relocation with incremental composite placement. The long-term results are acceptable but not comparable with those achieved by lengthening the clinical crown through periodontal surgery treatment *(I, II)*. Clinical and radiographic view after 12 years *(III–VI)*.

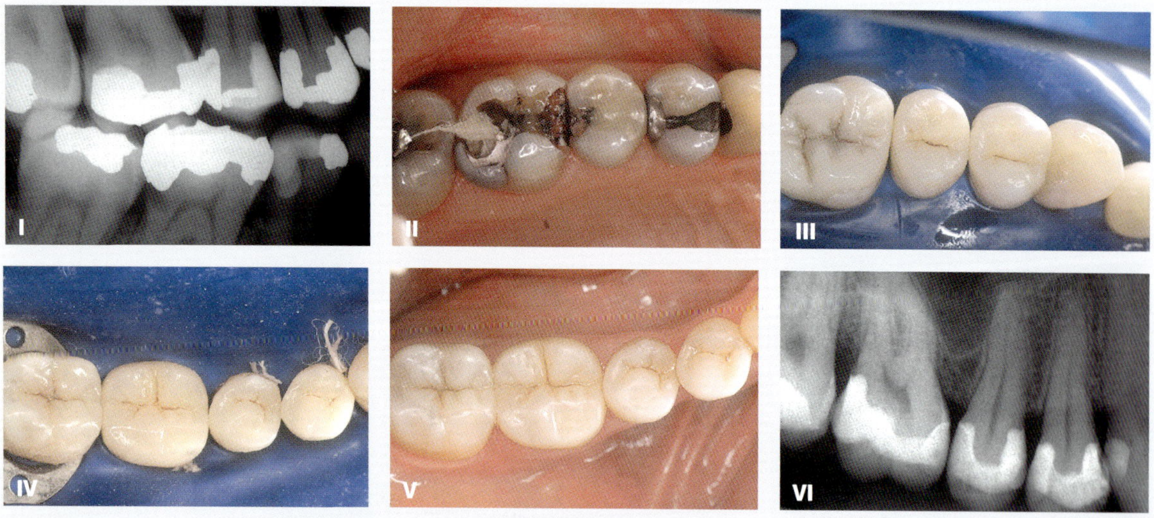

Fig 54 Another case of margin relocation, achieved without periodontal surgery, in both maxillary and the mandibular right quadrants *(I–X)* with associated clinical and radiographic follow-up after 10 years *(XI–XIII)*.

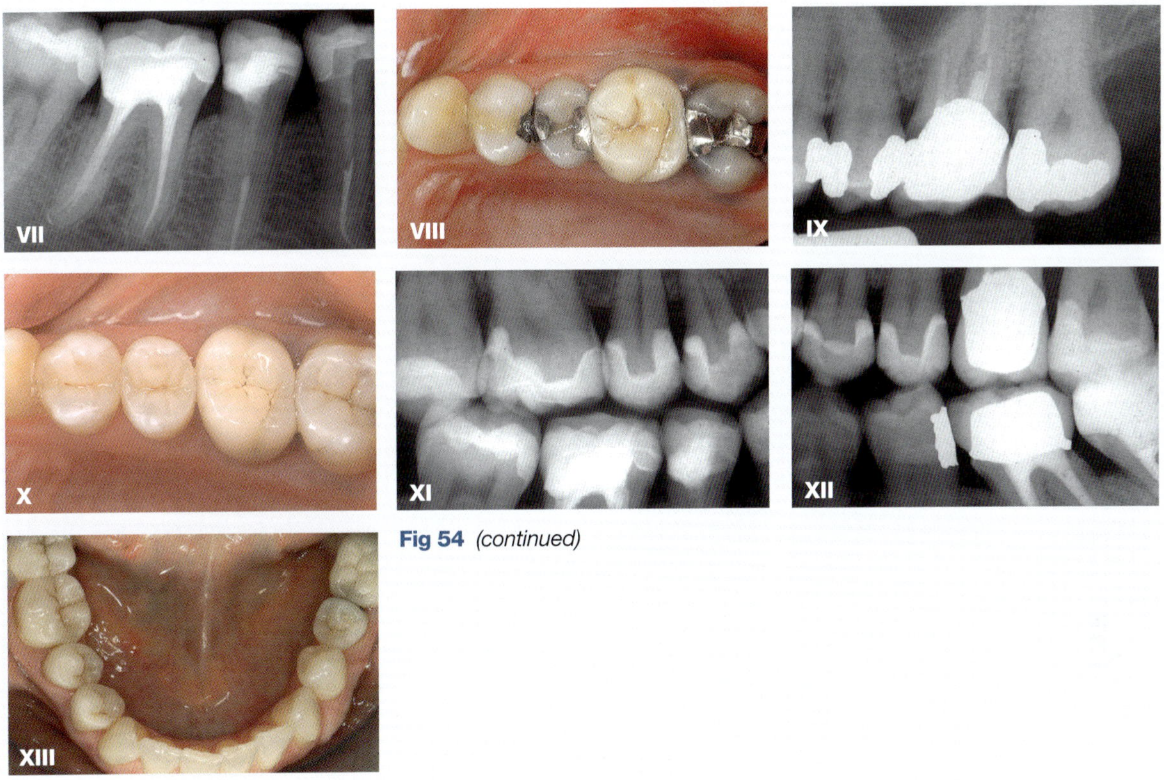

Fig 54 *(continued)*

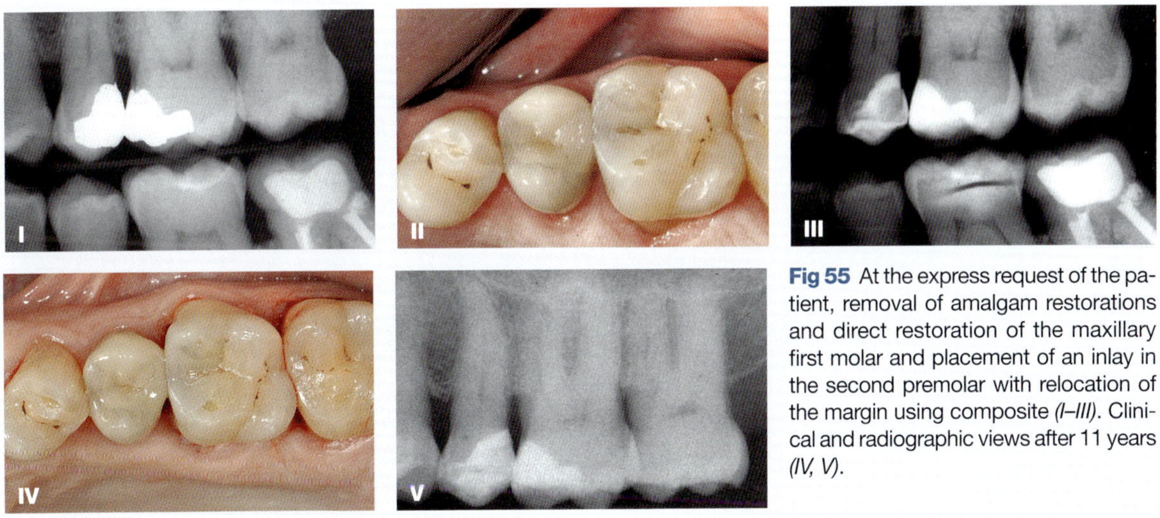

Fig 55 At the express request of the patient, removal of amalgam restorations and direct restoration of the maxillary first molar and placement of an inlay in the second premolar with relocation of the margin using composite *(I–III)*. Clinical and radiographic views after 11 years *(IV, V)*.

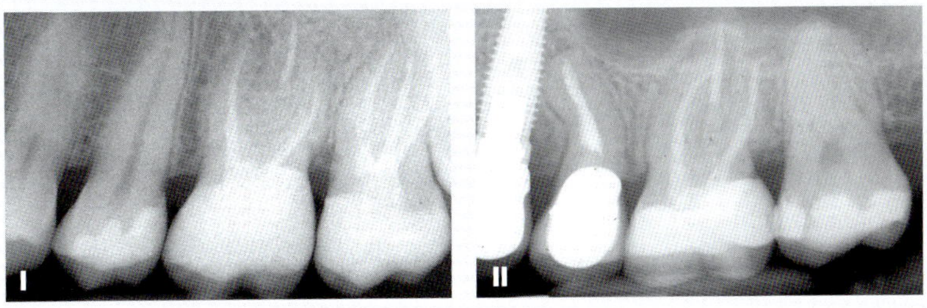

Fig 56 Radiographic view of marginal seals and emergence profiles of very deep indirect restorations following periodontal surgery *(I, II)*.

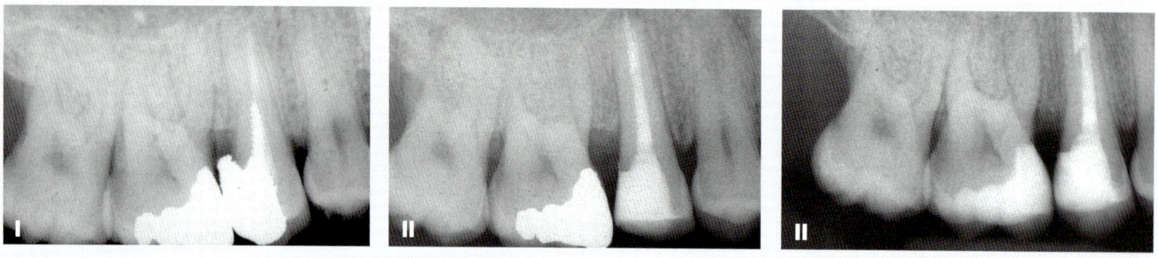

Fig 57 Infringement of the biologic space and restoration of correct parameters. The impact of reconstructive dentistry operations (eg, overcontouring) should be considered a factor of great etiologic importance with regard to the development of periodontal disease.

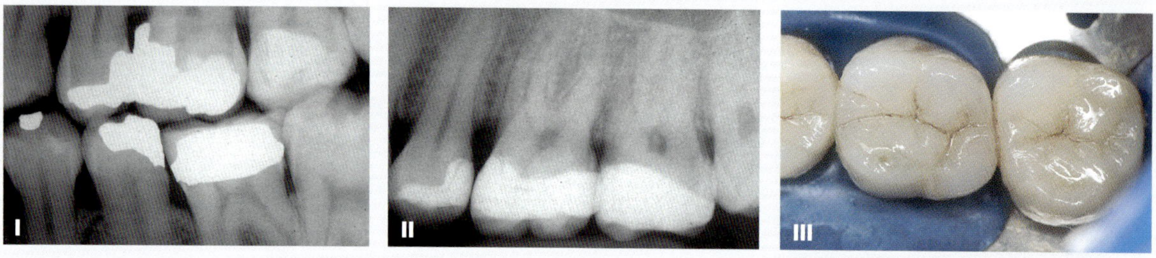

Fig 58 Radiographic and clinical view showing restoration of correct tooth morphology in the maxillary left quadrant.

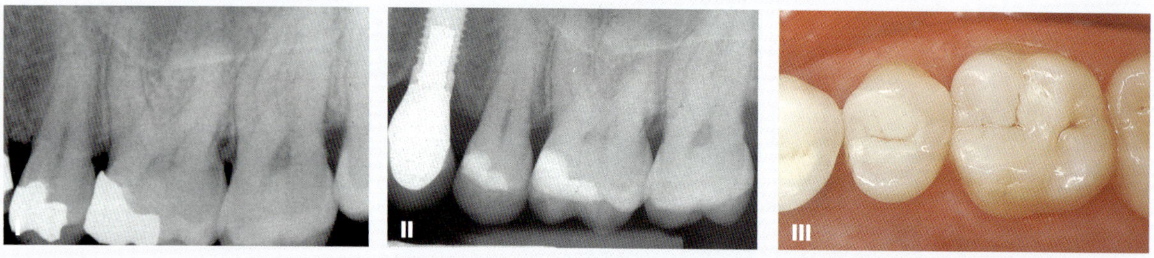

Fig 59 Removal of defective amalgam restorations *(I)* and replacement with indirect restorations that allow a return to correct anatomical configurations *(II, III)*.

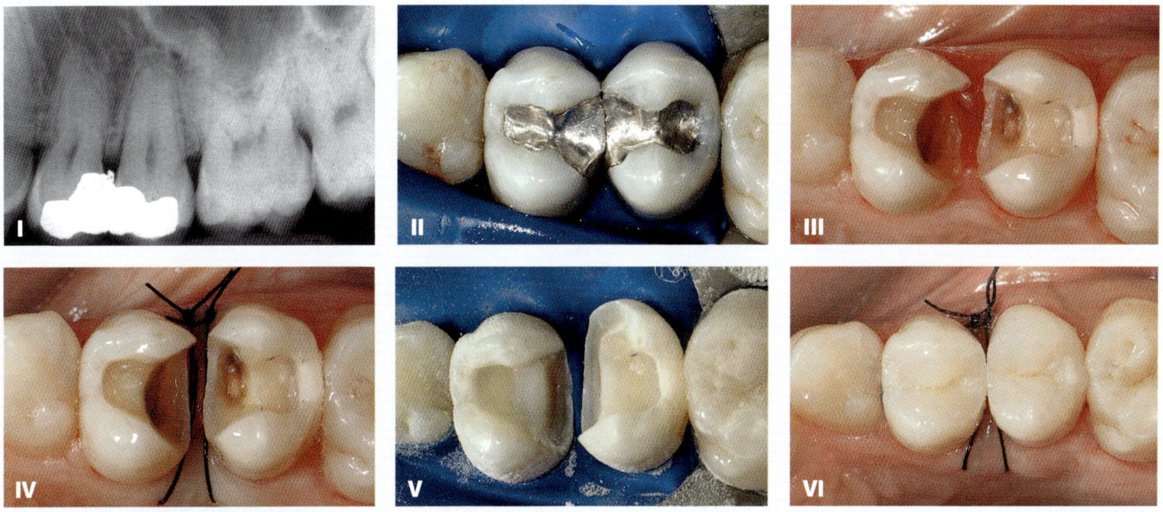

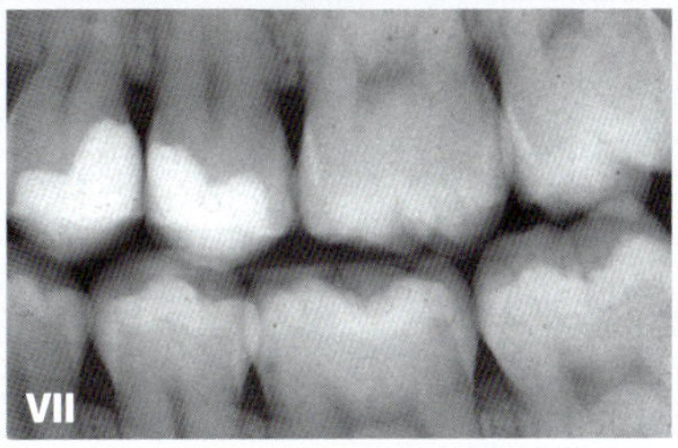

Fig 60 Significant inflammation of periodontal tissues caused by incorrect amalgam fillings *(I, II)*. Their removal, the surgical exposure of margins, and execution of two indirect composite restorations *(III–VI)* constitute the routine protocol for curing diseased tissue *(VII)*.

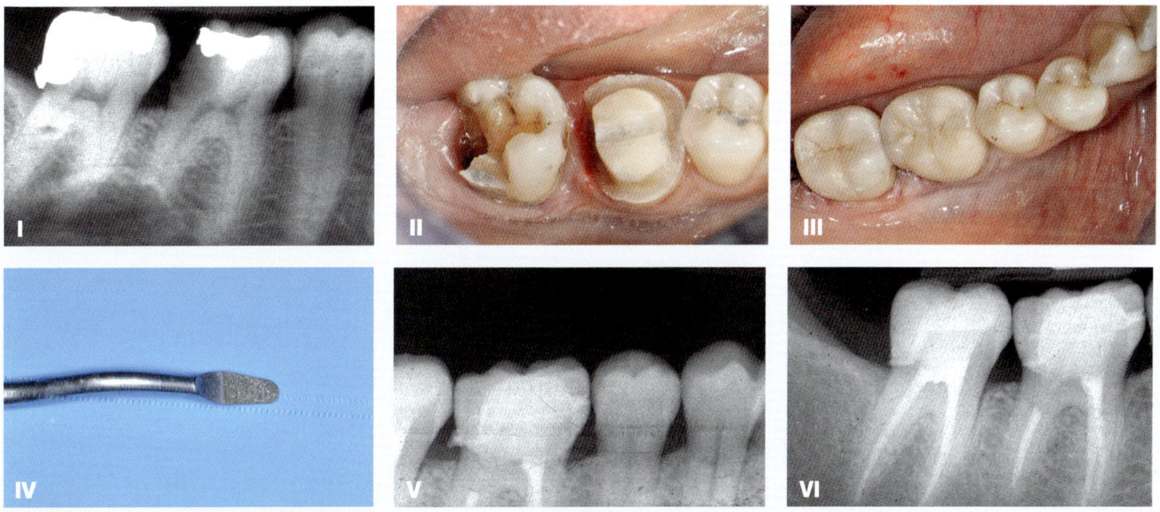

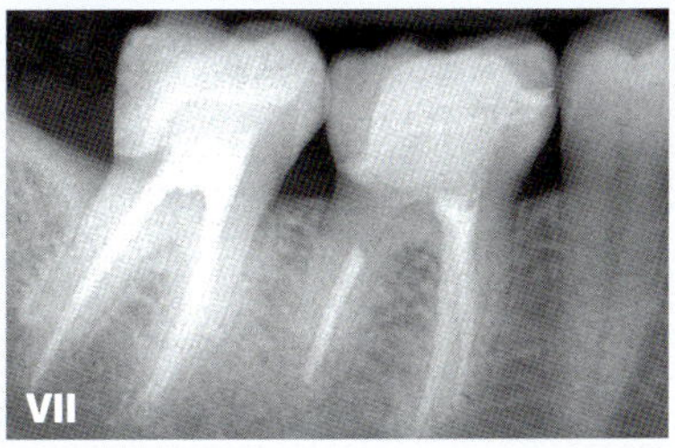

Fig 61 If excess composite is present following cementation in areas that are difficult to access *(I–III)*, subsonic instruments *(IV)* are ideal for removal and accurate finishing *(V–VII)*. Note that *VI* shows a very small amount of surplus composite at the tooth-restoration level in the distal part of the mandibular right second molar, and it has been removed in *VII*.

The bone septa are ruined, and the type of damage caused differs according to the anatomy of the septum affected.

If the septum is thick, an intraosseous defect is created; if it is thin, it may suffer irreversible damage with complete resorption of the bony tissue to an extent of 5 mm or more.

The gingival tissue shows signs of chronic inflammation or undergoes marked recession that exposes part of the root surface.

Adhesion allows the production of mainly partial restorations, with a great conservation of dental tissue that is respected by this particular preparation technique.

The restoration margins are mainly supragingival and therefore easier to control and accurately restore. They can also be more easily maintained by the patient (Fig 62). Even with deep decay, pulp vitality is often respected (Fig 63).

To conclude, it is possible to design a restorative-periodontal treatment plan at minimum biologic cost, and this constitutes one of the most worthwhile therapeutic goals.

Basic periodontal treatment, removal of inflammation and decay, and control of occlusion constitute the first stage of treatment.

Any regenerative periodontal techniques are applied at this stage.

The pre-restorative surgical-periodontal treatment plan is based on a detailed analysis of the support structures, the biotype, and the relationships present between the root structure, alveolar process, and soft tissue.

Probing, which is continuously correlated with the radiographic image, is critical and must be performed at all points of the tooth and gingival area with and without anaesthesia. It allows accurate definition of the topography of the alveolar crest and the clinical attachment level.

The anomalies and deformities present are thus identified, and it is possible to assess options for correcting them.

Particular attention should be paid to evaluating the periodontal architecture. In topographic terms, this must be strictly positive (otherwise it will tend to accumulate plaque) so that it can be maintained in the long term by means of simple oral hygiene procedures.

If the periodontal architecture displays negative features, these absolutely must be removed by means of ostectomy and osteoplasty procedures[7] (Fig 64).

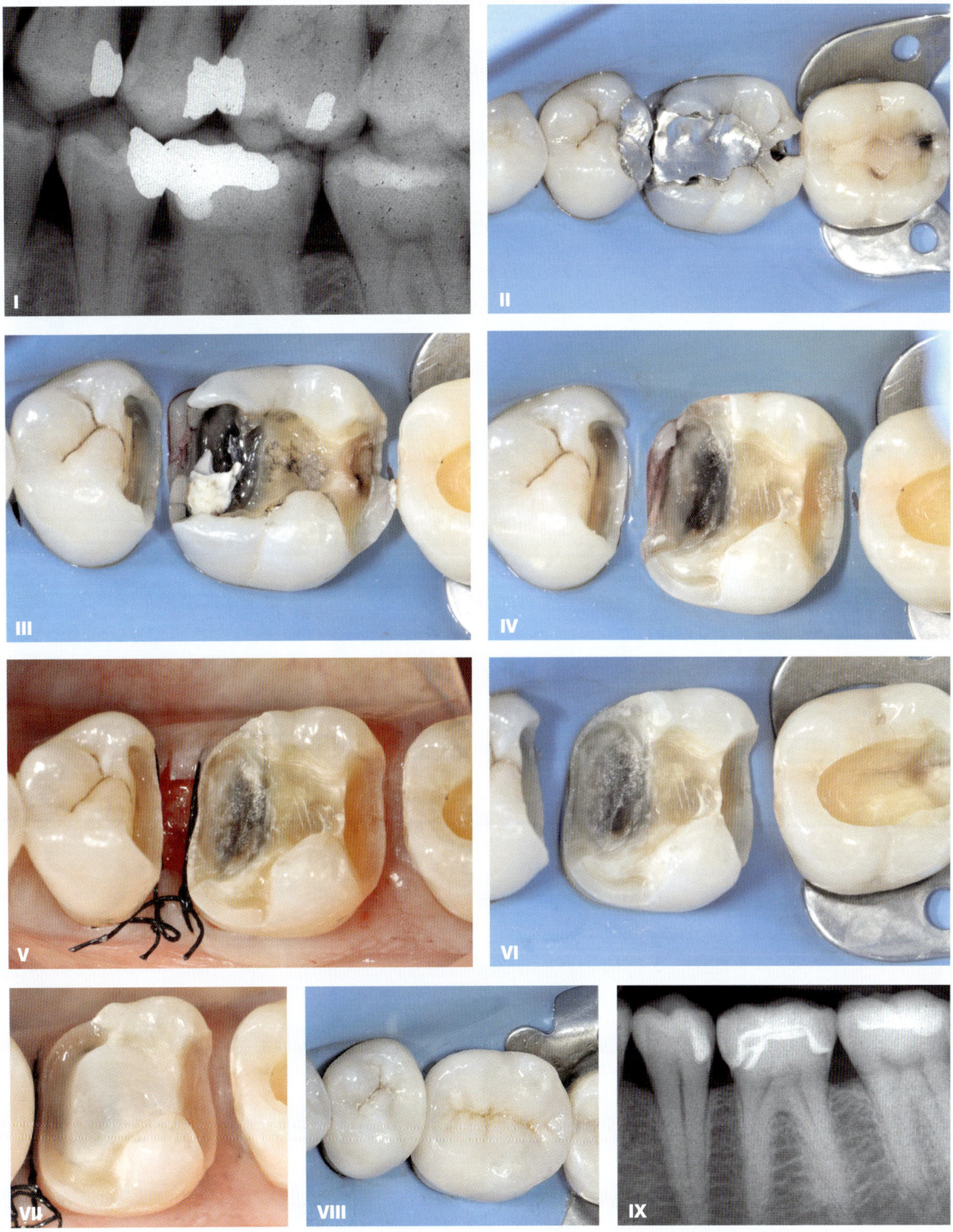

Fig 62 Resolving periodontal issues and caries lesions by means of multidisciplinary therapy.

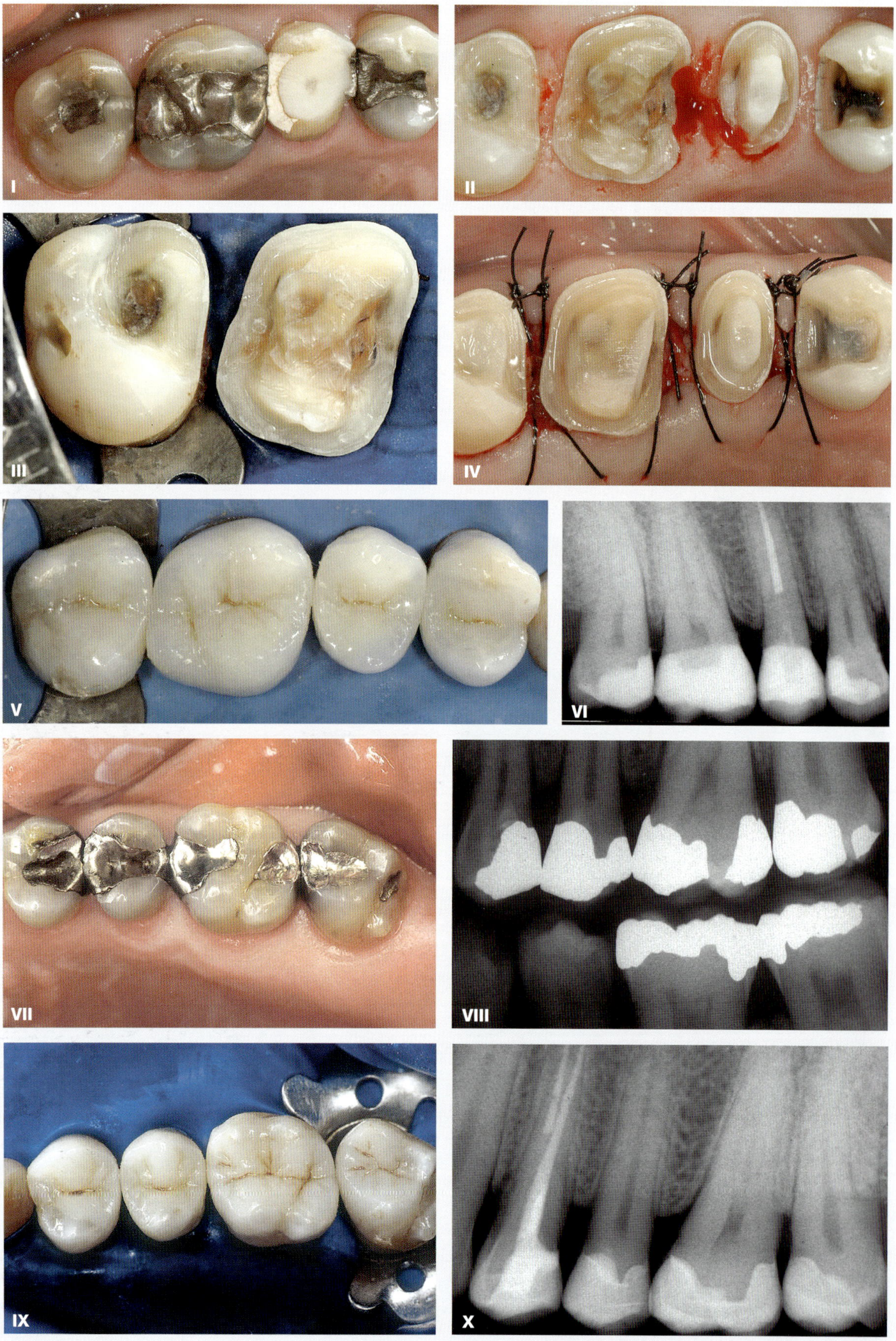

Fig 63 Surgical lengthening of clinical crowns involves all surfaces of the affected teeth. It is imperative to reconstruct a positive periodontal architecture. Ostectomy procedures make it possible to reestablish the appropriate biologic width. Osteoplasty procedures can be used to condition the morphology of soft tissues and obtain an ideal architecture *(I–X)*.

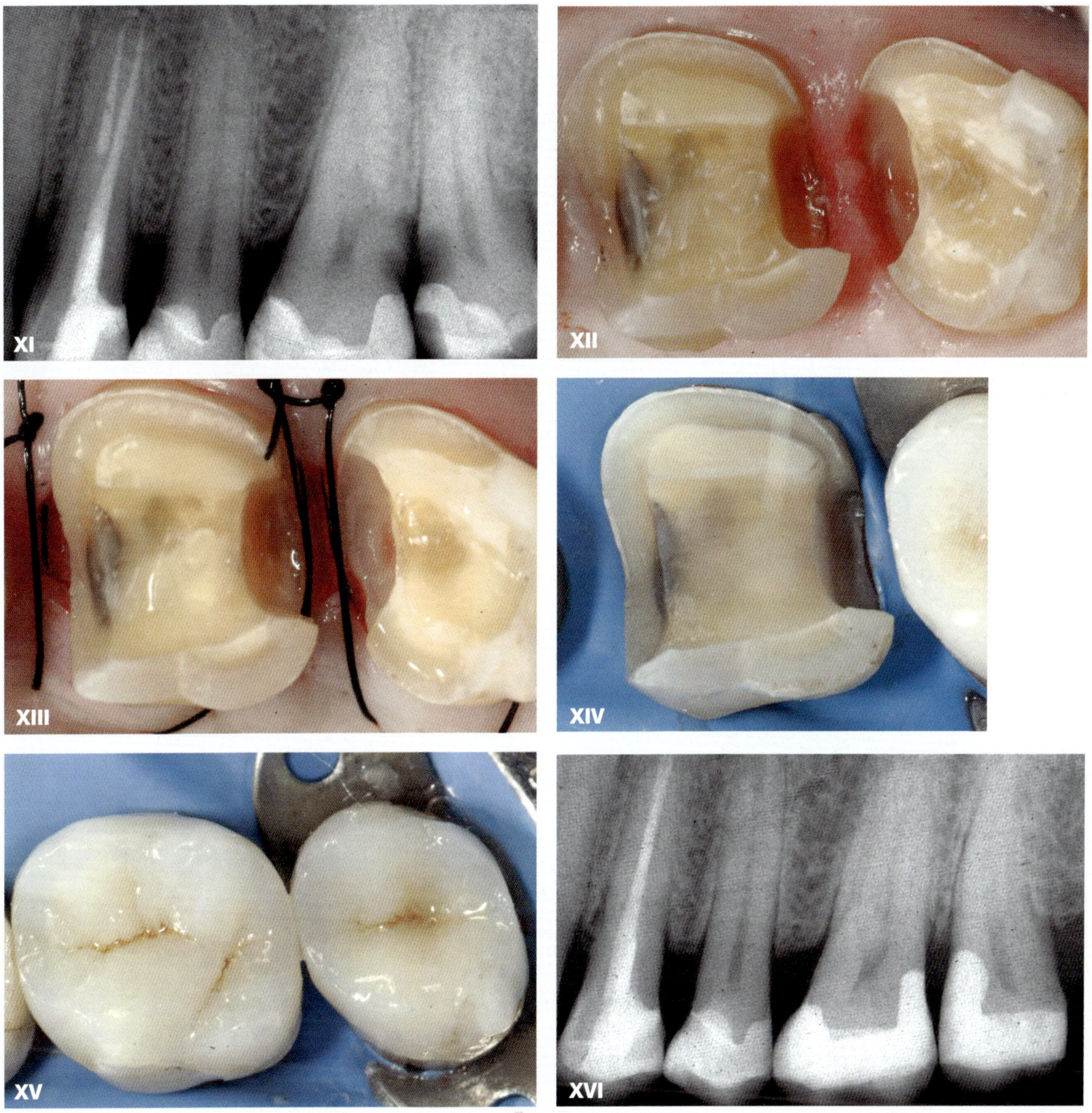

Fig 63 *(continued)* Recurrence of decay in the maxillary left first and second molars *(XI)* resolved using an interdisciplinary technique *(XII–XVI)*.

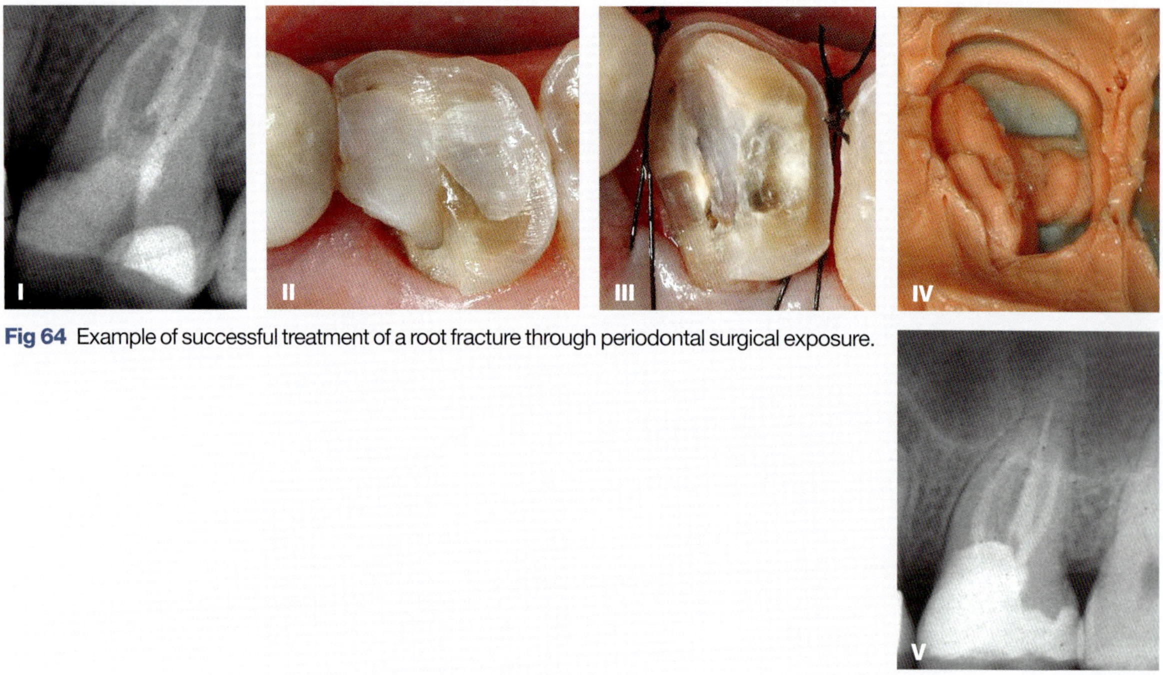

Fig 64 Example of successful treatment of a root fracture through periodontal surgical exposure.

Ostectomy can be used to reconstruct positive architecture. Osteoplasty can be used to condition and guide the morphology of the periodontal soft tissues in a favorable manner and achieve a minimum sulcus depth, thus allowing the patient and hygienist a situation of health that can be maintained over the long term.

The periodontal literature contains clear and detailed principles and techniques for carrying out all the surgical procedures necessary to correct any deformities present and reestablish the correct morphologic standards of positive architecture.

Particular attention should be paid to the concept of "fiber retention," which, following accurate and specific evaluation, allows considerable conservation of periodontal structures and allows a positive architecture to be recovered at a lower biologic cost by preserving all the fibers inserted in the root cement.

The flap must be designed with precision, and the surgical papillae should be extended to cover and protect the alveolar process. This maneuver is easier in wide interproximal spaces and more difficult in tight spaces. The flap is raised to partial thickness, and the blade must sculpt a flap of uniform thickness, with particular attention to corner lines. The periosteum must be maintained where possible to allow a surer and more precise anchorage for the suture, which performs the task of stabilizing the flap in its passive position. Ostectomy maneuvers can be performed quickly and accurately using handheld instruments. The instruments used for osteoplasty, which are useful for guiding and conditioning soft tissue morphology, are rotary, preferably with diamond burs.

Ultrasonic instruments offer an excellent alternative, and some studies have shown that they have a favorable impact on healing processes.

In any case, the periodontal surgery stage can be used to carry out restorative procedures in the same session with maximum control when following a customized protocol.

The visibility and accessibility of all preparation margins guaranteed by periodontal surgery create an ideal situation for the complex restorative maneuvers that can be performed in an optimal manner and, even more importantly, improve individual prognoses to the complete benefit of the patient. This is the "holy grail" of our routine work[8] (Fig 65).

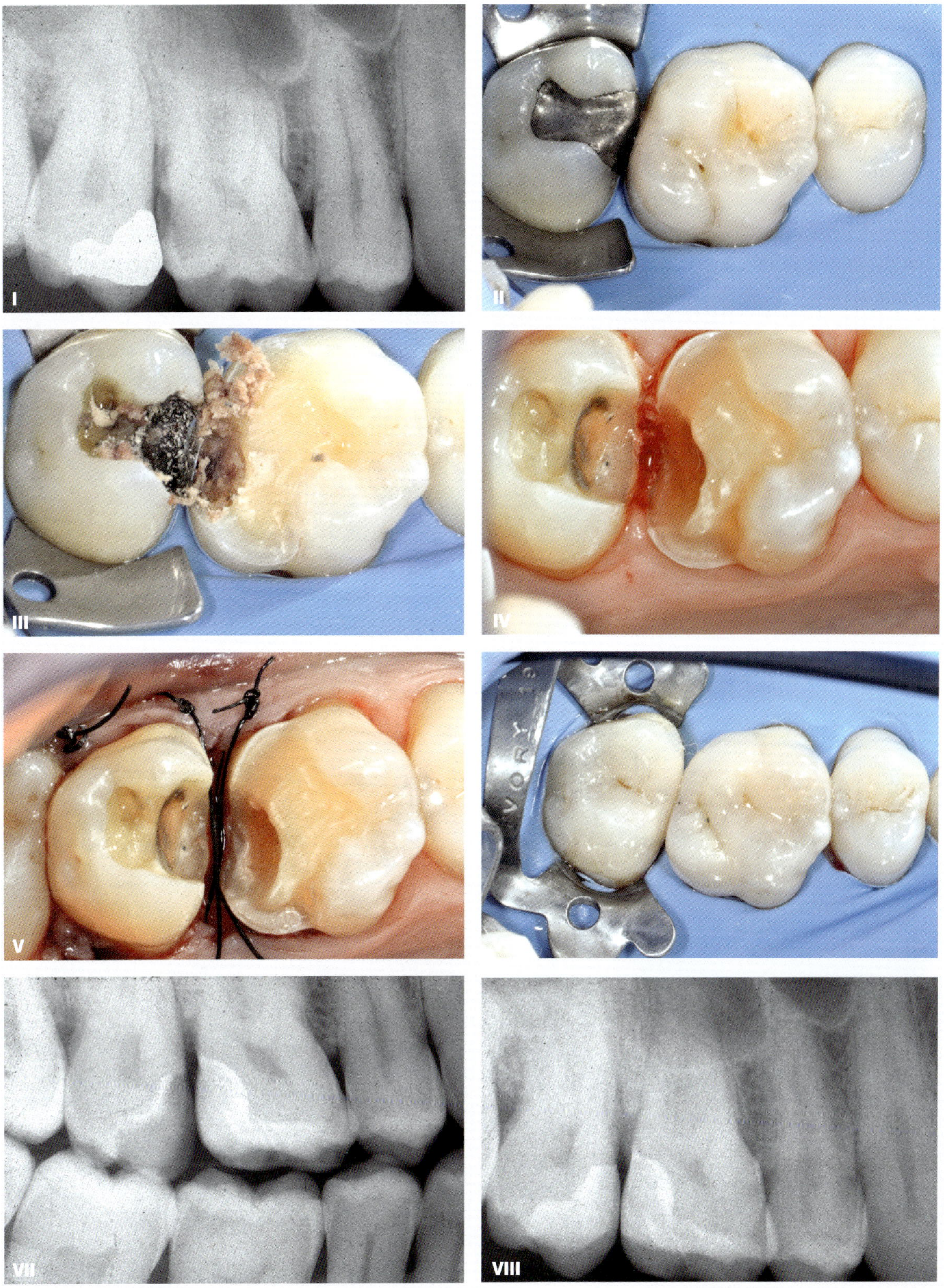

Fig 65 Another case example showing details of the outcome achieved through cooperation between a periodontist and a restorative dentist. (Courtesy of Dr Massimo De Paoli.)

Subgingival caries lesions located in furcation areas are particularly difficult to treat (Fig 66).
In such cases, the possibility of carrying out surgical lengthening of the clinical crown is limited and determined by root trunk length.
The advent of adhesive dentistry has allowed root structures to be maintained intact in such cases while still ensuring appropriate biologic width, while classic dentistry would have required root resection under all circumstances.
While restorative-periodontal treatment becomes more difficult near furcations, this complication is decidedly less severe in the mandibular region, where the furcations are buccal or lingual (Figs 67 to 69). It becomes considerably more significant in the maxillary arch, where the furcations face the interproximal region, no longer involving one tooth, as in the mandible, but two adjacent teeth, thus doubling the risk factors and increasing treatment difficulties.
The area that poses the most problems is the interproximal space located between the maxillary first and second molars (Figs 70 and 71).
This space is very restricted in a mesiodistal direction, somewhat extensive in a buccolingual direction, and very difficult to clean. Gingival epithelium is not keratinized and has a limited number of layers with reduced defensive capabilities. The roots tend to grow close to one another, making the septum very thin for a distance that may reach the apical third.
The area should be considered particularly vulnerable, with a high risk of periodontal and caries lesions.
Under such conditions, adhesive reconstruction and periodontal surgery make it possible to treat this difficult area with success.
With the possibility of maintaining an intact dental structure and also tooth vitality in most cases, clinicians can add an extremely worthwhile and effective therapeutic method to their arsenal that they could not even have dreamed of a few decades ago.
This treatment is all the more valuable when one considers that it is often indicated in young patients.

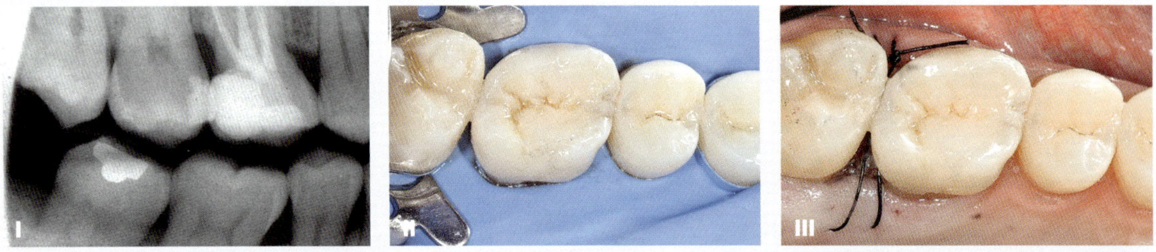

Fig 66 Deep distal decay of the maxillary right first molar. This case is also treated through cooperation between the periodontist and restorative dentist.

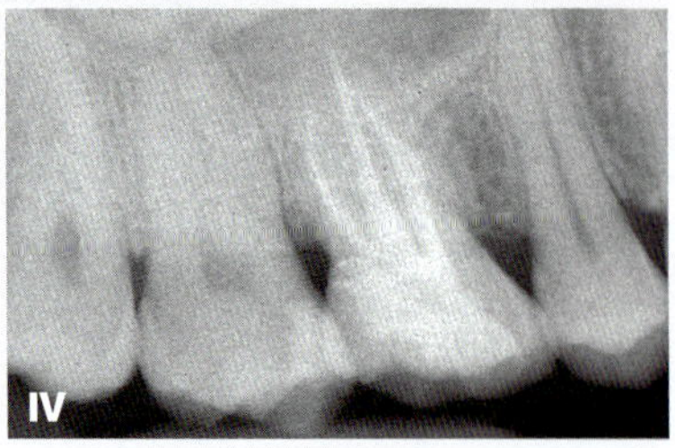

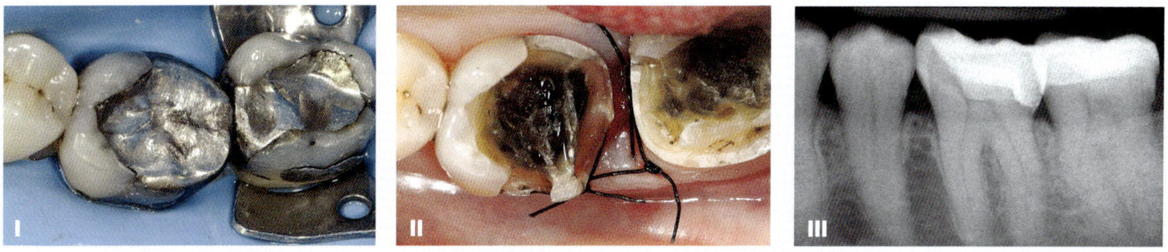

Fig 67 Clinical example showing restoration of severely compromised teeth. Periodontal surgery allows exposure of the margins, protection of the furcations, and development of proper biologic width. Selective flap design safeguards healthy periodontal areas that are not affected by dental disease.

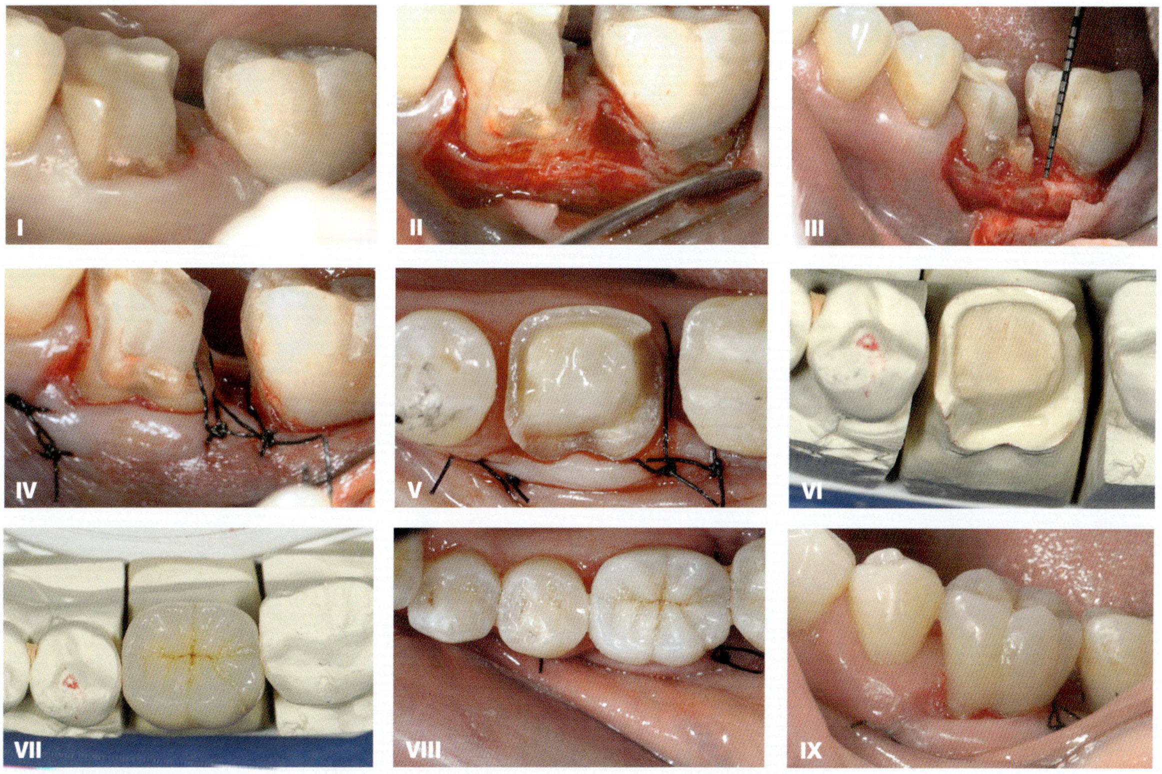

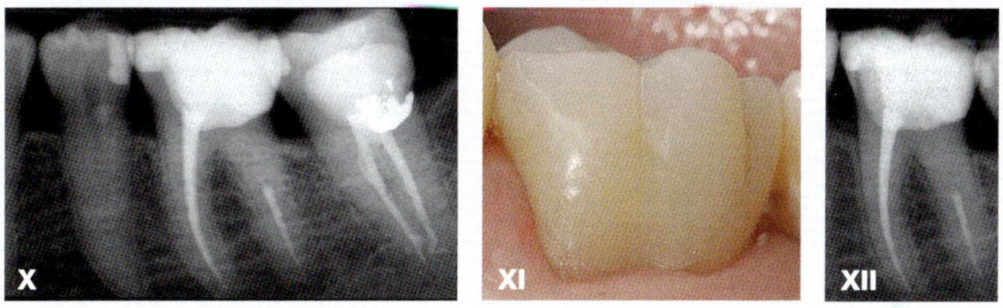

Fig 68 Complicated clinical case in which periodontal surgery was essential to expose the distobuccal margins *(I–V)*. The impression taken immediately after surgery and preparation produced a study cast that allowed the dental technician to work under the best conditions to produce the prosthesis *(VI–X)*. Clinical and radiographic 5-year follow-up *(XI, XII)*.

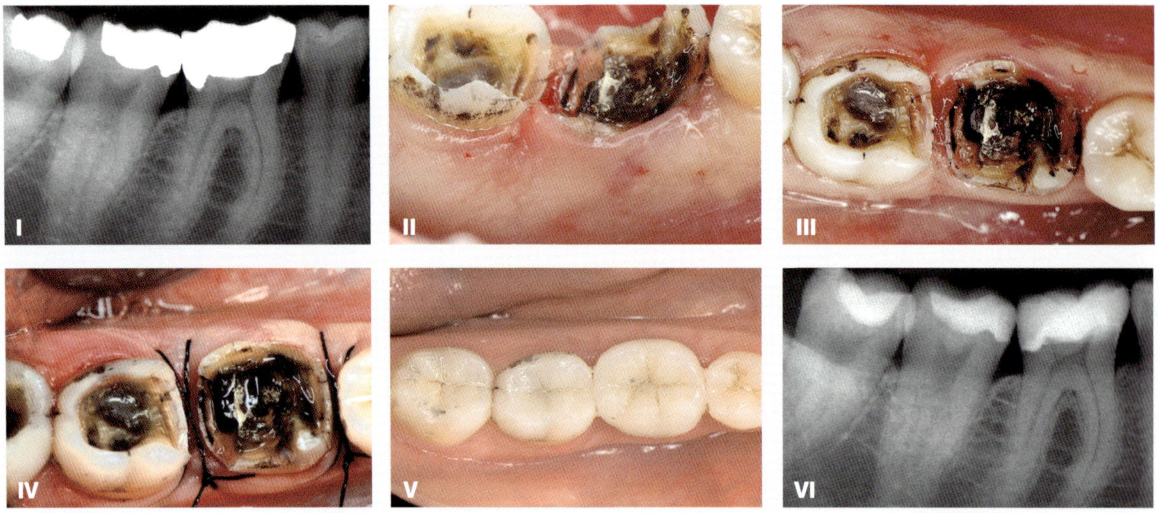

Fig 69 Another very complicated clinical situation that could never have been resolved without the aid of a periodontist. The reason for replacing the amalgam restorations was fracture of the mandibular right first molar restoration. Inlays were placed in the first and second molars, and a direct technique was used for the third molar.

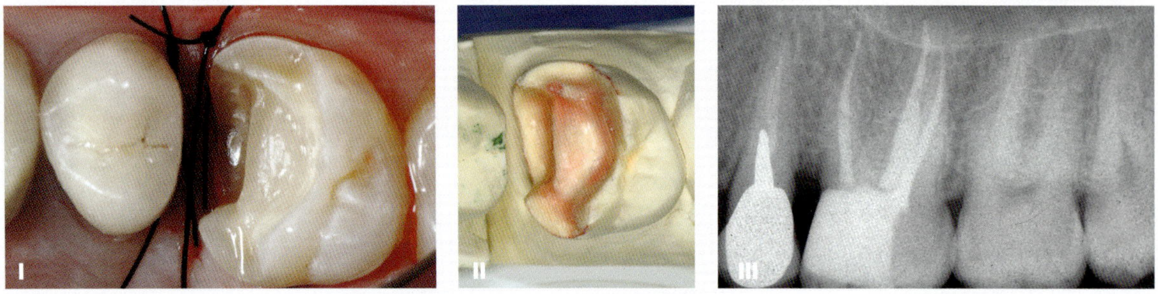

Fig 70 Surgical lengthening of the clinical crown allowed restoration of a critical area *(I, II)*. Follow-up radiographs after 4 years *(III)*.

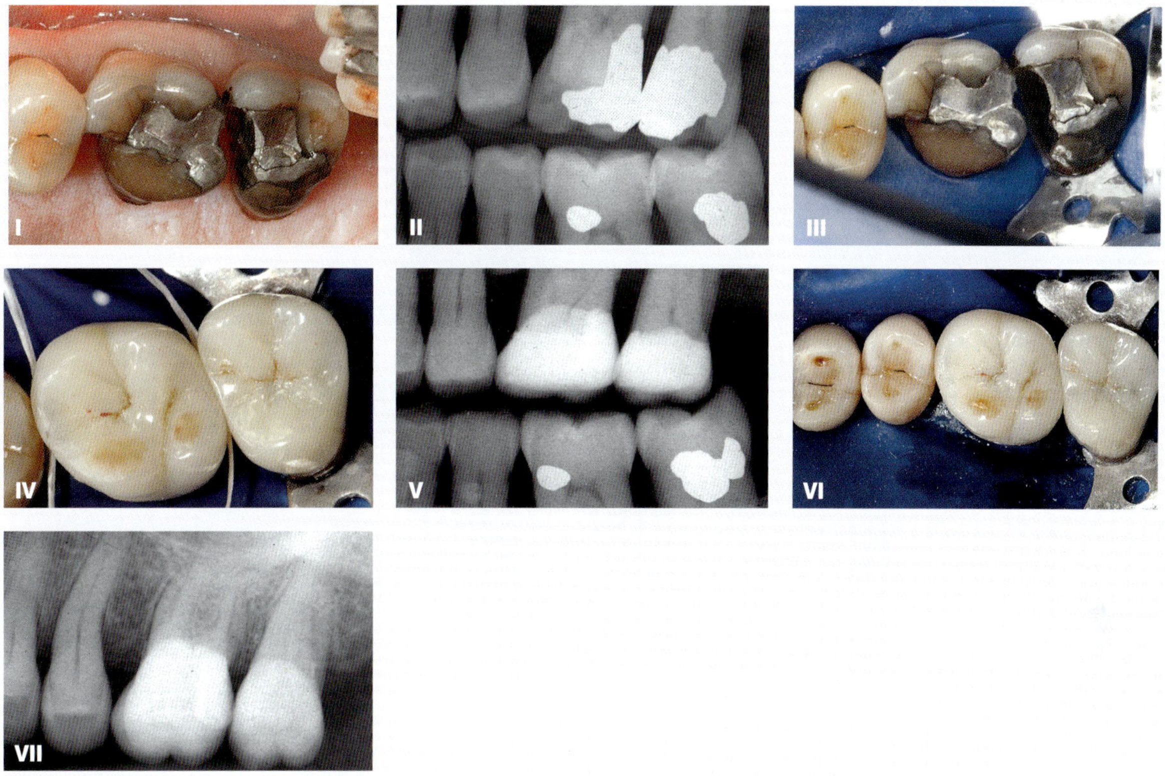

Fig 71 Recovery of deep coronal fractures *(I–VI)*. Radiograph at 8-year follow-up *(VII)*.

The complex clinical cases presented in Figs 72 to 76 and the clinical examples in Fig 77 illustrate the practical application of the concepts described above.

Clinical cases

Clinical case 1

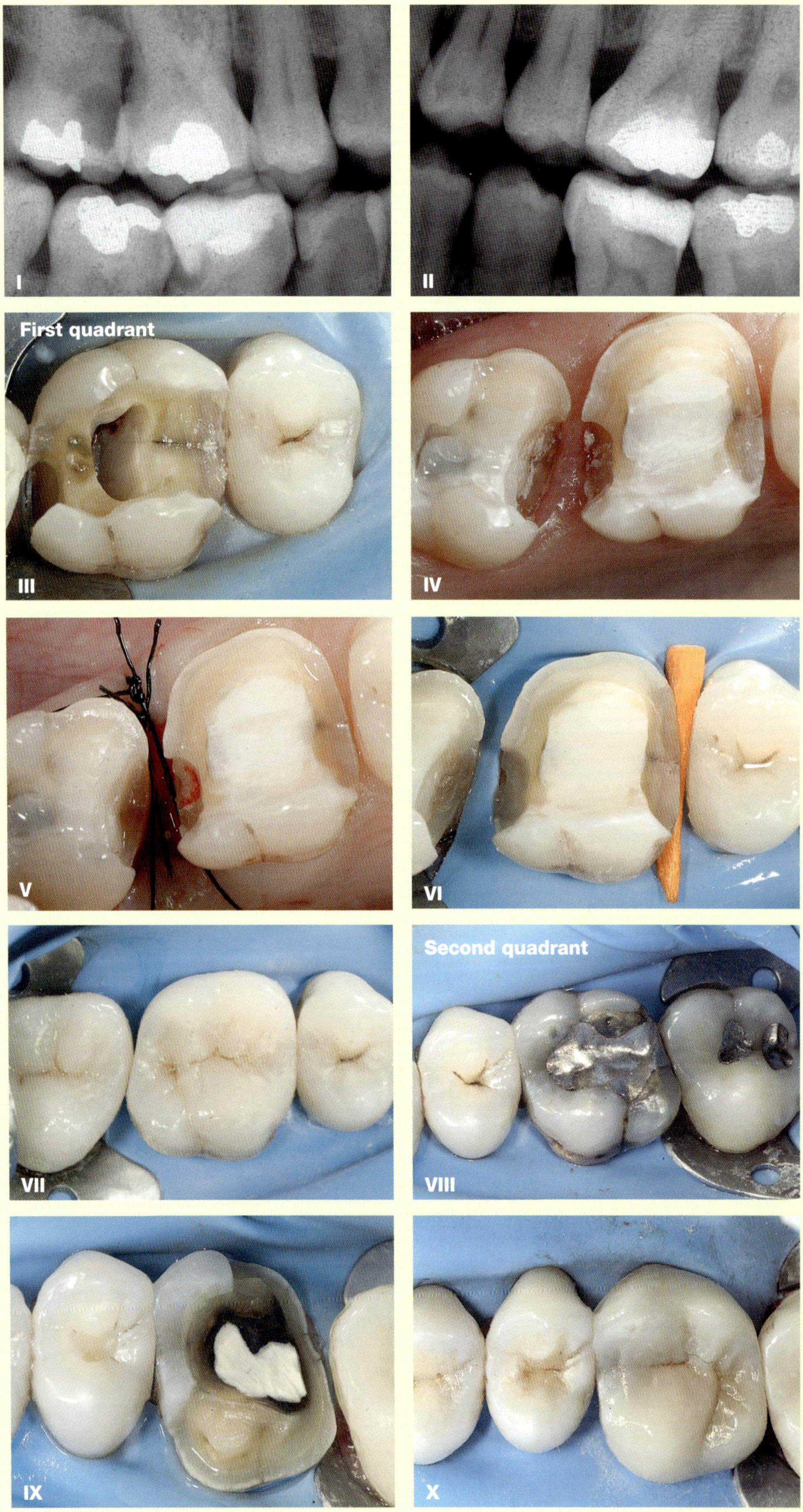

Fig 72 Bitewing radiographs revealed the presence of deep caries lesions *(I, II)*. In the maxillary right (first) quadrant, presence of a significant fracture line running from the margin toward the pulp chamber in the first molar *(III)* and view of the interproximal space between the first and second molars before and after periodontal surgery *(IV, V)*. Cemented inlays *(VI, VII)*. In the maxillary left (second) quadrant, intraoperative stages of preparation of the first molar under rubber dam *(VIII, IX)* and cemented restoration *(X)*. Occlusal and radiographic views of the mandible of the same patient *(XI–XIII)*. In the mandibular left (third) quadrant, after endodontic treatment due to pulpitis of the first molar, the multidisciplinary stage continued with preparation of an onlay for that tooth and periodontal surgery and removal of mesial and occlusal decayed tissue in the second molar *(XIV–XIX)*. Direct restorations in the second molar and cementation of an onlay in the first molar *(XX–XXII)*. Multidisciplinary treatment was also carried out in the mandibular right (fourth) quadrant with the placement of inlays *(XXIII–XXVII)*. Follow-up radiographs in the mandibular arch reveal removal of a significant surplus of composite after cementation of the right first molar, marginal seals, and emergence profiles, and a clinical occlusal view of the arch shows the cemented restorations *(XXVIII–XXXII)*. Clinical and radiographic follow-up after 4 years *(XXXIII–XXXVI)*.

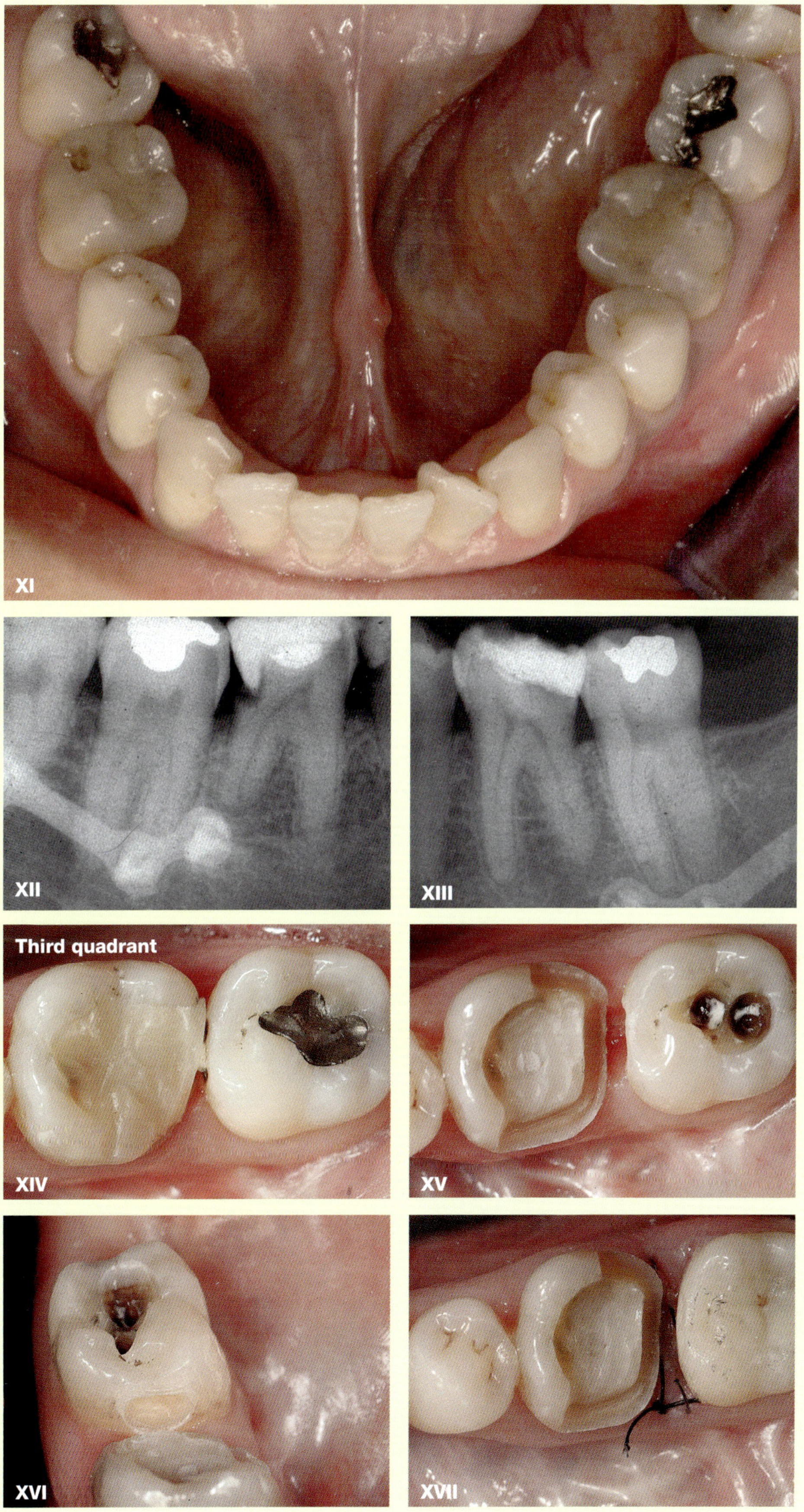

Fig 72 *(continued)*

Fig 72 *(continued)*

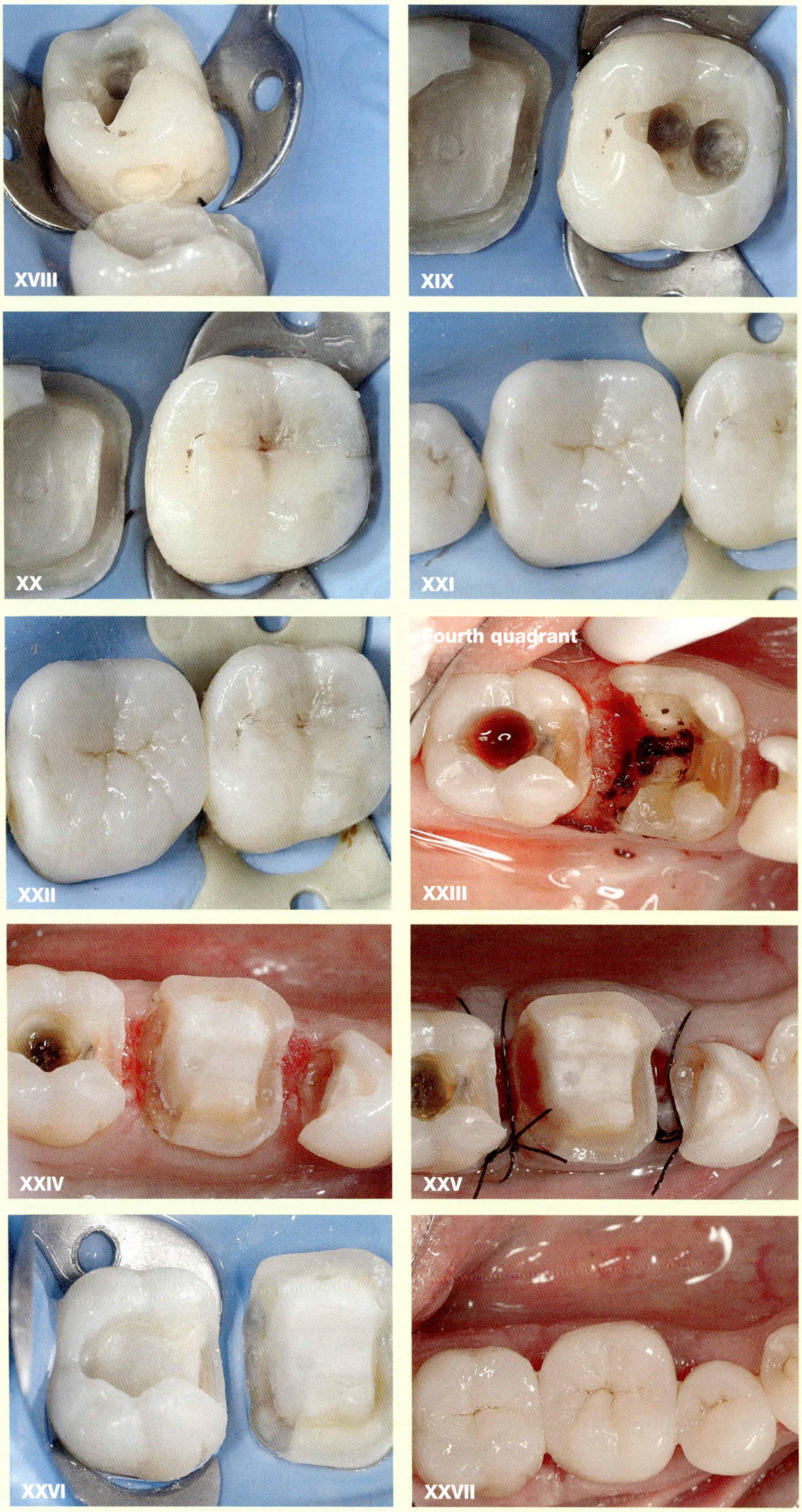

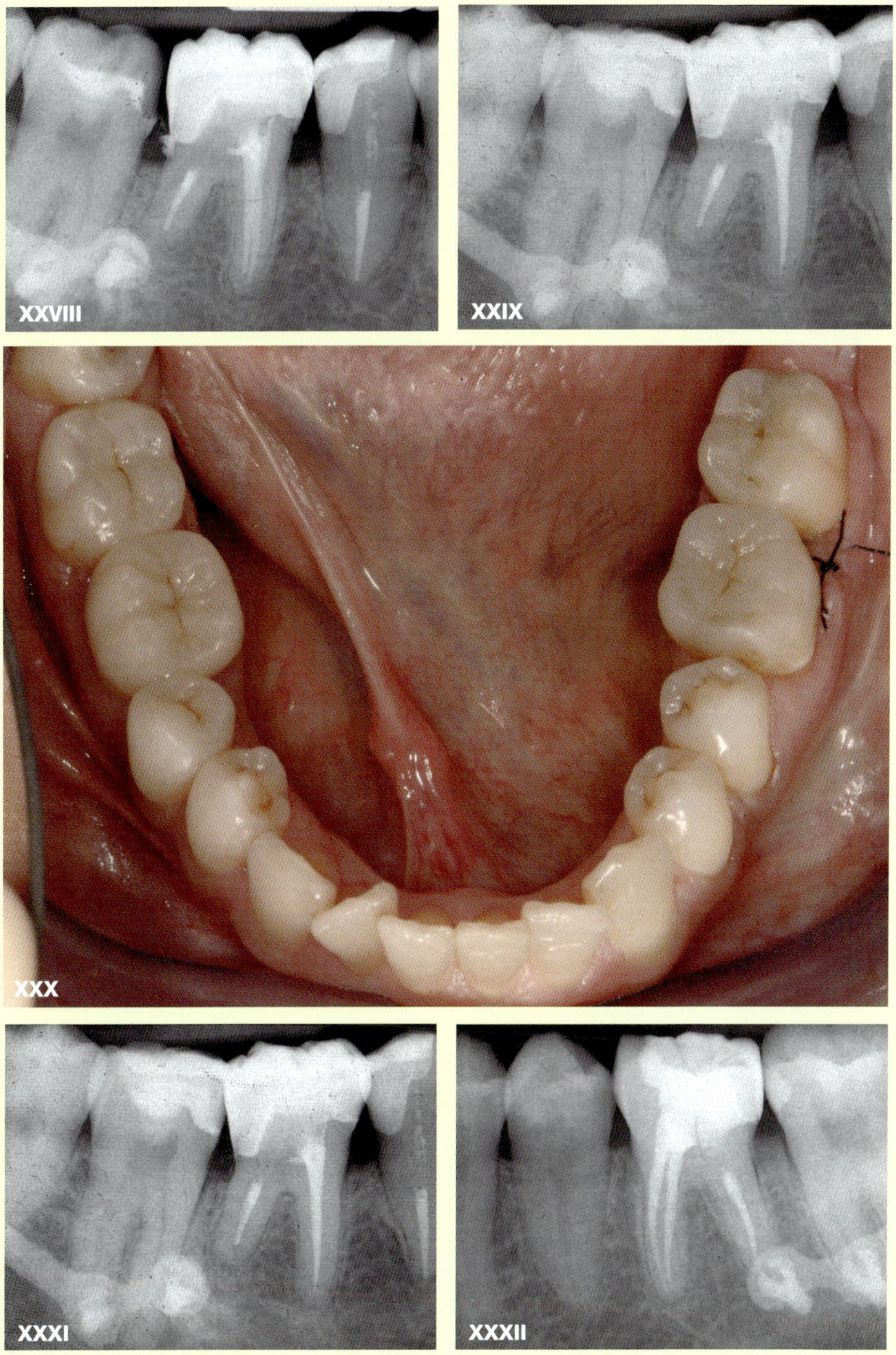

Fig 72 *(continued)*

Fig 72 *(continued)*

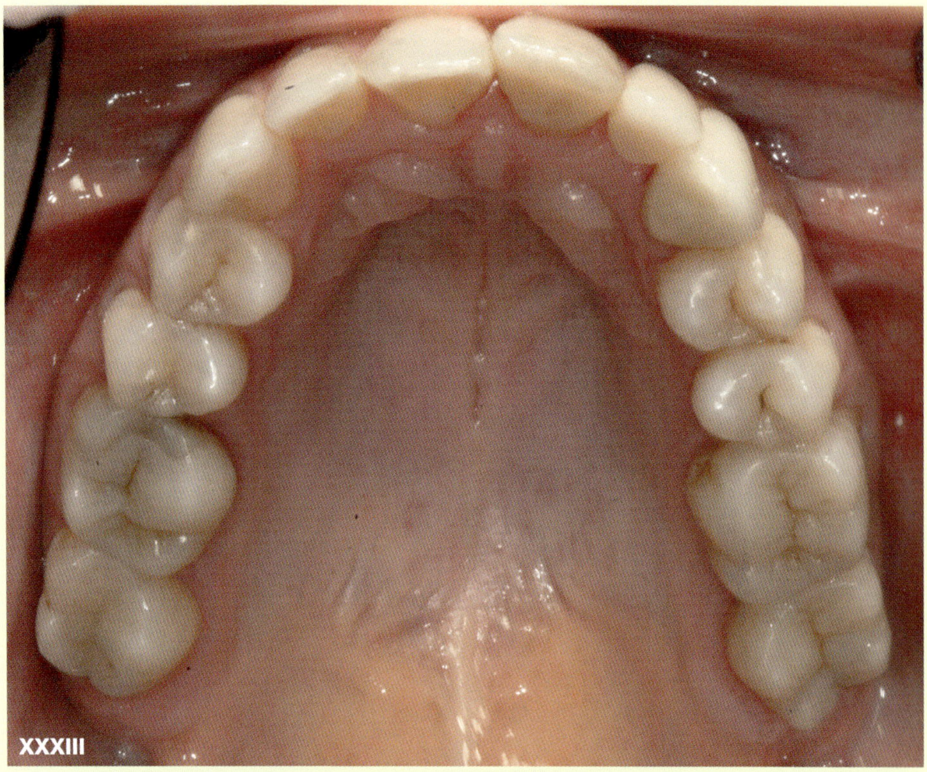

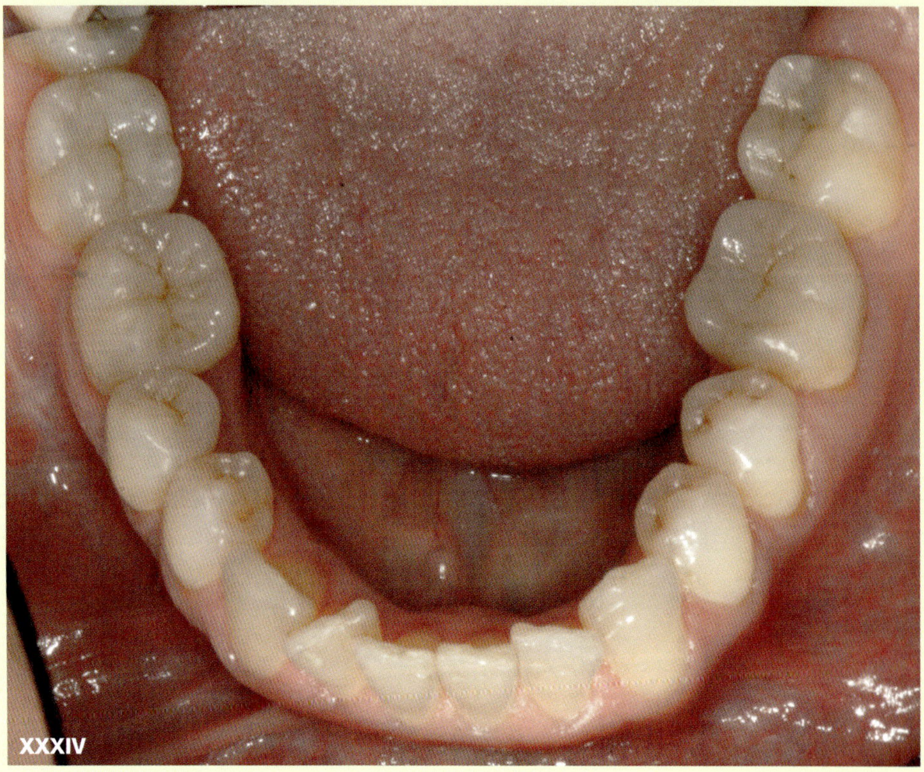

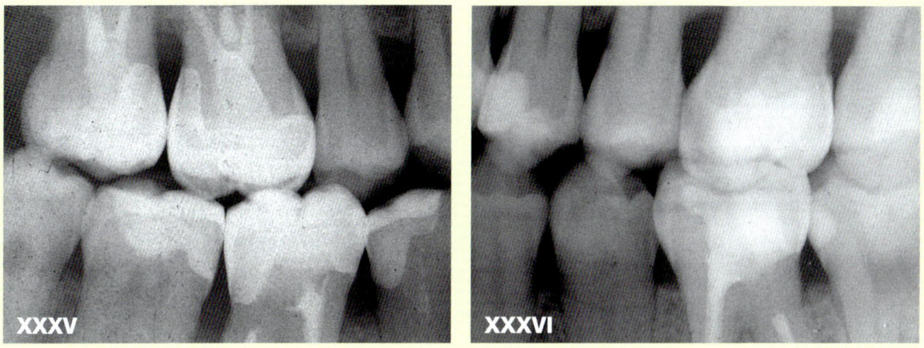

Fig 72 *(continued)*

Clinical case 2

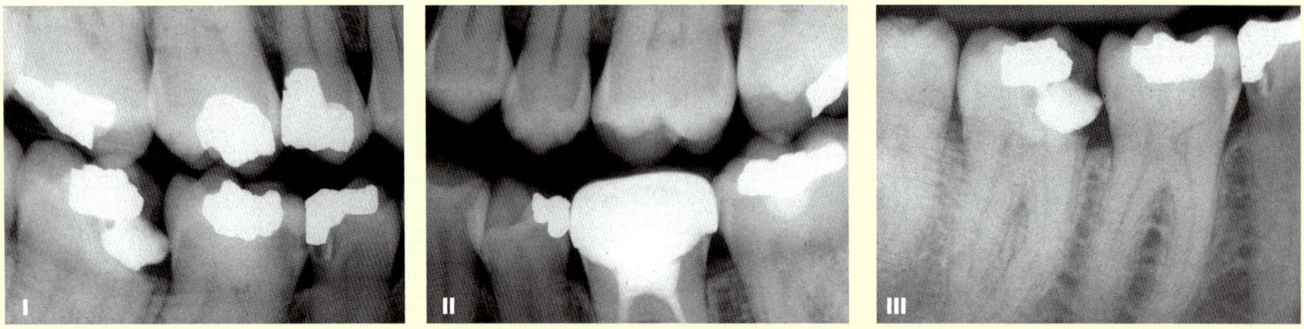

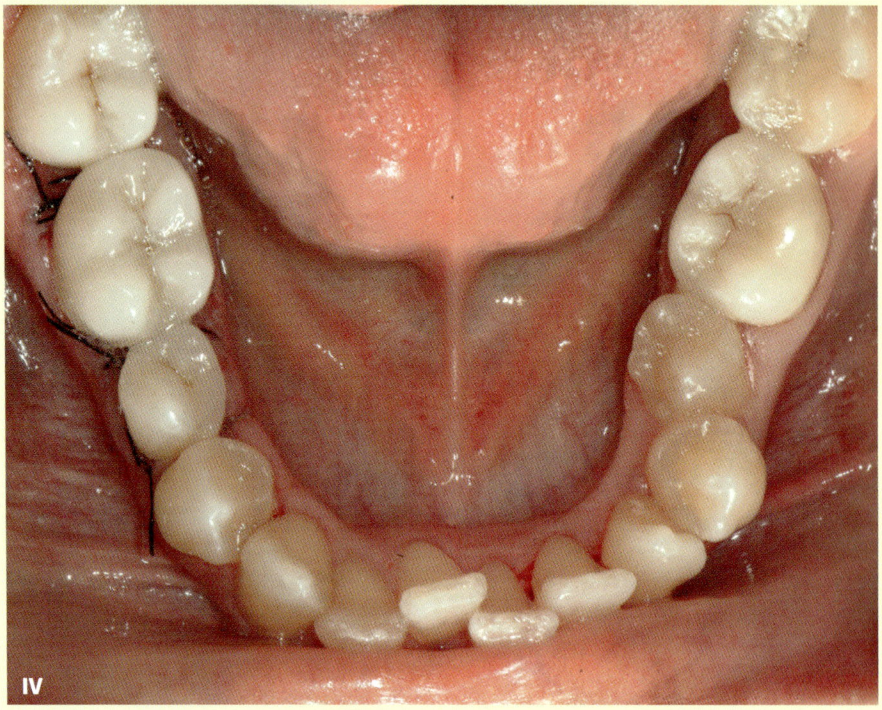

Fig 73 The patient presented with severe pain in the mandibular right quadrant, where radiographic examination *(I–III)* revealed penetrating decay in the second molar and deep decay in the second premolar and first molar. Caries lesions were found in the other quadrants. Interdisciplinary treatment is especially essential in such cases. After endodontic treatment of the mandibular right second molar, the second premolar and first molar were finished with indirect restorations *(IV)*. The accuracy of the marginal seals was achieved through surgical periodontal treatment. Note that, despite guaranteeing biologic width, the restoration margin on the second molar looks very close to the alveolar ridge due to anatomical reasons related to the vertical axis of the radiographic examination *(V, VII)*. The relationship between the restorations and the alveolar ridge is shown to be stable at a 4-year follow-up *(IX)*. As usual, in the absence of irreversible pulp disease, pulp vitality was maintained in the mandibular right first molar, while the presence of decay and an old restoration in the maxillary right second premolar prompted endodontic treatment. In the mandibular left quadrant, it was possible to replace an incorrect prosthetic crown with a full-coverage restoration with supragingival margins *(VI, VIII)*. The patient was strongly encouraged to pursue an orthodontic approach but declined.

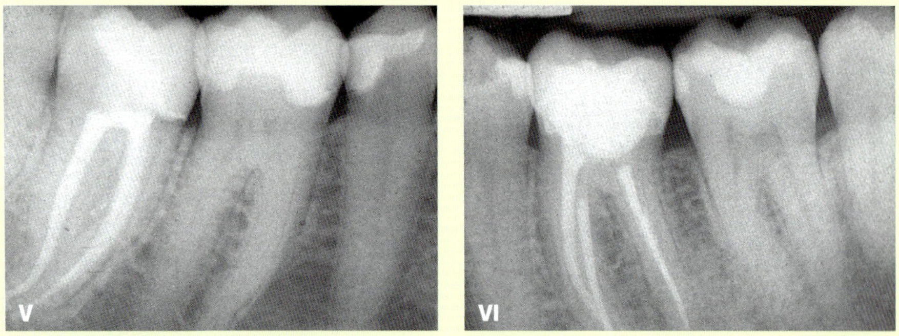

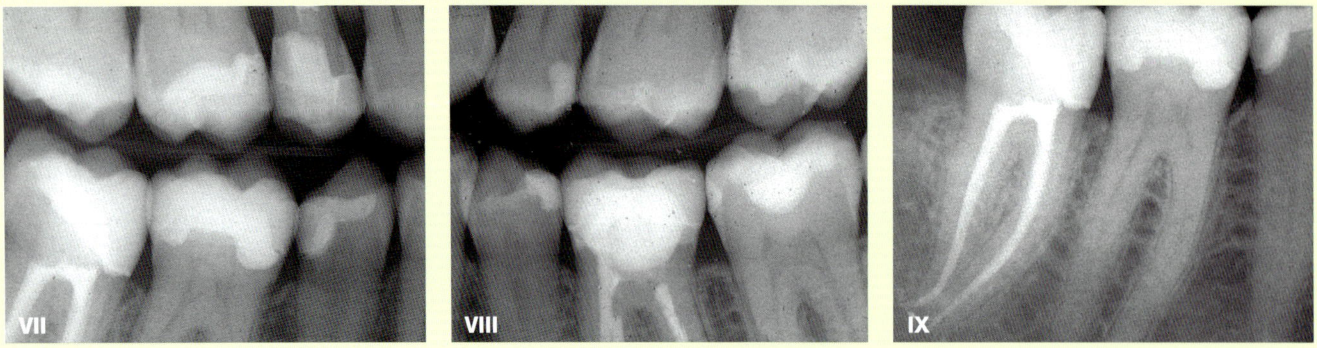

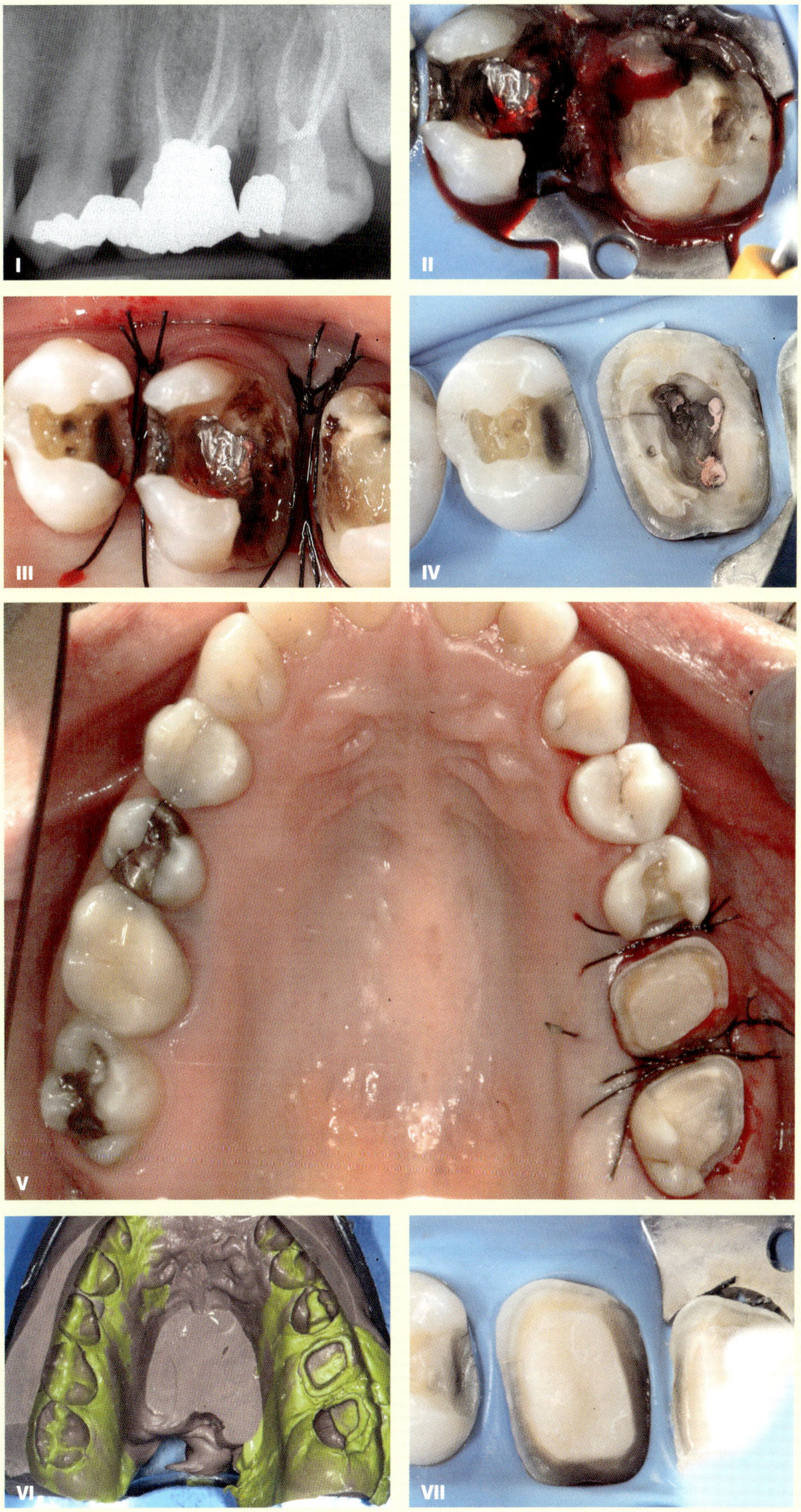

Clinical case 3

Fig 74 Reconstruction of a maxillary arch showing that the endodontically treated left first molar contains an amalgam filling and has a very defective marginal seal *(I)*. The difference between the tooth-periodontal relationships during the pre- and postsurgical stages is striking *(II–XI)*. At one stage of the cementation of restorations, rubber dam was removed *(IX)* in order to finish the distal margin of the first molar as accurately as possible *(XII)*. Clinical views of the maxillary left quadrant on the day that the sutures were removed *(XIII)* and 1 month later *(XIV)*. Occlusal view of the mandible *(XV)* and intraoperative stages showing management of the mandibular left quadrant *(XVI–XX)*.

Fig 74 *(continued)*

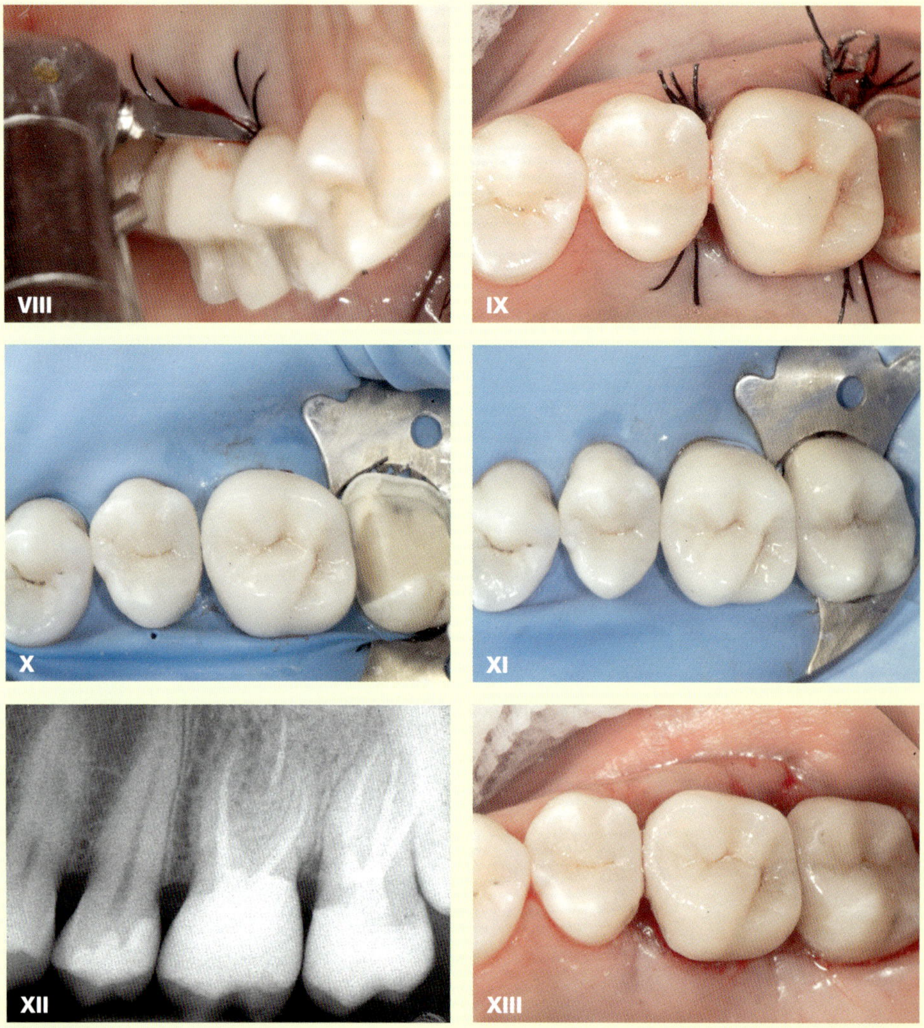

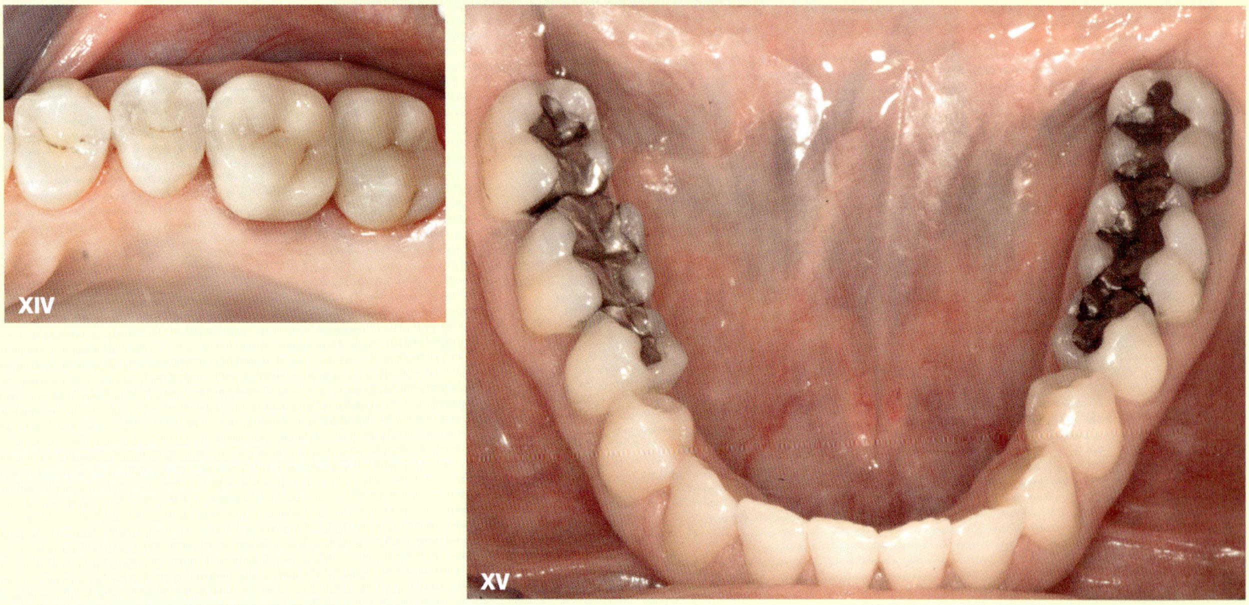

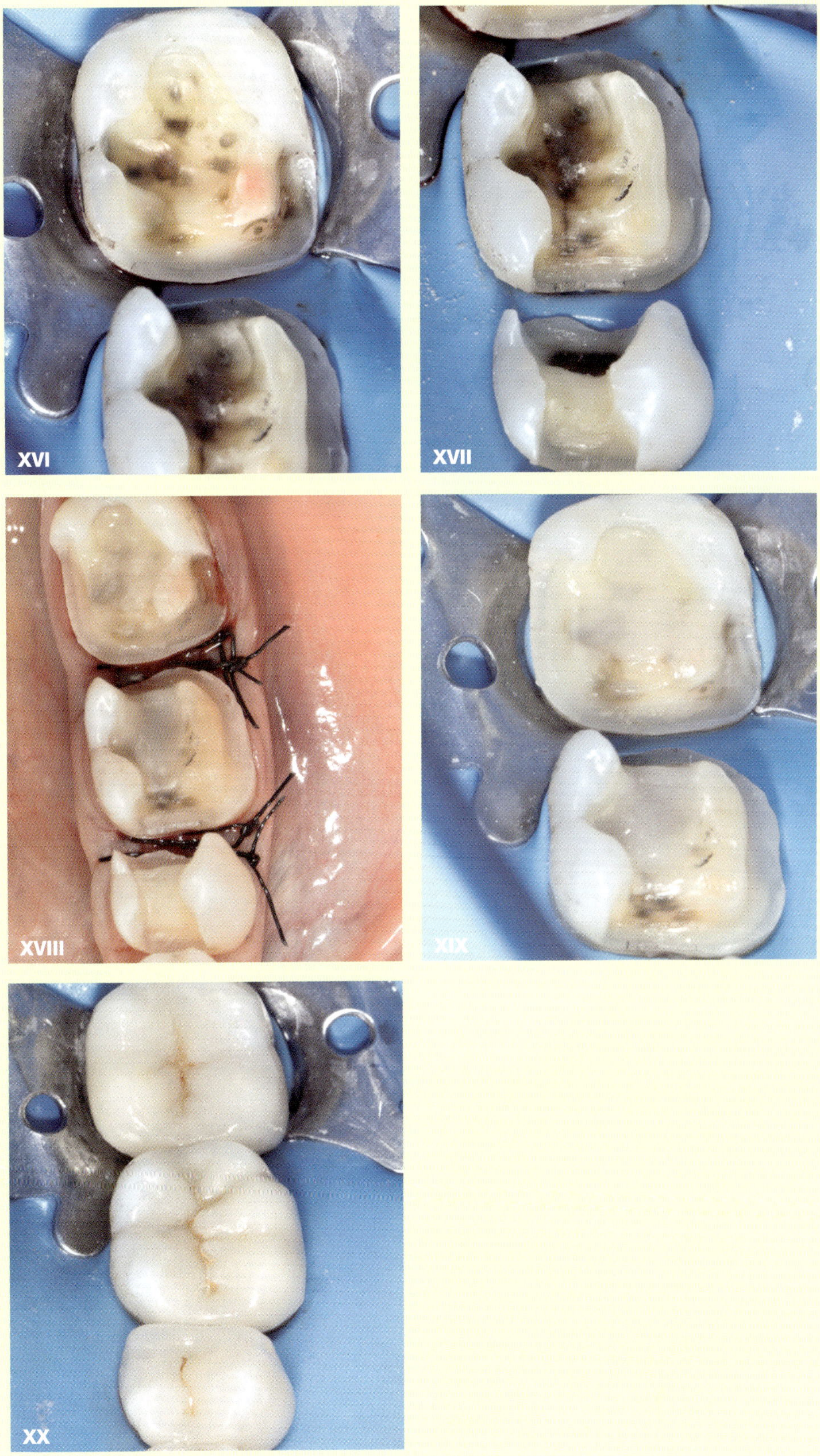

Fig 74 *(continued)*

Clinical case 4

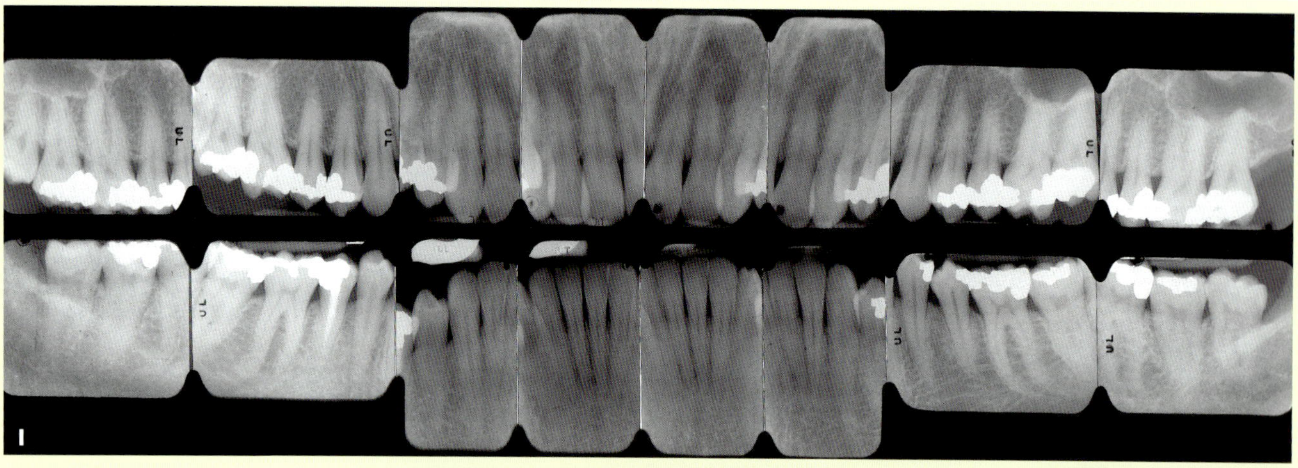

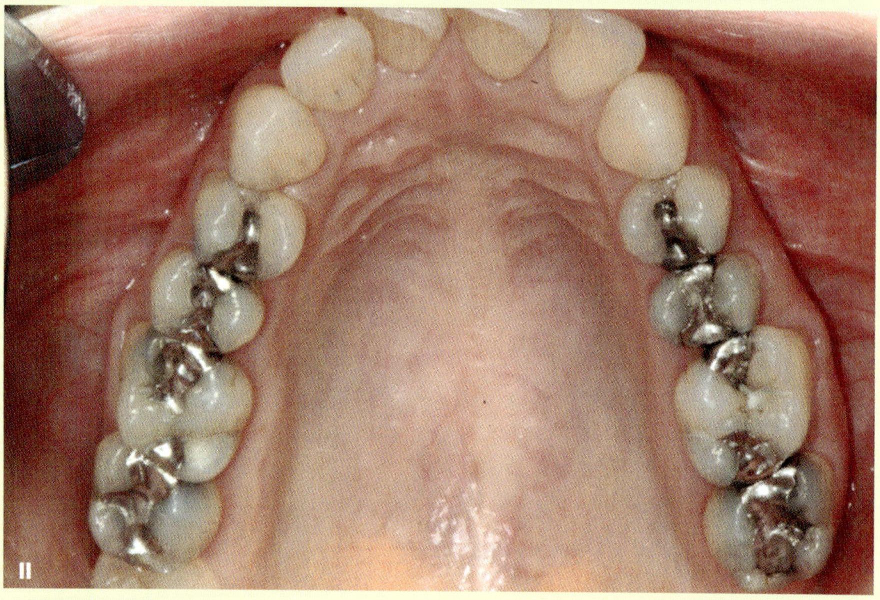

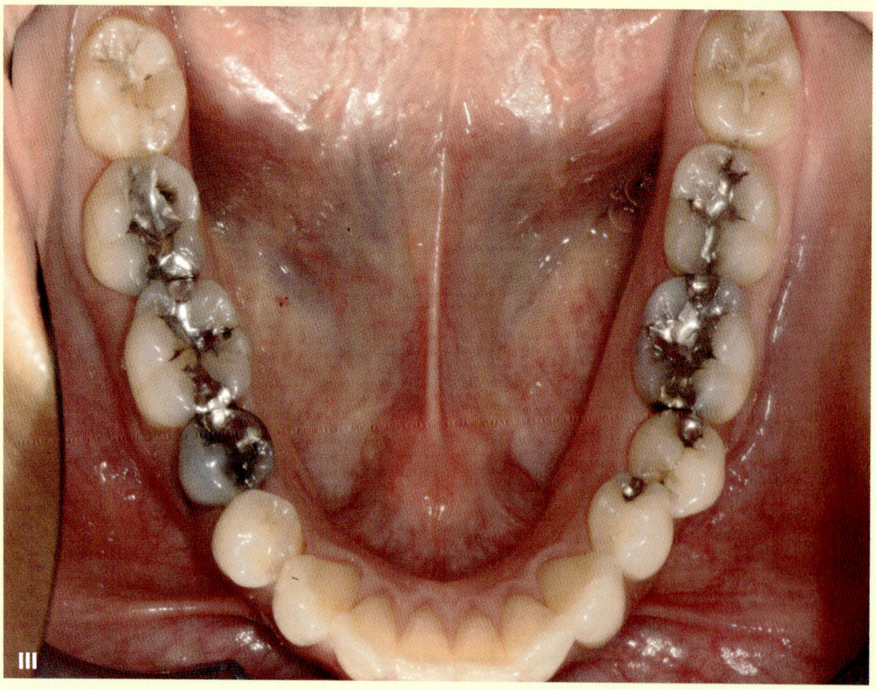

Fig 75 Radiographic and clinical views of both arches with amalgam restorations *(I–III)*. Treatment was carried out at the request of the patient for esthetic reasons. Multidisciplinary intraoperative stages during restoration of the mandibular left (third) quadrant *(IV–VII)*. In the maxillary right (first) quadrant, views showing rubber dam torn during removal of the metal restorations *(VIII–XI)*, the pre- and postsurgical stages *(XII, XIII)*, repositioning of dam during the same session in order to carry out internal reconstruction *(XIV, XV)*, preparations *(XVI, XVII)*, working cast *(XVIII)*, and the cemented indirect restorations *(XIX)*. Clinical views showing some multidisciplinary stages of the restoration in the maxillary left (second) quadrant *(XX–XXV)* and occlusal views of both restored arches *(XXVI, XXVII)*.

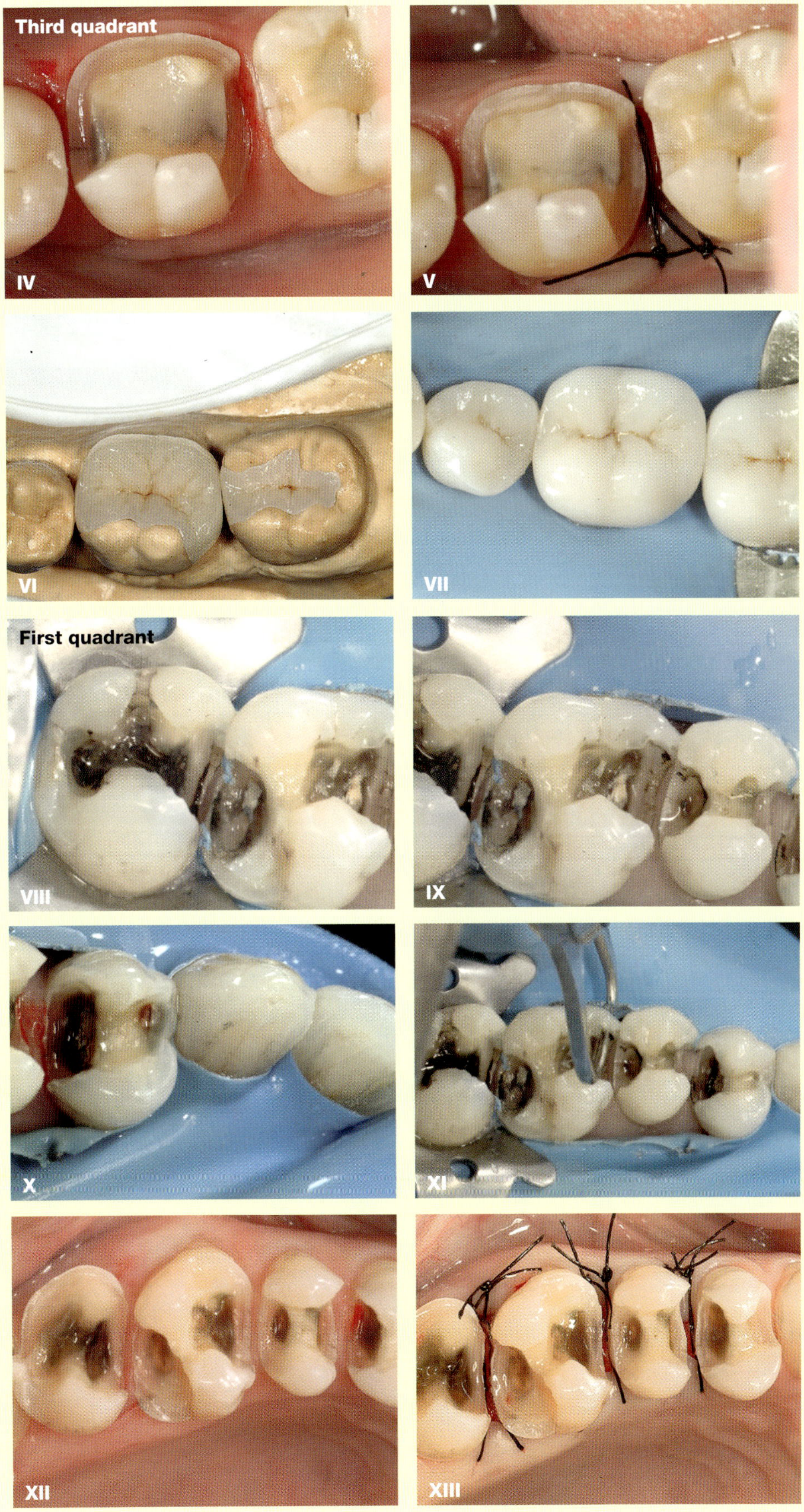

Fig 75 *(continued)*

Fig 75 *(continued)*

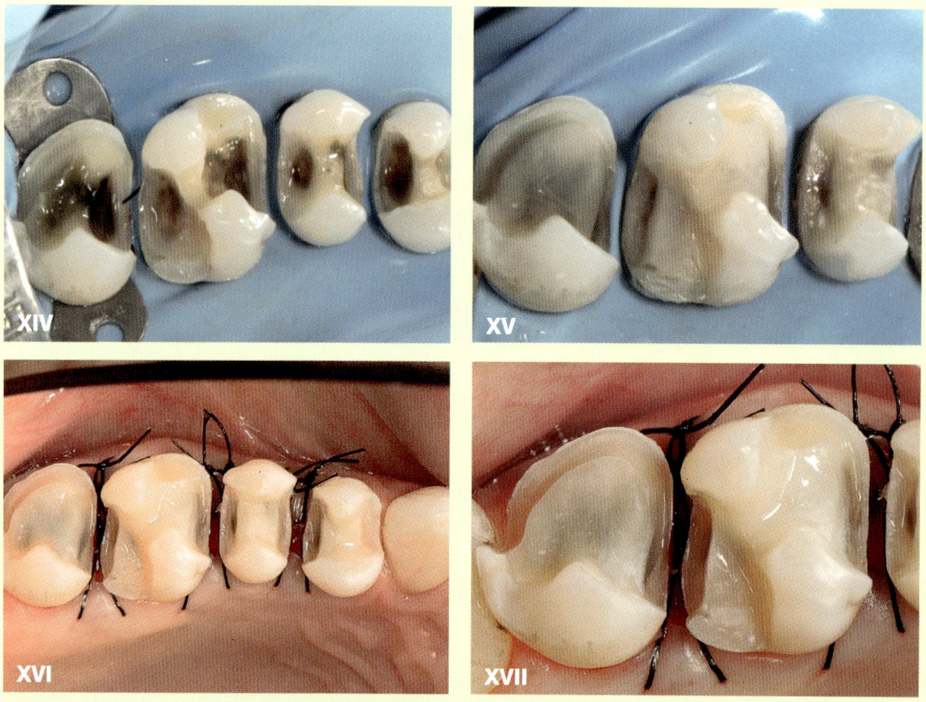

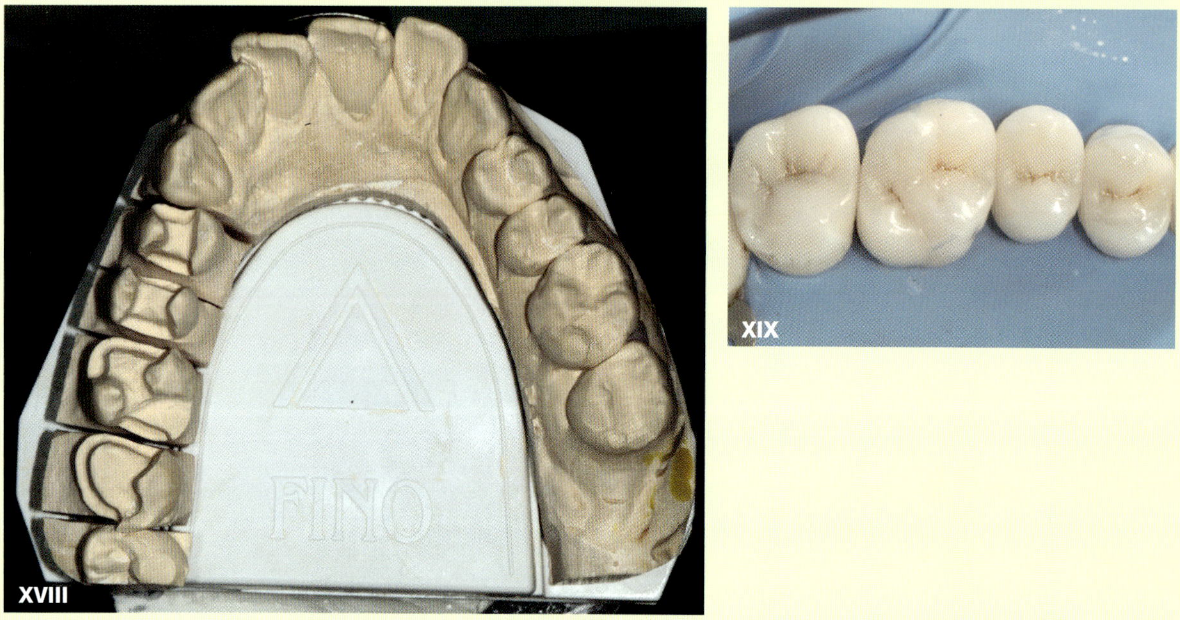

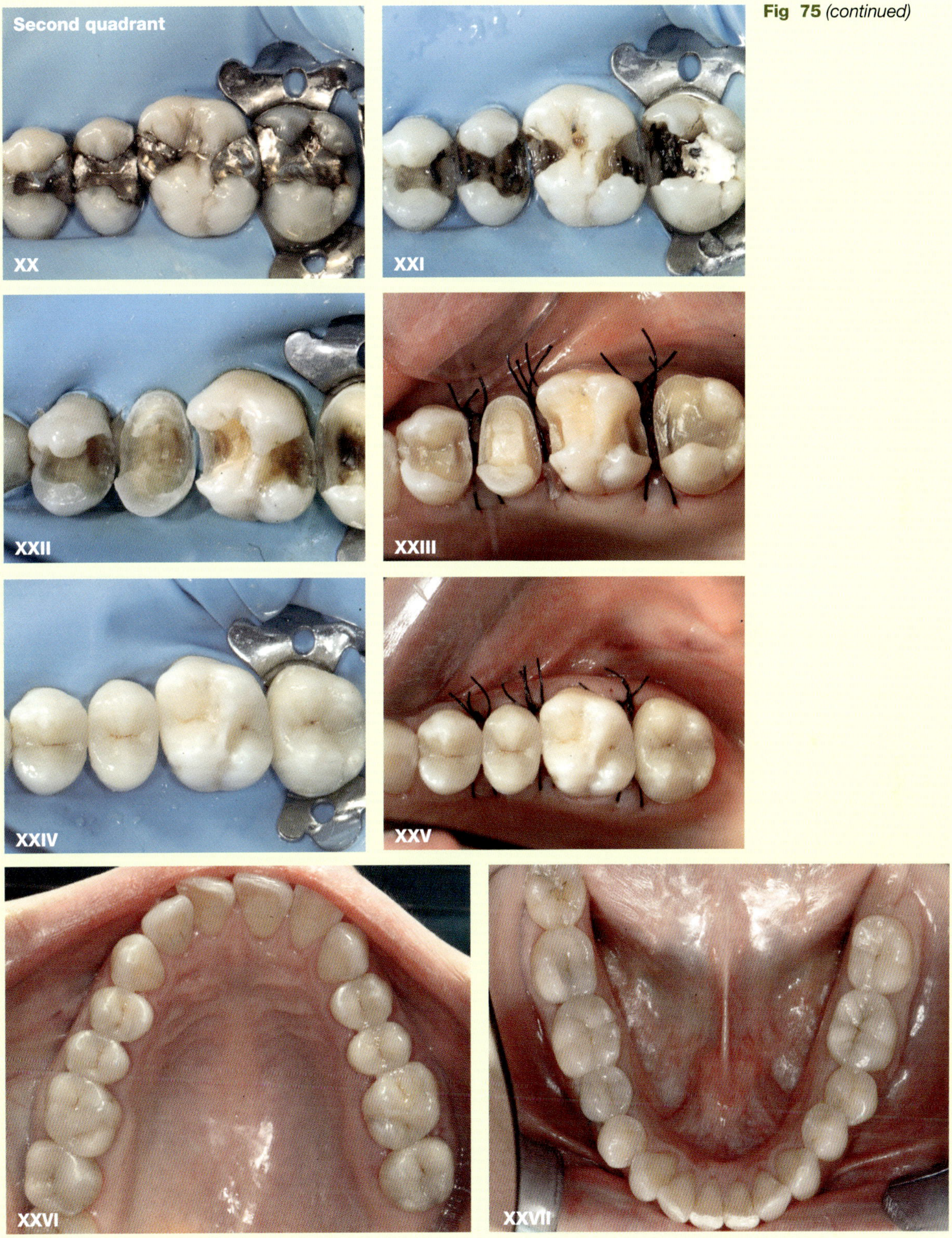

Fig 75 *(continued)*

Clinical case 5

Fig 76 Exposure of the margins and surgical lengthening of the clinical crown make it possible to apply an overlay to replace a previous metal-ceramic crown on the mandibular right first molar. In the new reconstruction, the margins are more accessible for hygiene procedures by the hygienist as well as the patient. One other benefit is the ease of instrumental and visual control by the practitioner. Preoperative radiographic view *(I)*. Removal of old restoration and decayed tissue from the mandibular right second molar *(II–IV)*. Removal of the metal-ceramic crown and evident decayed tissue *(V–VII)*. Formation of buildup and both molars after lengthening of the clinical crown *(VIII–XI)*. Occlusal and buccal views of cemented restorations *(XII–XIV)*. Follow-up radiographs before and after marginal finishing of both molars *(XV, XVI)*. Identical therapeutic approach for the mandibular left (third) quadrant *(XVII–XXIX)*. It should be emphasized that several blood spots may appear during finishing of the tooth-restoration margins under rubber dam once curing has been carried out and with surgical lengthening performed a few days earlier. In the author's opinion, it would be a sad state of affairs if new rubber dam had to be fitted merely to take an artificially pristine photograph. Occlusal view of the mandible and clinical and radiographic images of restorations in the mandibular left quadrant *(XXX–XXXII)*. Occlusal views at 4-year follow-up after a hygienist visit *(XXXIII, XXXIV)*.

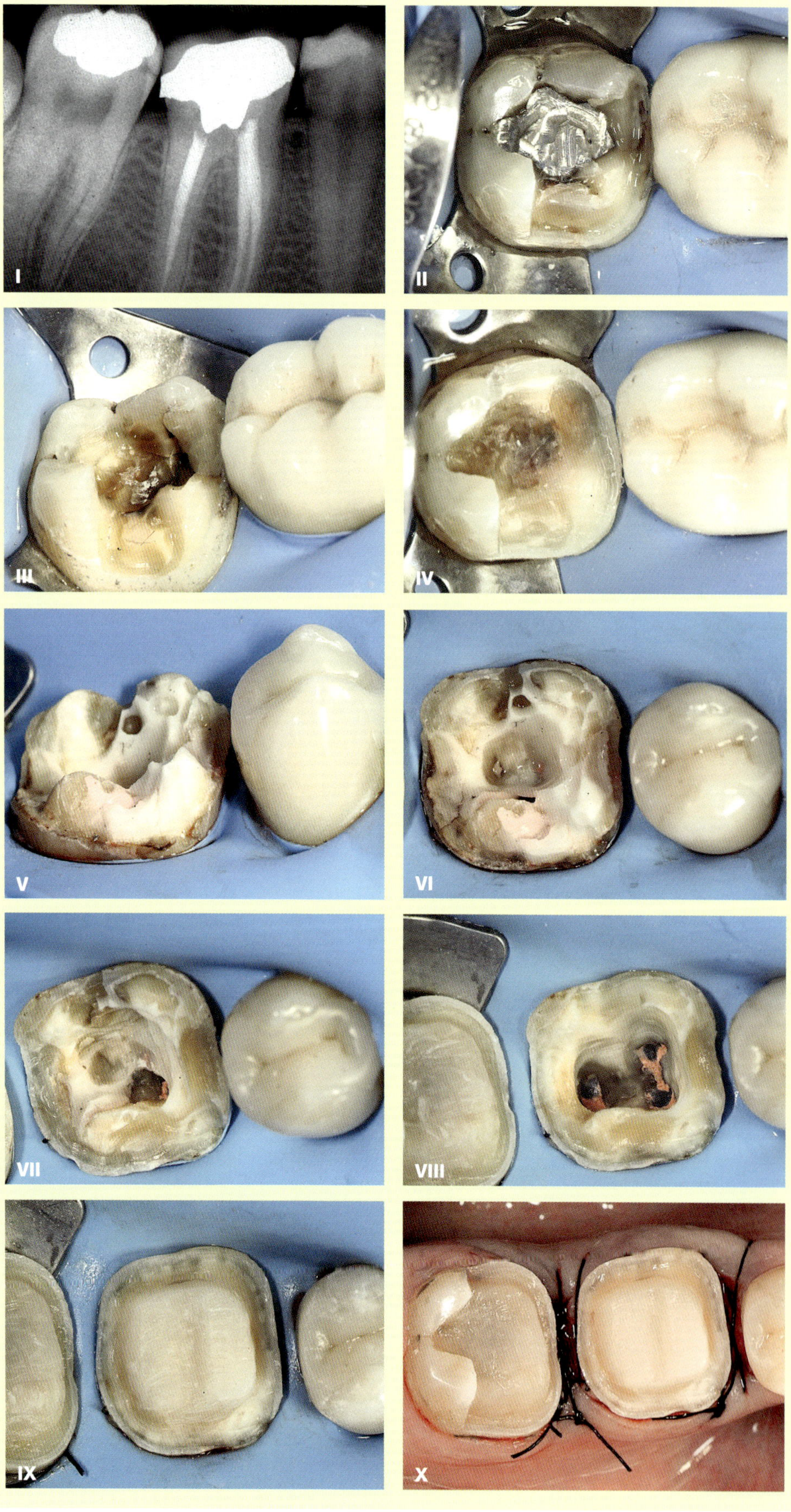

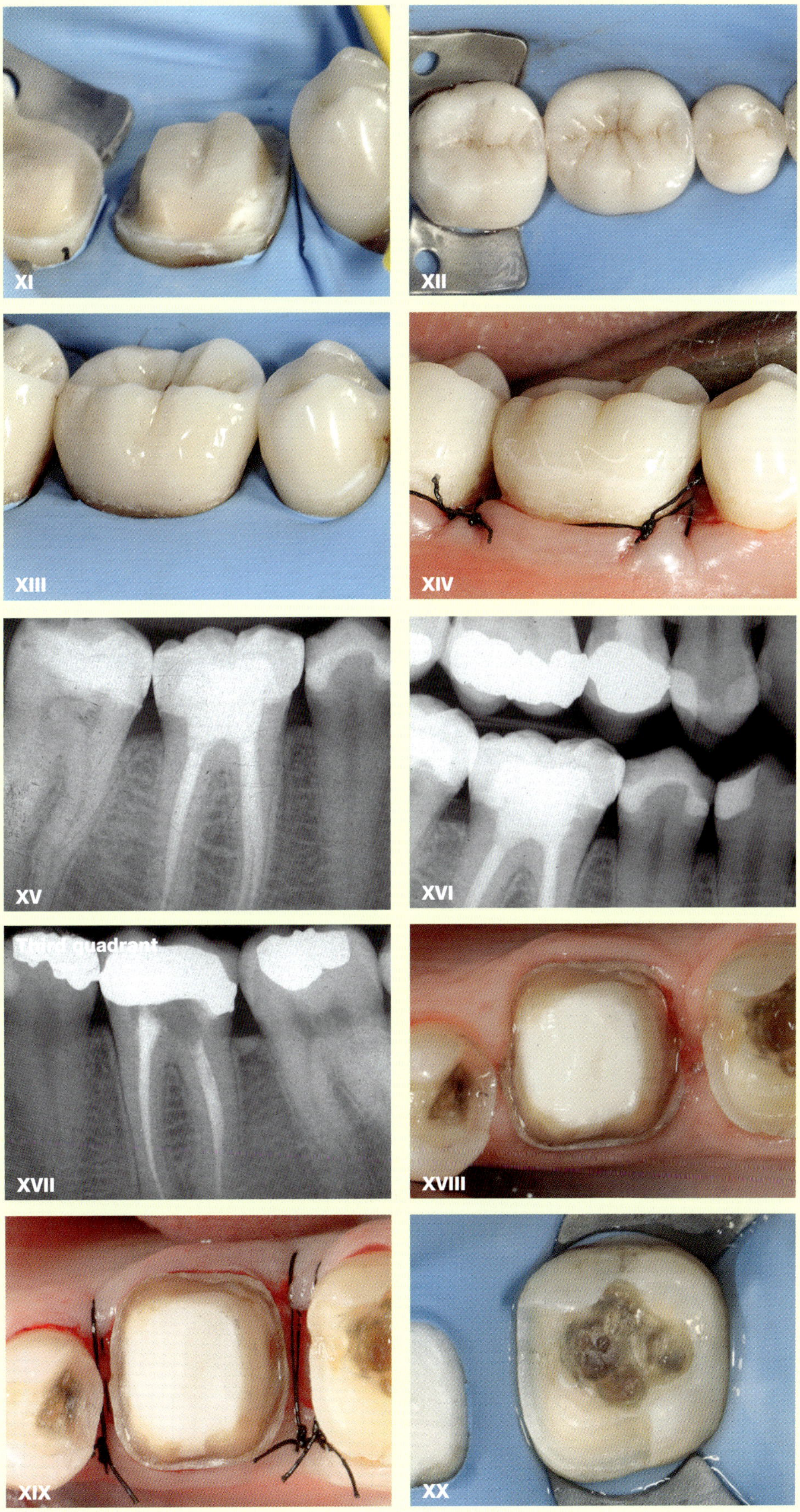

Fig 76 *(continued)*

Fig 76 *(continued)*

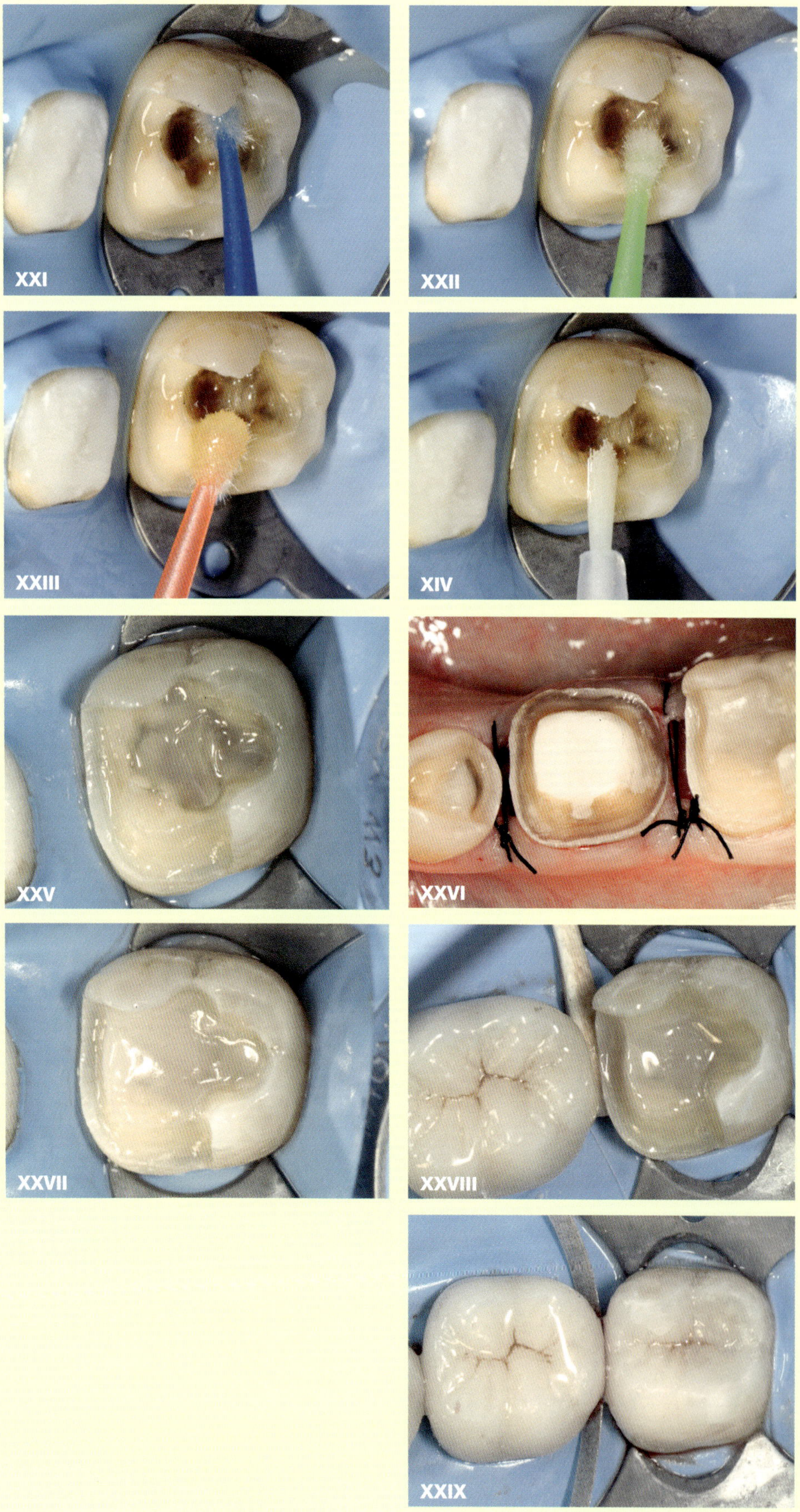

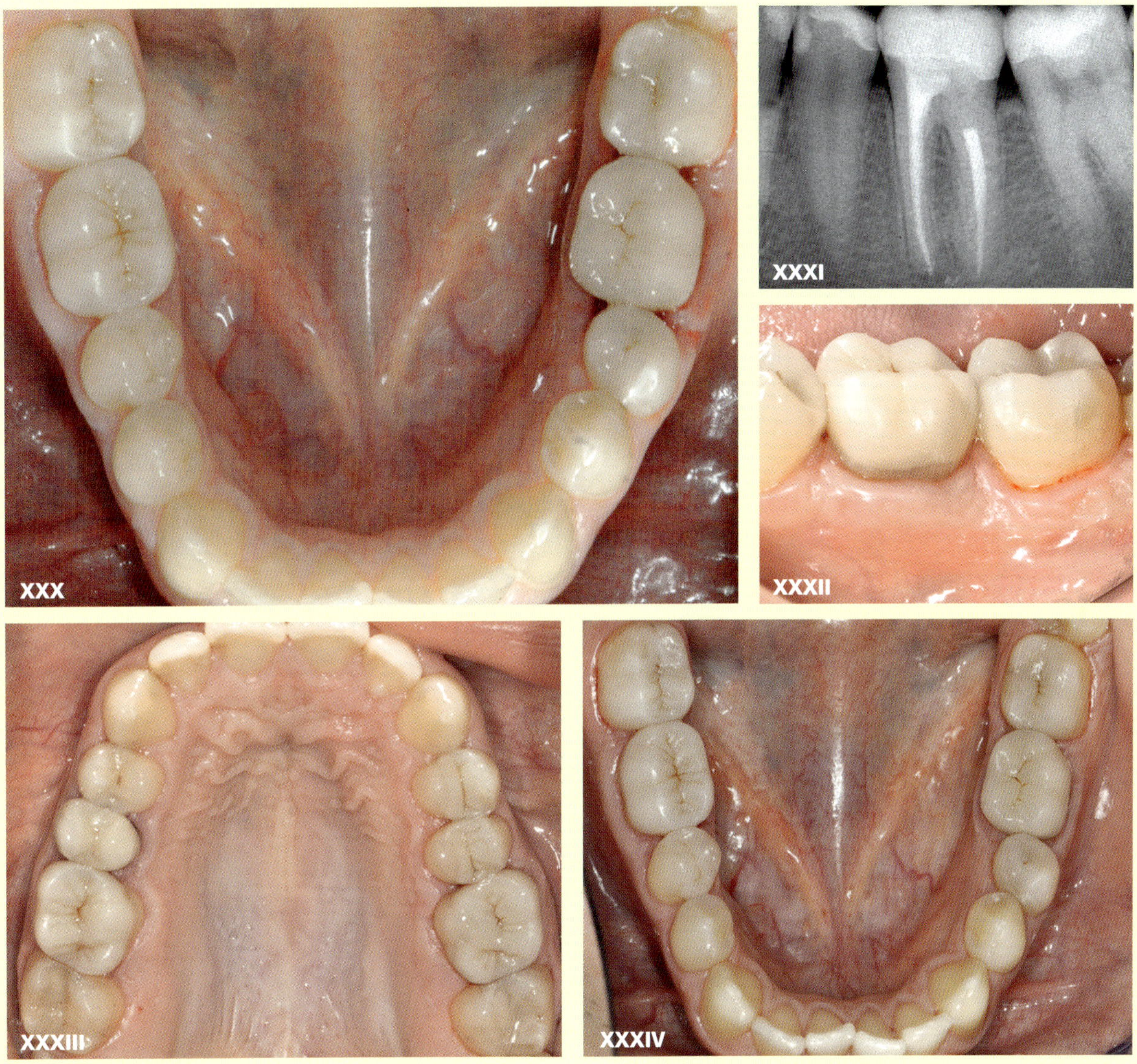

Fig 76 *(continued)*

Contacts, marginal seals, emergence profiles

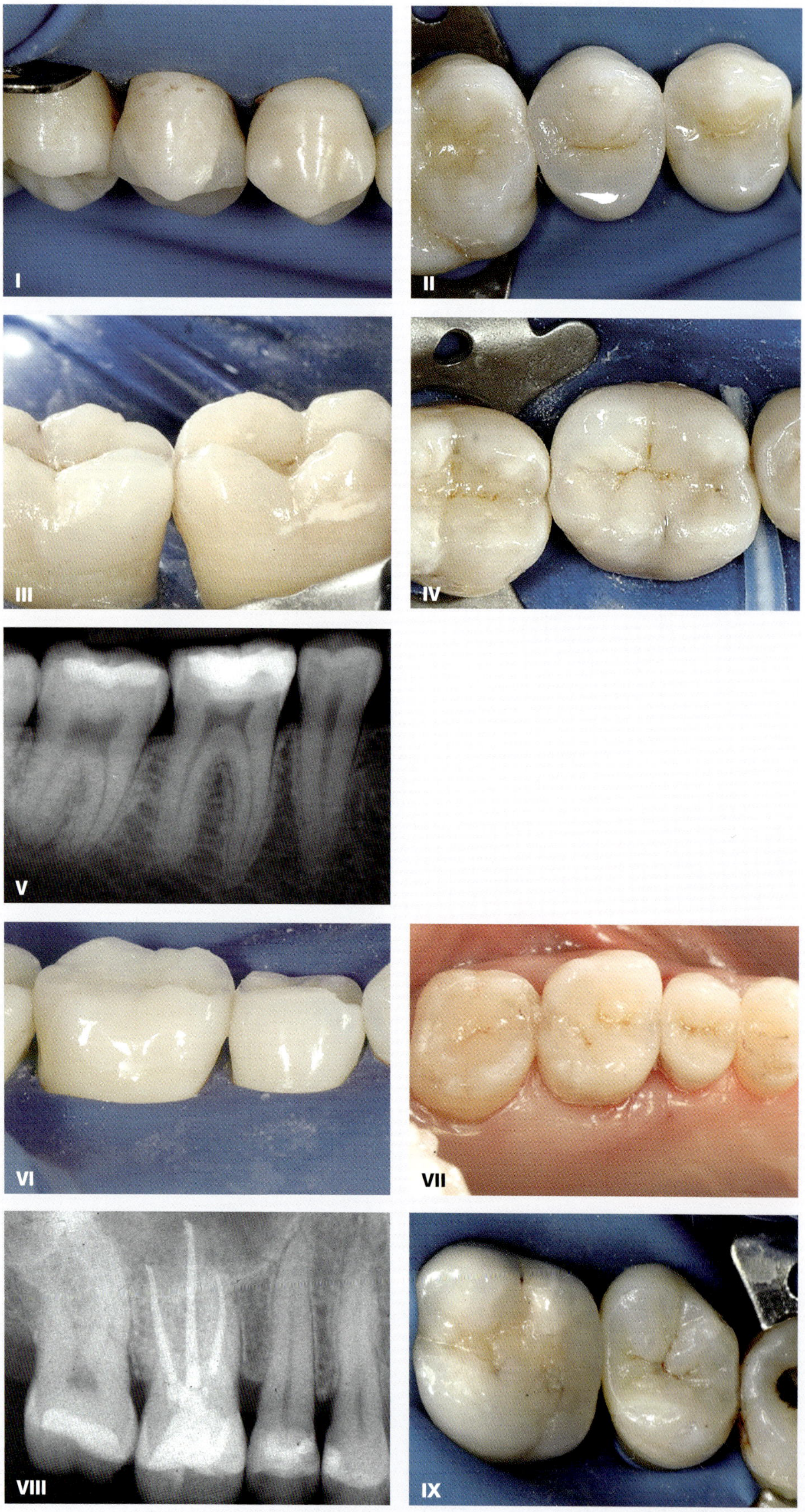

Fig 77 To conclude, a few important words to emphasize yet again the impact of interproximal contacts, marginal seals, and emergence profiles at the prognostic level. Whether the work involves ordinary amalgam or composite fillings, ceramic or composite partial restorations, or prosthetic crowns, the success of restorations is always conditioned by the accuracy or inaccuracy of these three parameters. Some clinical examples are shown in this figure.

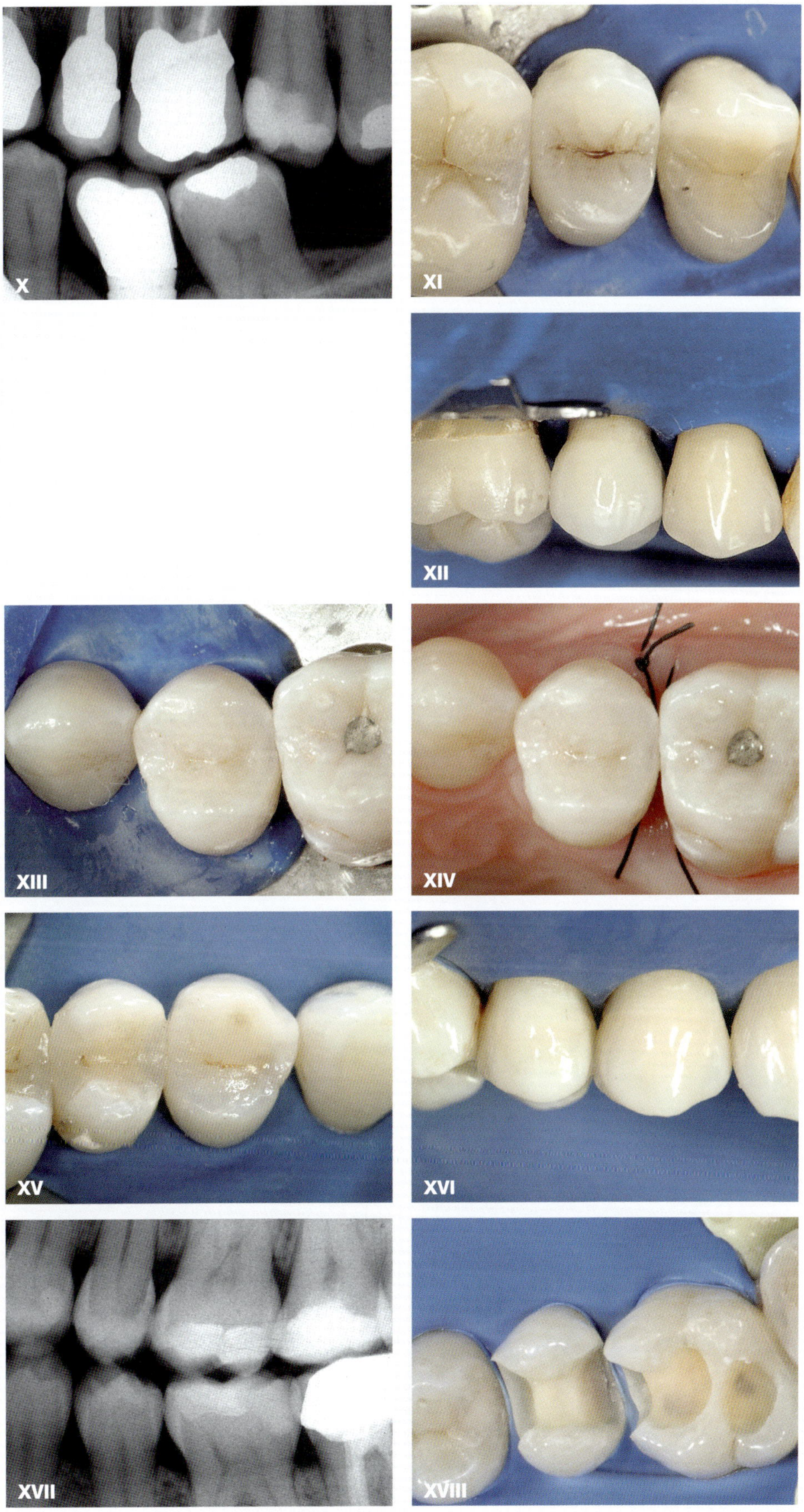

Fig 77 *(continued)*

Fig 77 *(continued)*

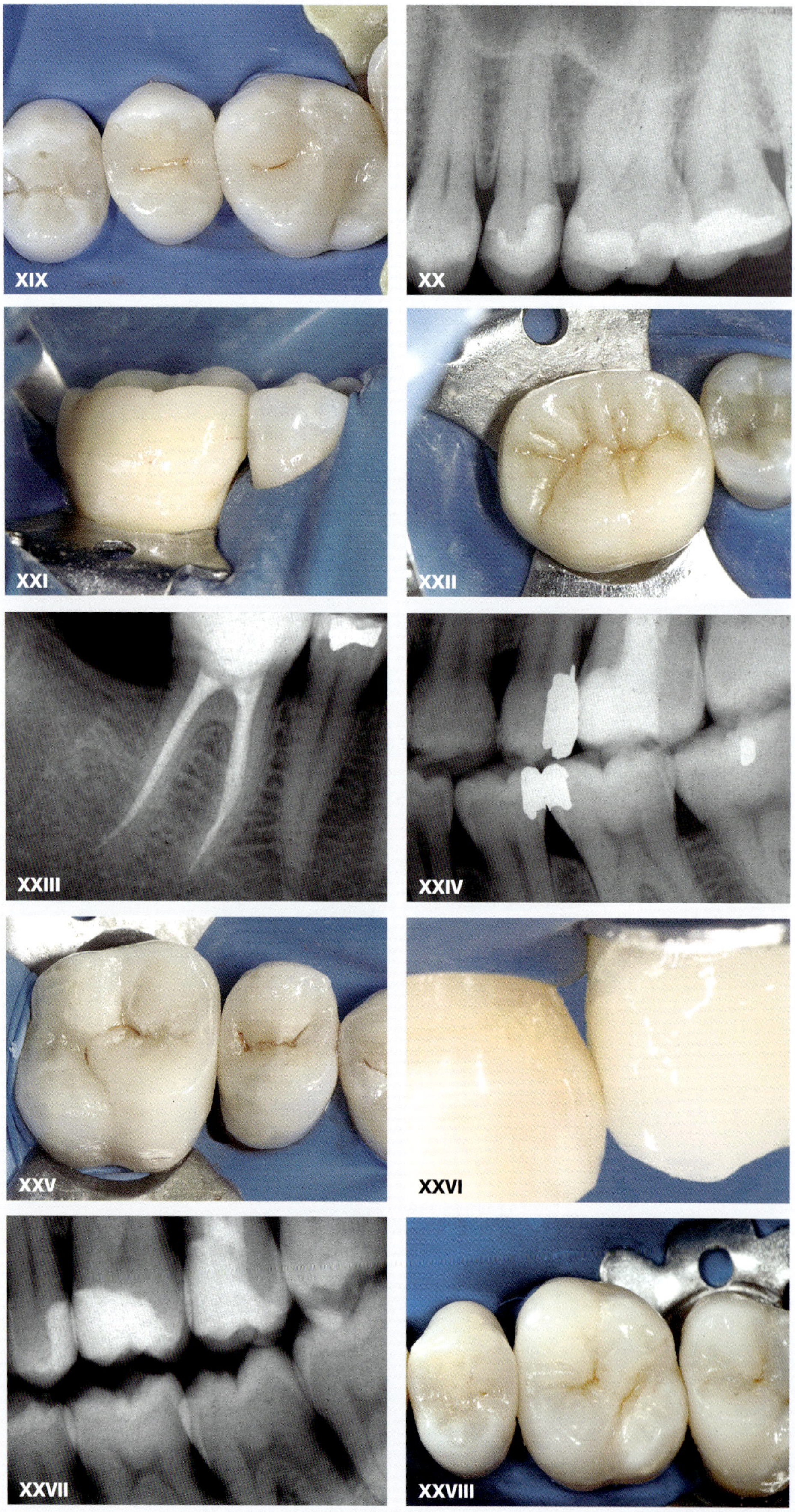

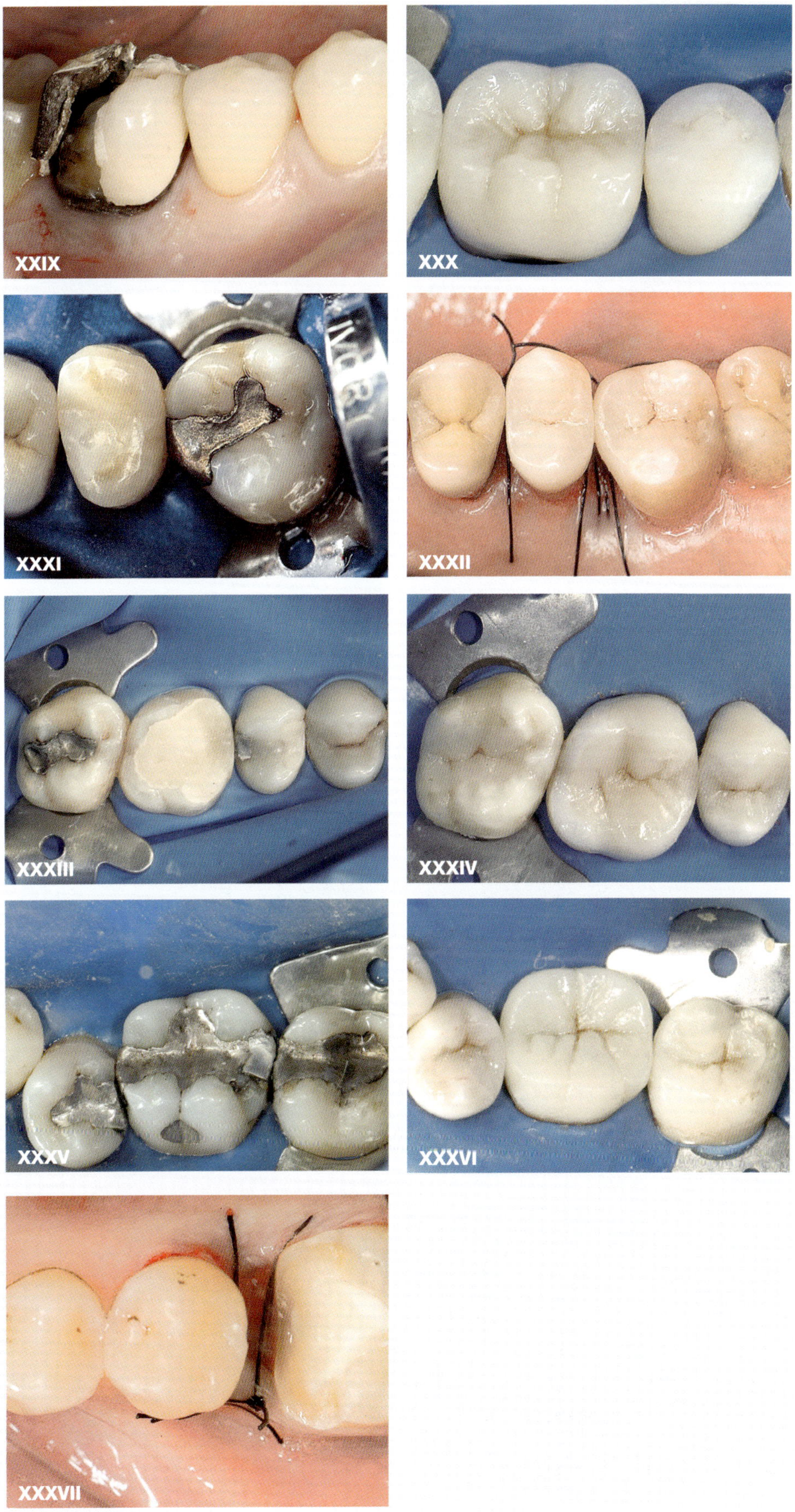

Fig 77 *(continued)*

Fig 77 *(continued)*

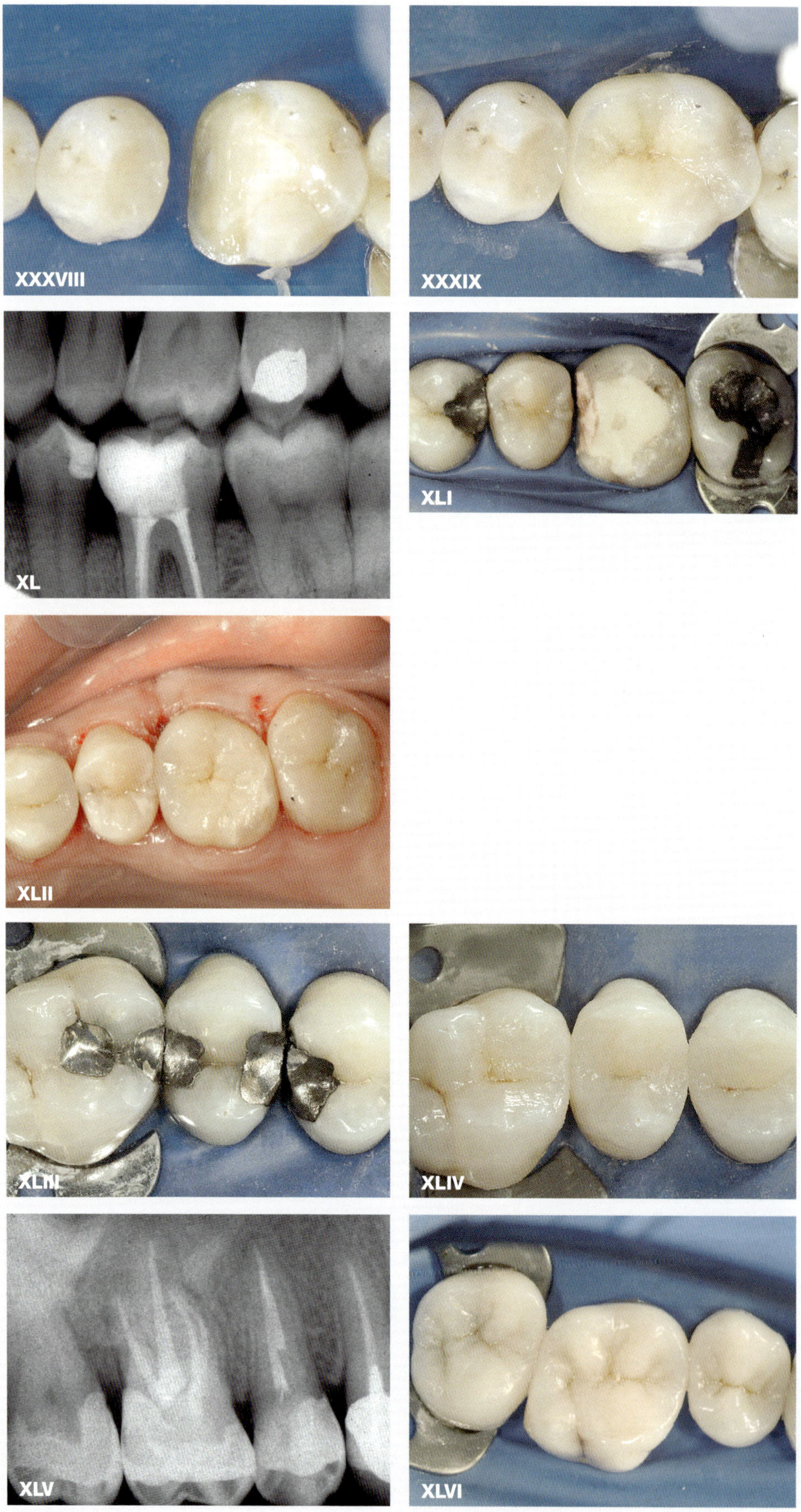

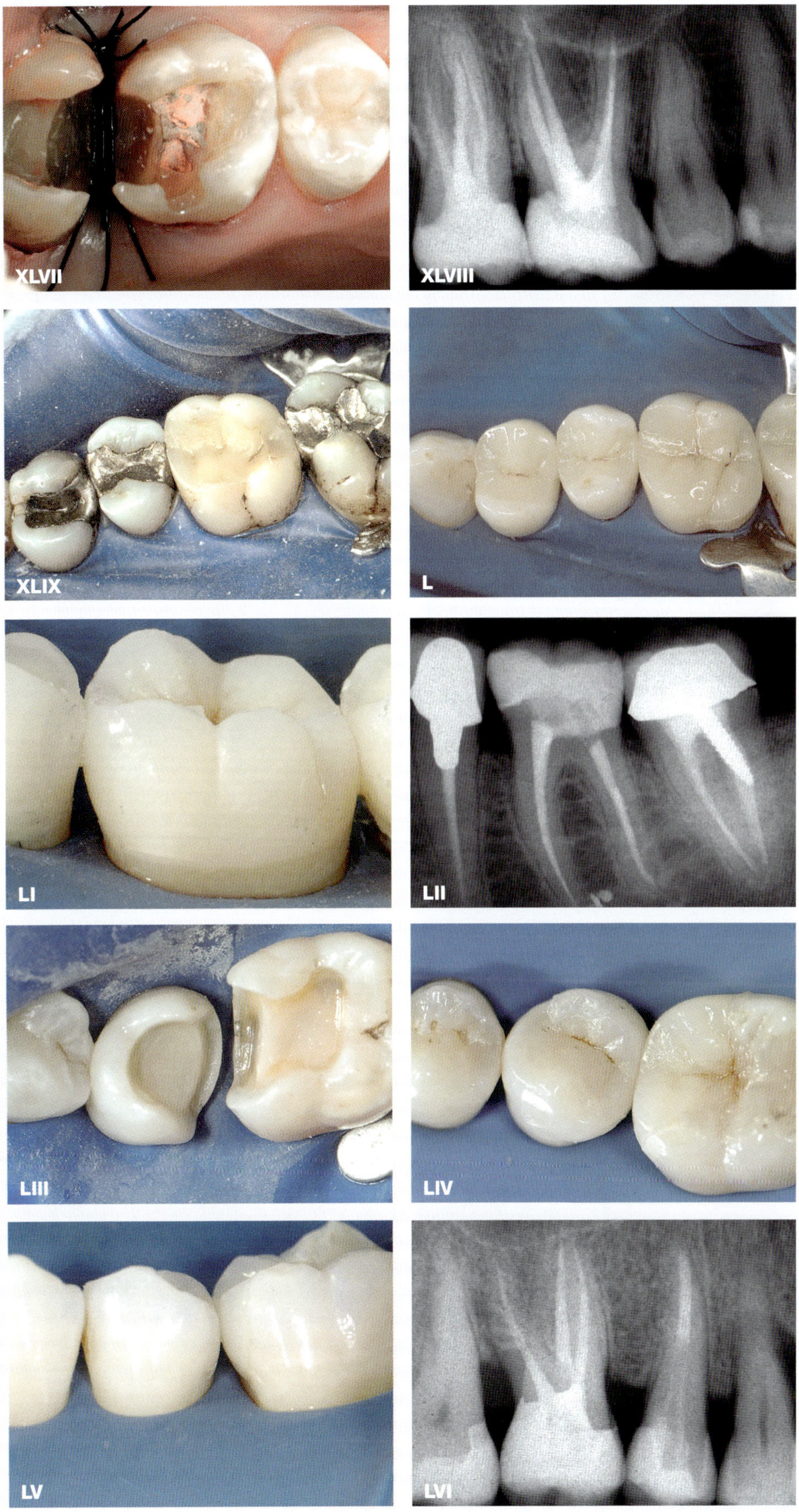

Fig 77 *(continued)*

Fig 77 *(continued)*

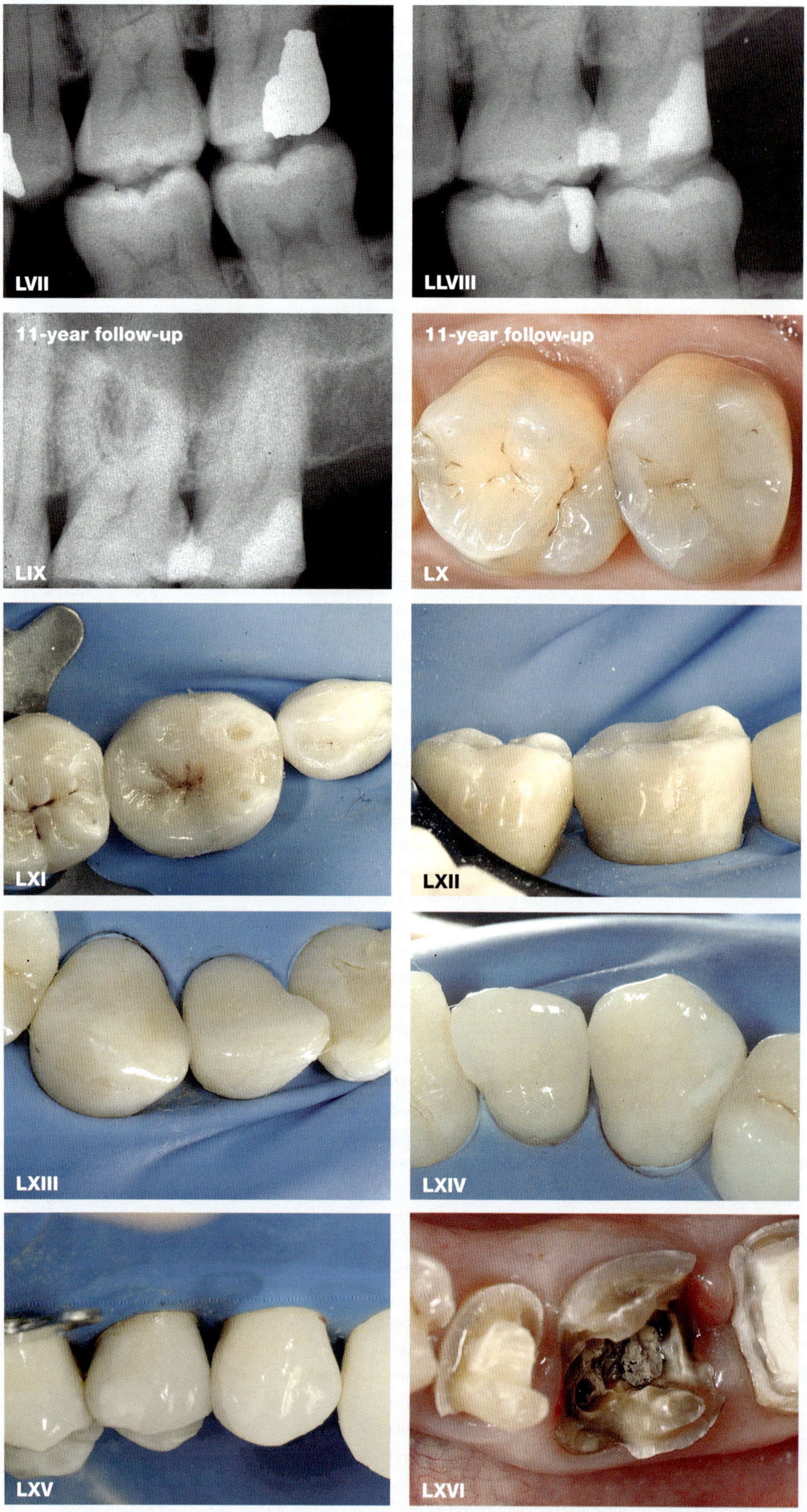

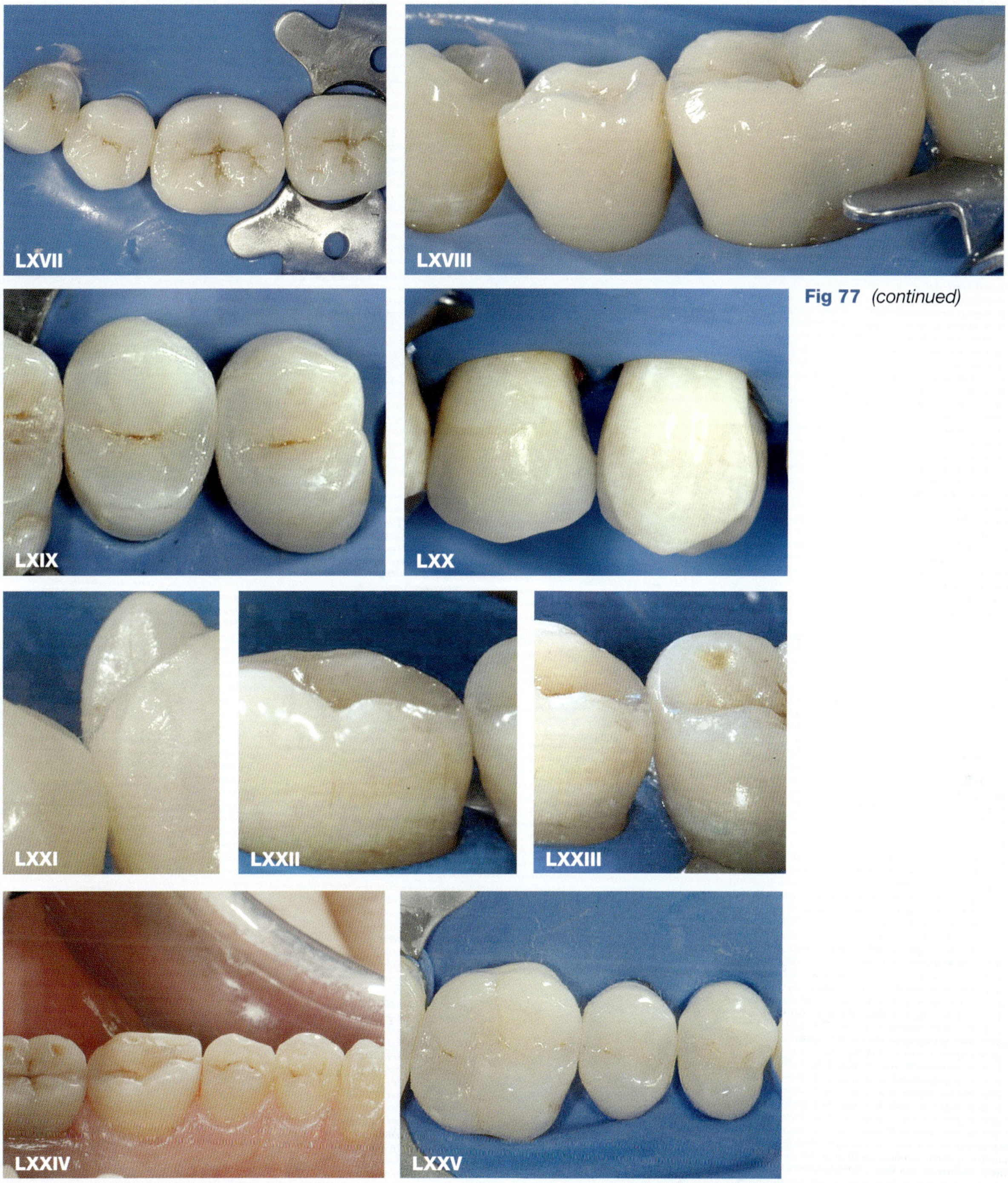

Fig 77 *(continued)*

References

1. Kramer GM. A consideration of root proximity. Int J Periodontics Restorative Dent 1987;7(6):8–33.
2. Löe H, Theilade E, Jensen SB. Experimental gingivitis in man. J Periodontol 1965;36:177–187.
3. Nevins M. Interproximal periodontal disease—The embrasure as an etiologic factor. Int J Periodontics Restorative Dent 1982;2(6):8–27.
4. Gargiulo AW, Wentz FM, Orban B. Dimensions and relations of the dento-gingival junction in humans. J Periodontol 1961;32:261–267.
5. Parma-Benfenati S, Fugazzotto PA, Ruben MP. The effect of restorative margins on the postsurgical development and nature of the periodontium. Part I. Int J Periodontics Restorative Dent 1985;5(6):30–51.
6. Parma-Benfenati S, Fugazzotto PA, Ferreira PM, Ruben MP, Kramer GM. The effect of restorative margins on the postsurgical development and nature of the periodontium. Part II. Anatomical considerations. Int J Periodontics Restorative Dent 1986;6(1):64–75.
7. Ochsenbein C. A primer for osseous surgery. Int J Periodontics Restorative Dent 1986;6(1):8–47.
8. Wilson RD, Maynard G. Intracrevicular restorative dentistry. Int J Periodontics Restorative Dent 1981;1(4):34–49.

Occlusion 5

The ultimate goal for all patients should be a fully healthy masticatory system that can be preserved in the long term.[1]
Traditional fixed prosthetic treatment ranges from the restoration of a single tooth to rehabilitation of the entire occlusion.
When missing teeth are replaced with fixed prostheses, the patient's masticatory effectiveness is restored, the health and integrity of the dental arches are protected, and often the patient's self-esteem is improved.[2]
By using fixed prosthetic restorations, even temporomandibular joint and neuromuscular problems can be corrected, with the knowledge that improper treatment of occlusion creates situations of disharmony and damage to the stomatognathic apparatus.[3]
A *crown* is a cemented extracoronal prosthetic restoration that covers the external surface of the natural tooth crown.
A *full crown* covers the entire clinical crown (Fig 1), and a *partial crown* is a coating that involves only portions of the clinical crown.
In this context, it is possible to introduce the concept of *inlays*, defined as the restoration of individual teeth due to limited proximo-occlusal lesions, and *onlays*, which cover one or more cusps for more extensive restorations.
Overlay is the term given to describe nearly full coverage of a tooth. It differs from a full crown in the fact that the margin location is supragingival (Fig 2).
If a conservative approach is adopted, restorations will be finalized by means of adhesively cemented partial restorations. The extent of the restorations can range, in simple cases, from a single tooth (Fig 3) or a few teeth up to restoration of full posterior quadrants in complex cases (Fig 4). The clinical and laboratory procedures naturally differ according to whether the case is simple or complex; therefore, the topic of occlusion is discussed separately for each case.

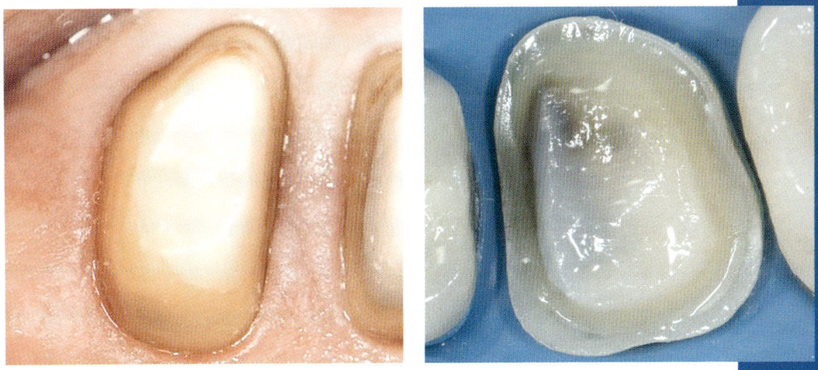

Figs 1 and 2 Note the difference in the positioning of the final preparation line between a full crown and an overlay.

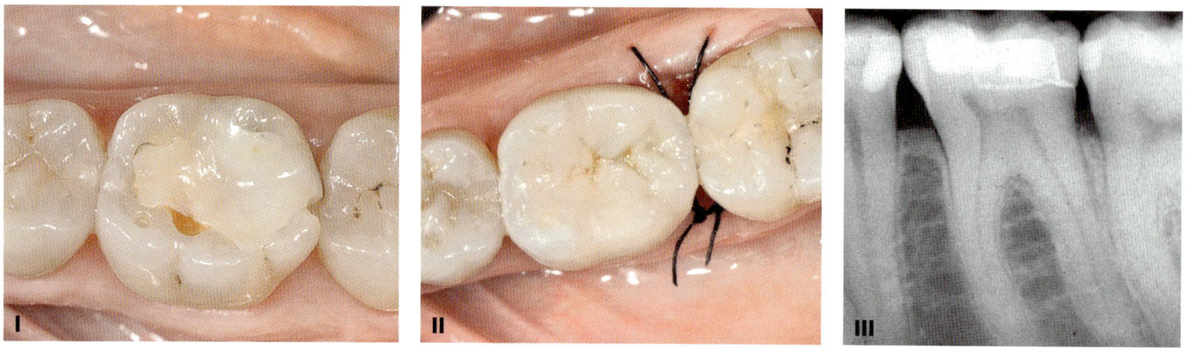

Fig 3 Example of a simple case limited to a single tooth.

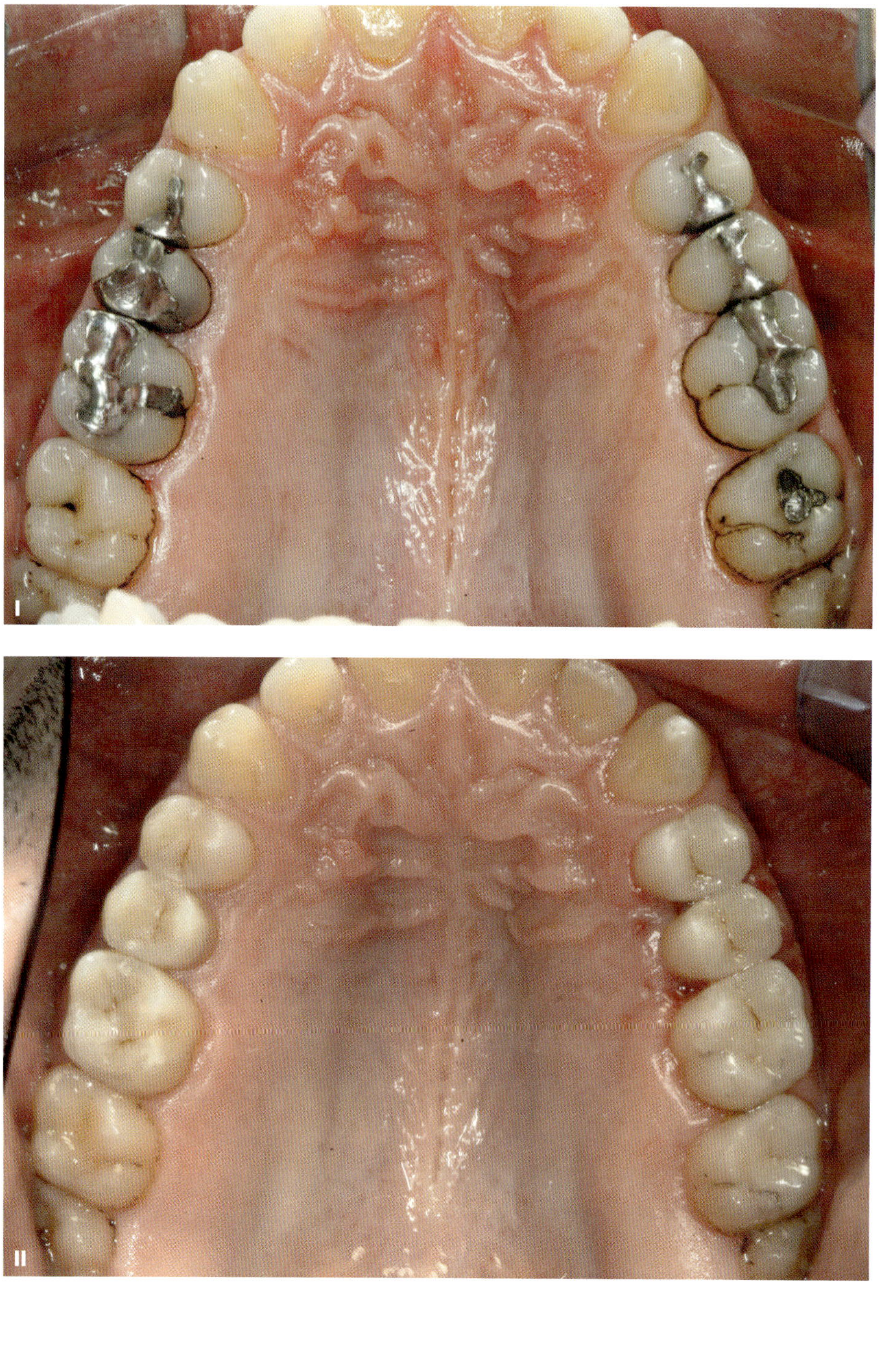

Fig 4 Example of a complex case concerning the restoration of both posterior quadrants of a maxillary arch.

The common premise is a quest for occlusal harmony, which is crucial to the long-term success of restorative treatment. Understanding the importance of occlusion and acquiring the experience necessary to resolve occlusal problems takes a long time, but clinicians must at least be able to diagnose and treat simple cases of occlusal disharmony and produce restorations that do not give rise to iatrogenic occlusal disorders.
The aim is to achieve posterior occlusal contacts that confer stability instead of creating deviant contacts that act to destabilize the mandibular position.
Occlusion must be carried out in a restoration in harmony with the optimum condylar position, the anterior and canine guidance, and the other factors affecting occlusion.

The author feels it incumbent to emphasize yet again the importance of accurate diagnosis: A comprehensive view of the teeth and their superficial and deep supporting structures allows formulation of a treatment plan that is ideal for a specific patient.
Shillingburg[2] presents the following factors as those that must be considered in order to come to a correct diagnosis:

- Medical history
- Evaluation of occlusion and the temporomandibular joint
- Intraoral examination
- Study casts
- General radiographic examination

After taking a thorough medical history, an occlusal and temporomandibular joint assessment provides important guidelines regarding whether or not to proceed with the planned restorations. If there are evident occlusal or joint abnormalities, the clinician must consider the need to correct parafunctions, premature contacts, muscular rigidity, popping, clicking, and movement limitations during opening, closure, or lateral excursion.
Palpation of the masseter, temporal, lateral pterygoid, trapezoid, and sternocleidomastoid muscles allows identification of any areas sensitive to pain.
This information will be crucial when it comes to deciding whether to begin restorative treatment immediately with the knowledge that implementation of treatment will lead to the solution of problems (eg, premature contacts that will be eliminated with new restorations), or whether it would be advisable to carry out another assessment using correction devices (such as a simple plate from canine to canine (hawley bite plane) rather than a bite correction (bite plane) or simple mouthguard (nightguard).
Regarding the intraoral examination, which has already been emphasized as very important, it is also worth summarizing specific details, such as observation of oral hygiene and the general periodontal condition, with particular reference to the presence or absence of adherent gingva around the teeth, in addition to the presence of gingival pockets and caries lesions, the quality of any endodontic treatments, whether or not the restorations present are defective, any infiltrations, and the presence of fracture lines in the marginal ridges and on the other coronal surfaces. If these fracture lines are not intercepted in time, they could progress to the point of fracture. As Dawson[1] points out, the signs of occlusal disease almost always precede the symptoms, and the severity of structural damage is usually progressive if not treated.
It would be unthinkable not to carry out an occlusal assessment in order to establish the presence of wear facets and interference on the nonworking side, just as it is useful to check any slide between the retrusive position and maximal intercuspation, the presence or absence of simultaneous contacts on both sides of the mouth, and the presence and width of the anterior guidance.

When the treatment plan involves two or at most three partial restorations, it is easy to check the occlusion, but in the restoration of entire arches, the protocol becomes more rigorous and requires the preparation of study casts that must accurately reproduce the maxilla and mandible. The purpose of these casts is to provide as much diagnostic information as possible, and to achieve this they must be fitted on an articulator by means of a facebow that is programmed with the aid of lateral bite registrations or interocclusal records. This will allow a sufficiently accurate simulation of arch movements.[4,5]

When restoring posterior elements, irrespective of whether the case is simple or complex, the following objectives must be pursued:

- Multiple and punctiform occlusal contacts
- Simultaneous occlusion on both sides
- Absence of interference in eccentric jaw movements.

As already stated, posterior restorations must be in harmony with the condylar and mandibular position. From a therapeutic viewpoint, there are two possibilities: perform the reconstruction in the normal mandibular position (conformist approach) or attempt to reestablish a new occlusal balance by repositioning the condyles in a centric relationship (rehabilitation approach).
The choice of using one or other of the mandibular positions is dictated by the practitioner's need, in extensive rehabilitations, to find a reproducible position for the condyles once all the teeth have been filed or, in some often dysfunctional cases, to extensively reorganize the occlusal surface.[6,7]
The mandibular position of reference in conservative treatment is therefore the habitual closure position or the position of maximal intercuspation, where many of the occlusal contacts are already present in untreated tooth components since the preparations are partial, even though they extend to more than one tooth..

Treatment of simple cases

Simple cases refer to clinical cases where intervention is limited to a few teeth (Figs 5 I to VI).
Under these conditions, simplified clinical and laboratory procedures can be used because occlusion is mainly controlled by preexisting occlusal contacts.
The simplification involves using impression trays for interocclusal records when taking an impression (eg, Triple Tray Dual Arch Impression Tray, Premier), which allows the clinician to take an impression of a half-arch and the opposing half-arch, the bite registration, and the maximal intercuspation all at the same time (Fig 5 VII).
The procedure is also simplified in the laboratory by using dedicated articulators that make it possible to save time and materials while maintaining good occlusal accuracy.[8]
The system the author's team adopts, an Amann Girrbach articulator, has bases with pre-inserted pins for construction of the cast. It is very fast and accurate without the additional costs of other systems (Figs 5 VIII and IX).
Because an impression is a record of both arches, it must be cast in two separate stages, one stage for each arch, in order to provide two separate casts (Figs 5 X to XII).
The instrument is dedicated to this procedure and is mainly used to carry out movements in a vertical plane only. After mounting the casts, the device automatically provides an occlusal relationship, which is usually corrected[9,10] (Fig 5 XIII).

Simple clinical case

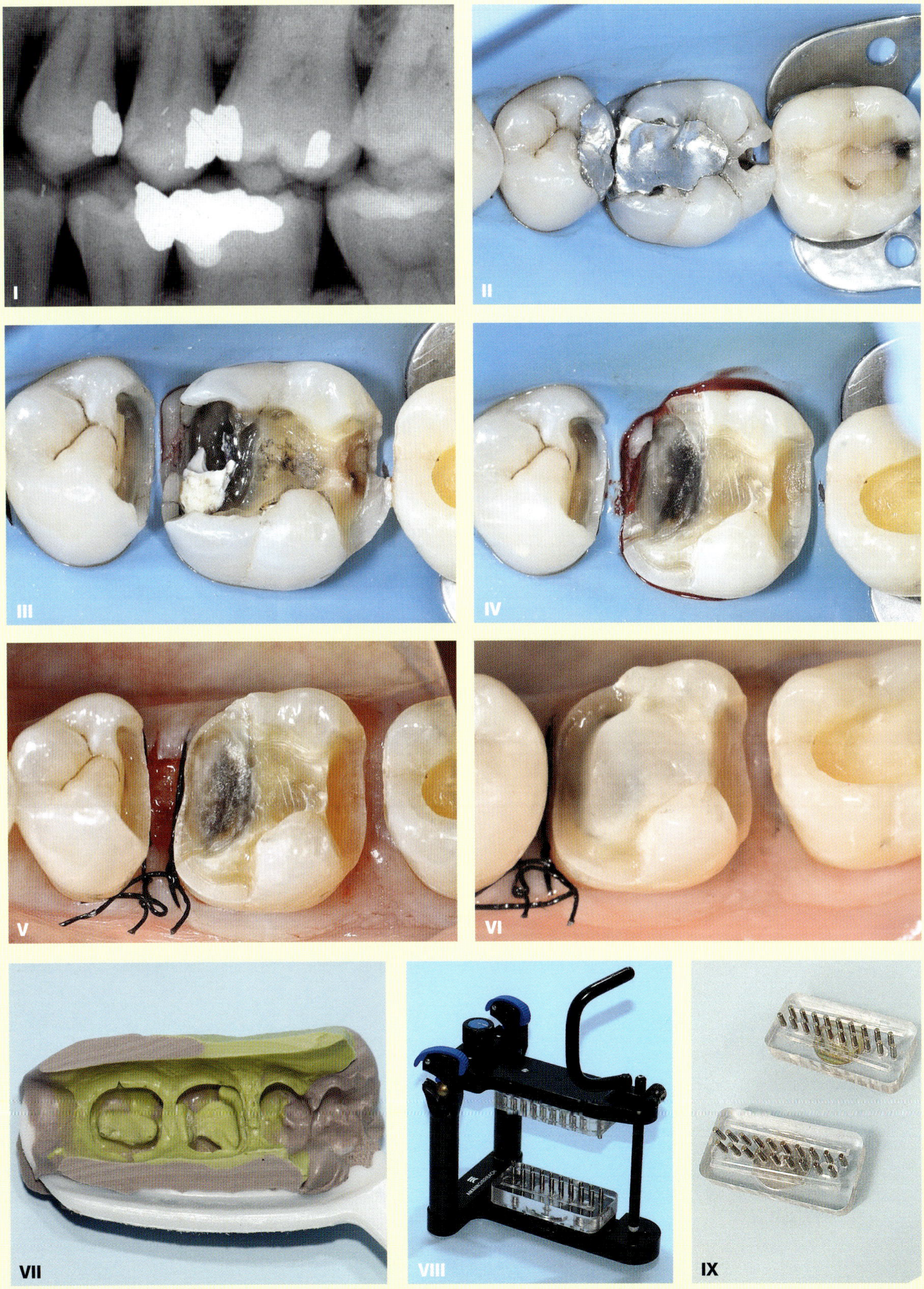

Fig 5 Simple clinical case. Even though three restorations are carried out, involvement of the occlusal surface is limited. Most of the occlusal contacts are on the cusps of natural teeth, guaranteeing occlusal stability and allowing the use if a simplified working method *(I–VI)*. Impression tray for interocclusal record *(VII)*. Amann Girrbach simplified articulator including mounting plates with pre-inserted fixed pins for segmentation of the plaster cast *(VIII, IX)*.

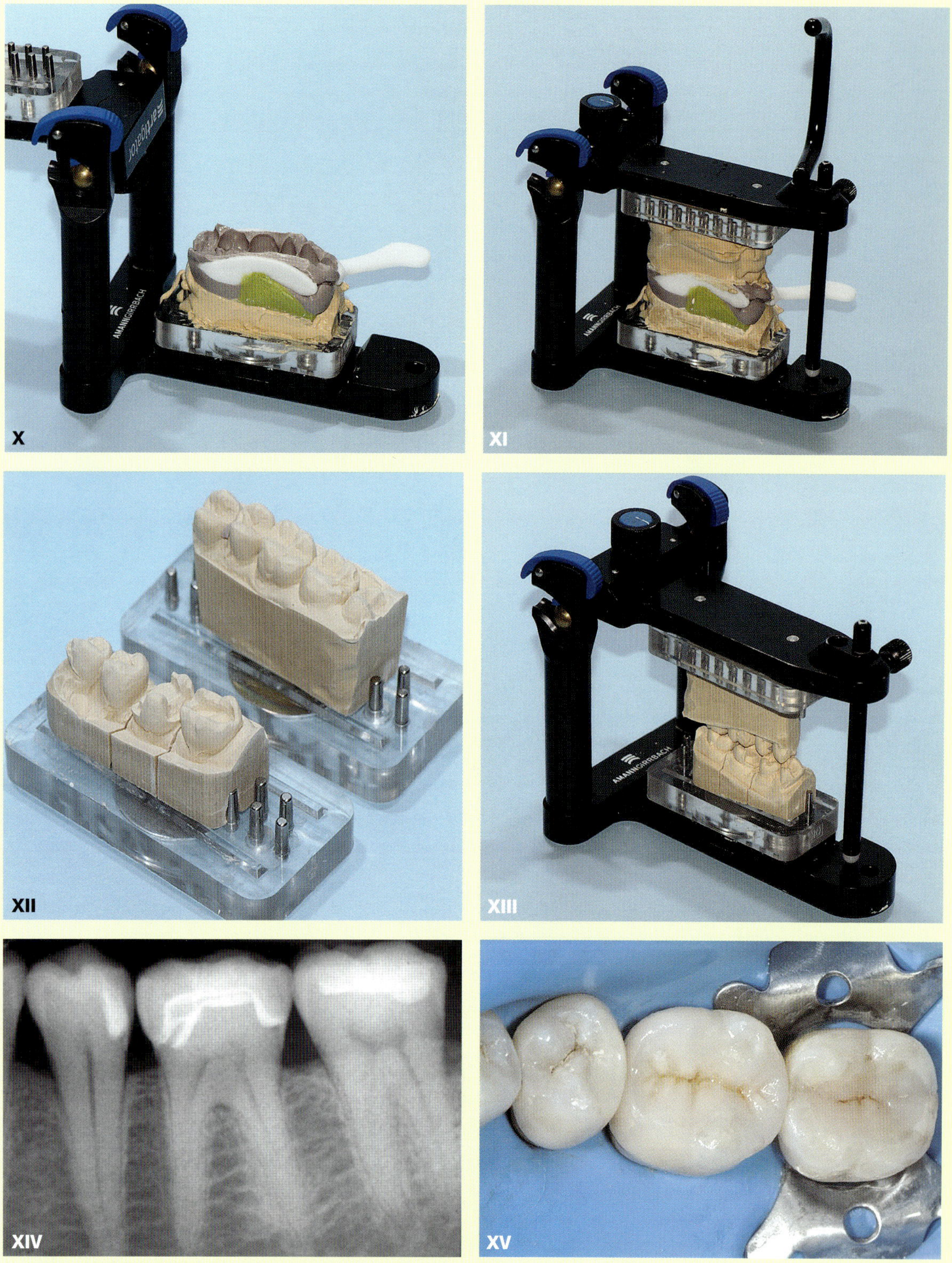

Fig 5 *(continued)* The impression is cast in two different stages, one for each arch, In order to prevent fusion of the two casts, which must be kept separate. If the impression was correctly taken, once the models have been cast they will be in the correct position of maximal intercuspation *(X–XIII)*. Finalization of the case and follow-up radiograph *(XIV, XV)*.

This procedure clearly can only be used safely in cases that are limited to a few teeth, but it is highly effective and efficient in such cases (Figs 5 XIV and XV).
This means significant simplification and saving of clinical and laboratory time while still offering sufficient accuracy to carry out the work correctly (Fig 6).
When developing the impression, the author's team used the plaster that they normally use in traditional prosthetic procedures. The material of choice is an extra-hard type IV die stone (Fujirock EP, GC).
The author's team always obtains two casts from the impression: the first "master" cast that is used to construct the restoration and a second cast that is not segmented and is used after constructing the inlays to check the contact surfaces.
The use of a double cast considerably reduces the time taken to adjust the seating of the inlay because the contact surfaces are always efficient and consistent with one another.

Simple clinical case: Laboratory stage

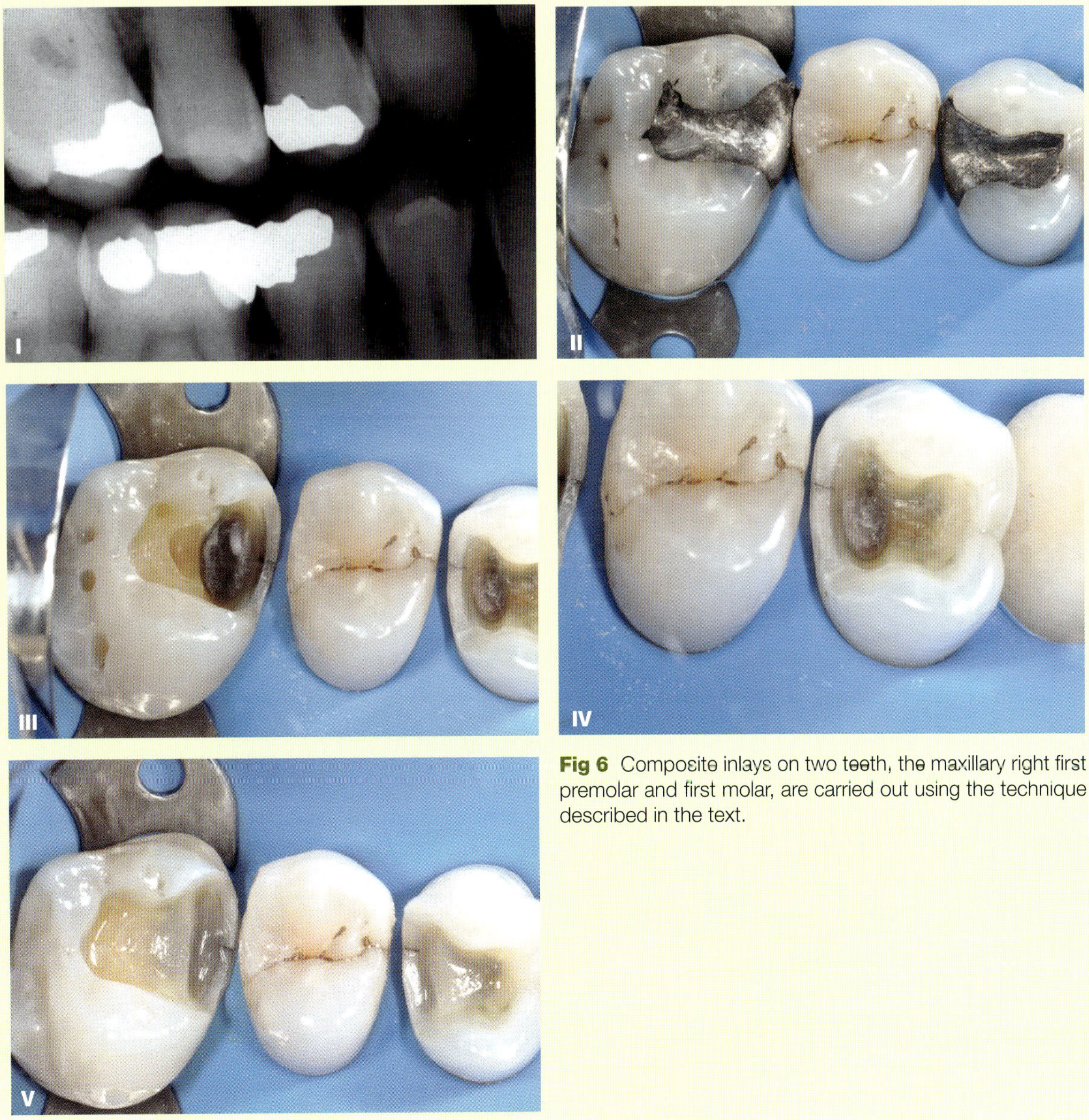

Fig 6 Composite inlays on two teeth, the maxillary right first premolar and first molar, are carried out using the technique described in the text.

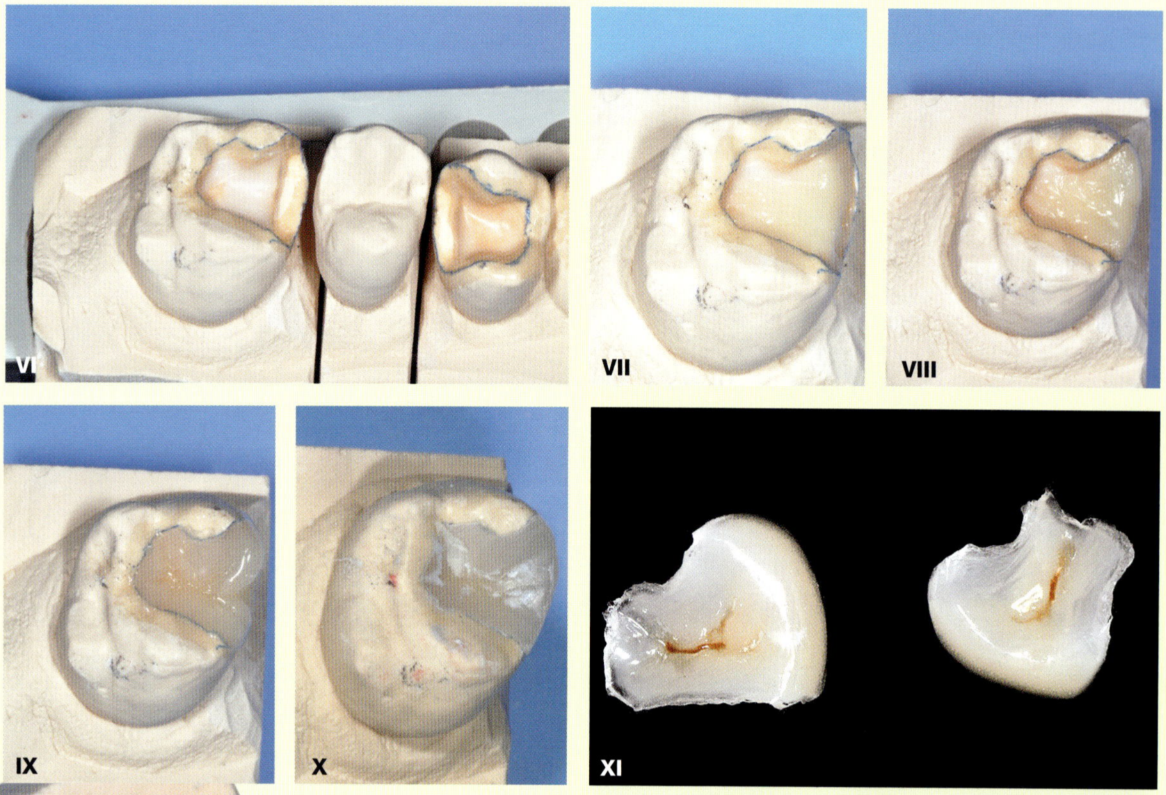

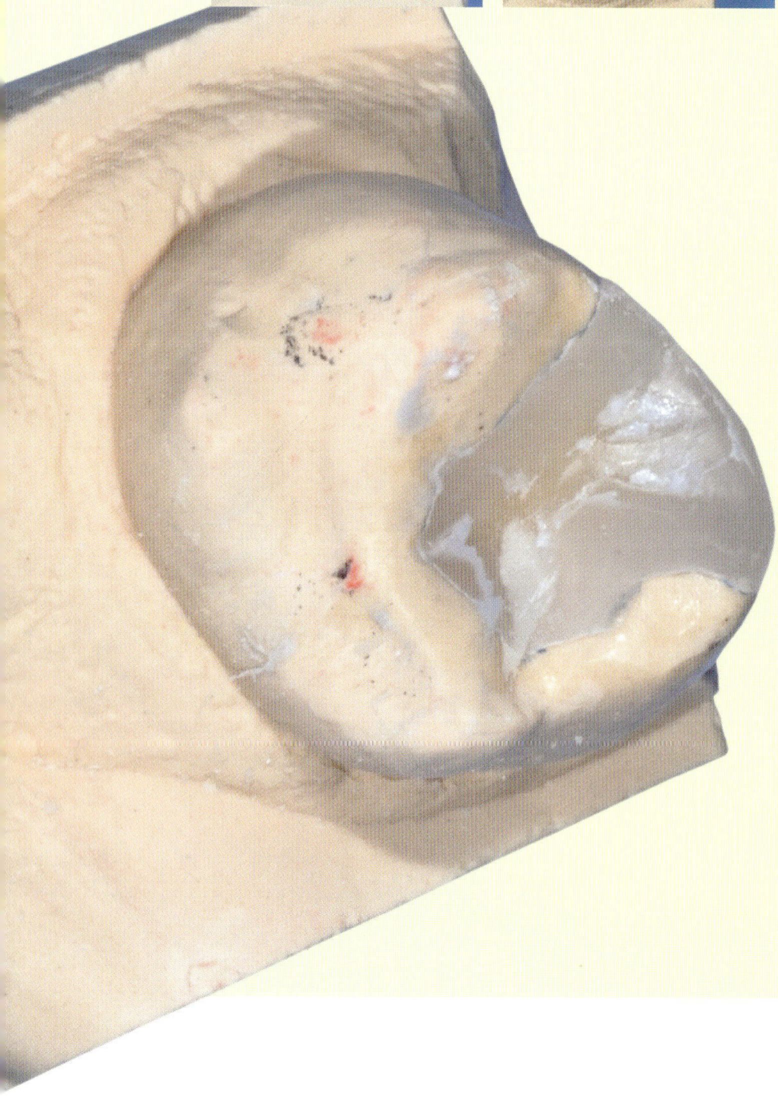

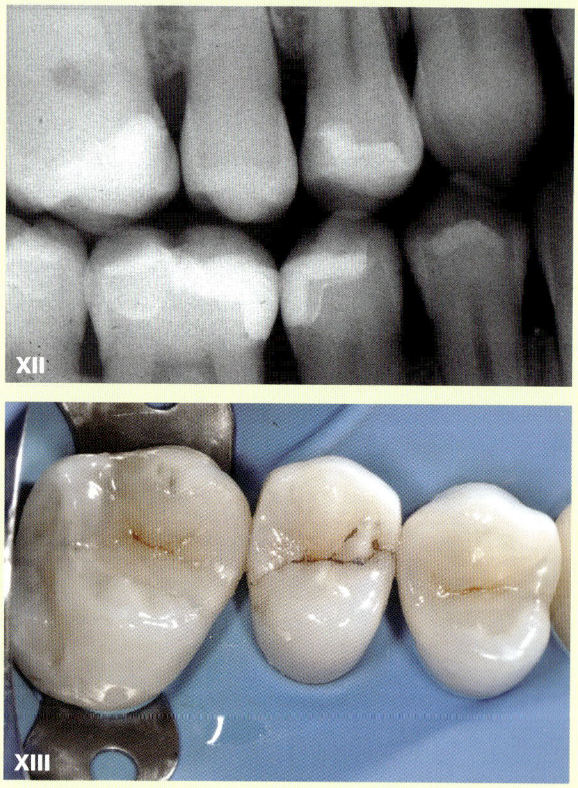

Fig 6 *(continued)*

The development of a master cast must follow rigid protocols in order to maintain the necessary precision; ie, casting time, cast segmentation, and mounting of the cast in dedicated mini-articulators must be carried out as a routine.
Once the casts have been mounted on the articulator bases, the affected area will be segmented; in other words, the individual teeth are separated.
This procedure is very important, not only in allowing the technician to work correctly but above all in controlling the plaster expansion reaction and guaranteeing a very precise cast. Even though the composite restoration offers very high fracture resistance, the product is nevertheless fragile during the construction procedures and must be treated with care until the time of cementation.
It must be remembered that after construction a composite restoration must comply with all standards of marginal precision, emergence profiles, material surface properties, and polish that are normally expected of a top-quality prosthetic product.

Treatment of complex cases

Complex cases (Figs 7 I to IV) are those in which greater commitment is required because of either a greater number of teeth to be treated or the need to correct preexisting occlusal problems, differences in occlusal plane levels, presence of premature contacts and interferences, or tooth extrusion or inclination. In such cases, the treatment procedure becomes more complicated and more like a traditional prosthetic procedure. Initial study casts are essential for a preliminary study of occlusion and can be used to reveal wear facets, malpositioning, rotations, extrusions, and inclinations that may be corrected during the restorative treatment.
It is essential for casts to be mounted on a semi-adjustable articulator and appropriately recorded based on patient function. This makes it possible to more effectively analyze any occlusal problems. The work will also be carried out in the articulator using full impressions in order to achieve greater accuracy at the occlusal level.

Normally the author's team works by quadrants even in complex cases, which makes for easier clinical management of the case. We should nevertheless remember that it is important to work on opposing quadrants in order to be able to alter and correct the occlusal plane.
The following materials are required for this procedure:

- Facebow
- Semi-adjustable articulator
- Material for bite registration
- Study casts
- Complete-arch impressions during treatment stages

The facebow method that the author's team uses is a simplified procedure introduced by John Kois: the Kois Dento-Facial Analyzer (Panadent). This instrument is very fast to use, only taking a few seconds, and allows positioning of the maxillary cast in an articulator with a good level of accuracy (Figs 7 V to VII).

The system is based on research that Kois conducted on a patient sample that was highly varied in terms of ethnic origin and sex, where the distance between the intercondylar axis and the central incisor margin was found to be 100 mm in approximately 80% of patients, with a tolerance of 5 mm.

Complex clinical case

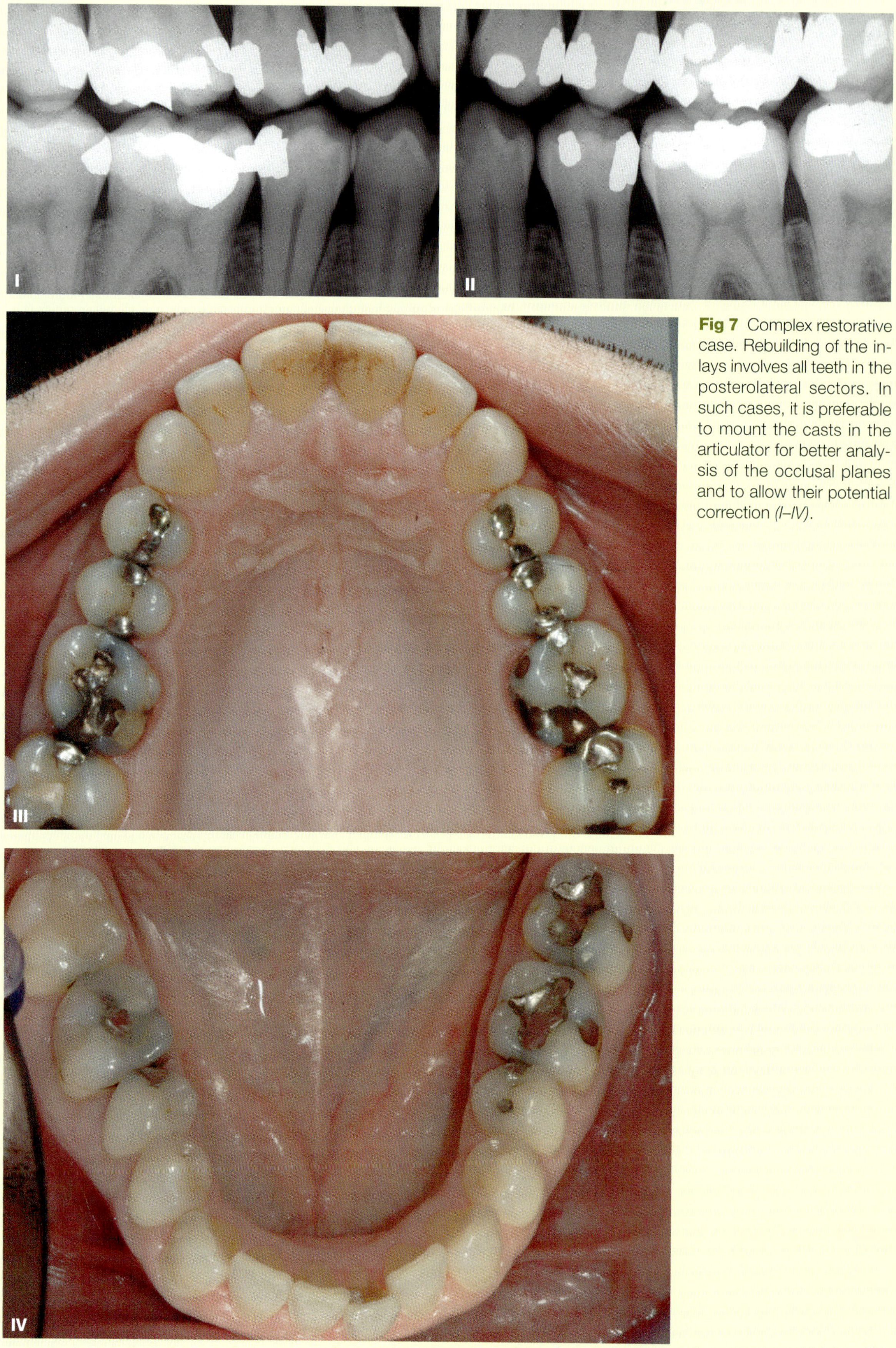

Fig 7 Complex restorative case. Rebuilding of the inlays involves all teeth in the posterolateral sectors. In such cases, it is preferable to mount the casts in the articulator for better analysis of the occlusal planes and to allow their potential correction *(I–IV)*.

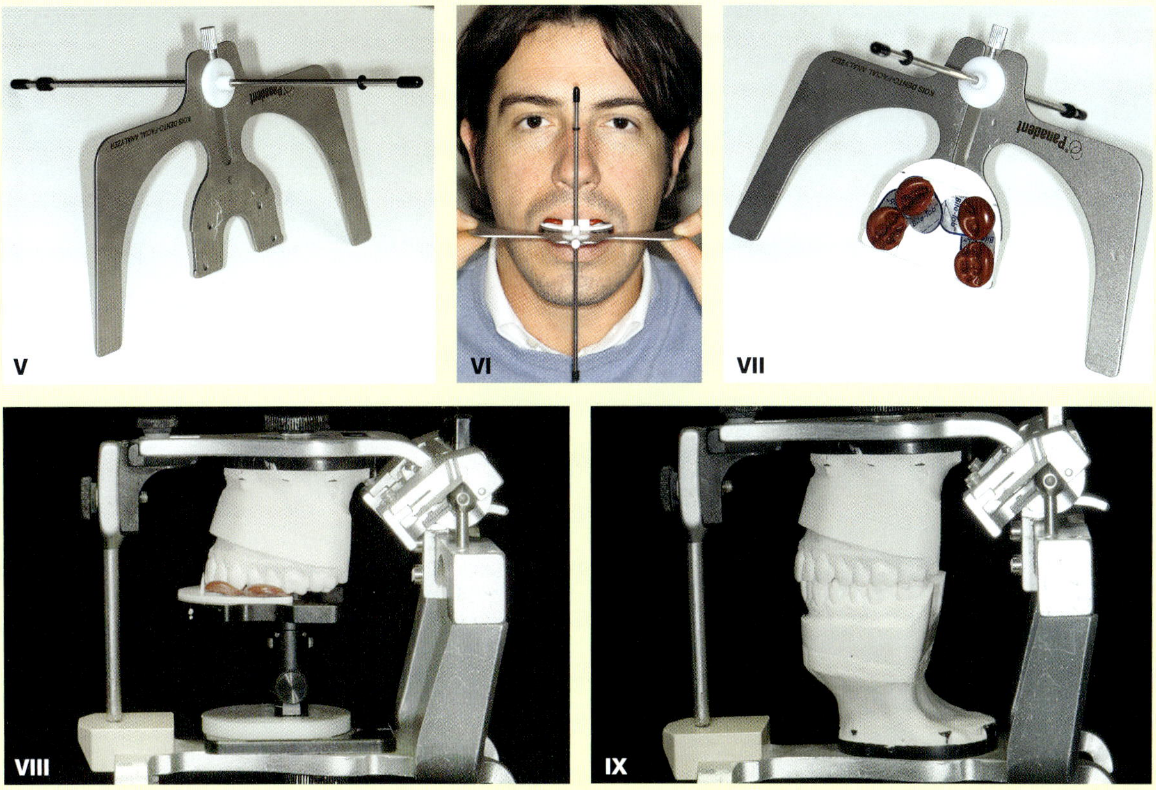

Fig 7 *(continued)* Kois Dento-Facial Analyzer *(V)*: the facial bow is recorded by using the pupillary line as a frontal plane reference *(VI)*. The plastic registration plate is removed from the dental analyzer and positioned on a special support *(VII)*. Mounting a maxillary cast in the correct position on the articulator by means of a special mounting aid *(VIII)*. Once the maxillary cast has been mounted, the mandibular cast can be mounted. This may be done in a position of maximal intercuspation or in centric relation according to clinical needs *(IX)*.

This is more or less the same error range achieved with arbitrary facebows that require positioning within the acoustic meatus.

Even when setting the articulator, the author's team uses a method that is simpler than the one normally used for a fixed prosthesis. The only recording performed is the protrusive mandibular position, which allows the condylar eminence value to be set in the articulator. The other settings are average values[11,12] (Figs 7 VIII and IX).

This procedure provides sufficient information for accurate restoration of entire occlusal quadrants (Figs 7 X to XXXII).

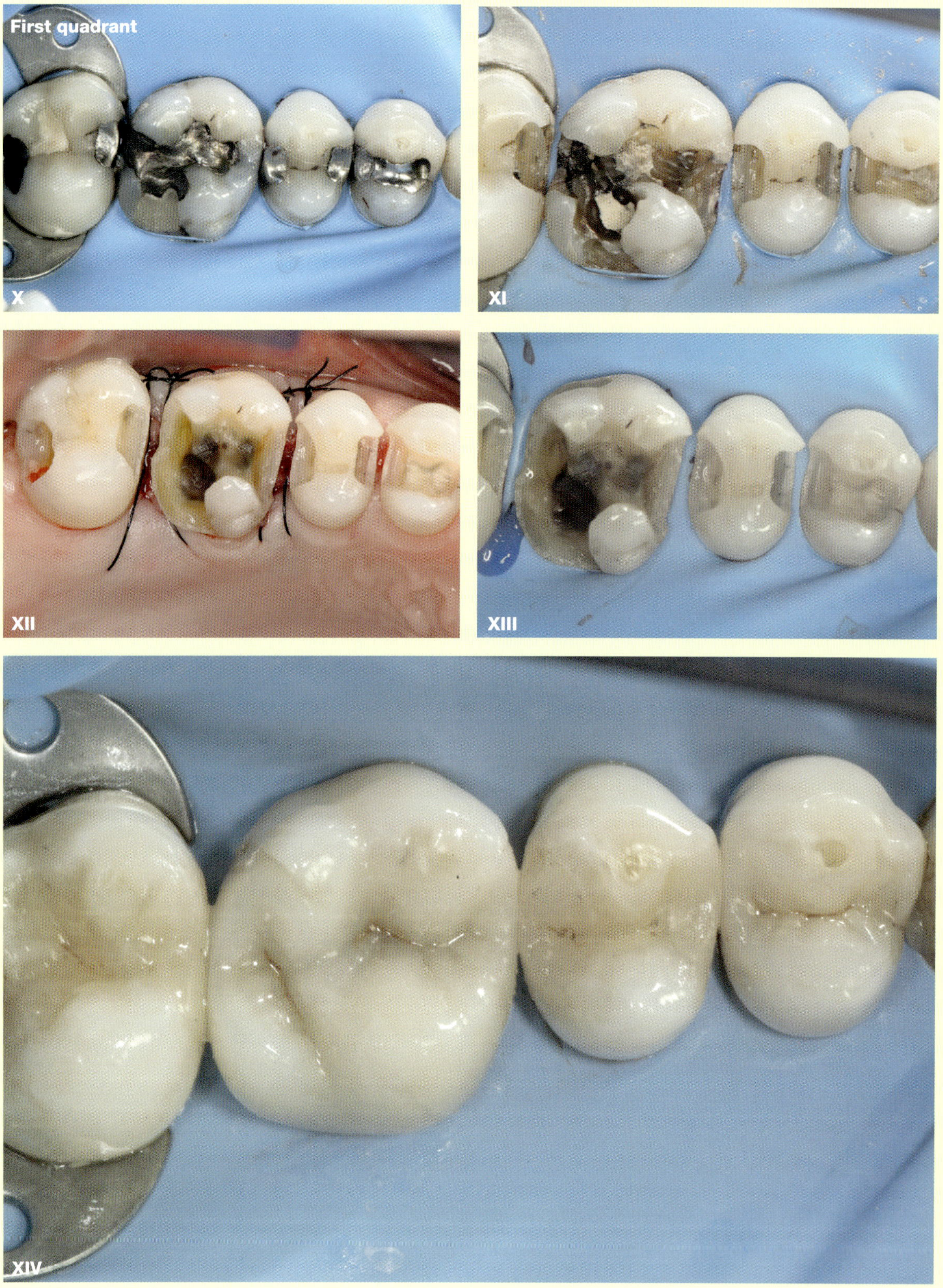
First quadrant
X
XI
XII
XIII
XIV

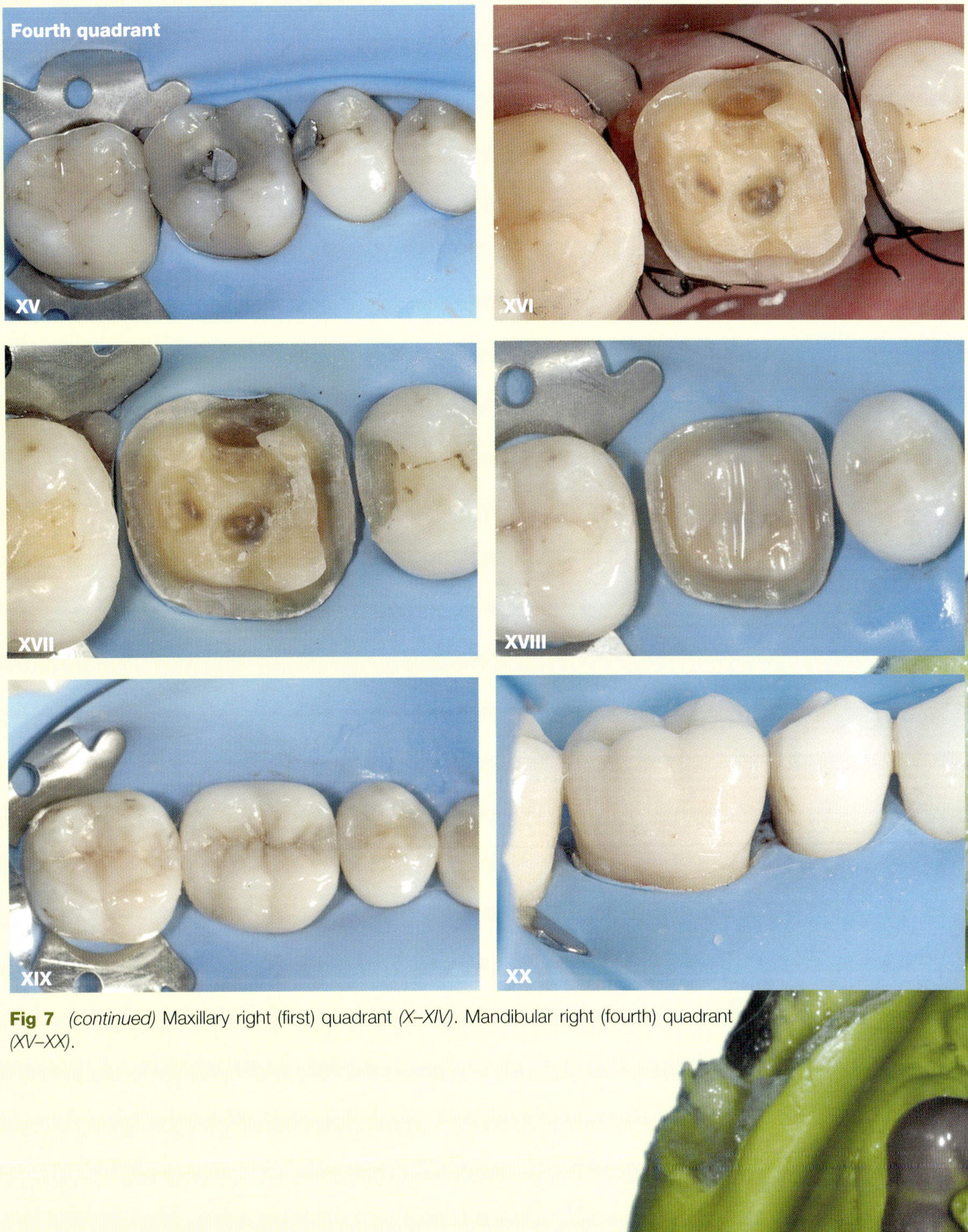

Fig 7 *(continued)* Maxillary right (first) quadrant *(X–XIV)*. Mandibular right (fourth) quadrant *(XV–XX)*.

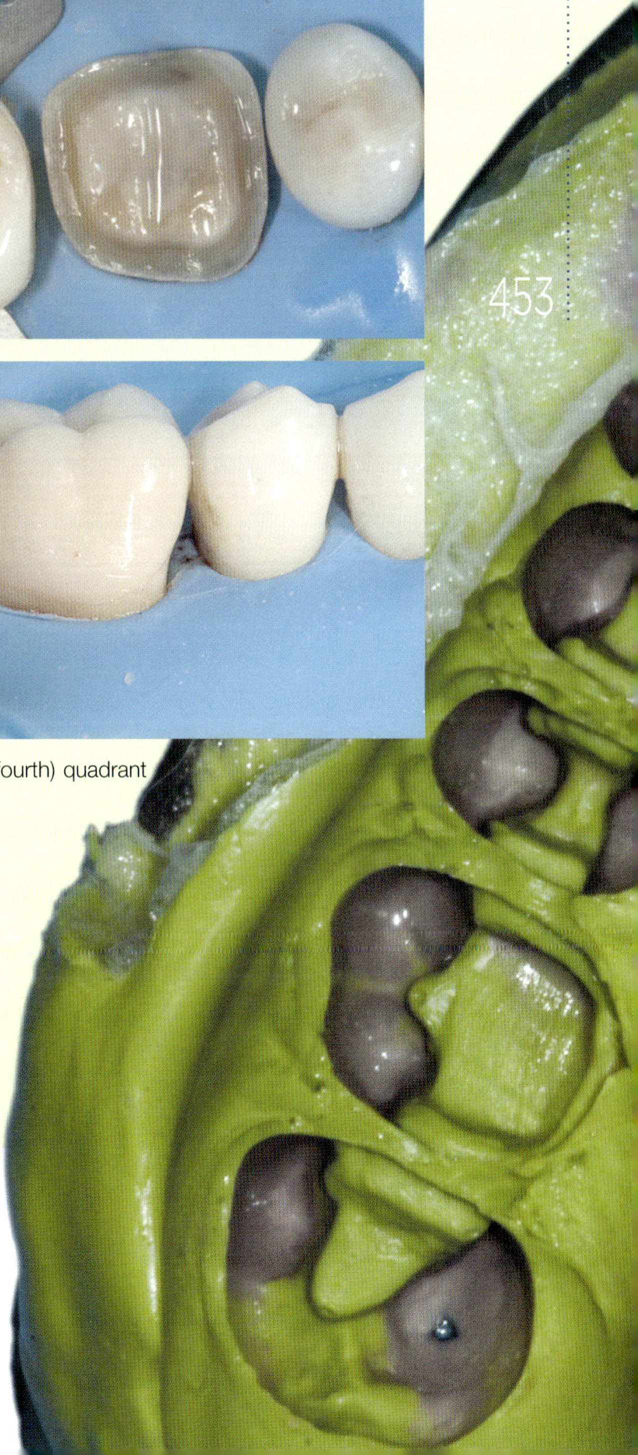

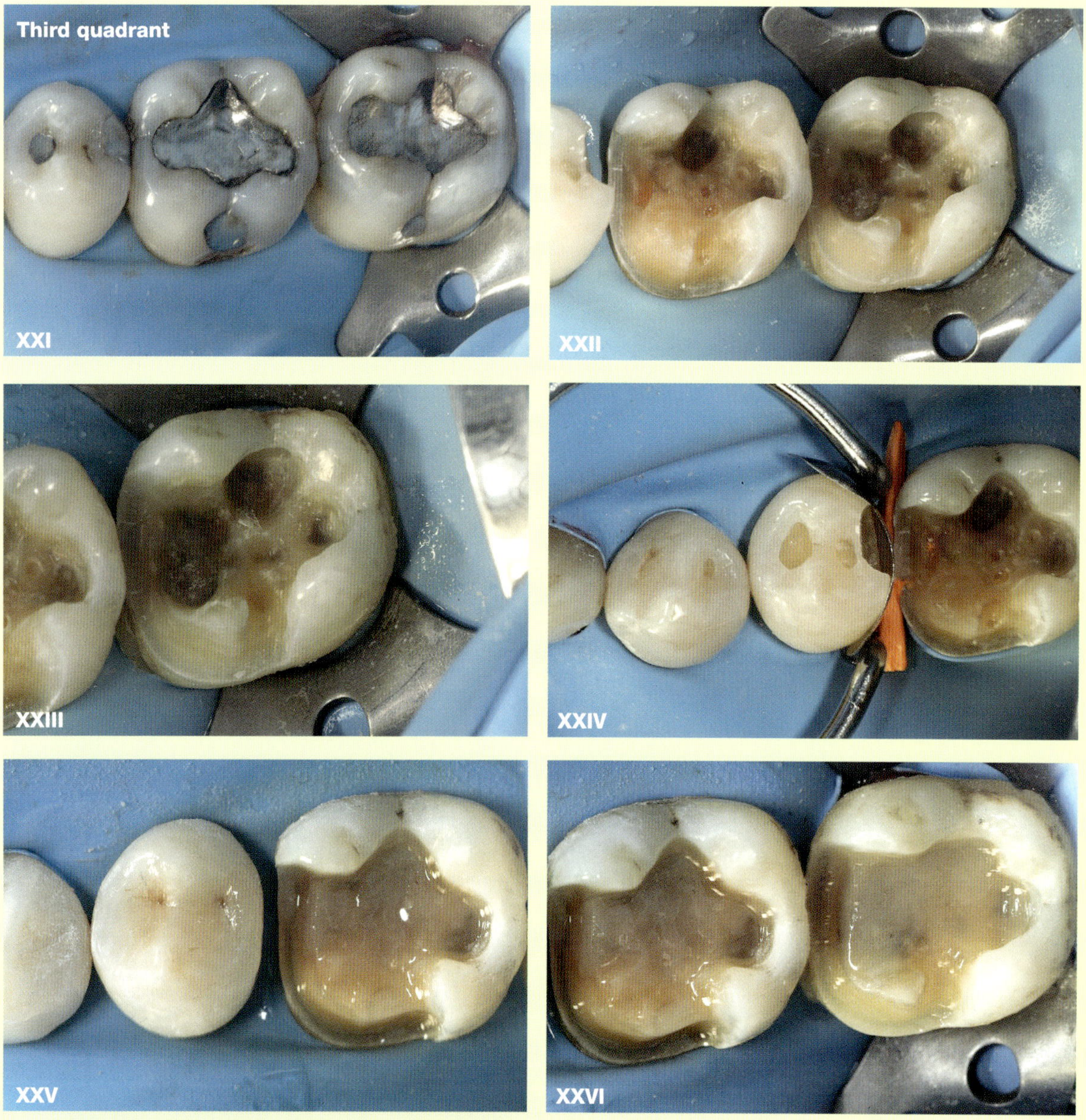

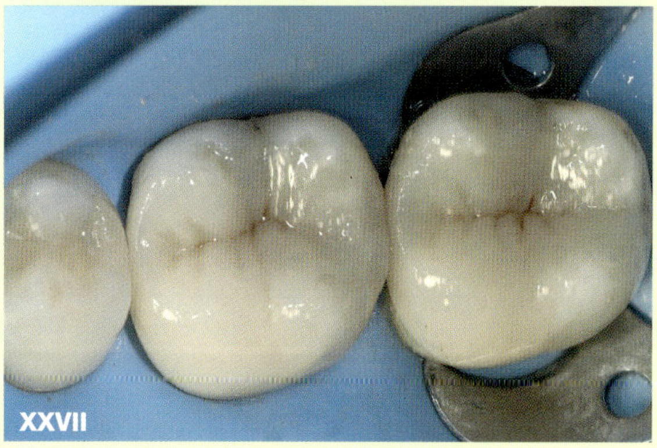

Fig 7 *(continued)* Mandibular left (third) quadrant *(XXI–XXVII)*.

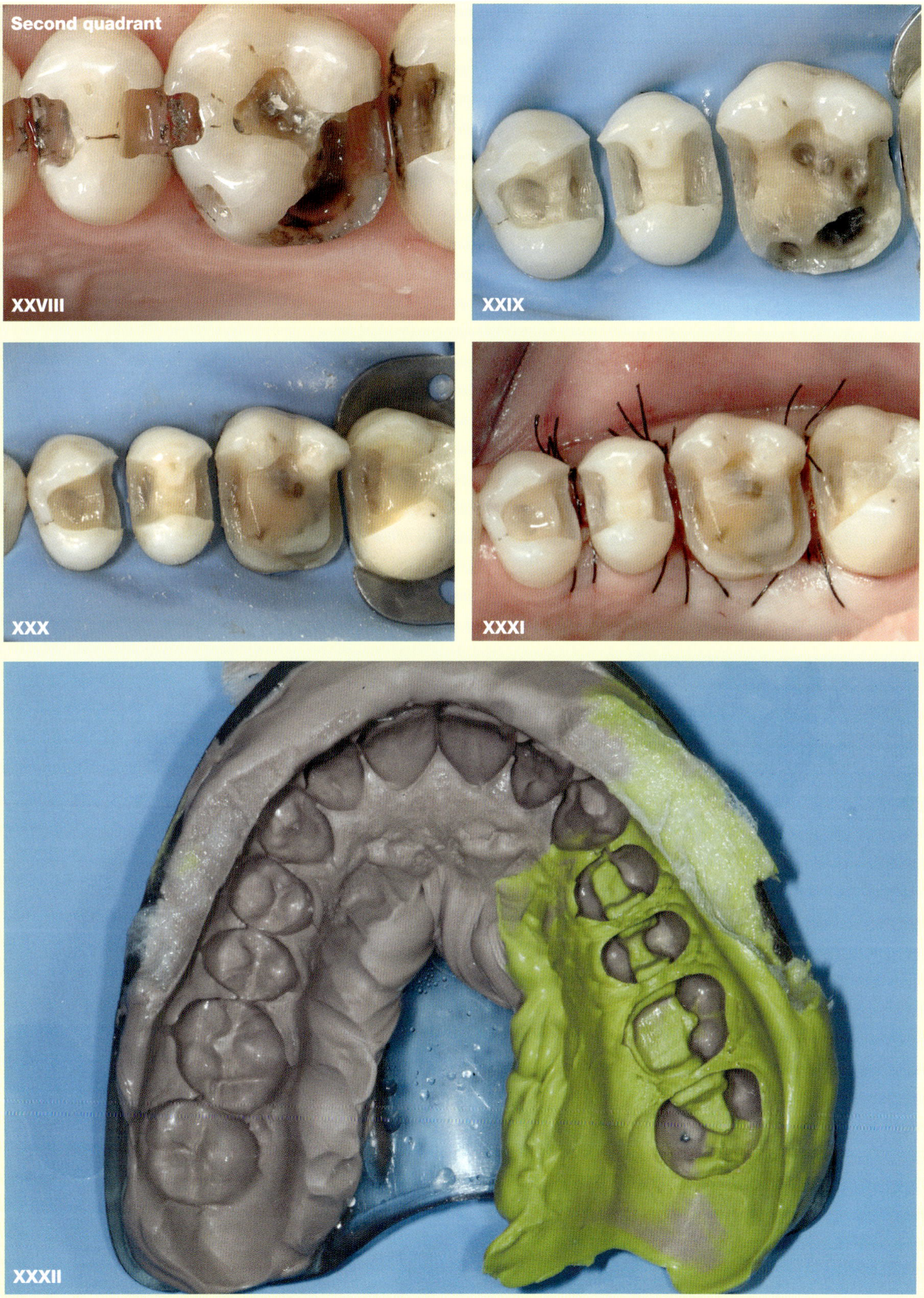

Fig 7 *(continued)* Maxillary left (second) quadrant. Clinical case with preparations completed and ready for the impression, which is taken once dam is removed *(XXVIII–XXXII)*.

Laboratory procedures

Normally the author's team works by quadrants even in complex cases, which makes for easier clinical management of the case. It should nevertheless be remembered that it is important to work on opposing quadrants in order to be able to alter and correct the occlusal plane.

The laboratory procedure involves various steps (described below):

- Cast preparation
- Margin preparation
- Internal spacing
- Stratification and modeling technique
- Curing
- Finishing and polishing

Cast preparation

The author's team uses the plaster that is normally used in traditional prosthetic procedures to take an impression: an extra-hard type IV die stone (Fujirock EP).

Margin preparation

At this point, the next step is to use a stereomicroscope to remove the plaster cast of the gingival tissues in order to free the margin and allow a correct reading. This is a procedure that must be carried out very carefully in order not to impair the precision of the master cast, and great care must be taken not to touch the preparation margin with the bur (Figs 8 I and II). In order to display the preparation margin correctly, the technician uses a soft wax pencil (Figs 8 III and IV) to mark the limit of the preparation around its entire perimeter. In order to fix the resulting mark, the author's team applies a cyanoacrylate-based product (Liquicol, Renfert) very accurately with an air jet to the margin portion only (Figs 8 V to VIII) in order to avoid buildup in the area where maximum precision should be ensured. One consequence of using a cyanoacrylate is a mechanical improvement in the plaster. This means that the margin is strengthened and the plaster is allowed to remain intact, without abrasions or alterations, until the end of the procedure.

Internal spacing

This section on the spacing procedure is included because the method used differs from that normally used for fixed prostheses. A spacer must be present on the cast in order to allow space for the cement in the reconstruction, which is important because the reconstruction will be raised occlusally after cementing without proper spacing. When making prostheses, the author's team normally uses a 20- to 25-µm spacer that allows sufficient space for the cement used to fix the crowns. For inlays, they prefer to use the same microhybrid composite used to produce the inlay for the cement. This is a material that offers much better filling properties than normal cement, and the compressibility limit of the composite is much higher. This means that more space needs to be created, and the author's team uses wax for the spacing, effectively creating a space that measures more than 100 µm on average and allows the elimination of any undercuts. The wax is positioned approximately 1.5 to 2.0 mm away from the preparation margin (Figs 8 IX and X).

Stratification and modeling

Both dentin layers and enamel layers are used to stratify the microhybrid composite, beginning with more chromatic layers in the center of the tooth and then desaturating the color through the application of subsequent layers. The restoration is completed by adding characterizations and coating with enamel material. The first step is to position the most chromatic dentin at the cervical and occlusal floor level. This will make it possible to increase the effect of restoration depth and confer a more natural appearance. The color is more saturated than normal in dentistry, and the next stage is to begin to desaturate the color in successive layers in order to finish off with the filter afforded by the enamel layer (Figs 8 XI and XII). This is done in the quest for a natural appearance, in which a contrast is sought between the various layers that, together with the opalescent effect of the enamel, make it possible to produce reconstructions that blend very well into the oral cavity.

The enamel layer must be relatively thin, not exceeding a thickness of 1.0 to 1.5 mm; otherwise restoration quality will suffer, and the final result will be less glossy and have a grayish effect (Figs 8 XIII and XIV).

Curing

The final structure is further cured in a special heater that uses both light and heat; adding heat makes it possible to achieve a higher level of conversion than when light alone is used, and this leads to an improvement in both mechanical and physical properties[13,14] (Fig 8 XV).

Finishing and polishing

Finishing is carried out with diamond burs and points. The aim when using burs is to emphasize the design of grooves and natural depressions in the tooth in order to optimize the anatomical design of the tooth, which may be further characterized by adding tints (optiglaze C, GC) to the groove (Fig 8 XVI).

Diamond points are essential for finishing the margin. The entire process is monitored through a stereomi-

Complex clinical case: Laboratory stage

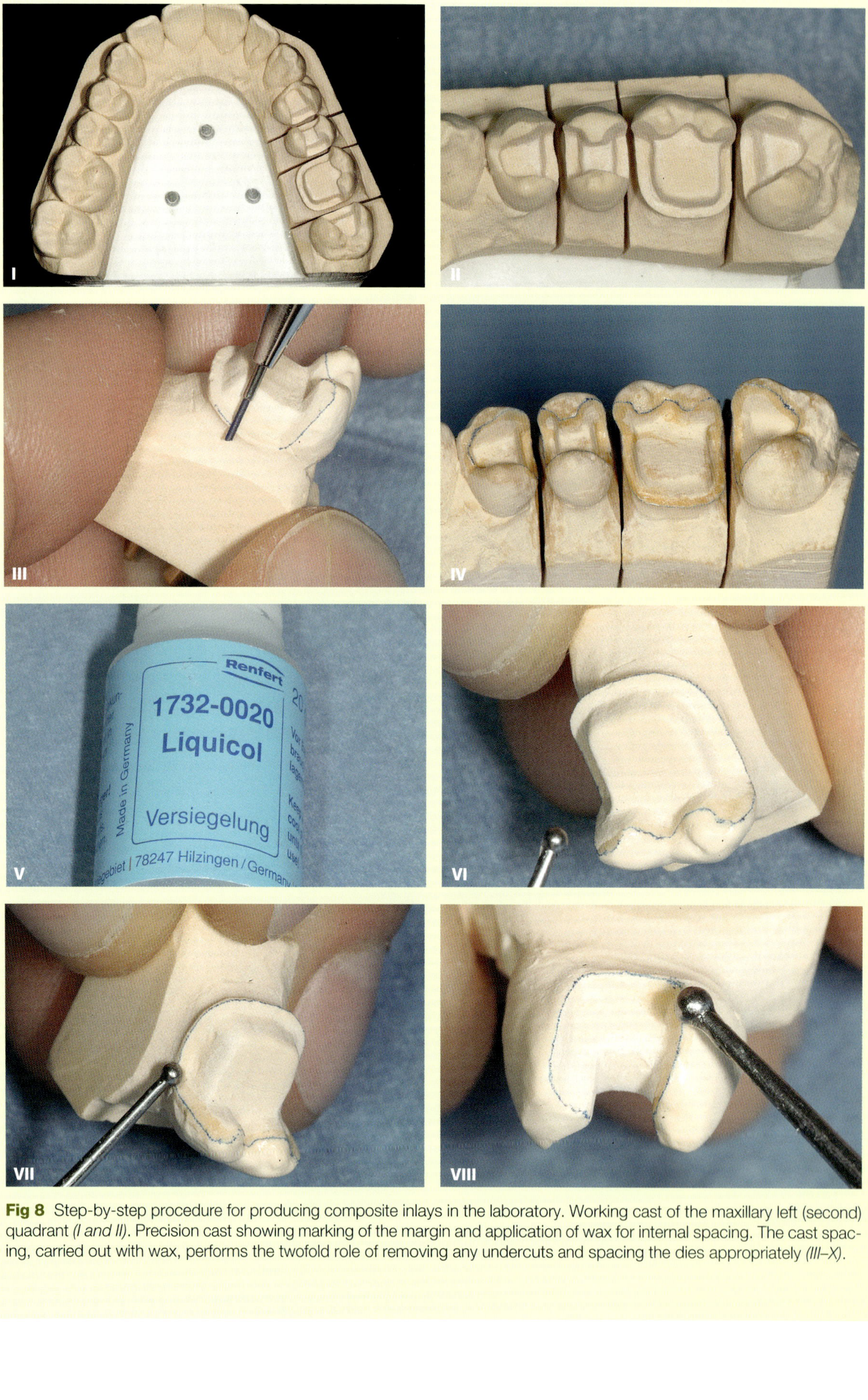

Fig 8 Step-by-step procedure for producing composite inlays in the laboratory. Working cast of the maxillary left (second) quadrant *(I and II)*. Precision cast showing marking of the margin and application of wax for internal spacing. The cast spacing, carried out with wax, performs the twofold role of removing any undercuts and spacing the dies appropriately *(III–X)*.

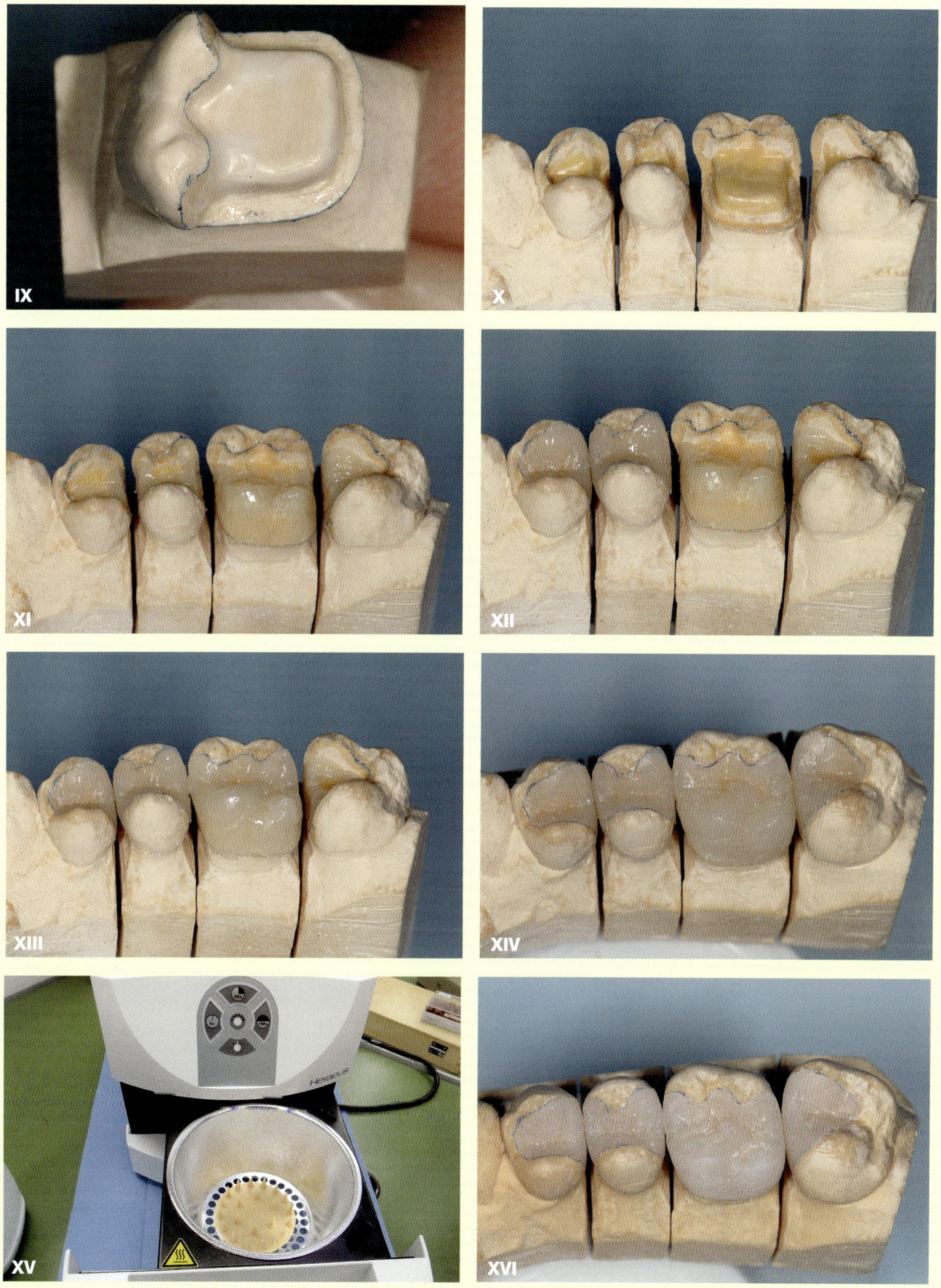

Fig 8 *(continued)* Application of the first layer of higher chromaticity dentin on the preparation base *(XI)*. Application of the second layer of dentin, beginning to desaturate the color using a layer with lower chromaticity than the previous layer *(XII)*. Layer of enamel material used to complete the stratification with an opalescent filter and initial reproduction of occlusal morphology *(XIII, XIV)*. Heater for curing *(XV)*. Inlays completed with the use of burs to maximally improve the reproduction of occlusal details *(XVI)*.

croscope, which makes it possible to achieve high marginal precision, a fundamental feature of all types of restoration.

Polishing must be carried out without altering the anatomical structure of the inlay and without affecting marginal precision.

The process starts with diamond paste applied in two decreasing 5- and 3-µm steps with a brush, and then the entire surface is gently treated in a gradual manner.

Final polishing is carried out using a soft brush and aluminum oxide paste, which gives the restoration a glossy appearance.

The author's team does not use light-cured glazes because they are unstable in the long term and are subject to color changes that detract from the esthetic appearance of the restoration (Figs 8 XVII to XXVII).

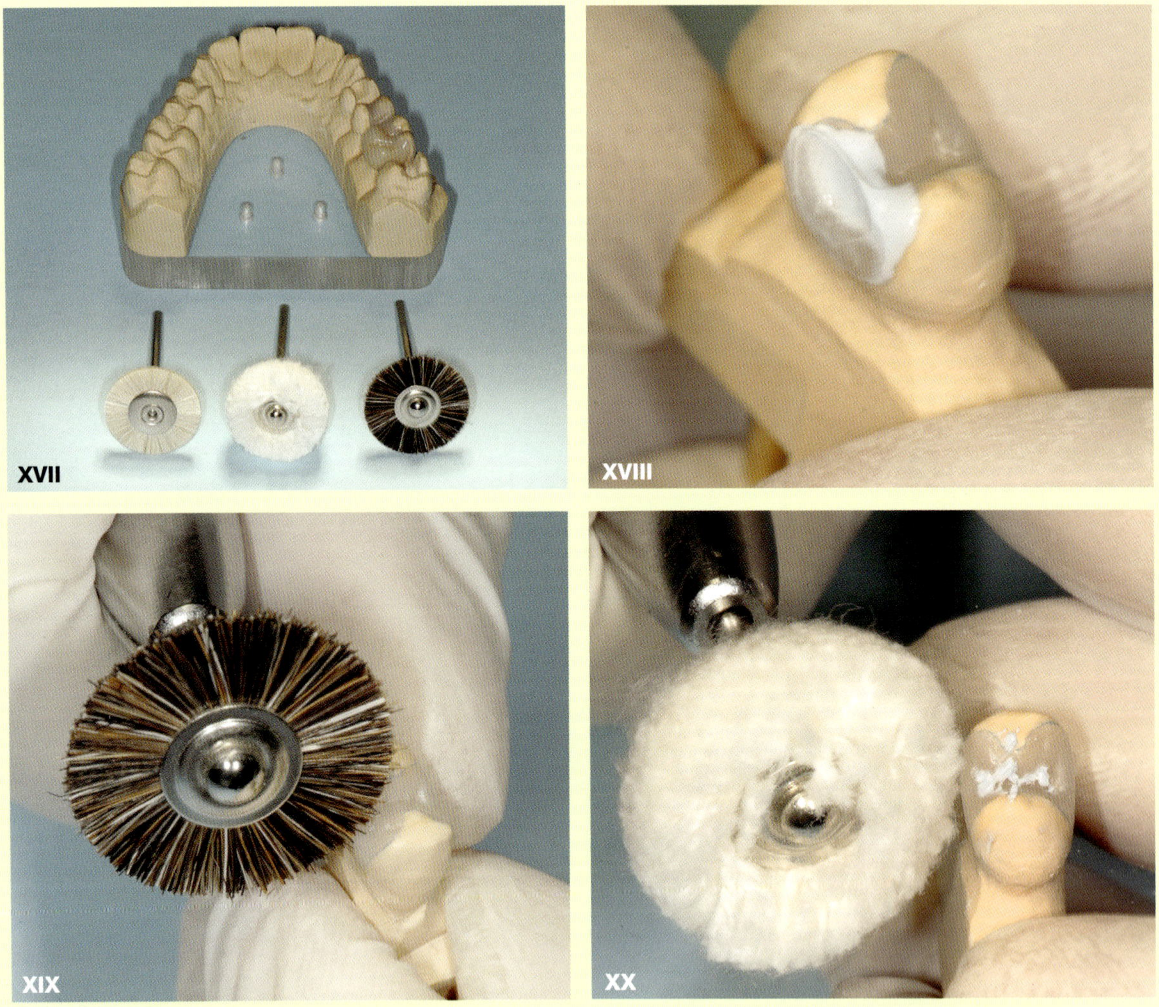

Fig 8 *(continued)* For final polishing, brushes, points, and diamond pastes are used in sequence for effective polishing of the composite without altering its morphology *(XVII–XX)*.

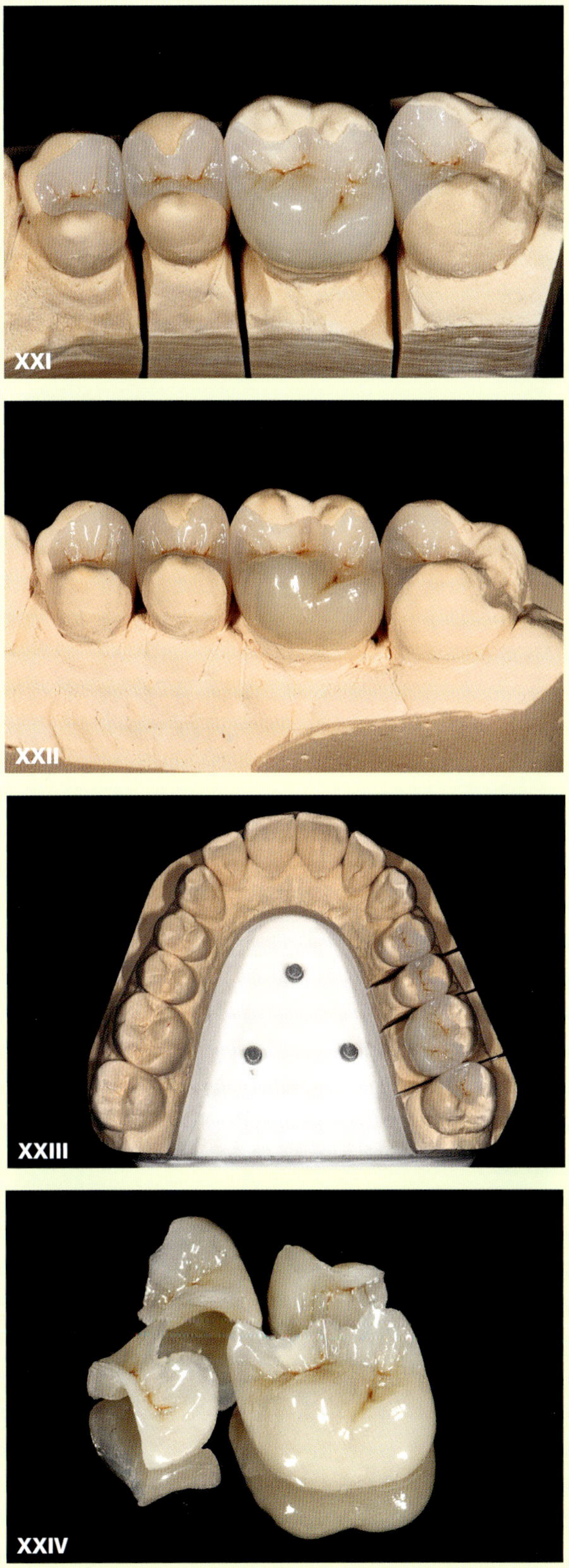

Fig 8 *(continued)* Inlays completed following characterization and polishing *(XXI–XXIV)*.

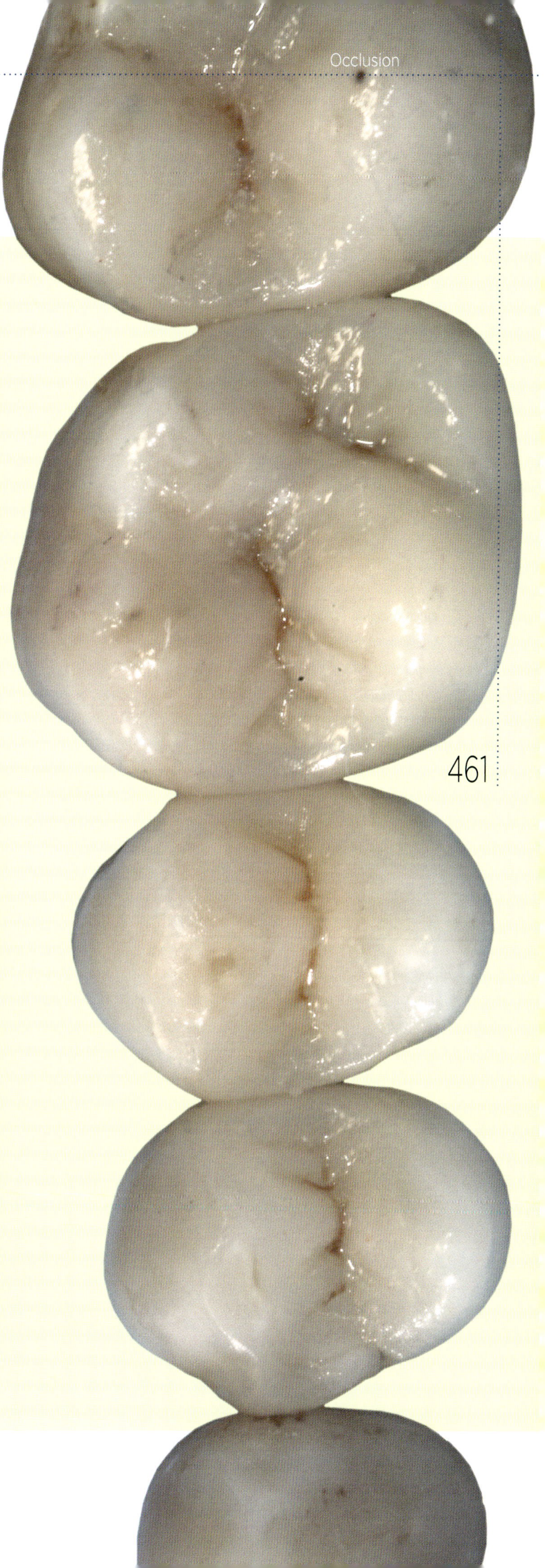

Occlusal adjustments

One particularly delicate and essential step for ensuring the success of treatment is checking the occlusion after cementing the inlays.

Occlusal contacts, the importance of which was previously emphasized, must meet the following requirements:

- Multiple and punctiform
- Simultaneous on both sides
- Absence of interference in eccentric jaw movements

The occlusion check is never random, but must observe specific repetitive and repeatable rules as follows. Firstly, occlusal adjustment is the final stage of the treatment that started by studying the occlusion and possibly involved wax-ups in complex cases. It is important to remember that by this stage any disharmony should have been corrected and conservative treatment should have been abandoned in cases that actually required more complex rehabilitation work.
The author prefers to explain this by saying that conservative treatment may be contraindicated following occlusal assessment. More complex treatment is indeed required in more than a few cases in order to achieve success.
It should be remembered that in occlusal abnormalities, success is achieved by re-creating harmony between factors determining the occlusion. During the initial analysis it is therefore always very important to identify all cases where a conservative approach is not possible.

Contraindications to exclusively conservative treatment:

- Bruxism with extensive occlusal wear
- Dysfunctional abnormalities of the temporomandibular joint
- Insufficient anterior guidance
- Open bite
- Collapse of posterior vertical dimension of occlusion

Working in an exclusively conservative manner in the above cases could easily lead to failure, with premature wear or fracture of the restorations. In the cases mentioned, inlays could be used as a therapeutic procedure, but as part of a more complex occlusal rehabilitation process.
It is often tempting to attribute failure and material fracture or wear to the ceramic or composite material, but often in such cases failure is really caused by poor management of the occlusal problem and having adopted a conformist approach instead of a rehabilitation approach, seeking new occlusal harmonies.

From a technical viewpoint, when checking the occlusion, the clinician must ensure that good support has been provided with maximal intercuspation and all occlusal interferences during eccentric jaw movements have been eliminated.

One common mistake made at this stage is that of not respecting a preestablished operating sequence and instead proceeding randomly, filing off a little here and a little there and ending up with a deficient vertical dimension of occlusion.
It is essential to remove only interferences, respecting and maintaining the contacts with maximal intercuspation.

The author's team achieves this by using the following sequence[15]:

- Removing protrusive interferences
- Adapting the working and nonworking side simultaneously for each lateral mandibular excursion
- Never filing the tip of the cusps but rather the groove in the opposing tooth when possible
- Checking the centric relationship and the maximal intercuspation only when all the interferences have been removed

The rationale behind this approach is that of not losing contacts with the correct bite and finding ourselves with multiple, synchronous, and bilateral contacts following occlusal adjustment with no interference in eccentric movements.
Centric interferences are removed last because they form part of the eccentric interferences. By proceeding in this way, minimal retouching is required at this stage because most have been removed previously during the removal of eccentric interferences.
One other important aspect of this approach is respect for tooth and restoration anatomy because filing the teeth on the cusp side and opening the occlusal grooves more effectively maintains the shape that the technician created in the laboratory, the anatomy, and, above all, the function by not losing the correct vertical dimension of occlusion despite removing all occlusal interferences.

From a practical viewpoint, the author's team uses fine articulating paper (AccuFilm II, Parkell) in two colors: red and black.
They usually mark eccentric movements using red paper and use black paper to mark centric stops or maximal intercuspation (Figs 8 XXVIII to XXXIII).
The patient is instructed to carry out the correct jaw movements to the limit and is partly aided by the practitioner to ensure they are performed correctly.
When working with inlays that have been thoroughly polished in the laboratory, it may be difficult to obtain the correct occlusal markers. As an aid in such cases, the author's team spreads a fine layer of petroleum jelly on the paper and then waits for a few minutes. The petroleum jelly acts as a solvent on the occlusal paper, allowing marking of the contacts more effectively with all the attendant benefits to the practitioner (Figs 8 XXXIV to XXXVIII).

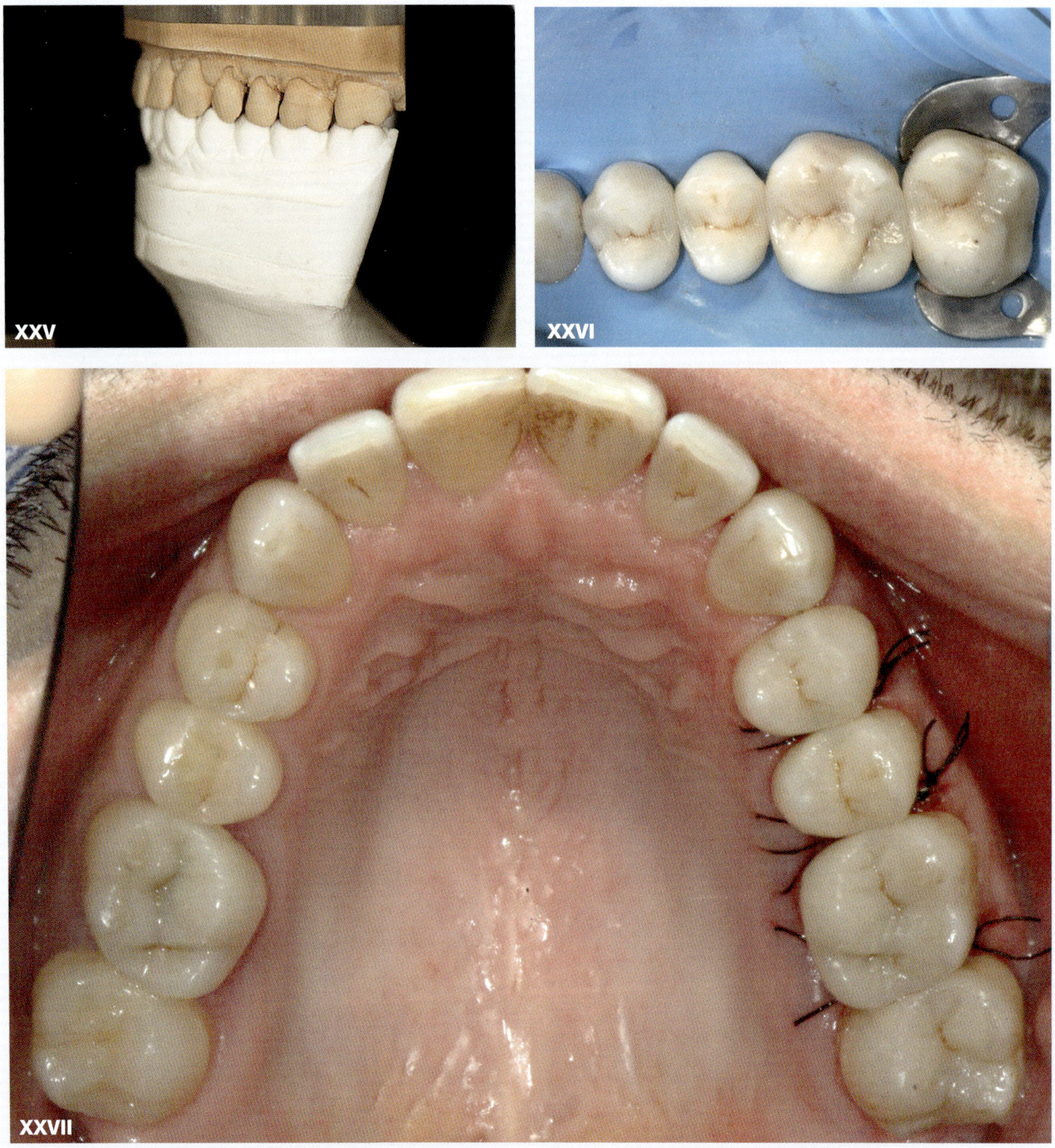

Fig 8 *(continued)* Step-by-step process of producing composite inlays in the laboratory. With a contrasting black background it is possible to see the effects of the stratification described. There is a visible difference in translucency and opacity between central and peripheral areas of the inlays. Tints have also been added to the surface to increase the three-dimensional effect of the reconstruction, which will make the restoration look very natural after cementation. Working cast with inlays in an articulator *(XXV)*. Final effect of the inlays after cementation. The restorations not only have a natural effect but also blend very well with the rest of the dentition. The slight color difference visible is due to dehydration of the teeth under rubber dam *(XXVI)*. A couple of hours after removing the dam, the improved final effect may be admired. In the quadrant in question, the sutures were still in place on the day of cementation and were removed the following week *(XXVII)*. Following periodontal surgery, it was easy to isolate the preparations properly using dam, allowing correct cementation.

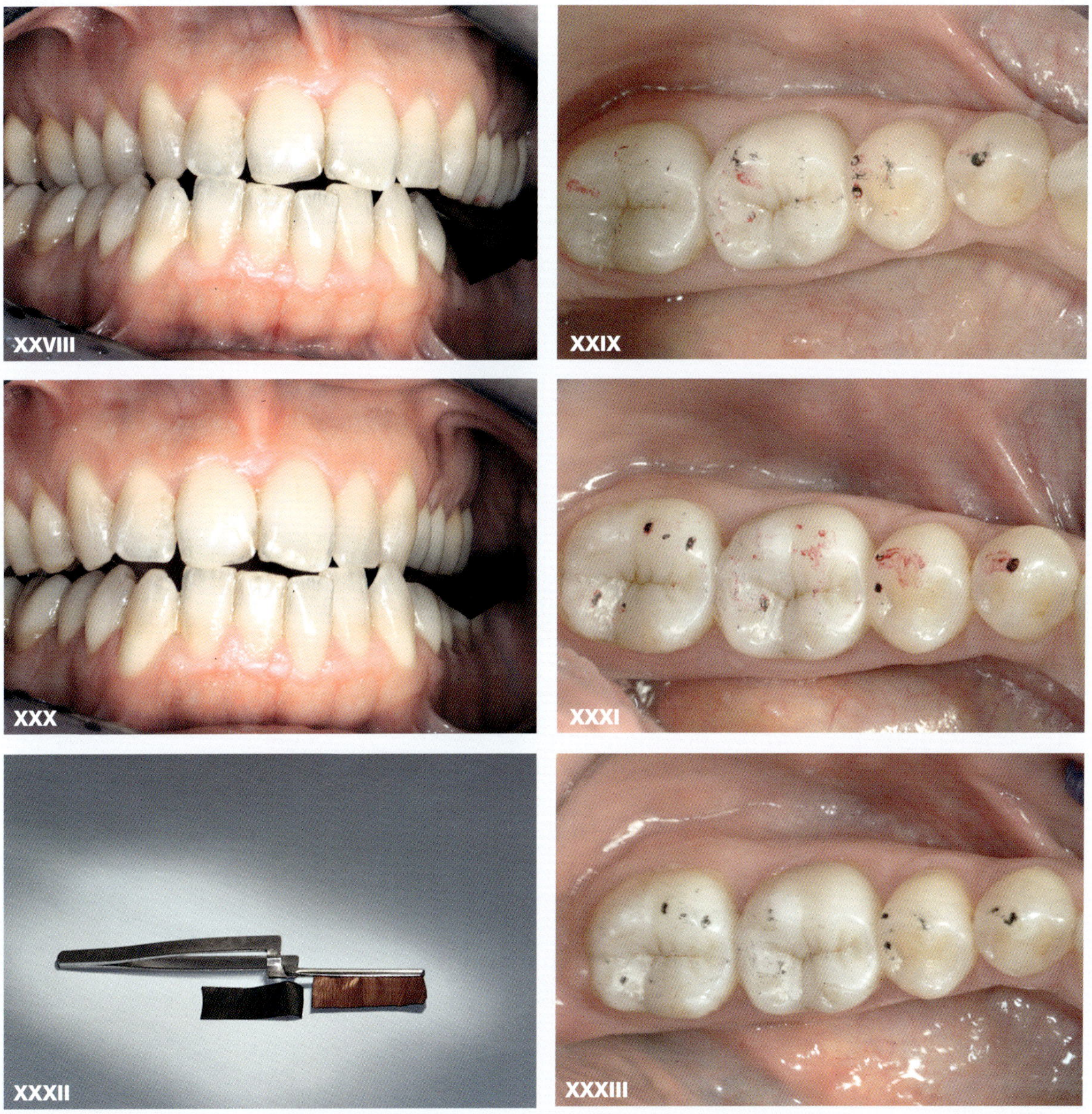

Fig 8 *(continued)* Checking the occlusion begins by testing the lateral movement performed by the side opposite to the restored side. This allows identification of any interferences in the nonworking movement, referred to as *balancing interferences*. These are the most dangerous interferences and must be completely removed *(XXVIII)*. The red marks are the signs left by the balancing interferences and must be completely removed without touching the black dots, which are the contacts in maximal intercuspation that must be maintained. In order to remove the interferences, a diamond bur with a granule size of 50 µm is used to avoid ruining the surface of the inlay and to ensure that it can then be easily repolished. These checks must be carried out several times until all the interferences are completely removed *(XXIX)*. Next mandibular movement to ward the side where the restorations are present, or the working side, is tested *(XXX)*. This patient's occlusal pattern includes insufficient canine guidance, meaning that the red contacts visible on the buccal cusps of the mandibular teeth are actually part of an ipsilateral group function and therefore must not be removed *(XXXI)*. Nevertheless, it should be noted that the presence of these dynamic contacts is not as dangerous as the balancing interferences from a functional viewpoint. This means that their removal is not always necessary and depends, as in this case, on the type of occlusal pattern present in the patient's mouth. The type of articulating paper that the author's team uses is very fine (approximately 12 µm) and very precise. When checking eccentric mandibular movements, they use it in a double layer for more effective recording of any interferences and premature contacts, while they use it in a single layer to record maximal intercuspation *(XXXII)*. Lastly, they test the maximal intercuspation position, recording the presence of multiple, synchronous, and punctiform contacts, which guarantee the stability of mandibular position *(XXXIII)*.

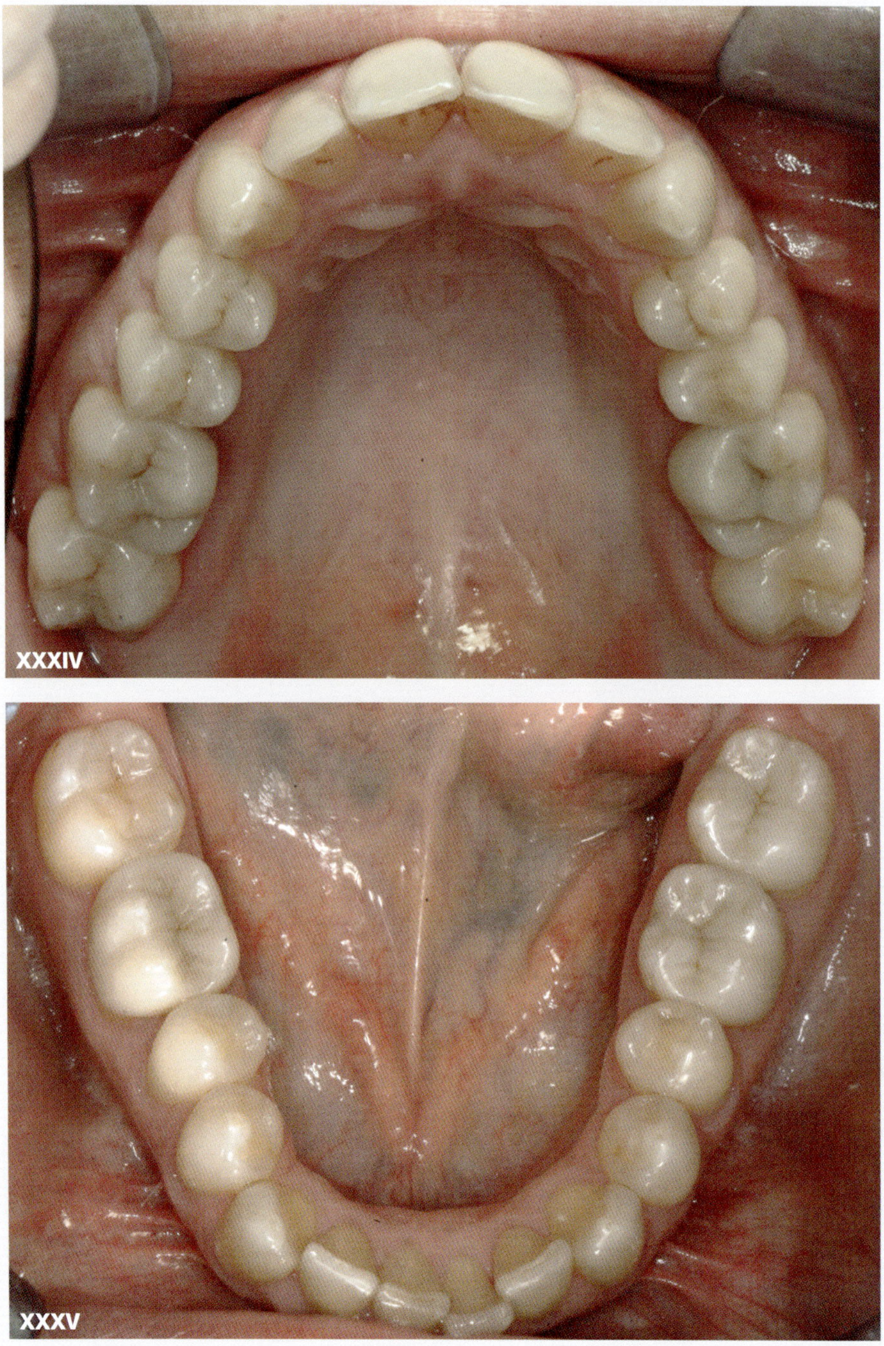

Fig 8 *(continued)* Complex restoration case. Both arches completely restored with composite inlays, radiographic status, and final bitewing radiographs of restorations *(XXXIV–XXX–VIII)*.

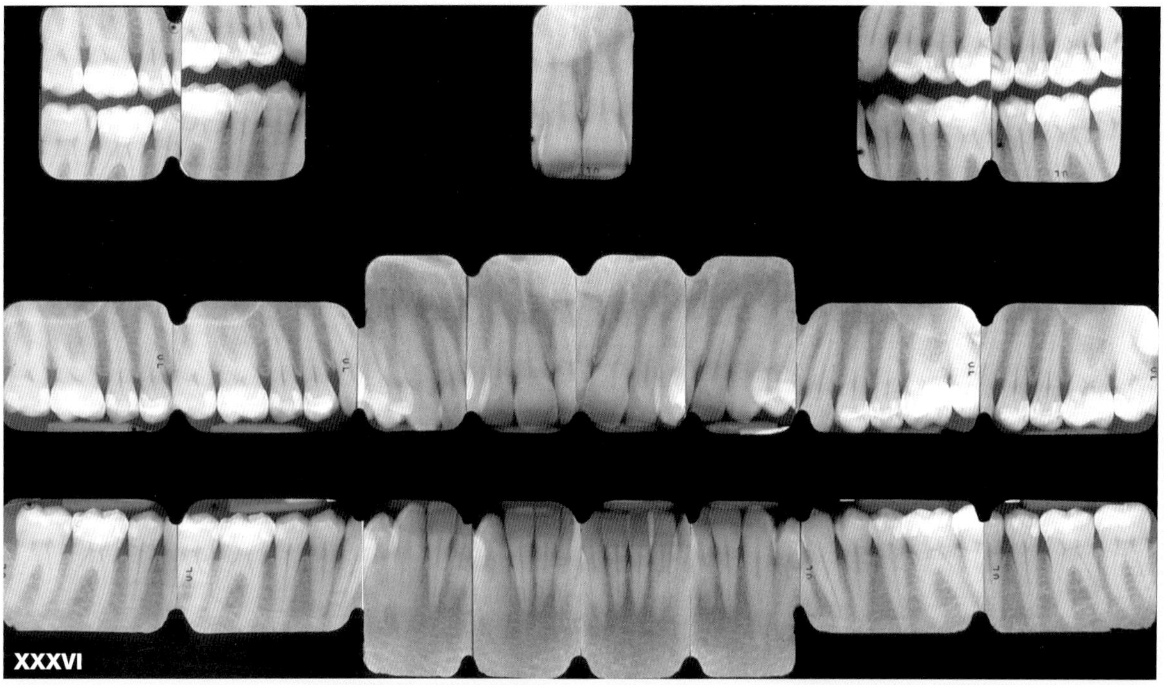
XXXVI

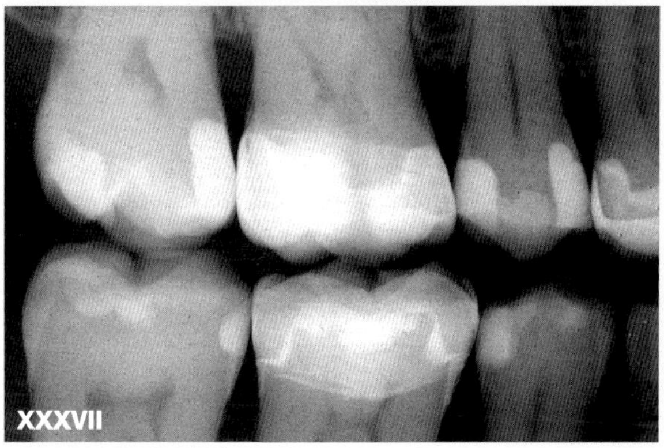
XXXVII

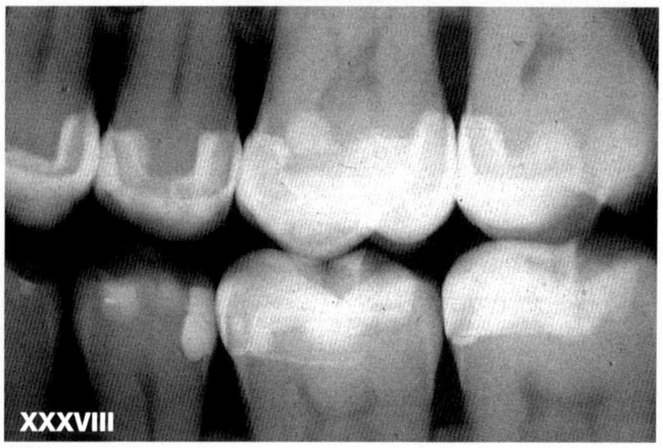
XXXVIII

References

1. Dawson PE. Functional Occlusion, from TMJ to Smile Design. St Louis: Mosby, 2007.
2. Shillingburg HT. Fundamentals of Fixed Prosthodontics, ed 3. Chicago: Quintessence, 1997.
3. Schiffman EL, Fricton JR, Haley D. The relationship of occlusion, parafunctional habits and recent life events to mandibular dysfunction in a non-patient population. J Oral Rehabil 1992;19:201–223.
4. Gracis S. Clinical considerations and rationale for the use of simplified instrumentation in occlusal rehabilitation. Part 1: Mounting of the models on the articulator. Int J Periodontics Restorative Dent 2003;23:57–67.
5. Gracis S. Clinical considerations and rationale for the use of simplified instrumentation in occlusal rehabilitation. Part 2: Setting of the articulator and occlusal optimization. Int J Periodontics Restorative Dent 2003;23:139–145.
6. Keough B. Occlusion-based treatment planning for complex dental restorations: Part 1. Int J Periodontics Restorative Dent 2003;23:237–247.
7. Keough B. Occlusion-based treatment planning for complex dental restorations: Part 2. Int J Periodontics Restorative Dent 2003;23:325–335.
8. Wöstmann B, Rehmann P, Balkenhol M. Accuracy of impressions obtained with dual-arch trays. Int J Prosthodont 2009;22:158–160.
9. Ceyhan JA, Johnson GH, Lepe X, Phillips KM. A clinical study comparing the three-dimensional accuracy of a working die generated from two dual-arch trays and a complete-arch custom tray. J Prosthet Dent 2003;90:228–234.
10. Ceyhan JA, Johnson GH, Lepe X. The effect of tray selection, viscosity of impression material, and sequence of pour on the accuracy of dies made from dual-arch impressions. J Prosthet Dent 2003;90:143–149 [erratum 2007;97:38].
11. Lundeen HC, Shryock EF, Gibbs CH. An evaluation of mandibular border movements: Their character and significance. J Prosthet Dent 1978;40:442–452.
12. Hart JK, Sakamura JS. Mandibular lateral side shift and the need of gnathological instrumentation. J Prosthet Dent 1985;54:415–420.
13. Park SH. Comparison of degree of conversion for light-cured and additionally heat-cured composites. J Prosthet Dent 1996;76:613–618.
14. Ferracane JL, Condon JR. Post-cure heat treatments for composites: Properties and fractography. Dent Mater 1992;8:290–295.
15. Solnit A, Curnutte DC. Occlusal Correction: Principles and Practice. Chicago: Quintessence, 1988.

Cracked tooth syndrome 6

Cracked tooth syndrome, described by Cameron in 1976,[1] was defined in 1988 by Frank et al[2] as an infraction or interruption in the continuity of the tooth surface without any perceptible separation. Today, a dentinal fracture line represents an increasingly widespread clinical event that is extremely difficult to manage.

The most important factor associated with dentinal fracture lines is also the most obvious: knowing of their existence (Figs 1 to 4). Krell and Rivera[3] observed 8,175 teeth in 6 years, identifying 796 cracks (9.7%), of which 30% affected the mandibular second molars, 29% the mandibular first molars, and 21% the maxillary first molars.

Williams[4] classified them as follows:

- Class I: Incomplete vertical fracture of the enamel and dentin without pulpal involvement
- Class II: Pulpal involvement
- Class III: Attachment involvement
- Class IV: Complete separation of fragments
- Class V: Retrograde root fracture

In 2003, Martin and Machtou[5] classified them as:

- Crack in the enamel
- Crack in the enamel and dentin, without signs of pulpitis
- Crack in the enamel and dentin with signs of pulpitis (subacute or acute)
- Coronal crack with pulp necrosis

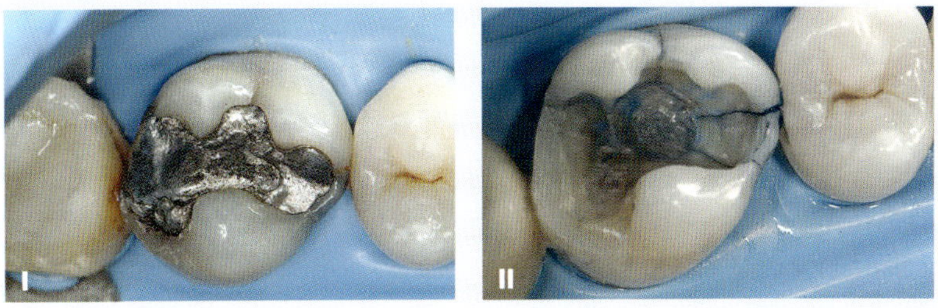

Fig 1 Large dentinal fracture lines visible after removing an amalgam restoration.

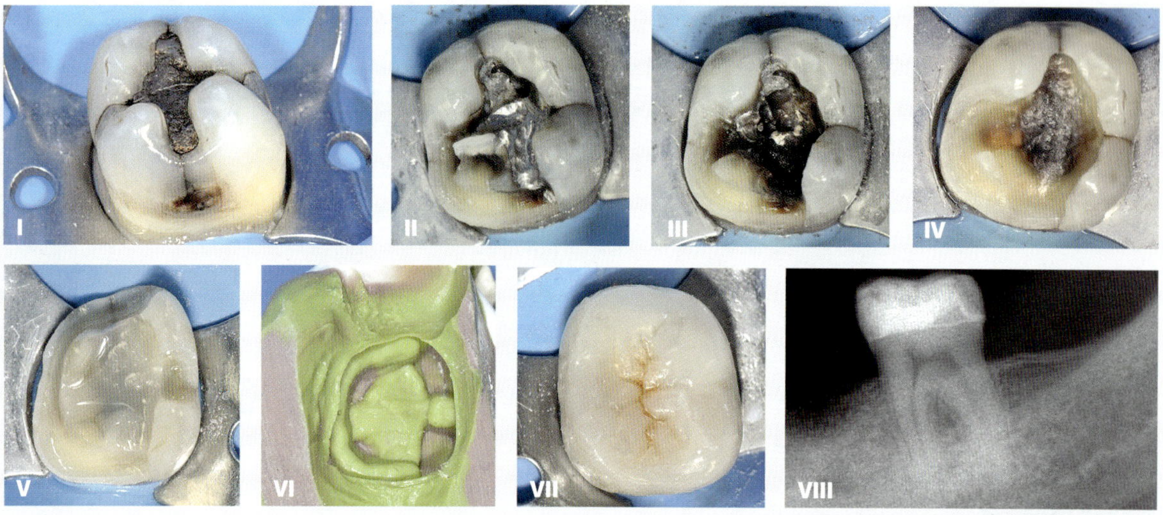

Fig 2 Preparation and cementation of an adhesive restoration in a mandibular molar with highly evident fracture lines. The missing proximal molar concentrates the load excessively on the tooth in question.

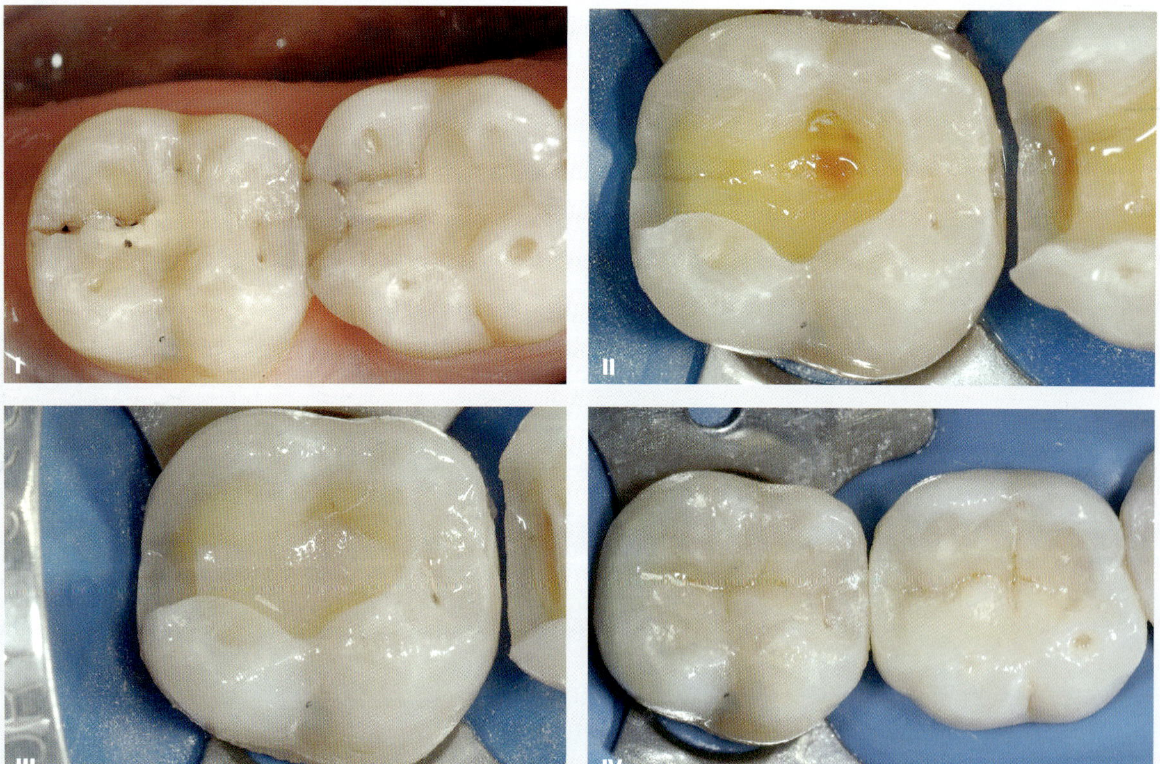

Fig 3 Small fracture line in a mandibular molar of a patient with parafunctions. Regular use of a bite guard is required for this reason.

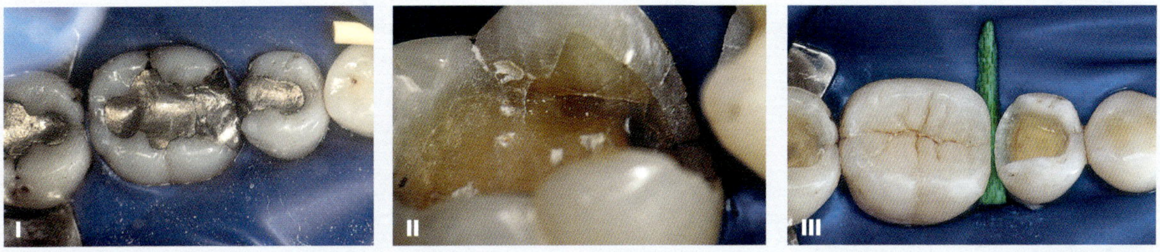

Fig 4 Fracture lines undermining the mesiolingual wall of a mandibular molar and execution of an onlay after wall removal.

Patients consult their dentist, usually complaining of twinges, sporadic at the beginning, while chewing. They also report a general sense of discomfort, which then develops into sensitivity to cold, followed over time by pain on chewing, which leads more or less inexorably to diffuse and discontinuous pain before reaching the point of intense, radiant pain—this is cracked tooth syndrome (Figs 5 to 10).
The crack causes pain due to pulp inflammation; a large number of dentinal tubules are open to the oral environment. The pain originates from the tooth without clinical, let alone radiographic, signs.
From a microbiologic viewpoint, Kahler et al[6] observed the presence of cocchi, bacilli, filamentous forms, and dividing bacteria in such cracks.
It goes without saying that these bacteria become responsible for irreversible pulp inflammation when the fracture fully involves the dentin, establishing direct communication between the oral environment and the pulp.[7]
In order to make a diagnosis, the clinician must refer to the patient's medical history, the symptoms described above, and their development, also examining the clinical appearance of the teeth with the aim of pinpointing these annoying fracture lines.

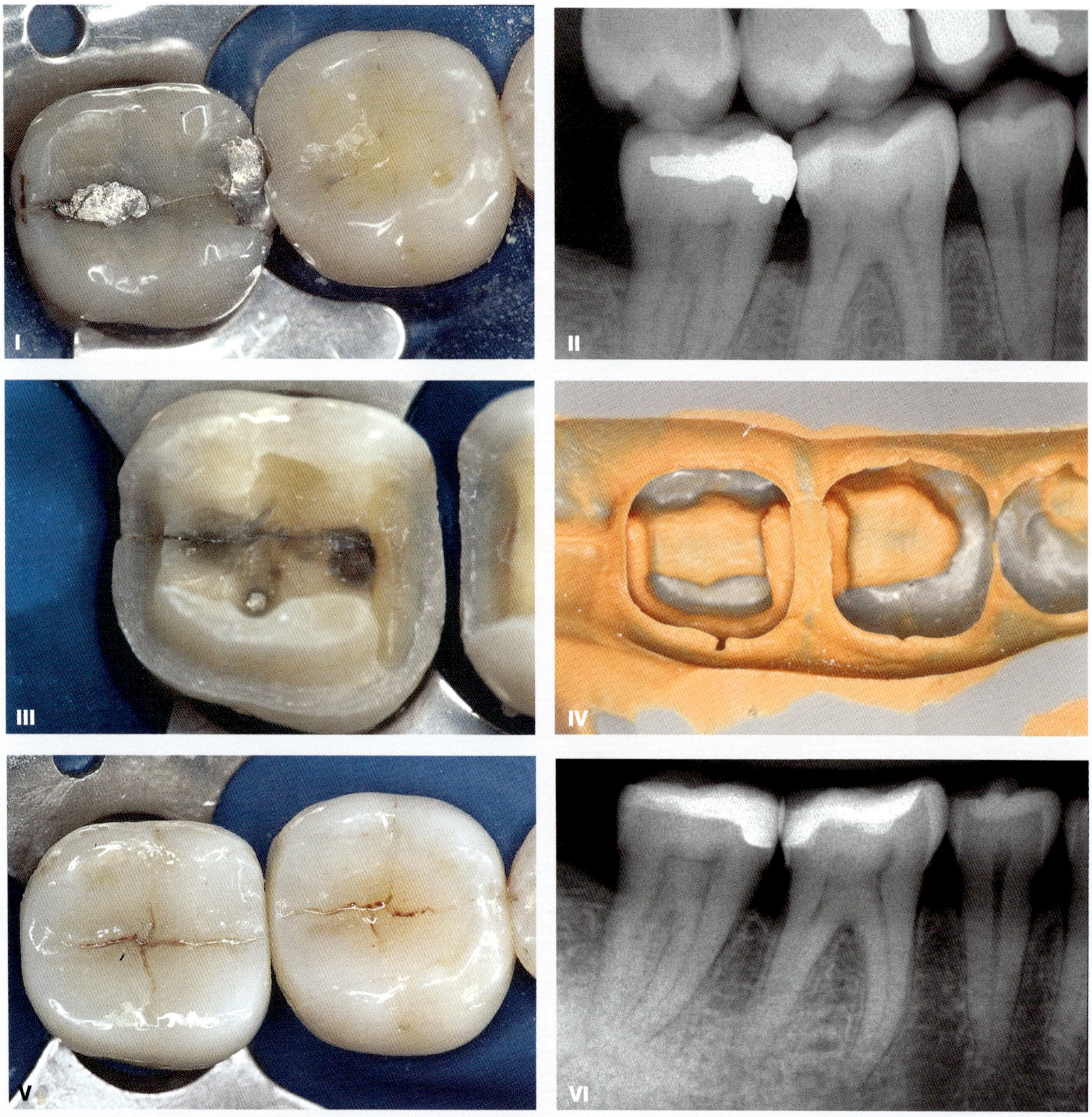

Fig 5 A mesio-occlusodistal fracture line in the mandibular right second molar made it impossible for the patient to chew. After cleaning the fracture line, followed by adhesion and buildup, reconstruction of the compromised tooth was completed by a composite onlay *(I–V)*. After a few months, the painful symptoms disappeared altogether, and a radiographic checkup 9 years later *(VI)* revealed the absence of periradicular lesions. A pulp vitality test was positive.

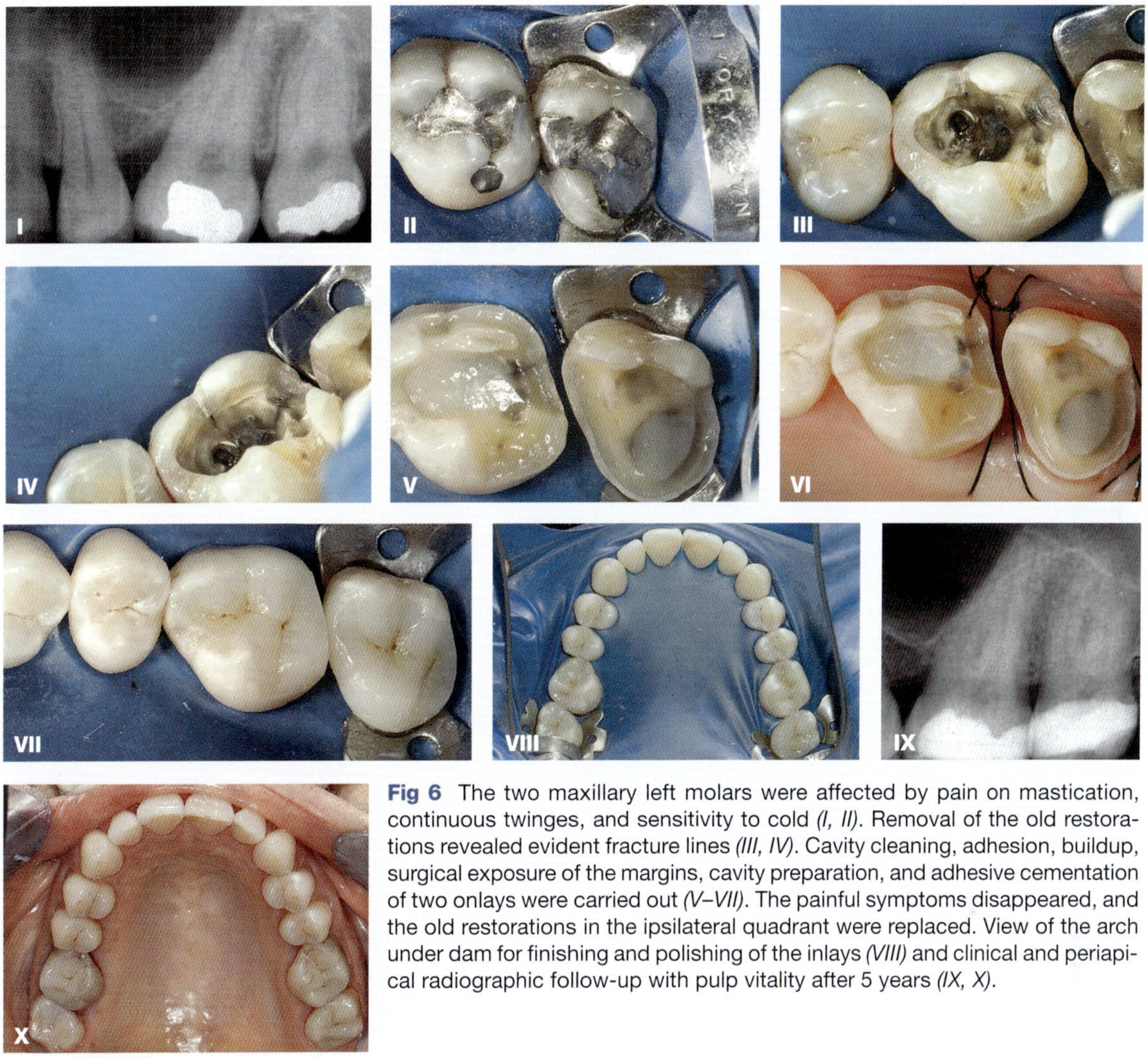

Fig 6 The two maxillary left molars were affected by pain on mastication, continuous twinges, and sensitivity to cold *(I, II)*. Removal of the old restorations revealed evident fracture lines *(III, IV)*. Cavity cleaning, adhesion, buildup, surgical exposure of the margins, cavity preparation, and adhesive cementation of two onlays were carried out *(V–VII)*. The painful symptoms disappeared, and the old restorations in the ipsilateral quadrant were replaced. View of the arch under dam for finishing and polishing of the inlays *(VIII)* and clinical and periapical radiographic follow-up with pulp vitality after 5 years *(IX, X)*.

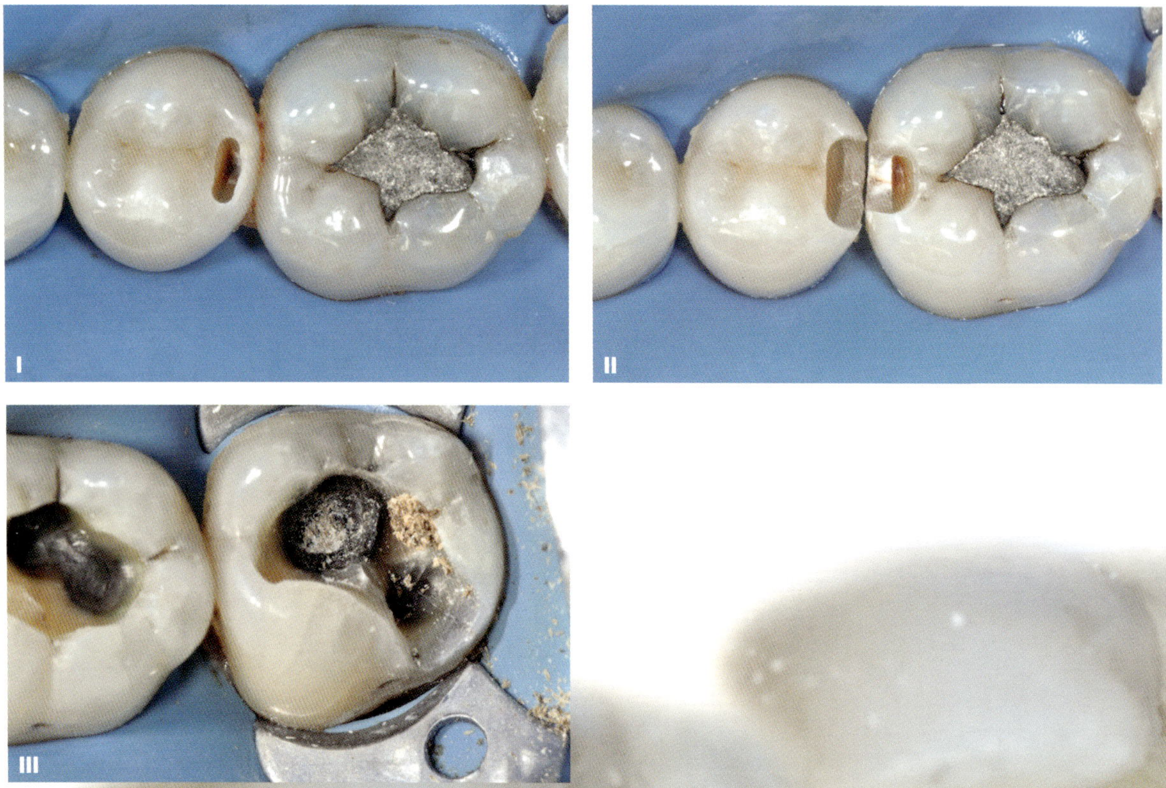
I
II
III

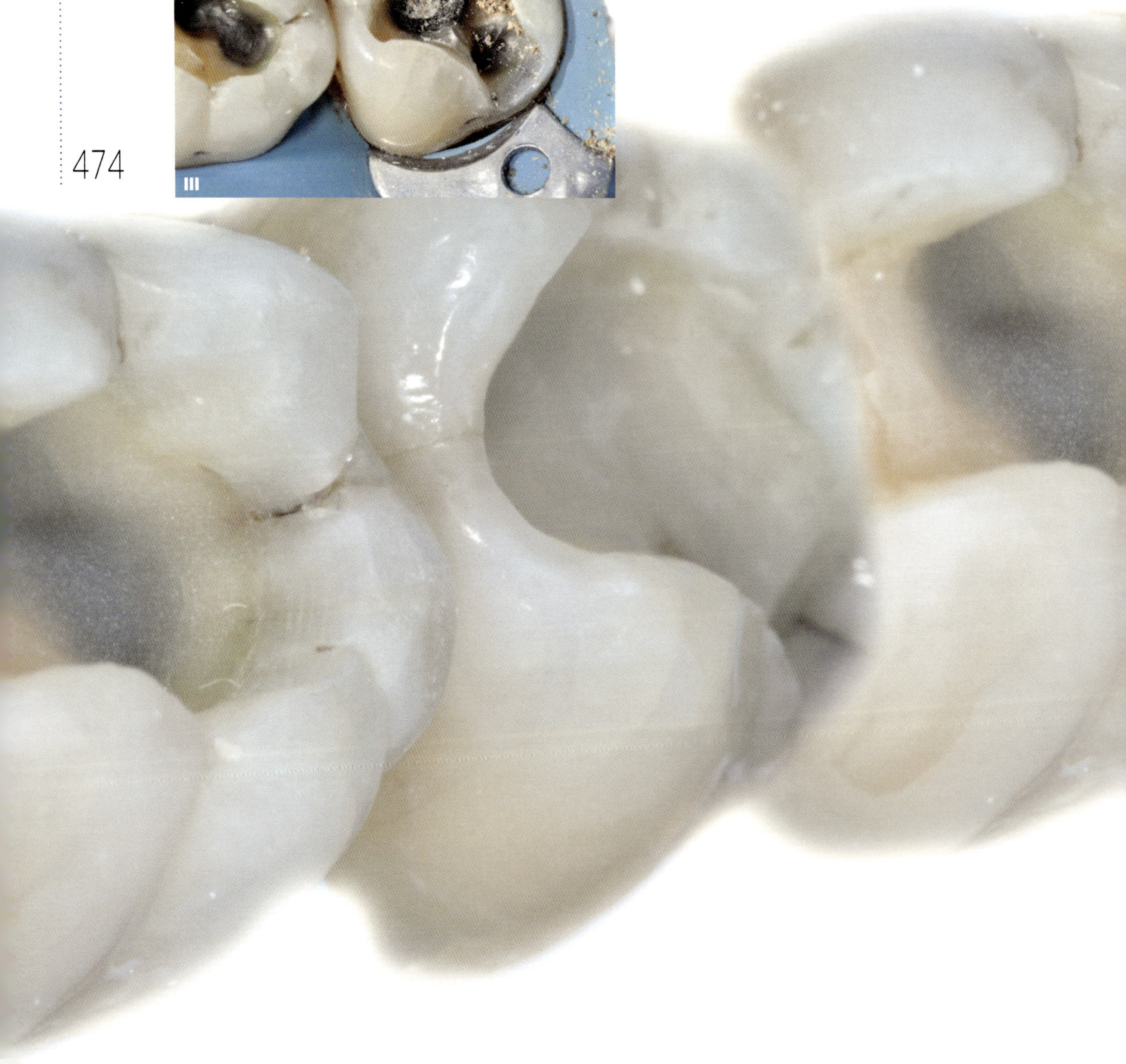

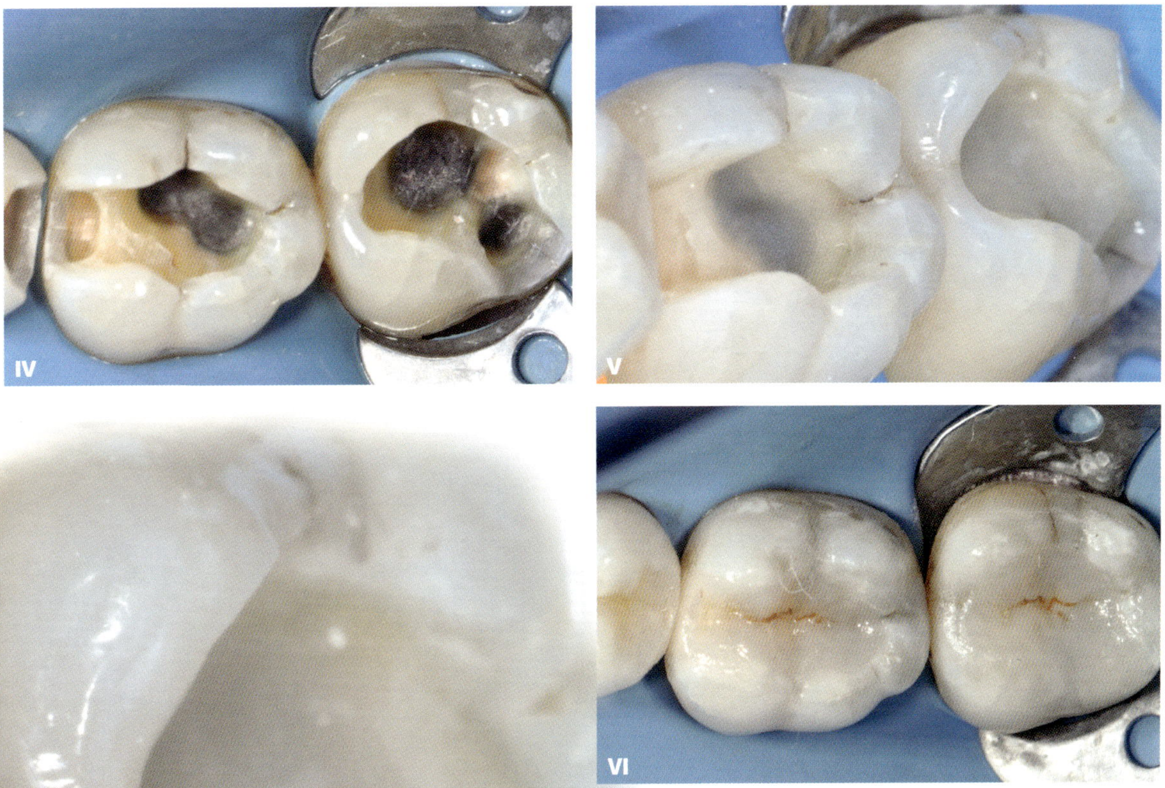

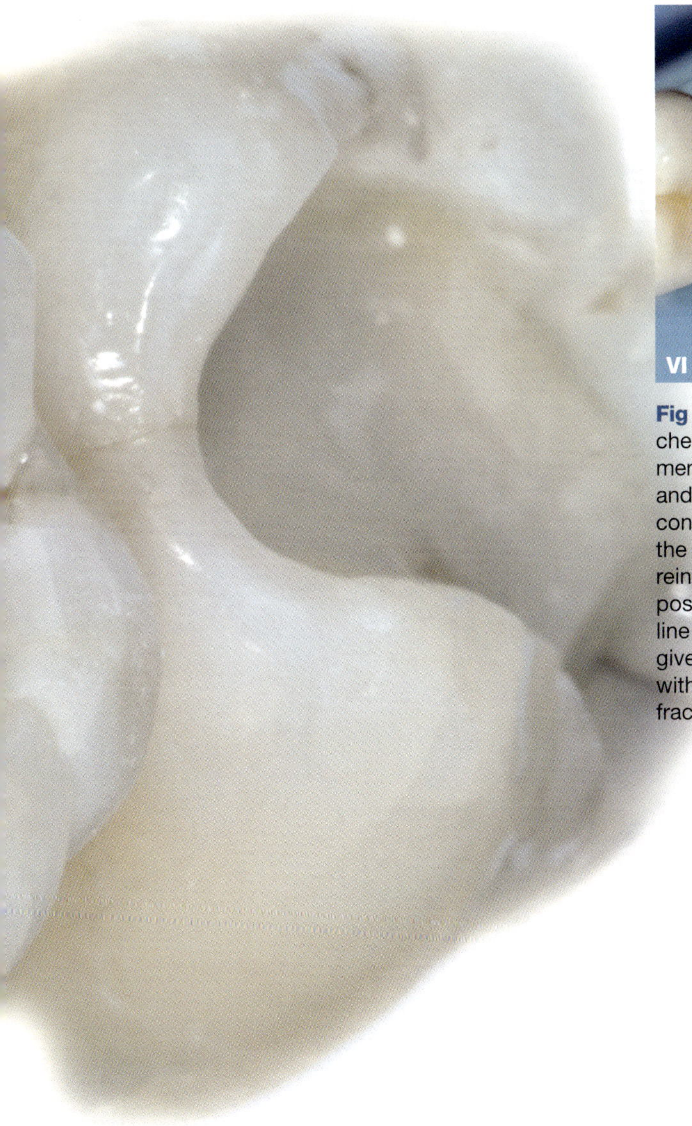

Fig 7 Caries lesions and slight sporadic discomfort on chewing in the mandibular left quadrant guided the treatment plan toward direct (second premolar) and indirect (first and second molars) restorations with the patient's informed consent *(I–IV)*. Despite the evident fracture line present in the distal wall of the first molar *(V)*, the latter was saved by reinforcing with flowable composite and traditional composite after removing decayed tissue within the fracture line *(VI)*. As shown in this case sample, this procedure has given and continues to give extremely encouraging results with regard to the durability of walls affected by moderate fracture lines.

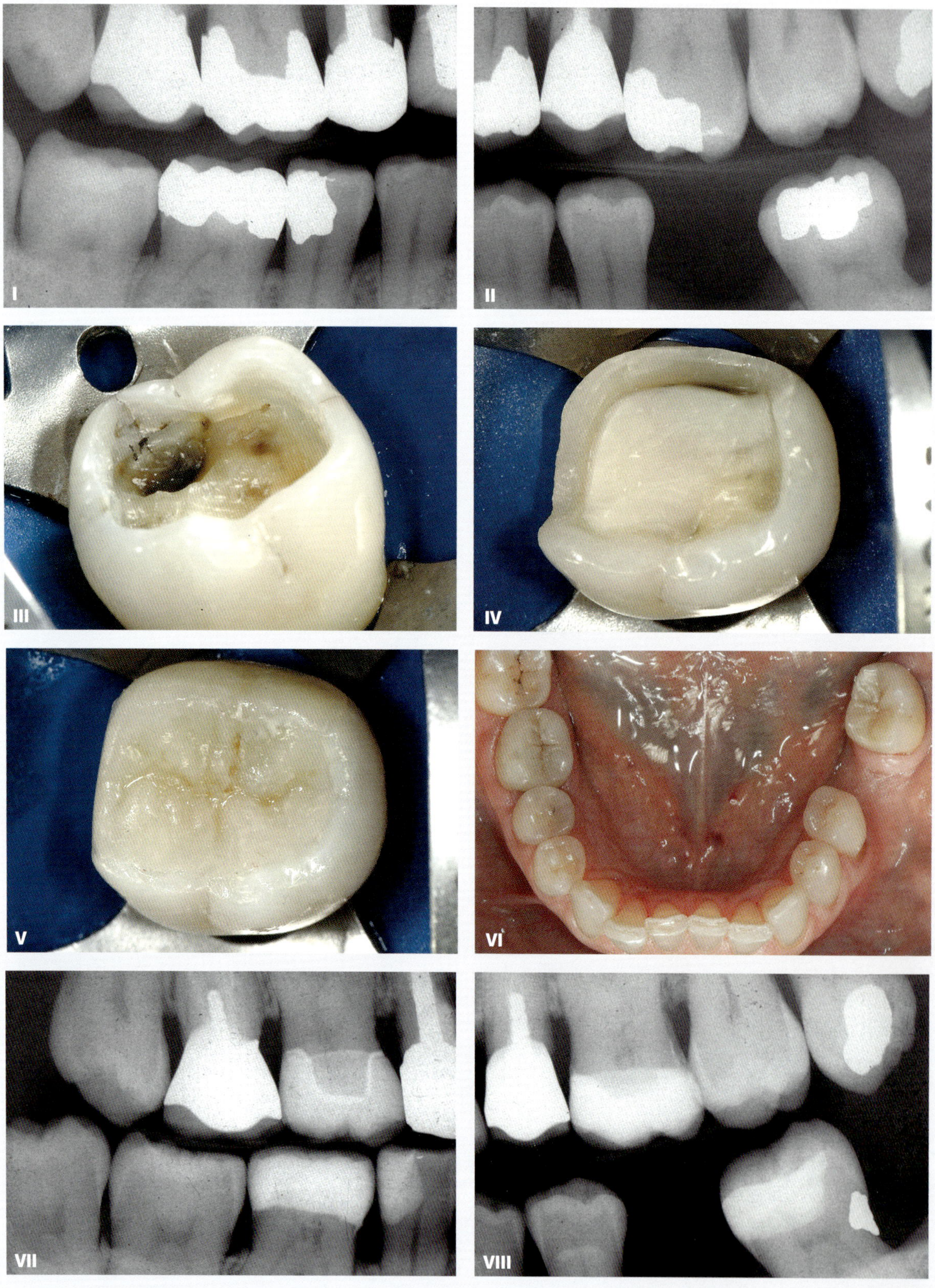

Fig 8 Preoperative bitewing radiographs and view of lingual fracture line of the wall of the mandibular left second molar and inadequate wall thicknesses, treated with an onlay *(I–V)*. Arch completed with direct and indirect restorations after 7 years and follow-up radiograph *(VI–VIII)*. A Class 5 restoration remains to be carried out on the mandibular left second premolar.

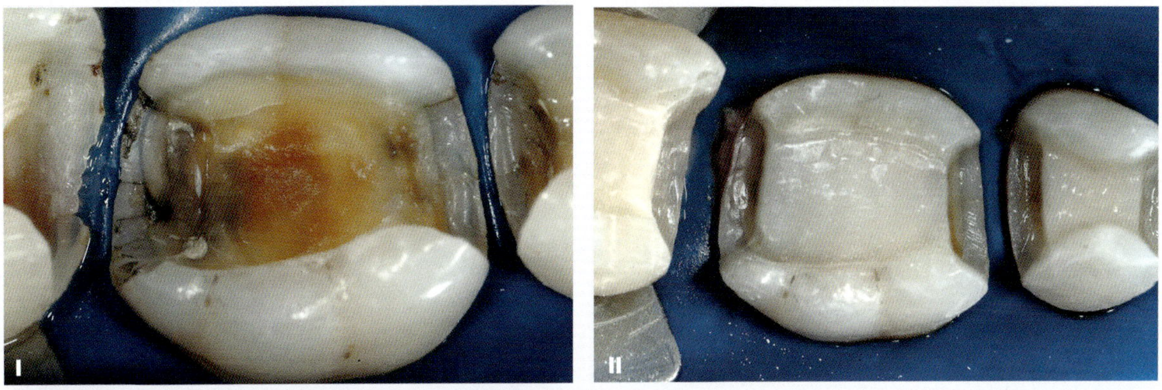

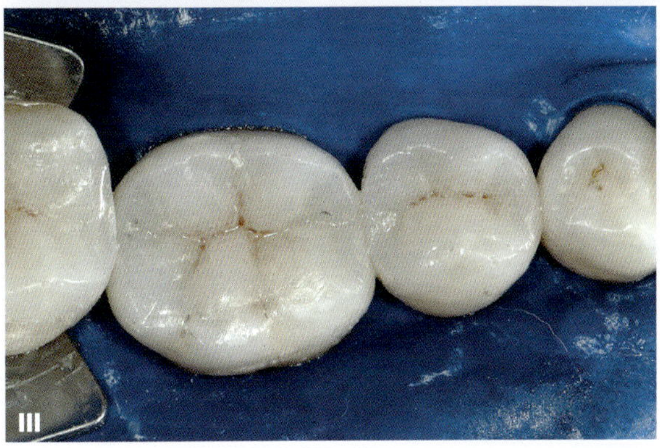

Fig 9 Horizontal fracture line of the mandibular right first molar, preparation of an onlay, and adhesive restorations in the entire quadrant.

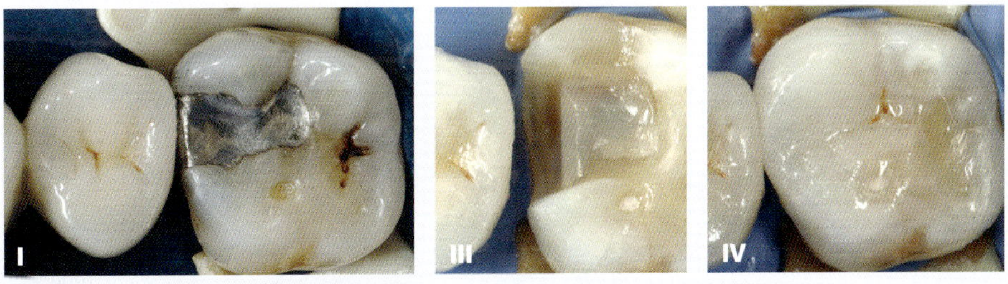

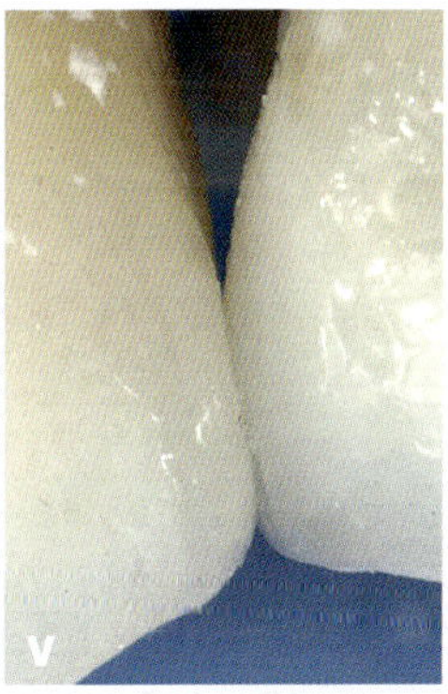

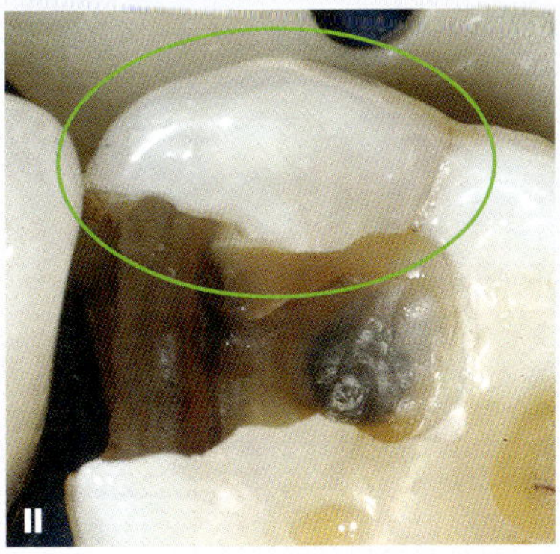

Fig 10 Pain on pressure and replacement of the amalgam filling in the maxillary left first molar with a composite inlay *(I)*. The fracture lines are evident *(II)*. Pain disappeared after cementation of the restoration *(III–V)*.

Magnification, transillumination, and dyes will be a great help when formulating a diagnosis (Figs 11 to 13).

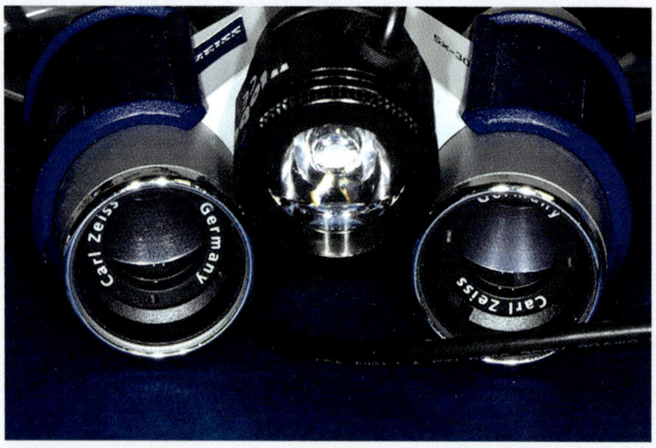

Fig 11

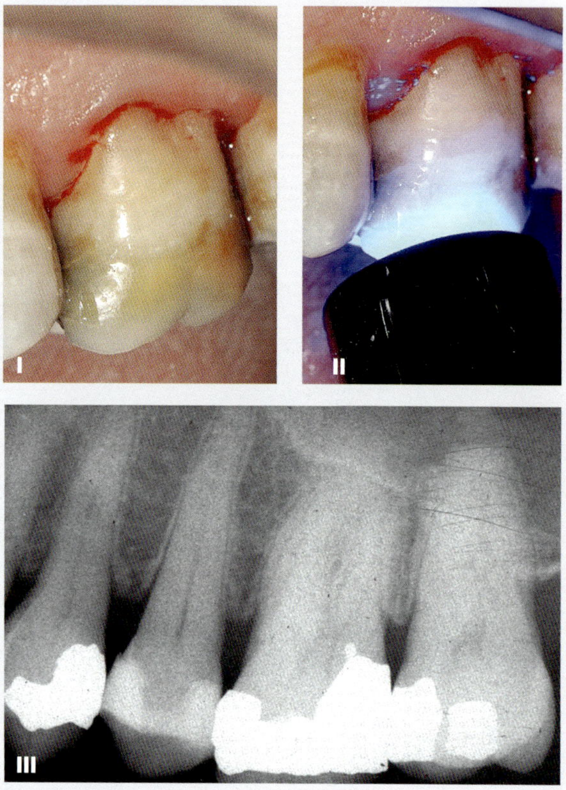

Fig 12

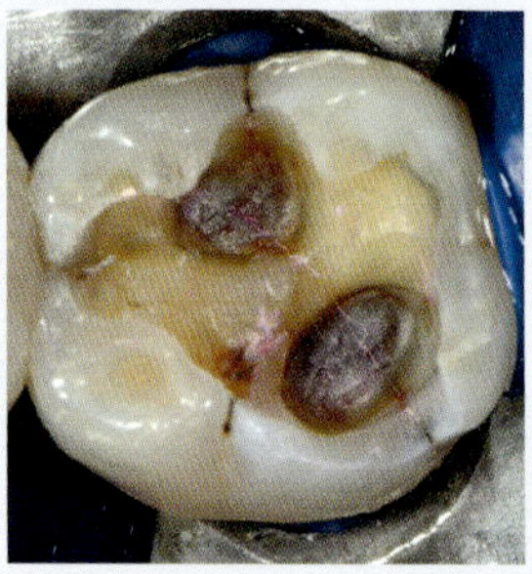

Fig 13

Figs 11 to 13 Instruments that are of great help in the clinical diagnosis of enamel and dentinal fractures include magnifying systems (Fig 11), transillumination (Fig 12), and dyes (Fig 13).

A chewing test carried out using a moist cotton roll offers a simple and effective means of diagnosis: When patients bite down, they will complain of pain on reopening and not on closure. They will actually feel a sense of relief at the moment of closure and acute pain on reopening because during closure the dentinal fluids are aspirated from the cusps, which are moving apart, while during reopening the same fluids will be compressed as the cusps move together (Fig 14).

Pressure on a cracked tooth causes the cusps on both sides to move apart and together, which causes the hydrodynamic effects responsible for stimulating the peripheral pulp receptors.[5,8] During this diagnostic stage, it is always advisable to carry out a pulp vitality test on the suspect tooth or teeth, while periodontal probing is essential to establish the presence or absence of a vertical root fracture (Fig 15).

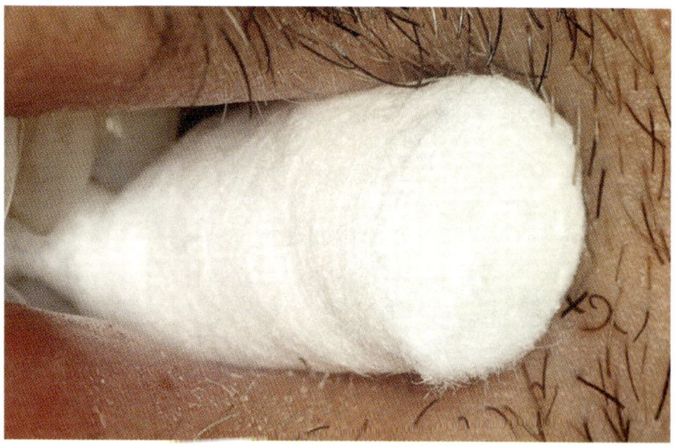

Fig 14 Chewing test with a moist cotton roll, beginning with the teeth that appeared to be less involved.

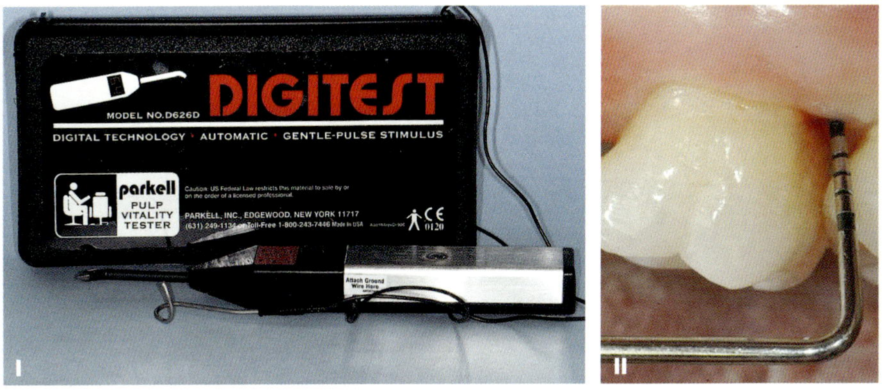

Fig 15 Electric instrument for pulp vitality test *(I)*. Periodontal probing should be performed in all cases, especially when vertical fracture lines in the root are suspected *(II)*.

It is important to be aware that radiographic examinations will be of no use at all. It goes without saying that early diagnosis is important because in many cases this will prevent the crack from progressing into a fracture.

Initial cracks in the enamel and dentin that go undiagnosed—either because they do not give rise to painful symptoms or because they are unintentionally overlooked during surface checks at hygienist appointments—can develop into a coronal fracture and/or cusp separation. This is an event that occurs in intact teeth and those with previous restorations. This certainly makes for easy diagnosis, but treatment and prognosis are a little more difficult (Fig 16). Early diagnosis of cracks in the enamel and dentin is not elementary, and the need for endodontic treatment in cracked teeth, if correctly indicated, requires the patient to be informed of alternative treatments due to uncertainty over the prognosis[9] (Fig 17). The author strongly supports this approach. In light of his clinical experience, the author heartily agrees with the assertions made by Paul et al,[9] who also confirm emphatically that the patient should be kept well-informed because of uncertainty over the prognosis.

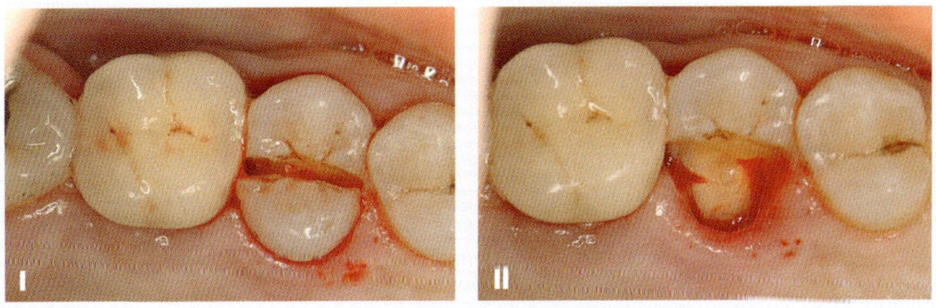

Fig 16 Fracture of the crown of the maxillary right second premolar without any previous restoration.

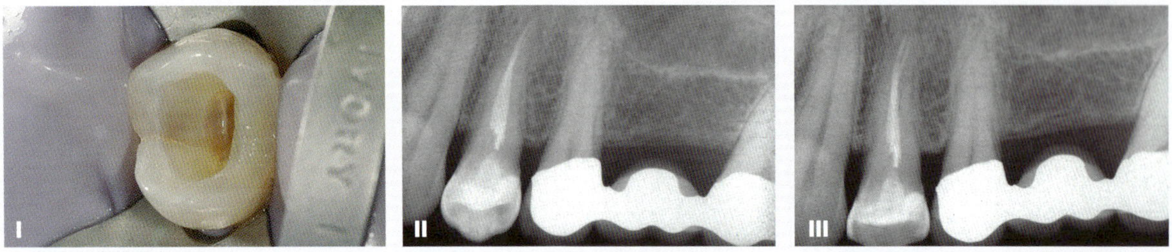

Fig 17 Vertical fracture of a maxillary left first premolar. Endodontic treatment and a subsequent inlay have an extremely relative prognostic value *(I, II)*. The patient must be informed and give written consent. Follow-up radiograph after 3 years *(III)*.

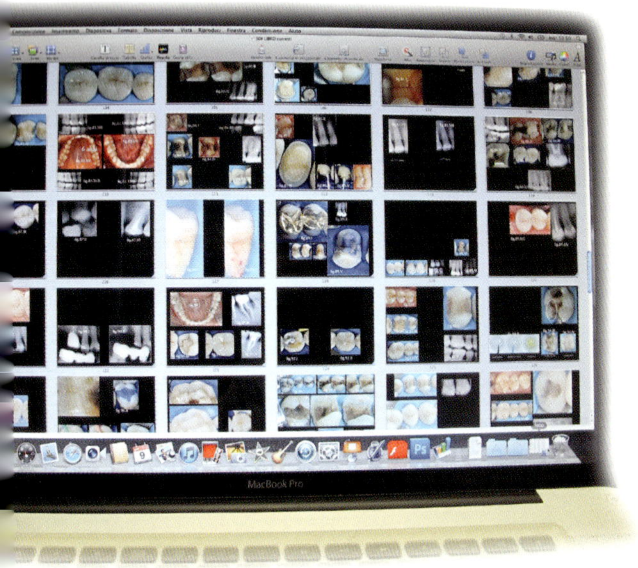

Fig 18 Patients should be informed through the presentation of clinical cases involving a course of treatment that is as similar as possible to the treatment that they are about to undergo.

Before any therapeutic procedure, it is important to provide the patient with as much information as possible, information that is not based on hearsay but on many photographs of clinical cases stored on the clinician's computer, because an image is indeed worth a thousand words (Fig 18).

At this stage, after scrolling through the photographs of cracks, which may range from a tiny crack on a marginal ridge to a huge crack that is revealed after opening a cavity, clinician and patient can decide together the course to be taken. In order to do this, the clinician could perhaps show the patient long-term follow-up photographs of treated clinical cases, emphasizing the variety of possible outcomes for dentinal fracture lines (Figs 19 and 20).

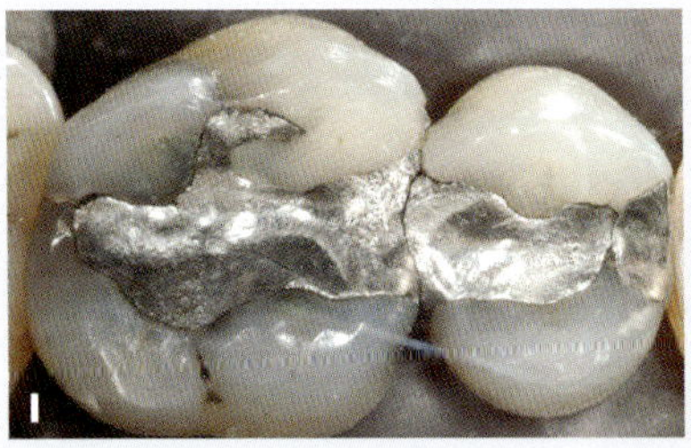

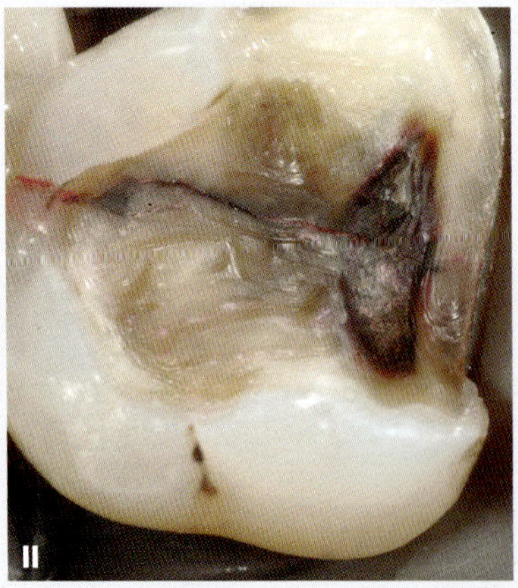

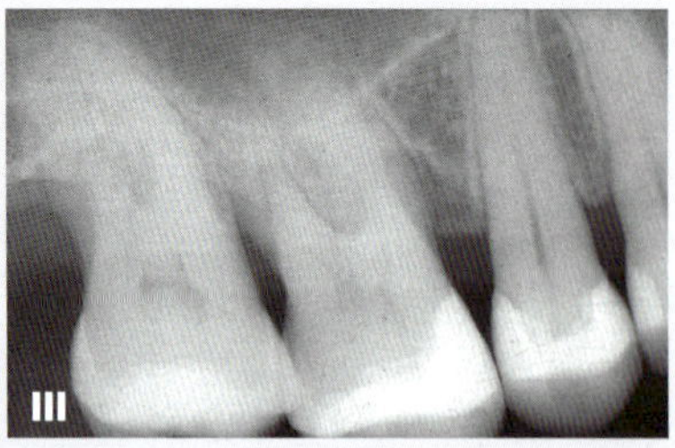

Fig 19 Very small distal crack in the maxillary right first molar; however, the fracture line revealed after removing the old restoration is very large *(I, II)*. Follow-up radiograps after 4 years *(III)* during which the patient did not experience the least discomfort when chewing or any sensitivity to heat. The periapical radiograph shows a state of health, an impeccable tooth-restoration margin, and stability of the suboptimal periodontal situation due to rigorous hygienist visits. Pulp vitality tests were absolutely normal.

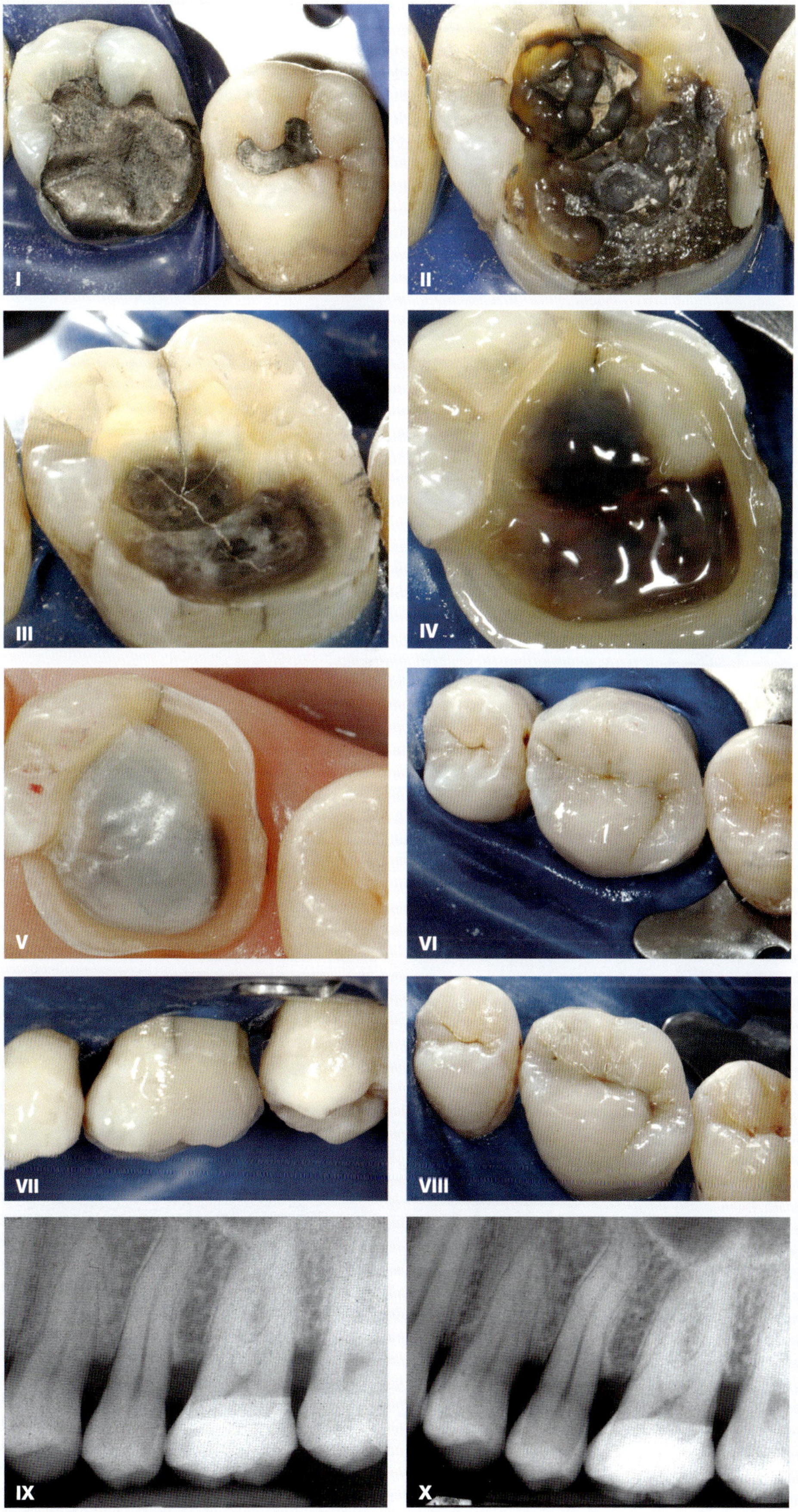

Fig 20 Another clinical case governed by fracture lines: elimination of decay, adhesion, preparation, and cemented restoration *(I–IX)*. Follow-up radiograph after 5 years *(X)*.

This is crucial, because it may be possible to resolve the problem—and fortunately this is often the case—by a simple indirect or direct restoration (Figs 21 and 22) or even endodontic treatment if the pain persists. If the tooth in question contains a vertical fracture, it may need to be removed and possibly replaced by an artificial root (ie, implant) (Figs 23 and 24).

The clinician is obliged to explain all of this to the patient before beginning treatment, and the patient is fully entitled to be informed. During this awareness-raising stage, the clinician will also obtain very useful information about the patient's psychologic makeup.

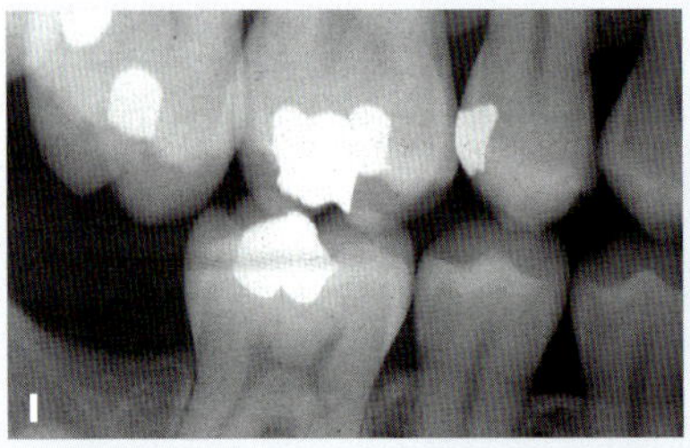
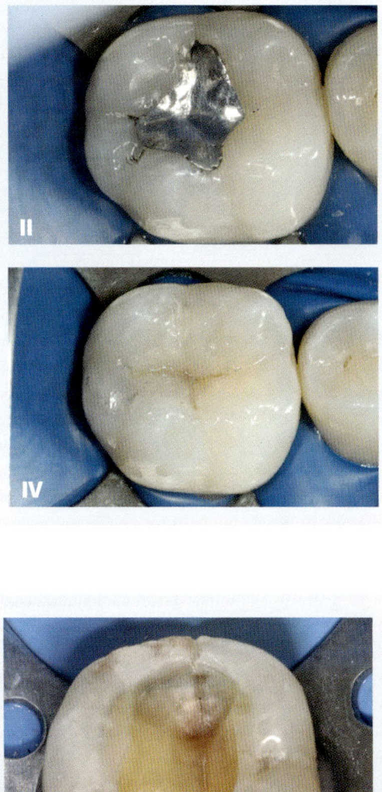
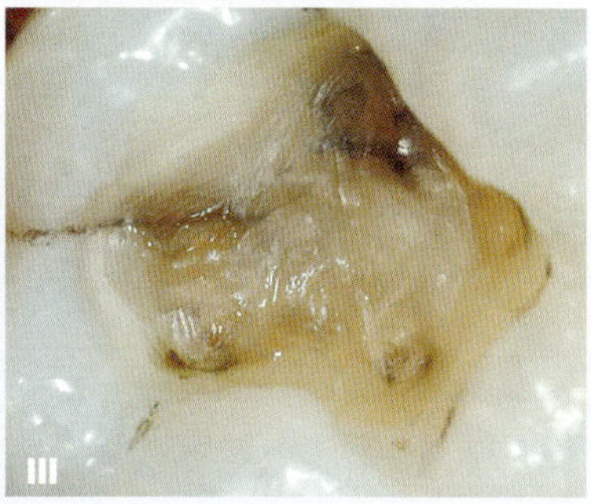

Fig 21 Class 1 restorations with evident fracture lines. In the author's experience, this clinical solution has offered an extremely encouraging long-term outcome.

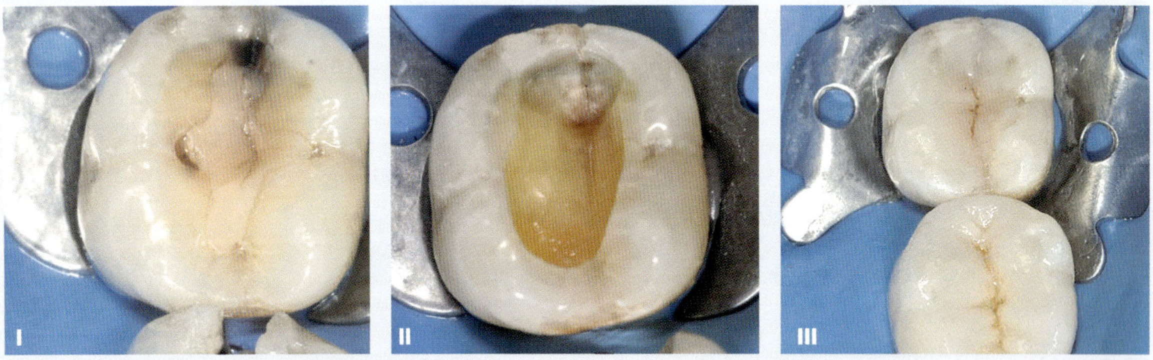
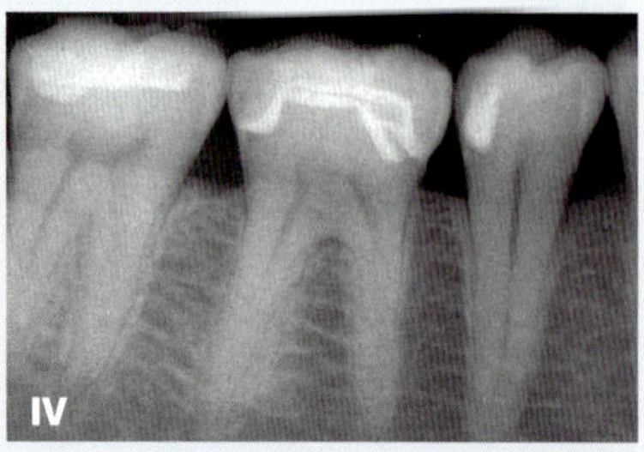

Fig 22 The fracture line in the mandibular right second molar is evident after removing decayed tissue *(I, II)*. The distal wall was saved after duly removing fragments of soft tissue within the fracture line. Because the treatment plan involved applying an indirect restoration to the adjacent first molar, the author preferred to opt for an indirect restoration for the second molar as well, making use of the same impression. Of course the distal wall was reinforced by adding flowable composite and traditional composite before taking an impression. Clinical and radiographic view of the cemented restorations *(III, IV)*.

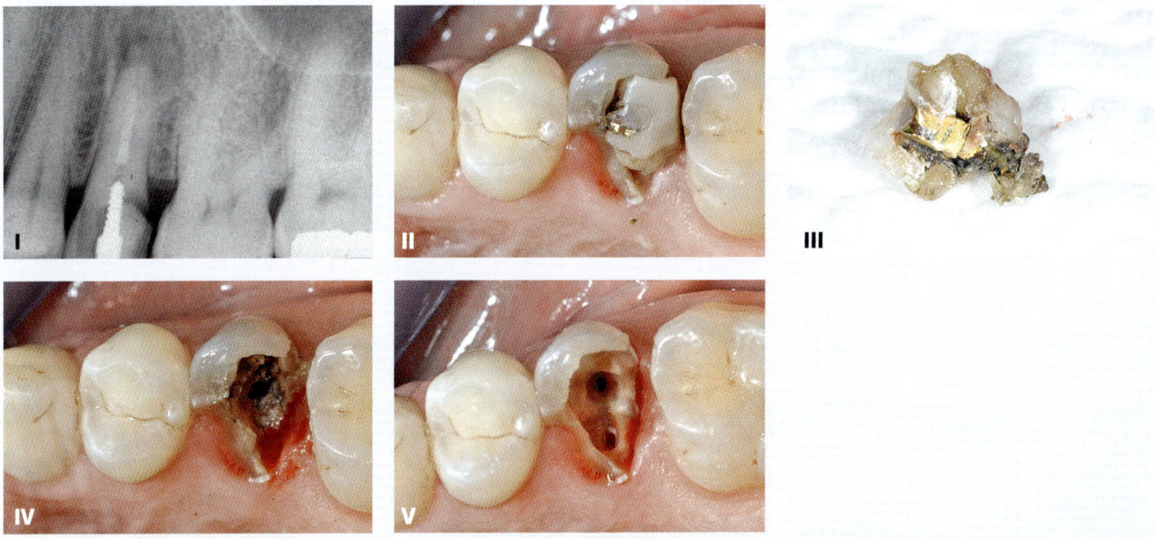

Fig 23 As previously stated, preparing a treatment plan after removal of the defective restorations and decay and a radiographic view of the tooth involved is essential. In this case, the healthy remaining tooth tissue was unable to guarantee a good prognosis. Orthodontic extrusion and/or lengthening of the clinical crown and endodontic re-treatment were inevitable. Last but not least, the problem was exacerbated by a mesiodistal fracture line. All these considerations resulted in a treatment plan that involved replacing the severely compromised tooth with an implant.

When the problem can be resolved by a simple direct or indirect restoration, everything is fine, but what happens if all the stages of restoration are required—ie, a restoration with periodontal treatment when necessary, followed by endodontic treatment—and then ultimately the problem can only be resolved by removal of the treated tooth?

When the only way to resolve the problem turns out to be an implant, the author believes that for ethical reasons clinicians should routinely deduct the cost of previous treatment from the cost of the implant because they are only too well aware of the uncertain outcome.

Returning to a previous discussion, the literature states that the presence of a mesio-occlusodistal (MOD) restoration is the greatest predisposing factor for dental fracture and that the presence of Class 1 or 2 restorations increases the risk of cracks 20-fold.[10–13] In light of this, whenever dealing with MOD restorations, eg, large amalgam fillings, the author believes it is advisable to remove the old restorations and replace them for preventive reasons with composite inlays with a modulus of elasticity that is considerably closer to that of the dentin[14] (Figs 25 and 26).

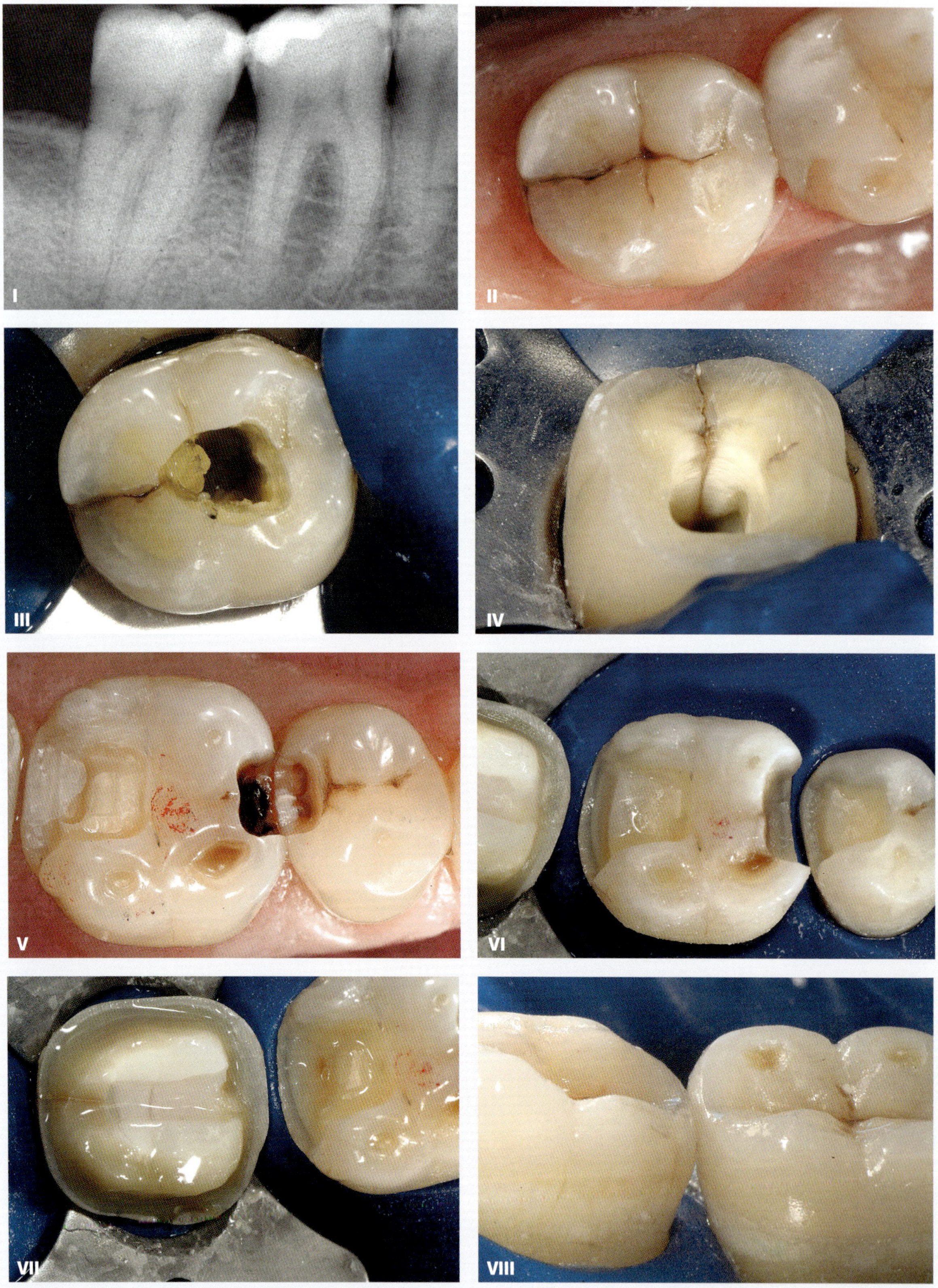

Fig 24 Vertical fracture line in the mandibular right second molar with pain on pressure. The fracture affected the distal root and was very deep *(I–III)*. Despite the absence of periodontal probing, the patient was informed that the prognosis could be poor in such cases, but the tooth was endodontically treated and reconstructed with an overlay in composite by mutual agreement *(IV–XI)*.

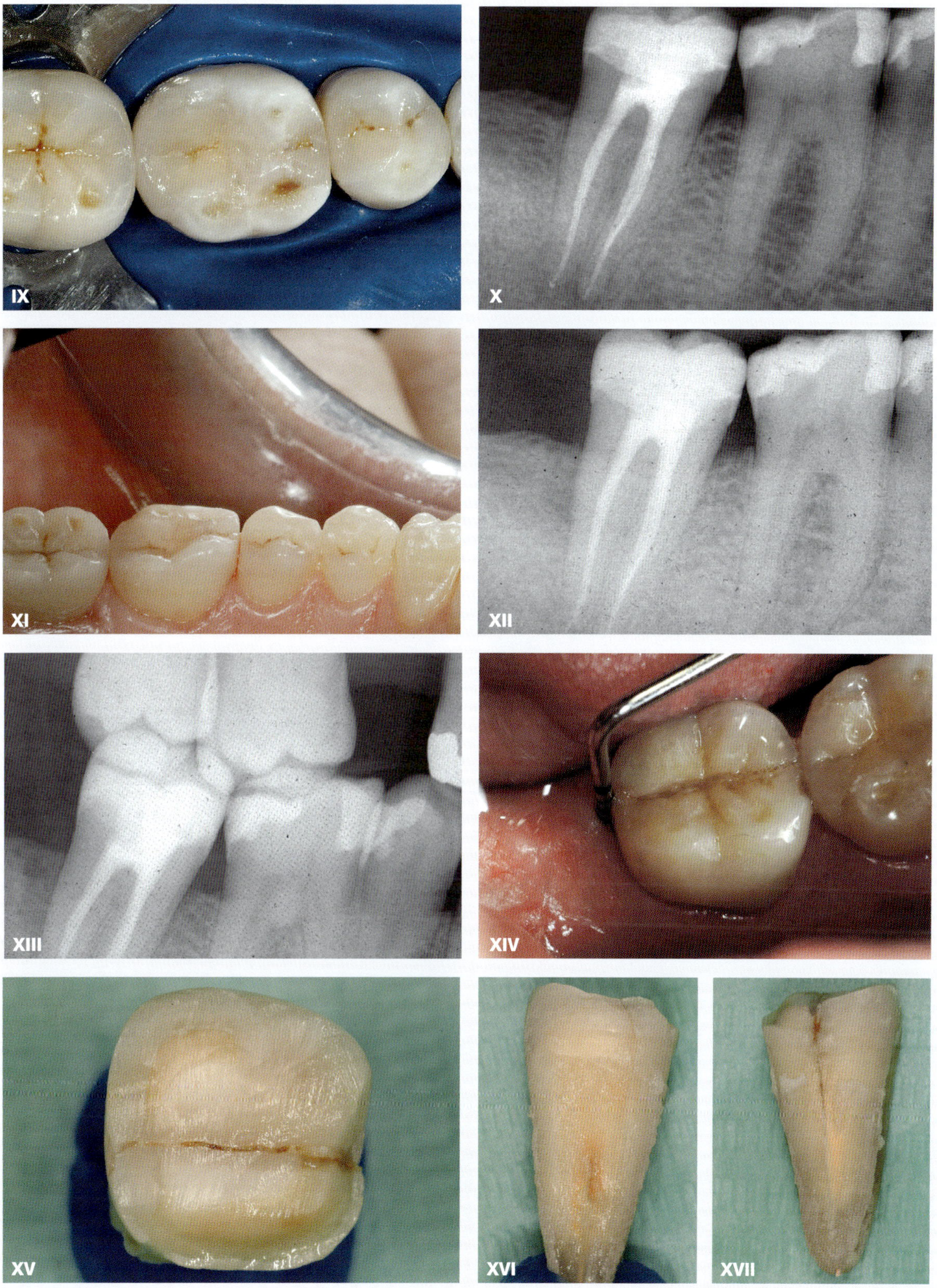

Fig 24 *(continued)* The first outcome was disappearance of the painful symptoms in the tooth in question; then a clinical and radiographic follow-up *(XII, XIII)* 14 months later revealed progression of the fracture line that was diagnosed by periodontal probing of 12 mm *(XIV)*. After the tooth was removed, the mesio-occlusodistal progression of the fracture in its occlusal aspect was revealed *(XV)*, despite the fact that it only involved the distal part in an occlusal direction at the outset. The full depth of the vertical fracture also became apparent *(XVI, XVII)*.

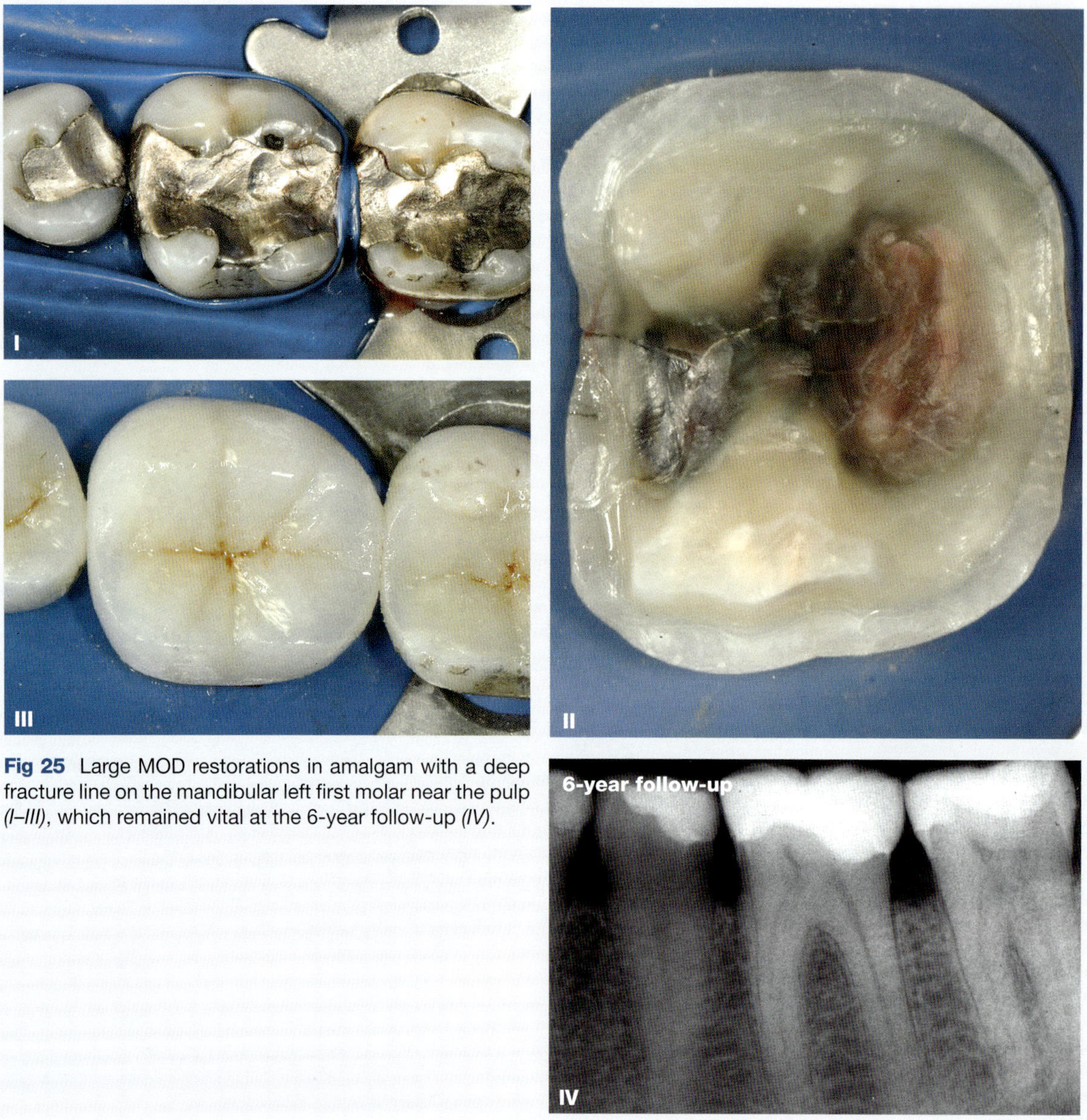

Fig 25 Large MOD restorations in amalgam with a deep fracture line on the mandibular left first molar near the pulp *(I–III)*, which remained vital at the 6-year follow-up *(IV)*.

The author has often heard worthy colleagues claim that when carrying out Class 1 restorations they have found very few fracture lines inside these cavities following their removal; the author's clinical experience is entirely different in this respect (Figs 27 to 29).

As already stated, a crack in the enamel is entirely asymptomatic, but its early diagnosis has a very significant impact on the treatment plan, which more often than not will be extremely conservative. The author has found in his clinical experience that cracks limited to the enamel alone are extremely rare, although it goes without saying that without an early diagnosis, the crack extends to the dentin and is responsible for pain caused by stimulation of the pulpal nerve fibers following the hydrodynamic effect determined by cusp opening and closure.

As accurately reported by Martin and Machtou,[5] if untreated, the bacteria penetrate into the dentinal tubules, giving rise to chronic pulpal inflammation, characterized by discontinuous pain that may be followed by a flare-up of chronic inflammation (Figs 30 and 31).

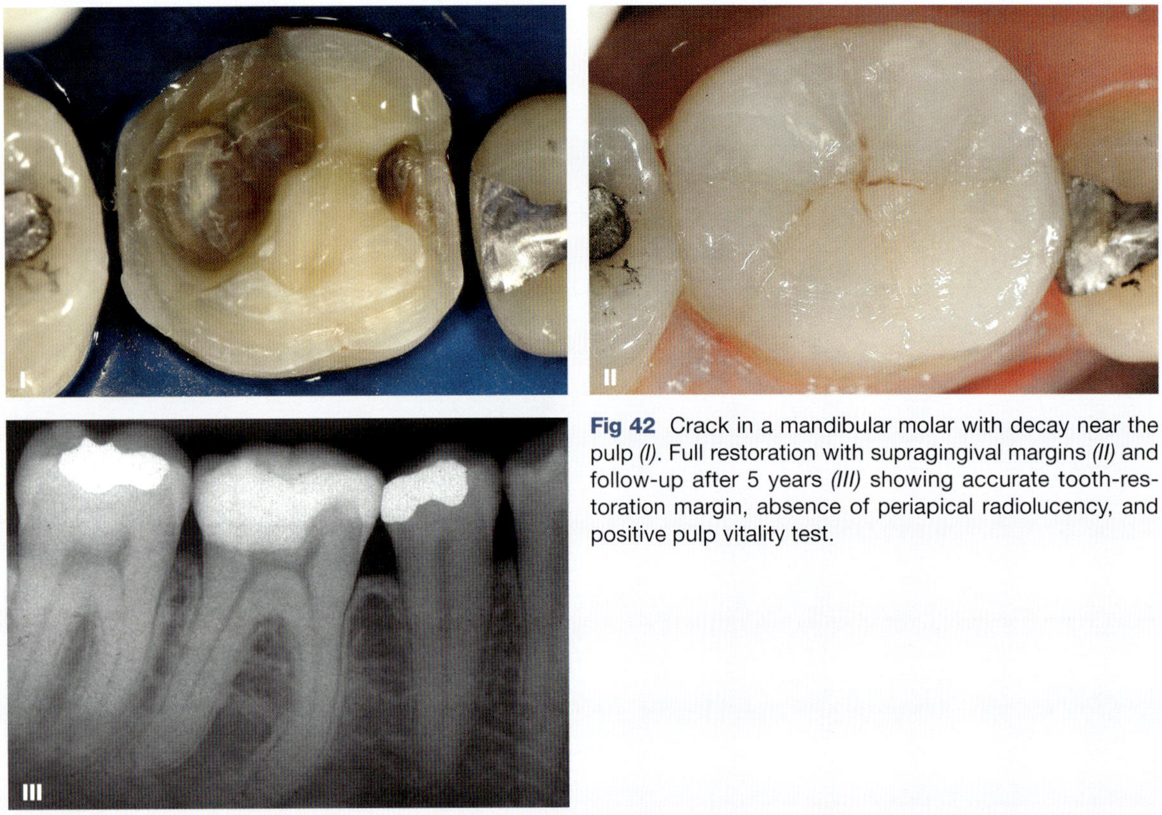

Fig 42 Crack in a mandibular molar with decay near the pulp *(I)*. Full restoration with supragingival margins *(II)* and follow-up after 5 years *(III)* showing accurate tooth-restoration margin, absence of periapical radiolucency, and positive pulp vitality test.

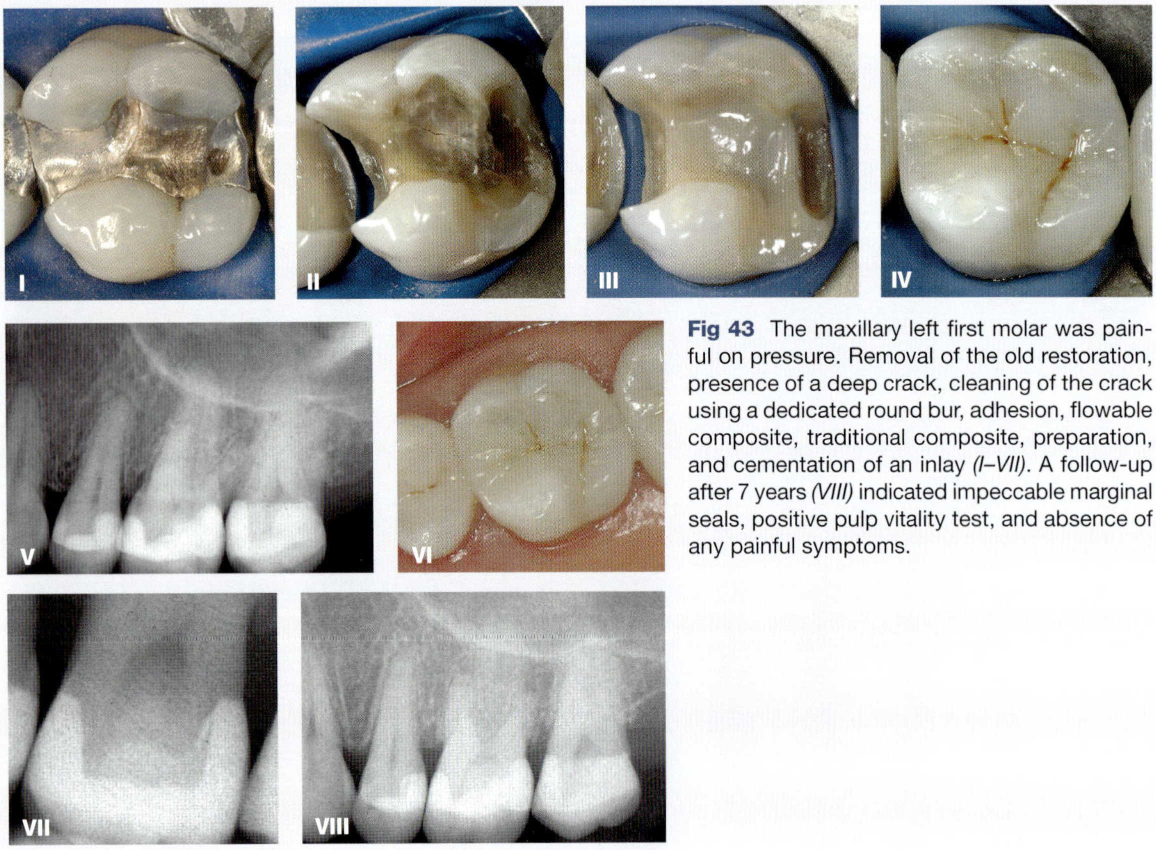

Fig 43 The maxillary left first molar was painful on pressure. Removal of the old restoration, presence of a deep crack, cleaning of the crack using a dedicated round bur, adhesion, flowable composite, traditional composite, preparation, and cementation of an inlay *(I–VII)*. A follow-up after 7 years *(VIII)* indicated impeccable marginal seals, positive pulp vitality test, and absence of any painful symptoms.

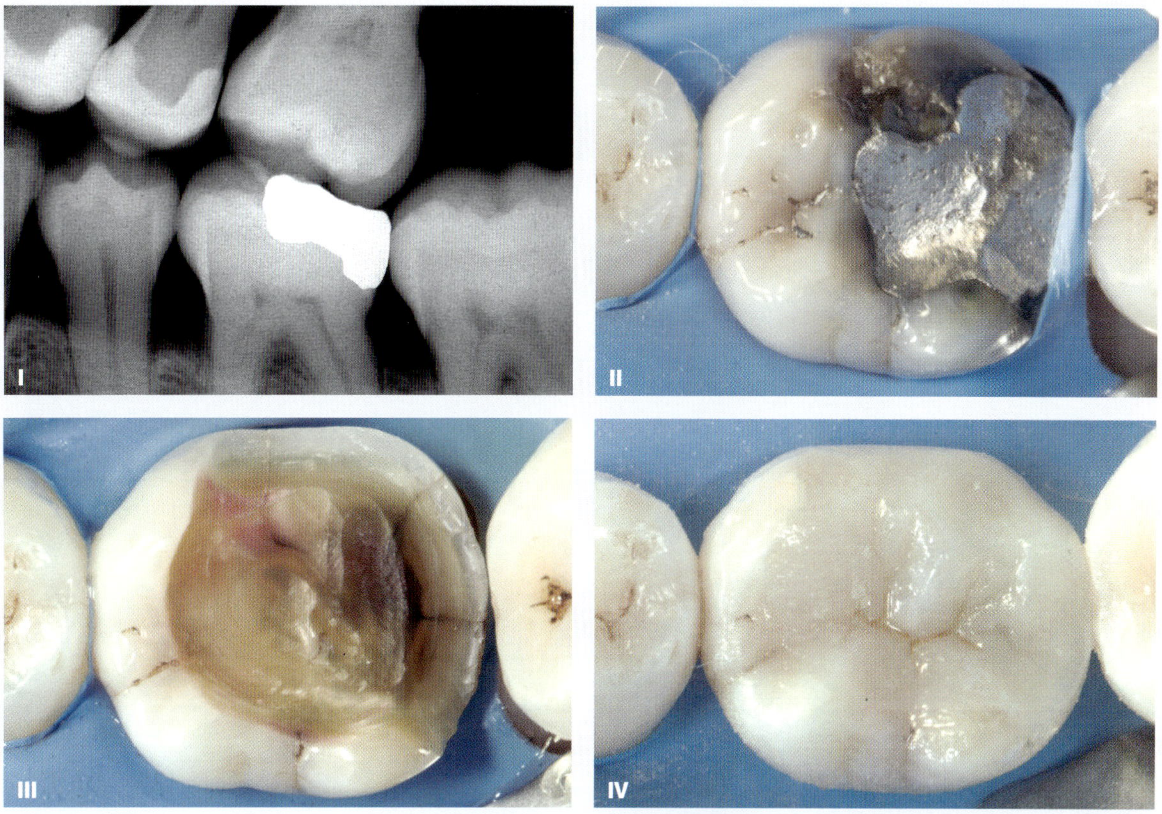

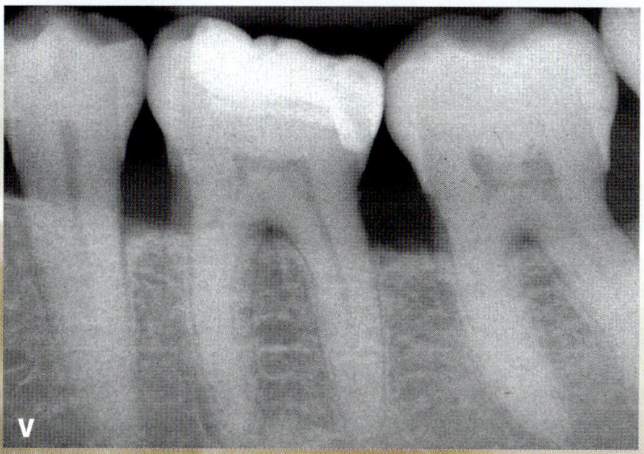

Fig 44 Leaky defective restoration with secondary decay caused pain when chewing *(I, II)*, leading to its removal. Significant fracture lines were revealed *(III)*. View of the composite restoration and post-cementation radiograph *(IV, V)*.

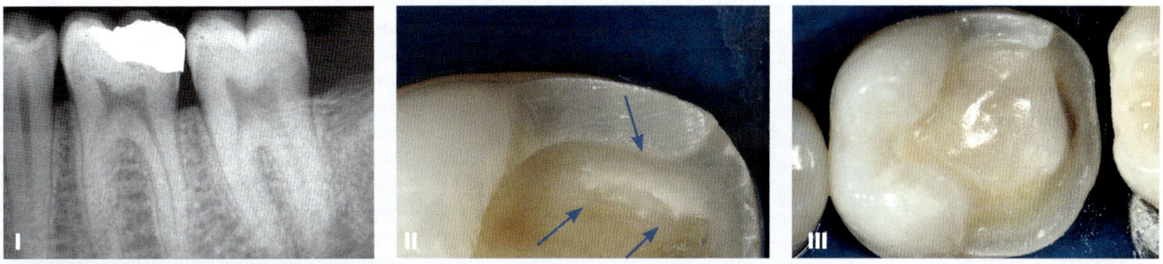

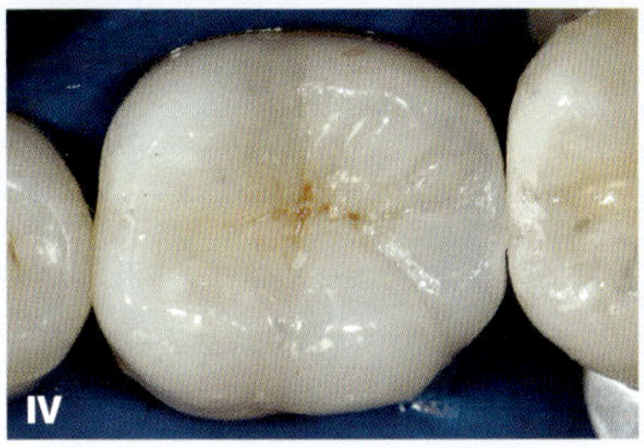

Fig 45 Mandibular molar with pain on chewing that disappeared after reconstruction with an adhesive restoration.

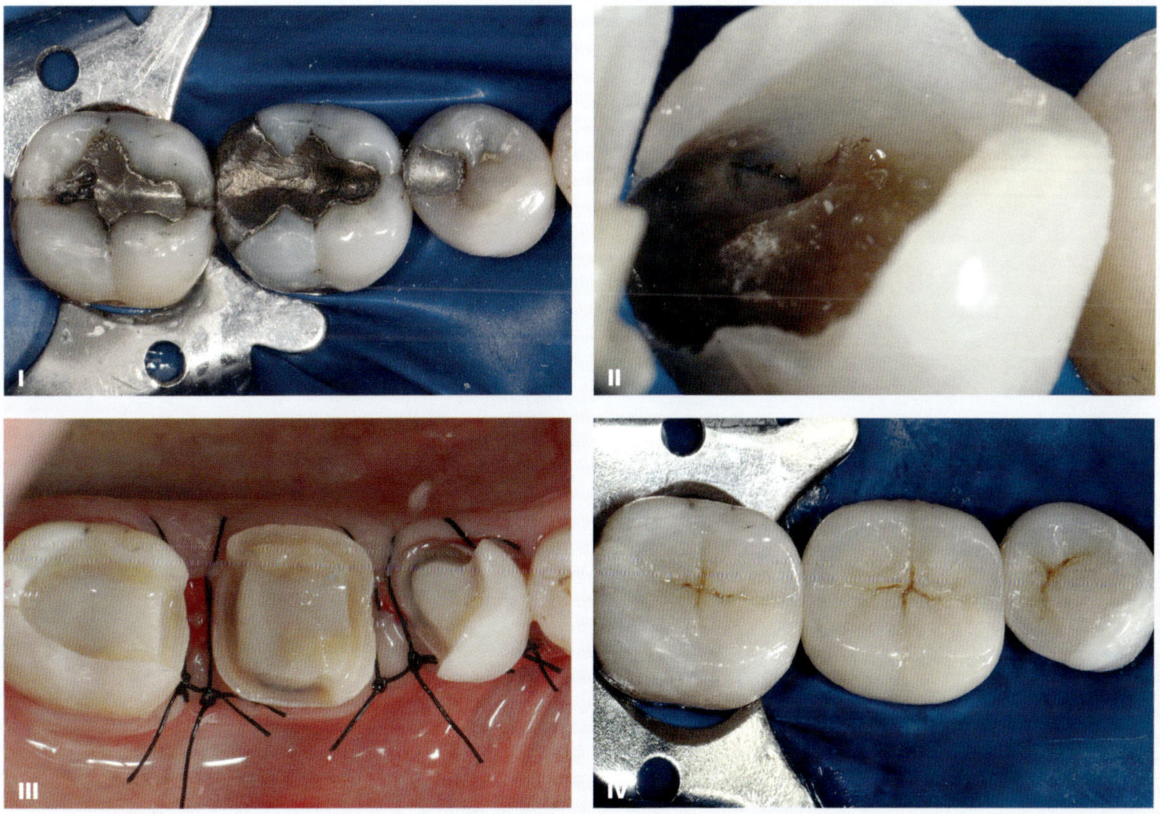

Fig 46 Pain on pressure and sensitivity to heat justified removal of old restorations in the mandibular right quadrant *(I)*. A deep crack was evident in the second premolar *(II)*. Three inlays were positioned following the usual protocol *(III, IV)*, and the painful symptoms disappeared.

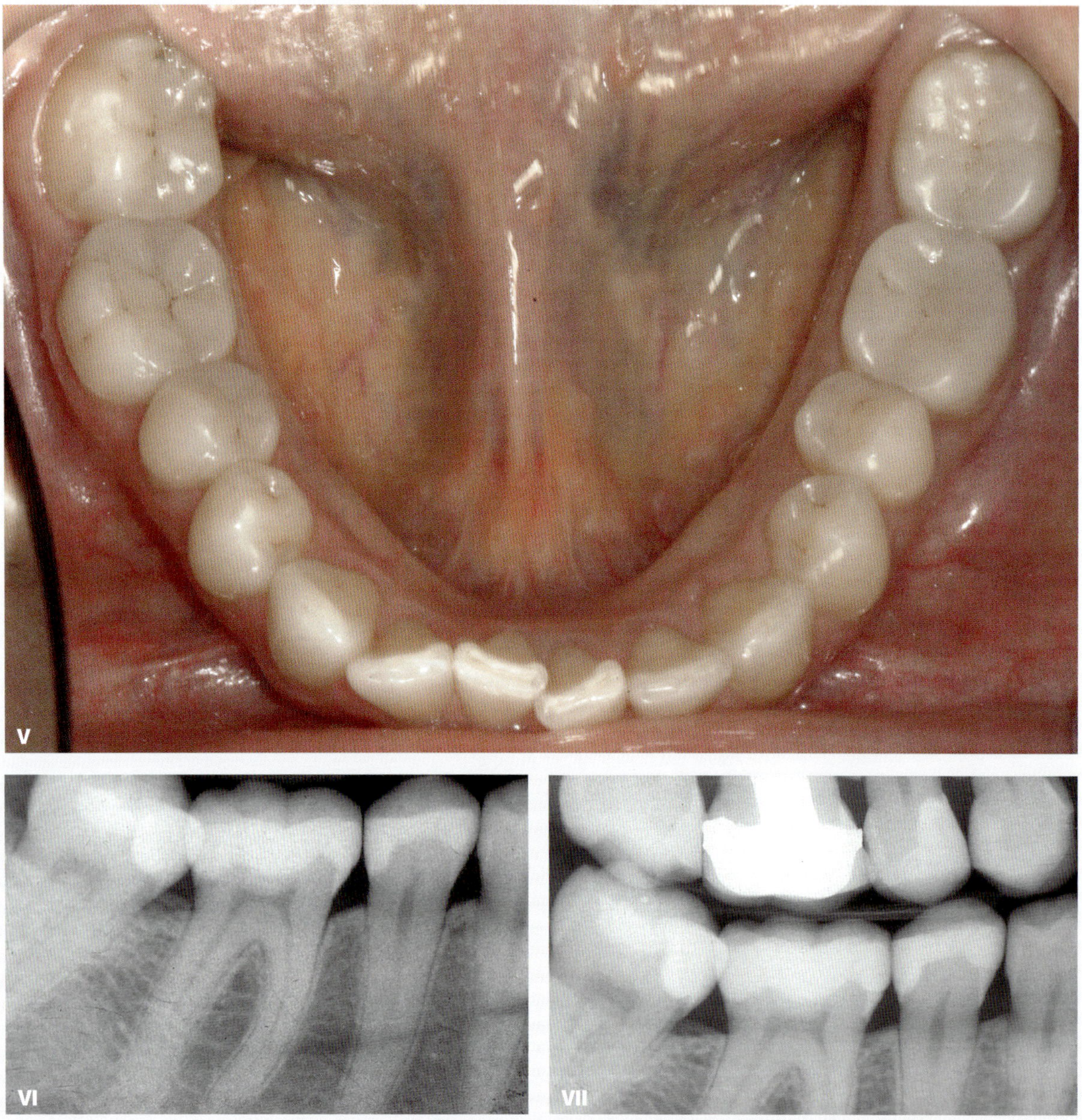

Fig 46 *(continued)* Radiographic and clinical follow-up after 5 years *(V–VII)*.

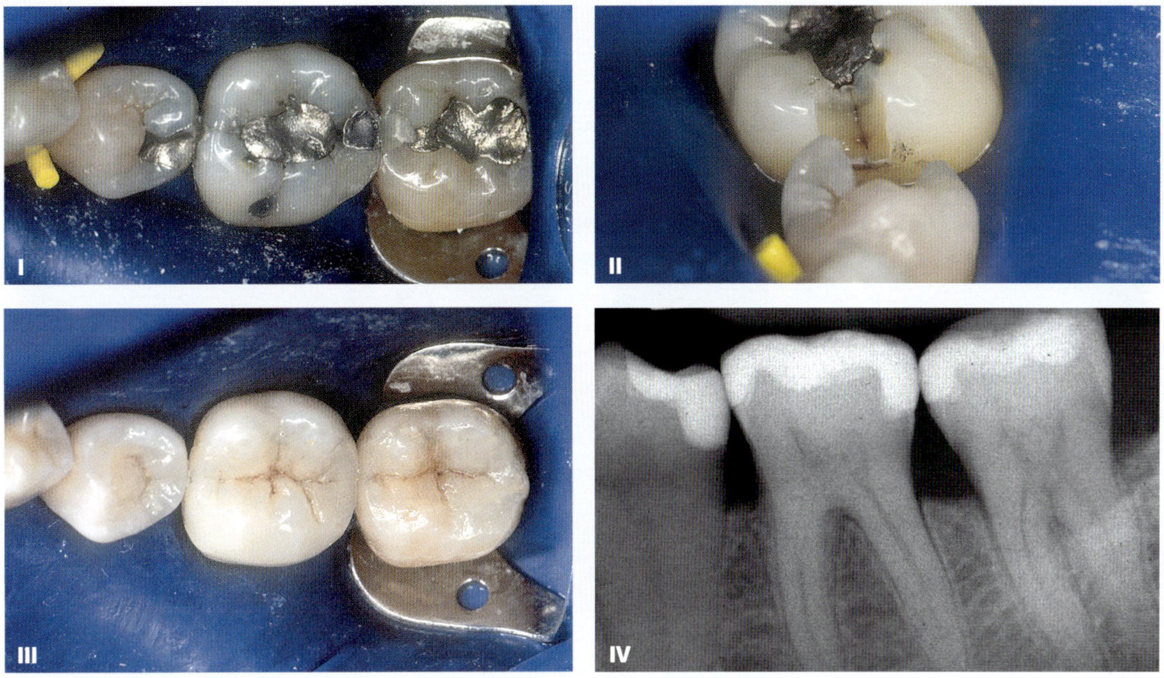

Fig 47 Vertical fracture line in the mandibular left first molar with the usual pain on chewing and subsequent restoration *(I–III)*. Follow-up after 9 years *(IV)*, during which time the patient experienced no problems.

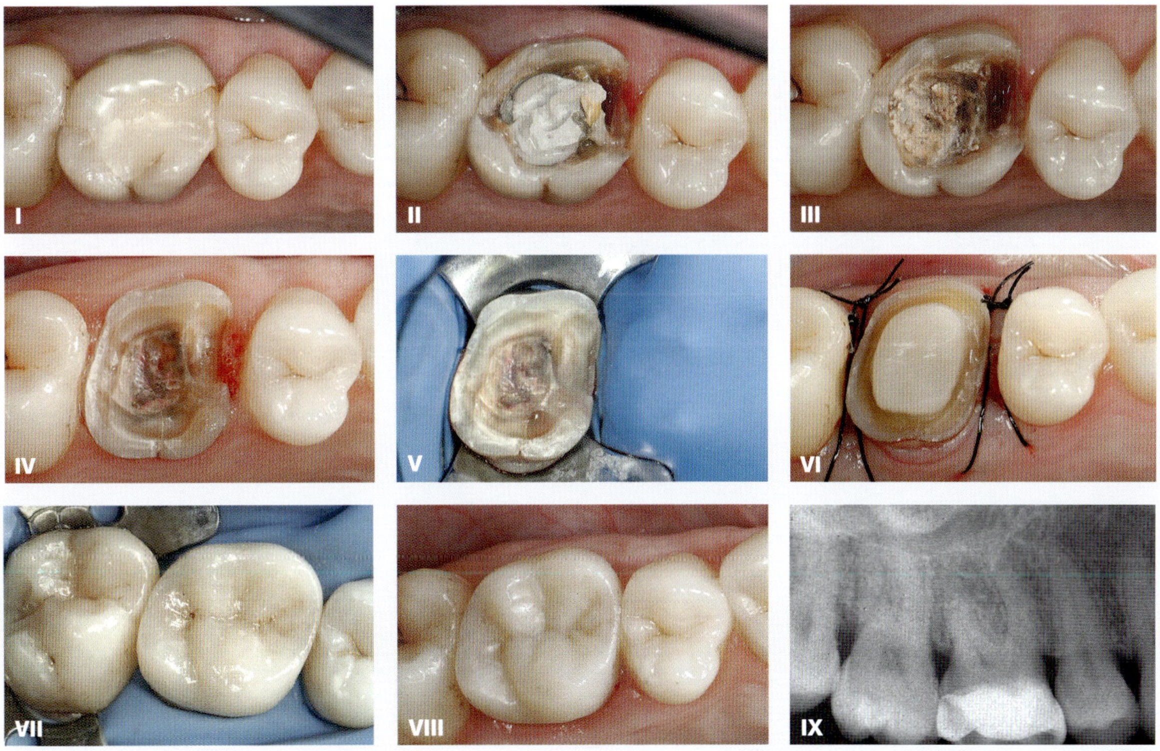

Fig 48 Borderline case due to depth of the caries lesion and dentinal cracks. After receiving the patient's informed consent, the tooth was reconstructed without endodontic treatment, trusting in the great potential of the adhesion *(I–VII)*. A medium-term follow-up (3 years later) showed entirely satisfactory results with accurate margins and a positive pulp vitality test *(VIII, IX)*. It must always be remembered that when signs and symptoms of irreversible pulp disease are present, endodontic treatment and intraradicular anchorages are necessary and should be carried out in a single session. This will extend the life of a tooth for a very long time, even when so badly compromised.

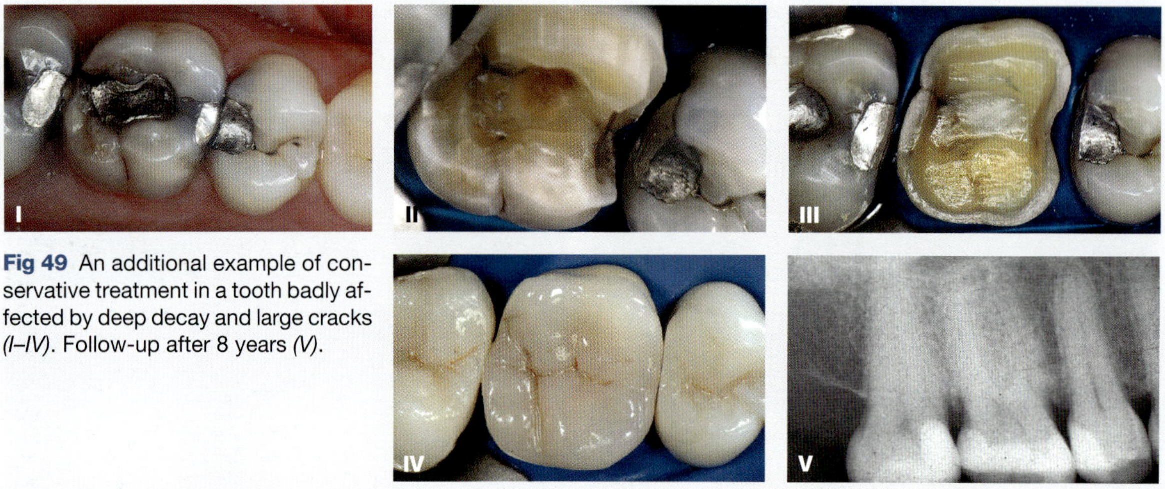

Fig 49 An additional example of conservative treatment in a tooth badly affected by deep decay and large cracks *(I–IV)*. Follow-up after 8 years *(V)*.

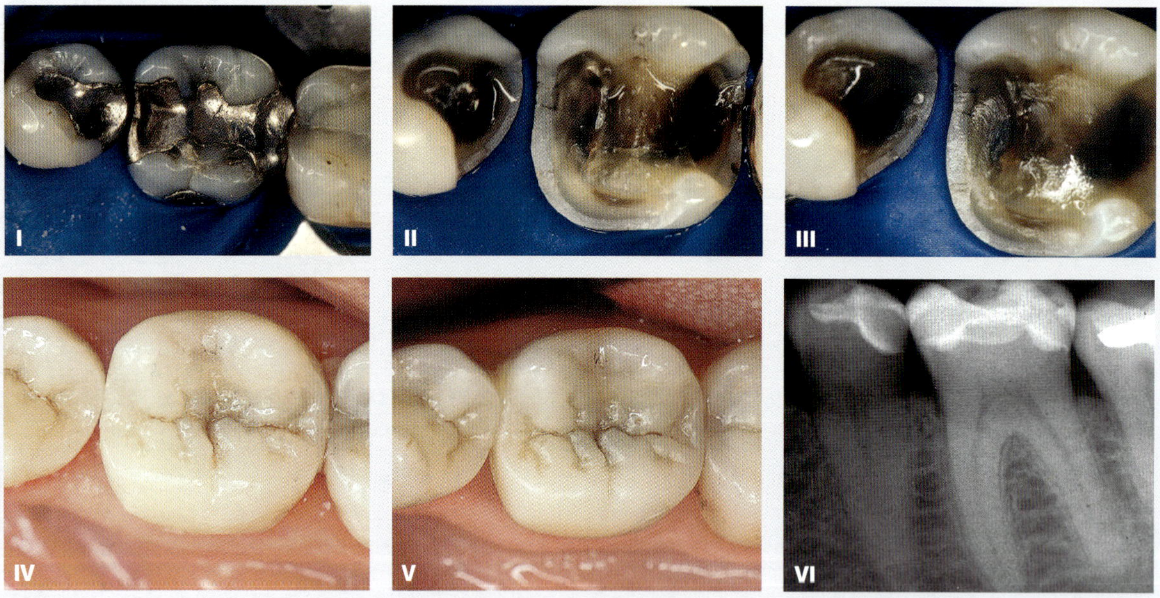

Fig 50 Very intense pain on pressure addressed using the usual treatment protocol, resulting in complete disappearance of the pain *(I–IV)*. Clinical and radiographic follow-up after 5 years *(V, VI)*.

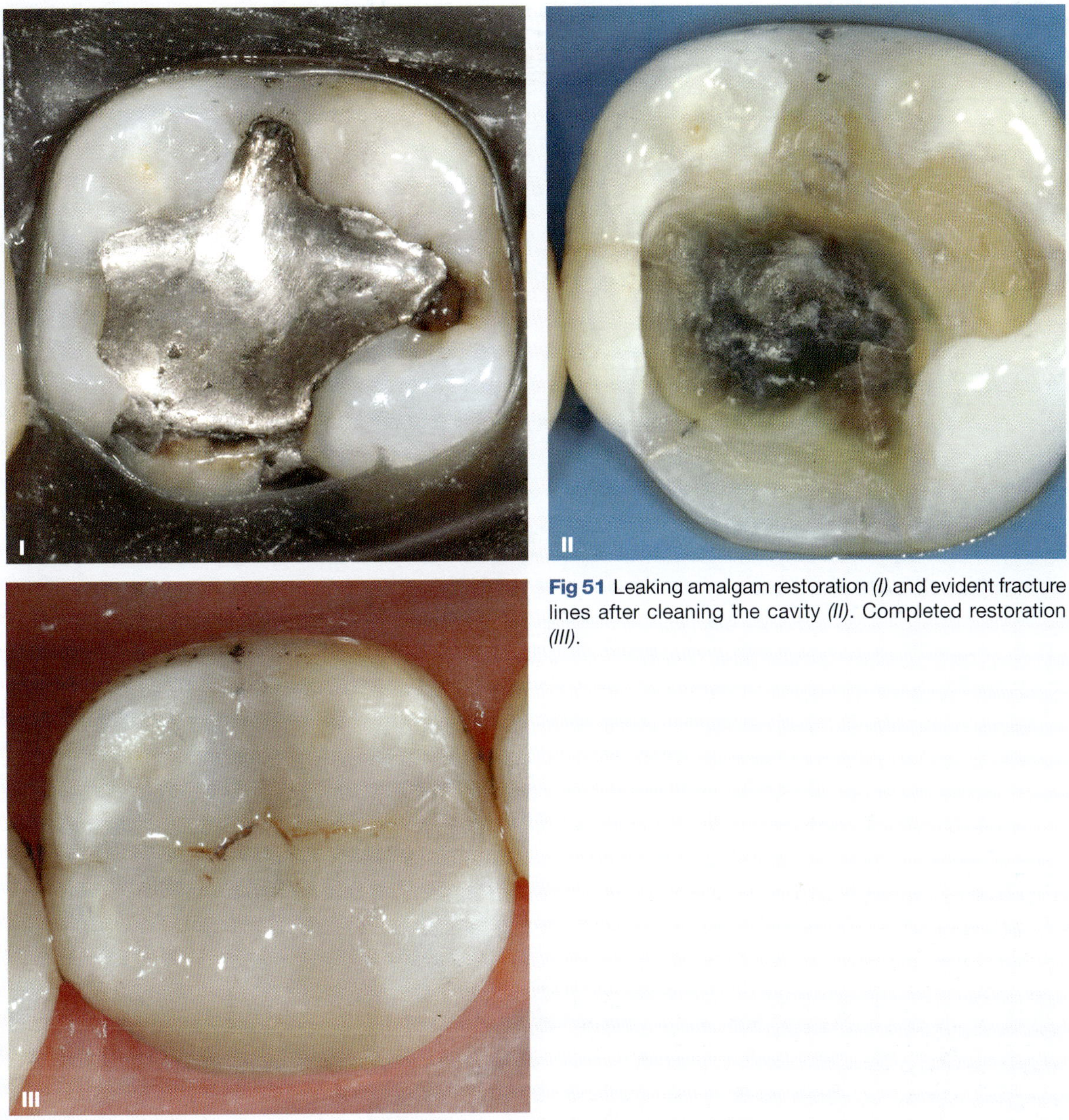

Fig 51 Leaking amalgam restoration *(I)* and evident fracture lines after cleaning the cavity *(II)*. Completed restoration *(III)*.

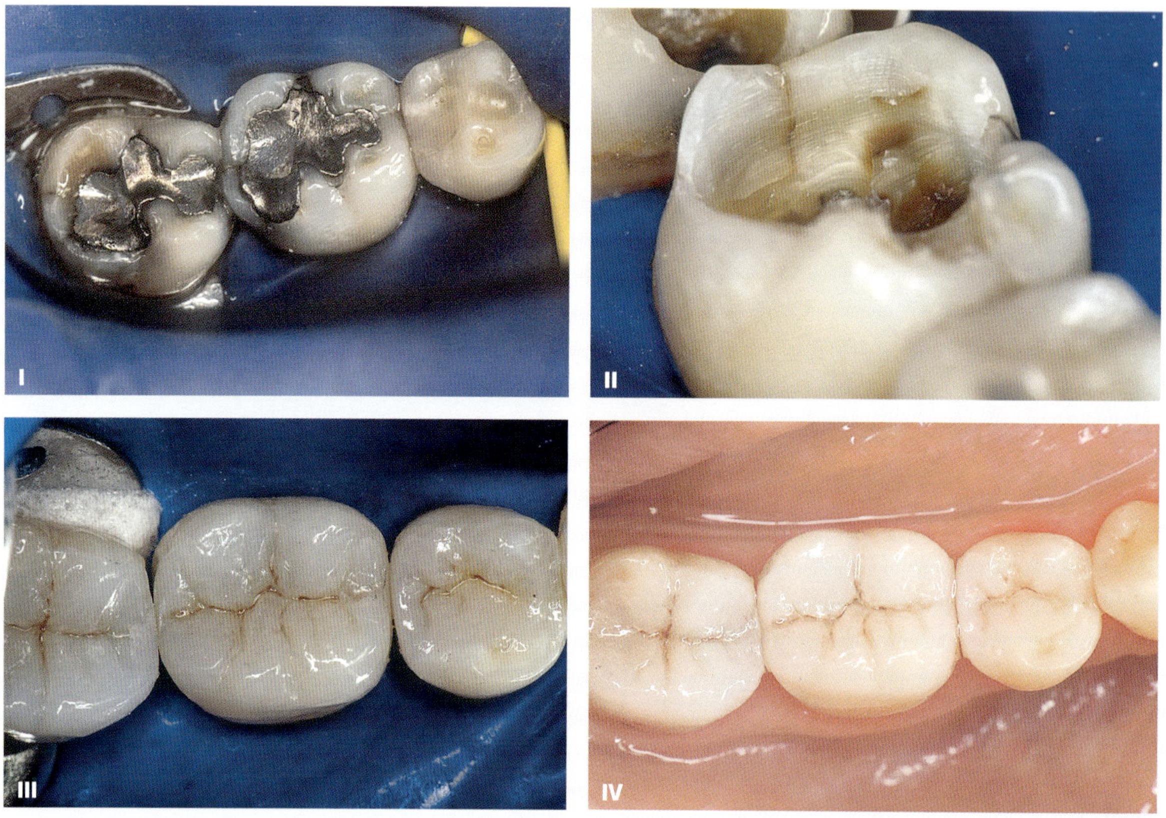

Fig 52 Fracture line in the distal wall of a mandibular right first molar *(I, II)* and views of cemented indirect restorations *(III, IV)*.

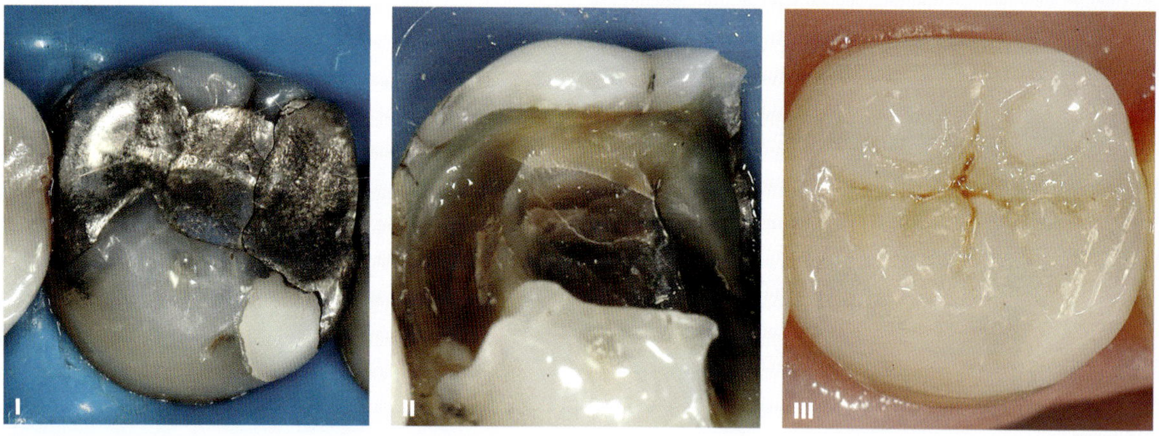

Fig 53 Fractured mandibular molar showing presence of significant fracture lines, restored with composite inlay covering all the cusps after assessing cusp thicknesses.

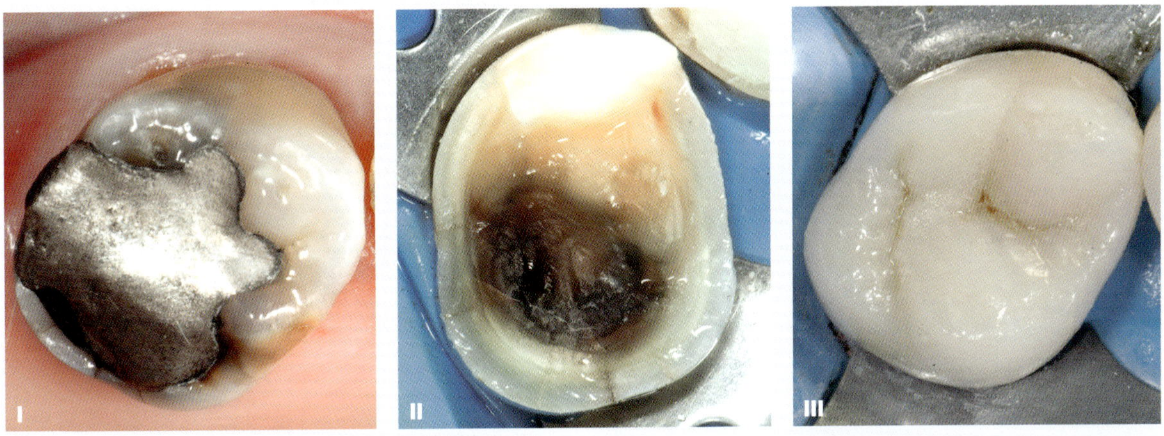

Fig 54 Reconstruction involving indirect restoration of a maxillary molar with a leaky amalgam filling and underlying fracture lines.

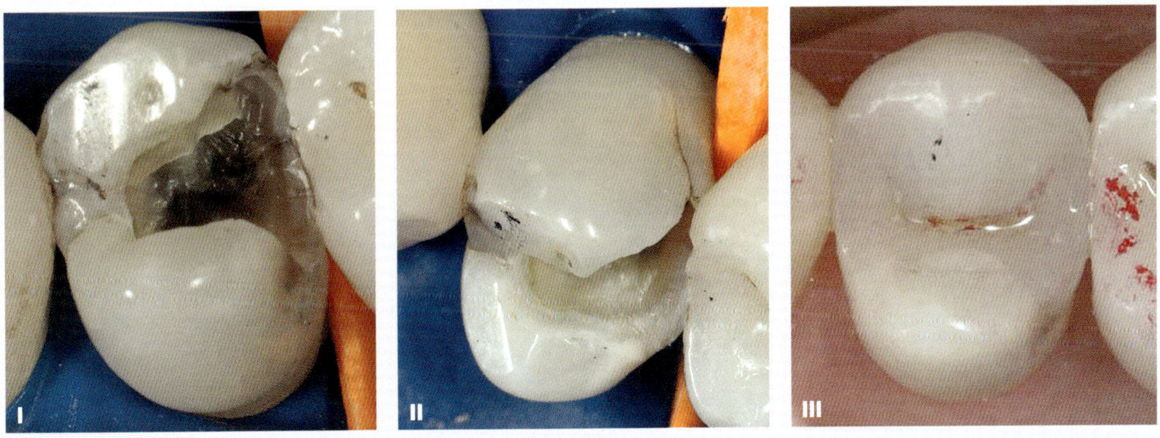

Fig 55 Classic fracture line coinciding with the corner of the box due to an old amalgam filling.

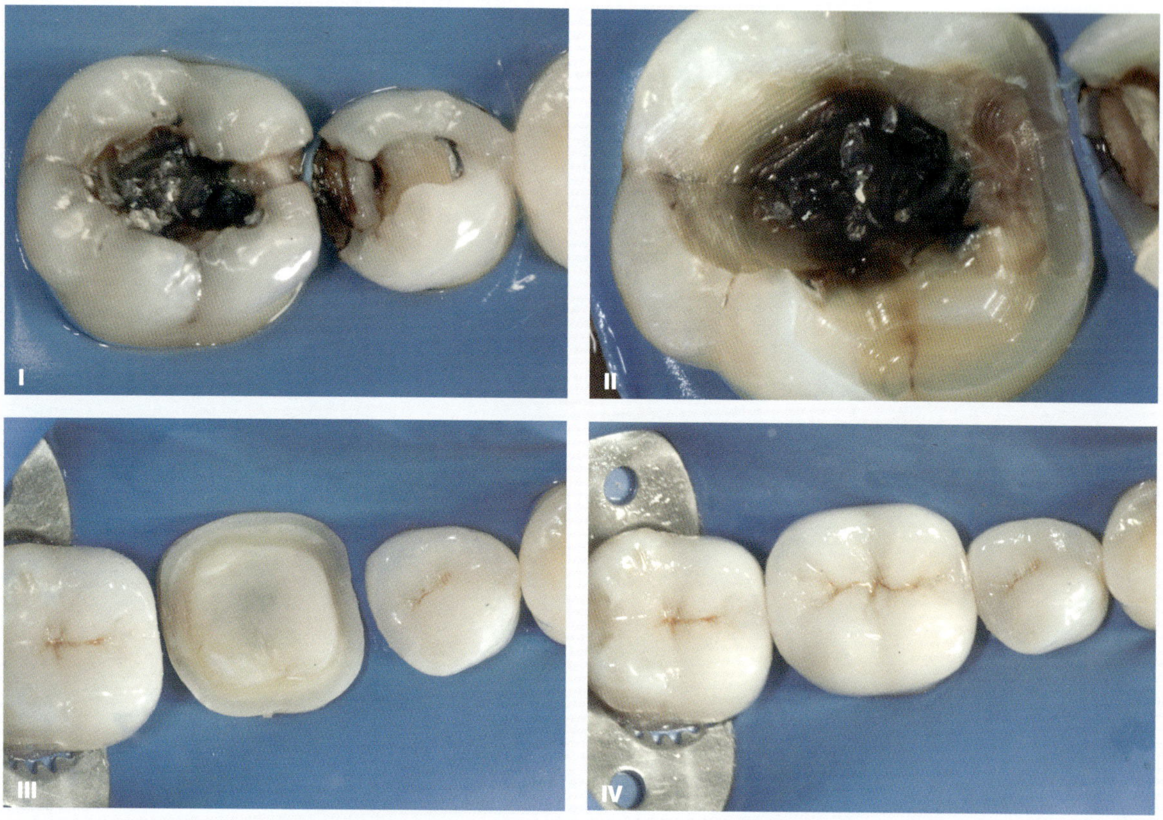

Fig 56 Fracture lines *(I, II)* undermining the mechanical strength of all the walls of the mandibular right first molar. Restoration with full coverage of the cusps *(III, IV)*.

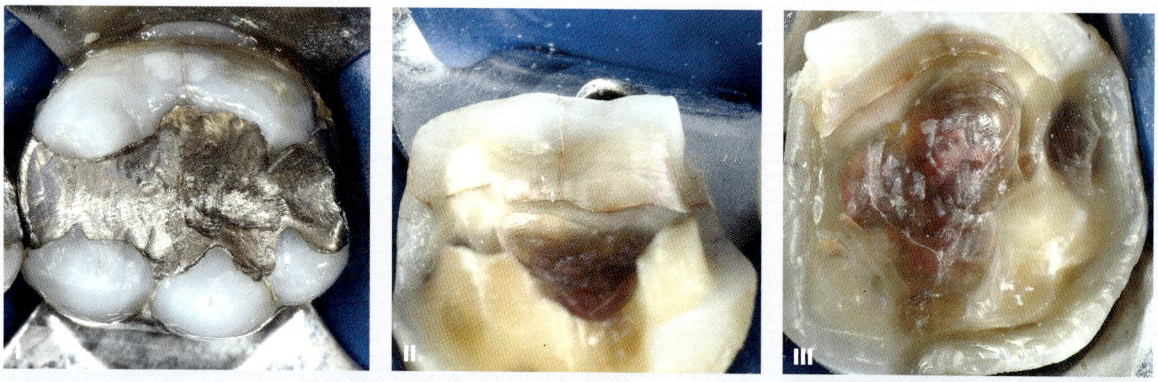

Fig 57 It comes as no surprise to see how much this MOD restoration has undermined the underlying dental structure *(I–III)*. This case was also restored with an inlay with full coverage of the cusps *(IV)*.

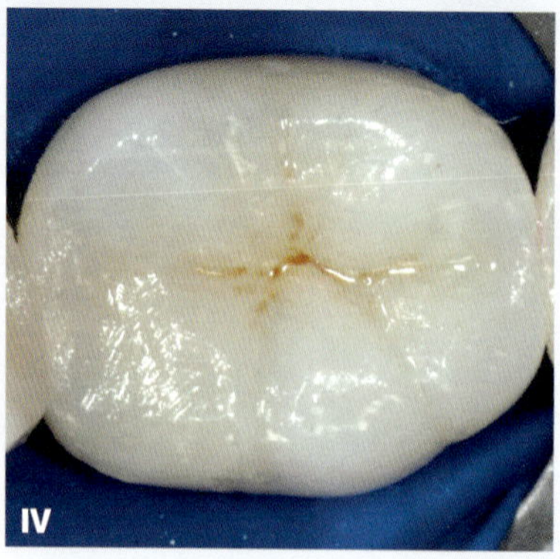

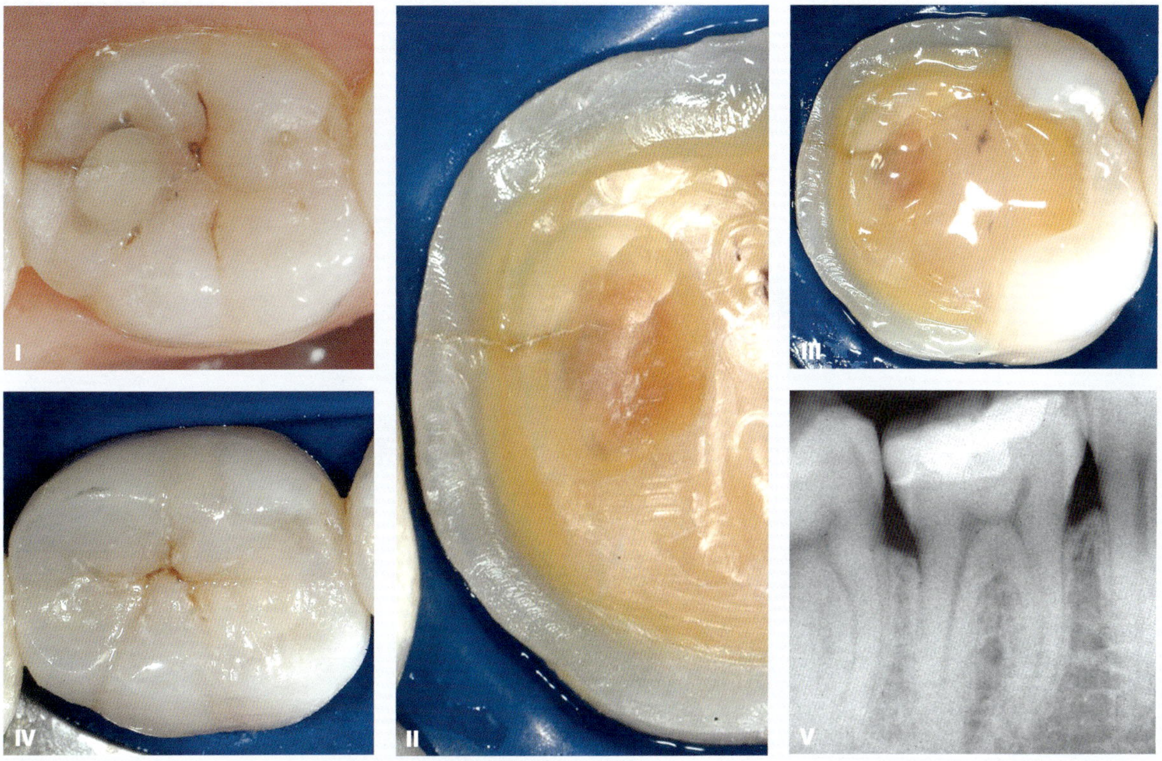

Fig 58 Upon removal of an old leaking composite restoration *(I)*, which was causing pain on chewing, the presence of a dentinal fracture line was noted *(II, III)*. A concomitant occlusal caries lesion extending buccally and lingually required cavity preparation for an onlay. All the painful symptoms completely disappeared a few weeks after cementing the onlay. View of the cemented onlay and postoperative radiograph *(IV, V)*.

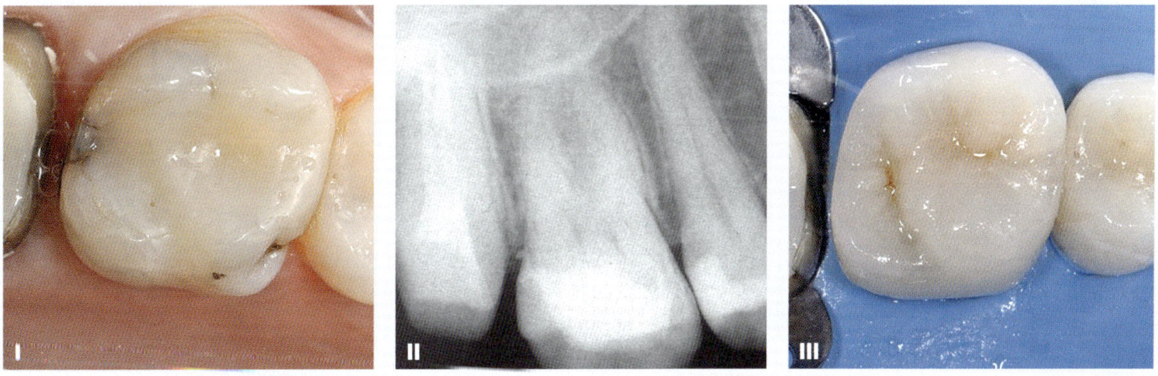

Fig 59 Presence of a fracture in the distal wall of the maxillary right first molar and reconstruction of a defective restoration.

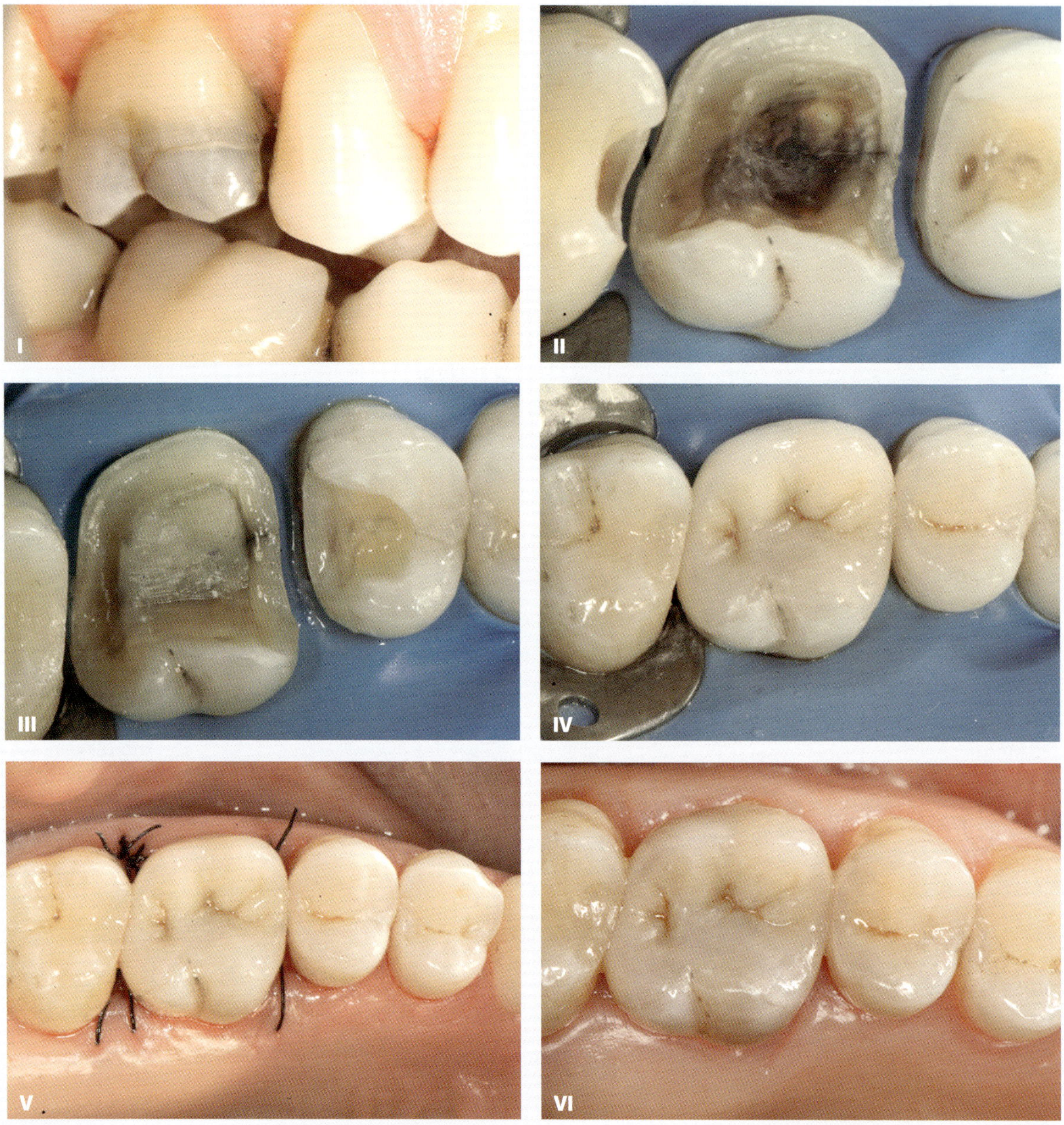

Fig 60 Very evident buccal fracture line in a maxillary right first molar *(I)* and presence of another mesial fracture line *(II)*. Cavity preparation for an onlay with maintenance of the palatal wall *(III)*. View of cemented inlay *(IV)* and sutures *(V)*, which were removed 1 week after periodontal surgery *(VI)*.

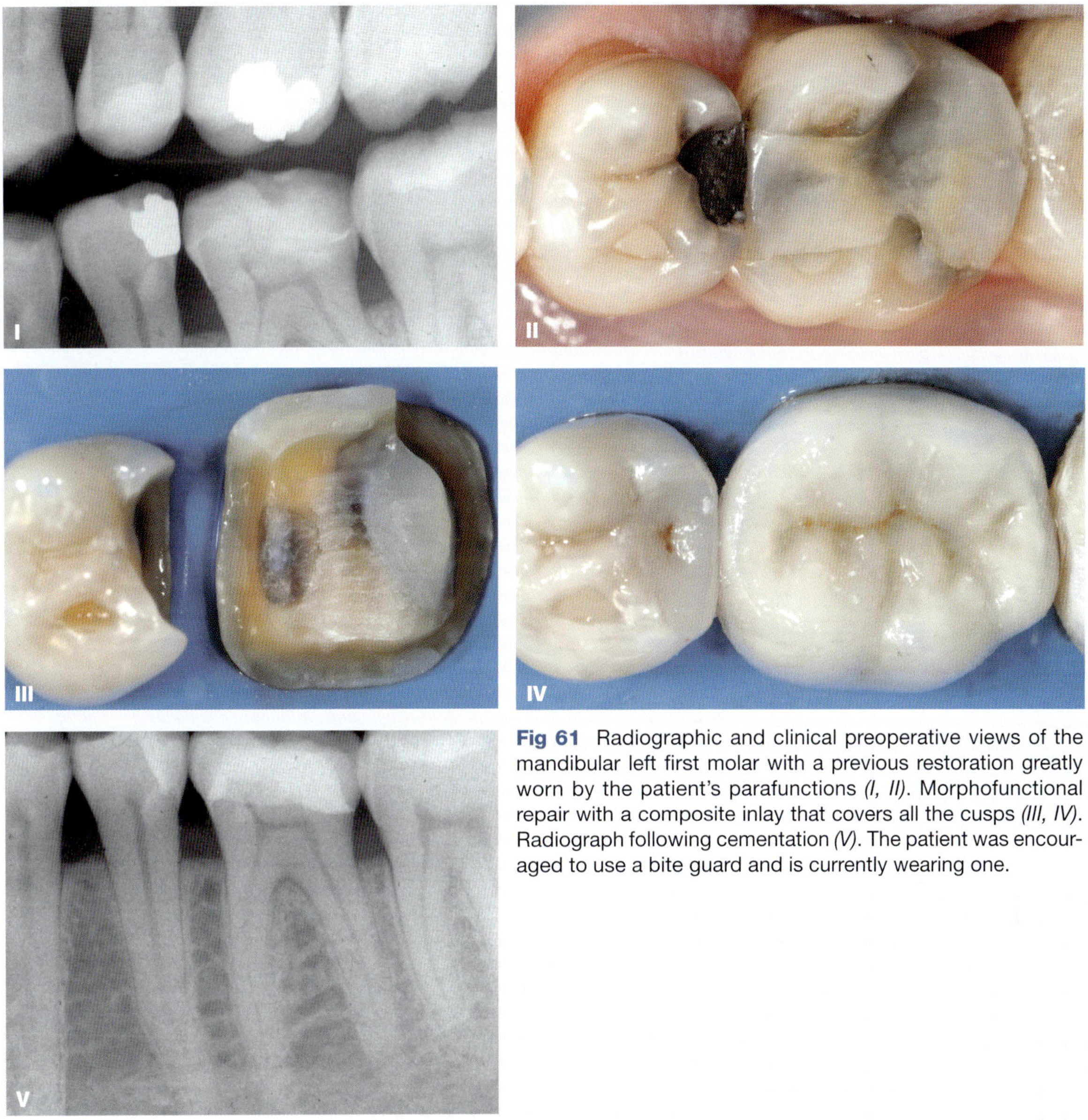

Fig 61 Radiographic and clinical preoperative views of the mandibular left first molar with a previous restoration greatly worn by the patient's parafunctions *(I, II)*. Morphofunctional repair with a composite inlay that covers all the cusps *(III, IV)*. Radiograph following cementation *(V)*. The patient was encouraged to use a bite guard and is currently wearing one.

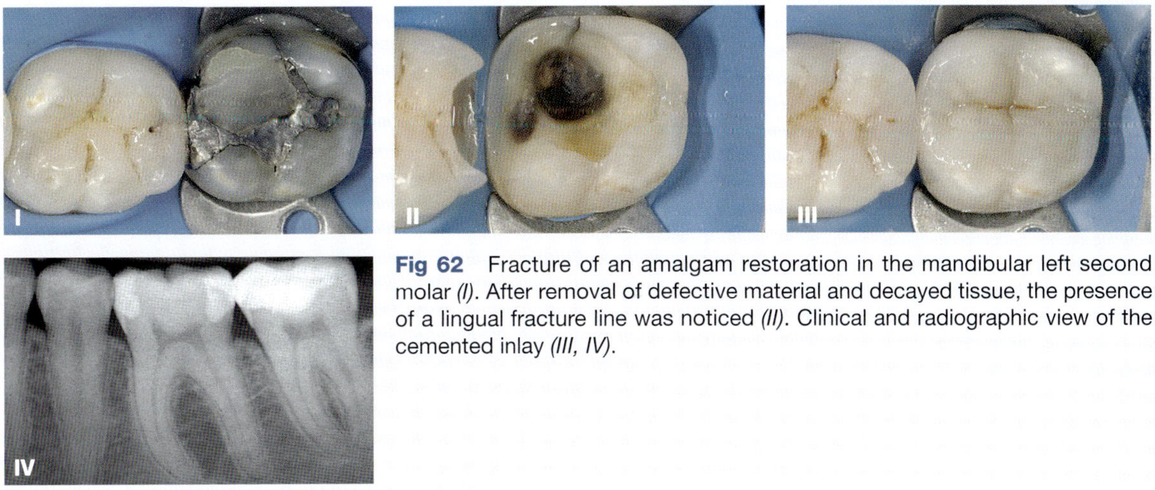

Fig 62 Fracture of an amalgam restoration in the mandibular left second molar *(I)*. After removal of defective material and decayed tissue, the presence of a lingual fracture line was noticed *(II)*. Clinical and radiographic view of the cemented inlay *(III, IV)*.

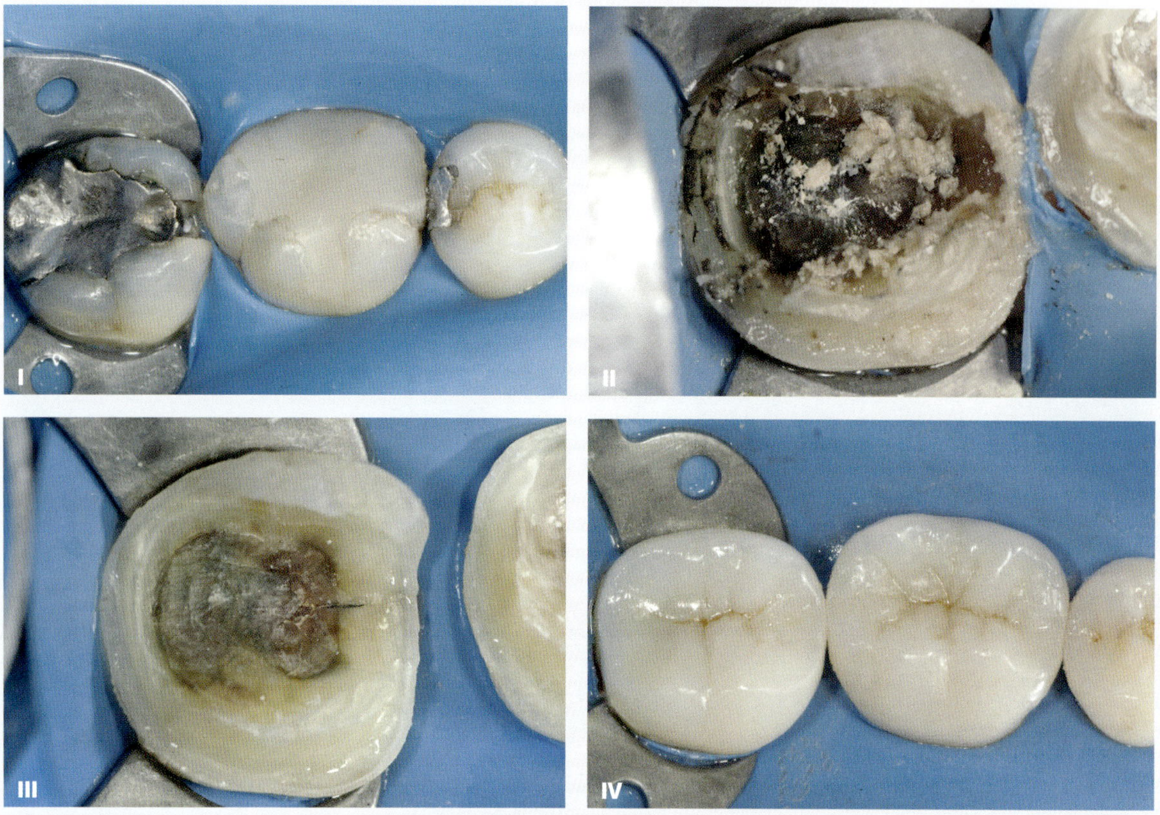

Fig 63 Reconstruction of restorations in the mandibular right quadrant. When cleaning the cavity, rubber dam may become torn. If this happens, new dam is simply positioned before carrying out the adhesive and buildup stage. View showing depth of the decay and a mesial fracture line in the second molar *(III)* and cemented inlays *(IV)*.

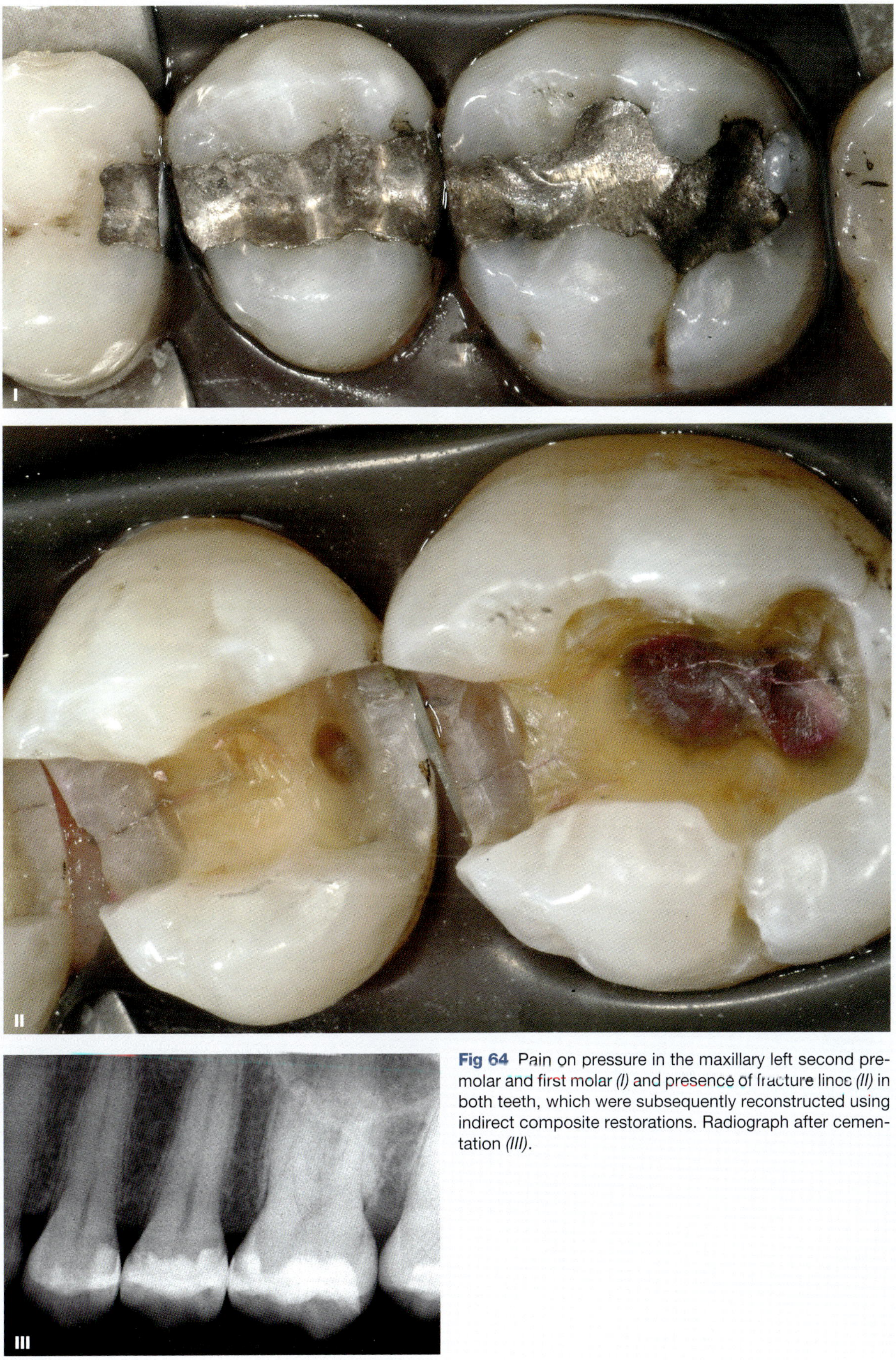

Fig 64 Pain on pressure in the maxillary left second premolar and first molar *(I)* and presence of fracture lines *(II)* in both teeth, which were subsequently reconstructed using indirect composite restorations. Radiograph after cementation *(III)*.

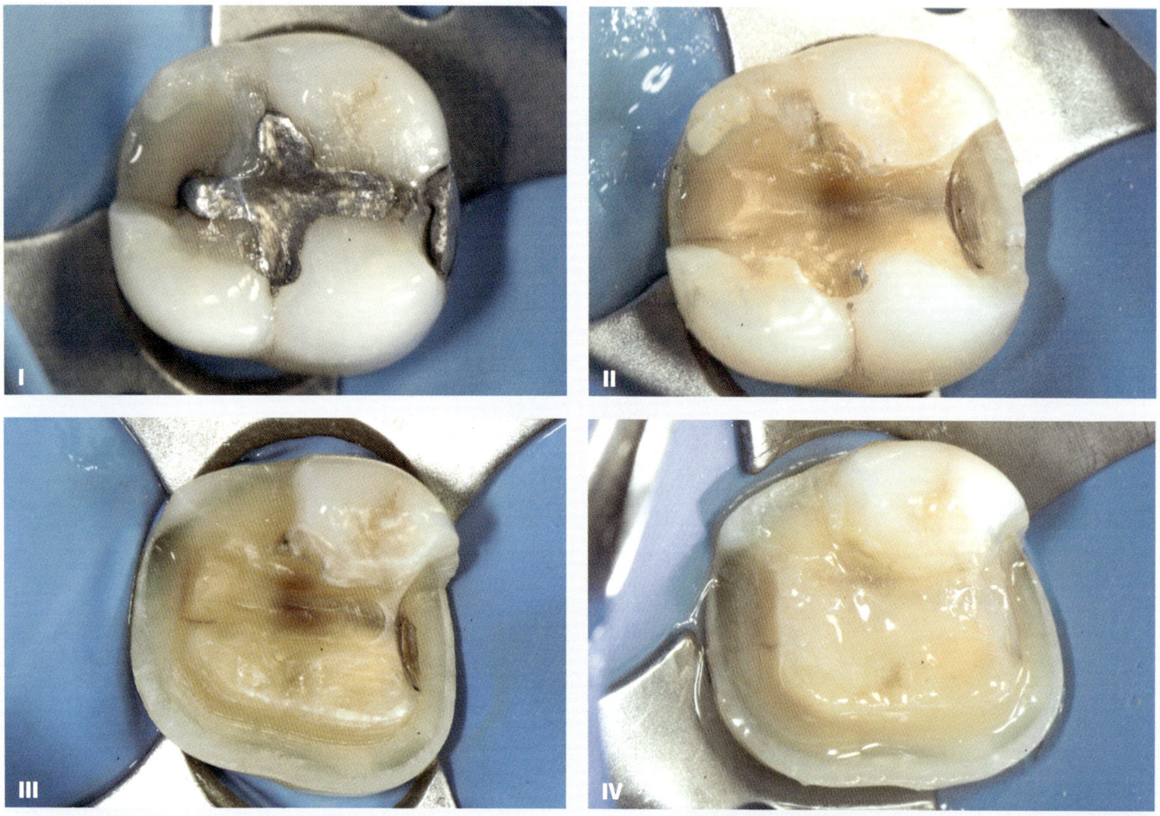

Fig 65 Inevitable fracture of a molar that had to withstand excessive loads because of the lack of adjacent teeth *(I, II)*. The presence of fracture lines is hardly surprising *(III)*. View of buildup and cemented onlay *(IV, V)*.

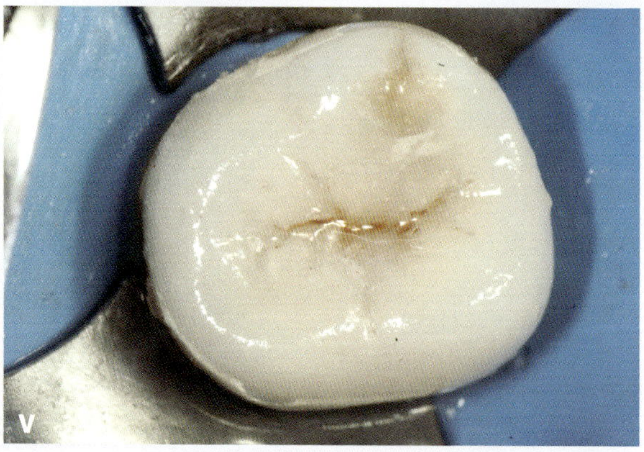

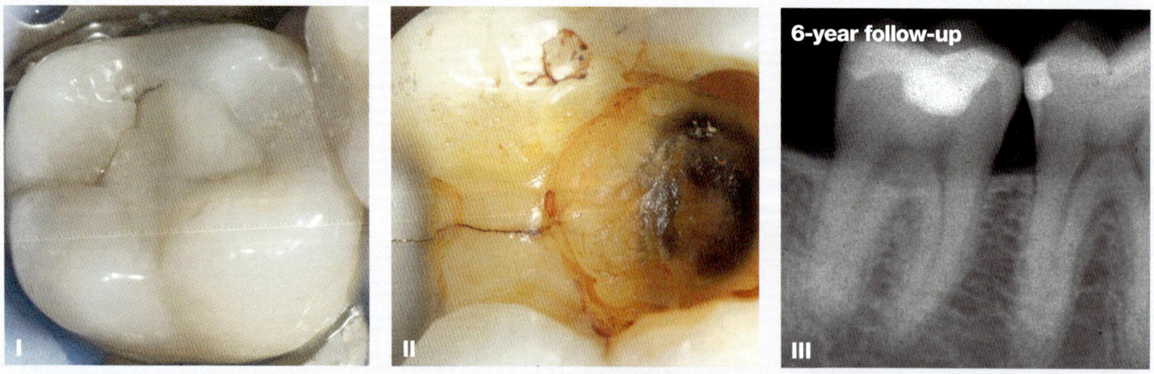

Fig 66 Pain on pressure affecting the mandibular right second molar in a patient with bruxism *(I)*. Presence of an occlusodistal fracture line *(II)* and follow-up radiograph after 6 years *(III)*. There was total disappearance of painful symptoms.

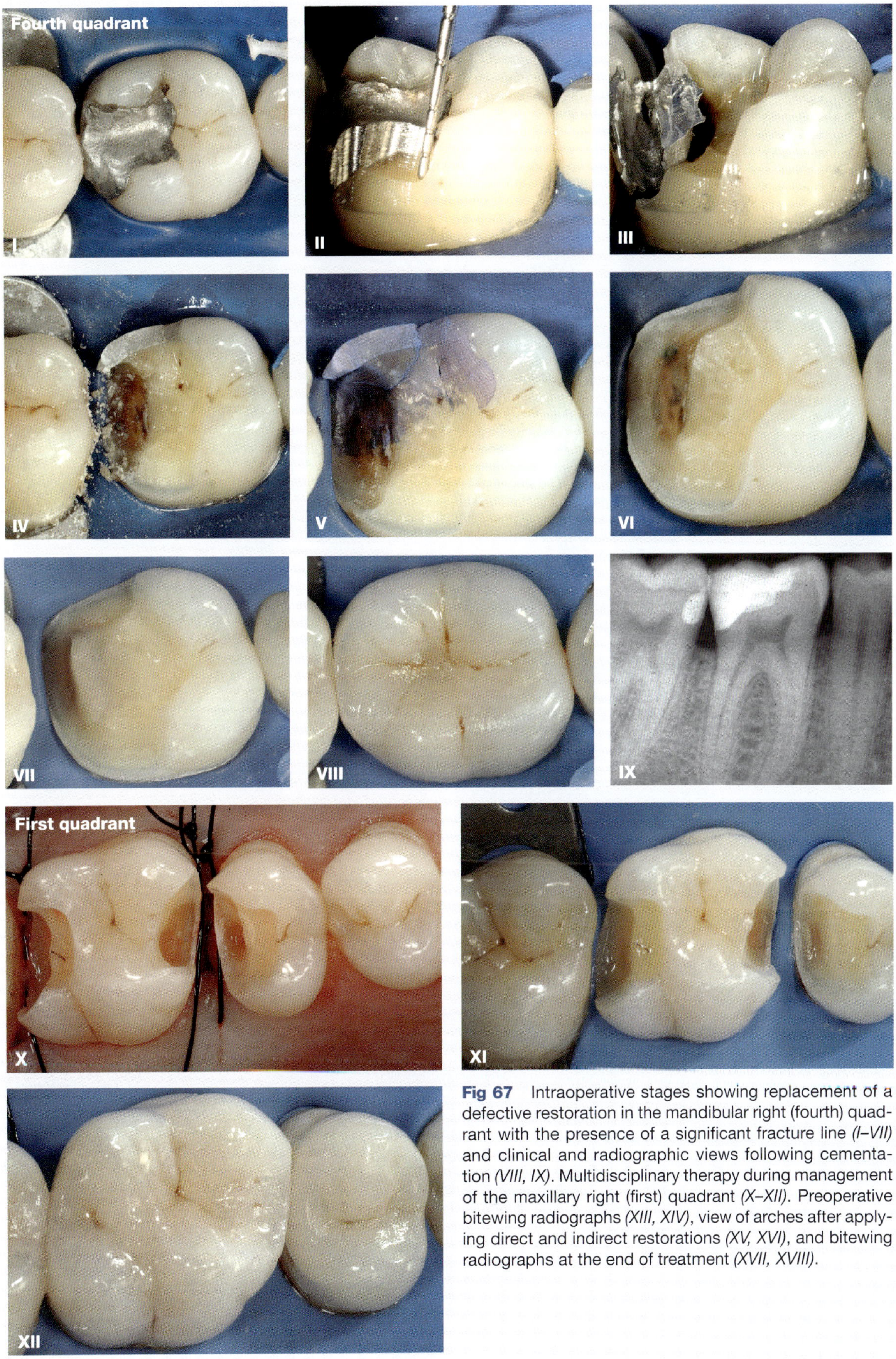

Fig 67 Intraoperative stages showing replacement of a defective restoration in the mandibular right (fourth) quadrant with the presence of a significant fracture line *(I–VII)* and clinical and radiographic views following cementation *(VIII, IX)*. Multidisciplinary therapy during management of the maxillary right (first) quadrant *(X–XII)*. Preoperative bitewing radiographs *(XIII, XIV)*, view of arches after applying direct and indirect restorations *(XV, XVI)*, and bitewing radiographs at the end of treatment *(XVII, XVIII)*.

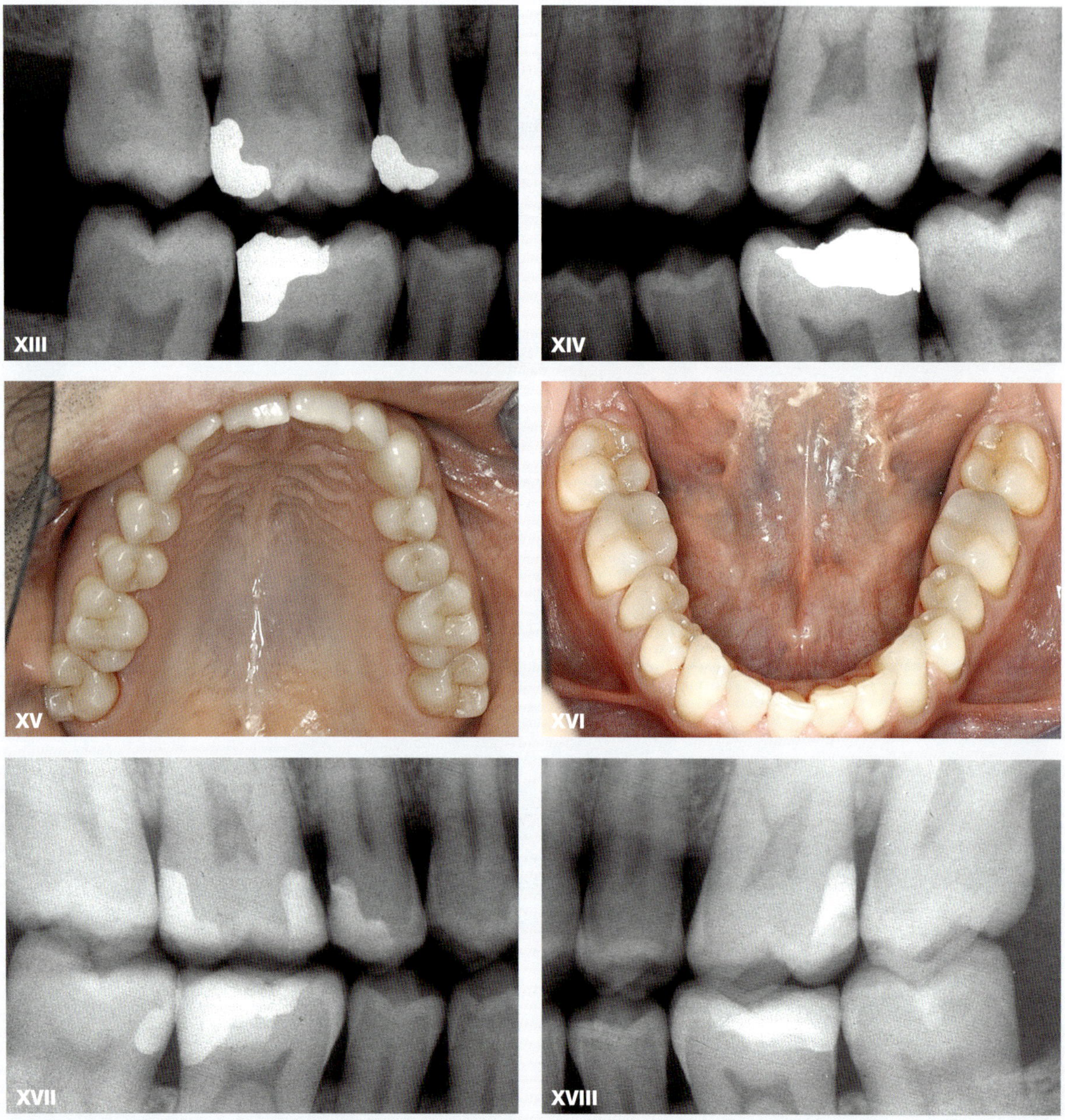

Fig 67 *(continued)*

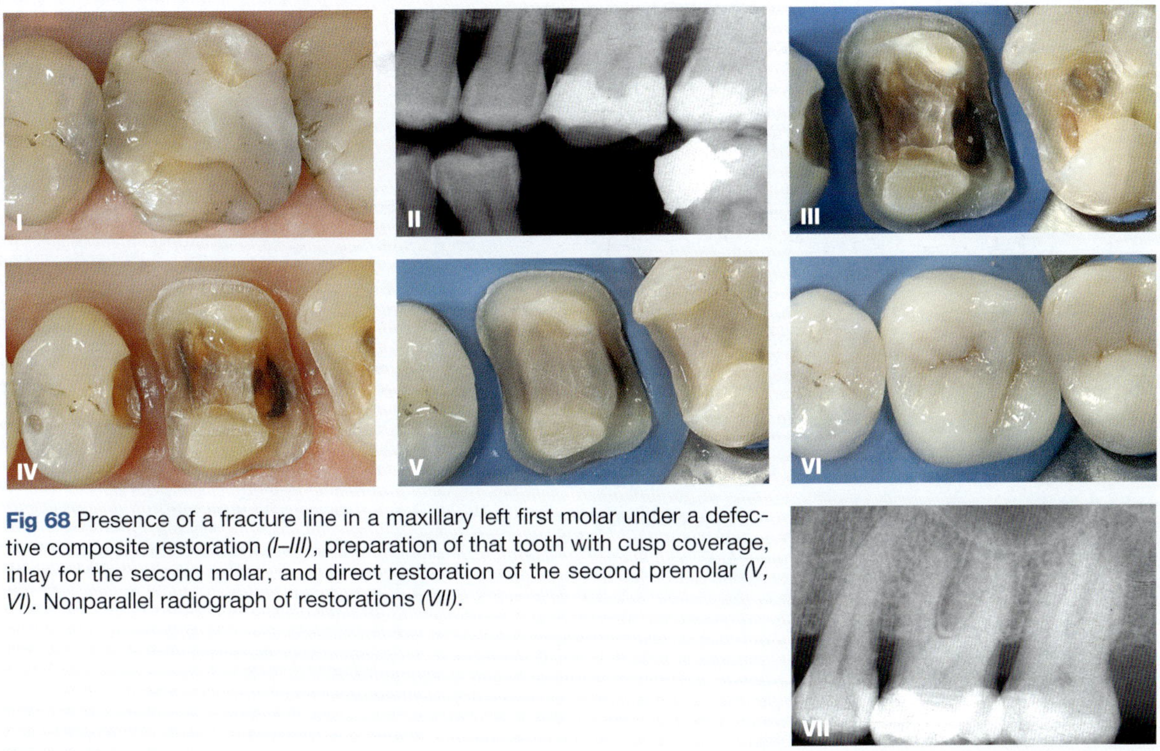

Fig 68 Presence of a fracture line in a maxillary left first molar under a defective composite restoration *(I–III)*, preparation of that tooth with cusp coverage, inlay for the second molar, and direct restoration of the second premolar *(V, VI)*. Nonparallel radiograph of restorations *(VII)*.

Significant problems are posed by cavity design in teeth without decay and without previous restorations but affected by multiple cracks, often of pre-fracture size, which may even be asymptomatic. What approach should be taken in this case (Fig 69)?

The real question is how to persuade the patient of the need to intervene in order to prevent worse damage in the future when the treatment is for a tooth that the patient quite rightly considers healthy. Indeed, the previously asymptomatic tooth might cause symptoms after surgery, in which case the clinician will hear the classic refrain, "It didn't give me any problems until you touched it."

There is obviously no right answer: many things must be considered, including the patient's receptiveness and motivation and the clinician's ability to leverage his or her experience, aided by presenting photographs showing step-by-step clinical cases. Alternatively, patient and clinician could mutually agree to wait to see if painful symptoms appear rather than a fracture.

Often doing nothing may constitute a treatment plan, and it is often not the worst choice.

It is a problem, but nothing can be done about it.

Conversely, if signs and symptoms are present, the author can offer some simple, easily understandable guidelines.

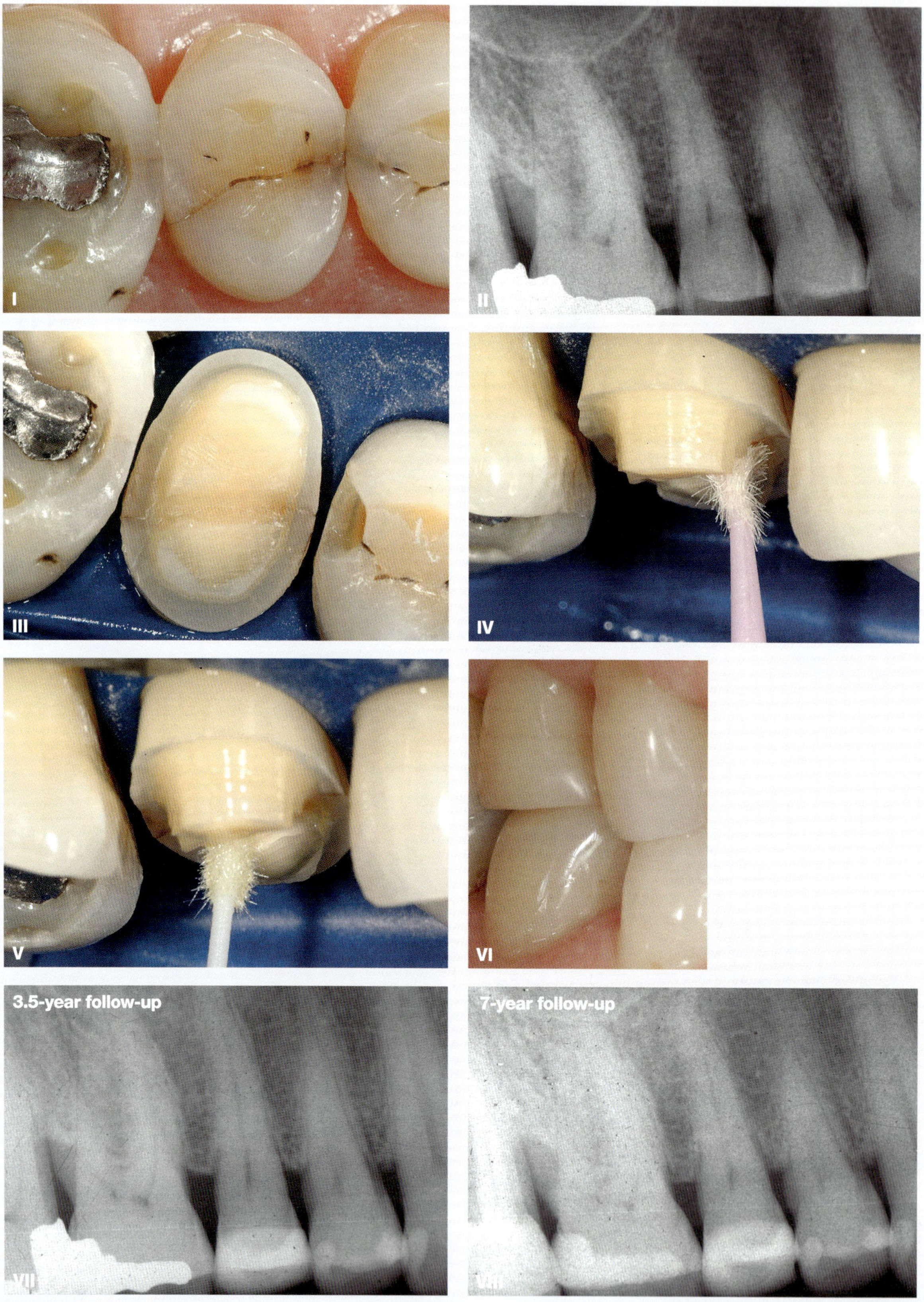

Fig 69 Very intense pain upon pressure in the maxillary right second premolar with a fracture line on a tooth without restorations *(I–III)* prompted the patient to request immediate removal. The author's team patiently convinced him to make an attempt to save the tooth, which was treated by an indirect restoration with coverage of two cusps *(IV–VI)*. Follow-up radiographs after 3.5 *(VII)* and 7 years *(VIII)*. The pulp vitality/sensitivity test was positive at long-term follow-up.

Guidelines for dentinal cracks:

- Preoperative periapical radiograph
- Pulp vitality test (thermal, electric, and cavity test)
- Chewing test (moist cotton wool roll)
- Gnathologic check
- Removal of defective restorations and any caries lesions
- Removal of decayed tissue that is often present within the fracture line: long-standing if pigmented, recently formed if white
- Disinfection with chlorhexidine
- Adhesive procedures
- New direct or indirect restoration in composite
- Long-term follow-ups (radiographs and vitality test)

Patient information

From a clinical and therapeutic viewpoint, it is useful to place operative procedures recommended for the treatment of dentinal cracks in order based on a scale of magnitude:

- Direct restoration, when indicated
- Indirect restoration (inlay, onlay, overlay)
- Orthodontic treatment, always and only when indicated
- Extraction
- Implant

Following some misunderstandings with patients, which have fortunately been very few but nonetheless unpleasant, the author finds it useful to introduce informed consent for this purpose (Figs 70 to 73).
According to the very fine article by Martin and Machtou,[5] the therapeutic options are determined by the etiology and the level of pulp inflammation and coronal damage.
A traumatic factor is often responsible for the crack, and if this factor is sporadic, it almost always goes away on its own: an effective restoration will resolve the problem. If the problem is a malocclusion, this must be the focus of treatment.
When the cause is associated with parafunctions, the situation is more complicated because such problems are notoriously difficult to manage, particularly bruxism (Fig 74).
With regard to pulp inflammation, treatment[20] will always be aimed at maintaining vitality, and good hybridization of the crack will prevent bacteria from the oral cavity penetrating the open dentinal tubules (Figs 75 to 82).

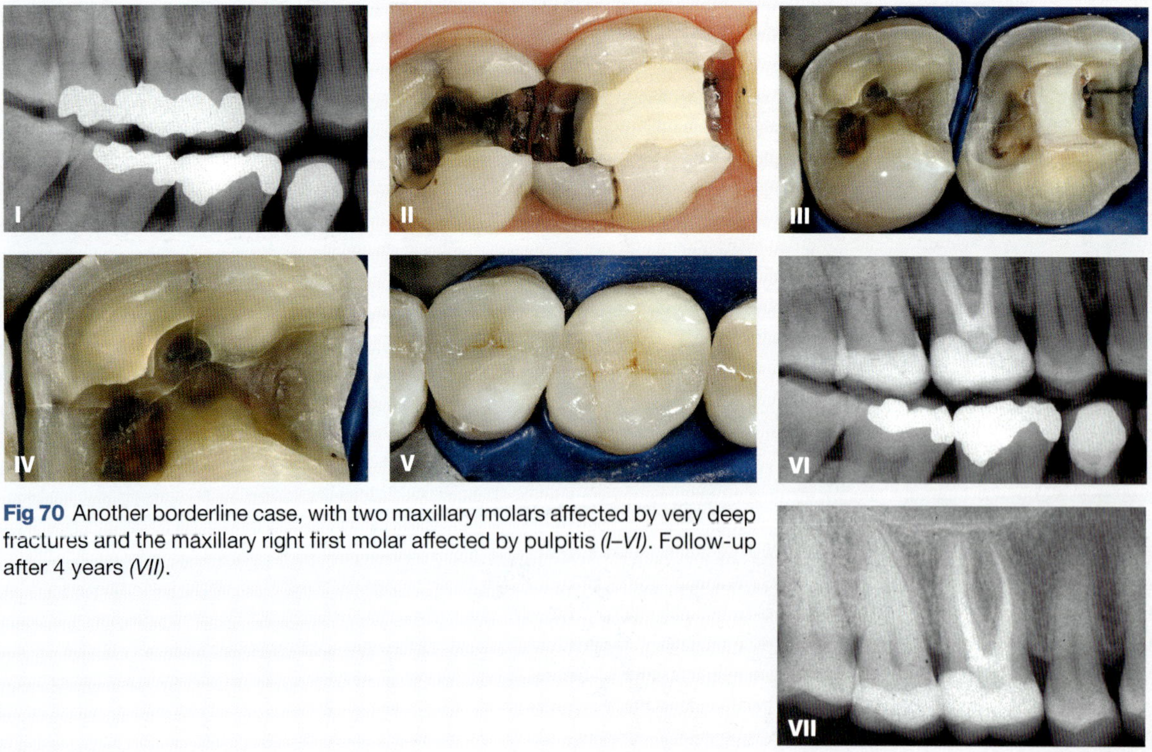

Fig 70 Another borderline case, with two maxillary molars affected by very deep fractures and the maxillary right first molar affected by pulpitis *(I–VI)*. Follow-up after 4 years *(VII)*.

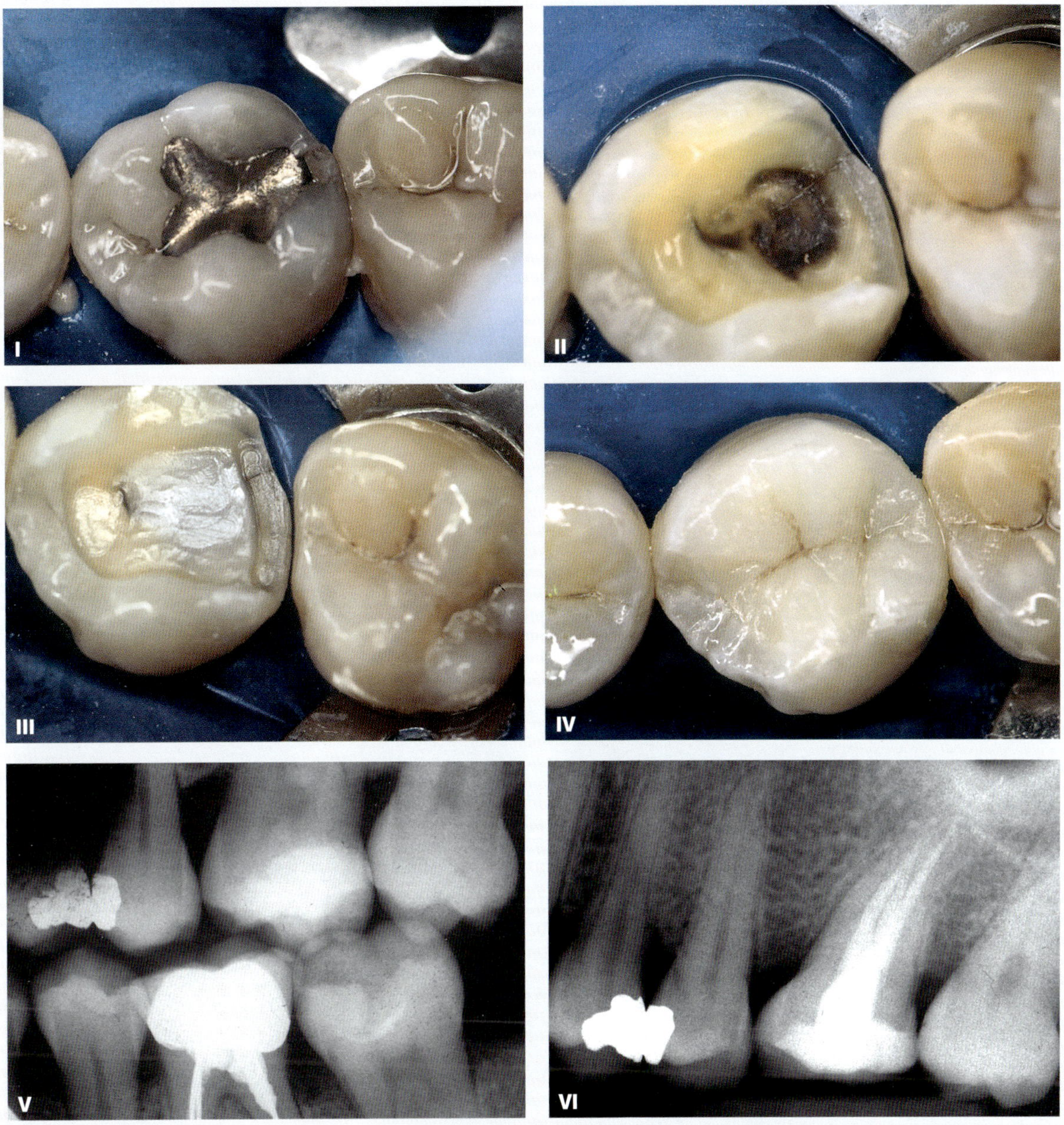

Fig 71 A small amalgam restoration caused constant pain and twinges during chewing. When the restoration was removed, deep decay and a dentinal crack were revealed *(I, II)*. After cementing an inlay, the painful symptoms disappeared altogether *(III–V)*. A few months later, pulpitis was diagnosed, and the tooth was endodontically treated *(VI)*.

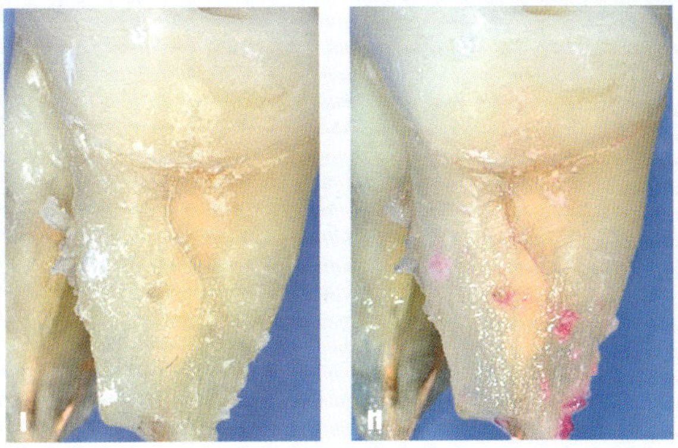

Fig 72 Example of vertical progression of a fracture line.

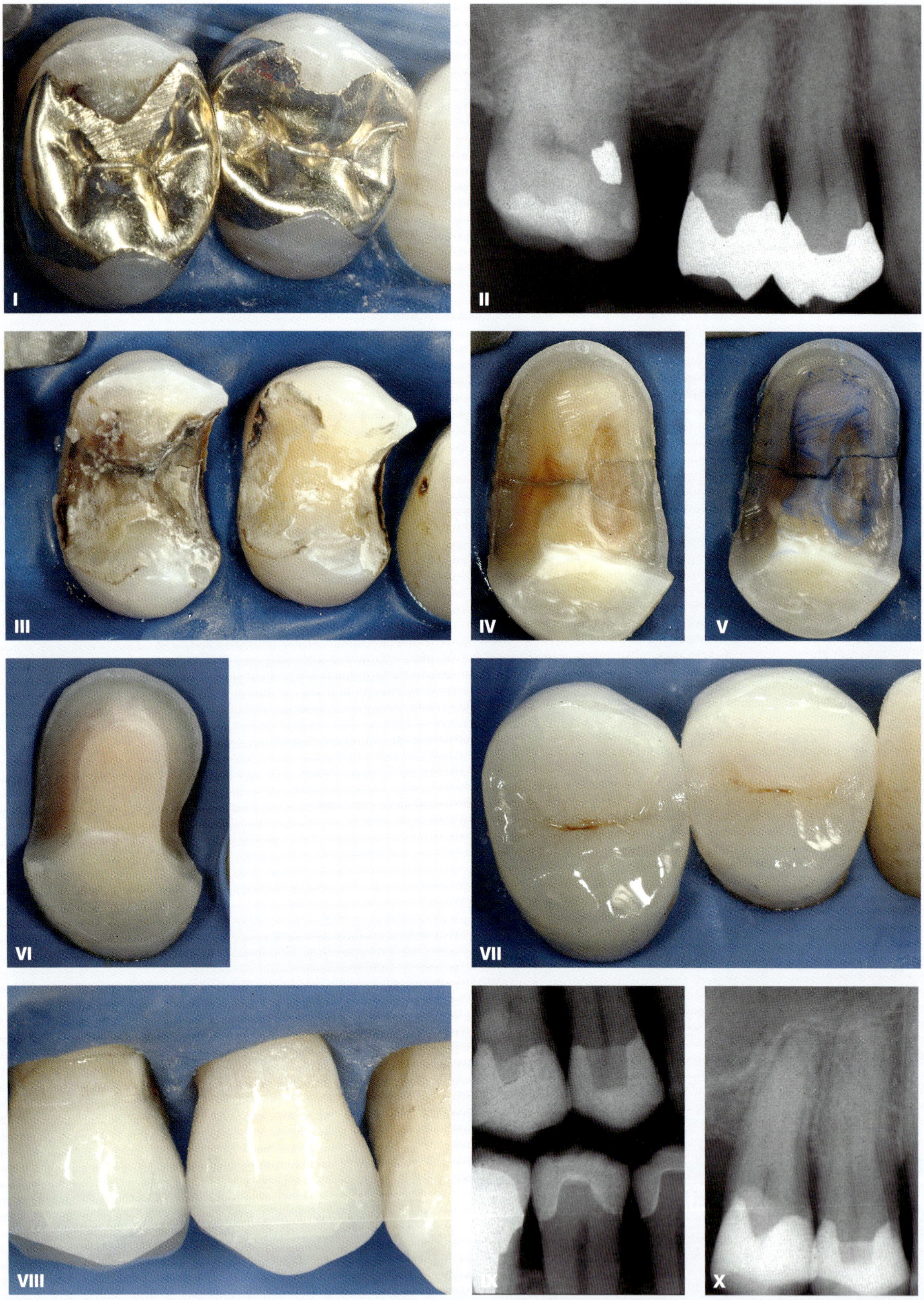

Fig 73 Pain on pressure in the maxillary right second premolar after removal of old gold inlays. An MOD fracture line is evident in the second premolar *(I–III)*. When duly informed of the uncertainty of the outcome, the patient agreed to have the inlays rebuilt in composite *(IV–X)*. At a follow-up after 1 year, the result of a pulp vitality test for the second premolar was negative, and because pain was also present on pressure, a need for endodontic treatment was identified *(XI)*.

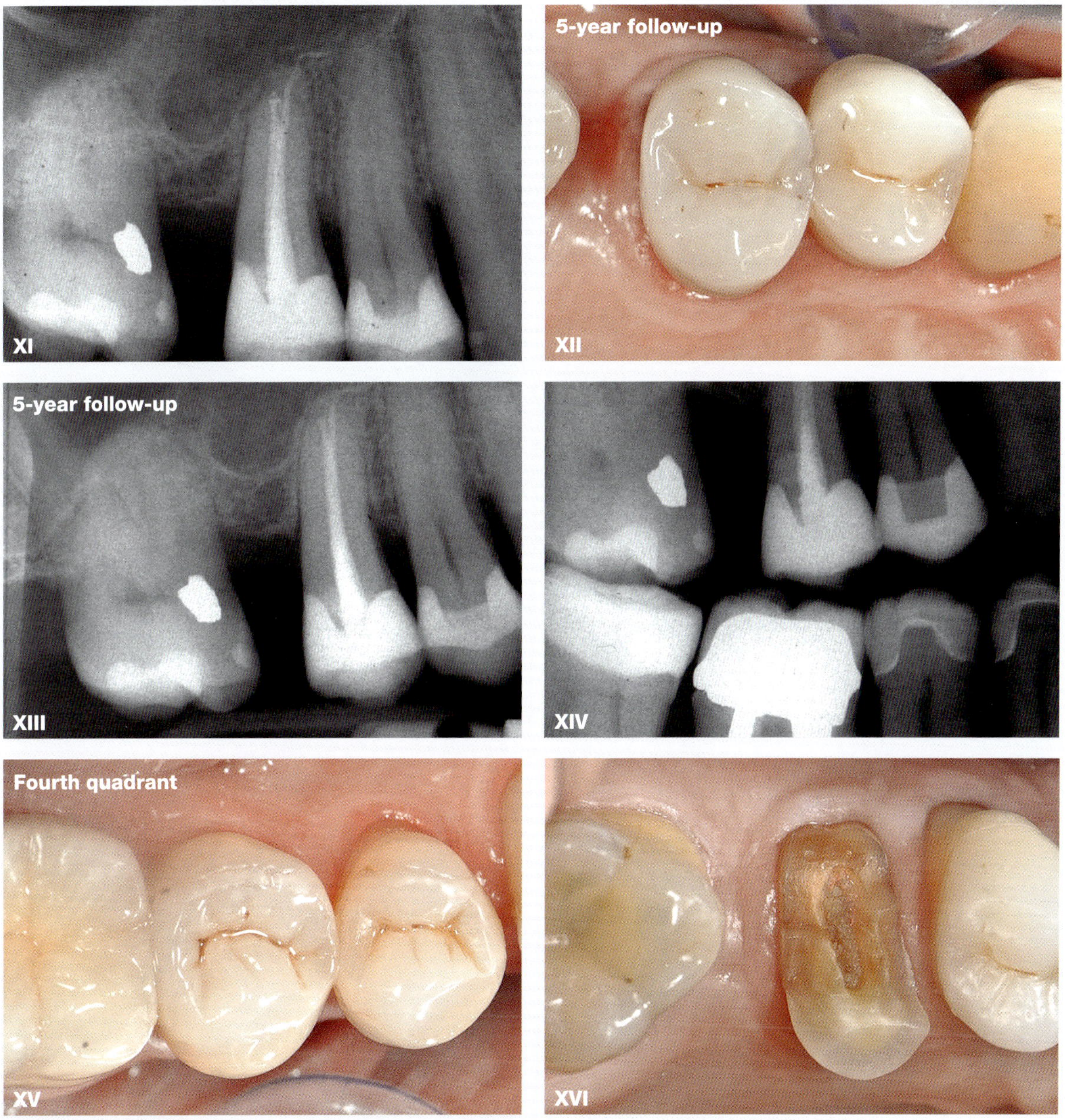

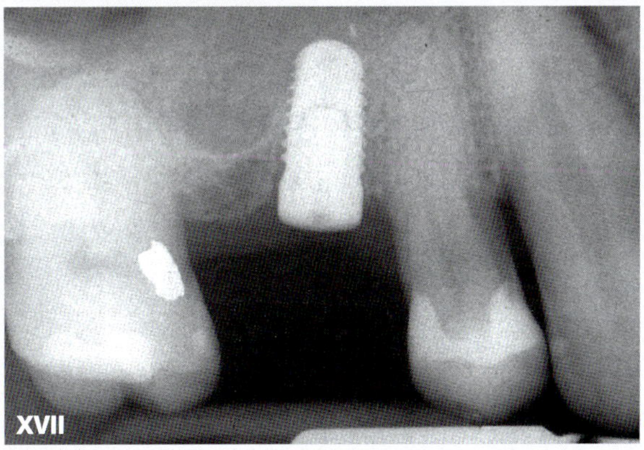

Fig 73 *(continued)* The follow-up after 5 years *(XII, XIII)* was entirely satisfactory, as was the 9-year follow-up on the opposing mandibular right (fourth) quadrant *(XIV, XV)*. After 10 years, coronal fracture of the maxillary right second premolar with deep periodontal probing led to replacement of the tooth with an implant *(XVI, XVII)*

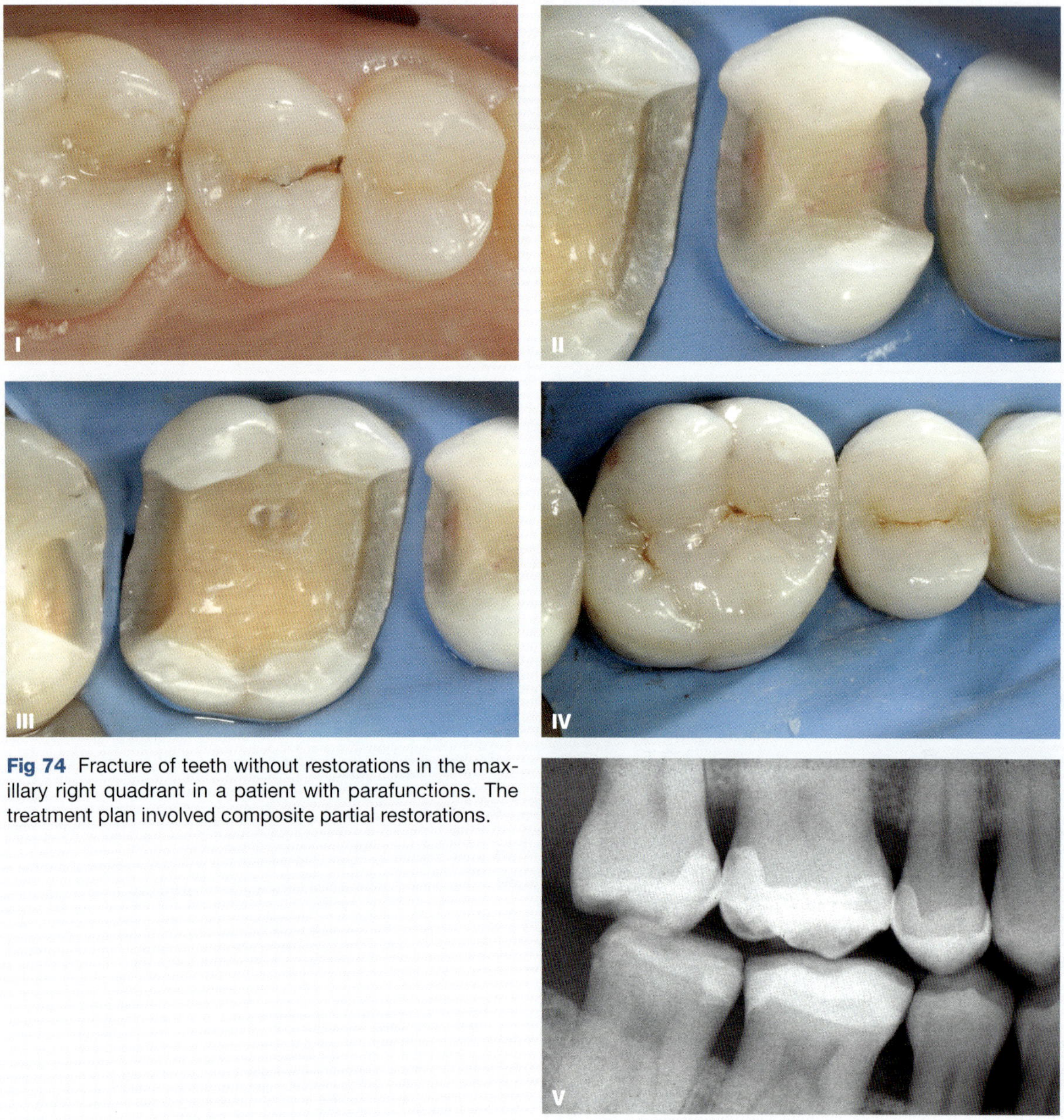

Fig 74 Fracture of teeth without restorations in the maxillary right quadrant in a patient with parafunctions. The treatment plan involved composite partial restorations.

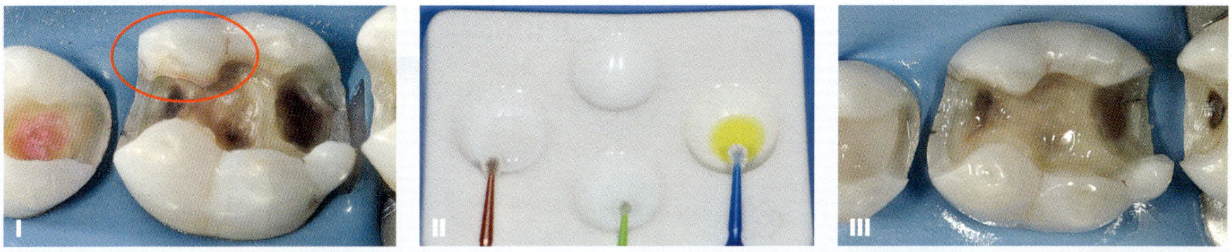

Fig 75 Cracking at the base of the mesiolingual cusp in a mandibular left first molar *(I)*. Adequate thicknesses led to the preparation of a cavity without wall removal, and the tooth was reconstructed with a simple inlay. Two-step adhesive system *(II, left to right*: chlorhexidine, etching-primer, bonding), flowable composite *(III)*, and traditional composite *(IV)*.

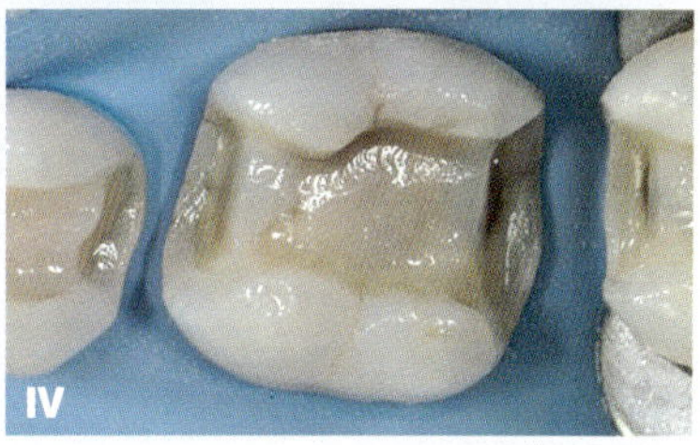

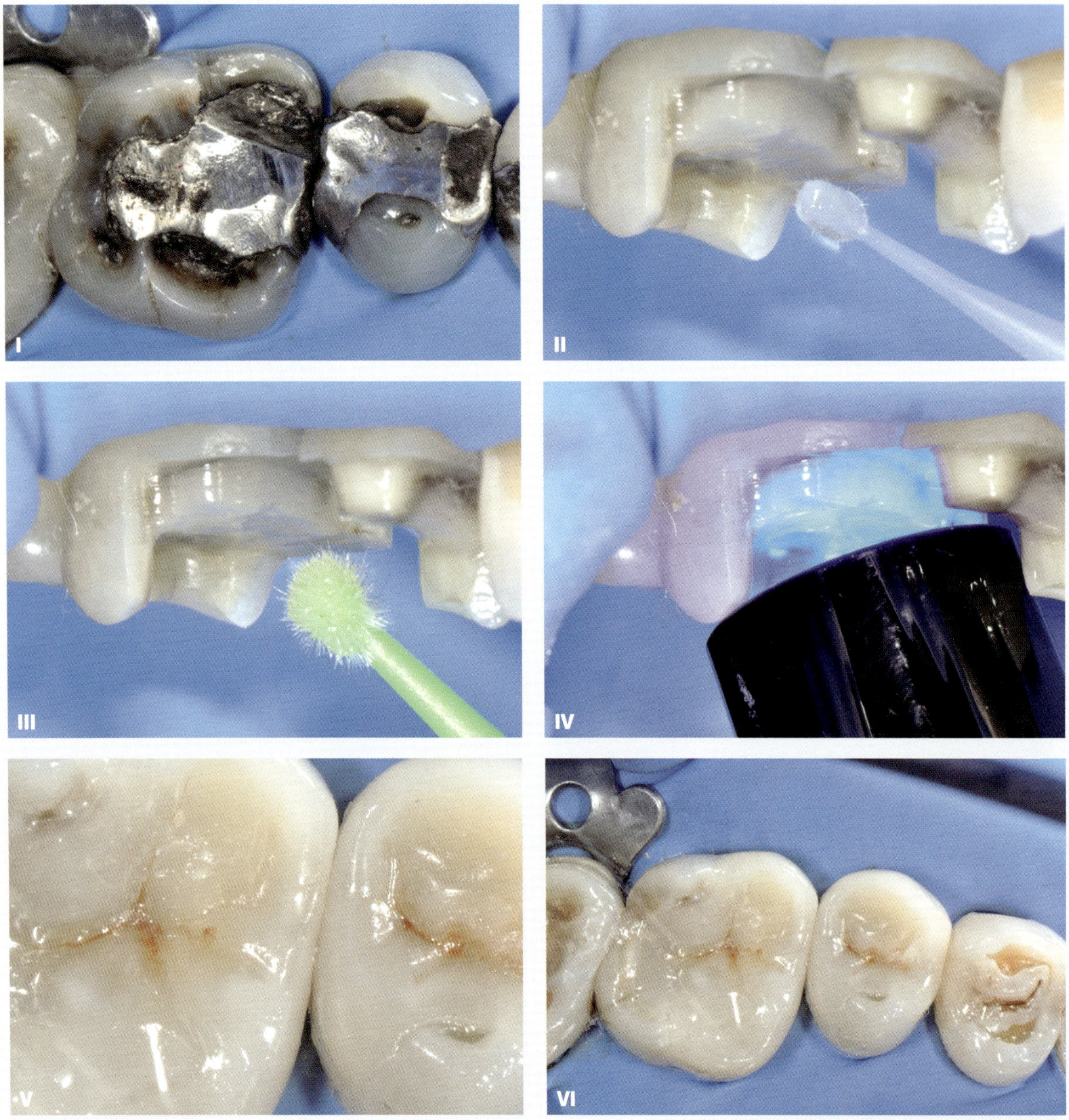

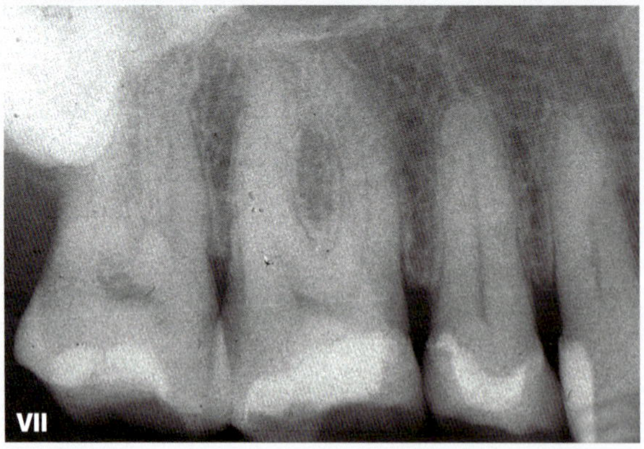

Fig 76 Cracking caused by parafunctions and a very deep cavity. Maintenance of pulp vitality.

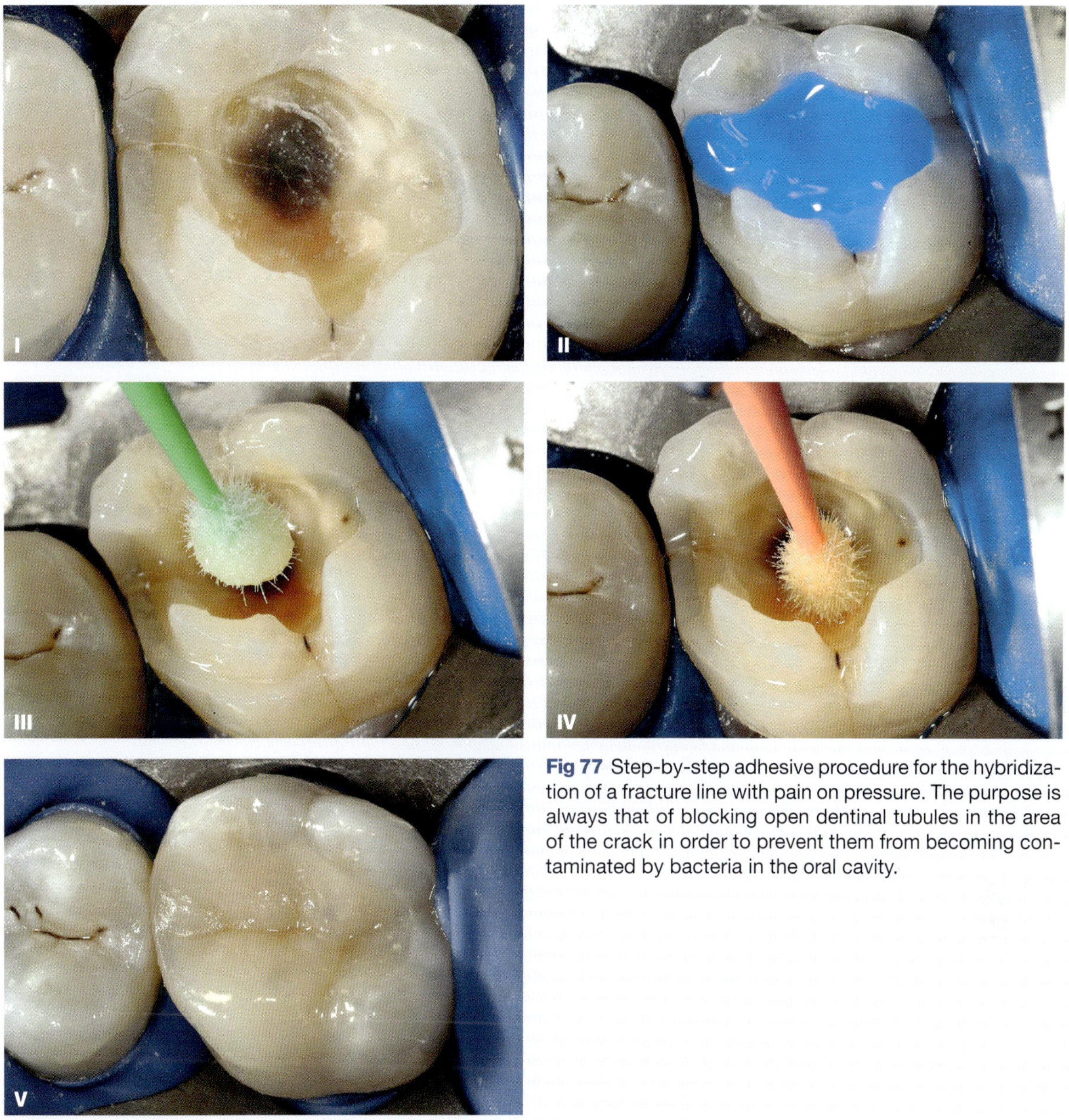

Fig 77 Step-by-step adhesive procedure for the hybridization of a fracture line with pain on pressure. The purpose is always that of blocking open dentinal tubules in the area of the crack in order to prevent them from becoming contaminated by bacteria in the oral cavity.

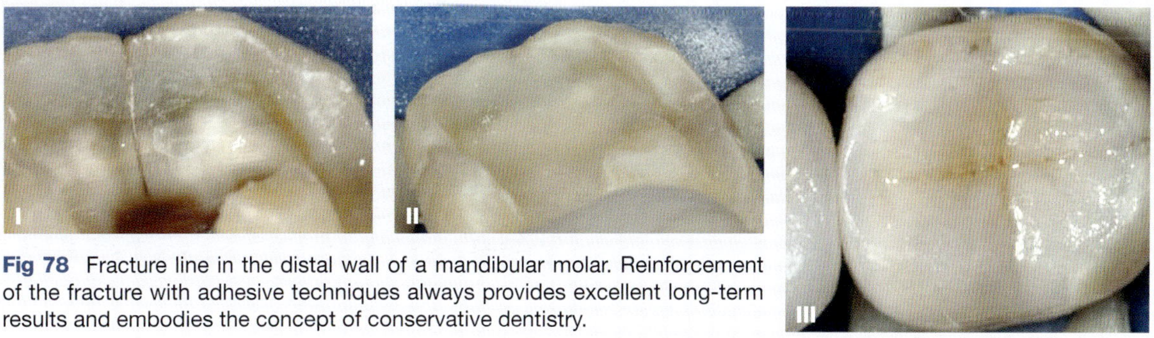

Fig 78 Fracture line in the distal wall of a mandibular molar. Reinforcement of the fracture with adhesive techniques always provides excellent long-term results and embodies the concept of conservative dentistry.

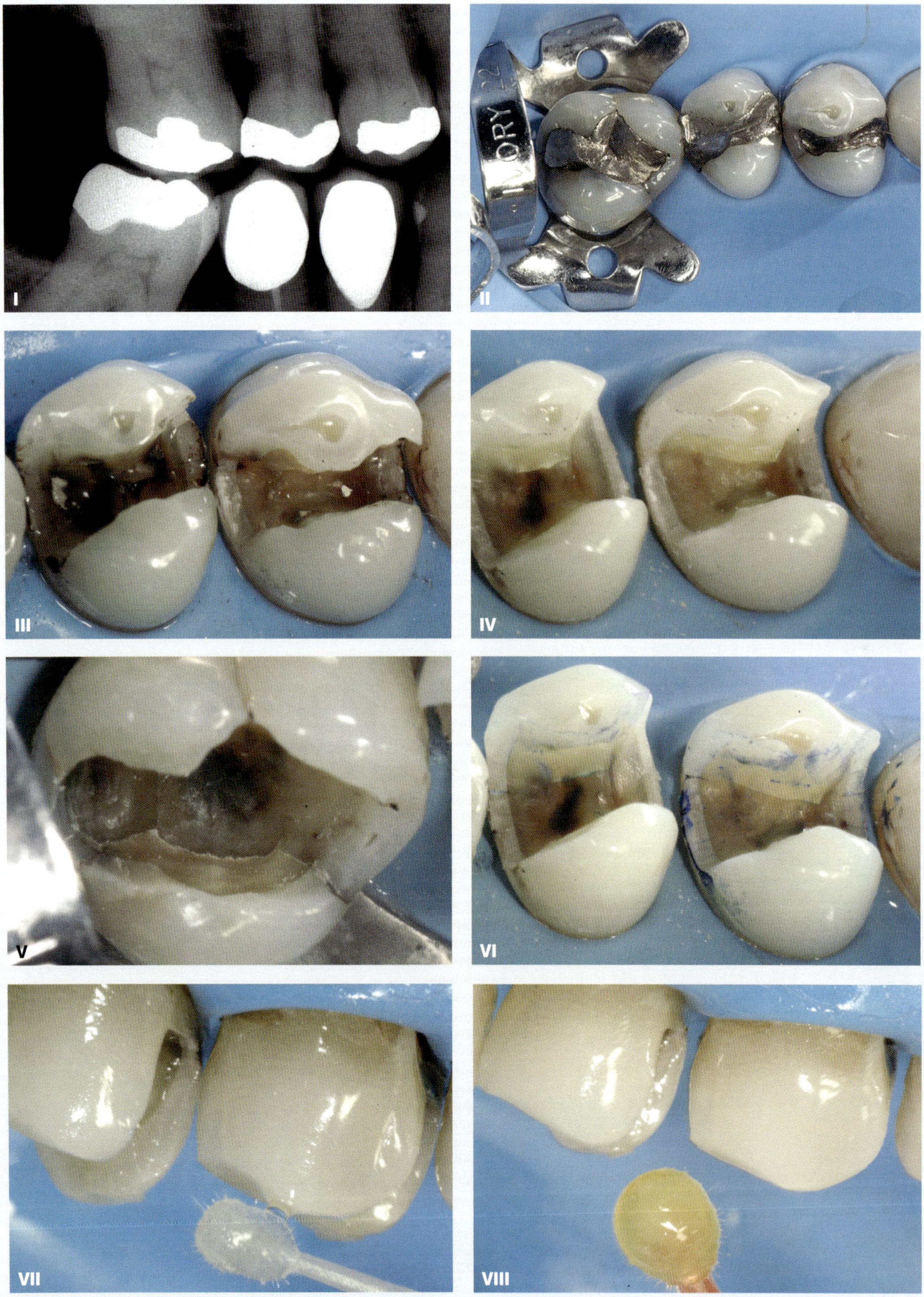

Fig 79 Fracture lines involve the maxillary right premolars and first molar. Three adhesive restorations resolve the problem in the most conservative way possible.

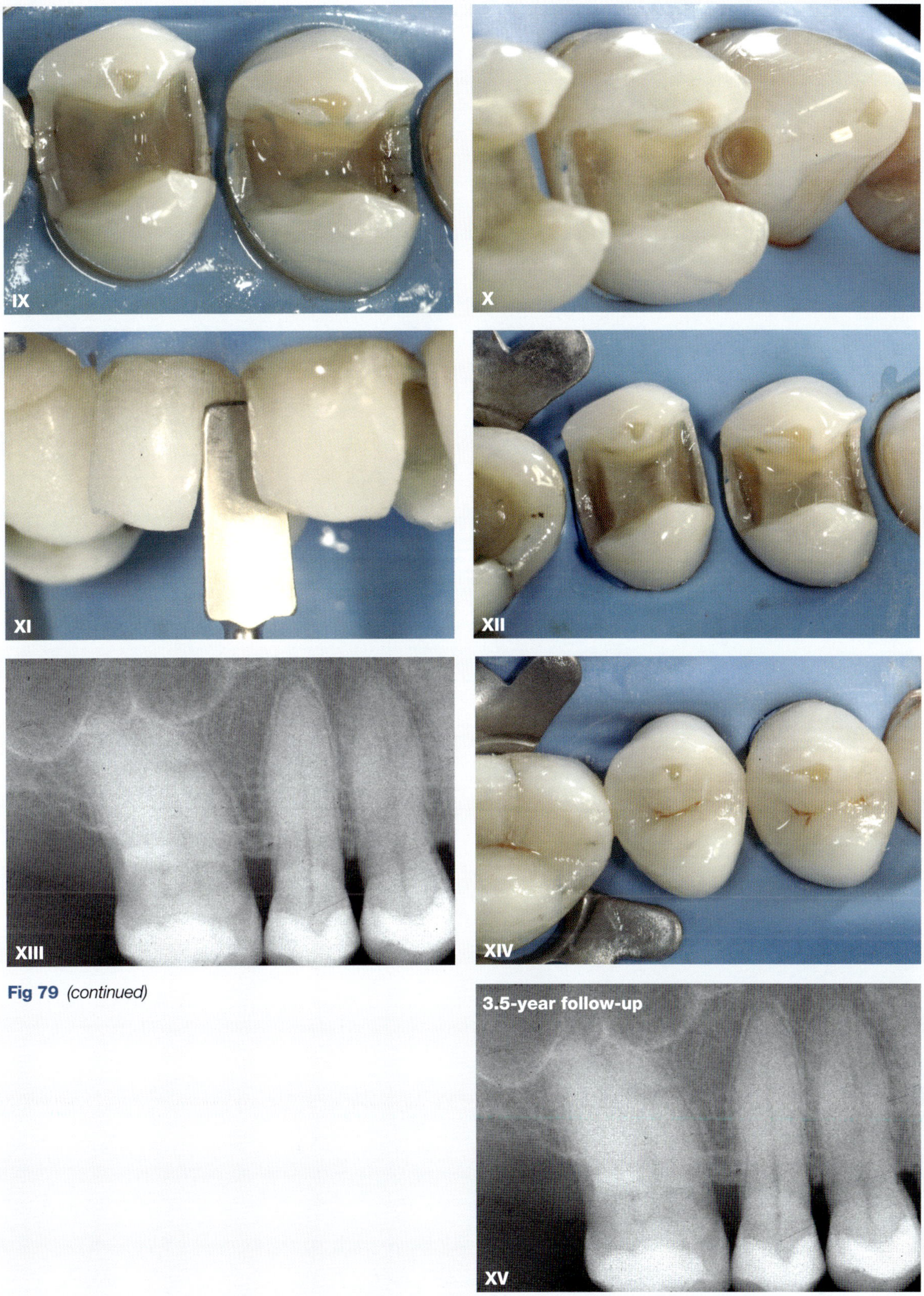

Fig 79 *(continued)*

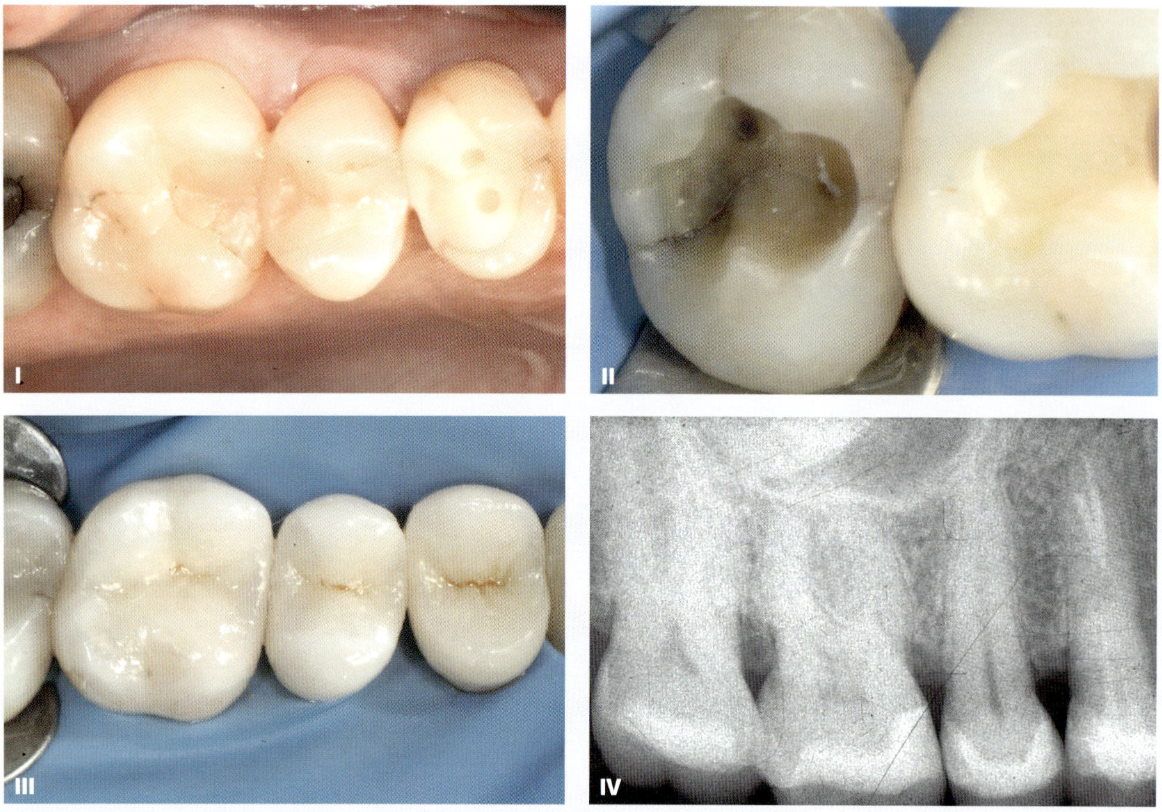

Fig 80 Optimization of the maxillary right quadrant with partial restorations in composite. Maintenance of the distal wall of the second molar despite the fracture line.

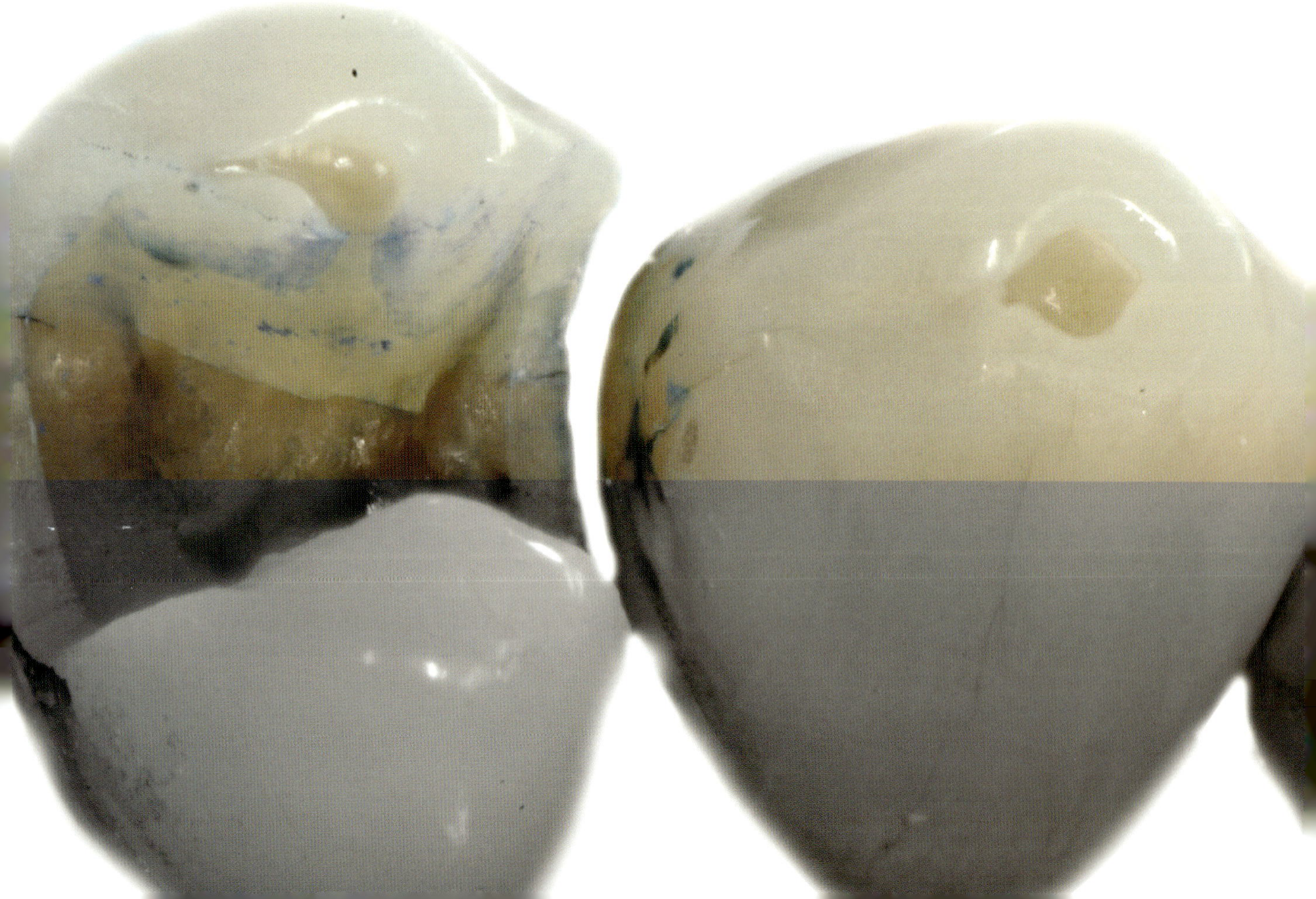

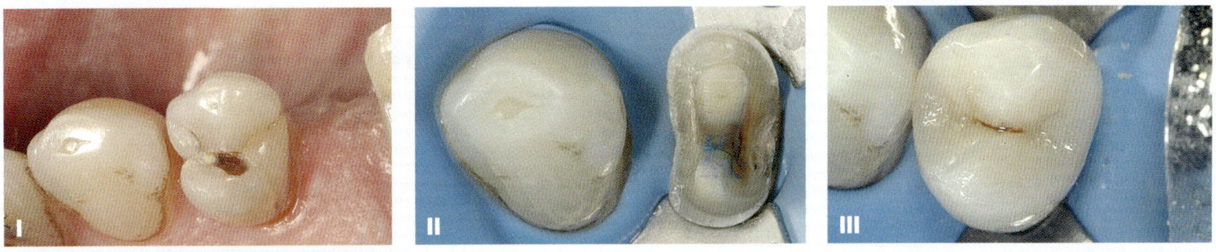

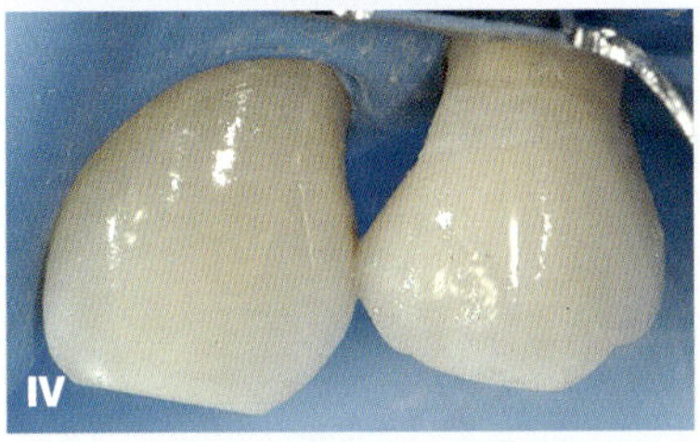

Fig 81 Deep decay and fracture line in an maxillary premolar.

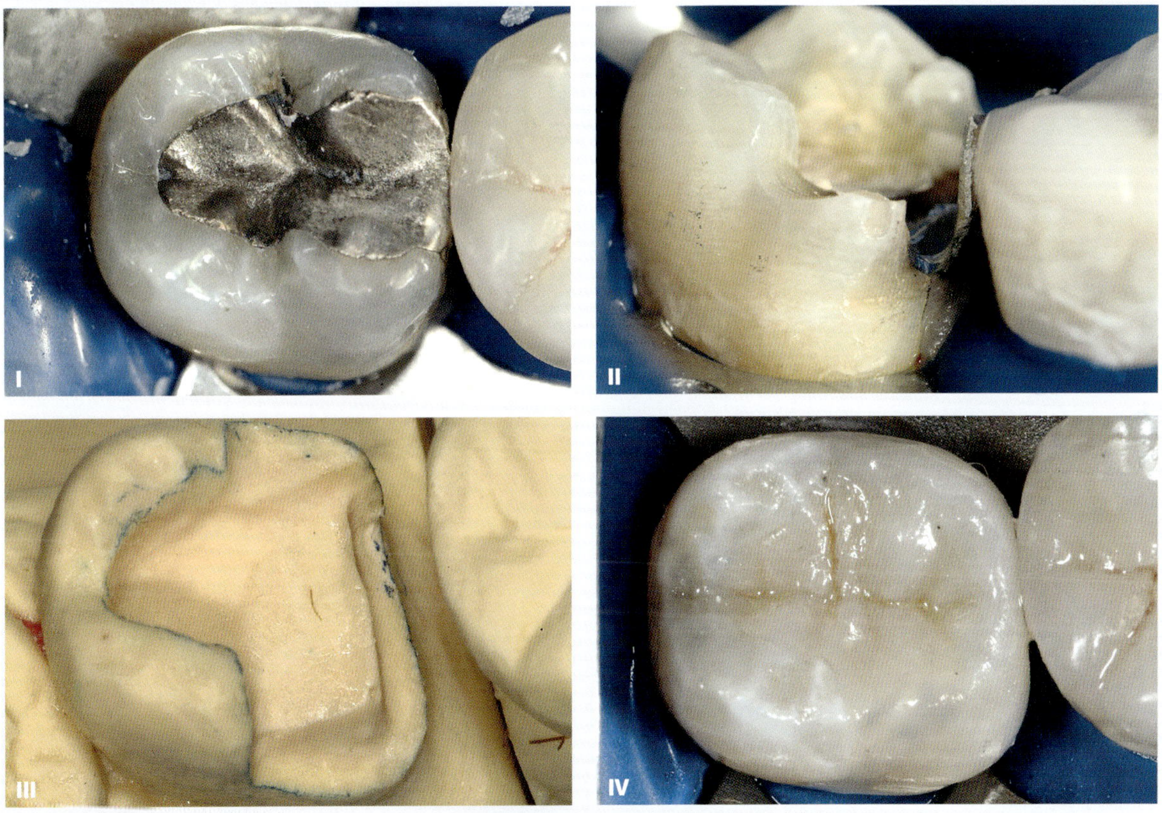

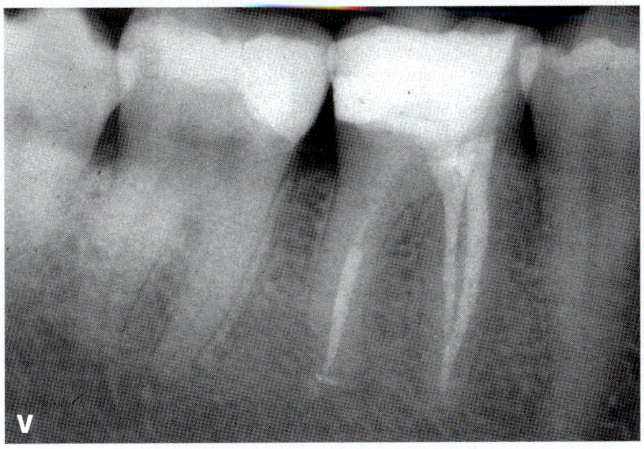

Fig 82 Vertical fracture line in the mandibular right second molar with periodontal probing within normal limits *(I, II)*. Composite onlay *(III, IV)* and follow-up after 5 years (V).

In the event of irreversible pulp inflammation, the patient first must be thoroughly informed of the risks associated with the instrumentation involved in this treatment because the teeth will have been made even more fragile by cracks that often reach the pulp chamber. The endodontist must then be sensitive enough to carry out the most conservative treatment possible with the aim of not exacerbating a dental structure that is already weak and saving as much root dentin as possible, resorting to the use of intraradicular anchorage only if strictly indicated, and naturally restricting endodontic re-treatment only to cases where this is strongly advisable (Figs 83 to 97).

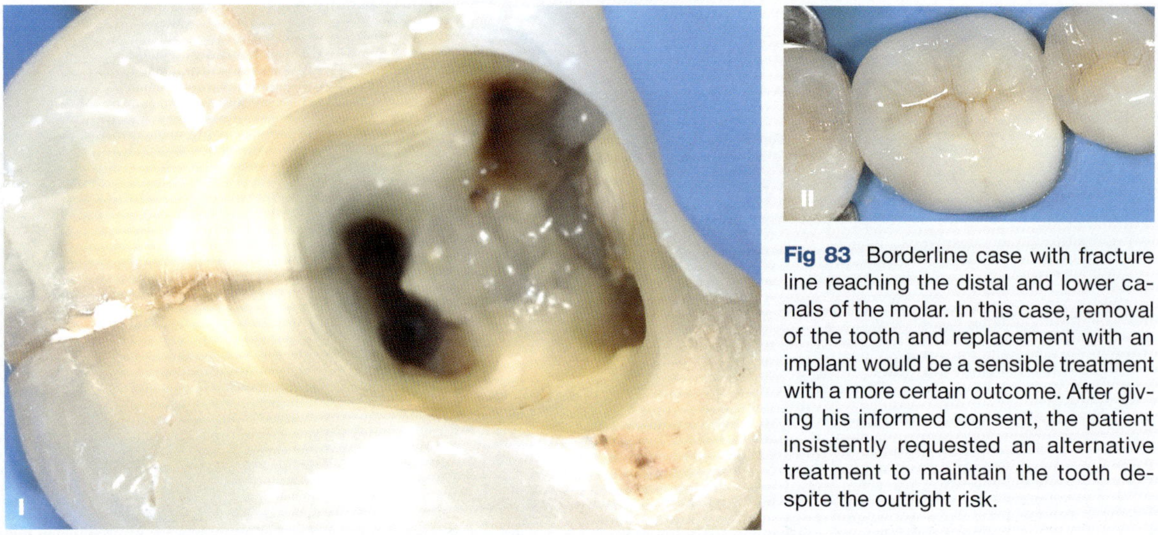

Fig 83 Borderline case with fracture line reaching the distal and lower canals of the molar. In this case, removal of the tooth and replacement with an implant would be a sensible treatment with a more certain outcome. After giving his informed consent, the patient insistently requested an alternative treatment to maintain the tooth despite the outright risk.

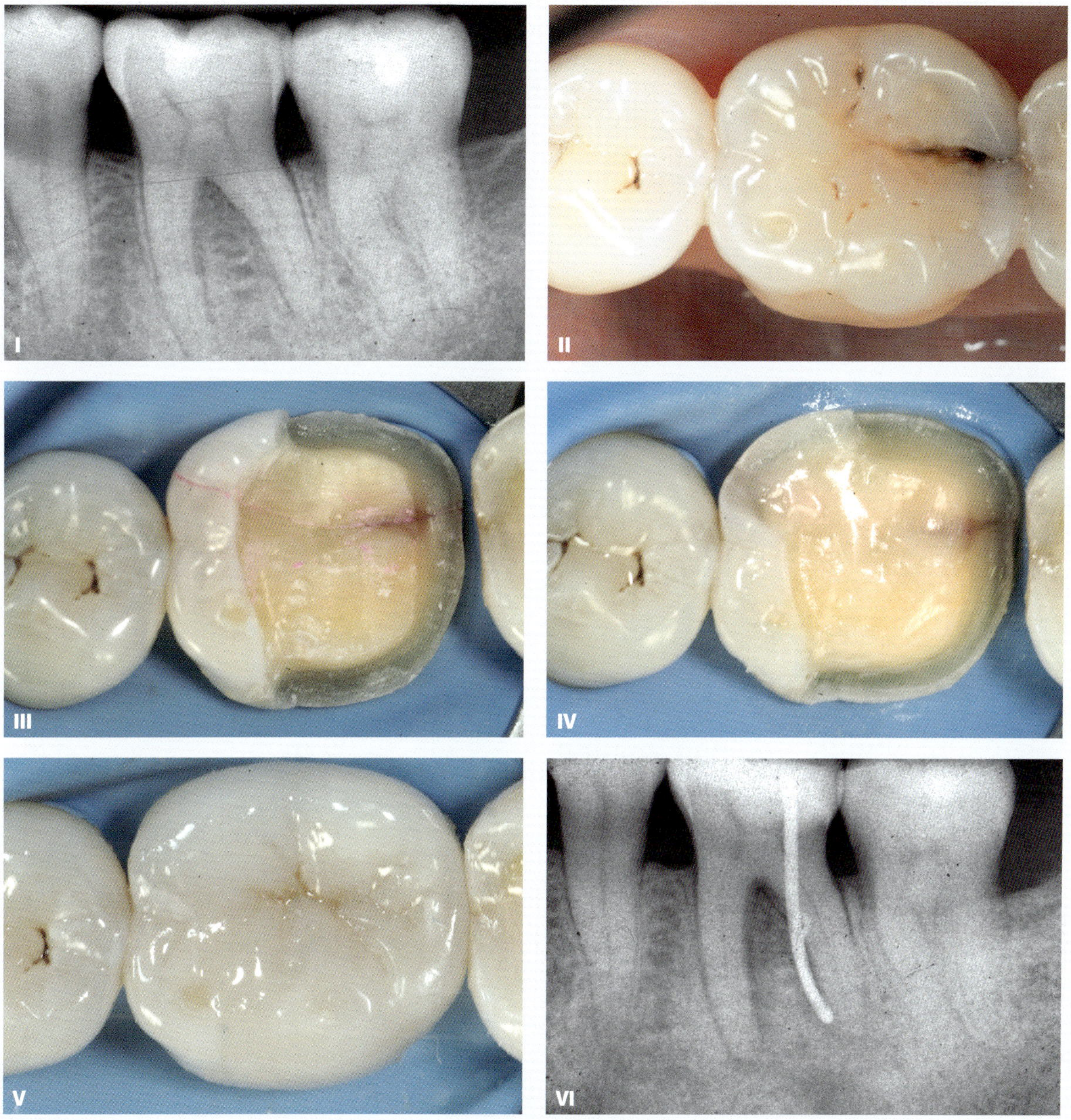

Fig 84 A mandibular left first molar with pain on chewing and very accentuated fracture lines starting from the occlusal plane *(I, II)*. A few weeks after cementing an onlay *(III–V)*, a fistula arose, and radiographic imaging determined a need for endodontic treatment *(VI, VII)*. The access cavity was treated with a simple direct restoration *(VIII, IX)*. The clinical and radiographic follow-up 1 year later revealed complete healing *(X, XI)*.

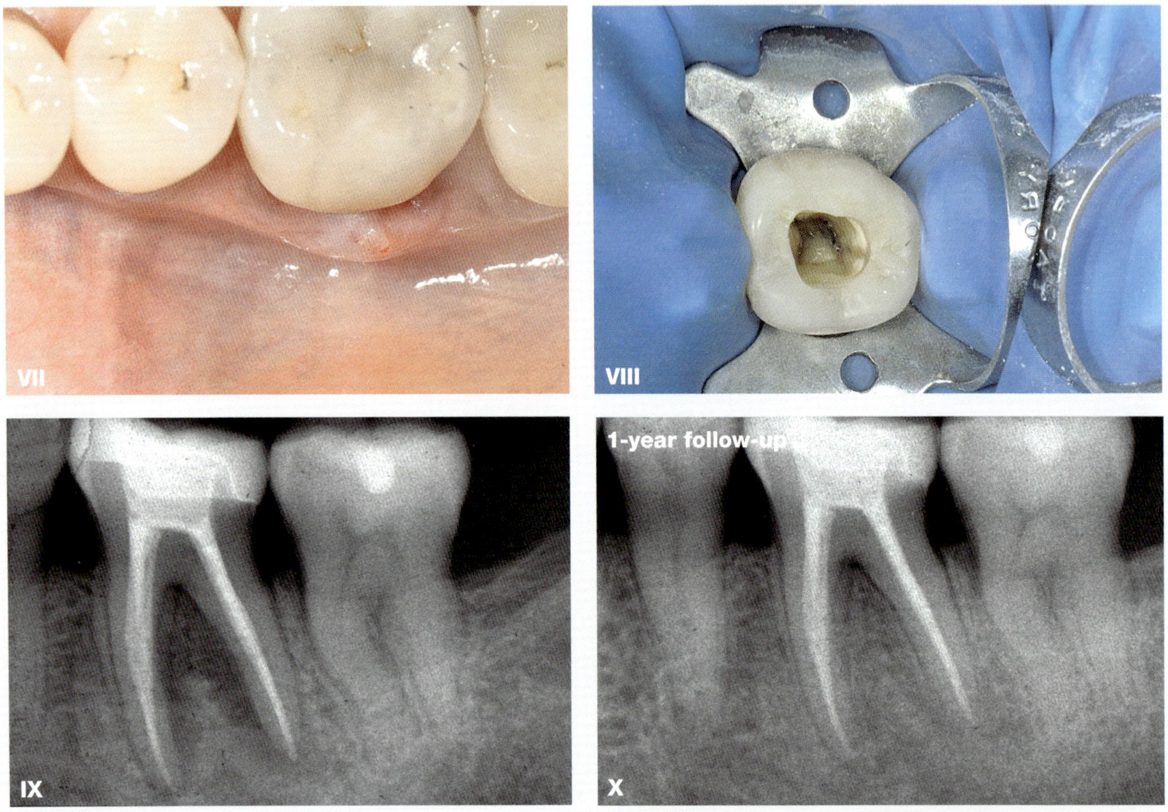

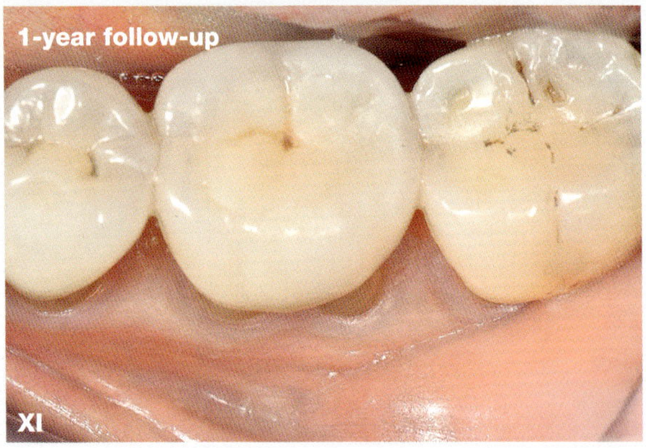

Fig 84 *(continued)*

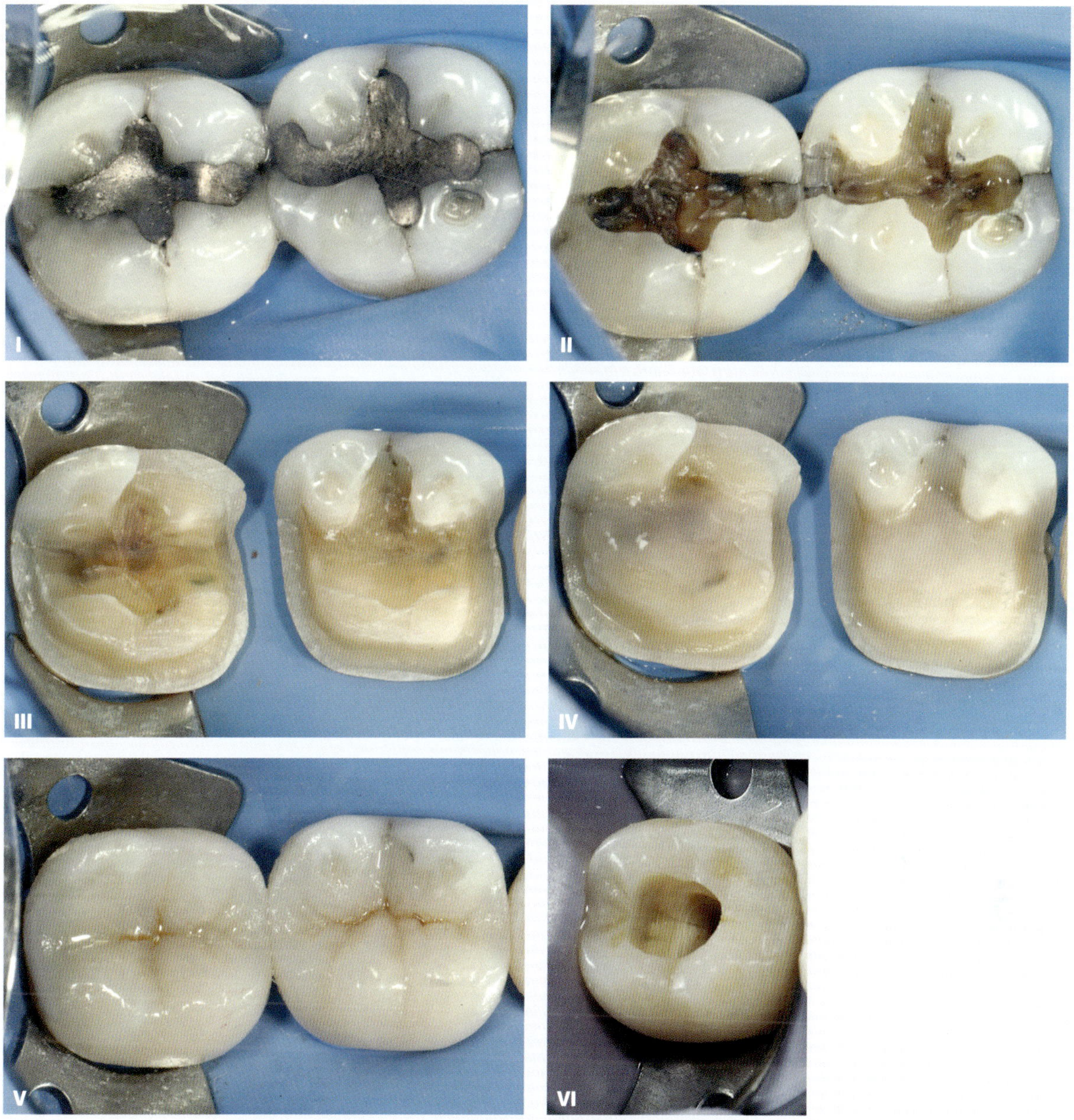

Fig 85 Mandible characterized by multiple fracture lines in the molars on both sides *(I, II)*. Usual therapeutic protocol with adhesive techniques *(III–VIII)* and clinical follow-up at 3 and 4 years *(IX, X)*. Both second molars were treated endodontically because of the persistence of painful symptoms on chewing.

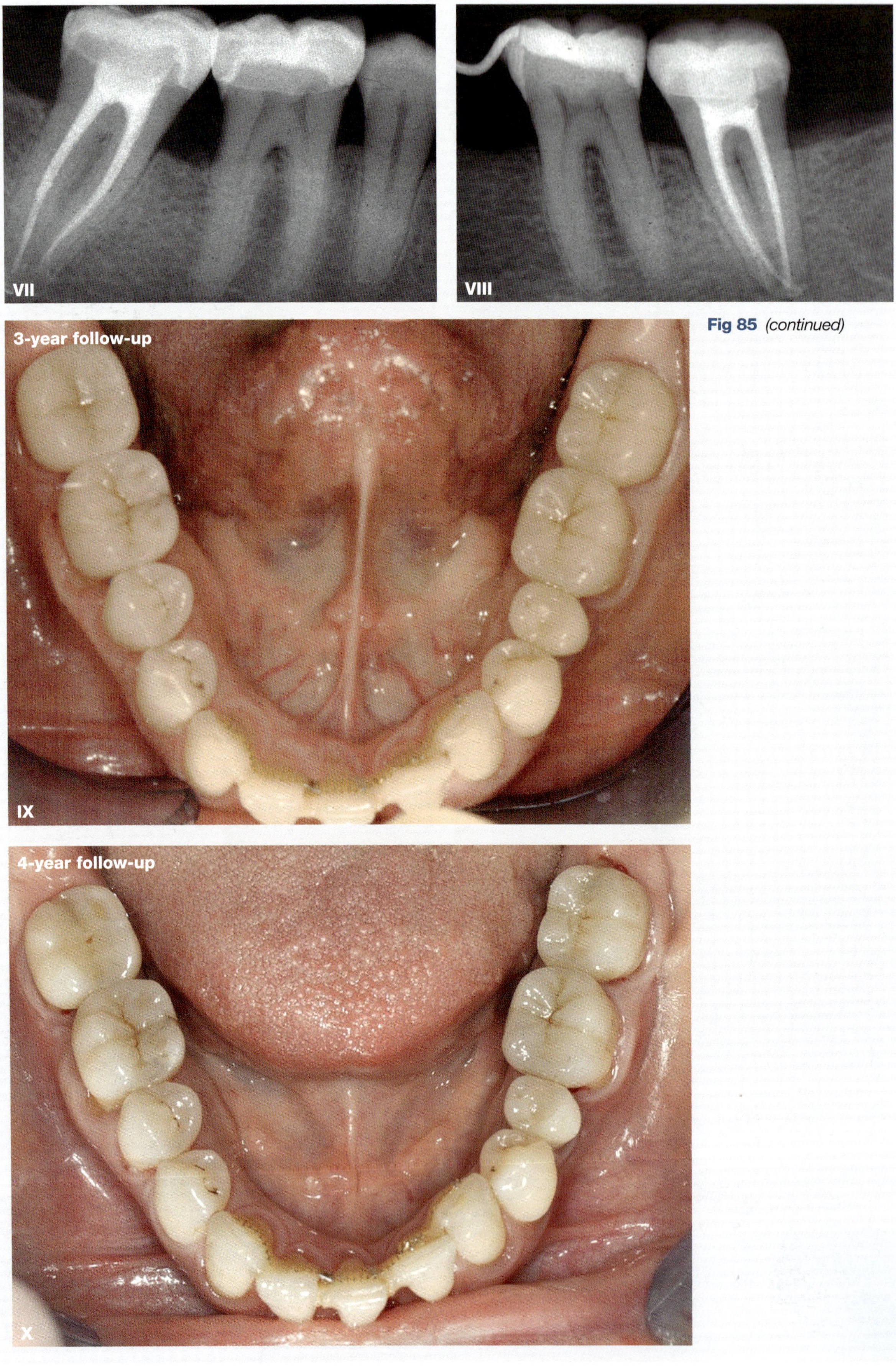

Fig 85 *(continued)*

Fig 86 An endodontically treated molar with a fracture line that continues into the distal canal *(I)*. Seven-year follow-up *(II)*.

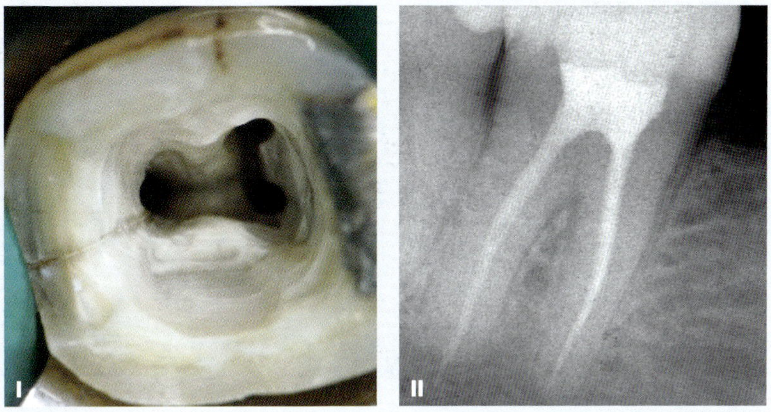

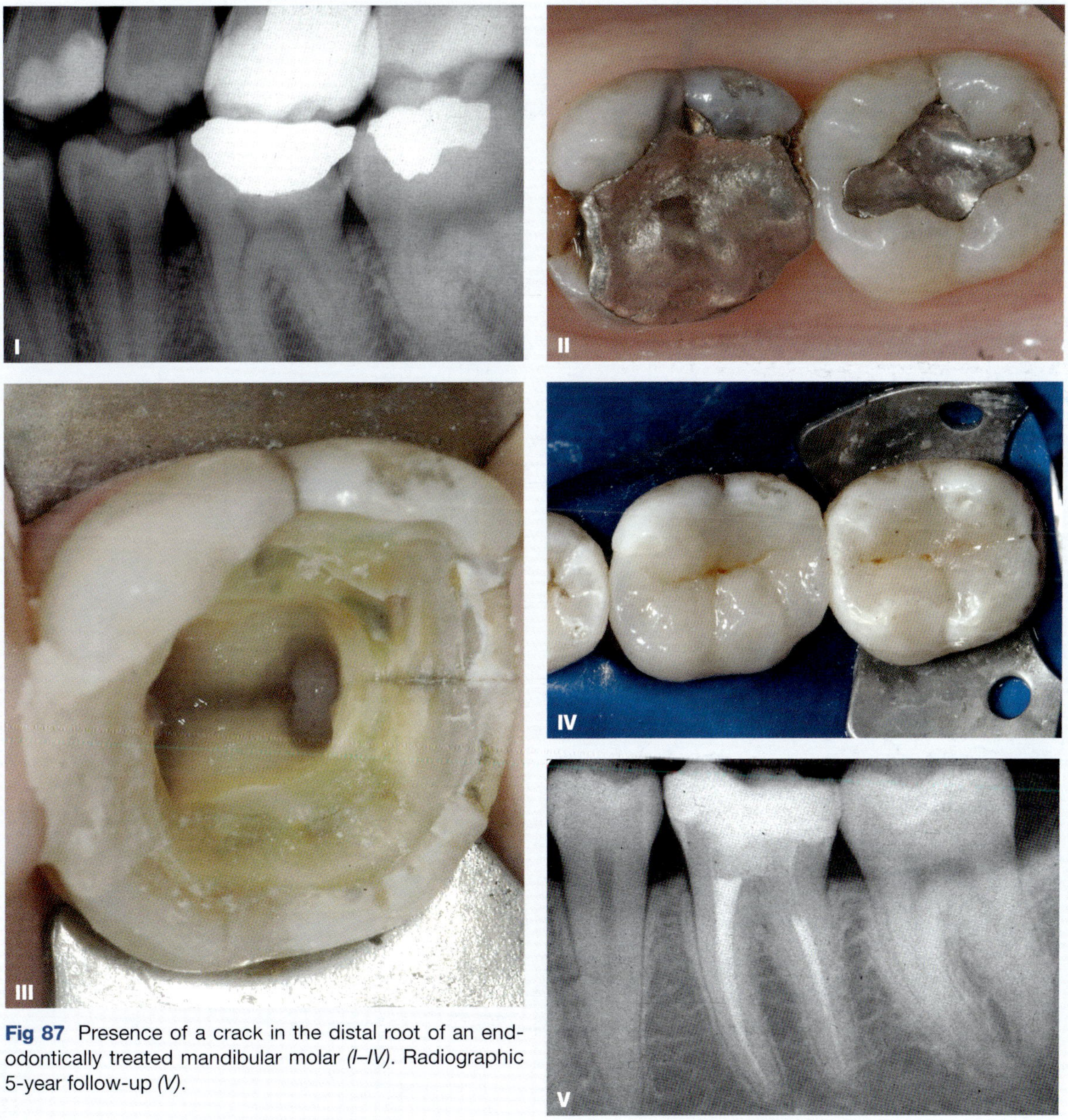

Fig 87 Presence of a crack in the distal root of an endodontically treated mandibular molar *(I–IV)*. Radiographic 5-year follow-up *(V)*.

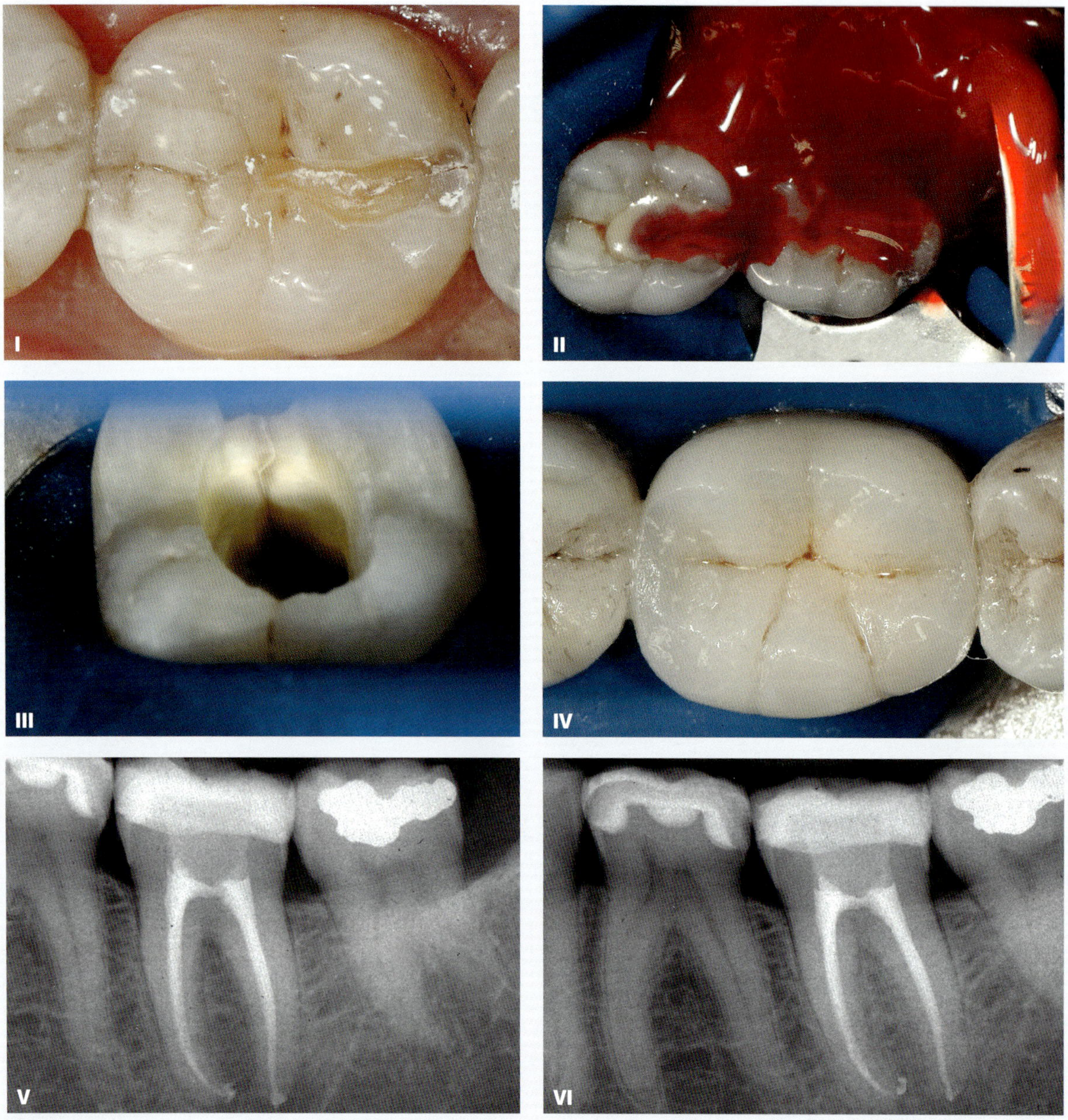

Fig 88 Minimal fracture line propagating to the distal canal of a mandibular left second molar *(I)*. Acute alveolar abscess, endodontic treatment, and overlay in composite *(II–V)*. Follow-up after 7 years *(VI)*.

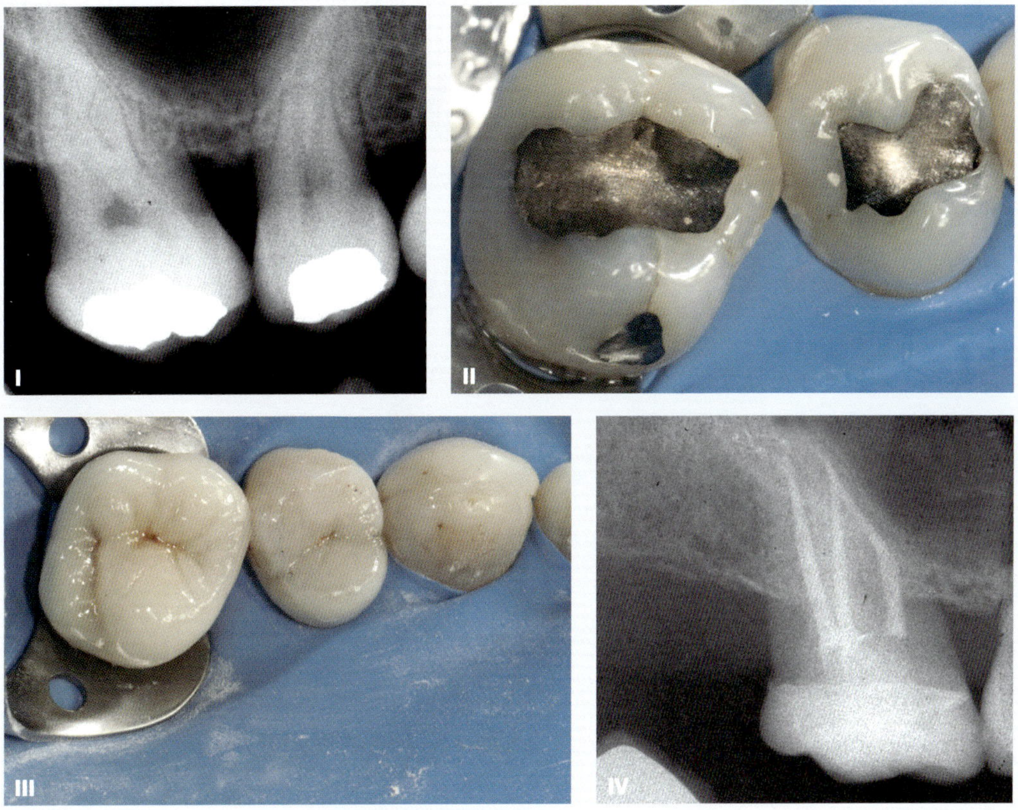

Fig 89 Multiple occlusal fracture lines, pulpitis, and overlay.

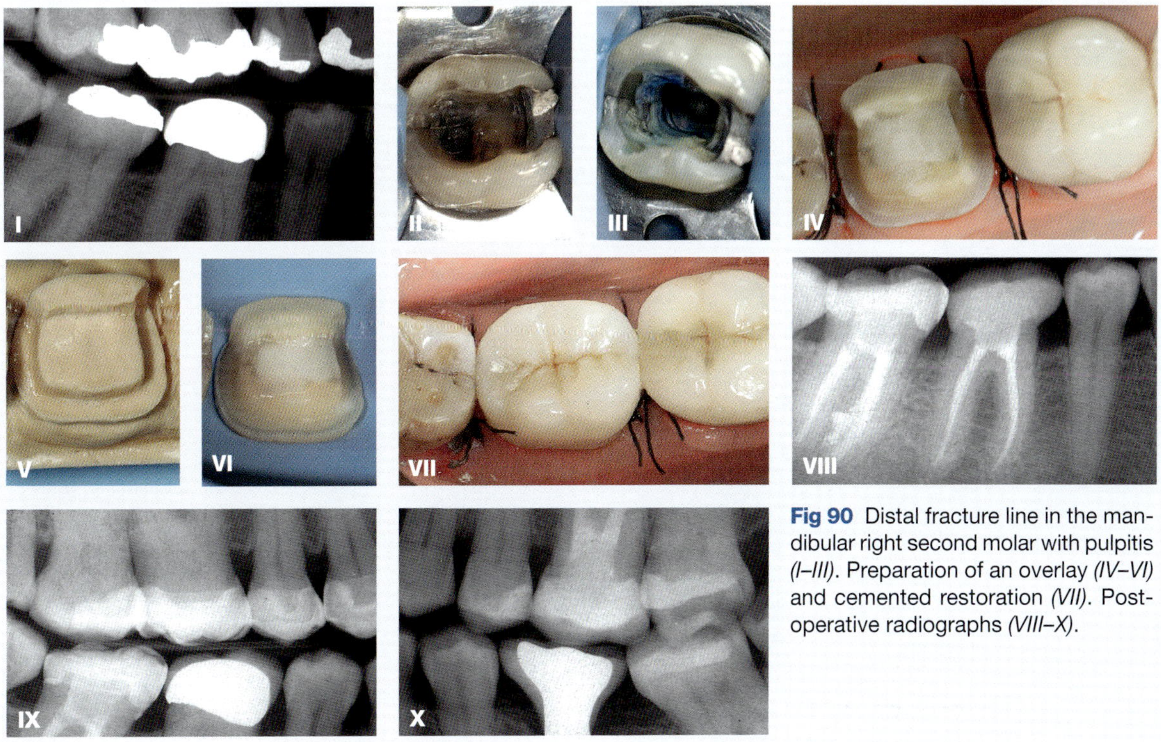

Fig 90 Distal fracture line in the mandibular right second molar with pulpitis *(I–III)*. Preparation of an overlay *(IV–VI)* and cemented restoration *(VII)*. Postoperative radiographs *(VIII–X)*.

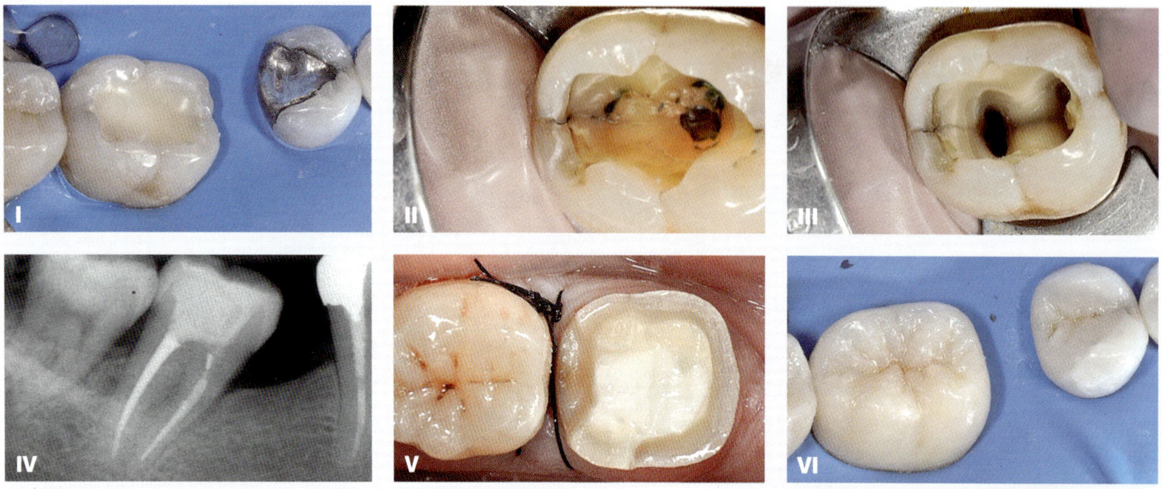

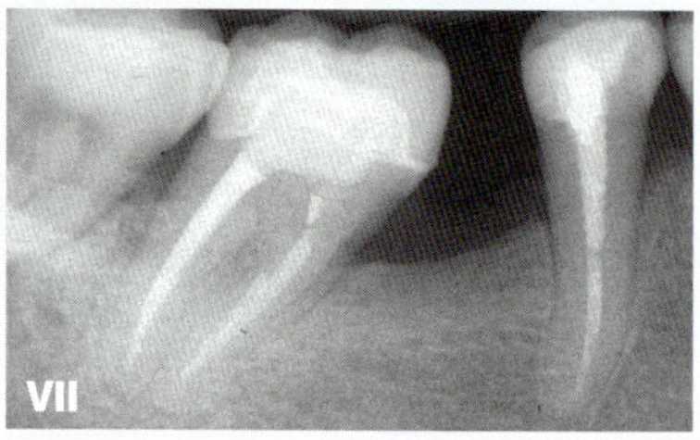

Fig 91 MOD fracture line in the mandibular right second molar. The decay reaches the pulp, requiring endodontic treatment and an overlay.

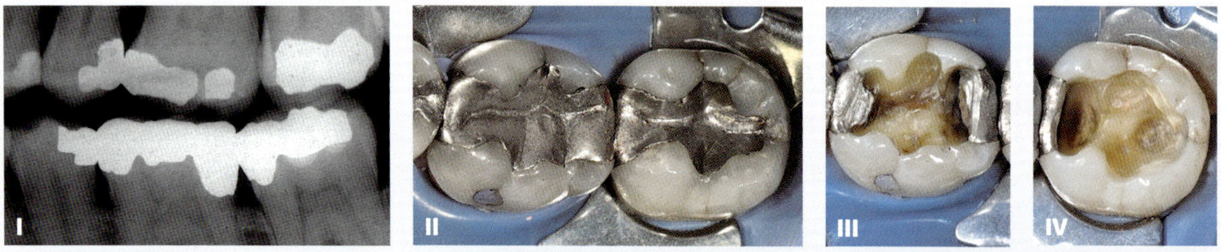

Fig 92 Pain on pressure in the mandibular left first and second molars. Very deep fracture line in the first molar, endodontic treatment of molars, and reconstruction with two overlays.

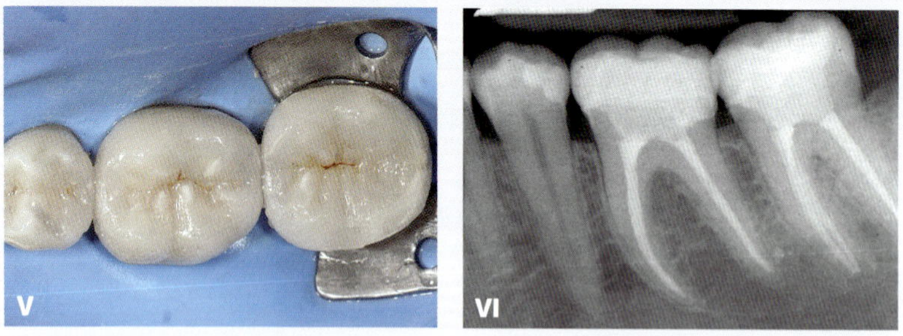

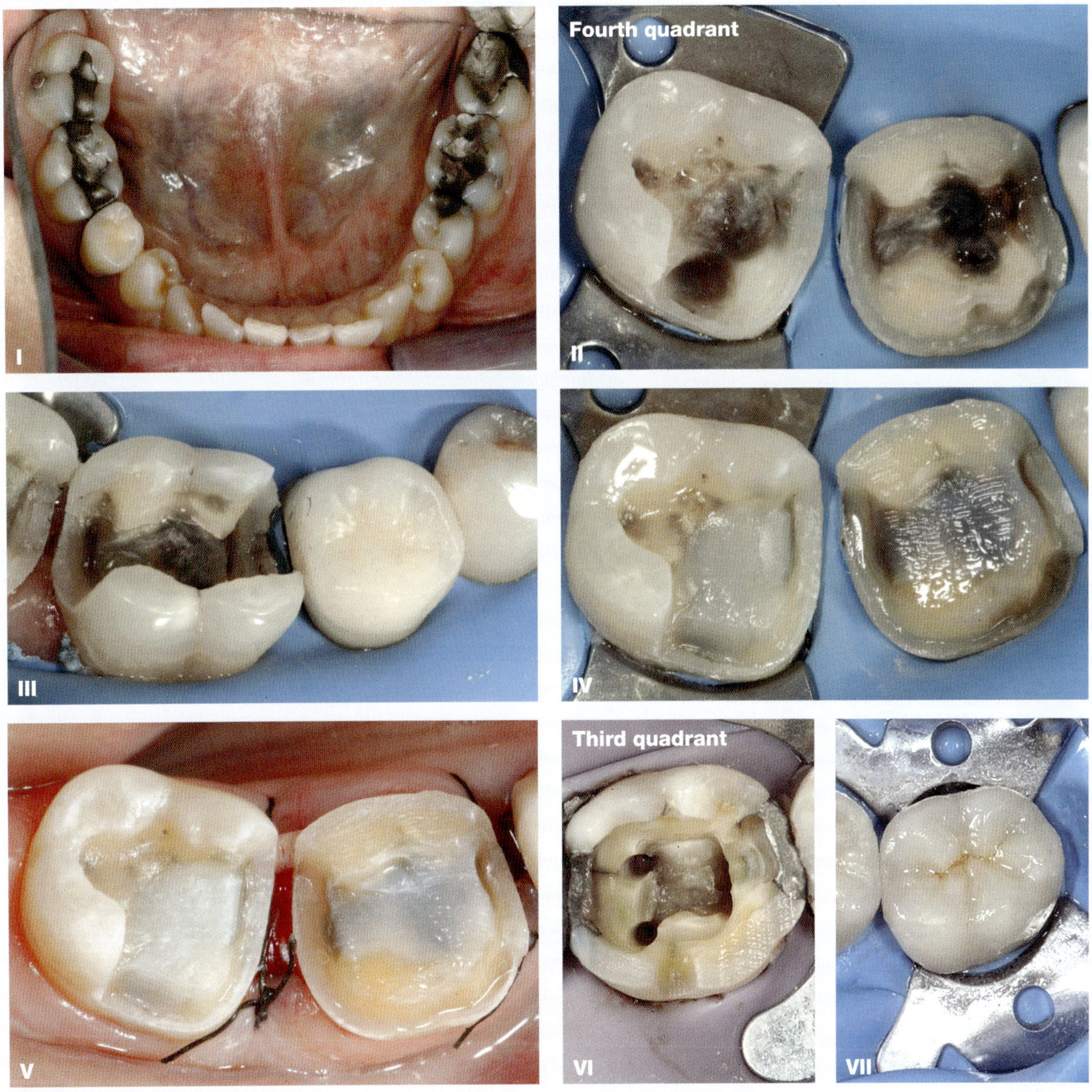

Fig 93 Deep decay and cracks make chewing impossible in the mandibular left (third) and right (fourth) quadrants. Interdisciplinary treatment of the entire arch and radiographic follow-up.

Fig 93 *(continued)*

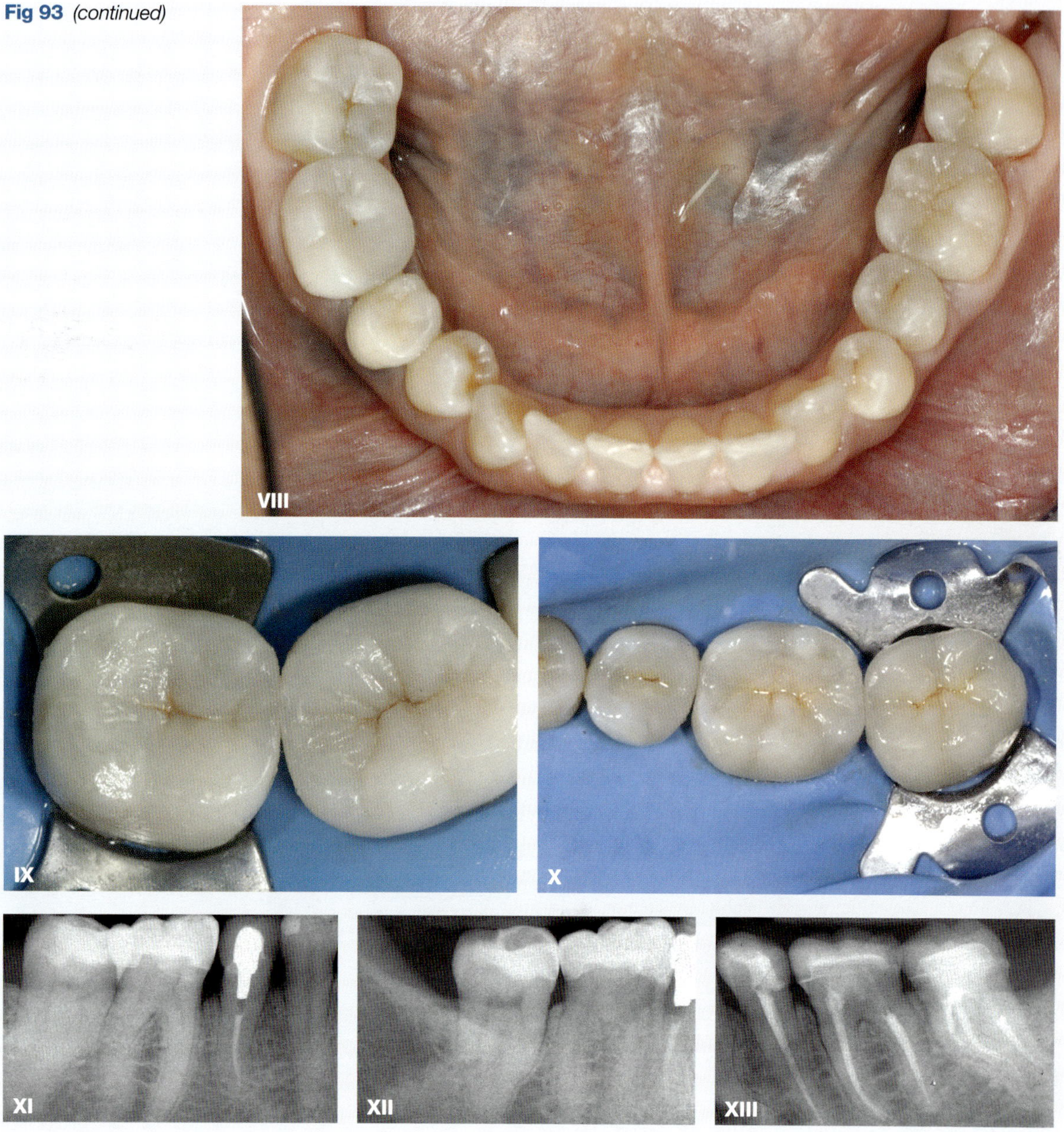

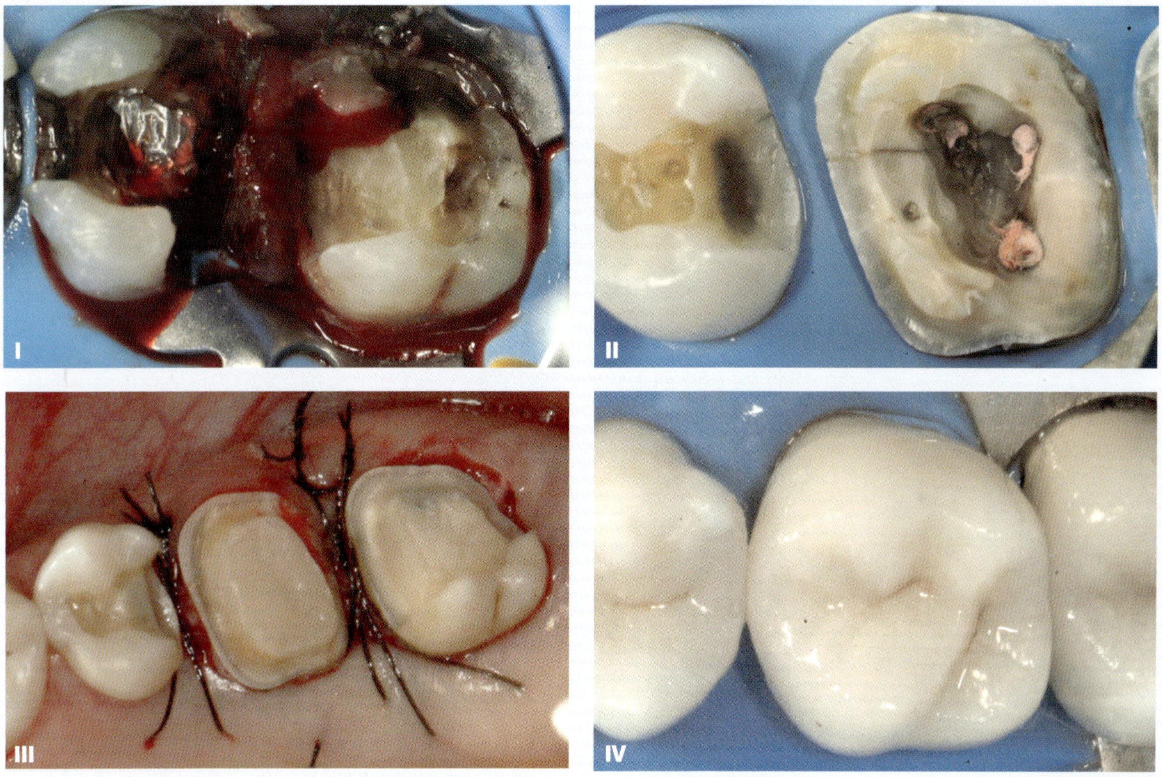

Fig 94 Periodontal treatment is essential in two extremely compromised molars with a deep fracture line in the maxillary left first molar.

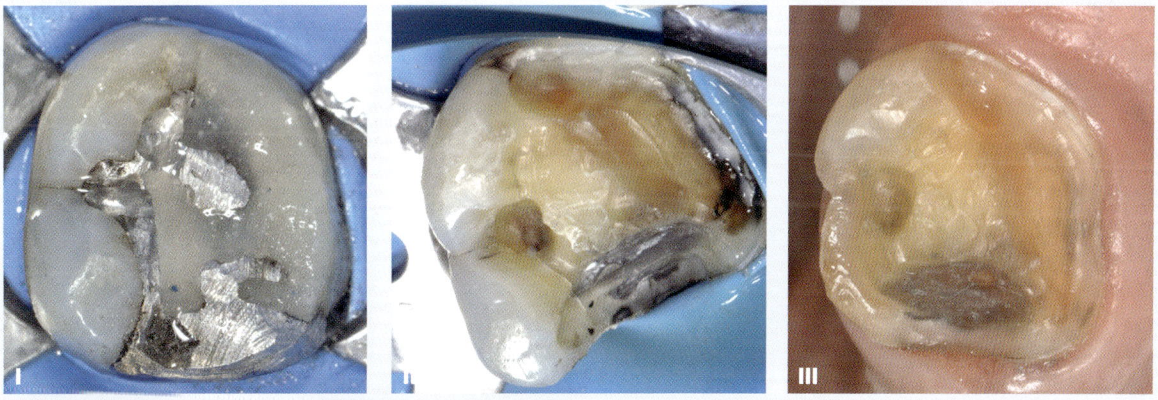

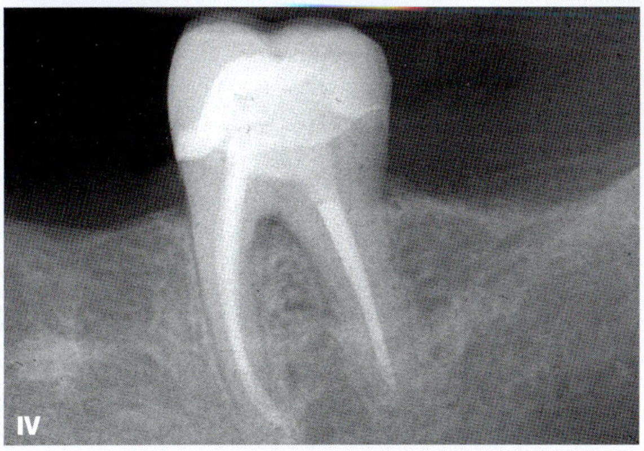

Fig 95 Reconstruction of an endodontically treated molar with an overlay. In this clinical situation, the patient must be informed that a single tooth is unable to support the loads of an entire quadrant, and it would therefore be extremely useful to place implants.

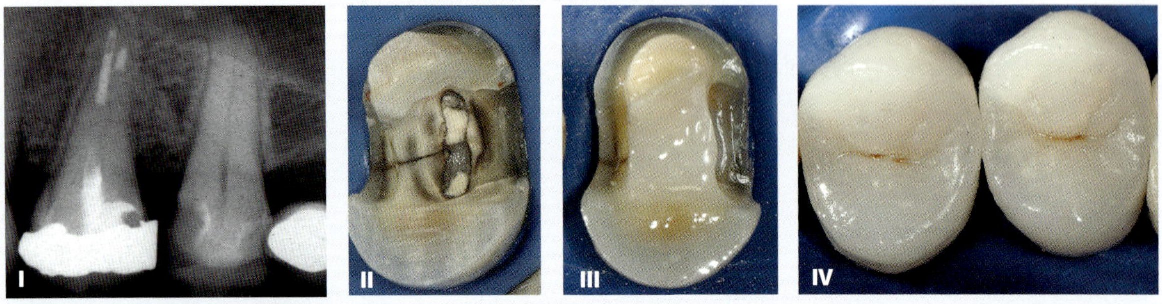

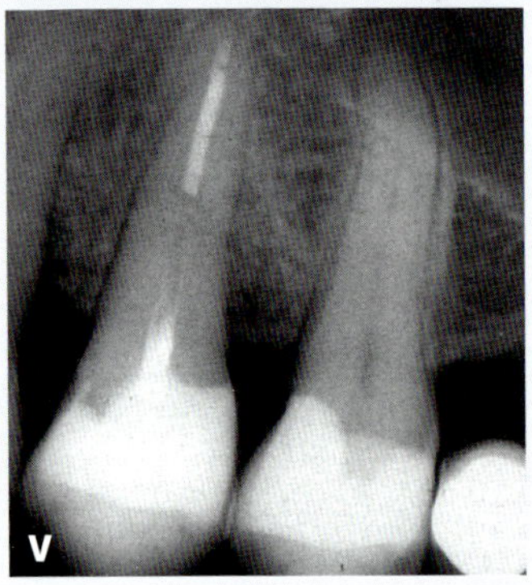

Fig 96 Very compromised premolar with MOD fracture line and defective endodontic treatment. The absence of periapical lesions after many years and the risk of the fracture exacerbating in the case of endodontic re-treatment nevertheless meant that it was not advisable to re-treat the tooth, of course with the full agreement of the patient.

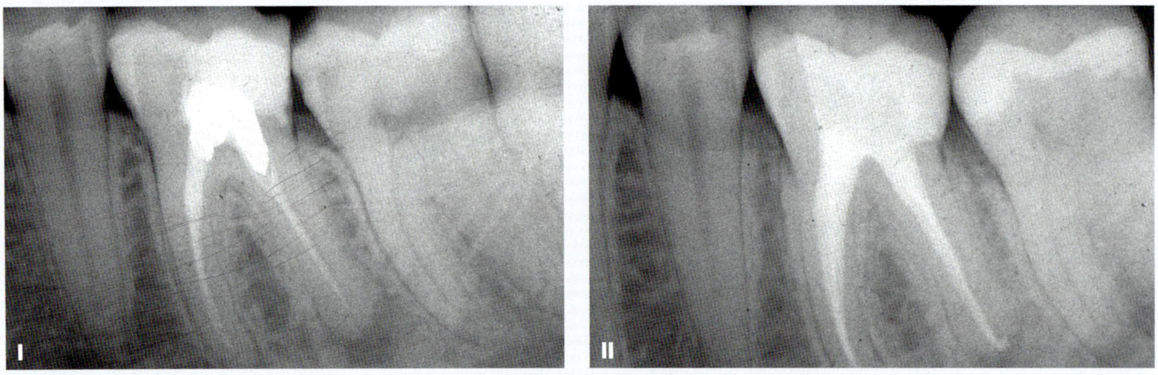

Fig 97 Endodontic re-treatment of the mandibular left first molar and protective onlay.

In the author's case sample of teeth with significant fracture lines treated endodontically, the number of endodontic and structural failures has been very small, and the results are supported by medium- and long-term radiographic follow-up of the teeth that are most at risk because of cracks and the small amount of healthy remaining tooth structure supporting restorations.

For preventive purposes, when large amalgam restorations are present, for example, in MOD cavities, it is important to restore elasticity to the teeth in order to prevent the formation of dentinal cracks (Figs 98 to 100).

Lastly, a word about timing: When the treatment plan involves endodontic, periodontal, and restorative treatment, the endodontic treatment, lengthening of the clinical crown, buildup, cavity preparation, and impression should be carried out as quickly as possible with the aim of finalizing cementation and hence protecting the compromised tooth.

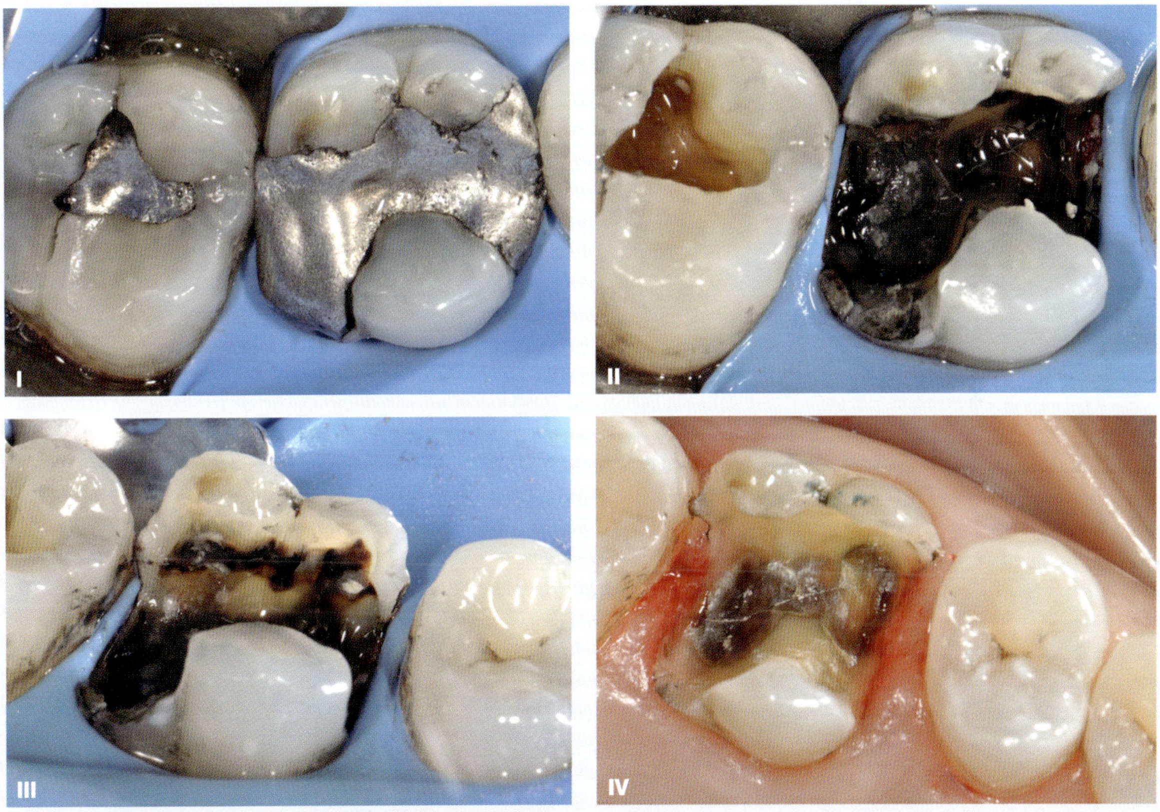

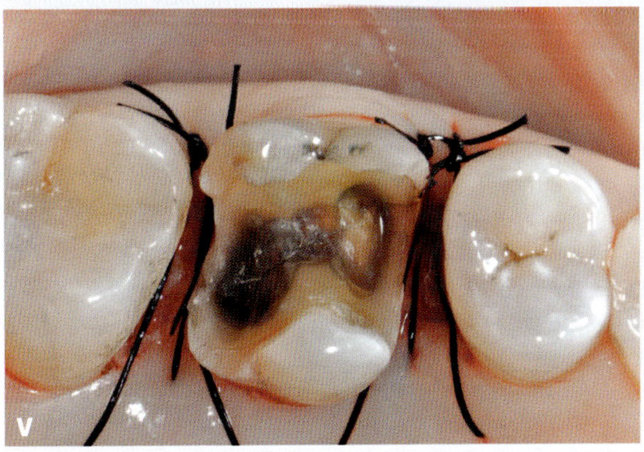

Fig 98 Significant fracture lines appeared after removing a leaking restoration in the maxillary right first molar and ablation of the underlying decayed tissue *(I–III)*. The pulp sensitivity test was positive. Preparation of an overlay *(IV–IX)* and radiographic check after 4 years *(X)*. A subsequent pulp vitality test was still positive.

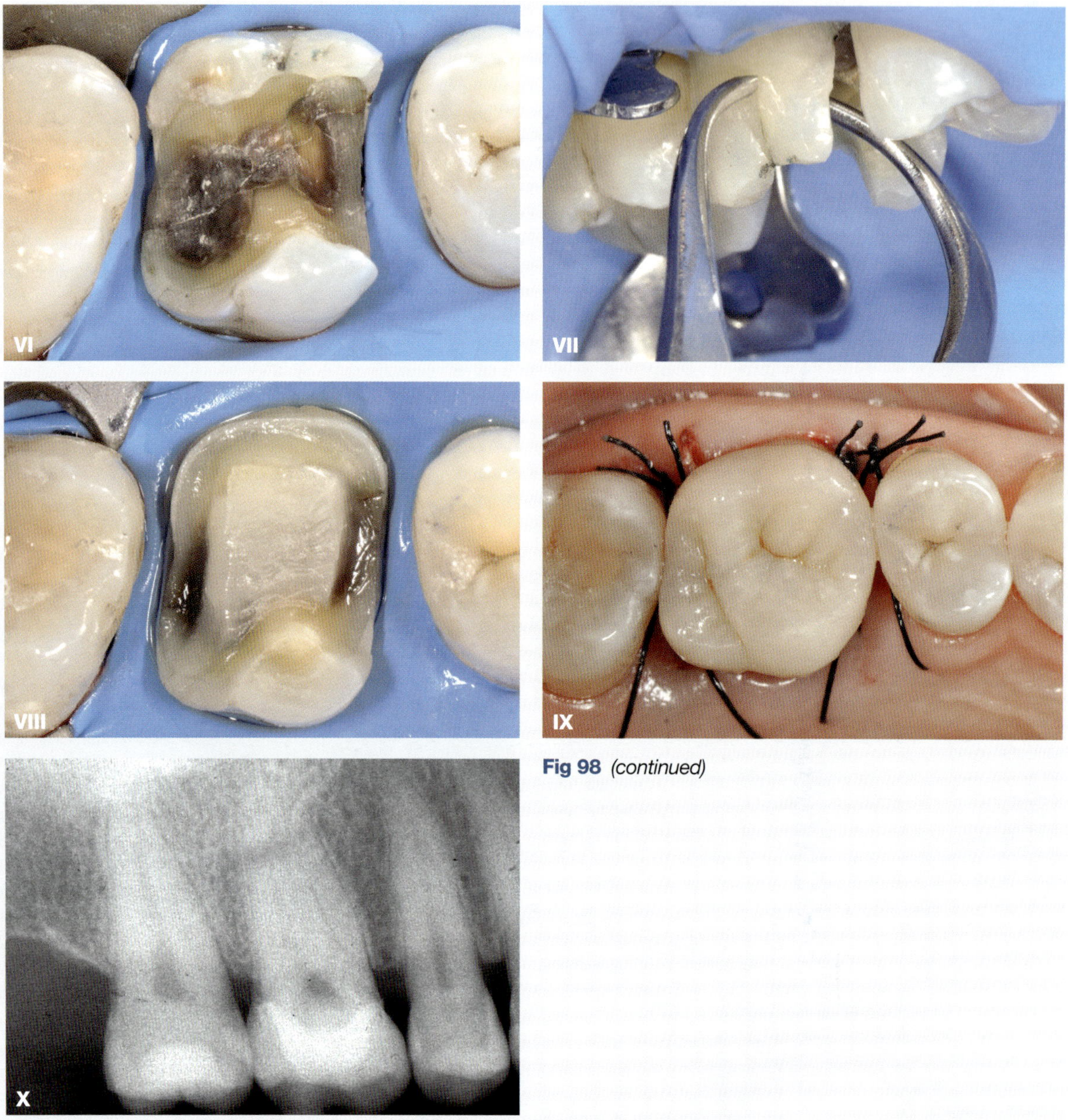

Fig 98 *(continued)*

This timing is routinely proposed and implemented to the satisfaction of the patient as well as the practitioners. It is naturally also applied under "normal" clinical situations and perhaps represents the greatest incentive for teamwork. Having said this, the author always attempts, with the consent of the duly informed patient, to minimize the insertion of implants, which as stated previously is all too often doomed to failure. This can be avoided above all by applying composite onlays and overlays that remain the supreme solution for the restoration of seriously compromised teeth and, as may be seen from the clinical and radiographic photographs, the results are absolutely encouraging provided the author's simple yet very rigorous adhesive protocol is followed to the letter. To avoid misunderstandings, it should be emphasized that patients with significant parafunctions must be treated by colleagues who are experts in prosthodontics and the masticatory system, given the number of failures (eg, adhesive and cohesive fractures, decementations) encountered when practitioners attempt to resolve the problem using adhesive techniques in patients who are inveterate bruxism sufferers. Case examples are presented in Figs 101 to 105.

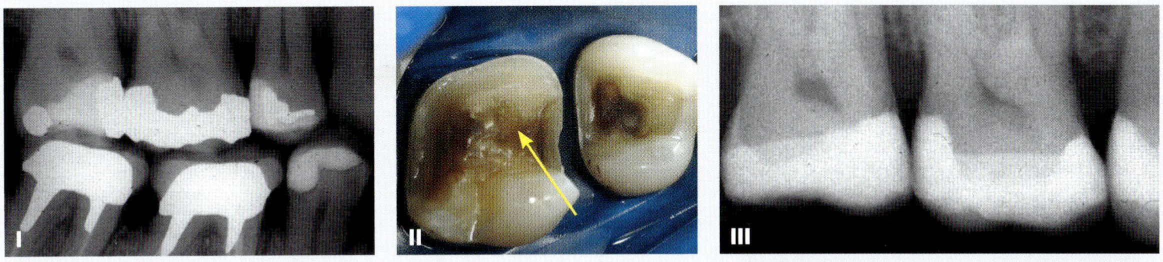

Fig 99 Pain on pressure in the molar, which had a very small crack that was not visible without magnification *(arrow)*. The painful symptoms ceased immediately after cementation of the onlay.

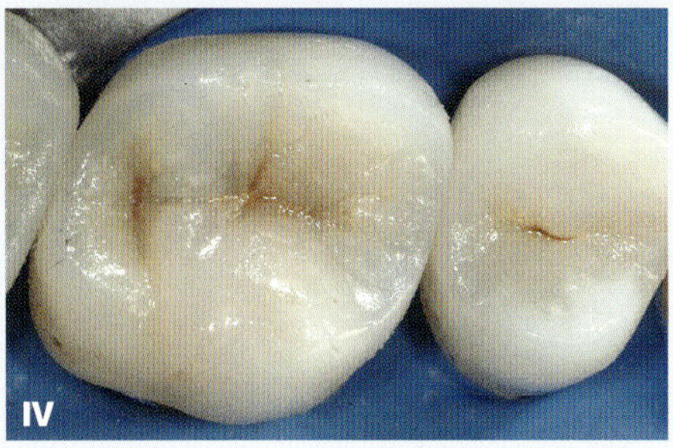

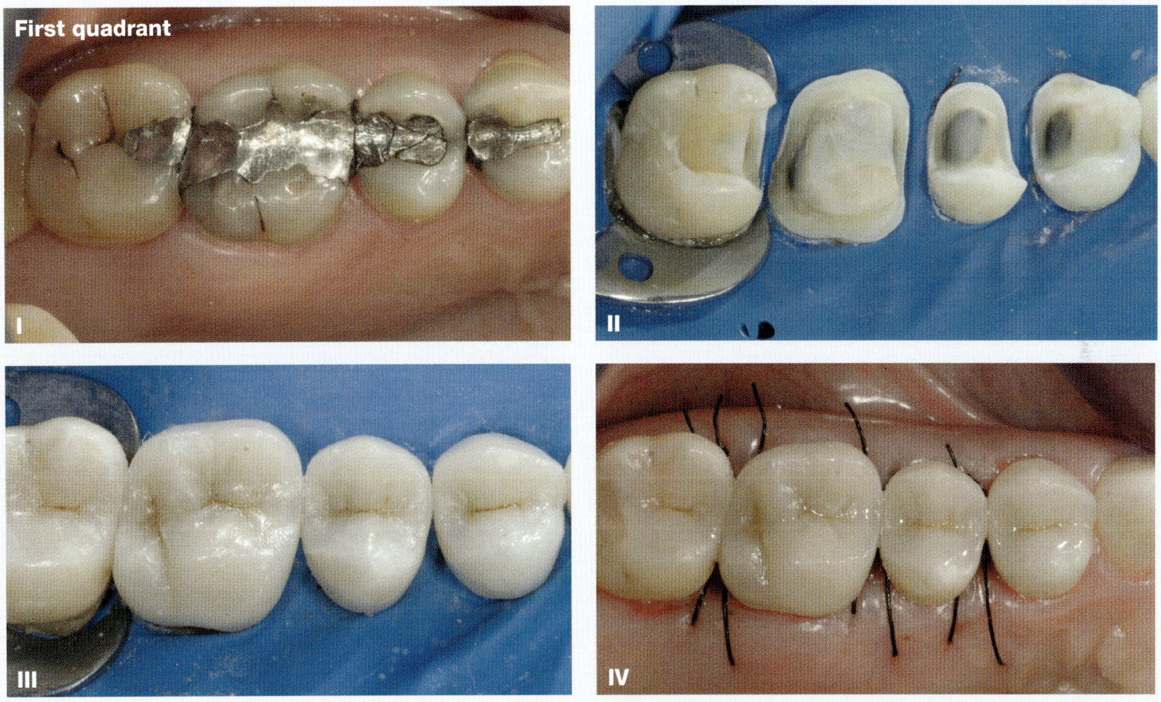

Fig 100 Execution and cementation of inlay, onlay, and overlay in 48 hours in the maxillary right (first) quadrant *(I–V)*. In the maxillary left (second) quadrant, a very accentuated crack was noted in the first molar, and endodontic treatment was inevitable due to the persistence of pain on pressure *(VI–XI)*. View of the arch before and after cementation of restorations *(XII, XIII)* and radiographic follow-up *(XIV, XV)*.

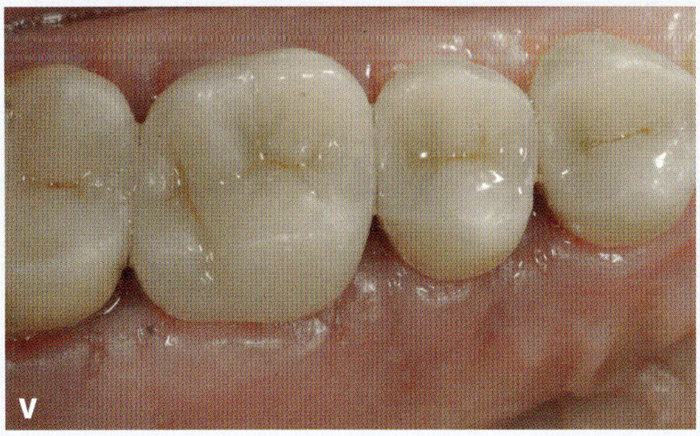

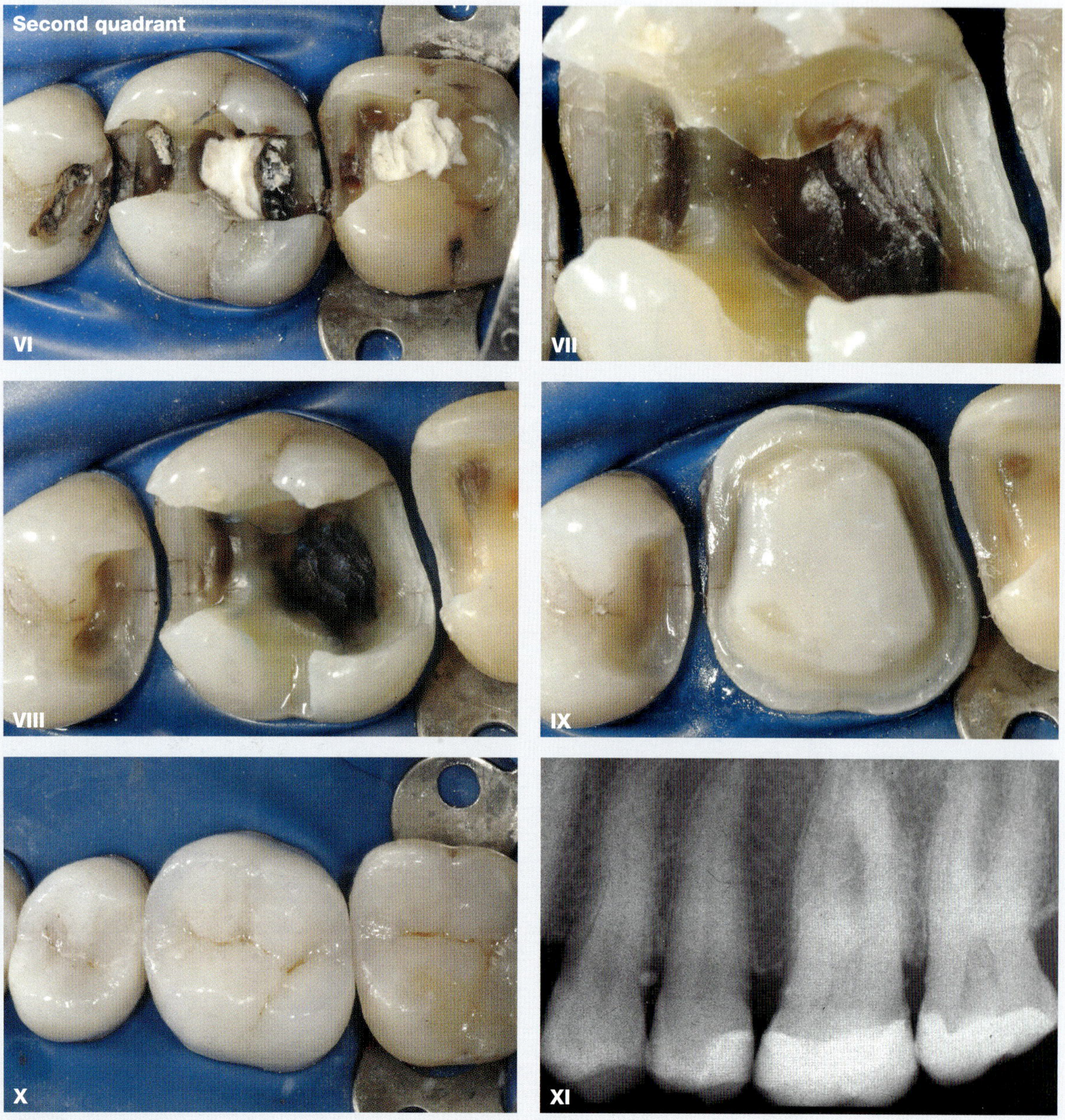

Fig 100 *(continued)*

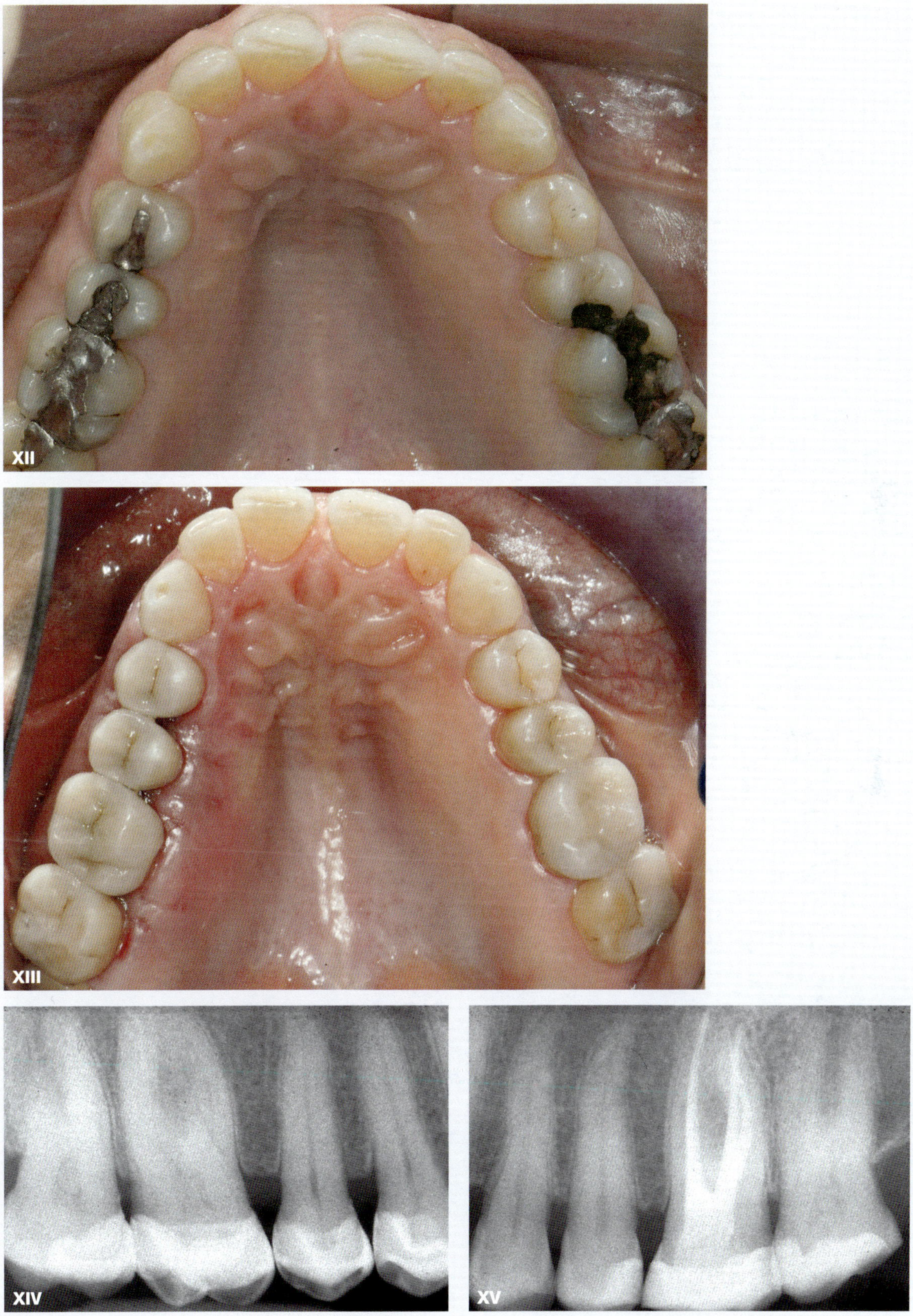

Fig 100 *(continued)*

Clinical cases

Clinical case 1

Fig 101 The patient presented with difficulty chewing on both the left and right sides, sporadic twinges, and very strong sensitivity to heat *(I–III)*. The tooth causing the most discomfort on pressure was identified as the mandibular right first molar. After removal of the old restoration, deep decay and multiple fracture lines made endodontic treatment essential, and a simple inlay was performed for the adjacent second premolar *(IV–VIII)*. The fracture lines underlying an old amalgam filling in the mandibular left first molar *(IX, X)* were so radical that removal and implants were discussed.

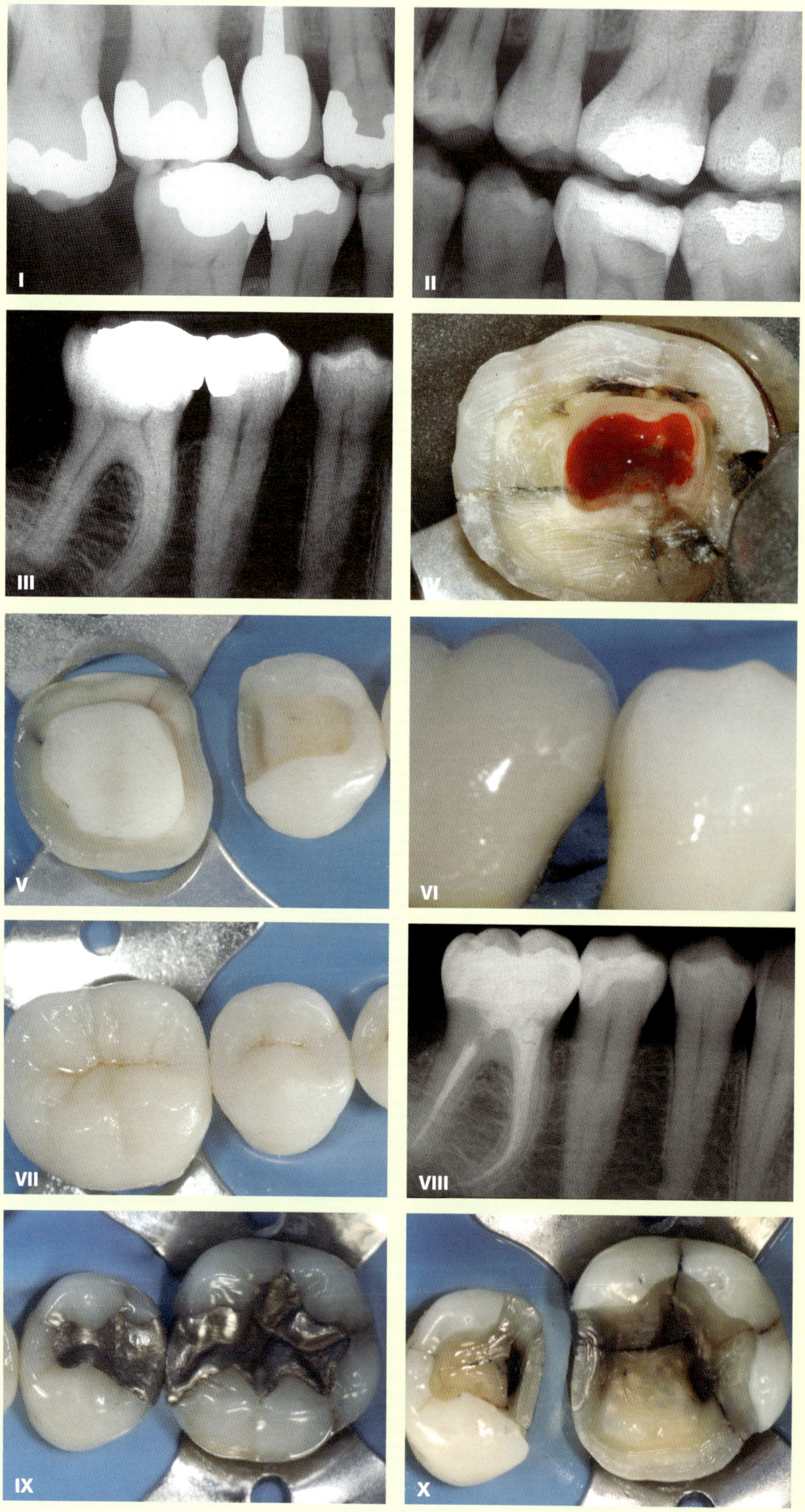

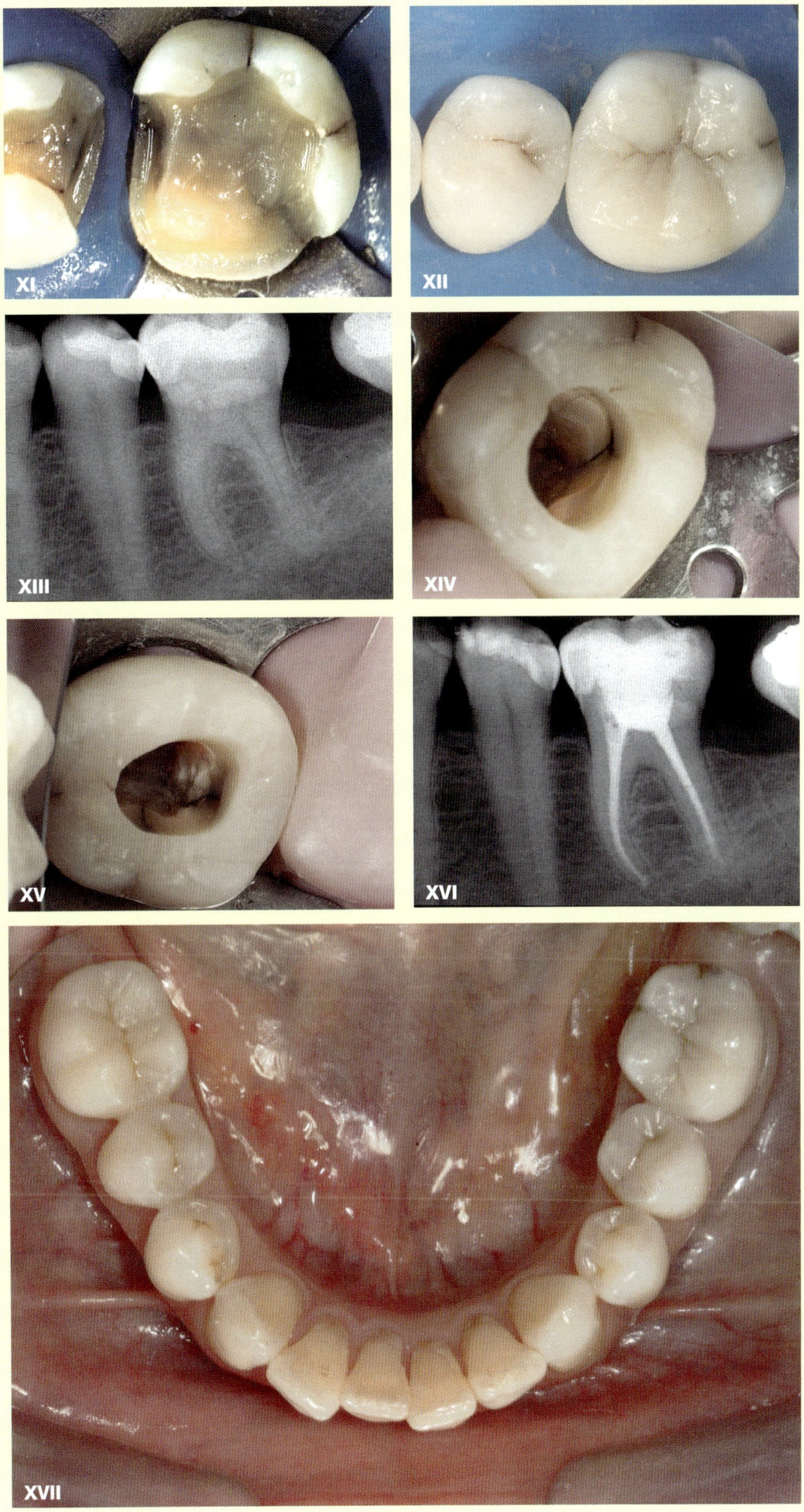

Fig 101 *(continued)* The patient was thoroughly informed of the risks and opted for conservative treatment, which meant partial restoration in composite for the first molar and the proximal premolar *(XI–XIII)*. Two weeks later pulpitis developed, which resulted in endodontic treatment of the first molar *(XIV–XVI)*. View of the mandible with cemented inlays *(XVII)*.

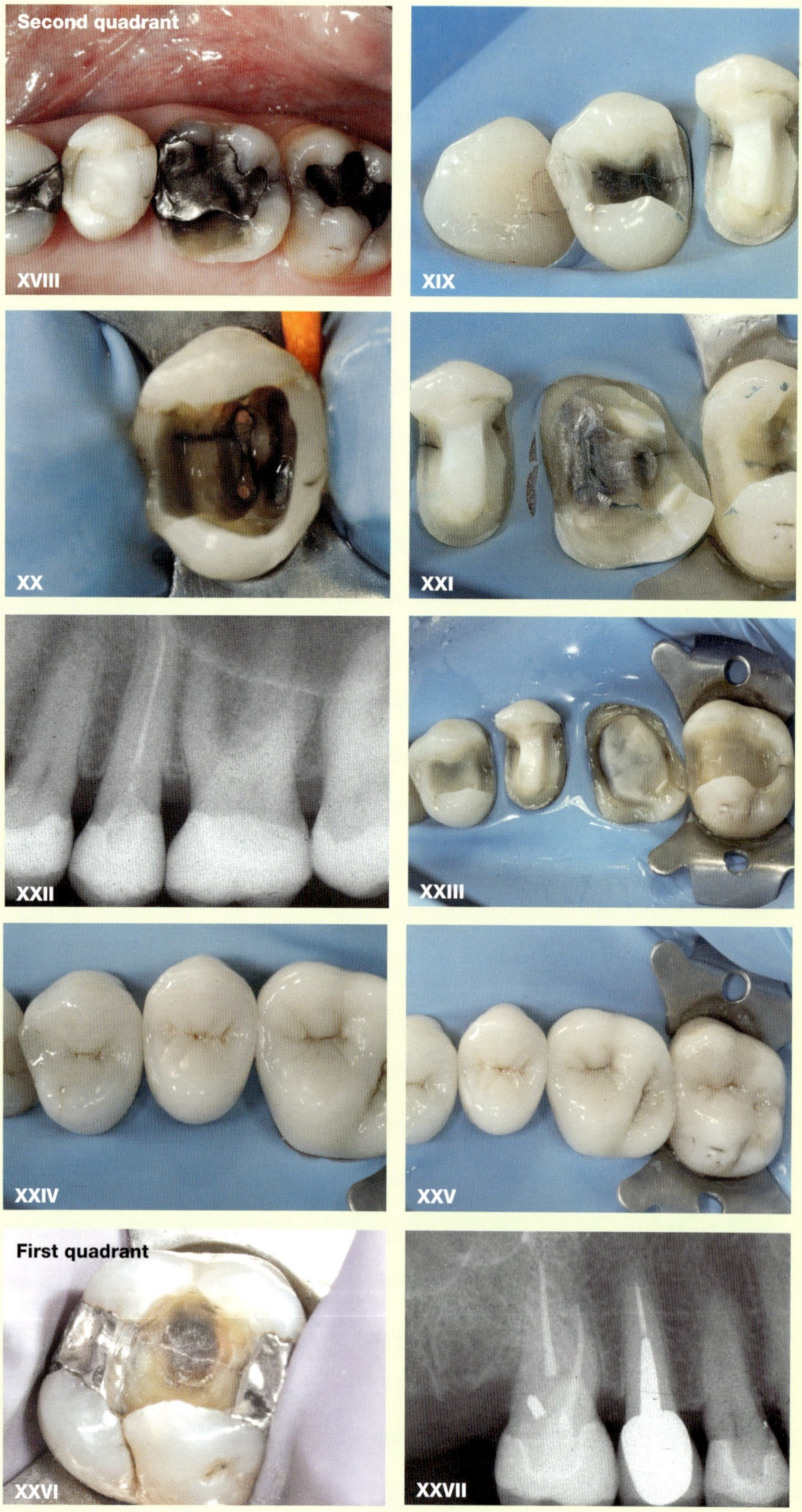

Fig 101 *(continued)* In the maxillary left (second) quadrant, coronal fractures and cracks under the old restorations guided the treatment plan toward the execution of an inlay, an onlay, and an overlay in accordance with the indications *(XVIII–XXV)*. The maxillary right (first) quadrant was managed with an overlay after endodontic treatment and removal of the distal root, justified by periodontal problems, in the first molar and an inlay for the first premolar *(XXVI, XXVII)*.

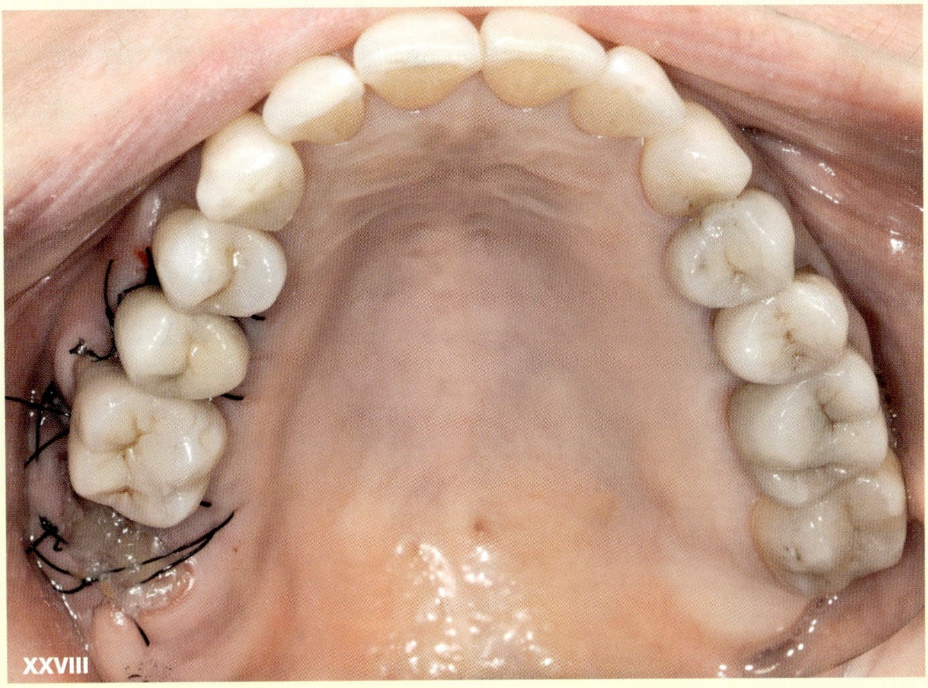

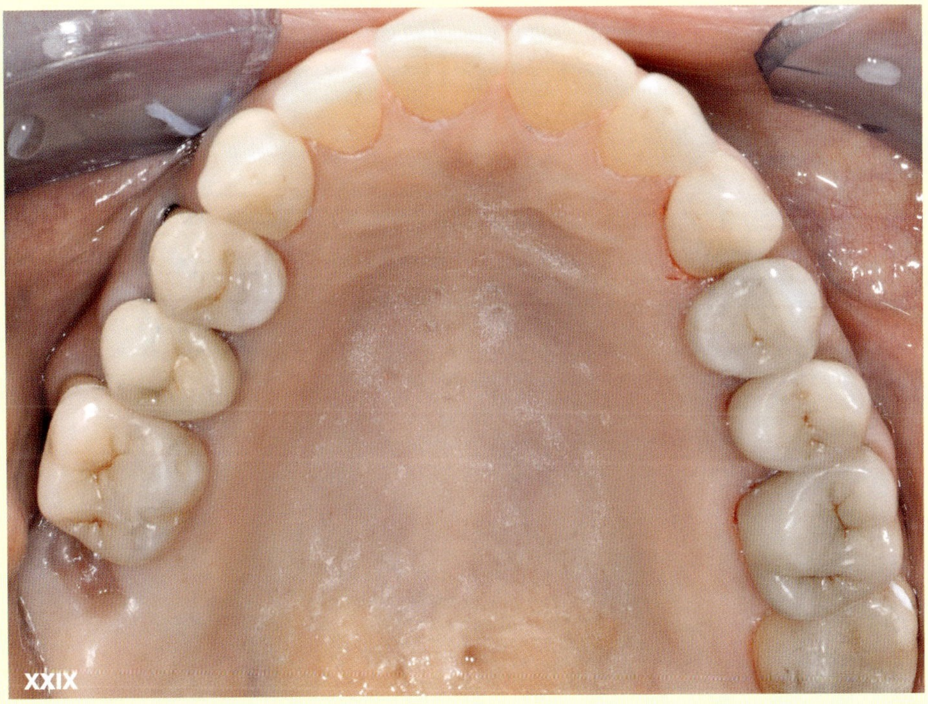

Fig 101 *(continued)* View of the maxilla at the end of treatment *(XXVIII, XXIX)*. As extensively discussed in the text, this therapeutic option should be backed by an informed consent signed by the patient. Above all, the patient must be made aware from the beginning of the risks of this treatment plan in the long term given the absolutely uncertain outcome in cases such as this. It goes without saying that removal of teeth with such characteristics does not in any way preclude the future insertion of implants.

Clinical case 2

Fig 102 Clinical case demonstrating the great potential of adhesive techniques. Three teeth with macroscopic fracture lines restored using adhesive techniques that perfectly illustrate the concept of conservative dentistry *(I–VII)*. After 8 years of function, they display structural integrity, perfect marginal seals, and pulp vitality *(VIII)*.

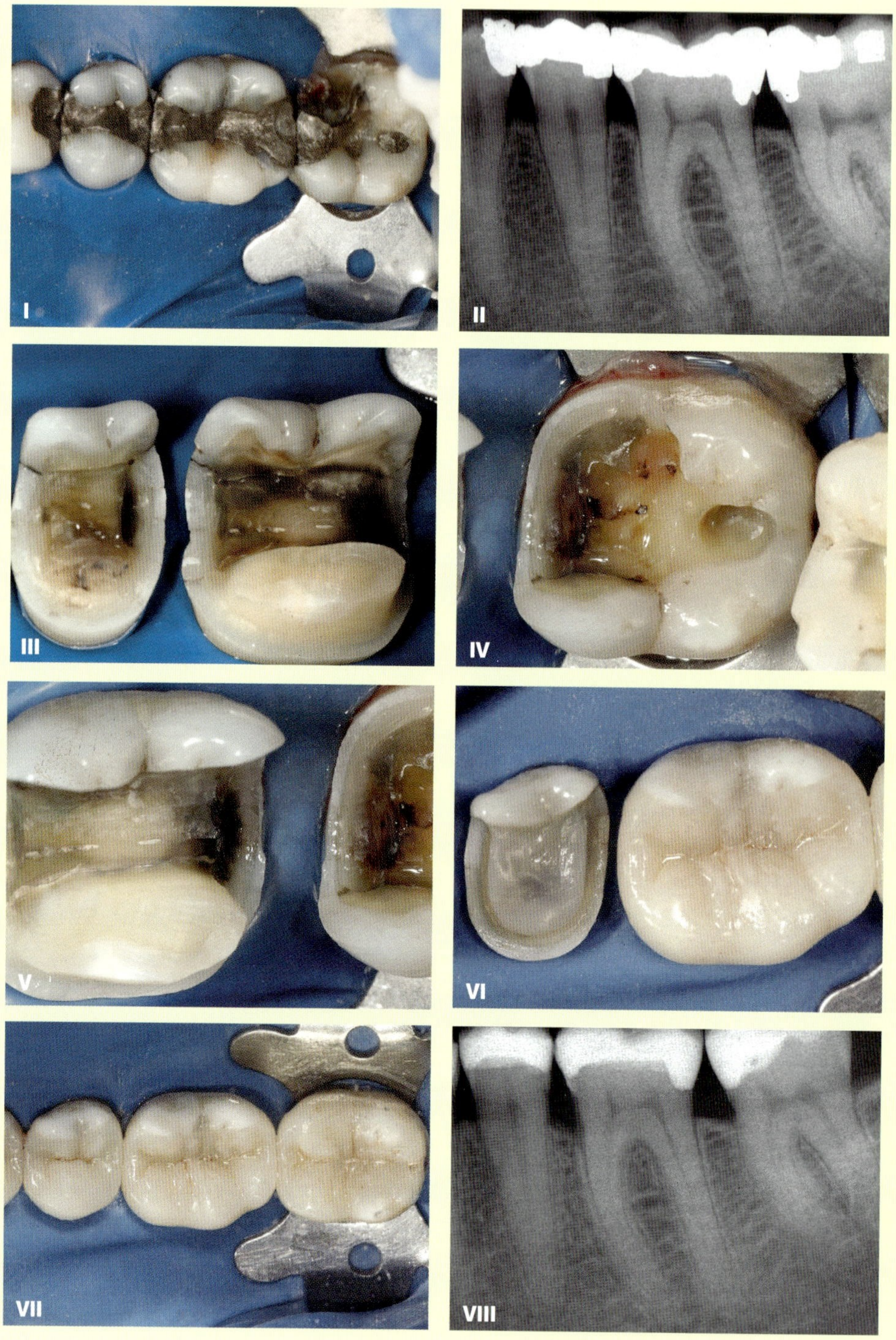

Clinical case 3

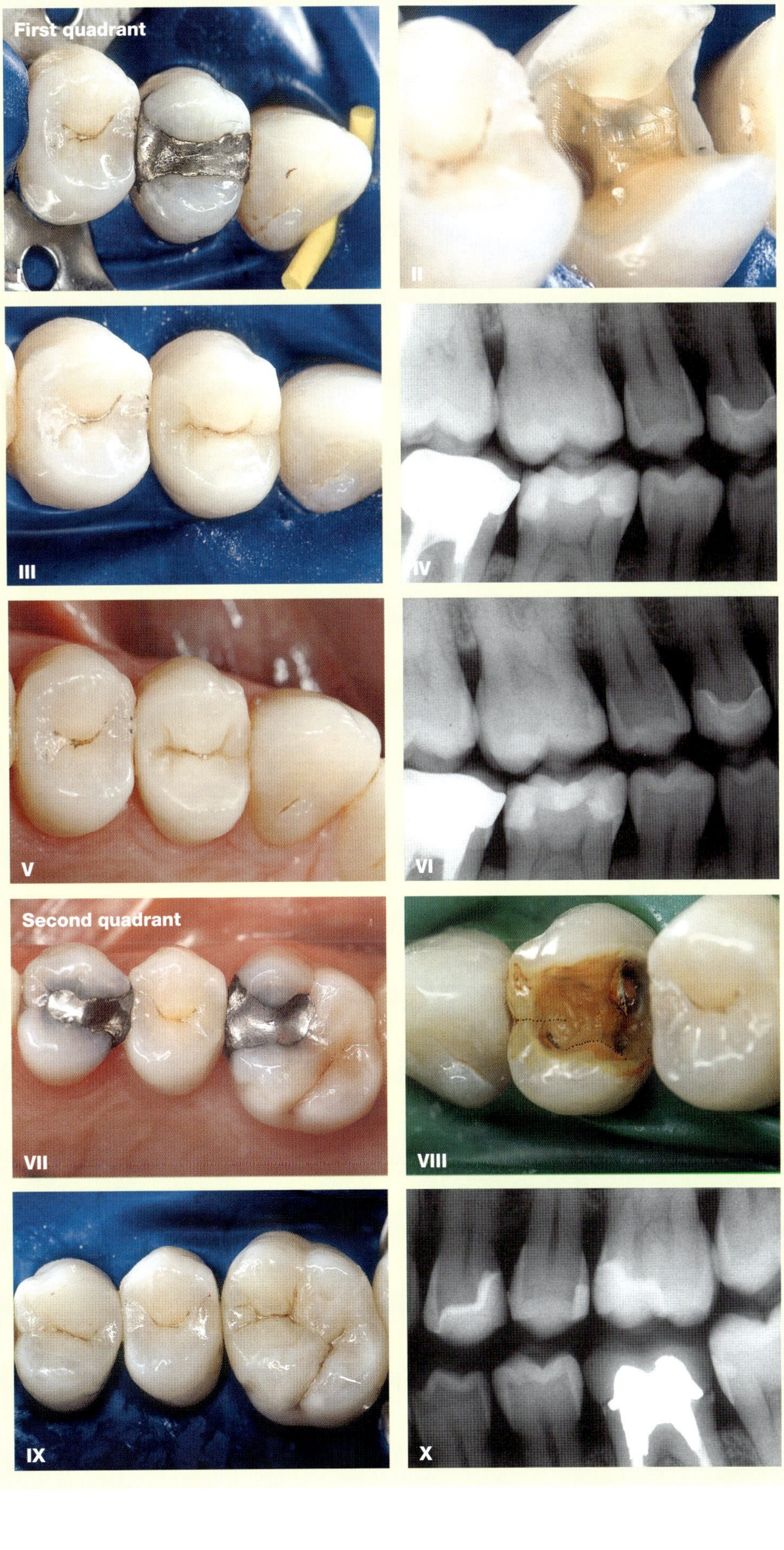

Fig 103 Maxillary premolars with minor fracture lines restored using inlays. With regard to horizontal fracture lines, clinical experience has shown such excellent long-term results that even thin walls affected by this type of abnormality can be retained with complete peace of mind *(I-XII)*. View of maxilla 7 years after applying inlays to the premolars and molars *(XIII)*.

Fig 103 *(continued)*

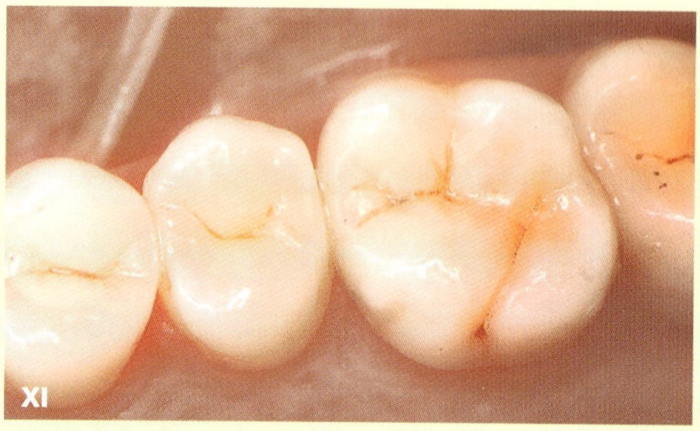

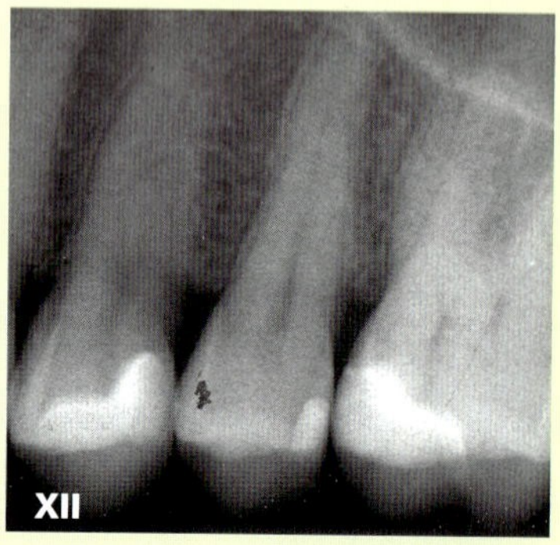

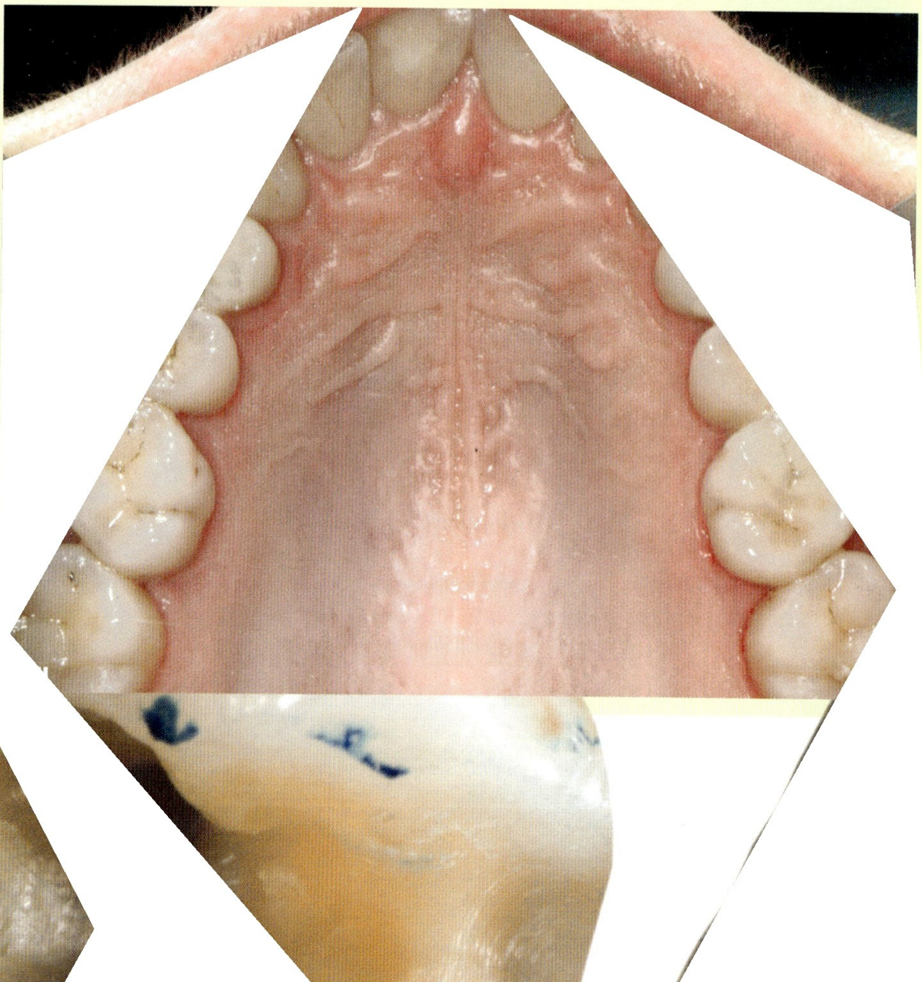

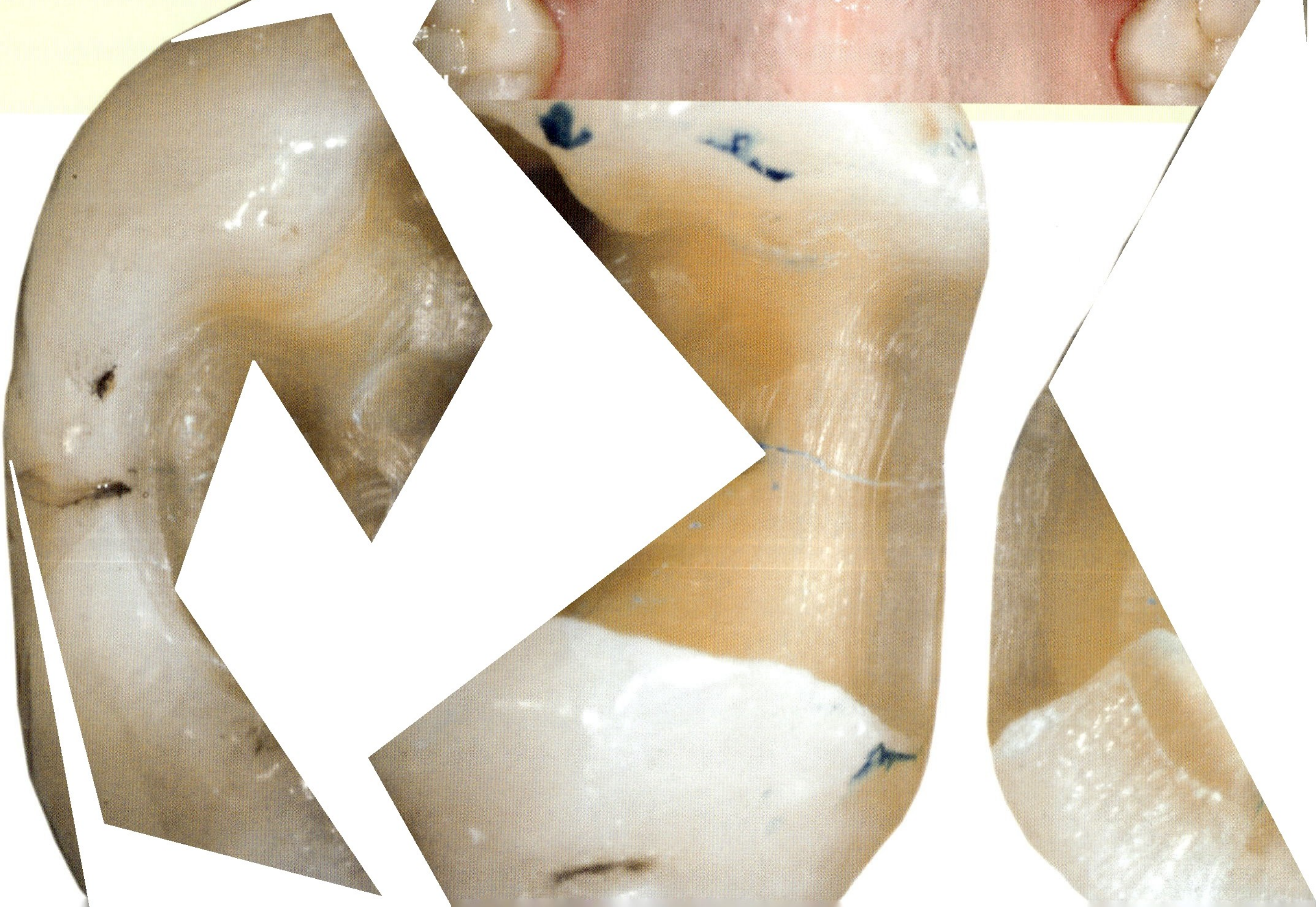

Clinical case 4

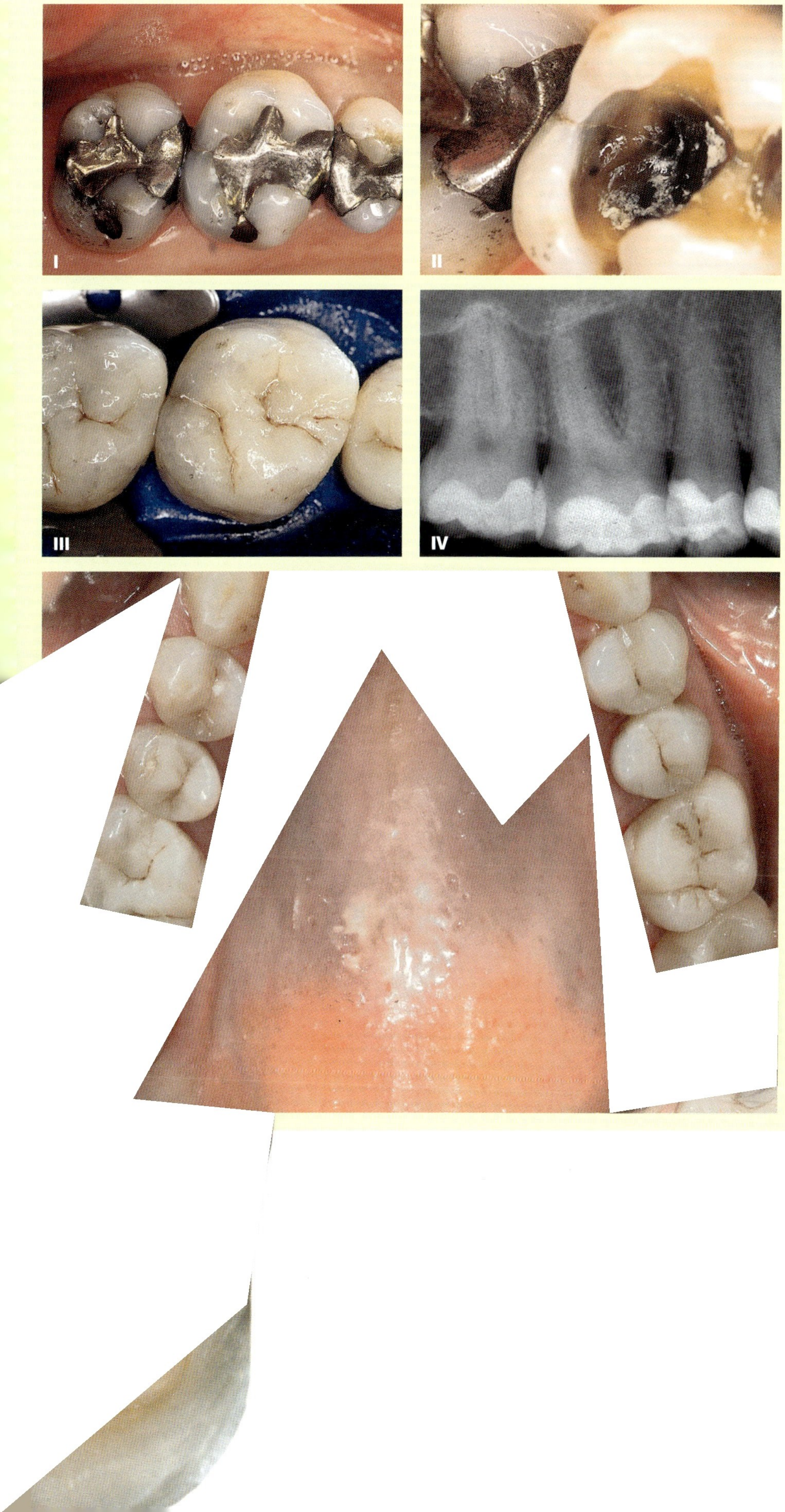

Fig 104 Maxillary right first molar with a small fracture line on the distal marginal ridge. Fracture depth is revealed after removing the amalgam *(I, II)*. Restoration with composite inlays *(III, IV)*. View of the arch after 6 years *(V)*.

Clinical case 5

Fig 105 The patient presented with pain on chewing in both arches. After removing two deep amalgam restorations in the first and second molars in the maxillary right (first) quadrant, significant fracture lines were evident. Following agreement with the patient, who was very receptive, an attempt was made to maintain all four walls in both teeth. This attempt was immediately thwarted by pulpitis in the second molar, which required endodontic treatment *(I–X)*. In the maxillary left (second) quadrant, a very deep fracture line was observed in the distal wall of the first molar while removing the old restoration. Treatment included endodontic retreatment, total preparation of the first molar, and partial preparation of the second molar due to carious infiltration of the latter. The respective adhesive restorations were then cemented *(XI–XVIII)*. In the mandibular left (third) quadrant, adhesive restorations were applied to the mandibular first and second molars *(XIX–XXVI)*. Views of the arches after completion of treatment *(XXVII, XXVIII)* and bitewing and periapical radiographs of the endodontically treated teeth *(XXIX–XXXII)*.

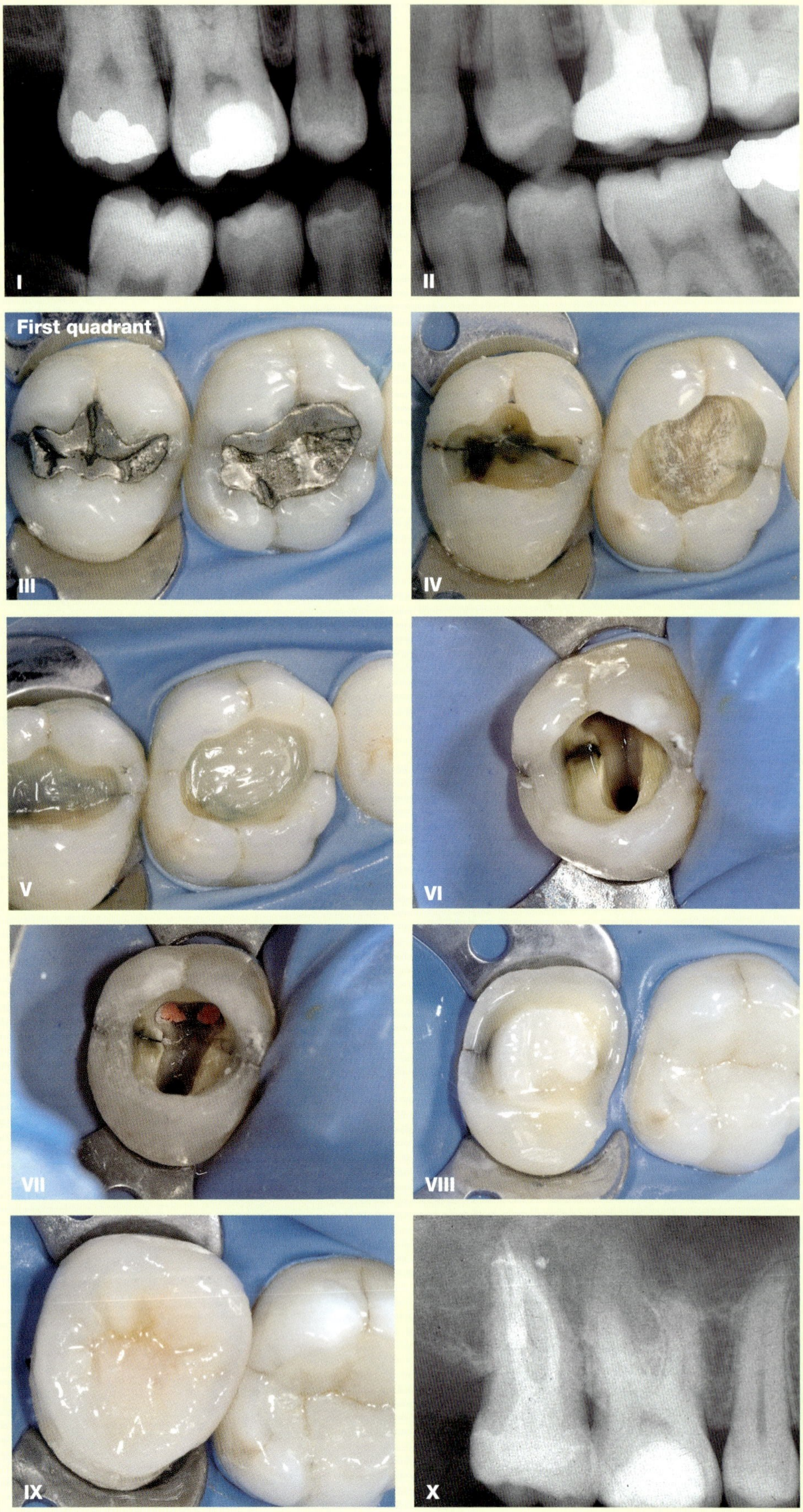

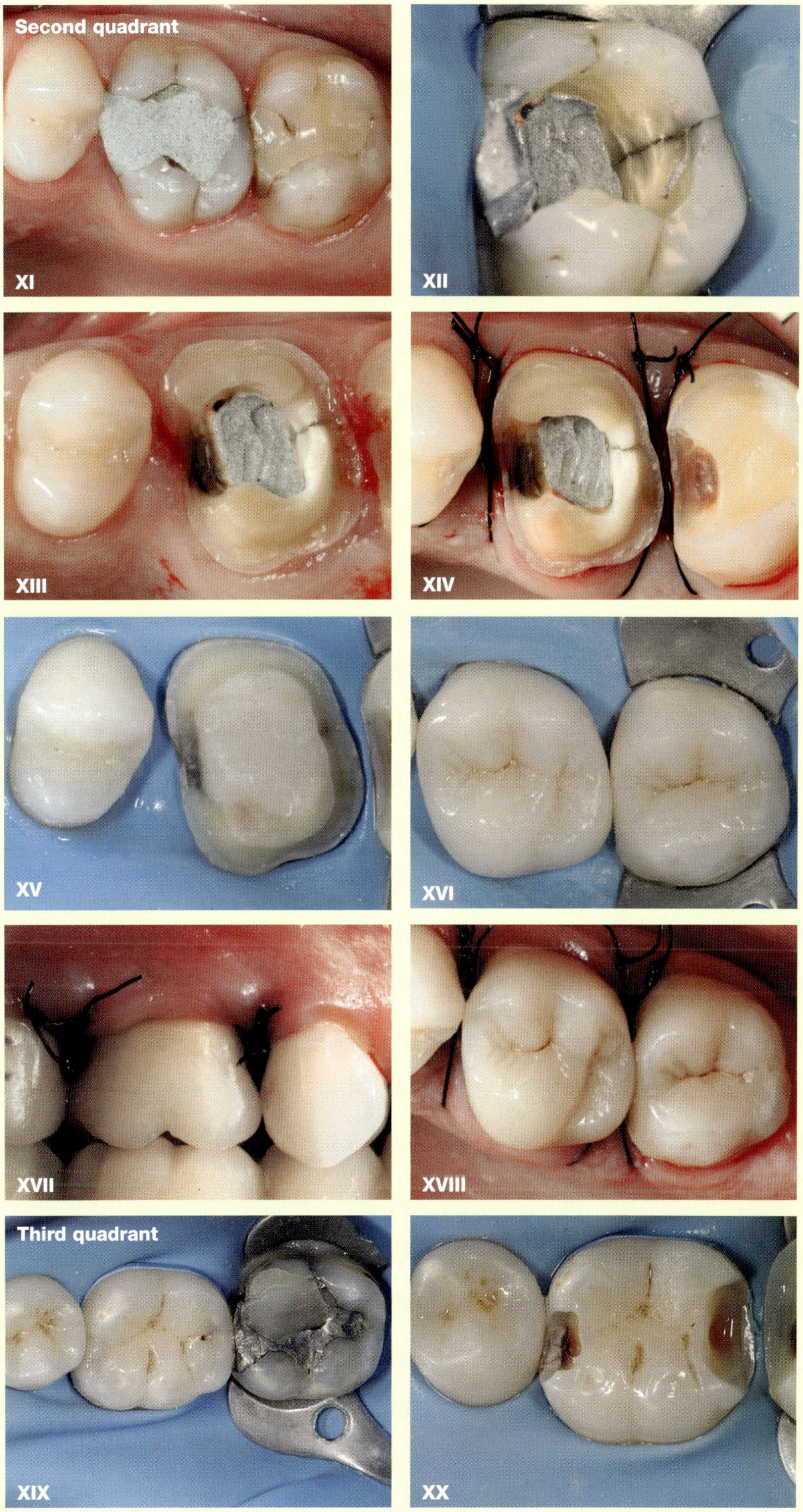

Fig 105 *(continued)*

Fig 105 *(continued)*

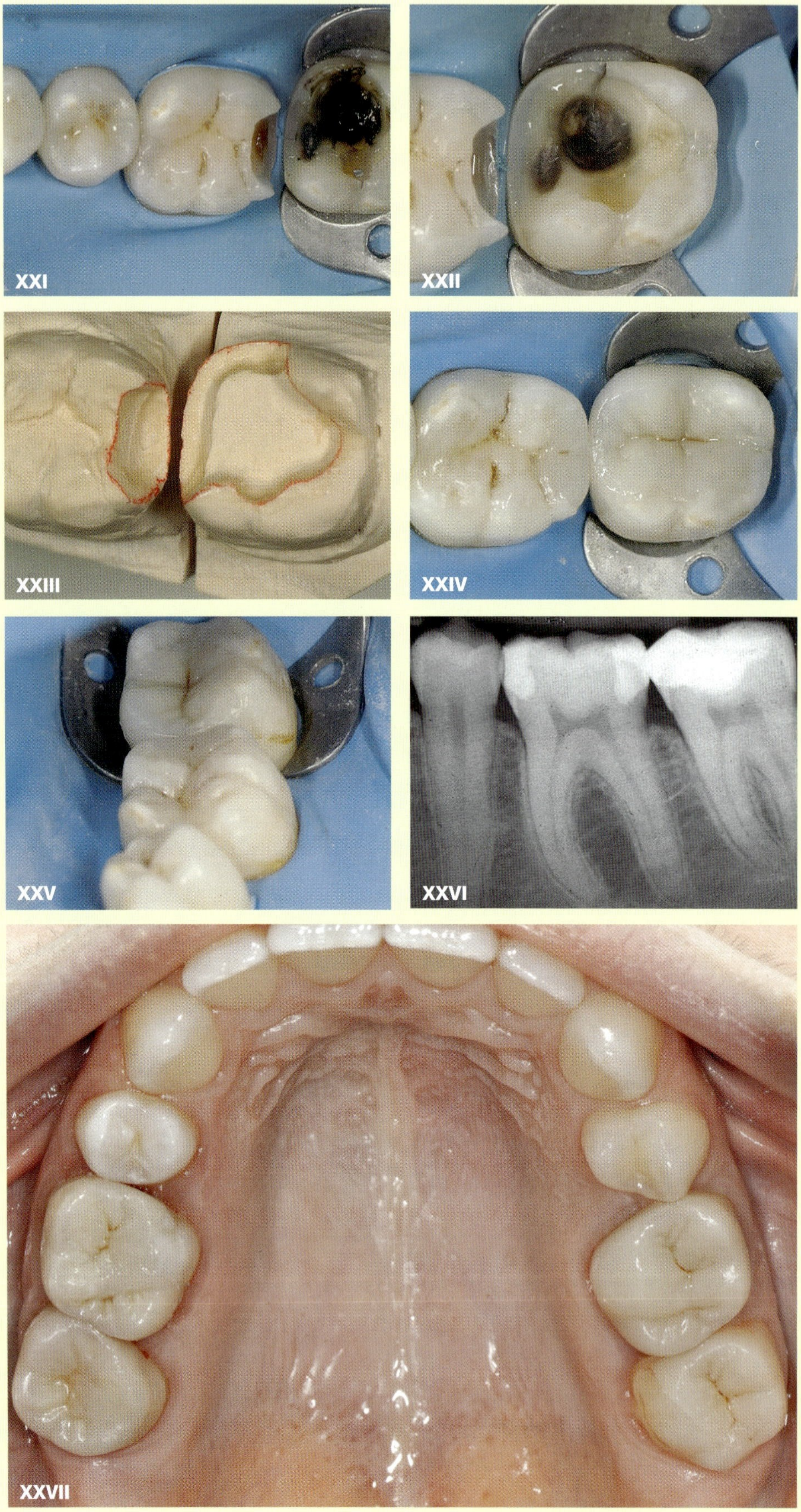

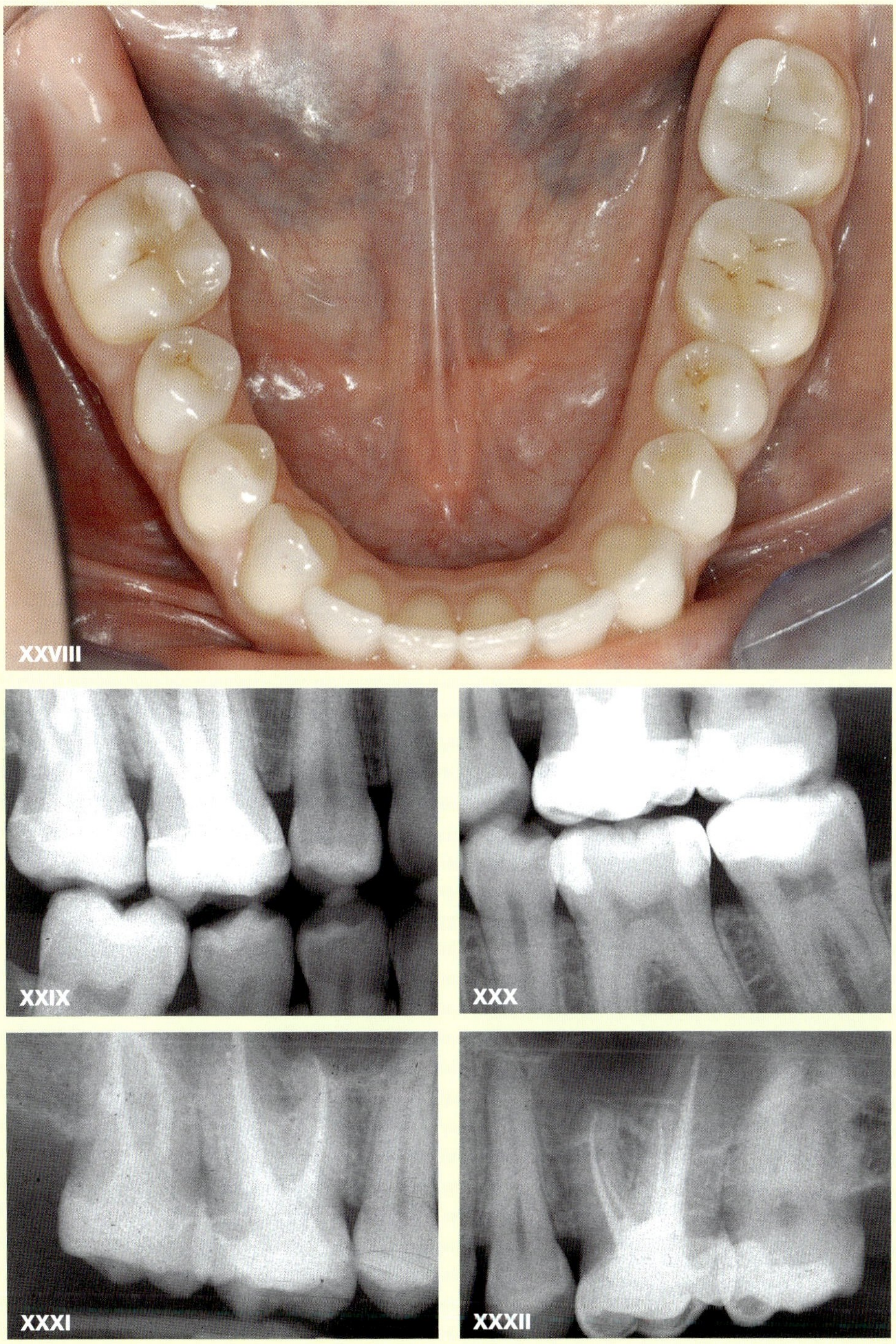

Fig 105 *(continued)*

References

1. Cameron CE. The cracked tooth syndrome: Additional findings. J Am Dent Assoc 1976;93:971–975.
2. Frank A, Simon JHS, Abou-Rass M, Glick DH. Endodonzia clinica e chirurgia. Concetti pratici. Padova, Italy: Piccin, 1988.
3. Krell KV, Rivera EM. A six year evaluation of cracked teeth diagnosed with reversible pulpitis: Treatment and prognosis. J Endod 2007;33:1405–1407.
4. Williams JJ. Cracked tooth syndrome: A new classification. Dent Today 1993;June/July:34–39.
5. Martin D, Matchou P. La dent fissurée: le traitement. L'information dentaire 2003;11:675–681.
6. Kahler B, Moule A, Stenzel D. Bacterial contamination of cracks in symptomatic vital teeth. Aust Endod J 2000;26:115–118.
7. Ricucci D. Patologia e Clinica Endodontica. Bologna, Italy: Martina, 2009.
8. Brännström M, Lindén LA, Aström A. The hydrodynamics of the dental tubule and of pulp fluid. A discussion of its significance in relation to dentinal sensitivity. Caries Res 1967;1:310–317.
9. Paul RA, Tamse A, Rosenberg E. Cracked and broken teeth–Definitions, differential diagnosis and treatment. Refuat Hapeh Vehashinayim 2007;24(2):7-12,68.
10. Patel DK, Burke FJ. Fractures of posterior teeth: A review and analysis of associated factors. Prim Dent Care 1995;2:6–10.
11. Benenati FW. Coping with cracked tooth syndrome. J Okla Dent Assoc 1996;86(3):16–18.
12. Homewood CI. Cracked tooth syndrome—Incidence, clinical findings and treatment. Aust Dent J 1998;43:217–222.
13. Ratcliff S, Becker IM, Quinn L. Type and incidence of cracks in posterior teeth. J Prosthet Dent 2001;86:168–172.
14. Hood JA. Biomechanics of the intact, prepared and restored tooth: Some clinical implications. Int Dent J 1991;41:25–32.
15. Hiatt WH. Incomplete crown-root fracture in pulpal-periodontal disease. J Periodontol 1973;44:369–379.
16. Cavel WT, Kelsey WP, Blankenau RJ. An in vivo study of cuspal fracture. J Prosthet Dent 1985;53:38–42.
17. Maxwell EH, Braly BV. Incomplete tooth fracture. Prediction and prevention. CDA J 1977;5(6):51–55.
18. Sasaki K, Hannam AG, Wood WW. Relationships between the size, position, and angulation of human jaw muscles and unilateral first molar bite force. J Dent Res 1989;68:499–503.
19. Fleiter B, Martin D. Il dente incrinato. L'informatore endodontico 2003;6(4):14–21.
20. Willemsen WL, van der Meer WJ. Repair and revision 4. Cracked tooth and crown fractures: Diagnostics and treatment [in Dutch]. Ned Tijdschr Tandheelkd 2001;108(5):170–172.